cpt® CODING ESSENTIALS

Ophthalmology | 2022

CPT® Coding Essentials Ophthalmology 2022

Printed in the United States of America

ISBN: 978-1-64016-143-6
OP259222

Additional copies of this book or other AMA products may be ordered by calling 612-435-6065 or visiting the AMA Store at amastore.com. Refer to product number OP259222.

AMA publication and product updates, errata, and addendum can be found at *amaproductupdates.org.*

Published by DecisionHealth, an HCPro brand
100 Winners Circle, Suite 300
Brentwood, TN 37027
www.codingbooks.com

Contents

Codes List

The CPT surgery and ancillary codes and code ranges that appear in this book are listed below.

Surgery Codes

15820-15821
15822-15823
21385
21386
21387
21390
21395
21400-21401
21406
21407
21408
65091-65093
65101-65105
65110-65114
65125
65130
65135-65140
65150-65155
65175
65205-65210
65220-65222
65235
65260-65265
65270
65272-65273
65275
65280
65285
65286
65290
65400
65410
65420-65426
65430
65435-65436
65450
65600
65710
65730
65750-65755
65756
65757
65760
65765
65767
65770
65771
65772
65775
65778-65779
65780
65781
65782
65785
65800
65810
65815
65820
65850
65855
65860
65865-65880
65900
65920
65930
66020-66030
66130
66150
66155
66160
66170-66172
66174-66175
66179-66180
66183
66184-66185
66225
66250
66500-66505
66600-66605
66625-66630
66635
66680
66682
66700
66710-66711
66720
66740
66761
66762
66770
66820-66821
66825
66830
66840
66850
66852
66920-66930
66940
66982
66983
66984
66985
66986
66987
66988
66989
66990
66991
67005-67010
67015
67025
67027
67028
67030
67031
67036-67040
67041
67042
67043
67101-67105
67107
67108
67110
67113
67115
67120
67121
67141-67145
67208-67210
67218
67220
67221-67225
67227
67228
67229
67250-67255
67311-67316
67318
67320
67331-67332
67334-67335
67340
67343
67345
67346
67400-67405
67412-67413
67414
67415
67420-67430
67440
67445
67450
67500-67505
67515
67550-67560
67570
67700
67710
67715
67800-67808
67810
67820-67835
67840
67850
67875
67880-67882
67900
67901-67902
67903-67904
67906

67908
67909
67911
67912
67914-67915
67916-67917
67921-67922
67923-67924
67930-67935
67938
67950
67961-67966
67971-67975
68020
68040
68100
68110-68130
68135
68200
68320-68325
68326-68328
68330-68340
68360-68362
68371
68400-68420
68440
68500-68505
68510
68520
68525
68530
68540-68550
68700
68705
68720
68745-68750
68760-68761
68770
68801
68810-68816
68840
68841
68850

Ancillary Codes

76510-76512
76513
76514
76516-76519
76529
80158
81290
81434
81460
81465
81552
83861
84590
86609
86628
86682
86738
87101-87103
87106-87107
87109
87118
87205
87206
87207-87209
87590-87592
87809
87850
92002
92004
92012
92014
92015
92018-92019
92020
92025
92060
92065
92071-92072
92081
92082
92083
92100
92132
92133-92134
92136
92145
92201-92202
92227-92229
92230
92235-92242
92250
92260
92265
92270
92273-92274
92283
92284
92285
92286-92287
92310-92313
92314-92317
92325
92326
92340-92342
92352-92353
92354-92355
92358
92370-92371
92534
92540
92544
92545
92546
99024
99071
99151-99153
99155-99157
99172
99173
99174
99177
0100T
0198T
0207T
0253T
0308T
0329T
0330T
0333T
0378T-0379T
0402T
0444T-0445T
0449T-0450T
0464T
0465T
0469T
0472T-0473T
0474T
0506T
0507T
0509T
0514T
0563T
0604T-0606T
0616T-0618T
0621T-0622T
0671T
0699T
0704T
0705T
0706T

Introduction

Unlike other specialty coding books on the market, *CPT® Coding Essentials for Ophthalmology 2022* combines ophthalmology-specific procedural coding and reimbursement information with verbatim guidelines and parenthetical information from the Current Procedural Terminology (CPT®) codebook. In addition, *CPT® Coding Essentials for Ophthalmology 2022* enhances that CPT-specific information by displaying pertinent diagnostic codes, procedural descriptions, illustrations, relative value units (RVUs), and more on the same page as the CPT code being explained. This one book provides ophthalmology coding and billing knowledge that otherwise might take years of experience or multiple resources to accumulate. It sets a foundation for ophthalmology coders and subspecialty coding experts that facilitates correct code assignment.

This book includes reporting rules for CPT code submission as written and enforced by the Centers for Medicare & Medicaid Services (CMS). *CPT® Coding Essentials for Ophthalmology 2022* is not intended to equip coders with information to make medical decisions or to determine diagnoses or treatments; rather, it is intended to aid correct code selection that is supported by physician or other qualified health care professional (QHP) documentation. This reference work does not replace the need for a CPT codebook.

IMPORTANT: The RVU file that contains the modifier values for new CPT codes was not released as the *2022 CPT Coding Essentials* specialty books went to press. Once the data are available, the file will be posted at www.amaproductupdates.com.

The pending RVU modifier data affect the following new 2022 codes: 33267-33268, 33269, 33370, 33509, 33894-33895, 33897, 43497, 53451-53454, 63052-63053, 64628-64629, 66989, 66991, 68841

About the *CPT® Coding Essentials* Editorial Team and Content Selection

The *CPT® Coding Essentials* series is developed by a team of veteran clinical technical editors and certified medical coders. When developing the content of this book, the team members consider all annual new, revised, and deleted medical codes. They adhere to authoritative medical research; medical policies; and official guidelines, conventions, and rules to determine the final content presented within this book. In addition, the team monitors utilization and denial trends when selecting the codes highlighted in *CPT® Coding Essentials for Ophthalmology 2022.*

The main section of *CPT® Coding Essentials for Ophthalmology 2022* is titled "CPT® Procedural Coding." This section is organized for ease of use and simple lookup by displaying CPT codes in numeric order. Each code-detail page of this section presents a single code or multiple codes representing a code family concept.

The procedures featured are those commonly performed by an ophthalmologist, but more difficult for coders to understand or often miscoded in claims reporting. This book does not provide a comprehensive list of all services performed in the specialty, nor all sites within eye system. Similarly, the CPT to ICD-10-CM crosswalks are intended to illustrate those conditions that would most commonly present relative to the procedure and the specialist. The crosswalks are not designed to be an exhaustive list of all possible conditions for each procedure, nor medical necessity reasons for coverage.

The "CPT® Procedural Coding" section is complemented by other sections that review ophthalmology terminology and anatomy, ICD-10-CM conventions and coding, ICD-10-CM documentation tips, and ICD-10-PCS procedure coding and format. The appendices contain data from the CMS National Correct Coding Initiative, multiple ICD-10-CM compliant ophthalmological conditions documentation checklists, and the evaluation and management (E/M) documentation guidelines.

Sections Contained Within This Book

What follows is a section-by-section explanation of *CPT® Coding Essentials for Ophthalmology 2022.*

Terminology, Abbreviations, and Basic Anatomy

This section provides a quick reference tool for coders who may come across unfamiliar terminology in medical record documentation. This review of basic terminology displays lists of alphabetized Greek and Latin root words, prefixes, and suffixes associated with ophthalmology.

The combination of root words with prefixes and suffixes is the basis of medical terminology and enables readers to deduce the meaning of new words by understanding the components. For example, *neuro* is a root word for *nerve,* and *–algia* is a suffix for *pain*; thus, *neuralgia* describes nerve pain.

Also included in this section are a glossary of ophthalmology-specific terms and a list of acronyms and abbreviations. Keep in mind that these glossary definitions are specific to ophthalmology. The same word may have a different meaning in a different specialty. In some cases, a parenthetical note after the term may provide the reader with a common acronym or synonym for that term. Pay particular attention to the use of capitalization in the abbreviation and acronym list, as the same letters sometimes have varied meaning in clinical nomenclature, depending on capitalization.

Introduction to ICD-10-CM and ICD-10-PCS

For coders who want a review, *CPT® Coding Essentials for Ophthalmology 2022* recaps the development of the ICD-10-CM and ICD-10-PCS code sets and outlines important concepts pertaining to both.

Lists of common ICD-10-CM diagnoses and conditions for each selected CPT code or code range may be found within the "CPT® Procedural Coding" section.

The *ICD-10-CM* content provided within this book complements your use of the *ICD-10-CM 2022* codebook. This section provides a chapter-by-chapter overview of ICD-10-CM that includes common new diagnoses and their codes, as well as identification of new or substantially changed chapter-specific guidelines for 2022.

ICD-10-PCS is not used for reporting physician services; however, an understanding of ICD-10-PCS is essential to physician practices because physician inpatient surgical documentation is used by hospitals for the abstraction of ICD-10-PCS codes for hospital billing. An overview of this structure is reviewed in this section.

ICD-10-CM Anatomy and Physiology

Advanced understanding of the eye and ocular adnexa is essential to accurate coding for ophthalmology. A detailed study of the anatomy and physiology gives beginner or intermediate coders the information boost they may need to abstract the medical record accurately.

Anatomy of the Eye

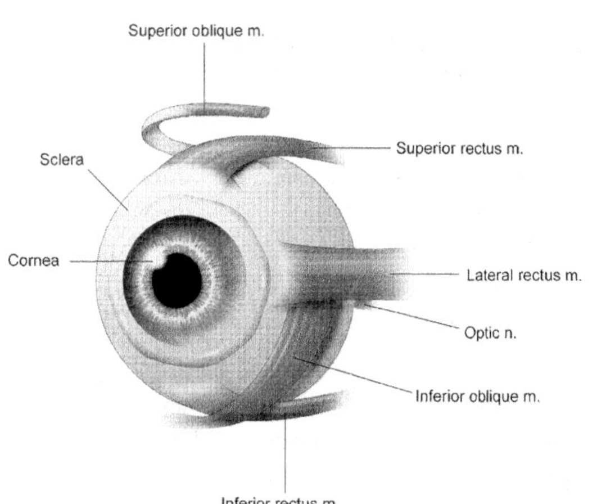

The anatomy and physiology explanations are accompanied by labeled and detailed illustrations for ophthalmology, beginning at the cellular level and extending to the functions and interactions of the various body parts and tissues. This chapter also includes discussion of common disorders affecting the eye and ocular adnexa, their pathophysiology, as well as coding exercises to assess mastery of the coding topic.

ICD-10-CM Documentation

Accurate, complete coding of diseases, disorders, injuries, conditions, and even signs and symptoms using ICD-10-CM codes requires extensive patient encounter documentation. This section highlights commonly encountered conditions that require a high level of specificity for documentation and coding.

The documentation information is presented in an easy-to-understand bulleted format that enables the physician, other QHP, and/or coder to identify quickly the specificity of documentation required for accurate ICD-10-CM code abstraction. This section also includes coding exercises to assess mastery of the documentation topic.

CPT® Procedural Coding for Ophthalmology

"CPT® Procedural Coding" is the main section of this book and displays pertinent coding and reimbursement data for each targeted CPT code or code family on code-detail pages. The following is presented within each surgical code detail page:

- CPT code and verbatim description with icons (when required)
- Parentheticals (when they exist)
- Official CPT coding guidelines
- Plain English descriptions
- Illustrations
- ICD-10-CM diagnostic codes
- AMA *CPT® Assistant* newsletter references
- CMS Pub 100 references
- CMS relative value units
- CMS global periods
- CMS modifier edits

Category III codes and codes from diagnostic (ancillary) sections will contain a truncated version of the code-detail page content, as diagnostic tests are too broad for all data elements contained in the surgical code detail pages.

CPT Coding Guidelines

The guidelines and parenthetical instructions included in the CPT codebook provide coders with insight into how the CPT Editorial Panel and CPT Advisory Committee intend the codes to be used. This information is critical to correct code selection, and until now, has been unavailable in books other than official AMA CPT codebooks.

Section guidelines for the pertinent sections of the CPT code set (Surgery, Radiology, Pathology, and Medicine) appear before the code-detail pages associated with the respective CPT section. Guidelines that appear elsewhere within a CPT code set section are displayed on the code-detail pages, whenever appropriate. The reproduction of ophthalmology coding guidelines and parenthetical information in *CPT® Coding Essentials for Ophthalmology 2022* is verbatim from the AMA CPT codebook.

CPT Codes and Descriptions

CPT codes are listed in numerical order and include anesthesia, surgery, radiology, pathology and laboratory, medicine, and Category III codes pertinent to ophthalmology.

The CPT code set has been developed as stand-alone descriptions of medical services. However, not all descriptions of CPT codes are presented in their complete form within the code set. In some cases, one or more abbreviated code descriptions (known as *child codes*) appear indented and without an initial capital letter. Such codes refer back to a common portion of the preceding code description (known as a *parent code*) that includes a semi-colon (;) and includes all of the text prior to the semi-colon. An example of this parent–child code system is as follows:

65710 Keratoplasty (corneal transplant); anterior lamellar
65730 penetrating (except in aphakia or pseudophakia)
65750 penetrating (in aphakia)
65755 penetrating (in pseudophakia)

The full descriptions for indented codes 65730, 65750, and 65755 are:

65730 Keratoplasty (corneal transplant); penetrating (except in aphakia or pseudophakia)
65750 Keratoplasty (corneal transplant); penetrating (in aphakia)
65755 Keratoplasty (corneal transplant); penetrating (in pseudophakia)

On the code-detail pages, a code may be indented beneath the preceding parent code, as shown in the first code grouping. Alternately, a full description of the indented code, as shown in the second code grouping, may be displayed if the parent code is not included on the same code-detail page.

Icons

Icons on the code-detail page may affect ICD or CPT codes. The male (♂) and female (♀) edit icons are applied to ICD codes. New or revised CPT codes are identified with a bullet (●) or triangle (▲), respectively. The plus sign (✚) identifies add-on codes. Add-on codes may never be reported alone, but are always reported in addition to the main procedure, and should never be reported with modifier 51, *Multiple Procedures*.

A bullet with the numeral 7 within it (❼) is displayed next to ICD-10-CM codes that require a seventh character. Consult the ICD-10-CM codebook for appropriate seventh characters.

The bolt symbol (⚡) identifies CPT codes for vaccines pending FDA approval.

The star symbol (★) identifies CPT codes that may be used to report telemedicine services when appended by modifier 95.

The right/left arrows symbol (⇄) identifies where the full range of lateral codes would be appropriate. To conserve space in the *CPT® Coding Essentials* series, we have chosen to use this icon to denote laterality.

The cell phone icon (▯) denotes the *CPT® QuickRef*, a mobile app created by the AMA and available from the App Store and Google Play. The icon indicates that additional dynamic information can be accessed within the app (in-app purchases required).

Parenthetical Information

The CPT code set sometimes provides guidance in the form of a parenthetical note. For example:

(For repair of iris or ciliary body, use 66680)

Code-detail pages include parenthetical instructions specific to both the code and the section within which the code is placed within the CPT code set. Not all codes and/or sections have associated parenthetical notes.

CPT® Assistant References

CPT® Assistant is a monthly newsletter published by the AMA to provide supplemental guidance to the CPT codebook. If a CPT code is the subject of discussion in a past issue of *CPT® Assistant,* the volume and page numbers are noted beneath the code to direct readers to the relevant newsletter archives to keep abreast of compliant coding rules.

Plain English Description

A simple description of what is included in the service represented by each CPT code is provided as a guide for coders to select the correct CPT code while reading the medical record. Not all approaches or methodologies are described in the Plain English Description; rather, the most common approaches or methodologies are provided. In some cases, the description provides an overview to more than one code, as some code-detail pages have multiple codes listed.

Illustrations

Streamlined line drawings demonstrate the anatomical site of the procedure, illustrating the basics of the procedure to assist in code selection. In some cases, not all codes on code-detail pages and not all approaches or methodologies are captured in the single illustration.

Diagnostic Code Crosswalk

ICD-10-CM codes commonly associated with the service represented on the code-detail pages are listed with their official code descriptions. These crosswalk codes were selected by trained coding professionals based on their knowledge and experience. The most common and medically related ICD-10-CM codes appropriate to the procedure or services represented on the code-detail pages are provided within space constraints. The intent is not to provide a list of codes that are deemed medically necessary or relate to payment policies.

When a seventh character is required for a code, a bullet with the numeral 7 within it (❼) alerts the coder. Sometimes, a seventh character is appended to a code with only three, four, or five characters. In those cases, "X" placeholders are to be appended to the codes so that only the seventh character must be added. For example, the following ICD-10-CM diagnosis code:

T85.21 Breakdown (mechanical) of intraocular lens requires a seventh character; therefore, it is displayed with six characters in this manner:

❼T85.21X Breakdown (mechanical) of intraocular lens

Within ICD-10-CM, many diagnoses have different codes based on laterality (for example, right retina, left retina, bilateral retina). Due to space constraints, not every laterality code is listed. Rather, a representative code is listed along with an icon indicating that other laterality code versions are available.

The provided crosswalks are not meant to replace your ICD-10-CM codebook. Please consult your manual for all seventh characters needed to complete listed codes and additional laterality choices, as well as ICD-10-CM coding conventions essential to proper use.

Pub 100

CMS Pub 100 (Publication 100-04; "Medicare Claims Processing Manual") is an online resource of federal coding regulations that often relate to CPT coding. If a CPT code or its associated procedure is the topic of discussion in a CMS Pub 100 entry, the Pub 100 reference is noted so that coders may access it at www.cms.gov/Regulations-and-Guidance/Guidance/Manuals/Internet-Only-Manuals-IOMs.

Payment Grids

Information in the payment grids that appear on code-detail pages comes from CMS. These grids identify the relative value of providing a specific professional service in relation to the value of other services, the number of postoperative follow-up days associated with each CPT code, and other reimbursement edits. All data displayed in the payment grids are relevant to physicians participating in Medicare.

Global Period

During the follow-up, or global surgery period, any routine care associated with the original service is bundled into the original service. This means that, for example, an E/M visit to check the surgical wound would not be billable if it occurs during the global surgery period.

Possible global periods under Medicare are 0, 10, and 90 days. "XXX" indicates that the global period concept does not apply to the service.

Relative Value Units (RVUs)

RVU data show the breakout of work, practice expense (PE), and malpractice expense (MP) associated with a code, and provide a breakout for the service depending on whether it was performed in the physician's office or in a facility not belonging to the physician. Understandably, the physician payment for a surgical procedure is reduced if a procedure is hosted by a facility, as the facility would expect payment to cover its share of costs. A physician who performs the surgery in his or her own office is not subject to the same cost-sharing. This cost difference is shown in the PE column.

The payment information provided is sometimes used to set rates or anticipate payments. Payment information may be affected by modifiers appended to the CPT code.

Modifiers

Sometimes, modifiers developed by the AMA and CMS may be appended to CPT codes to indicate that the services represented by the codes have been altered in some way. For example, modifier 26 reports the professional component (PC) of a service that has both a professional and a technical component (TC). A patient who undergoes an ultrasound might have a technician perform the ultrasound itself, while the physician interprets the ultrasound results to determine a diagnosis. The technician's service would be reported with the same ultrasound CPT code as the physician, but the physician would use modifier 26 to indicate the PC only, and the technician would report modifier TC, which is a Healthcare Common Procedure Coding System (HCPCS; pronounced as "hick-picks") Level II modifier identifying the service as the technical portion only. If the physician performs the ultrasound and interprets the results, no modifier is required.

When such circumstances affect the code, users may find the payment information provided for the full code, the professional services–only code, and the technical component–only code.

Many modifiers affect payment for services or with whom payment is shared when multiple providers or procedures are involved in a single surgical encounter. CMS provides definitions for the payments, based on the number listed in the modifier's field.

Modifier 50 (Bilateral Procedure)

This modifier indicates which payment-adjustment rule for bilateral procedures applies to the service.

0 150% payment adjustment for bilateral procedures does not apply. If a procedure is reported with modifier 50 or with modifiers RT and LT, Medicare bases payment for the two sides on the lower of (a) the total actual charge for both sides or (b) 100% of the fee-schedule amount for a single code. For example the fee-schedule amount for code XXXXX is $125. The physician reports code XXXXX-LT with an actual charge of $100 and XXXXX-RT with an actual charge of $100.

Payment would be based on the fee-schedule amount ($125) because it is lower than the total actual charges for the left and right sides ($200). The bilateral adjustment is inappropriate for codes in this category (a) due to physiology or anatomy or (b) because the code descriptor specifically states that it is a unilateral procedure and there is an existing code for the bilateral procedure.

1 150% payment adjustment for bilateral procedures applies. If a code is billed with the bilateral modifier or is reported twice on the same day by any other means (such as with RT and LT modifiers or with a "2" in the units field), payment is based for these codes when reported as bilateral procedures on the lower of (a) the total actual charge for both sides or (b) 150% of the fee-schedule amount for a single code. If a code is reported as a bilateral procedure and is reported with other procedure codes on the same day, the bilateral adjustment is applied before any applicable multiple procedure rules are applied.

2 150% payment adjustment for bilateral procedure does not apply. RVUs are already based on the procedure being performed as a bilateral procedure. If a procedure is reported with modifier 50, or is reported twice on the same day by any other means (such as with RT and LT modifiers with a "2" in the units field), payment is based for both sides on the lower of (a) the total actual charges by the physician for both sides or (b) 100% of the fee-schedule amount for a single code. For example, the fee-schedule amount for code YYYYY is $125. The physician reports code YYYYY-LT with an actual charge of $100 and YYYYY-RT with an actual charge of $100.

Payment would be based on the fee-schedule amount ($125) because it is lower than the total actual charges for the left and right sides ($200). The RVUs are based on a bilateral procedure because (a) the code descriptor specifically states that the procedure is bilateral, (b) the code descriptor states that the procedure may be performed either unilaterally or bilaterally, or (c) the procedure is usually performed as a bilateral procedure.

3 The usual payment adjustment for bilateral procedures does not apply. If a procedure is reported with modifier 50, or is reported for both sides on the same day by any other means (such as with RT and LT modifiers or with a "2" in the units field), Medicare bases payment for each side or organ or site of a paired organ on the lower of (a) the actual charge for each side or (b) 100% of the fee-schedule amount for each side. If a procedure is reported as a bilateral procedure and with other procedure codes on the same day, the fee-schedule amount for a bilateral procedure is determined before any applicable multiple procedure rules are applied. Services in this category are generally radiology procedures or other diagnostic tests that are not subject to the special payment rules for other bilateral procedures.

9 Concept does not apply.

Modifier 51 (Multiple Procedures)

This modifier indicates which payment-adjustment rule for multiple procedures applies to the service.

0 No payment-adjustment rules for multiple procedures apply. If the procedure is reported on the same day as another procedure, payment is based on the lower of (a) the actual charge or (b) the fee-schedule amount for the procedure.

1 This indicator is only applied to codes with a procedure status of "D." If a procedure is reported on the same day as another procedure with an indicator of "1," "2," or "3," Medicare ranks the procedures by the fee-schedule amount, and the appropriate reduction to this code is applied (100%, 50%, 25%, 25%, 25%, and by report). Carriers and Medicare Administrative Contractors (MACs) base payment on the lower of (a) the actual charge or (b) the fee-schedule amount reduced by the appropriate percentage.

2 Standard payment-adjustment rules for multiple procedures apply. If the procedure is reported on the same day as another procedure with an indicator of "1," "2," or "3," carriers and MACs rank the procedures by the fee-schedule amount and apply the appropriate reduction to this code (100%, 50%, 50%, 50%, 50%, and by report). MACs base payment on the lower of (a) the actual charge or (b) the fee-schedule amount reduced by the appropriate percentage.

3 Special rules for multiple endoscopic procedures apply if a procedure is billed with another endoscopy in the same family (ie, another endoscopy that has the same base procedure). The base procedure for each code with this indicator is identified in field 31G of Form CMS-1500 or its electronic equivalent claim. The multiple endoscopy rules apply to a family before ranking the family with other procedures performed on the same day (for example, if multiple endoscopies in the same family are reported on the same day as endoscopies in another family or on the same day as a non-endoscopic procedure). If an endoscopic procedure is reported with only its base procedure, the base procedure is not separately paid. Payment for the base procedure is included in the payment for the other endoscopy.

4 Diagnostic imaging services are subject to multiple procedure payment reduction (MPPR) methodology. Technical component (TC) of diagnostic imaging services is subject to a 50% reduction of the second and subsequent imaging services furnished by the same physician (or by multiple physicians in the same group practice using the same group national provider identifier [NPI]) to the same beneficiary on the same day, effective for services July 1, 2010, and after. Physician component (PC) of diagnostic imaging services are subject to a 25% payment reduction of the second and subsequent imaging services effective January 1, 2012.

5 Selected therapy services are subject to MPPR methodology. Therapy services are subject to 20% of the PE component for certain therapy services furnished in office or other non-institutional settings, and a 25% reduction of the PE component for certain therapy services furnished in institutional settings. Therapy services are subject to 50% reduction of the PE component for certain therapy services furnished in both institutional and non-institutional settings.

6 Diagnostic ophthalmology services are subject to the MPPR methodology. Full payment is made for the TC service with the highest payment under the Medicare physician fee schedule (MPFS). Payment is made at 75% for subsequent TC services furnished by the same physician (or by multiple physicians in the same group practice using the same group NPI) to the same beneficiary on the same day.

7 Diagnostic ophthalmology services are subject to the MPPR methodology. Full payment is made for the TC service with the highest payment under the MPFS. Payment is made at 80% for subsequent TC services furnished by the same physician (or by multiple physicians in the same group practice using the same group NPI) to the same beneficiary on the same day.

9 Concept does not apply.

Modifier 62 (Two Surgeons)

This modifier indicates services for which two surgeons, each in a different specialty, may be paid.

0 Co-surgeons not permitted for this procedure.

1 Co-surgeons could be paid. Supporting documentation is required to establish medical necessity of two surgeons for the procedure.

2 Co-surgeons permitted. No documentation is required if two specialty requirements are met.

9 Concept does not apply.

Modifier 66 (Surgical Team)

This modifier indicates services for which a surgical team may be paid.

0 Team surgeons not permitted for this procedure.

1 Team surgeons could be paid. Supporting documentation is required to establish medical necessity of a team; paid by report.

2 Team surgeons permitted; paid by report.

9 Concept does not apply.

Modifier 80 (Assistant Surgeon)

This modifier indicates services for which an assistant at surgery is never paid.

0 Payment restriction for assistants at surgery applies to this procedure unless supporting documentation is submitted to establish medical necessity.

1 Statutory payment restriction for assistants at surgery applies to this procedure. Assistants at surgery may not be paid.

2 Payment restriction for assistants at surgery does not apply to this procedure. Assistants at surgery may be paid.

9 Concept does not apply.

Because many of the services represented by CPT codes in the Radiology, Pathology, and Medicine sections of the CPT code set are diagnostic in nature, crosswalks to the ICD-10-CM code set are too numerous to list. Instead, a narrative description of the service is followed by RVU, modifier, and global information. The official CPT parenthetical information associated with the CPT code is included as well.

The following page presents a guide to the information contained within a code-detail page.

HCPCS Level II Codes

The HCPCS Level II code set is a collection of codes that are used to report health care procedures, supplies, and services. HCPCS Level I codes are CPT codes, developed and copyrighted by the AMA. HCPCS Level II codes include alphanumeric codes developed by CMS to report services, procedures, and supplies that are not reported with CPT codes. These codes include: ambulance services; durable medical equipment; prosthetics, orthotics, and supplies (DMEPOS); drugs; and quality-measure reporting. HCPCS Level II codes also include two-character modifiers used to identify anatomic sites, describe the provider of care or supplies, or describe specific clinical findings.

Modifiers

HCPCS Level II and CPT modifiers appropriate to ophthalmology coding are included in this chapter. A modifier provides the means to report or indicate that a service reported with a CPT or HCPCS Level II code has been altered by some specific circumstance but unchanged in its definition or code. The service may have been greater, or lesser, or may have been performed by multiple physicians who will share in reimbursement for the service. Modifiers also enable health care professionals to effectively respond to payment policy requirements established by other entities, and often affect reimbursement.

Modifiers may be part of the CPT code set or part of the HCPCS Level II code set. Both types are included in this chapter. CMS rules specific to the assignment of modifiers are presented in numeric (CPT modifiers) or alphanumeric order (HCPCS Level II modifiers).

Appendices

What follows is an explanation the appendices contained within *CPT® Coding Essentials for Ophthalmology 2022.*

Appendix A: National Correct Coding Initiative Edits

The National Correct Coding Initiative (CCI) was developed by CMS to restrict the reporting of inappropriate code combinations and reduce inappropriate payments to providers. The CCI edits essentially identify when a lesser code should be bundled into the parent code and not separately reported, and when two codes are mutually exclusive. In either case, only one of the codes is eligible for reimbursement. In other cases, it is only appropriate to report both codes concurrently if modifier 59 is appended to identify that one of the codes reported is a distinct procedural service.

Each of the CCI edits presented in this appendix includes a superscript that identifies how the edit should be applied. With a superscript of 0 (12001^0), the two codes may never be reported together. With a superscript of 1 (12001^1), a modifier may be applied and both codes reported, if appropriate. A superscript of 9 (12001^9) indicates that the modifier issue is not applicable to this code pairing, and the two codes should not be reported together. Remember, the modifier can only be used when the paired codes represent distinct procedural services. The modifier would be appended to the lesser of the two codes, as defined by their RVUs.

The CCI edits for each of the CPT codes found in this guide are included in in this appendix, listed in numeric order for simple lookup. CCI edits are updated quarterly. Those listed in this guide are effective January 1, 2022 through March 31, 2022. Future quarterly CCI edits can be found at www.cms.gov/Medicare/Coding/NationalCorrectCodInitEd/Version_Update_Changes.

Appendix B: Clinical Documentation Checklist

One of the greatest challenges of ICD-10-CM coding is ensuring that the clinical documentation from providers is sufficient.

The Clinical Documentation Checklists were developed to be used as a communication tool between coder and physician, or as a document that can be reproduced as a template for documentation by the physician. Essentially, the checklist identifies those documentation details required for complete and accurate code selection. For example, in ICD-10-CM, secondary diabetes is divided into diabetes due to underlying condition (E08) and diabetes induced by drugs or chemicals (E09). Furthermore, another category, other specified diabetes mellitus (E13), has been added. This category is selected for patients who have postsurgical or postpancreatectomy diabetes, or when the cause of secondary diabetes is not documented. Type 1 is reported with E10 codes, and type 2 with E11 codes.

Appendix C: Documentation Guidelines for Evaluation and Management (E/M) Services

As the author and owner of E/M codes found in the CPT code set, the AMA has developed detailed guidelines on how to determine which code is appropriate to report, based on the medical record for the encounter. These guidelines look at the quality and quantity of the data in the record:

- History
- Examination
- Medical decision making
- Counseling
- Coordination of care
- Nature of the presenting problem
- Length of the visit.

In 1995, CMS published its own documentation guidelines (DGs). Recognizing that the 1995 DGs did not appropriately reflect the work performed in some specialties, CMS published a second set of DGs in 1997. Both sets are still in use. The 1995 DGs are appropriate for multi-system examinations (eg, internal medicine physician). The 1997 DGs are appropriate for in-depth, single-system examinations, (eg, retinal specialist).

For Medicare and Medicaid, either the 1995 or 1997 DGs is to be followed, depending on the preference of the provider or

Master code or code family for this code-detail page. All information on this page links to or crosswalks to this code(s).

thalmology 2022 65855

CPT® Procedural Coding

65855

65855 Trabeculoplasty by laser surgery

(Do not report 65855 in conjunction with 65860, 65865, 65870, 65875, 65880)

(For trabeculectomy, use 66170)

Parenthetical instructions that are part of the official CPT codebook give crucial direction to prevent coding errors.

ing Notes

Procedures on the Eye and Adnexa

stic and treatment ophthal services, see Medicine, Ophthalmolog et seq)(Do not report code 69990 in a codes 65091-68850)

Official CPT code description(s) for the master code(s) enable coders to double-check their code selections.

AMA *CPT Assistant* ▢

65855: Mar 98: 7, Mar 03: 23

Citations for *CPT® Assistant* are provided so coders know when to seek further information from this authoritative reference.

Plain English Description

The procedure may also be referred to as argon laser trabeculoplasty (ALT) or selective laser ... This procedure is performed ... e glaucoma, pseudoexfoliation ... ntary dispersion syndrome. ... stered to constrict the pupil, ... of fluid in the eyes, and prevent elevation of eye pressure. A slit lamp and gonioscopy lens are used to guide the laser beam into the trabecular meshwork. The laser is activated and small burns are made in the trabecular ... ment typically involves creating ... 180 degrees of trabecular

Plain English Descriptions of the procedure or service explain what the master code represents, enabling the coder to verify code selections against the medical record.

isty by laser surgery

Gonioscopy lens

Guided laser beam

Simple line illustrations bring clarity and understanding to complex procedures.

ICD-10-CM Diagnostic Codes

⇄	H18.041	Kayser-Fleischer ring, right eye
⇄	H21.231	Degeneration of iris (pigmentary), right eye
⇄	H25.11	Age-related nuclear cataract, right eye
	H25.89	Other age-related cataract
⇄	H40.001	Preglaucoma, unspecified, right eye
⇄	H40.011	Open angle with borderline findings, low risk, right eye
⇄	H40.031	Anatomical narrow angle, right eye
⇄	H40.051	Ocular hypertension, right eye
❼	H40.10	Unspecified open-angle glaucoma
❼⇄	H40.111	Primary open-angle glaucoma, right eye
❼⇄	H40.112	Primary open-angle glaucoma, left eye
❼⇄	H40.113	Primary open-angle glaucoma, bilateral
❼⇄	H40.121	Low-tension glaucoma, right eye
❼⇄	H40.131	Pigmentary glaucoma, right eye
❼⇄	H40.141	Capsular glaucoma with pseudoexfoliation of lens, right eye
⇄	H40.152	Residual stage of open-angle glaucoma, left eye
❼⇄	H40.221	Chronic angle-closure glaucoma, right eye
	).31	Glaucoma secondary to eye trauma, right eye
	).41	Glaucoma secondary to eye inflammation, right eye
	).51	Glaucoma secondary to other eye disorders, right eye
	).61	Glaucoma secondary to drugs, right eye
⇄	H40.831	Aqueous misdirection, right eye
⇄	H54.0X33	Blindness right eye category 3, blindness left eye category 3
⇄	H54.0X34	Blindness right eye category 3, blindness left eye category 4
⇄	H54.0X35	Blindness right eye category 3, blindness left eye category 5
⇄	H54.0X43	Blindness right eye category 4, blindness left eye category 3
⇄	H54.0X44	Blindness right eye category 4, blindness left eye category 4
⇄	H54.0X45	Blindness right eye category 4, blindness left eye category 5
⇄	H54.0X53	Blindness right eye category 5, blindness left eye category 3
⇄	H54.0X54	Blindness right eye category 5, blindness left eye category 4
⇄	H54.0X55	Blindness right eye category 5, blindness left eye category 5
⇄	H54.1131	Blindness right eye category 3, low vision left eye category 1
⇄	H54.1132	Blindness right eye category 3, low vision left eye category 2
⇄	H54.1141	Blindness right eye category 4, low vision left eye category 1
⇄	H54.1142	Blindness right eye category 4, low vision left eye category 2
⇄	H54.1151	Blindness right eye category 5, low vision left eye category 1
⇄	H54.1152	Blindness right eye category 5, low vision left eye category 2
⇄	H54.1213	Low vision right eye category 1, blindness left eye category 3
⇄	H54.1214	Low vision right eye category 1,
⇄	H54.2X22	Low vision right eye category 2, low vision left eye category 2
⇄	H54.413A	Blindness right eye category 3, normal vision left eye
⇄	H54.414A	Blindness right eye category 4, normal vision left eye
⇄	H54.415A	Blindness right eye category 5, normal vision left eye
⇄	H54.42A3	Blindness left eye category 3, normal vision right eye
⇄	H54.42A4	Blindness left eye category 4, normal vision right eye
⇄	H54.42A5	Blindness left eye category 5, normal vision right eye
⇄	H54.511A	Low vision right eye categor normal vision left eye
⇄	H54.512A	Low vision right eye categor normal vision left eye
⇄	H54.52A1	Low vision left eye category normal vision right eye
⇄	H54.52A2	Low vision left eye category normal vision right eye

Common diagnoses associated with the procedure are linked to the ICD-10-CM code set. Icons identify when a seventh character is required, and Xs have been added to codes as placeholders to prevent errors when assigning the seventh character. Diagnoses that are limited to one sex are noted with an icon. Diagnoses that apply to multiple sides/regions of the body are noted with an icon.

Citations for the CMS' Pub 100 billing guidance is provided so coders know when to seek further information from this authoritative reference.

ICD-10-CM Coding Notes

For codes requiring a 7th character extensi to your ICD-10-CM book. Review the chara descriptions and coding guidelines for prop selection. For some procedures, only certai characters will apply.

CCI Edits

Refer to Appendix A for CCI edits.

Pub 100

65855: Pub 100-03, 1, 140.5

From the CMS database, key CPT code modifiers affecting relative values when they indicate multiple procedures or multiple providers, as in co-surgery, team surgery, or assistant surgery are listed here.

Facility RVUs ▢

Code	Work	PE Facility	MP
65855	3.00	2.71	0.22

Non-facility RVUs ▢

Code	Work	PE Non-Facility	MP
65855	3.00	3.78	0.22

RVUs are national Medicare relative value units, or a breakdown of the costs of medical care based on CPT code. Physician work, practice expense, malpractice expense, and total expense differ for facility and nonfacility, so both are listed. RVUs may be used to predict or set fees for physician payment. RVUs shown are for physicians participating in the Medicare program.

Modifiers (PAR) ▢

Code	Mod 50	Mod 51	Mod 62	66	80
65855	1	2	1	1	1

Global Period

Code	Days
65855	010

The Medicare global period indicates the number of postoperative days during which any routine care associated with the original service is bundled into the original service. Possible global periods are 0, 10, and 90 days.

● New ▲ Revised ✚ Add On ⊘Modifier 51 Exempt ★Telemedicine ▢ CPT QuickRef ⁄FDA Pending ⇄ Laterality ❼ Seventh Character ♂Male ♀Female

 161

coder. The CPT guidelines, while largely incorporated into the 1995 and 1997 DGs, still have unique features accepted by some private payers. Unabridged copies of all three sets of DGs are presented in Appendix C.

Terminology, Abbreviations, and Basic Anatomy

The Terminology, Abbreviations, and Basic Anatomy chapter can be used as a reference tool if there is confusion when reading medical record documentation and when a more extensive understanding of medical terminology is needed. The following includes terms, abbreviations, symbols, prefixes, suffixes, and anatomical illustrations that will help clarify some of the more difficult issues, and give a firmer understanding of information, that is in medical record documentation.

Medical Terminology

Majority of medical terms are composed of Greek and Latin word parts and are broken down into different elements. One element is the root word. The root word is the foundation of the medical term and contains the fundamental meaning of the word. All medical terms have one or more roots.

Examples:

hydr = water

lith = stone

path = disease

Combining forms (or vowel, usually "o") links the root word to the suffix or to another root word. This combining vowel does not have a meaning on its own; it only joins one part of a word to another.

Prefixes and suffixes are two of the other elements used in medical terminology and consist of one or more syllables (prepositions or adverbs) placed before or after root words to show various kinds of relationships. Prefixes are before the root word and suffixes are after the root word and consist of one or more letters grouped together. They are never used independently; however, they can modify the meaning of the other word parts. Many prefixes and suffixes are added to other words with a hyphen, but medical dictionary publishers are opting to drop the hyphen on many of the more common prefixed medical words.

Examples:

Prefixes:

micro = small

peri = surrounding

Suffixes:

algia = pain

an = pertaining to

The following are lists of prefixes and suffixes typically seen in Ophthalmology:

Root Words/Combining Forms

acous/o	hearing
acr/o	extremities, top, extreme point
aden/o	gland
adip/o	fat
andr/o	male
ankyl/o	stiff, bent, crooked
anter/o	front
arthr/o	joint
ather/o	yellowish, fatty plaque
audi/o	hearing
aur/o	ear
aut/o	self
bi/o	life
blast/o	developing cell
blephar/o	eyelid
bronch/o	bronchial tubes
canth/o	canthus
capsul/o	capsule
carcin/o	cancer
cardi/o	heart
cheil/o	lip
chondr/o	cartilage
cis/o	to cut
conjuctiv/o	conjunctiva
coron/o	heart
crani/o	skull
cry/o	cold
cutane/o	skin
cyan/o	blue
cyt/o	cell
dacry/o	tear duct, tear
derm/o	skin
dermat/o	skin
dextr/o	right
dipl/o	double, two
dips/o	thirst
dist/o	distant, far
ech/o	sound
encephal/o	brain
erythr/o	red

erythem/o	red
eti/o	cause of disease
gloss/o	tongue
gluc/o	sugar
glyc/o	sugar
gravid/o	pregnancy
gynec/o	female, woman
hemat/o	blood
hidr/o	sweat
hist/o	tissue
hom/o	sameness
irid/o	iris
isch/o	to hold back
kal/o	potassium
kerat/o	cornea
lei/o	smooth
leuk/o	white
irid/o	iris
lith/o	stone
melan/o	black
ment/o	mind
morph/o	shape, form
my/o	muscle
myc/o	fungus
myel/o	spinal cord
myring/o	eardrum
natr/o	sodium
necr/o	death
nephr/o	kidney
neur/o	nerve
noct/o	night
odont/o	tooth
odyn/o	pain, distress
olig/o	few, scanty
onc/o	tumor
opt/o	eye
ophthalm/o	eye
or/o	mouth
orth/o	straight
oste/o	bone
ot/o	ear
pachy/o	thick
path/o	disease
phac/o	lens
phag/o	to eat, swallow
phak/o	lens
phleb/o	vein
phot/o	light
phren/o	diaphragm
plas/o	formation, development
psych/o	mind
py/o	pus
quadr/o	four
rhin/o	nose
rhytid/o	wrinkle
rhiz/o	nerve root
sial/o	salivary gland
sarc/o	flesh
sect/o	to cut
spir/o	breathing
spondyl/o	vertebra
squam/o	scale-like
staphyl/o	clusters
steat/o	fat
strept/o	twisted chains
terat/o	monster
thec/o	sheath
thromb/o	clot
trich/o	hair
tympan/o	eardrum
vas/o	vessel
ven/o	vein
viscer/o	internal organs
xanth/o	yellow
xer/o	dry

Prefixes

a(d)-	towards
a(n)-	without
ab-	from
ab(s)-	away from
ad-	towards
allo-	other, another
ambi-	both
amphi-	on both sides, around
ana-	up to, back, again, movement from
aniso-	different, unequal
ante-	before, forwards
anti-	against, opposite
ap-, apo-	from, back, again
bi(s)-	twice, double
bio-	life
brachy-	short
cata-	down
circum-	around
con-	together
contra-	against
cyte-	cell
de-	from, away from, down from
deca-	ten
di(s)-	two
dia-	through, complete
di(a)s	separation

diplo-	double
dolicho-	long
dur-	hard, firm
dys-	bad, abnormal
e-, ec-, ek-	out, from out of
ecto-	outside, external
em-	in
en-	into
endo-	into
ent-	within
epi-	on, up, against, high
eso-	will carry
eu-	well, abundant, prosperous
eury-	broad, wide
ex-, exo-	out, from out of
extra-	outside, beyond, in addition
haplo-	single
hapto-	bind to
hemi-	half
hept-	seven
hetero-	different
hex-	six
homo-	same
hyper-	above, excessive
hypo-	below, deficient
im-, in-	not
in-	into, to
infra-	below, underneath
inter-	among, between
intra-	within, inside, during
intro-	inward, during
iso-	equal, same
juxta-	adjacent to
kata-	down, down from
macro-	large
magno-	large
medi-	middle
mega-	large
megalo-	very large
meso-	middle
meta-	beyond, between
micro-	small
neo-	new
non-	not
ob-	before, against
octa-	eight
octo-	eight
oligo-	few
pachy-	thick
pan-	all
para-	beside, to the side of, wrong
pent-	five
per-	by, through, throughout
peri-	around, round-about
pleo-	more than usual
poly	many
post-	behind, after
pre-	before, in front, very
pros-	besides
prox-	besides
pseudo-	false, fake
quar(r)-	four
re, red-	back, again
retro-	backwards, behind
semi-	half
sex-	six
sept-	seven
sub-	under, beneath
super-	above, in addition, over
supra-	above, on the upper side
syn-	together, with
sys-	together, with
tetra-	four
thio-	sulfur
trans-	across, beyond
tri-	three
uni-	one
ultra-	beyond, besides, over

Suffixes

-ase	enzyme
-cele	hernia
-cide	killing
-ectasia	dilation
-ectomy	removal of, cut out
-edema	swelling
-form	shaped like
-ia	pathological condition
-iasis	infestation, pathological state
-ile	little version
-illa	little version
-illus	little version
-in	stuff
-ism	condition indicated by root/prefix
-itis	inflammation
-ium	structure; tissue
-ize	do
-logy	study of, reasoning about
-megaly	large
-noid	mind, spirit
-oid	resembling, image of
-ogen	precursor
-ol(e)	alcohol

-ole	little version
-oma	tumor (usually)
-opia, -opsia	vision
-osis	full of
-ostomy	artificial opening
-pathy	disease of, suffering
-penia	lack
-pexy	fix in place
-plasty	re-shaping
-philia	affection for
-rhage	burst out
-rhea	discharge, flowing out
-rrhexis	shredding, rupture
-pagus	Siamese twins
-sis	idea
-thrix	hair
-tomy	cut; incise
-ule	little version
-um	thing

Ophthalmology Terms

The following definitions are medical terms commonly seen while coding and billing for Ophthalmology:

Accommodation – In younger people, under age forty, the lens is adjusted by the ciliary muscles to focus clearly for near as well as far vision. With age the lens is less able to change, eventually requiring reading glasses or bifocals for close work.

Achromatopsia – Characterized by a lack of color vision with poor visual acuity, nystagmus, and sensitivity to sunlight. No treatment is available except, for example, sunglasses for the sensitivity to light.

Age-Related Macular Degeneration – The most common form of macular degeneration is Age-Related Macular Degeneration (ARMD). It is believed that one contributing factor of ARMD is excessive light exposure over a person's lifetime. Limiting excessive light exposure (e.g., wearing sunglasses and a hat outside) and a diet rich in antioxidants as well as zinc may prevent or retard the development of ARMD. In general, the lighter a person's complexion, the greater the risk of ARMD.

Albinism – A hereditary condition in which darker pigment fails to form in the eye, hair and skin. In ocular albinism, visual acuity ranges from 20/40 to 20/200 (legal blindness), the eyes may dance (nystagmus) and the person is very sensitive to sunlight. No treatment is available, except dark sunglasses for the photophobia.

Amblyopia – Commonly known as lazy eye. A loss of vision in a young child due to the eye not being used. The eye is normal but the brain tends to suppress or ignore the image received by the amblyopic eye. The most common causes include a muscle imbalance, a focusing problem, or a problem such as a cataract or corneal scar. Sometimes both eyes can be affected.

Amsler Grid – A chart featuring horizontal and vertical lines used to test vision.

Angioid Streaks – Fragmentation of Bruch's membrane due to the degeneration of the elastic layers and development of subretinal fibrovascular tissue. Sometimes does not cause vision problems; however, can cause a reduction of visual acuity leading to legal blindness. Often associated with another disease such as sickle cell disease and certain syndromes.

Aniridia – A hereditary eye problem in which the iris, the colored part of the eye, is absent. There is poor vision, sensitivity to sunlight, nystagmus, and a tendency to develop glaucoma.

Anisocoria – A difference in the size of the two pupils. It is present in about 5% of normal children. The most serious cause of an acquired Anisocoria follows a head injury with some brain or nerve damage; a disease such as a tumor also causes it.

Anisometropia – A difference in the focusing power of the two eyes. One of the major causes of amblyopia; the brain is not able to clearly focus both eyes simultaneously. This is a "hidden" cause of amblyopia and very difficult to detect without an eye exam.

Aphakia – The loss or absence of the lens of an eye.

Aqueous Humor – A colorless watery fluid filling the space between the lens and the cornea. It maintains the shape of the front of the eye.

Astigmatism – Irregular curvature of either the cornea (front of the eye) or the lens. If either structure is shaped more like a football rather than a basketball, light is not sharply focused on the retina. This results in blurry vision for both distance and near.

Atrophy – Decay or wasting away. Dying.

Best's Disease – Also called Vitelliform macular dystrophy. Causes atrophy of the Retinal Pigment Epithelium (RPE) and photoreceptors in the macula. Late in the disease there is a loss of visual acuity to legal blindness and a blind spot in central vision. No treatment is available.

Binocular Vision – The blending of the separate images seen by each eye into a single image; allows images to be seen with depth.

Bispectral Index (BIS) – A calculation based on certain readings of an EEG. Used to measure the hypnotic state/sedation level of a patient.

Blepharitis – Inflammation of the eyelids or lid margins. It is often caused by an infection. A chronic form produces a scaling or crusting of the lid margins. This is treatable by an eye doctor.

Blind Spot – Area of the retina that contains no light receptor cells (rods and cones). If the light from an object falls on the blind spot, that object will not be seen.

Blindness – Legal blindness is defined as: (1) visual acuity of 20/200 (only being able to see the big E on the eye chart) or less in the best eye even with the eyes corrected by glasses or contact lenses; or (2) The peripheral visual field is reduced to 20 degrees of visual angle or less. Twenty degrees of visual angle is about the size of a one-foot ruler held at arm's length.

CAM Treatment – CAM is an abbreviation for Cambridge (England) where a new therapy for amblyopia was proposed that used rotating gratings (series of black and white bars). Patients would view the rotating gratings while they performed various drawing tasks on top of the rotating gratings. Research has shown, however, that CAM treatment is not effective at improving visual acuity in amblyopic children.

Carbidopa – A peripheral decarboxylase inhibitor. Dopa decarboxylase is an enzyme that converts levodopa into dopamine, a major neurotransmitter and neuromodular of cellular function. Carbidopa is sometimes used to prevent the peripheral conversion of levodopa into dopamine in peripheral sites such as the gut, thus allowing more levodopa to reach the brain where it can have therapeutic effects.

Cataract – Opacity or haziness of the lens of the eye. A cataract is noticed particularly at night when oncoming headlights produce glare disability or/and discomfort. It may or may not reduce the vision depending on size, density and location. If a cataract reduces visual acuity significantly, an ophthalmologist can replace the defective lens with an artificial lens.

Chalazion – In the eyelid, there are a number of glands that produce lubricants for the cornea and eyelid. A chalazion occurs when a gland become plugged, enlarged, or infected. The lid looks like it has a lump about the size of a small pea. Occasionally it occurs as a thickness within the lid. Warm compresses help some disappear; others require surgical removal by an ophthalmologist.

Chorioretinitis – An inflammation of the back of the eye involving the choroid and retina. It may be due to a number of different diseases, which affect the body such as toxoplasmosis, histoplasmosis, sarcoidosis, tuberculosis, and syphilis.

Choroid (Eye) – The thin vascular middle layer of the eye filled with blood vessels that is situated between the sclera and the retina and nourishes the retina; part of the uvea.

Choroideremia – Atrophy or decay of the choroid, choriocapillaris and Bruch's membrane of the eye, leading to a severe loss of vision. Usually progresses to light perception by 50 years of age. Leads to night blindness tunnel vision and reduced visual acuity. No treatment available.

Choroiditis – Inflammation of the back of the eye involving the choroid and retina. It may be due to a number of different diseases, which affect the body such as toxoplasmosis, histoplasmosis, sarcoidosis, tuberculosis and syphilis.

Ciliary Body – A body of tissue that connects the iris with the choroids and includes a group of muscles which act on the lens of the eye to change its shape.

Coloboma – A congenital (born with) problem with the eye that is related to a maldevelopment or underdevelopment of a part of the eye. It may involve the eyelid, or interior part of the eye (involving the choroid and occasionally the optic nerve). No treatment is available.

Cone – One of the two light receiving retinal cells (the other is the rod) that is responsible for daylight vision (e.g., color vision, high visual acuity, bright light vision). The area of the retina that provides central or reading vision, known as the fovea, contains only cones.

Cone Dystrophy – Also sometimes referred to as cone degeneration. The cones of the eye degenerate over time leading to visual acuity between 20/50 and 20/200 – legal blindness. There may be a progressive vision loss, abnormal color vision and photophobia. No treatment is available, except for dark sunglasses for the photophobia. Patients with cone dystrophies and cone degenerations benefit for rehabilitation services.

Cone Rod Degeneration – Also called cone-rod dystrophy. Leads to a loss of visual acuity between 20/25 to 20/400 – legal blindness. First there is a loss of cone photoreceptors followed by a loss of rod photoreceptors. Visual fields may be restricted, abnormal color vision and photophobia. No treatment is available.

Congenital – Existing at and usually before, birth, referring to conditions that are present at birth, regardless of their causation.

Congenital Cataract – A cataract or clouding of the lens of the eye, that occurs in the fetus at some time during pregnancy.

Conjunctiva – The membrane that lines the exposed eyeball and the inside of the eyelid.

Conjunctivitis – Inflammation of the membrane covering the surface of the eyeball. It can be a result of infection, irritation, or related to systemic diseases, such as Reiter's syndrome.

Cornea – The clear front window of the eye that transmits and focuses light into the eye.

Corneal Curvature – The shape of the front surface of the eye.

Cortex – The surface of the brain. The word cortex is derived from the Greek name meaning "bark" (like tree bark). The visual cortex contains 32 or more areas devoted to visual information processing. Two major cortical pathways are the "What" and the "Where" visual pathways, that are devoted to what an object is and where an object is.

Cortical Blindness – A person with cortical blindness will have normal eyes and normal optic nerves but, nevertheless, will not be able to see. The cause of the blindness is with the cortex or surface of the brain that contains 32 or more sites for visual information processing. More recently, the preferred term for such individuals is cortical visual impairment, because many people will not be totally blind but will exhibit unusual visual losses; for example, they may be blind to stationary objects but be able to see moving objects.

Cover Test – A test for a muscle imbalance. While the person is looking at a distant object, one eye is covered and then uncovered (cover-uncover). This is repeated on the other eye. Finally, it is performed on both eyes, covering one then the other (alternate-cover). If one or both eyes shift during this test, there is a problem with alignment of the eyes. The misalignment with the eyes often cannot be seen with both eyes opened.

Cupping of the Optic Disc – A depression of the optic nerve where the optic nerve leaves the eye. In glaucoma, the cup may be enlarged indicating damage to the nerves leading from the eye to the brain.

Cycloplegia – A paralysis of the ciliary muscles following the instillation of eye drops. This produces a loss of accommodation or focusing ability. With the lens relaxed, a better estimate of the refractive error is possible in most cases. Most cycloplegic eye drops also dilate the pupil. Cycloplegia may last from a few hours to several days, depending on certain factors such as skin color – the lighter the longer.

Degenerative Myopia – Pathologic progressive myopia. Causes Retinal Pigment Epithelium (RPE) and choriocapillaris atrophy and photoreceptor degeneration. Leads to reduced visual acuity, night blindness and retinal detachment, the latter requires retinal surgery.

Depth Perception – The ability to distinguish objects in a visual field.

Dermoid Cyst – A congenital (born with) tumor present in infancy as a yellowish swelling on the surface of the eye. It may enlarge during puberty. The dermoid cyst can be surgically removed by an ophthalmologist.

Detached Retina – A condition in which the retina separates from another layer of cells in the back of the eye, resulting in a decrease in nutrition and visual function. It may be due to a hemorrhage, trauma, tumor, vascular malformation or from traction of the vitreous to which it is attached. Sometimes, people with high myopia will develop a retinal detachment, which requires emergency surgery.

Diabetic Retinopathy – Pathologic changes in the back of the eye, retina, caused by diabetes. Background type is characterized by ongoing microaneurysms, retinal hemorrhages and swelling of the central part of the eye, known as the macula. The proliferate type involves the growth of abnormal blood vessels in the retina and optic disk, blood leaking into the jelly part of the eye, known as the vitreous, and detachment of the retina.

Dilation – A process by which the pupil is temporarily enlarged with special eye drops (mydriatic); allows the eye care specialist to better view the inside of the eye.

Diopter – The unit used to measure the amount of refractive or focusing power of the eye. It also refers to the strength of lens required to provide clear vision. In general, the higher the refractive error, as measured in diopters, the worse the eye.

Diplopia – Commonly known as double vision. In children, diplopia is often associated with a muscle imbalance such as esotropia. A refractive error may also cause enough blurring that a person sees two objects.

Dominant Progressive Foveal Dystrophy – Dominant Stargardt's disease. A degeneration of the Retinal Pigment Epithelium (RPE) and photoreceptors of the eye. Slowly progressive, leading to legal blindness later in life. Usually starts in the 20s to 40s. Results in decreased visual acuity, central scotoma and defective color vision. There is no treatment.

Drusen – Amorphous, sub-RPE material; probably the remains of the Retinal Pigment Epithelium (RPE)as a result of atrophy. Associated, sometimes with aging and with Age-Related Macular Degeneration (ARMD). There may be no symptoms present in the early stages and may lead to a reduction in visual acuity later in life.

Dyslexia – A learning problem in which a person has difficulty with letter or word recognition. Children often are of normal or above normal intelligence; however, they have difficulty reading and sometimes naming pictures of objects. More recent evidence suggests that dyslexia is a decoding problem based on phonemes – the basic language components. This is a higher cortical processing problem and NOT a vision or eye problem, per se.

Electrooculogram (EOG) – A test of the functional integrity of the Retinal Pigment Epithelium (RPE)– a layer of cells next to the retina of the eye. The EOG involves electrodes attached to the inner and outer corners of the eye and the patient is required to look back-and-forth between two small lights in a large white globe (ganzfeld) with bright lights on and off.

Electroretinogram (ERG) – A test that measures the functional integrity of the retina, including the rod and cone photoreceptors. Usually involves the use of dilating drops in the eye and use of a contact lens electrode.

Endophthalmitis – Inflammation involving the internal parts of the eye – i.e., choroid, retina, ciliary body, and iris. A very serious condition sometimes seen after an injury to the eye by a foreign object. Vision is severely threatened. Large doses of cortisone and antibiotics are often needed. May lead to the removal of the eye. Must be treated by an eye doctor ASAP.

Enucleation – An operation in which the whole eye and the front part of the optic nerve are removed. It is usually performed when the eye contains a tumor or is blind and very painful.

Esophoria – A tendency for an eye to turn inward a little bit. It occurs under certain conditions such as fatigue. Esophoria is sometimes uncovered by the cover test.

Esotropia – Cross-eyed or, in medical terms, convergent or internal strabismus.

Exophoria – A tendency for an eye to turn outward a little bit. Occurs sometimes under certain conditions such as fatigue, bright sunlight or prolonged use of the eyes.

Exophthalmos – Abnormal protrusion of the eyeball often caused by thyroid disease or a tumor behind the eye. Medical treatment is necessary.

Exotropia – Divergent gaze. Also known as external strabismus.

Eye – The organ of sight. The word "eye" comes from the Teutonic "auge." The eye has a number of components. These include the cornea, iris, pupil, lens, retina, macula, optic nerve and vitreous.

Farsightedness (Hyperopia) – Medically termed hyperopia; the ability to see distant objects more clearly than close objects.

Floaters – Small condensations of cells in the vitreous body, the fluid in the eye, which cast shadows on the back of the eye, known as the retina. This is normally associated with aging. Floaters may indicate a more serious problem such as a retinal detachment.

Fluorescein Angiography – A diagnostic test used to assess pathology that affects the retina, choroids and/or iris of the eye. Fluorescein angiography is used to assess the blood flow of the eye and abnormal states are referred to as either hyperfluorescence or hypofluorescence relative to the normal amount of fluorescence. Fluorescein angiography involves an intravenous injection of sodium Fluorescein (a dye) into the antecubital vein (a vein in the arm) and then photographs are taken of the eye as the dye enters and leaves the blood system of the eye. The doctor will evaluate prefilling (i.e., what the retina and choroid look like before the dye enters the eye), transit (i.e., first passage of dye through the retina and choroid), recirculation (i.e., fluorescein has become equally distributed throughout the eye and then starts to circulate through again) and later phase (i.e., as the fluorescein is eliminated from the body by the kidneys). The test lasts about 30 minutes. Nausea and vomiting are the most common side effects, occurring in about 5% or less of patients. Severe side effects (e.g., anaphylaxis, death) have been reported but are very rare.

Fovea – A small yellow spot, is the most sensitive part of the retina. It is situated in the center of the posterior region, directly behind and in line with the lens. The human eye perceives light stimuli by means of cones and rods that are present in the retina of the eye. Most of the cones and rods are found in the central fovea of the eye.

Fundus – The back part of the eye that can be seen with an instrument called an ophthalmoscope. Visible features include the retina with its blood vessels, the optic nerve and choroid. The fundus surrounds the fovea, that part of the eye used for reading.

Glaucoma – An eye condition in which the fluid pressure inside the eyes rises because of slowed fluid drainage from the eye. Untreated, it may damage the optic nerve and other parts of the eye, leading to vision loss or even blindness.

Glaucoma Treatment (Medical) – Although glaucoma cannot be cured, it can usually be controlled. Medical treatment can be in the form of eyedrops or pills. Some drugs are designed to reduce pressure by slowing the flow of fluid into the eye, while others help to improve fluid drainage.

Gonioscopy – The examination of the internal angle between the iris and cornea. This is accomplished by placing a contact lens over the cornea. It is vital in all cases of suspected glaucoma.

Gyrate Atrophy – Diffuse total choroid vascular atrophy of the eye. Leads to night blindness, tunnel vision, cataracts and reduced visual acuity. Patients are usually myopic. Treatment involves pyridoxine; arginine free diet to reduce ornithinemia. Poor prognosis and usually leads to legal blindness by the age of 40 years.

Hemianopia – A loss of one-half of the field of vision; for example, all of the right side of vision is gone. This is sometimes seen in older people with vascular problems, in certain types of brain tumors or after head trauma.

Hemorrhage – Bleeding or the abnormal flow of blood.

Humor, Aqueous – In medicine, humor refers to a fluid (or semifluid) substance. Thus, the aqueous humor is the fluid normally present in the front and rear chambers of the eye. It is a clear, watery fluid that flows between and nourishes the lens and the cornea; it is secreted by the ciliary processes.

Hyaloid Canal – Narrow passageway that allows blood to flow through the eye.

Hyperopia – Commonly known as farsightedness. Most children are hyperopic and see things in the distance better than very close things.

Hyperphoria – A tendency for one eye to drift upward. A vertical type of muscle imbalance between the eyes.

Hypertropia – A muscle imbalance in which one eye is straight and the other is turned upward.

Hyphema – Blood in the aqueous fluid - front part of the eye, often caused by an injury. Patient should seek immediate medical attention since a hyphema may lead to glaucoma and permanent loss of vision.

Intraocular Pressure (IOP) – The pressure the fluid (vitreous) contained within the eye, exerts on the globe (lining of the eyeball). Increased intraocular pressure is a feature of glaucoma.

Iridocyclitis – Inflammation of the iris and ciliary body. It may be due to a disease within the eye or occur as a reaction to an injury or disease elsewhere in the body.

Iris – The colored part of the eye that helps regulate the amount of light that enters the eye.

Iritis – Inflammation of the iris, usually marked by pain, congestion in the ciliary region, photophobia, contraction of the pupil and discoloration of the iris.

Keratitis – An inflammation of the cornea often caused by a virus or bacteria. Scarring and loss of vision may result.

Keratoconus – Inherited disease where the cornea becomes progressively shaped like a cone. Wearing a contact lens may slow the progression of the disease. Corneal transplant surgery may be required.

Keratoplasty – A corneal transplant.

Lacrimal Gland – The tear gland located under the upper eyelid at the outer corner of the eye. The fluid it secretes cleans and provides moisture for the cornea. It is responsible for tearing during emotional stimulation or following corneal irritation by a foreign body or chemical.

Lacrimal Sac – The tear sac located on the side of the nose adjacent to the inner corner of the eye. Tears normally drain from the eye into the tear duct and then through the sac, finally leaving by a drain which enters the nose. The tear sac remains filled with tears when an infant has a blocked tear duct. An infection of the tear sac is called a dacryocystitis.

LASIK – LASIK (Laser in-Situ Keratomileusis) combines the precision of the excimer laser delivery system with the benefits of Lamellar Keratoplasty (LK) which has been proven to treat a wide range of refractive errors. Using the accuracy and precision of the excimer laser, LASIK changes the shape of the cornea to improve the way light is focused or "refracted" by the eye. First, a thin corneal flap is created, as an instrument called a microkeratome glides across the cornea. Then, in just seconds, ultraviolet light and high-energy pulses from the excimer laser reshape the internal cornea with accuracy up to 0.25 microns. By adjusting the pattern of the laser beam, it is possible to treat high levels of nearsightedness and moderate amounts of farsightedness and astigmatism.

Lazy Eye – A term often used instead of amblyopia. A loss of visual function, usually measured by visual acuity, in one or both eyes that cannot be explained by identifiable causes(s) such as a cataract or retinal disease. An eye that turns in (esotropia) or out (exotropia) may have a certain degree of central visual loss (amblyopia). A lazy eye is often treated by placing a patch over the stronger eye and forcing use of the lazy eye. The earlier the detection of the lazy eye the better for recovery of central vision with patching. If left untreated, after the age of about 8 or 9 years, patching therapy is no longer effective and the child will have a permanent loss of vision and loss of binocular vision and depth perception.

Leber's Disease (Leber's Congenital Amaurosis) – A severe form of rod-cone degeneration present at birth. Infants have very poor visual acuity, photophobia and nystagmus. Infant's with Leber's will often constantly rub their eyes with their fists and poke their eyes with their fingers and thumb. No treatment is available.

Lens – The lens is the transparent structure inside the eye that focuses light rays onto the retina.

Lens Capsule – A membrane that surrounds the lens of the eye. In cataract surgery, the lens is usually replaced with an intraocular lens but the lens capsule remains in the eye.

Levodopa – A precursor for the neurotransmitter/neuromodular dopamine. Levodopa is usually referred to as "L-dopa" and is often used to treat older adults with Parkinson's disease. Through enzymatic action of Dopa Decarboxylase, levodopa is converted into dopamine. However, levodopa can be converted to dopamine in peripheral sites such as the gut and then will not be able to cross the blood-brain barrier for central therapeutic effects. To prevent peripheral conversion of levodopa to dopamine, a peripheral decarboxylase inhibitor, such as carbidopa, is combined with levodopa to increase the amount of levodopa into the brain where it is then converted to dopamine. Carbidopa cannot cross the blood-brain barrier.

Macula – A small area in the retina that contains special light-sensitive cells and allows us to see fine details clearly.

Macular Degeneration – A degeneration or loss of the macula of the eye, usually hereditary. The most common form of macular degeneration is Age-related Macular Degeneration (ARMD). It is believed that one contributing factor for ARMD is excessive light exposure over a person's lifetime. Limiting excessive light exposure (e.g., wearing sunglasses and a hat outside) and a diet rich in antioxidants as well as zinc may prevent or retard the development of ARMD. In general, the lighter a person's complexion the greater the risk of ARMD.

Microphthalmia – An unnatural smallness of the eyes, occurring as the result of disease or of imperfect development.

Mydriasis – Dilation of the pupil.

Mydriatic – A drug that dilates the pupil (see cycloplegia). Sometimes used to treat amblyopia, particularly if the child will not wear an eye patch over the stronger eye.

Myopia – Commonly known as nearsightedness. A refractive error in which the light rays focus in front of the retina producing blurry distance vision. External optical correction (glasses or contact lenses) are required for clear distance vision. It is now believed that myopia is partly hereditary; you're more likely to become myopic if your parents are myopic. Also, near work can lead to a further worsening of the myopia. If the myopia is greater than 6 diopters, a condition known as high myopia, the possibility of retinal detachment is increased.

Near Point of Accommodation – The closest point in front of the eyes that an object may be clearly focused.

Near Point of Convergence – The maximum extent the two eyes can be turned inward.

Nearsightedness (Myopia) – The ability to see near objects more clearly than distant objects. Also called myopia. Myopia can be caused by a longer-than-normal eyeball or by any condition that prevents light rays from focusing on the retina.

Nystagmus – Rapid rhythmic repetitious involuntary (unwilled) eye movements. Nystagmus can be horizontal, vertical or rotary.

Ocular Hypertension – High (greater than 21 mm Hg) intraocular pressure.

Ocular Dexter (OD) – Right eye.

Oculus Sinister (OS) – Left eye.

Oculus Uterque (OU) – Both eyes.

Ophthalmologist – A physician (MD) who specializes in the diagnosis and treatment of eye problems and diseases. The ophthalmologist works with the use of glasses, contact lenses, eye medication and surgery.

Ophthalmoscope – A lighted instrument used to examine the inside of the eye, including the retina and the optic nerve.

Ophthalmoscopy – Examination of the internal structure of the eye.

Optic Atrophy – A disease of the optic nerve in which the nerve fibers carrying the electrical impulses from the eye to the brain start to die off. In such cases the optic nerve has a pale or whitish appearance compared to the normal pink color. Optic atrophy is associated with poor reading vision and often the cause of legal blindness. May be associated with a serious medical condition and requires further medical examination to determine the cause of the atrophy.

Optic Cup – The white, cup-like area in the center of the optic disc.

Optic Disc – The visible part of the optic nerve inside the eye. The axons of the ganglion cells of the inner retina make-up the optic nerve.

Optic Nerve – A bundle of more than 1 million nerve fibers that connects the retina with the brain. The optic nerve is responsible for interpreting the impulses it receives into images.

Optic Nerve Hypoplasia – A small and underdeveloped optic nerve. Optic nerve hypoplasia is one of the leading causes of vision loss and blindness in infants and children. Optic nerve hypoplasia occurs in the early stages of fetal development, when the eyes are forming. The optic nerve never fully develops or, once developed, dies-off and reduces in size for unknown reasons. Recent evidence suggests that ganglion cell axons, that make-up the optic nerve, are not able to grow through the optic nerve head because certain chemical messengers are not present for directional growth from the eye to the brain. Optic nerve hypoplasia is variable, and can result in only minor vision problems to complete blindness. Usually, if the infant has nystagmus the optic nerve hypoplasia is more severe and vision is very much reduced. If the infant does not have nystagmus, the likelihood for significant vision loss in less. All infants with optic nerve hypoplasia should have a CT scan or MRI to look for midline brain defects that can result in body growth problems. If the infant does not have nystagmus, the chance of midline brain defects is small. If the infant has nystagmus, the chance of midline defects is greater. Some infants have optic nerve hypoplasia in one eye only. If only in one eye, the chance of midline defects is very small and the physician may choose not to do a CT scan or MRI, depending on other factors.

Optic Neuritis – An inflammation of the optic nerve usually with some loss of sight (may be temporary). It may signify a more serious neurological condition. A leading cause of optic neuritis is multiple sclerosis (MS).

Optician – A technician who fits a person for glasses. He/she does not test for glasses. Some opticians also fit contact lenses.

Optometrist (OD) – A licensed non-physician educated to detect eye problems with special emphasis on correcting refractive errors. Depending on training, an optometrist may use diagnostic and therapeutic medicines. An optometrist does not perform surgery.

Orbit – In medicine, the orbit is the bony cavity in which the eyeball sits.

Orthokeratology – The use of contact lenses to change the shape of the cornea in order to correct refractive error.

Peripheral Vision – Side vision; the ability to see objects and movement outside of the direct line of vision.

Persistent Hyperplastic Primary Vitreous (PHPV) – Persistent Hyperplastic Primary Vitreous (PHPV) is a developmental abnormality of the eye alone. During intrauterine eye formation, the growing lens of the eye has a blood supply. After the lens has reached full intrauterine development, the blood supply regresses (shrivels away) so that at birth no blood vessels exist around the lens. If the lens development and blood vessel regression do not proceed normally, PHPV can result. PHPV is not known to be associated with any specific intrauterine insult. Problems such as maternal infection or ingestion of toxic substances generally affect BOTH eyes and cause cataracts which do not resemble PHPV. Typically, a pediatric ophthalmologist would not order any specific laboratory or radiology tests on a baby with PHPV cataract. It is just bad luck. Fortunately, with prompt management, modern microsurgical techniques have allowed many (although not all) children with PHPV to develop usable vision.

Photophobia – Sensitivity to light. Severe discomfort to bright lights. Usually a symptom of eye disease, such as glaucoma, in an infant or retinal disease in a child or adult. Sometimes treated with dark sunglasses.

Photorefractive Keratectomy (PRK) – PRK stands for Photo Refractive Keratectomy which is a form of refractive surgery to correct a refractive error such as myopia. A laser is used to remove a front layer of cells of the cornea to change the refractive state of the eye so that glasses are no longer needed. Complications include under or over correction of the refractive error and glare problems, particularly at night with oncoming headlights. If serious infection occurs, blindness might result.

Pinguecula – Irritation caused by the degeneration of the conjunctiva.

Posterior Chamber – The back section of the eye's interior.

Posterior Optical Segment – Portion of the eye located behind the crystalline lens, and including vitreous, choroid retina, and optic nerve.

Posterior Vitreous Detachment (PVD) – The separation of the vitreous from the retina.

Presbyopia – The normal decrease in focusing power (accommodation) of the eye which occurs with aging. It begins about age twelve but becomes most noticeable to the average farsighted person after age forty. Bifocals or reading glasses are required for clear near vision.

Pseudostrabismus – A child's eyes appear to be out-of-alignment, and usually one eye appears to turn in. In infants this appearance is especially noticeable when there is excessive skin on either side of the nose that covers the inner corner of each eye. As the child looks to one side, part of the eye disappears under this skin and looks crossed.

Pterygium – A triangular membrane with blood vessels which grows from the sclera toward the cornea. It occurs more often on the nasal side of the eye. It is more common in dusty and windy climates. Surgery is often necessary.

Ptosis – A drooping of the upper eyelid. In children it is usually a congenital problem. It rarely causes amblyopia. Most children simply hold their heads back if the droop is severe. Surgery, the only treatment, is usually suggested prior to starting school when the appearance is cosmetically unacceptable.

Pupil – The dark aperture in the iris that determines how much light is let into the eye.

Pupillary Response – The constriction or dilation of the pupil as stimulated by light.

Radial Keratotomy – A surgical procedure in which incisions are made into the epithelium of the cornea to correct refractive error.

Refraction – In ophthalmology, the bending of light that takes place within the human eye. Refractive errors include nearsightedness (myopia), farsightedness (hyperopia), and astigmatism. Lenses can be used to control the amount of refraction, correcting those errors.

Refractive Error – The degree to which light reaches the back of the eye—myopia, hyperopia, astigmatism.

Retina – The retina is the nerve layer that lines the back of the eye, senses light and creates impulses that travel through the optic nerve to the brain.

Retinal Detachment – A retina that separates from its connection at the back of the eye. The process of retinal detachment is usually due to a tear (a rip) in the retina, often when the vitreous gel pulls loose or separates from its attachment to the retina, most commonly along the outside edge of the eye. This rip is sometimes accompanied by bleeding if a blood vessel is also torn. After the retina has torn, liquid from the vitreous gel passes through the tear and accumulates behind the retina. The buildup of fluid behind the retina is what separates (detaches) the retina from the back of the eye. As more of the liquid vitreous collects behind the retina, the extent of the retinal detachment can progress and involve the entire retina, leading to a total retinal detachment. A retinal detachment almost always affects only one eye. The second eye, however, must be checked thoroughly for any signs of the problem.

Retinal Pigment Epithelium – The pigment cell layer that nourishes the retinal cells; located just outside the retina and attached to the choroid.

Retinitis Pigmentosa (RP) – A hereditary degeneration of the retina which leads to a severe loss of vision, usually legal blindness. Progressive symptoms include night blindness, loss of side vision leading to tunnel vision and decreased central vision and visual acuity. Visual acuity may be compromised early by the formation of cataracts, requiring cataract surgery. There are three main forms of RP based on heredity: dominant, X-linked and recessive. In the dominant form, about 50% of all family members have the disease. In the X-linked form, RP skips every other generation because females are carriers and males get the RP. In the recessive form, there is no family history or only sporadic occurrences of the disease. If one member of the family (e.g., older son) is diagnosed with recessive RP there is a 25% chance that the other brothers and sisters, with the same mother and father, have the disease. About 1 in every 3600 people have RP. A possible treatment to slow down the progression of the disease is the use of vitamin A palmitate (15,000 IUs/day). However, Vitamin A therapy for RP is controversial and women of childbearing age must NOT get pregnant while on vitamin A because of an association with birth defects.

Retinoblastoma – The most common cancer in the eye occurring in early childhood. A parent or doctor may first suspect a problem by detecting whiteness in the normally dark pupil. Occasionally it leads to a wandering eye, (strabismus). It does not spread from one eye to the other but about 25% have a tumor in each eye. Immediate medical treatment is necessary. Sometimes the eye(s) must be removed to prevent spreading of the tumor into the brain.

Retrobulbar Neuritis – Inflammation of the optic nerve. It causes a loss in vision. It is sometimes indicative of a neurological disease.

Rod Cone Dystrophy – A number of retina diseases in which the rod photoreceptors first start to degenerate followed by the cone photoreceptors. Other parts of the retina and Retinal Pigment Epithelium (RPE)are also adversely affected. Symptoms include loss of side vision and night blindness followed by the loss of central vision. RP is the most common form of rod-cone degeneration. Some forms occur at birth while other forms may start much later in life. Generally very poor prognosis.

Rods – Visual cells of the retina that are important for night vision and peripheral vision. The rods are the first affected in rod-cone degenerations such as RP.

Sclera – Tough, white outer coat of the eyeball.

Sclerotic – The essential parts of the eye are enclosed in a tough outer coat, the sclerotic, to which the muscles moving it are attached, and which in front changes into the transparent cornea.

Scotoma – An absence of vision in part of the visual field. It is present in such conditions as glaucoma, or in more serious diseases within the brain. Often detected by a visual field test.

Slit Lamp – A special type of examination of the anterior structures of the eye. These include the conjunctiva, sclera, lids, iris, cornea and anterior chamber.

Snellen Chart – The familiar eye chart with larger letters at the top and smaller ones at the bottom. It is used for measuring central vision.

Staphyloma – An abnormal bulging of the cornea or sclera. It is usually a congenital problem.

Stargardt's Disease – Also called Juvenile macular degeneration. Early, in the course of the disease, the retina may look normal to the eye doctor. Later in the disease process, there is a total loss of the Retinal Pigment Epithelium (RPE) and photoreceptors in the macula. Disease progression is rapid leading to a central scotoma, reduced central vision leading to legal blindness and some loss of color vision by the age of 20 years. Patients sometime become photophobic.

Stereopsis – Also known as depth perception. The separation between the eyes provides for slightly different views of an object by each eye. The brain, for the purpose of telling the location of an object in 3D space, uses this difference in views between the eyes or disparity.

Strabismus – A condition in which the visual axes of the eyes are not parallel and the eyes appear to be looking in different directions.

Suspensory Ligament of Lens – A series of fibers that connect the ciliary body of the eye with the lens, holding it in place.

Tear Duct – Part of the drainage system for the tears. The dilated part of the tear duct is called the lacrimal sac. An obstruction along the tear duct in infancy will cause a watery or draining eye. A warm compress is sometimes used to open a blocked tear duct. A tear duct probing surgery may be necessary to relieve the blockage.

Tonometer – An instrument used to measure the pressure within the eye. This is one of several factors used in diagnosis of glaucoma. The results may also be used to follow the response of treatment to this disease.

Tonometry – The standard to determine the fluid pressure inside the eye (Intraocular Pressure - IOP).

Trachoma – A viral infection of the cornea and conjunctiva which may produce scarring and impaired vision.

Trichiasis – The inward turning of an eyelash. If it scratches the cornea, there is discomfort similar to a foreign body sensation.

Tunnel Vision – A reduced visual field in which the eyes only see straight ahead (no peripheral vision). It may be due to certain eye diseases, such as glaucoma or RP.

Ultrasound – High-frequency sound waves. Ultrasound waves can be bounced off of tissues using special devices. The echoes are then converted into a picture called a sonogram. Ultrasound imaging, referred to as ultrasonography, allows physicians and patients to get an inside view of soft tissues and body cavities, without using invasive techniques.

Unilateral – Having, or relating to, one side. Unilateral is as opposed, for example, to bilateral (which means having, or relating to, two sides).

Usher's Syndrome – Characterized by a severe sensori-neural hearing loss at birth and followed by the development of Retinitis Pigmentosa. Usher's syndrome is the leading cause of deaf-blindness. Occurs in about 1 in 33,000 births. However, in the deaf population about 1 in 50 have Usher's syndrome.

Uvea – Part of the eye, the uvea collectively refers to the iris, the choroid of the eye, and the ciliary body.

Uveal Tract – The entire vascular coat of the eye composed of the iris, ciliary body, and choroid.

Uveitis – Inflammation of the uveal tract. It may be anterior involving the iris and ciliary body (iridocyclitis), or posterior involving the choroid (choroiditis).

Vision Therapy – Refers to a mixture of therapies that employ eye movement tasks, eye-hand coordination tasks, 3D tasks, etc., which purportedly improve everything from golf games to dyslexia to reading problems in children and adults.

Visual Acuity – The clarity or clearness of the vision, a measure of how well a person sees. The ability to distinguish details and shapes of objects; also called central vision.

Visual Evoked Potential (VEP) – See Visual Evoked Response.

Visual Evoked Response (VER) – A test of the function of the visual pathways from the retina, along the optic nerve and optic tract to the early parts of the visual centers of the brain. Usually, EEG electrodes are placed on the head and the patient is required to view a flashing light and an alternating pattern (e.g., stripes or checks) on a TV. The VER is a diagnostic test for such things as Multiple Sclerosis, optic neuritis, optic neuropathies, cortical visual impairment and certain types of brain tumors. The pattern VER can also provide an objective estimate of a patient's visual acuity, even if the patient is nonverbal (e.g., too young, comatose or mentally impaired).

Visual Suppression – This occurs when the brain ignores the visual image being transmitted from one eye. It is not voluntary. In the younger child, it is associated with strabismus and amblyopia. An eye that is misaligned or is out of focus is likely to be suppressed by the child.

Vitreous Humor – The vitreous humor is a clear, jelly-like substance that fills the middle of the eye.

Yag Laser Surgery – The use of a laser to punch a hole in the iris to relieve increased pressure within the eye as, for example, from acute angle-closure glaucoma. Can be used to cut away secondary membranes that sometimes form after cataract surgery.

Abbreviations/Acronyms

The following definitions are medical terms commonly seen while coding for Ophthalmology:

A	before meals
A	without, lack of
A & P	anterior and posterior; auscultation and percussion
Ab	antibody
Ab	away from
abd	abdomen
ABG	arterial blood gases
ABP	arterial blood pressure
Ac	before meals
AC	anterior chamber
AC/A	accommodative convergence/accommodation ratio
ACT	anticoagulant therapy; active motion
Ad	to, toward, near to
Ad lib	as desired
ADH	antidiuretic hormone
ADL	activities of daily living
AES	anterior eye segment
AET	alternate esotropia
AHC	acute hemorrhagic conjunctivitis
AIDS	acquired immune deficiency syndrome
AK	astigmatic keratotomy
AKC	allergic keratoconjunctivitis
ALK	automated lamellar keratoplasty
ALT	argon laser trabeculoplasty
AMA	against medical advice
AMB	ambulatory
Ambi	both
Amphi	about, on both sides, both
Ampho	both
Ana	up, back, again, excessive
Ant	before, forward, in front of
Anti	against, opposed to
App	applanation tonometry

AR Syndrome	Axenfeld-Rieger syndrome
ARMD,AMD	age-related macular degeneration
ARN	acute retinal necrosis
ASC	anterior subcapsular cataract
ASHD	arteriosclerotic heart disease
ATN	acute tubular necrosis
AU	both ears
AXT	alternate exotropia
B/K	below knee
BBS	bilateral breath sounds
BDR	background diabetic retinopathy
BG	blood glucose
BI	brain injury
bi	twice, double
BID	twice a day
bilat	bilateral
BLR	bilateral lateral rectus
BMR	basal metabolic rate
BMR	bilateral medial rectus
BP	blood pressure
BRAO	branch retinal artery occlusion
BRM	biologic response modifiers
BRVO	branch retinal vein occlusion
BSA	body surface area
BSS	balanced salt solution
BUN	blood urea nitrogen
BUT	(tear) break up time
bx	biopsy
C	Celsius (centigrade)
c (C)	with
C & S	culture and sensitivity
c/o	complaint of
C3F8	perfluoropropane gas
Ca	calcium, cancer, carcinoma
CA	cardiac arrest
CACG	chronic angle closure glaucoma
CAT	computerized tomography scan
Cata	down, according to, complete
CBC	complete blood count
CBR	complete bed rest
CC	chief complaint
CCF	carotid cavernous fistula
CCS	carotid cavernous shunt
CDCR	canaliculodacryocystorhinostomy
Circum	around, about
CJDCR	conjunctivodacryocystorhinostomy
CMS	circulation, motion, sensation
CO	cardiac output
CO2	carbon dioxide
COAG	chronic open angle glaucoma
Com	with, together
Con	with, together
Contra	against, opposite
CP	chest pain, cleft palate
CRAO	central retinal artery occlusion
CRRR	corneal rust ring remover

CRT	capillary refill time
CRVO	central retinal vein occlusion
CSC,CSR	central serous (chorio) retinopathy
CSF	cerebrospinal fluid, colony stimulating factors
CT	chest tube, computed tomography
CVA	cerebral vascular accident, costovertebral angle
CVP	central venous pressure
CX	circumflex
Cx'd	cancelled
CXR	chest x-ray
D5LR	dextrose 5% with lactated ringers
D5W	dextrose 5% in water
DAT	diet as tolerated
DBP	diastolic blood pressure
DC (dc)	discontinue
DCR	dacryocystorhinostomy
DDVD	double dissociated vertical deviation
De	away from
DEX (DXT)	blood sugar
DHD	dissociated horizontal deviation
Di	twice, double
Dia	through, apart, across, completely
Dis	reversal, apart from, separation
DKA	diabetic ketoacidosis
DM	diabetes mellitus
DNA	deoxyribonucleic acid
DNR	do not resuscitate
DR	diabetic retinopathy
DRS	diabetic retinopathy study
DVD	dissociated vertical deviation
Dx	diagnosis
Dys	bad, difficult, disordered
E	esophoria
E, ex	out, away from
Ec	out from
ECCE	extracapsular cataract extraction
ECF	extracellular fluid, extended care facility
ECG (EKG)	electrocardiogram/electrocardiograph
Ecto	on outer side, situated on
EENT	eye, ear, nose and throat
EKC	epidemic keratoconjunctivitis
EL	endolaser
Em, en	empyema (pus in); encephalon (in the head)
EMM	epimacular membrane
Endo	within
Epi	upon, on
EPRP	endopanretinal photocoagulation
ERM	epiretinal membrane
ESRD	end stage renal disease
ET	esotropia
ET	endotracheal tube
ETDRS	early treatment diabetic retinopathy study
Exo	outside, on outer side, outer layer
Extra	outside
FAX	fluid-air exchange
FD	fatal dose, focal distance

FDA	Food & Drug Administration
FGX	fluid-gas exchange
FP	fibrous proliferation
FUO	fever of unknown origin
FVD	fluid volume deficit
GOT	glutamic oxalic transaminase
h/o	history of
HA	headache
Hb	hemoglobin
HCO3	bicarbonate
HCT	hematocrit
HDL	high density lipoprotein
HEENT	head, eye, ear, nose and throat
Hemi	half
Hgb	hemoglobin
HIV	human immunodeficiency virus
HPI	history of present illness
HRT	hormone replacement therapy
HS	hour of sleep
HSK	herpes simplex keratitis
HSV	herpes simplex virus
HTN (BP)	hypertension
Hx	history
Hyper	over, above, excessive
Hypo	under, below, deficient
HZO	herpes zoster ophthalmicus
I&A	irrigation and aspiration
I&O	intake and output
IBW	ideal body weight
ICCE	intracapsular cataract extraction
ICE	iridocorneal endothelial (syndrome)
ICP	intracranial pressure
IDDM	insulin dependent diabetes mellitus
IM	intramuscular
Im, in	in, Into
Imp	impression
Infra	below
Inter	between
Intra	within
Intro	into, within
IO	inferior oblique
IOL	intraocular lens
IPCV	idiopathic polypoidal choroidal vasculopathy
IR	inferior rectus
IRMA	intraretinal microvascular abnormality
IV	intravenous
JAMA	Journal of the American Medical Association
JVP	jugular venous pressure
K	potassium
KCl	potassium chloride
KCS	keratoconjunctivitis sicca
KI	potassium iodide
KM	keratomileusis
KPE	Kelman phacoemulsification
KPs	keratic precipitates
KVO	keep vein open

L & A	light and accommodation
LASIK	laser in situ keratomileusis
LDVD	left dissociated vertical deviation
LHT	left hypertropia
LK	lamellar keratoplasty
LLQ	left lower quadrant
LR	lateral rectus
LUQ	left upper quadrant
Lytes	electrolytes
MA	microaneurysm
MAP	mean arterial pressure
MAR	medication administration record
MB	muscle balance
MDI	multiple daily vitamin
Meta	beyond, after, change
MH	macular hole
MM	mucous membrane
MP	membrane peeling
MR	medial rectus
MR	manifest refraction
MRI	magnetic resonance imaging
MS	multiple sclerosis, morphine sulfate
MVR	microvitreoretinal
Na	sodium
NaCl	sodium chloride
NAD	no apparent distress
NED	no evidence of disease
Neg	negative
NIDDM	non-insulin-dependent diabetes mellitus
NKA	no known allergies
NKMA	no known medication allergies
noc	night
NPDR	non-proliferative diabetic retinopathy
NPO	nothing by mouth
NS	nuclear sclerosis
NS	normal saline
NS (NIS)	normal saline
NSAID	nonsteroidal anti-inflammatory drug
NSR	normal sinus rhythm
NV	nausea & vomiting
NV	neovascularization
NVD	neovascularization at disc
NVE	neovascularization elsewhere
NVG	neovascular glaucoma
NVI	neovascularization of iris (rubeosis iridis)
NYD	not yet diagnosed
O2	oxygen
OA	overaction (eg. muscle)
OD	oculus dexter (right eye)
OOB	out of bed
Opistho	behind, backward
OS	oculus sinister (left eye)
OT	ocular tension
OU	oculus uterque (both eyes)
p	after
P	pulse

PACG	primary angle closure glaucoma
PAG	perennial allergic conjunctivitis
Para	beside, beyond, near to
PAS	peripheral anterior synechiae
PCF	pharyngoconjunctival fever
PCO	posterior capsule opacity
PDD	pervasive development disorder
PDR	physician's desk reference
PDR	proliferative diabetic retinopathy
PE	physical examination
PED	pigment epithelial detachment
PED	persistent epithelial defect
Peri	around
PERL	pupils equal, react to light
Permeate	pass through
PERRLA	pupils equal, round, react to light, accommodation
PFCL	perfluorocarbon liquid
PH	pinhole
PH	past history
PHPV	persistent hyperplastic primary vitreous
PI	present illness
PK,PKP	penetrating keratoplasty
PLCO	posterior lens capsule opacity
PMH	past medical history
PNH	paroxysmal nocturnal hemoglobinuria
PO	by mouth
POAG	primary open angle glaucoma
Post	after, behind
post op	post-operative
PPL	pars plana lensectomy
PPMD	posterior polymorphous dystrophy
PPV	pars plana vitrectomy
PR	pneumatic retinopexy
Pre	before, in front of
pre op	pre-operative
prep	preparation
PRK	photorefractive keratectomy
PRN	as needed
Pro	before, in front of
PRP	panretinal photocoagulation
PS	posterior synechiae
PSC	posterior subcapsular cataract
PT	prothrombin time
PTK	phototherapeutic keratectomy
PTT	partial thromboplastin time
PVD	peripheral vascular disease
PVD	posterior vitreous detachment
PVR	proliferative vitreoretinopathy
PXG	pseudoexfoliation glaucoma
PXS	pseudoexfoliation syndrome
Q	every
Q2H	every 2 hours
QD	everyday
QH	every hour
QID	four times a day
qns	quantity not sufficient

QOD	every other day
Qs	quantity sufficient, quantity required
R	respirations
R/R	resection and recession
RAPD	relative afferent pupillary defect
RBC	red blood cells
RD	retinal detachment
RDVD	right dissociated vertical deviation
RDW	red cell distribution width
Re	back, again, contrary
REEDA	redness, edema, ecchymosis, drainage, approximation
Retro	backward, located behind
RHT	right hypertropia
RK	radial keratotomy
RLF	retrolental fibroplasia
RLQ	right lower quadrant
RO	rule out
ROP	retinopathy of prematurity
ROS	review of systems
RP	retinitis pigmentosa
RRD	rhegmatogenous retinal detachment
RT or R	right
RUQ	right upper quadrant
Rx	prescription, pharmacy
S	without
S (s)	without
s C	without correction
S/S	signs & symptoms
SAC	seasonal allergic conjunctivitis
SBP	Scleral buckling procedure
SC	senile cataract
Semi	half
SF	scleral fixation
SF6	sulfur hexafluoride (gas)
SLE	slit lamp examination
SLK	superior limbic keratoconjunctivitis
SMD	senile macular degeneration
SNF	skilled nursing facility
SO	silicone oil
SO	superior oblique
SO	sympathetic ophthalmia
SOB	shortness of breath
SOBOE	shortness of breath on exertion
SOP	standard operating procedure
SR	sinus rhythm
SRF	subretinal fluid
STAT	immediately
Sub	under
Super	above, upper, excessive
Supra	above, upper, excessive
Sx	symptoms
Sym	together, with
T	temperature
TIA	transient ischemic attack
TID	three times a day
Tn	tension (ocular)

TPN	total parenteral nutrition
TPR	temperature, pulse, respiration
Trans	across, through, beyond
TRD	tractional retinal detachment
TSCPC	transscleral cyclophotocoagulation
Tx	treatment, traction
UA	urinalysis
UA	underaction (eg. muscle)
UBW	usual body weight
UGA	under general anesthesia
Ultra	beyond, in excess
up ad lib	up as desired
US	ultrasonic, ultrasound
VA	visual acuity
VBP	venous blood pressure
VENT	ventral
VF	visual field
VH	vitreous hemorrhage
VKH	Vogt-Koyanagi-Harada syndrome
VLDL	very low density lipoprotein
VP	venous pressure, venipuncture
VS	vital signs
VT/Vtach	ventricular tachycardia
VW	vessel wall, vascular wall
WBC	white blood cell
WD	well developed
WHO	World Health Organization
WN	well nourished
WNL	within normal limits
X	times
X	exophoria
XT	exotropia

Anatomy

Anatomy is the science of the structure of the body. This section will address systemic, regional, and clinical anatomy as it applies to coding in the Ophthalmology setting. Anatomical terms have distinct meanings and are a major part of medical terminology.

Anatomical Positions

Often in medical records, anatomical positional terms are used to identify specific areas of body parts and body positions. The following list is commonly used terms that may be found in medical documentation:

- Superior = Nearer to head
- Inferior (caudal) = Nearer to feet
- Anterior (ventral) = Nearer to front
- Proximal = Nearer to trunk or point of origin (e.g., of a limb)
- Distal = Farther from trunk or point of origin (e.g., of a limb)
- Superficial = Nearer to or on surface
- Deep = Farther from surface
- Posterior (dorsal) = Nearer to back
- Medial = Nearer to median plane
- Lateral = Farther from median plane

Anatomical Planes

Anatomical descriptions are based on four anatomical planes that pass through the body in the anatomical position:

- Median plane (midsagittal plane) is the vertical plane passing longitudinally through the body, dividing it into right and left halves
- Sagittal planes are vertical planes passing through the body at right angles to the median plane, dividing it into anterior (front) and posterior (back) portions
- Horizontal planes are transverse planes passing through the body at right angles to the median and coronal planes; a horizontal plane divides the body into superior (upper) and inferior (lower) parts (it is helpful to give a reference point such as a horizontal plane through the umbilicus).

Anatomical Movement Terms

Various terms are used to describe movements of the eye. Eye movements are controlled by muscles innervated by cranial nerves III, IV, and VI. The oculomotor nerve controls the pupil. The extraocular muscle movements of the eye include:

Adduction	The medial rectus extraocular muscle moves the eye so the pupil is directed towards the nose.
Abduction	The pupil is directed laterally.
Elevation	The pupil is directed up. The superior rectus muscle moves the eye upwards.
Depression	The pupil is directed down, controlled by the inferior rectus muscle.
Intorsion	The superior oblique muscle rotates the top of eye towards the nose.
Extorsion	The inferior oblique muscle rotates the superior aspect of the eye away from the nose.

Ophthalmology Anatomy

Anatomy of the Eye

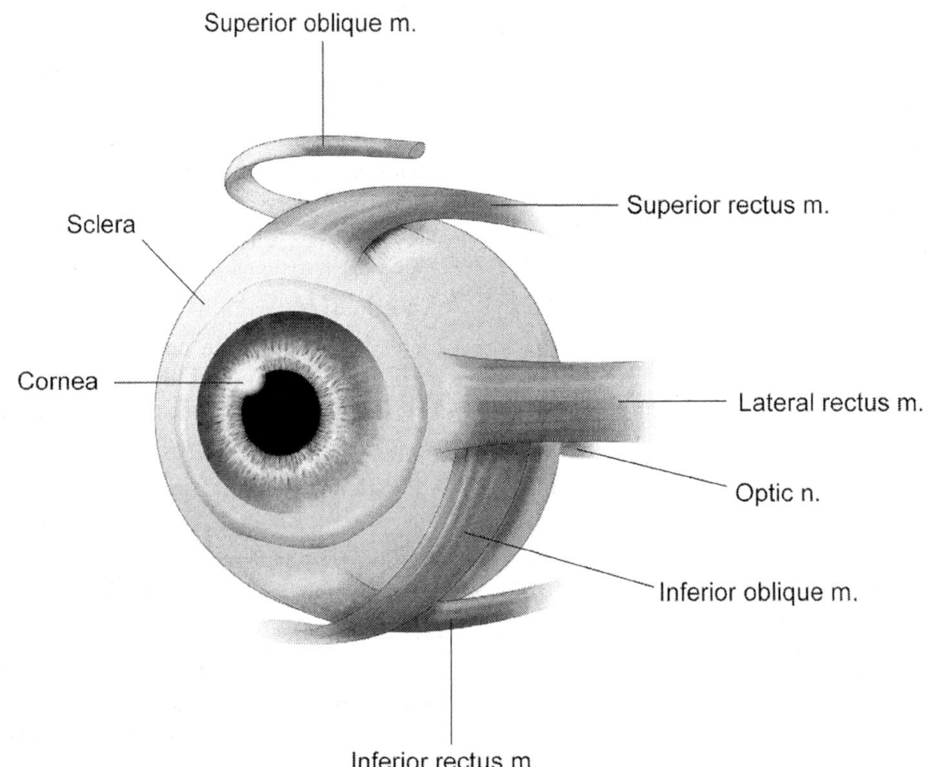

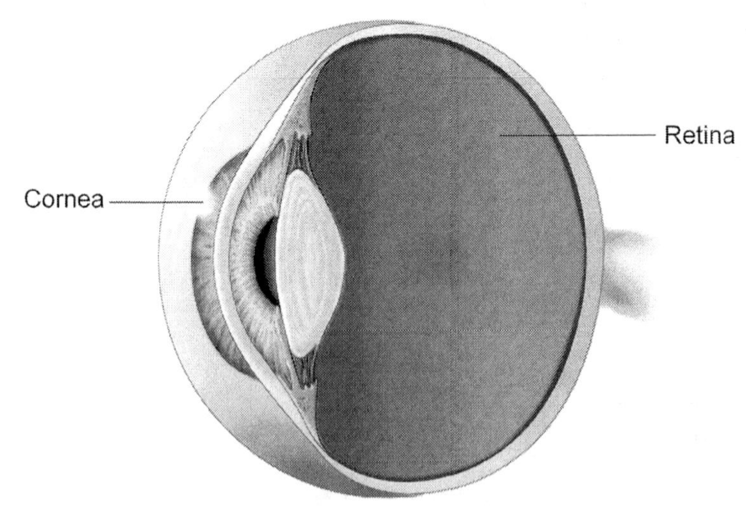

The Right Eye
(Transverse Section)

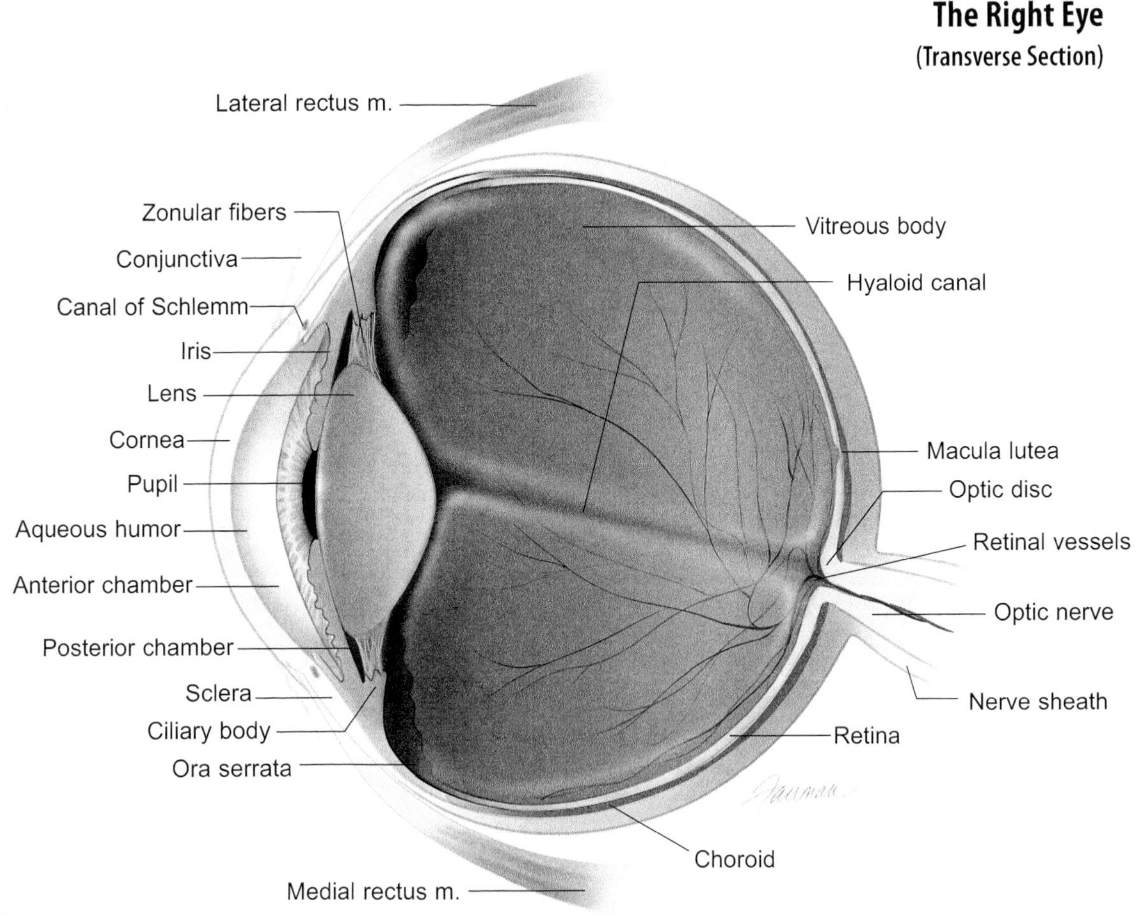

Introduction to ICD-10-CM and ICD-10-PCS Coding

ICD-10

The International Classification of Diseases (ICD) is designed to promote international comparability in the collection, processing, classification, and presentation of mortality statistics. This includes providing a format for reporting causes of death on the death certificate. The reported conditions are translated into medical codes through use of the classification structure and the selection and modification rules contained in the applicable revision of the ICD, published by the World Health Organization (WHO). These coding rules improve the usefulness of mortality statistics by giving preference to certain categories, consolidating conditions, and systematically selecting a single cause of death from a reported sequence of conditions.

ICD-10 is used to code and classify mortality data from death certificates, having replaced ICD-9 for this purpose as of January 1, 1999. The ICD-10 is copyrighted by the WHO, which owns and publishes the classification. WHO has authorized the development of an adaptation of ICD-10 for use in the United States for U.S. government purposes.

Development of ICD-10-CM

The National Center for Health Statistics (NCHS) is the Federal agency responsible for use of the *International Statistical Classification of Diseases and Related Health Problems,* 10th revision (ICD-10) in the United States. The NCHS has developed ICD-10-CM, a clinical modification of the classification for morbidity purposes. As agreed, all modifications must conform to WHO conventions for the ICD. ICD-10-CM was developed following a thorough evaluation by a Technical Advisory Panel and extensive additional consultation with physicians, clinical coders, and others, including public comments, to assure clinical accuracy and utility.

On August 22, 2008, the Department of Health and Human Services (DHHS) published a proposed rule to adopt ICD-10-CM (and ICD-10-PCS) to replace ICD-9-CM in HIPAA transactions. On January 16, 2009, the final rule on adoption of ICD-10-CM and ICD-10-PCS was published. The final initial implementation date was October 1, 2015.

The ICD-10-CM Coordination and Maintenance Committee

Annual modifications are made through the ICD-10-CM Coordination and Maintenance Committee. The Committee is made up of representatives from two Federal Government agencies, the National Center for Health Statistics (NCHS) and the Centers for Medicare and Medicaid Services (CMS). The Committee holds meetings twice a year which are open to the public. Modification proposals submitted to the Committee for consideration are presented at the meetings for public discussion. Approved modification proposals are incorporated into the official government version and become effective for use October 1.

ICD-10-CM Coding for Ophthalmology

Chapter 7 addresses diseases of the eye and adnexa, including categories H00-H59. Disorders in of the eyelid, lacrimal system, conjunctiva, sclera, cornea, ciliary body, iris, lens, retina, choroid, globe, optic nerve, vitreous body, visual pathways, ocular muscles, plus glaucoma, blindness, and complications of the eye and adnexa are discussed.

- H00-H05 Disorders of Eyelid, Lacrimal System, and Orbit –Conditions include hordeolum, chalazion, eyelid inflammation, disorders of the lacrimal system, and orbit issues.
- H10-H11 Disorders of Conjunctiva - Conditions conjunctivitis, conjunctival degenerations and deposits, pterygium, scars of the conjunctiva, conjunctival hemorrhage, and conjunctivochalasis.
- H15-H22 Disorders of Sclera, Cornea, Iris, and Ciliary Body - Conditions include corneal scars, opacities of the cornea, scleral disorders, keratitis, iridocyclitis, and disorders of the iris and ciliary body.
- H25-H28 Disorders of Lens - Conditions include various forms of cataracts, trauma to the lens, and other lens-specific disorders.
- H30-H36 Disorders of Choroid and Retina - Conditions include chorioretinal inflammation, chorioretinal scars, choroidal degeneration, choroidal hemorrhage, and choroidal dystrophy.
- H40-H42 Glaucoma - Conditions include various types of glaucoma.
- H43-H44 Disorders of Vitreous Body and Globe - Conditions include disorders of the vitreous body, such as opacities and prolapses, as well as disorders of the globe, such as myopia and purulent endophthalmitis.
- H46-H47 Disorders of Optic Nerve and Visual Pathways - Conditions include optic neuritis, retrobulbar neuritis, nutritional optic neuropathy, and optic papillitis.
- H49-H52 Disorders of Ocular Muscles, Binocular Movement, Accommodation, and Refraction - Conditions include strabismus, disorders of eye movement, refraction, and accommodation, and problems with eye muscles.

- H53-H54 Visual Disturbances and Blindness - Conditions include diplopia, visual field defects, color blindness, night blindness, and other visual disturbances.
- H55-H57 Other Disorders of Eye and Adnexa - Conditions include various type of nystagmus and various types of irregular eye movements.
- H59 Intraoperative and Postprocedural Complications NEC - Conditions include various types of intraoperative and postprocedural complications and disorders of the eye and adnexa (Grebner & Suarez, 2013).

Example:

Condition	ICD-10-CM
Diabetic cataract, right eye	E11.36 Type 2 diabetes mellitus with diabetic cataract

ICD-10-CM Official Guidelines for Coding and Reporting

The structure and format of the Guidelines for Coding and Reporting are as follows:

- Section I. Conventions, general coding guidelines and chapter-specific guidelines
- Section II. Selection of principal diagnosis
- Section III. Reporting additional diagnoses
- Section IV. Diagnostic coding and reporting guidelines for outpatient services
- Appendix I. Present on admission reporting guidelines

Section I – Conventions, General Coding Guidelines and Chapter-Specific Guidelines

Section I of the Guidelines is divided into three general areas:

A. Conventions of the ICD-10-CM
B. General Coding Guidelines
C. Chapter-Specific Coding Guidelines

Conventions

The conventions for the ICD-10-CM are the general rules for its use independent of the guidelines. These conventions are incorporated within the Alphabetic Index and the Tabular List as instructional notes, which take precedence over general guidelines.

The Alphabetic Index and Tabular List

The ICD-10-CM is divided into the Alphabetic Index of terms and their corresponding code, and the Tabular List, a chronological list of codes divided into chapters based on body system or condition. The Alphabetic Index contains the Index of Diseases and Injury, the Index of External Causes of Injury, the Table of Neoplasms, and the Table of Drugs and Chemicals.

Format and Structure

The ICD-10-CM Tabular List contains categories, subcategories, and codes made up of characters that are either a letter or a number. All categories are 3 characters. A three-character category with no further subdivision is equivalent to a code. Subcategories are either 4 or 5 characters. Valid codes may consist of 3, 4, 5, 6 or 7 characters. Each level of subdivision after a category is a subcategory. The final level of subdivision is the valid code. Codes that have applicable 7th characters are still referred to as codes, not subcategories. A code that requires an applicable 7th character is considered invalid without the 7th character.

When locating a code in ICD-10-CM, it is important to note that the 7th characters do not appear in the Alphabetic Index. The Tabular List must be checked to determine whether a 7th character should be assigned, and if so, which one to select.

7th Characters

Certain categories have applicable 7th characters. The meanings of the 7th character are dependent on the chapters, and in some cases the categories, in which they are used. The applicable 7th characters and their definitions are found under each category or subcategory to which they apply in the Tabular List. When 7th character designations are listed under a category or subcategory, the 7th character is required for all codes in that category or subcategory. Failing to assign a 7th character results in an invalid diagnosis code that will not be recognized by payers. Because the 7th character must always be in the 7th place in the data field, codes that are not 6 characters in length require the use of the placeholder 'X' to fill the empty characters. There are a number of chapters that make use of 7th characters including:

- Chapter 7 – Diseases of the Eye and Adnexa (H00-H59). The 7th character is used for glaucoma codes to designate the stage of the glaucoma.
- Chapter 13 – Diseases of the Musculoskeletal System and Connective Tissue (M00-M99). A 7th character is required for chronic gout codes to identify the condition as with or without tophus. The 7th character is also used for stress fractures and pathological fractures due to osteoporosis, neoplastic or other disease to identify the episode of care (initial, subsequent, sequela). For subsequent encounters, the 7th character also provides information on healing (routine, delayed, with nonunion, with malunion).
- Chapter 15 – Pregnancy, Childbirth, and the Puerperium (O00-O9A). The 7th character identifies the fetus for those conditions that may affect one or more fetuses in a multiple gestation pregnancy. The 7th character identifies the specific fetus as fetus 1, fetus 2, fetus 3, and so on – NOT the number of fetuses.
- Chapter 18 – Symptoms, Signs and Abnormal Clinical/Laboratory Findings, NOS (R00-R99). There are subcategories for coma that identify elements from the coma scale and the 7th character provides information on when the coma scale assessment was performed.
- Chapter 19 – Injury, Poisoning and Certain Other Consequences of External Causes (S00-T88). The 7th character is used to identify the episode of care (initial, subsequent, sequela). For fractures, it identifies the episode of care, the status of the fracture as open or closed, and fracture healing for subsequent encounters as routine, delayed, nonunion, or malunion.

- Chapter 20 – External Causes of Morbidity (V01-Y99). The 7th character is used to identify the episode of care (initial, subsequent, sequela).

Examples of codes with applicable 7th characters:

- M48.46XA Fatigue fracture of vertebra, lumbar region, initial encounter for fracture
- M80.051D Age-related osteoporosis with current pathological fracture, right femur, subsequent encounter for fracture with routine healing
- O33.4XX0 Maternal care for disproportion of mixed maternal and fetal origin, fetus not applicable or unspecified. Note: 7th character 0 is used for single gestation
- O36.5932 Maternal care for other known or suspected poor fetal growth, third trimester, fetus 2
- S52.121A Displaced fracture of head of right radius, initial encounter for closed fracture
- T88.2XXS Shock due to anesthesia, sequela
- W11.XXXA Fall on and from ladder, initial encounter

Note the use of the placeholder 'X' for those codes that are less than 6 characters in the examples above.

Excludes Notes

There are two types of excludes notes in ICD-10-CM which are designated as Excludes1 and Excludes2. The definitions of the two types differ, but both types indicate that the excluded codes are independent of each other. A type 1 Excludes note, identified in the Tabular as ***Excludes1***, is a pure excludes. It means that the condition referenced is "NOT CODED HERE." For an Excludes1 the two codes are never reported together because the two conditions cannot occur together, such as a congenital and acquired form of the same condition. An exception to the Excludes1 definition is the circumstance when the two conditions are unrelated to each other. If it is not clear whether the two conditions involving an Excludes1 note are related or not, query the provider. For example, code F45.8, Other somatoform disorders, has an Excludes1 note for "sleep related teeth grinding (G47.63)," because "teeth grinding" is an inclusion term under F45.8. Only one of these two codes should be assigned for teeth grinding. However psychogenic dysmenorrhea is also an inclusion term under F45.8, and a patient could have both this condition and sleep related teeth grinding. In this case, the two conditions are clearly unrelated to each other, and so it would be appropriate to report F45.8 and G47.63 together.

A type 2 Excludes note, identified in the Tabular as ***Excludes2***, indicates that the excluded condition is "NOT INCLUDED HERE." This means that the excluded condition is not part of the condition represented by the code, but the patient may have both conditions at the same time and the two codes may be reported together when the patient has both conditions.

General Coding Guidelines

Locating a Code in the ICD-10-CM

To select a code in the classification that corresponds to a diagnosis or reason for visit documented in a medical record, first locate the term in the Alphabetic Index, and then verify the code in the Tabular List. Read and be guided by instructional notations that appear in both the Alphabetic Index and the Tabular List.

It is essential to use both the Alphabetic Index and Tabular List when locating and assigning a code. The Alphabetic Index does not always provide the full code. Selection of the full code, including laterality and any applicable 7th character can only be done in the Tabular List. A dash (-) at the end of an Alphabetic Index entry indicates that additional characters are required. Even if a dash is not included at the Alphabetic Index entry, it is necessary to refer to the Tabular List to verify that no 7th character is required.

Each unique ICD-10-CM diagnosis code may be reported only once for an encounter. This applies to bilateral conditions when there are no distinct codes identifying laterality or two different conditions classified to the same ICD-10-CM diagnosis code.

Laterality

Some ICD-10-CM codes indicate laterality, specifying whether the condition occurs on the left, right or is bilateral. If no bilateral code is provided and the condition is bilateral, assign separate codes for both the left and right side. When laterality is not documented by the provider, code assignment for the affected side may be based on documentation from other clinicians. If there is conflicting documentation regarding the affected side, the patient's attending provider should be queried for clarification. Codes for "unspecified" side should rarely be used, such as when the documentation in the record is insufficient to determine the affected side and it is not possible to obtain clarification.

Documentation by Clinicians Other than the Patient's Provider

The assignment of a diagnosis code is based on the provider's (i.e., physician or other qualified healthcare practitioner legally accountable for establishing the patient's diagnosis) documentation that the condition exists. The few exceptions include codes for body mass index, pressure ulcer stage, depth of non-pressure ulcers, coma scale, NIH stroke scale, laterality, blood alcohol level, and social determinants of health. This information may be documented by "clinicians" other than the patient's provider, such as healthcare professionals who are permitted, based on regulatory or accreditation requirements, to document in the medical record. The provider's statement that the patient has a particular condition is sufficient. Code assignment is not based on clinical criteria used by the provider to establish the diagnosis.

Chapter-Specific Coding Guidelines

The information that follows provides an overview of each chapter and highlights some of the more significant aspects of the guidelines. Using this overview is a good starting point for learning about ICD-10-CM; however, this resource must be combined with more intensive training using the Official Guidelines for Coding and Reporting and the current code set in order to attain the proficiency needed to assign ICD-10-CM codes accurately to the highest level of specificity.

Chapter 1 – Certain Infectious and Parasitic Diseases (A00-B99)

Infectious and parasitic diseases are those that are generally recognized as communicable or transmissible. Examples of diseases in Chapter 1 include: human immunodeficiency virus, scarlet fever, sepsis due to infectious organisms, meningococcal infection, and genitourinary tract infections. It should be noted that not all infectious and parasitic diseases are found in Chapter 1. Localized infections are found in the body system chapters. Examples of localized infections found in other chapters include strep throat, pneumonia, influenza, and otitis media.

Chapter Guidelines

Guidelines in Chapter 1 relate to coding of infections that are classified in chapters other than Chapter 1 and for infections resistant to antibiotics. Note that only severe sepsis and septic shock require additional codes from Chapter 18 – Symptoms, Signs, and Abnormal Clinical Findings NOS. Exceptions include sepsis complicating pregnancy, childbirth and the puerperium and congenital/newborn sepsis which are found in Chapters 15 and 16 respectively. In order to report sepsis, severe sepsis, and septic shock accurately, both the guidelines and coding instructions in the Tabular List must be followed.

Some infections are classified in chapters based on the body system that is affected rather than in Chapter 1. For infections that are classified in other chapters that do not identify the infectious organism, it is necessary to assign an additional code from the following categories in Chapter 1:

- B95 Streptococcus, Staphylococcus, and Enterococcus as the cause of diseases classified elsewhere
- B96 Other bacterial agents as the cause of diseases classified elsewhere
- B97 Viral agents as the cause of diseases classified elsewhere

Codes for infections classified to other chapters that require an additional code from Chapter 1 are easily identified by the instructional note, "Use additional code (B95-B97) to identify infectious agent."

In addition to the extensive guidelines related to MRSA infections, there are also guidelines for reporting bacterial infections that are resistant to current antibiotics. An additional code from category Z16 is required for all bacterial infections documented as antibiotic resistant for which the infection code does not also capture the drug resistance.

Chapter 2 – Neoplasms (C00-D49)

Codes for all neoplasms are located in Chapter 2. Neoplasms are classified primarily by site and then by behavior (benign, carcinoma in-situ, malignant, uncertain behavior, and unspecified). In some cases, the morphology (histologic type) is also included in the code descriptor. Many neoplasm codes have more specific site designations and laterality (right, left) is a component of codes for paired organs and the extremities. In addition, there are more malignant neoplasm codes that capture morphology.

Chapter Guidelines

Careful review of the guidelines related to neoplasms, conditions associated with malignancy, and adverse effects of treatment for malignancies is required. The guidelines provide instructions for coding primary malignancies that are contiguous sites versus primary malignancies of two sites where two codes are required. Another coding challenge related to neoplasms is determining when the code for personal history should be used rather than the malignant neoplasm code. For blood cancers, this is further complicated because it is necessary to determine whether the code for "in remission" or "personal history" should be assigned.

Primary malignancies that overlap two or more sites that are next to each other (contiguous) are classified to subcategory/code .8 except in instances where there is a combination code that is specifically indexed elsewhere. When there are two primary sites that are not contiguous, a code is assigned for each specific site. For example, a large (primary) malignant mass in the right breast (female) that extends from the upper outer quadrant to the lower outer quadrant would be reported with code C50.811 Malignant neoplasm of overlapping sites of right female breast. However, if there are two distinct lesions in the right breast (female), a 0.5 cm lesion in the upper outer quadrant and a non-contiguous 1 cm lesion in the lower outer quadrant, two codes would be required, C50.411 for the 0.5 cm lesion in the upper outer quadrant and C50.511 for the 1 cm lesion in the lower outer quadrant.

Malignant neoplasms of ectopic tissue are coded to the site of origin. For example, ectopic pancreatic malignancy involving the stomach is assigned code C25.9 Malignant neoplasm of pancreas, unspecified.

There are guidelines for anemia associated with malignancy and for anemia associated with treatment. When an admission or encounter is for the management of anemia associated with a malignant neoplasm, the code for the malignancy is sequenced first followed by the appropriate anemia code, such as D63.0 Anemia in neoplastic disease. For anemia associated with chemotherapy or immunotherapy, when the treatment is for the anemia only, the anemia code is sequenced first followed by the appropriate code for the neoplasm and code T45.1X5- Adverse effect of antineoplastic and immunosuppressive drugs. For anemia associated with an adverse effect of radiotherapy, the anemia should be sequenced first, followed by the code for the neoplasm and code Y84.2 Radiological procedure and radiotherapy as the cause of abnormal reaction in the patient.

Code C80.0 Disseminated malignant neoplasm, unspecified is reported only when the patient has advanced metastatic disease with no known primary or secondary sites specified. It should not be used in place of assigning codes for the primary site and all known secondary sites. Cancer unspecified is reported with code C80.1 Malignant (primary) neoplasm, unspecified. This code should be used only when no determination can be made as to the primary site of the malignancy. This code would rarely be used in the inpatient setting.

The guidelines provide detailed information on sequencing of neoplasm codes for various scenarios, such as sequencing for an encounter for a malignant neoplasm during pregnancy. Be sure to review the Official Guidelines for Coding and Reporting for this chapter before assigning a code.

Coding for a current malignancy versus a personal history of malignancy is dependent on two factors. First, it must be determined whether the malignancy has been excised or eradicated. Next, it must be determined whether any additional treatment is being directed to the site of the primary malignancy.

Primary malignancy excised/or eradicated?	Still receiving treatment directed at primary site?	Code Assignment
No	Yes	Use the malignant neoplasm code
Yes	Yes	Use the malignant neoplasm code
Yes	No	Use a code from category Z85 Personal history of primary or secondary malignant neoplasm

There are also guidelines related to coding for leukemia in remission versus coding for personal history of leukemia. These guidelines also apply to multiple myeloma and malignant plasma cell neoplasms. Categories with codes for "in remission" include:

- C90 Multiple myeloma and malignant plasma cell neoplasms
- C91 Lymphoid leukemia
- C92 Myeloid leukemia
- C93 Monocytic leukemia
- C94 Other leukemias of specified cell type

Coding for these neoplasms requires first determining, based on the documentation, whether or not the patient is in remission. If the documentation is unclear as to whether the patient has achieved remission, the physician should be queried.

Coding is further complicated because it must also be determined whether a patient who has achieved and maintained remission is now "cured," in which case the applicable code for personal history of leukemia or personal history of other malignant neoplasms of lymphoid, hematopoietic and related tissues should be assigned. If the documentation is not clear, the physician should be queried. Categories that report a history of these neoplasms include:

- Z85.6 Personal history of leukemia
- Z85.79 Personal history of other malignant neoplasms of lymphoid, hematopoietic and related tissues

Multiple myeloma, malignant plasma cell neoplasm, leukemia eradicated?	Still receiving treatment for the neoplasm?	Documentation that patient is currently in remission or has maintained remission and is now "cured"?	Code Assignment
No	Yes	No	Use the malignant neoplasm code with fifth character '0' for not having achieved remission or fifth character '2' for in relapse
Yes	No	In remission	Use the malignant neoplasm code with fifth character '1' for in remission
Yes	No	Maintained remission/cured	Use a code from category Z85 Personal history of primary or secondary malignant neoplasm

Chapter 3 – Diseases of the Blood and Blood-Forming Organs and Certain Disorders Involving the Immune Mechanism (D50-D89)

Diseases of the blood and blood-forming organs include disorders involving the bone marrow, lymphatic tissue, platelets, and coagulation factors. Certain disorders involving the immune mechanism such as immunodeficiency disorders (except HIV/AIDS) are also classified to Chapter 3.

Chapter Guidelines

There are no chapter-specific guidelines for Chapter 3. However, Chapter 2 guidelines should be reviewed for anemia associated with a malignancy or with treatment of a malignancy.

Chapter 4 – Endocrine, Nutritional, and Metabolic Diseases (E00-E89)

Chapter 4 covers diseases and conditions of the endocrine glands which include the pituitary, thyroid, parathyroids, adrenals, pancreas, ovaries/testes, pineal gland, and thymus; malnutrition and other nutritional deficiencies; overweight and obesity; and metabolic disorders such as lactose intolerance, hyperlipidemia, dehydration, and electrolyte imbalances. One of the most frequently treated conditions, diabetes mellitus, is found in this chapter.

Diabetes Mellitus

Diabetes mellitus, one of the most common diseases treated by physicians, is classified in Chapter 4 and since complications of diabetes can affect one or more body systems, all physician specialties must be familiar with diabetes coding. Two significant concepts to note in diabetes coding include 1) the code categories, and 2) most codes are combination codes that capture the type of diabetes, the body system affected as well as the specific manifestations/complications. However, some categories include instructional notes to assign additional codes from other chapters for added specificity. Diabetes mellitus code categories include:

- E08 Diabetes mellitus due to an underlying condition. Examples of underlying conditions include:
  - Congenital rubella
  - Cushing's syndrome
  - Cystic fibrosis
  - Malignant neoplasm
  - Malnutrition
  - Pancreatitis and other diseases of the pancreas
- E09 Drug or chemical induced diabetes mellitus
- E10 Type 1 diabetes mellitus
- E11 Type 2 diabetes mellitus
- E13 Other specified diabetes mellitus. This category includes diabetes mellitus:
  - Due to genetic defects of beta-cell function
  - Due to genetic defects in insulin action
  - Postpancreatectomy
  - Postprocedural
  - Secondary diabetes not elsewhere classified

Combination codes capture information about the body system affected and specific complications/manifestations affecting that body system. Specific information regarding some types of complications may be captured in a single code:

- Ketoacidosis which is further differentiated as with or without coma
- Kidney complications with specific codes for diabetic nephropathy, diabetic chronic kidney disease, and other diabetic kidney complications
- Ophthalmic complications with specific codes for diabetic retinopathy including severity (nonproliferative - mild, moderate, severe; proliferative; unspecified) and whether there is any associated macular edema or retinal detachment; diabetic cataract; and other ophthalmic complications
- Diabetic neurological complications with specific codes for amyotrophy, autonomic (poly)neuropathy, mononeuropathy, polyneuropathy, other specified neurological complication
- Diabetic circulatory complications with specific codes for peripheral angiopathy differentiated as with gangrene or without gangrene
- Diabetic arthropathy with specific codes for neuropathic arthropathy and other arthropathy
- Diabetic skin complication with specific codes for dermatitis, foot ulcer, other skin ulcer, and other skin complication
- Diabetic oral complications with specific codes for periodontal disease and other oral complications
- Hypoglycemia which is further differentiated as with or without coma

"Uncontrolled" and "not stated as uncontrolled" are not components of the diabetes codes. 'Uncontrolled' diabetes may mean either with hyperglycemia or hypoglycemia per the Alphabetic Index. Terms such as 'poorly controlled', 'out of control', or 'inadequately controlled' default to the specified type of diabetes with hyperglycemia. Therefore, diabetes with hyperglycemia should be based only on the documentation to avoid reporting cases of uncontrolled diabetes meant with hypoglycemia incorrectly.

Chapter Guidelines

All chapter-specific guidelines for Chapter 4 relate to coding diabetes mellitus. Some of the guidelines are discussed below.

Diabetics may have no complications, a single complication or multiple complications related to their diabetes. For diabetics with multiple complications it is necessary to report as many codes within a particular category (E08-E13) as are necessary to describe all the complications of the diabetes mellitus. Sequencing is based on the reason for the encounter. In addition, as many codes from each subcategory as are necessary to completely identify all of the associated conditions that the patient has should be assigned. For example, if an ophthalmologist is evaluating a patient with type 1 diabetes who has mild nonproliferative diabetic retinopathy without macular edema and diabetic cataracts, two codes from the subcategory for type 1 diabetes with ophthalmic complications must be assigned, code E10.329 for mild nonproliferative retinopathy without macular edema and code E10.36 to capture the diabetic cataracts.

The physician should always be queried when the type of diabetes is not documented. However, the guidelines do provide instructions for reporting diabetes when the type is not documented. Guidelines state that when the type of diabetes mellitus is not documented in the medical record the default is E11 Type 2 diabetes mellitus. In addition, when the type of diabetes is not documented but there is documentation of long-term insulin or hypoglycemic drug use, a code from category E11 Type 2 diabetes mellitus is assigned along with code Z79.4 Long-term (current) use of insulin or Z79.84, Long term (current) use of oral hypoglycemic drugs.

If both oral hypoglycemic medication and insulin use is documented, assign code Z79.4 Long term (current) use of insulin and code Z79.84 Long term (current) use of oral hypoglycemic drugs.

If the patient is treated with both insulin and an injectable non-insulin antidiabetic drug, assign code Z79.4 Long term (current) use of insulin and code Z79.899 Other long term (current) drug therapy.

If the patient is treated with both oral hypoglycemic drugs and an injectable non-insulin antidiabetic drug, assign codes Z79.84 Long term (current) use of oral hypoglycemic drugs and Z79.899 Other long term (current) drug therapy.

Diabetes mellitus in pregnancy and gestational diabetes are reported with codes from Chapter 15 Pregnancy, Childbirth, and the Puerperium as the first listed diagnosis. For pre-existing diabetes mellitus, an additional code from Chapter 4 is reported to identify the specific type and any systemic complications or manifestations.

Complications of insulin pump malfunction may involve either overdosing or underdosing of insulin. Underdosing of insulin or other medications is captured by the addition of a column and codes in the Table of Drugs and Chemicals specifically for underdosing. Underdosing of insulin due to insulin pump failure requires a minimum of three codes. The principal or first-listed diagnosis code is the code for the mechanical complication which is found in subcategory T85.6-. Fifth, sixth and seventh characters are required to capture the specific type of mechanical breakdown or failure (fifth character), the type of device which in this case is an insulin pump (sixth character '4'), and the episode of care (seventh character). The second code T38.3X6- captures underdosing of insulin and oral hypoglycemic [antidiabetic] drugs. A seventh character is required to capture the episode of care. Then additional codes are assigned to identify the type of diabetes mellitus and any associated complications due to the underdosing.

Secondary diabetes mellitus is always caused by another condition or event. Categories for secondary diabetes mellitus include: E08 Diabetes mellitus due to underlying condition, E09 Drug and chemical induced diabetes mellitus, and E13 Other specified diabetes mellitus. For patients with secondary diabetes who routinely use insulin or hypoglycemic drugs, code Z79.4 Long-term (current) use of insulin or Z79.84, Long term (current) use of oral hypoglycemic drugs should be reported. Code Z79.4 is not reported for temporary use of insulin to bring a patient's blood sugar under control during an encounter. Coding and sequencing for secondary diabetes requires review of the guidelines as well as the instructions found in the tabular. For example, a diagnosis of diabetes due to partial pancreatectomy with postpancreatectomy hypoinsulinemia requires three codes. Code E89.1 Postprocedural hypoinsulinemia is the principal or first-listed diagnosis followed by a code or codes from category E13 that identifies the type of diabetes as "other specified" and the complications or manifestations, and lastly code Z90.411 is reported for the acquired partial absence of the pancreas.

Chapter 5 – Mental and Behavioral Disorders (F01-F99)

Mental disorders are alterations in thinking, mood, or behavior associated with distress and impaired functioning. Many mental disorders are organic in origin, where disease or injury causes the mental or behavioral condition. Examples of conditions classified in Chapter 5 include: schizophrenia, mood (affective) disorders such as major depression, anxiety and other nonpsychotic mental disorders, personality disorders, and intellectual disabilities.

Chapter Guidelines

Detailed guidelines are provided for coding certain conditions classified in Chapter 5, including pain disorders with related psychological factors, and mental and behavioral disorders due to psychoactive substance use, abuse, and dependence.

Pain related to psychological disorders may be due exclusively to the psychological disorder, or may be due to another cause that is exacerbated by the psychological factors. Documentation of any psychological component associated with acute or chronic pain is essential for correct code assignment. Pain exclusively related to psychological factors is reported with code F45.41, which is the only code that is assigned. Acute or chronic pain disorders with related psychological factors are reported with code F45.42 Pain disorder with related psychological factors and a second code from category G89 Pain not elsewhere classified for documented acute or chronic pain disorder.

Mental and behavioral disorders due to psychoactive substance use are reported with codes in categories F10-F19. Both the guidelines and tabular instructions must be followed to code mental and behavioral disorders due to psychoactive substance use correctly. As with all other diagnoses, the codes for psychoactive substance use, abuse, and dependence may only be assigned based on provider documentation and only if the condition meets the definition of a reportable diagnosis. In addition, psychoactive substance use codes are reported only when the condition is associated with a mental or behavioral disorder and a relationship between the substance use and the mental or behavioral disorder is documented by the physician.

The codes for mental and behavioral disorders caused by psychoactive substance use are specific as to substance; selecting the correct code requires an understanding of the differences between use, abuse, and dependence. Physicians may use the terms use, abuse and/or dependence interchangeably; however only one code should be reported for each behavioral disorder documented when the documentation refers to use, abuse and dependence of a specific substance. When these terms are used together or interchangeably in the documentation the guidelines are as follows:

- If both use and abuse are documented, assign only the code for abuse
- If both use and dependence are documented, assign only the code for dependence
- If use, abuse and dependence are all documented, assign only the code for dependence
- If both abuse and dependence are documented, assign only the code for dependence

Coding guidelines also provide instruction on correct reporting of psychoactive substance dependence described as "in remission." Selection of "in remission" codes in categories F10-F19 requires the physician's clinical judgment. Codes for "in remission" are assigned only with supporting provider documentation. If the documentation is not clear, the physician should be queried.

Chapter 6 – Diseases of Nervous System (G00-G99)

Diseases of the Nervous System include disorders of the brain and spinal cord (the central nervous system) such as cerebral degeneration or Parkinson's disease, and diseases of the peripheral nervous system, such as polyneuropathy, myasthenia gravis, and muscular dystrophy. Codes for some of the more commonly treated pain diagnoses are also found in Chapter 6 including: migraine and other headache syndromes (categories G43-G44); causalgia (complex regional pain syndrome II) (CRPS II) (G56.4-, G57.7-); complex regional pain syndrome I (CRPS I) (G90.5-); neuralgia and other nerve, nerve root and plexus disorders (categories G50-G59); and pain, not elsewhere classified (category G89).

Chapter Guidelines

Chapter-specific coding guidelines for the nervous system and sense organs cover dominant/nondominant side for hemiplegia and monoplegia, and pain conditions reported with code G89 Pain not elsewhere classified.

Codes for hemiplegia and hemiparesis (category G81) and monoplegia of the lower limb (G83.1-), upper limb (G83.2-), and unspecified limb (G83.3-) are specific to the side affected and whether that side is dominant or non-dominant. Conditions in these categories/subcategories are classified as:

- Unspecified side
- Right dominant side
- Left dominant side
- Right non-dominant side
- Left non-dominant side

When documentation does not specify the condition as affecting the dominant or non-dominant side the guidelines provide specific instructions on how dominant and non-dominant should be determined. For ambidextrous patients, the default is dominant. If the left side is affected, the default is non-dominant. If the right side is affected, the default is dominant.

There are extensive guidelines for reporting pain codes in category G89, including sequencing rules and when to report a code from category G89 as an additional code. It should be noted that pain not specified as acute or chronic, post-thoracotomy, post-procedural, or neoplasm-related is not reported with a code from category G89. Codes from category G89 are also not assigned when the underlying or definitive diagnosis is known, unless the reason for the encounter is pain management rather than management of the underlying condition. For example, when a patient experiencing acute pain due to vertebral fracture is admitted for spinal fusion to treat the vertebral fracture, the code for the vertebral fracture is assigned as the principal diagnosis, but no pain code is assigned. When pain control or pain management is the reason for the admission/encounter, a code from category G89 is assigned and in this case the G89 code is listed as the principal or first-listed diagnosis. For example, when a patient with nerve impingement and severe back pain is seen for a spinal canal steroid injection, the appropriate pain code is assigned as the principal or first-listed diagnosis. However, when an admission or encounter is for treatment of the underlying condition and a neurostimulator is also inserted for pain control during the same episode of care, the underlying condition is reported as the principal diagnosis and a code from category G89 is reported as a secondary diagnosis. Pain codes from category G89 may be used in conjunction with site-specific pain codes that identify the site of pain (including codes from chapter 18) when the code provides additional diagnostic information such as describing whether the pain is acute or chronic. In addition to the general guidelines for assignment of codes in category G89, there are also specific guidelines for postoperative pain, chronic pain, neoplasm related pain and chronic pain syndrome.

Postoperative pain may be acute or chronic. There are four codes for postoperative pain: G89.12 Acute post-thoracotomy pain, G89.18 Other acute post-procedural pain, G89.22 Chronic post-thoracotomy pain, and G89.28 Other chronic post-procedural pain. Coding of postoperative pain is driven by the provider's documentation. One important thing to remember is that routine or expected postoperative pain occurring immediately after surgery is not coded. When the provider's documentation does support reporting a code for post-thoracotomy or other postoperative pain, but the pain is not specified as acute or chronic, the code for the acute form is the default. Only postoperative pain that is not associated with a specific postoperative complication is assigned a postoperative pain code in category G89. Postoperative pain associated with a specific postoperative complication such as painful wire sutures is coded to Chapter 19, Injury, Poisoning, and Certain Other Consequences of External Causes with an additional code from category G89 to identify acute or chronic pain.

Chronic pain is reported with codes in subcategory G89.2- and includes: G89.21 Chronic pain due to trauma, G89.22 Chronic post-thoracotomy pain, G89.28 Other chronic post-procedural pain, and G89.29 Other chronic pain. There is no time frame defining when pain becomes chronic pain. The provider's documentation directs the use of these codes. It is important to note that central pain syndrome (G89.0) and chronic pain syndrome (G89.4) are not the same as "chronic pain," so these codes should only be used when the provider has specifically documented these conditions.

Code G89.3 is assigned when the patient's pain is documented as being related to, associated with, or due to cancer, primary or secondary malignancy, or tumor. Code G89.3 is assigned regardless of whether the pain is documented as acute or chronic. Sequencing of code G89.3 is dependent on the reason for the admission/encounter. When the reason for the admission/encounter is documented as pain control/pain management, code G89.3 is assigned as the principal or first-listed code with the underlying neoplasm reported as an additional diagnosis. When the admission/encounter is for management of the neoplasm and the pain associated with the neoplasm is also documented, the neoplasm code is assigned as the principal or first-listed diagnosis and code G89.3 may be assigned as an additional diagnosis. It is not necessary to assign an additional code for the site of the pain.

Chapter 7 – Diseases of Eye and Adnexa (H00-H59)

Chapter 7 classifies diseases of the eye and the adnexa. The adnexa includes structures surrounding the eye, such as the tear (lacrimal) ducts and glands, the extraocular muscles, and the eyelids. Coding diseases of the eye and adnexa can be difficult due to the complex anatomic structures of the ocular system. Laterality is required for most eye conditions. For conditions affecting the eyelid, there are also specific codes for the upper and lower eyelids.

Not all eye conditions are found in Chapter 7. For example, some diseases that are coded to other chapters have associated eye manifestations, such as eye disorders associated with infectious diseases (Chapter 1) and diabetes (Chapter 4). There are also combination codes for conditions and common symptoms or manifestations. Most notable are combination codes for diabetes mellitus with eye conditions (E08.3-, E09.3-, E10.3-, E11.3-, E13.3-). Because the diabetes code captures the manifestation, these conditions do not require additional manifestation codes from Chapter 7.

Chapter Guidelines

All guidelines for Chapter 7 relate to assignment of codes for glaucoma. Glaucoma codes (category H40) are specific to type and, in most cases, laterality (right, left, bilateral) is a component of the code. For some types of glaucoma, the glaucoma stage is also a component of the code. Glaucoma stage is reported using a 7th character extension as follows:

- 0 – Stage unspecified
- 1 – Mild stage
- 2 – Moderate stage
- 3 – Severe stage
- 4 – Indeterminate stage

Indeterminate stage glaucoma identified by the 7th character 4 is assigned only when the stage of the glaucoma cannot be clinically determined. If the glaucoma stage is not documented, 7th character 0, stage unspecified, must be assigned.

Because laterality is a component of most glaucoma codes, it is possible to identify the specific stage for each eye when the type of glaucoma is the same, but the stages are different. When the patient has bilateral glaucoma that is the same type and same stage in both eyes, and there is a bilateral code, a single code is reported with the seventh character for the stage. When laterality is not a component of the code (H40.10-, H40.20-) and the patient has the same stage of glaucoma bilaterally, only one code for the type of glaucoma with the appropriate 7th character for stage is assigned. When the patient has bilateral glaucoma but different types or different stages in each eye and the classification distinguishes laterality, two codes are assigned to identify appropriate type and stage for each eye rather than the code for bilateral glaucoma. When there is not a code that distinguishes laterality (H40.10-, H40.20-) two codes are also reported, one for each type of glaucoma with the appropriate seventh character for stage. Should the glaucoma stage evolve during an admission, the code for the highest stage documented is assigned.

Chapter 8 – Diseases of the Ear and Mastoid Process (H60-H95)

Chapter 8 classifies diseases and conditions of the ear and mastoid process by site, starting with diseases of the external ear, followed by diseases of the middle ear and mastoid, then diseases of the inner ear. Several diseases with associated ear manifestations are classified in other chapters, such as otitis media in influenza (J09.X9, J10.83, J11.83), measles (B05.3), scarlet fever (A38.0), and tuberculosis (A18.6).

Chapter Guidelines

Currently, there are no chapter-specific guidelines for diseases of the ear and mastoid process.

Chapter 9 – Diseases of the Circulatory System (I00-I99)

This chapter conditions affecting the heart muscle and coronary arteries, diseases of the pulmonary artery and conditions affecting the pulmonary circulation, inflammatory disease processes such as pericarditis, valve disorders, arrhythmias and other conditions affecting the conductive system of the heart, heart failure, cerebrovascular diseases, and diseases of the peripheral vascular system.

Hypertension

Essential hypertension is reported with code I10 Essential hypertension and is not designated as benign, malignant or unspecified. The classification presumes a causal relationship between hypertension and heart involvement and between hypertension and kidney involvement, as the two conditions are linked by the term "with" in the Alphabetic Index. These conditions should be coded as related even in the absence of provider documentation explicitly linking them, unless the documentation clearly states the conditions are unrelated.

For hypertension and conditions not specifically linked by relational terms such as "with," "associated with" or "due to" in the classification, provider documentation must link the conditions in order to code them as related.

There are categories for hypertensive heart disease (I11), hypertensive chronic kidney disease (I12), hypertensive heart and chronic kidney disease (I13), and secondary hypertension (I15).

Myocardial Infarction

The period of time for initial treatment of acute myocardial infarction (AMI) is 4 weeks. Codes for the initial treatment should be used only for an AMI that is equal to or less than 4 weeks old (category I21). If care related to the AMI is required beyond 4 weeks, an aftercare code is reported. Codes for subsequent episode of care for AMI (category I22) are used only when the patient suffers a new AMI during the initial 4-week treatment period of a previous AMI. In addition, codes for initial treatment of acute type 1 ST elevation myocardial infarction (STEMI) are more specific to site requiring identification of the affected coronary artery. Type 1 anterior wall AMI is classified as involving the left main coronary artery (I21.01), left anterior descending artery (I21.02), and other coronary artery of anterior wall (I21.09). A type 1 AMI of the inferior wall is classified as involving the right coronary artery (I21.11) or other coronary artery of the inferior wall (I21.19). Codes for other specified sites for type 1 STEMI include an AMI involving the left circumflex coronary artery (I21.21) or other specified site (I21.29). There is also a code for an initial type 1 STEMI of an unspecified site (I21.3). Type 1 NSTEMI (I21.4) is not specific to site. A subsequent type 1 STEMI within 4 weeks of the first AMI is classified as involving the anterior wall (I22.0), inferior wall (I22.1), or other sites (I22.8). There is also a code for a subsequent type 1 STEMI of an unspecified site (I22.9). No site designation is required for a subsequent NSTEMI (I22.2).

ICD-10-CM provides codes for different types of myocardial infarction. Type 1 myocardial infarctions are assigned to codes I21.1-I21.4. Type 2 myocardial infarction, and myocardial infarction due to demand ischemia or secondary to ischemic balance, is assigned to code I21.A1, Myocardial infarction type 2 with a code for the underlying cause. Assign code I21.A1 when a type 2 AMI code is described as NSTEMI or STEMI. Acute myocardial infarctions type 3, 4a, 4b, 4c, and 5 are assigned to code I21.A9, Other myocardial infarction type. If the type of AMI is not documented, code I21.9 Acute myocardial infarction, unspecified would be assigned.

Coronary Atherosclerosis

Codes for coronary atherosclerosis (I25.1-, I25.7-, I25.81-) continue to be classified by vessel type, but codes also capture the presence or absence of angina pectoris.When angina is present the codes capture the type of angina (unstable, with documented spasm, other forms of angina, unspecified angina).

Nontraumatic Subarachnoid/Intracerebral Hemorrhage

These codes are specific to site. For nontraumatic subarachnoid hemorrhage (category I60), the specific artery must be identified, and laterality is also a component of the code. For example, code I60.11 reports nontraumatic subarachnoid hemorrhage from right middle cerebral hemorrhage. Nontraumatic intracerebral hemorrhage (category I61) is specific to site as well with the following site designations: subcortical hemisphere, cortical hemisphere, brain stem, cerebellum, intraventricular, multiple localized, other specified, and unspecified site.

Cerebral Infarction

Codes for cerebral infarction (category I63) are specific to type (thrombotic, embolic, unspecified occlusion or stenosis), site, and laterality. The site designations require identification of the specific precerebral or cerebral artery.

Chapter Guidelines

Guidelines for coding diseases of the circulatory system cover five conditions which include hypertension, acute myocardial infarction, atherosclerotic coronary artery disease and angina, intraoperative and postprocedural cerebrovascular accident, and sequelae of cerebrovascular disease.

As was stated earlier, hypertension is not classified as benign, malignant, or unspecified. Hypertension without associated heart or kidney disease is reported with the code I10 Essential hypertension.

There are combination codes for atherosclerotic coronary artery disease with angina pectoris. Documentation of the two conditions are reported with codes from subcategories I25.11- Atherosclerotic heart disease of native coronary artery with angina pectoris, and I25.7- Atherosclerosis of coronary artery bypass grafts and coronary artery of transplanted heart with angina pectoris. It is not necessary to assign a separate code for angina pectoris when both conditions are documented because the combination code captures both conditions. A causal relationship between the atherosclerosis and angina is assumed unless documentation specifically indicates that the angina is due to a condition other than atherosclerosis.

Intraoperative and postprocedural complications and disorders of the circulatory system are found in category I97. Codes from category I97 for intraoperative or postprocedural cerebrovascular accident are found in subcategory I97.8-. Guidelines state that a cause and effect relationship between a cerebrovascular accident (CVA) and a procedure cannot be assumed. The physician must document that a cause and effect relationship exists. Documentation must clearly identify the condition as an intraoperative or postoperative event. The condition must also be clearly documented as an infarction or hemorrhage. Intraoperative and postoperative cerebrovascular infarction (I97.81-, I97.82-) are classified in the circulatory system chapter while intraoperative and postoperative cerebrovascular hemorrhage (G97.3-, G97.5-) are classified in the nervous system chapter.

Category I69 Sequelae of cerebrovascular disease is used to report conditions classifiable to categories I60-I67 as the causes of late effects, specifically neurological deficits, which are classified elsewhere. Sequelae/late effects are conditions that persist after the initial onset of the conditions classifiable to categories I60-I67. The neurologic deficits may be present at the onset of the cerebrovascular disease or may arise at any time after the onset. If the patient has a current CVA and deficits from an old CVA, codes from category I69 and categories I60-I67 may be reported together. For a cerebral infarction without residual neurological deficits, code Z86.73 Personal history of transient ischemic attack (TIA) is reported instead of a code from category I69 to identify the history of the cerebrovascular disease.

Acute myocardial infarction (AMI) is reported with codes that identify type 1 AMI as ST elevation myocardial infarction (STEMI) and non ST elevation myocardial infarction (NSTEMI). Initial acute type 1 myocardial infarction is assigned a code from category I21 for STEMI/NSTEMI not documented as subsequent or not occurring within 28 days of a previous myocardial infarction. All encounters for care of the AMI during the first four weeks (equal to or less than 4 full weeks/28 days), are assigned a code from category I21. Encounters related to the myocardial infarction after 4 full weeks of care are reported with the appropriate aftercare code. Old or healed myocardial infarctions are assigned code I25.2 Old myocardial infarction.

Code I21.9 Acute myocardial infarction, unspecified is the default for unspecified acute myocardial infarction or unspecified type. If only type 1 STEMI or transmural MI without the site is documented, assign code I21.3 ST elevation (STEMI) myocardial infarction of un-specified site.

Subsequent type 1 or unspecified AMI occurring within 28 days of a previous AMI is assigned a code from category I22 for a new STEMI/NSTEMI documented as occurring within 4 weeks (28 days) of a previous myocardial infarction. The subsequent AMI may involve the same site as the initial AMI or a different site. Codes in category I22 are never reported alone. A code from category I21 must be reported in conjunction with the code from I22. Codes from categories I21 and I22 are sequenced based on the circumstances of the encounter.

Do not assign code I22 for subsequent myocardial infarctions other than type 1 or unspecified. For subsequent type 2 AMI assign only code I21.A1. For subsequent type 4 or type 5 AMI, assign only code I21.A9.

Chapter 10 – Diseases of the Respiratory System (J00-J99)

Diseases of the respiratory system include conditions affecting the nose and sinuses, throat, tonsils, larynx and trachea, bronchi, and lungs. Chapter 10 is organized by the general type of disease or condition and by site with diseases affecting primarily the upper respiratory system or the lower respiratory system in separate sections.

Chapter Guidelines

The respiratory system guidelines cover chronic obstructive pulmonary disease (COPD) and asthma, acute respiratory failure, influenza due to avian influenza virus, and ventilator associated pneumonia.

Codes for COPD in category J44 differentiate between uncomplicated cases and those with an acute exacerbation. For coding purposes an acute exacerbation is defined as a worsening or decompensation of a chronic condition. An acute exacerbation is not the same as an infection superimposed on a chronic condition, though an exacerbation may be triggered by an infection.

Guidelines for reporting acute respiratory failure (J96.0-) and acute and chronic respiratory failure (J96.2-) relate to sequencing of these codes. Depending on the documentation these codes may be either the principal or first-listed diagnosis or a secondary diagnosis. Careful review of the provider documentation and a clear understanding of the guidelines including the definition of principal diagnosis are required to sequence these codes correctly.

There are three code categories for reporting influenza which are as follows: J09 Influenza due to certain identified influenza viruses, J10 Influenza due to other identified influenza virus, and J11 Influenza due to unidentified influenza virus. All codes in category J09 report influenza due to identified novel influenza A virus with various complications or manifestations such as pneumonia, other respiratory conditions, gastrointestinal manifestations or other manifestations. Identified novel influenza A viruses include avian (bird) influenza, influenza A/H5N1, influenza of other animal origin (not bird or swine), and swine influenza. Codes from category J09 are reported only for confirmed cases of avian influenza and the other specific types of influenza identified in the code description. This is an exception to the inpatient guideline related to uncertain diagnoses. Confirmation does not require a positive laboratory finding. Documentation by the provider that the patient has avian influenza or influenza due other identified novel influenza A virus is sufficient to report a code from category J09. Documentation of "suspected," "possible," or "probable" avian influenza or other novel influenza A virus is reported with a code from category J10.

Ventilator associated pneumonia (VAP) is listed in category J95 Intraoperative and postprocedural complications and disorders of respiratory system not elsewhere classified, and is reported with code J95.851. As with all procedural and postprocedural complications, the provider must document the relationship between the conditions, in this case VAP, and the procedure. An additional code should be assigned to identify the organism. Codes for pneumonia classified in categories J12-J18 are not assigned additionally for VAP. However, when a patient is admitted with a different type of pneumonia and subsequently develops VAP, the appropriate code from J12-J18 is reported as the principal diagnosis and code J95.851 is reported as an additional diagnosis

Chapter 11 – Diseases of the Digestive System (K00-K95)

Diseases of the digestive system include conditions affecting the esophagus, stomach, small and large intestines, liver, and gallbladder. Some of the most frequently diagnosed digestive system diseases and conditions, such as cholecystitis and cholelithiasis, have specific elements incorporated into the codes. For example, cholecystitis is classified as acute, chronic, or acute and chronic regardless of whether the cholecystitis occurs alone or with cholelithiasis. Combination codes for cholelithiasis with cholecystitis identify the site of the calculus as being in the gallbladder and/or bile duct and the specific type of cholecystitis. Combination codes also report cholelithiasis of the bile duct with cholangitis. There are other digestive system conditions that require an acute or chronic designation as well as more combination codes that capture diseases of the gallbladder and associated complications.

Chapter Guidelines

Currently there are no guidelines for the digestive system.

Chapter 12 – Diseases of the Skin and Subcutaneous Tissue (L00-L99)

Diseases of the skin and subcutaneous tissue include diseases affecting the epidermis, dermis and hypodermis, subcutaneous tissue, nails, sebaceous glands, sweat glands, and hair and hair follicles. Common conditions of the skin and subcutaneous tissue include boils, cellulitis, abscess, pressure ulcers, lymphadenitis, and pilonidal cysts.

Chapter Guidelines

All guidelines related to coding of diseases of the skin and subcutaneous tissue relate to pressure ulcers and non pressure chronic ulcers. Codes from category L89 Pressure ulcer are combination codes that identify the site of the pressure ulcer as well as the stage of the ulcer. For patients with multiple pressure ulcers, multiple codes should be assigned to capture all pressure ulcer sites.

Pressure ulcer stages are based on severity. Severity is designated as:

- Stage 1 – Pressure ulcer skin changes limited to persistent focal edema
- Stage 2 – Pressure ulcer with abrasion, blister, partial thickness skin loss involving epidermis and/or dermis
- Stage 3 – Pressure ulcer with full thickness skin loss involving damage or necrosis of subcutaneous tissue
- Stage 4 – Pressure ulcer with necrosis of soft tissues through to underlying muscle, tendon, or bone
- Unstageable – Pressure ulcer stage cannot be clinically determined
- Unspecified – Pressure ulcer stage is not documented

Assignment of the pressure ulcer stage code should be guided by clinical documentation of the stage or documentation of the terms found in the Alphabetic Index. For clinical terms describing the stage that are not found in the Alphabetic Index and when there is no documentation of the stage, the provider should be queried. Assignment of the code for unstageable pressure ulcer (L89.--0) should be based on the clinical documentation. These codes are used for pressure ulcers whose stage cannot be clinically determined (e.g., the ulcer is covered by eschar or has been treated with a skin or muscle graft) and pressure ulcers that are documented as deep tissue injury, but not documented as due to trauma. Unstageable pressure ulcers should not be confused with the codes for unspecified stage (L89.--9). When there is no documentation regarding the stage of the pressure ulcer, the appropriate code for unspecified stage (L89.--9) is assigned.

The depth of non-pressure chronic ulcers and the stage of pressure ulcers may be coded from documentation provided by a clinician other than the patient's provider, such as a wound care nurse. The actual diagnosis must be made by the patient's provider. Code assignment for the specific type and site of the ulcer must be based on information in the provider's documentation.

Patients admitted with pressure ulcers documented as healing should be assigned the appropriate pressure ulcer stage code based on the documentation in the medical record. If the documentation does not provide information about the stage of the healing pressure ulcer, a code for unspecified stage is assigned. If the documentation is unclear as to whether the patient has a current (new) pressure ulcer or if the patient is being treated for a healing pressure ulcer, query the provider. No code is assigned if the documentation states that the pressure ulcer is completely healed.

If a patient is admitted with a pressure ulcer at one stage and it progresses to a higher stage, two separate codes should be assigned: one code for the site and stage of the ulcer on admission and a second code for the same ulcer site and the highest stage reported during the stay. For ulcers that were present on admission but healed at the time of discharge, assign the code for the site and stage of the pressure ulcer at the time of admission.

Non-pressure ulcers described as healing should be assigned the appropriate non-pressure ulcer code based on the documentation in the medical record. If the documentation does not provide information about the severity of the healing non-pressure ulcer, assign the appropriate code for unspecified severity. For ulcers that were present on admission but healed at the time of discharge, assign the code for the site and severity of the non-pressure ulcer at the time of admission.

If the patient is admitted with a non-pressure ulcer at one severity level and it progresses to a higher severity level, two separate codes should be assigned: one code for the site and severity level of the ulcer on admission and a second code for the same ulcer site and the highest severity level reported during the stay.

Chapter 13 – Diseases of the Musculoskeletal System and Connective Tissue (M00-M99)

Coding of musculoskeletal system and connective tissue conditions requires both precise site specificity and laterality. For example, conditions affecting the cervical spine require identification of the site as occipito-atlanto-axial, mid-cervical or cervicothoracic. Laterality is also included for most musculoskeletal and connective tissue conditions affecting the extremities. For some conditions only right and left are provided, but for other conditions that frequently affect both sides, codes for bilateral are also listed. For example, osteoarthritis of the hips has designations for bilateral primary osteoarthritis (M16.0), bilateral osteoarthritis resulting from hip dysplasia (M16.2), bilateral post-traumatic osteoarthritis (M16.4), and other bilateral secondary osteoarthritis of the hip (M16.6). In addition, there are 7th characters for some code categories.

7th Characters

In Chapter 13, 7th characters are required for chronic gout to identify the presence or absence of tophus (tophi). Tophi are solid deposits of monosodium urate (MSU) crystals that form in the joints, cartilage, bones, and elsewhere in the body. Chronic gout is reported with codes in category M1A. The required 7th characters identify chronic gout as without tophus (0) or with tophus (1).

Fatigue and compression fractures of the vertebra, stress fractures, and pathological fractures due to osteoporosis, neoplastic or other disease also require 7th characters to identify the episode of care. For fatigue fractures of the vertebra (M48.4-) and collapsed vertebra (M48.5-) the 7th character designates episode of care as: initial encounter for fracture (A), subsequent encounter for fracture with routine healing (D), subsequent encounter for fracture with delayed healing (G), and sequela (S). For age-related osteoporosis with current pathological fracture (M80.0-), other osteoporosis with current pathological fracture (M80.1-), stress fracture (M84.3-), pathological fracture not elsewhere classified (M84.4-), pathological fracture in neoplastic disease (M84.5-), and pathological fracture in other disease (M84.6-), 7th character designations include those listed for fatigue and compression fractures of the vertebra, and also include two additional 7th characters for subsequent encounter with nonunion (K) or malunion (P). The table below explains and defines the 7th characters used for fractures classified in Chapter 13.

Character	Definition	Explanation
A	Initial encounter for fracture	Use 'A' for as long as the patient is receiving active treatment for the pathologic fracture. Examples of active treatment are: surgical treatment, emergency department encounter, evaluation and treatment by a new physician
D	Subsequent encounter with routine fracture healing	For encounters after the patient has completed active treatment and when the fracture is healing normally
G	Subsequent encounter for fracture with delayed healing	For encounters when the physician has documented that healing is delayed or is not occurring as rapidly as normally expected
K	Subsequent encounter for fracture with nonunion	For encounters when the physician has documented that there is nonunion of the fracture or that the fracture has failed to heal. This is a serious fracture complication that requires additional intervention and treatment by the physician

Character	Definition	Explanation
P	Subsequent encounter for fracture with malunion	For encounters when the physician has documented that the fracture has healed in an abnormal or nonanatomic position. This is a serious fracture complication that requires additional intervention and treatment by the physician
S	Sequela	Use for complications or conditions that arise as a direct result of the pathological fracture, such as a leg length discrepancy following pathological fracture of the femur. The specific type of sequela is sequenced first followed by the pathological fracture code.

Chapter Guidelines

Chapter specific guidelines are provided for musculoskeletal system and connective tissue coding related to the following: site and laterality, acute traumatic versus chronic or recurrent musculoskeletal conditions, osteoporosis, and pathological fractures. Guidelines related to coding of pathological fractures relate to the use of 7th characters which are discussed above.

Most codes in Chapter 13 have site and laterality designations. Site represents either the bone, joint or muscle involved. For some conditions where more than one bone, joint, or muscle is commonly involved, such as osteoarthritis, there is a "multiple sites" code available. For categories where no multiple site code is provided and more than one bone, joint or muscle is involved, it is necessary to report multiple codes to indicate the different sites involved. Because some conditions involving the bones occur at the upper and/or lower ends at the joint, it is sometimes difficult to determine whether the code for the bone or joint should be reported. The guidelines indicate that when a condition involves the upper or lower ends of the bones, the site code assigned should be designated as the bone, not the joint.

Many musculoskeletal conditions are a result of a previous injury or trauma to a site, or are recurrent conditions. Musculoskeletal conditions are classified either in Chapter 13, Diseases of the Musculoskeletal System and Connective tissue or in Chapter 19, Injury, Poisoning, and Certain Other Consequences of External Causes. The table below identifies where various conditions/injuries are classified.

Condition	Chapter
Healed injury	Chapter 13
Recurrent bone, joint, or muscle condition	Chapter 13
Chronic or other recurrent conditions	Chapter 13
Current acute injury	Chapter 19

Osteoporosis is a systemic condition, meaning that all bones of the musculoskeletal system are affected. Therefore, site is not a component of the codes under category M81 Osteoporosis without current pathological fracture. The site codes under M80 Osteoporosis with current pathological fracture identify the site of the fracture not the osteoporosis. A code from category M80, not a traumatic fracture code, should be used for any patient with known osteoporosis who suffers a fracture, even if the patient had a minor fall or trauma, if that fall or trauma would not usually break a normal, healthy bone. For a patient with a history of osteoporosis fractures, status code Z87.31, Personal history of osteoporosis fracture should follow the code from category M81.

Chapter 14 – Diseases of the Genitourinary System (N00-N99)

The Genitourinary System includes the organs and anatomical structures involved with reproduction and urinary excretion in both males and females. Female genitourinary disorders include pelvic inflammatory diseases, vaginitis, salpingitis and oophoritis. Common male genitourinary disorders include prostatitis, benign prostatic hyperplasia, premature ejaculation and erectile dysfunction.

Chapter Guidelines

All coding guidelines relate to coding of chronic kidney disease. The guidelines cover stages of chronic kidney disease (CKD), CKD and kidney transplant status, and CKD with other conditions.

Chapter 15 – Pregnancy, Childbirth and the Puerperium (O00-O9A)

The majority of codes for complications that occur during pregnancy require identification of the trimester.

Trimester

The trimester is captured by the fourth, fifth or sixth character. The fourth, fifth or sixth character also captures the episode of care for complications that can occur at any point in the pregnancy, during childbirth or postpartum, such as eclampsia (O15). Some complications of pregnancy that typically occur or are treated only in a single trimester such as ectopic pregnancy (O00) do not identify the trimester. In addition, complications that occur only during childbirth or the puerperium contain that information in the code description, such as obstructed labor due to generally contracted pelvis (O65.1) or puerperal sepsis (O85).

7th Character

A 7th character identifying the fetus is required for certain categories. Some complications of pregnancy and childbirth occur more frequently in multiple gestation pregnancies. These complications may affect one or more fetuses and require a 7th character to identify the fetus or fetuses affected by the complication. The following categories/subcategories require identification of the fetus:

- O31 Complications specific to multiple gestation
- O32 Maternal care for malpresentation of fetus
- O33.3 Maternal care for disproportion due to outlet contraction of pelvis
- O33.4 Maternal care for disproportion of mixed maternal and fetal origin
- O33.5 Maternal care for disproportion due to unusually large fetus
- O33.6 Maternal care for disproportion due to hydrocephalic fetus

- O35 Maternal care for known or suspected fetal abnormality and damage
- O36 Maternal care for other fetal problems
- O40 Polyhydramnios
- O41 Other disorders of amniotic fluid and membranes
- O60.1 Preterm labor with preterm delivery
- O60.2 Term delivery with preterm labor
- O64 Obstructed labor due to malposition and malpresentation of fetus
- O69 Labor and delivery complicated by umbilical cord complications

The 7th character identifies the fetus to which the complication code applies. For a single gestation, when the documentation is insufficient, or when it is clinically impossible to identify the fetus, the 7th character '0' for not applicable/unspecified is assigned. For multiple gestations, each fetus should be identified with a number as fetus 1, fetus 2, fetus 3, etc. The fetus or fetuses affected by the condition should then be clearly identified using the number assigned to the fetus. For example, a triplet gestation in the third trimester with fetus 1 having no complications, fetus 2 in a separate amniotic sac having polyhydramnios, and fetus 3 having hydrocephalus with maternal pelvic disproportion would require reporting of the complications as follows: Fetus 1 – No codes; Fetus 2 – O40.3XX2, Polyhydramnios, third trimester, fetus 2; Fetus 3 – O33.6XX3, Maternal care for disproportion due to hydrocephalic fetus, fetus 3. An additional code identifying the triplet pregnancy would also be reported. Applicable 7th characters are:

- 0 – not applicable or unspecified
- 1 – fetus 1
- 2 – fetus 2
- 3 – fetus 3
- 4 – fetus 4
- 5 – fetus 5
- 9 – other fetus

Chapter Guidelines

Chapter 15 guidelines include information covering general rules and sequencing of codes and coding rules for specific conditions. Only guidelines related to trimester, pre-existing conditions versus conditions due to pregnancy, and gestational diabetes are discussed here. Consult the Official Guidelines for Coding and Reporting for the complete Chapter 15 guidelines.

Most codes for conditions and complications of pregnancy have a final character indicating the trimester. Assignment of the final character for trimester is based on the provider's documentation which may identify the trimester or the number of weeks of gestation for the current encounter. Trimesters are calculated using the first day of the last menstrual period and are as follows:

- First trimester – less than 14 weeks 0 days
- Second trimester – 14 weeks 0 days to less than 28 weeks 0 days
- Third trimester – 28 weeks 0 days to delivery

There are codes for unspecified trimester; however, these codes should be used only when the documentation is insufficient to determine the trimester and it is not possible to obtain clarification from the provider. If a delivery occurs during the admission and there is an "in childbirth" option for the complication, the code for "in childbirth" is assigned.

When an obstetric patient is admitted and delivers during that admission, the condition that prompted the admission should be sequenced as the principal diagnosis. If multiple conditions prompted the admission, sequence the one most related to the delivery as the principal diagnosis. A code for any complication of the delivery should be assigned as an additional diagnosis.

For inpatient services, when an inpatient admission encompasses more than one trimester, the code is assigned based on when the condition developed not when the discharge occurred. For example, if the condition developed during the second trimester and the patient was discharged during the third trimester, the code for the second trimester is assigned. If the condition being treated developed prior to the current admission/encounter or was a pre-existing condition, the trimester character at the time of the admission/encounter is used.

Certain categories in Chapter 15 distinguish between conditions that existed prior to pregnancy (pre-existing) and those that are a direct result of the pregnancy. Two examples are hypertension (O10, O11, O13) and diabetes mellitus (O24). The physician must provide clear documentation as to whether the condition existed prior to pregnancy or whether it developed during the pregnancy or as a result of the pregnancy. Categories that do not distinguish between pre-existing conditions and pregnancy related conditions may be used for either. If a puerperal complication develops during the delivery encounter and a specific code for the puerperal complication exists, the code for the puerperal complication may be reported with codes related to complications of pregnancy and childbirth.

Gestational diabetes can occur during the second and third trimesters in women without a pre-pregnancy diagnosis of diabetes mellitus. Gestational diabetes may cause complications similar to those in patients with pre-existing diabetes mellitus. Gestational diabetes is classified in category O24 along with pre-existing diabetes mellitus. Subcategory O24.4- Gestational diabetes mellitus, cannot be used with any other codes in category O24. Codes in subcategory O24.4- are combination codes that identify the condition as well as how it is being controlled. In order to assign the most specific code, the provider must document whether the gestational diabetes is being controlled by diet or insulin. If documentation indicates the gestational diabetes is being controlled with both diet and insulin, only the code for insulin-controlled is assigned. Code Z79.4 for long-term insulin use is not reported with codes in subcategory O24.4-. Codes for gestational diabetes are not used to report an abnormal glucose tolerance test which is reported with code O99.81 Abnormal glucose complicating pregnancy, childbirth, and the puerperium.

Chapter 16 – Newborn (Perinatal) Guidelines (P00-P96)

Perinatal conditions have their origin in the period beginning before birth and extending through the first 28 days after birth. Codes from this chapter are used only on the newborn medical record, never on the maternal medical record. These conditions must originate during this period but for some conditions morbidity may not be manifested or diagnosed until later. As long as the documentation supports the origin of the condition during the perinatal period, codes for perinatal conditions may be reported. Examples of conditions included in this chapter are maternal conditions that have affected or are suspected to have affected the fetus or newborn, prematurity, light for dates, birth injuries, and other conditions originating in the perinatal period and affecting specific body systems.

Chapter Guidelines

The principal diagnosis for the birth record is always a code from Chapter 21, category Z38 Liveborn according to place of birth and type of delivery. Additional diagnoses are assigned for all clinically significant conditions identified on the newborn examination. Other guidelines relate to prematurity, fetal growth retardation, low birth weight and immaturity status.

In determining prematurity, different providers may utilize different criteria. A code for prematurity should not be assigned unless specifically documented by the physician. Two code categories are provided for reporting prematurity and fetal growth retardation, P05 Disorders of newborn related to slow fetal growth and fetal malnutrition and P07 Disorders of newborn related to short gestation and low birth weight, not elsewhere classified. Assignment of codes in categories P05 and P07 should be based on the recorded birth weight and estimated gestational age.

To identify those instances when a healthy newborn is evaluated for a suspected condition that is determined after study not to be present, assign a code from category Z05, Observation and evaluation of newborns and infants for suspected conditions ruled out. Do not use a code from category Z05 when the patient has identified signs or symptoms of a suspected problem; in such cases code the sign or symptom. A code from category Z05 may also be assigned as a principal or first-listed code for readmissions or encounters when the code from category Z38 code no longer applies. Codes from category Z05 are for use only for healthy newborns and infants for which no condition after study is found to be present. On a birth record, a code from category Z05 is to be used as a secondary code after the code from category Z38, Liveborn infants according to place of birth and type of delivery.

Chapter 17 – Congenital Malformations, Deformations, and Chromosomal Abnormalities (Q00-Q99)

Congenital anomalies are conditions that are present at birth. Congenital anomalies include both congenital malformations, such as spina bifida, atrial and ventricular septal heart defects, undescended testes, and chromosomal abnormalities such as trisomy 21 also known as Down's syndrome. Chapter 17 is organized with congenital anomalies, malformations, or deformations grouped together by body system followed by other congenital conditions such as syndromes that affect multiple systems with the last block of codes being chromosomal abnormalities.

Codes for congenital malformations, deformations and chromosomal abnormalities require specificity. For example, codes for encephalocele (category Q01) are specific to site and must be documented as frontal, nasofrontal, occipital, or of other specific sites. Cleft lip and cleft palate (categories Q35-Q37) require documentation of the site of the opening in the palate as the hard or soft palate and the location of the cleft lip as unilateral, in the median, or bilateral.

Chapter Guidelines

When a malformation, deformation, or chromosomal abnormality is documented, the appropriate code from categories Q00-Q99 is assigned. A malformation, deformation, or chromosomal abnormality may be the principal or first-listed diagnosis or it may be a secondary diagnosis. For the birth admission, the principal diagnosis is always a code from category Z38 and any congenital anomalies documented in the birth record are reported additionally. In some instances, there may not be a specific diagnosis code for the malformation, deformation, or chromosomal abnormality. In this case the code for other specified is used and additional codes are assigned for any manifestations that are present. However, when there is a specific code available to report the congenital anomaly, manifestations that are an inherent component of the anomaly should not be coded separately. Additional codes may be reported for manifestations that are not an inherent component of the anomaly. Although present at birth the congenital malformation, deformation, or chromosomal abnormality may not be diagnosed until later in life and it is appropriate to assign a code from Chapter 17 when the physician documentation supports a diagnosis of a congenital anomaly. If the congenital malformation or deformity has been corrected, a personal history code should be used to identify the history of the malformation or deformity.

Chapter 18 – Symptoms, Signs, and Abnormal Clinical and Laboratory Findings, Not Elsewhere Classified (R00-R99)

Codes for symptoms, signs, abnormal results of laboratory or other investigative procedures, and ill-defined conditions without a diagnosis classified elsewhere are classified in Chapter 18. There are 7 code blocks that identify symptoms and signs for specific body systems followed by a code block for general symptoms and signs. The last 5 code blocks report abnormal findings for laboratory tests, imaging and function studies, and tumor markers. Examples of signs and symptoms related to specific body systems include: shortness of breath (R06.02), epigastric pain (R10.13), cyanosis (R23.0), ataxia (R27.0), and dysuria (R30.0). Examples of general signs and symptoms include: fever (R50.9), chronic fatigue (R53.82), abnormal weight loss (R63.4), systemic inflammatory response syndrome (SIRS) of non-infectious origin (R65.1-), and severe sepsis (R65.2-). Examples of abnormal findings include: red blood cell abnormalities (R71.-), proteinuria (R80-), abnormal cytological findings in specimens from cervix uteri (R87.61-), and inconclusive mammogram (R92.2).

Combination Codes

A number of codes identify both the definitive diagnosis and common symptoms of that diagnosis. When using these combination codes, an additional code should not be assigned for the symptom. For example, R18.8 Other ascites is not reported with the combination code K70.31 Alcoholic cirrhosis of the liver with ascites because code K70.31 identifies both the definitive diagnosis (alcoholic cirrhosis) and a common symptom of the condition (ascites).

Coma Scale

One significant ICD-10-CM coding concept relates the coma scale codes (R40.2-). Coma scale codes can be used by trauma registries in conjunction with traumatic brain injury codes, acute cerebrovascular disease, and sequela of cerebrovascular disease codes or to assess the status of the central nervous system. These codes can also be used for other non-trauma conditions, such as monitoring patients in the intensive care unit regardless of medical condition. The coma scale codes are sequenced after the diagnosis code(s).

The coma scale consists of three elements, eye opening (R40.21-), verbal response (R40.22-), and motor response (R40.23-) and a code from each subcategory must be assigned to complete the coma scale. If all three elements are documented, codes for the individual scores should be assigned. In addition, a 7th character indicates when the scale was recorded and the 7th character should match for all three codes. The 7th characters identify the time/place as follows:

- 0 – Unspecified time
- 1 – In the field (EMT/ambulance)
- 2 – At arrival in emergency department
- 3 – At hospital admission
- 4 – 24 hours or more after hospital admission

If all three elements are not known but the total Glasgow coma scale is documented, the code for the total Glasgow coma score is assigned. The Glasgow score is classified as follows:

- Glasgow score 13-15
- Glasgow score 9-12
- Glasgow score 3-8
- Other coma without documented Glasgow coma scale score or with partial score reported

Chapter Guidelines

There are a number of general guidelines for the use of symptom codes and combination codes that include symptoms as well as some specific guidelines related to repeated falls, the coma scale (discussed above), and systemic inflammatory response syndrome (SIRS) due to non-infectious process. There are also some guidelines referencing signs and symptoms in Section II Selection of Principal Diagnosis. For example, the first guideline related to the use of symptom codes indicates that these codes are acceptable for reporting purposes when a related definitive diagnosis has not been established (confirmed) by the provider. It may also be appropriate to report a sign or symptom code with a definitive diagnosis. However, this is dependent upon whether or not the symptom is routinely associated with the definitive diagnosis/disease process. When the sign or symptom is not routinely associated with the definitive diagnosis, the codes for signs and symptoms may be reported additionally. The definitive diagnosis should be sequenced before the symptom code. When the sign or symptom is routinely associated with the disease process, the sign or symptom code is not reported additionally unless instructions in the Tabular indicate otherwise.

There is a code for repeated falls (R29.6) and another code for history of falling (Z91.81). The code for repeated falls is assigned when a patient has recently fallen and the reason for the fall is being investigated. The code for history of falling is assigned when a patient has fallen in the past and is at risk for future falls. Both codes may be assigned when the patient has had a recent fall that is being investigated and also has a history of falling.

Guidelines related to SIRS due to a non-infectious process (R65.1-) relate to sequencing of codes. Also discussed is the need to verify whether any documented acute organ dysfunction is associated with the SIRS or due to the underlying condition that caused the SIRS or another related condition as this affects code assignment.

Chapter 19 – Injury, Poisoning, and Certain Other Consequences of External Causes (S00-T88)

Codes for injury, poisoning and certain other consequences of external causes are found in Chapter 19. One of the important characteristics to note is that injuries are organized first by body site and then by type of injury. Another is that laterality is included in the code descriptor. The vast majority of injuries to paired organs and the extremities identify the injury as the right or left. In addition, most injuries are specific to site. For example, codes for an open wound of the thorax (category S21), are specific to the right back wall, left back wall, right front wall or left front wall. For open wounds of the abdominal wall (S31.1-, S31.6-), the site must be identified as right upper quadrant, left upper quadrant, epigastric region, right lower quadrant, or left lower quadrant. Also, the vast majority of codes require a 7th character to identify episode of care. Episode of care designations have been discussed previously and many of the same designations are used in Chapter 13. However, there are some additional 7th characters for episode of care that are used only in this chapter for fractures of the long bones. Additionally, the codes for poisoning, adverse effects and toxic effects are combination codes that capture both the drug and the external cause. The Table of Drugs and Chemicals includes an underdosing column.

Application of 7th Characters

Most categories in the injury and poisoning chapter require assignment of a 7th character to identify the episode of care. For most categories there are three (3) 7th character values to select from: 'A' for initial encounter; 'B' for subsequent encounter and 'S' for sequela. Categories for fractures are an exception with fractures having 6 to 16 7th character values in order to capture additional information about the fracture including, whether the fracture is open or closed and whether the healing phase is routine or complicated by delayed healing, nonunion, or malunion. Detailed guidelines are provided related to selection of the 7th character value. Related guidelines and some examples of encounters representative of the three episodes of care 7th character values found in the majority of categories are as follows:

A Initial encounter. Initial encounter is defined as the period when the patient is receiving active treatment for the injury, poisoning, or other consequences of an external cause. An 'A' may be assigned on more than one claim. For example, if a patient is seen in the emergency department (ED) for a head injury that is first evaluated by the ED physician who requests a CT scan that is read by a radiologist and a consultation by a neurologist, the 7th character 'A' is used by all three physicians and also reported on the ED claim. If the patient required admission to an acute care hospital, the 7th character 'A' would be reported for the entire acute care hospital stay because the 7th character extension 'A' is used for the entire period that the patient receives active treatment for the injury.

D Subsequent encounter. This is an encounter after the patient has completed the active phase of treatment and is receiving routine care for the injury or poisoning during the period of healing or recovery. Unlike aftercare following medical or surgical services for other conditions which are reported with codes from Chapter 21, Factors Influencing Health Status and Contact with Health Services (Z00-Z99), aftercare for injuries and poisonings is captured by the 7th character D. For example, a patient with an ankle sprain may return to the office to have joint stability re-evaluated to ensure that the injury is healing properly. In this case, the 7th character 'D' would be assigned.

S Sequela. The 7th character extension 'S' is assigned for complications or conditions that arise as a direct result of an injury. An example of a sequela is a scar resulting from a burn.

Fracture Coding

Two things of note related to fracture coding include the 7th character extensions which differ from the 7th character extensions for other injuries, and the incorporation of information from certain fracture classification systems in the code descriptors. In fact, for open fractures of the long bones, correct assignment of the 7th character requires an understanding of the Gustilo classification system. For most fractures the 7th character extensions are the same as those detailed in Chapter 13 for pathological fractures. The designations are again summarized here and are as follows:

7th Character	Description
A	Initial encounter for closed fracture
B	Initial encounter for open fracture type
D	Subsequent encounter for fracture with routine healing
G	Subsequent encounter for fracture with delayed healing
K	Subsequent encounter for fracture with nonunion
P	Subsequent encounter for fracture with malunion
S	Sequela

For fractures of the shafts of the long bones, the 7th characters further describe the fracture as open or closed. When documentation does not indicate whether the fracture is open or closed, the default is closed. For open fractures, the 7th character also captures the severity of the injury using the Gustilo classification. The Gustilo classification applies to open fractures of the long bones including the humerus, radius, ulna, femur, tibia, and fibula. The Gustilo open fracture classification groups open fractures into three main categories designated as Type I, Type II and Type III with Type III injuries being further divided into Type IIIA, Type IIIB, and Type IIIC subcategories. The categories are defined by characteristics that include the mechanism of injury, extent of soft tissue damage, and degree of bone injury or involvement. The table below identifies key features of Gustilo fracture types. When the Gustilo classification type is not specified for an open fracture, the 7th character for open fracture type I or II should be assigned.

Type	Wound/ Contamination	Soft Tissue Damage	Type of Injury	Most Common Fracture Type(s)
Gustilo Type I	< 1 cm/Wound bed clean	Minimal	Low-energy	Simple transverse, short oblique, minimally comminuted
Gustilo Type II	> 1 cm/ Minimal or no contamination	Moderate	Low-energy	Simple transverse, short oblique, minimally comminuted
Gustilo Type III	> 1 cm/ Contaminated wound	Extensive Type IIIA – • Adequate soft tissue coverage open wound • No flap coverage required Type IIIB • Extensive soft tissue loss • Flap coverage required Type IIIC • Major arterial injury • Extensive repair • May require vascular surgeon for limb salvage	High-energy	Unstable fracture with multiple bone fragments including the following: • Open segmental fracture regardless of wound size • Gun-shot wounds with bone involvement • Open fractures with any type of neurovascular involvement • Severely contaminated open fractures • Traumatic amputations • Open fractures with delayed treatment (over 8 hours)

ICD-10-CM/PCS Coding

The applicable 7th character extensions for fractures of the shafts of the long bones are as follows:

7th Character	Description
A	Initial encounter for closed fracture
B	Initial encounter for open fracture type I or II
C	Initial encounter for open fracture type IIIA, IIIB, or IIIC
D	Subsequent encounter for closed fracture with routine healing
E	Subsequent encounter for open fracture type I or II with routine healing
F	Subsequent encounter for open fracture type IIIA, IIIB, or IIIC with routine healing
G	Subsequent encounter for closed fracture with delayed healing
H	Subsequent encounter for open fracture type I or II with delayed healing
J	Subsequent encounter for open fracture type IIIA, IIIB, or IIIC with delayed healing
K	Subsequent encounter for closed fracture with nonunion
M	Subsequent encounter for open fracture type I or II with nonunion
N	Subsequent encounter for open fracture type IIIA, IIIB, or IIIC with nonunion
P	Subsequent encounter for closed fracture with malunion
Q	Subsequent encounter for open fracture type I or II with malunion
R	Subsequent encounter for open fracture type IIIA, IIIB, or IIIC with malunion
S	Sequela

Chapter Guidelines

There are detailed guidelines for reporting of injury, poisoning and certain other consequences of external causes. The following topics are covered in the chapter-specific guidelines: application of 7th characters; coding of injuries, traumatic fractures, burns and corrosions; adverse effects, poisoning, underdosing and toxic effects; adult and child abuse, neglect and other maltreatment; and complications of care.

The principles for coding traumatic fractures are the same as coding of other injuries. Applicable 7th characters for fractures have already been discussed. Two additional guidelines of note provide default codes when certain information is not provided. A fracture not indicated as open or closed is coded as closed. A fracture not indicated as displaced or nondisplaced is coded as displaced.

Burns are classified first as corrosion or thermal burns and then by depth and extent. Corrosions are burns due to chemicals. Thermal burns are burns that come from a heat source but exclude sunburns. Examples of heat sources include: fire, hot appliance, electricity, and radiation.

The guidelines are the same for both corrosions and thermal burns with one exception: corrosions require identification of the chemical substance. The chemical substance that caused the corrosion is the first-listed diagnosis and is found in the Table of Drugs and Chemicals. Codes for drugs and chemicals are combination codes that identify the substance and the external cause or intent, so an external cause of injury code is not required. However, external cause codes should be assigned for the place of occurrence, activity, and external cause status when this information is available. The correct code for an accidental corrosion is found in the column for poisoning, accidental (unintentional).

Codes for adverse effects, poisoning, underdosing and toxic effects are combination codes that include both the substance taken and the intent. If the intent of the poisoning is unknown or unspecified, code the intent as accidental intent. The undetermined intent is only for use if the documentation in the record specifies that the intent cannot be determined. No additional external cause code is reported with these codes. Underdosing is defined as taking less of a medication than is prescribed by the provider or the manufacturer's instructions. Underdosing codes are never assigned as the principal or first-listed code. The code for the relapse or exacerbation of the medical condition for which the drug was prescribed is listed as the principal or first-listed code and the underdosing code is listed secondarily. An additional code from subcategories Z91.12- or Z91.13- , Z91.14- should also be assigned to identify the intent of the noncompliance if known. For example, code Z91.120 would be assigned for intentional underdosing due to financial hardship.

Complications of surgical and medical care not elsewhere classified are reported with codes from categories T80-T88. However, intraoperative and post-procedural complications are reported with codes from the body system chapters. For example, ventilator associated pneumonia is considered a procedural or post-procedural complication and is reported with code J95.851 Ventilator associated pneumonia from Chapter 10 – Diseases of the Respiratory System. Complication of care code assignment is based on the provider's documentation of the relationship between the condition and the care or procedure. Not all conditions that occur following medical or surgical treatment are classified as complications. Only conditions for which the provider has documented a cause-and-effect relationship between the care and the complication should be classified as complications of care. If the documentation is unclear, query the provider. Some complications of care codes include the external cause in the code. These codes include the nature of the complication as well as the type of procedure that caused the complication. An additional external cause code indicating the type of procedure is not necessary for these codes.

Pain due to medical devices, implants, or grafts requires two codes, one from the T-codes to identify the device causing the pain, such as T84.84- Pain due to internal orthopedic prosthetic devices, implants, and grafts and one from category G89 to identify acute or chronic pain due to presence of the device, implant, or graft.

Transplant complications are reported with codes from category T86. These codes should be used for both complications and rejection of transplanted organs. A transplant complication code is assigned only when the complication affects the function of the transplanted organ. Two codes are required to describe a transplant complication, one from category T86 and a secondary code that identifies the specific complication. Patients who have undergone a kidney transplant may have some form of chronic kidney disease (CKD) because the transplant may not fully restore kidney function. CKD is not considered to be a transplant complication unless the provider documents a transplant complication such as transplant failure or rejection. If the documentation is unclear, the provider should be queried. Other complications (other than CKD) that affect function of the kidney are assigned a code from subcategory T86.1- Complications of transplanted kidney and a secondary code that identifies the complication.

Chapter 20 – External Causes of Morbidity (V00-Y99)

Codes for external causes of morbidity are found in Chapter 20. External cause codes classify environmental events and other circumstances as the cause of injury and other adverse effects.

Codes in this chapter are always reported as a secondary code with the nature of the condition or injury reported as the first-listed diagnosis. Codes for external causes of morbidity relate to all aspects of external cause coding including: cause, intent, place of occurrence, and activity at the time of the injury or other health condition.

External cause codes are most frequently reported with codes in Chapter 19, Injury, Poisoning and Certain Other Consequences of External Causes (S00-T88). There are conditions in other chapters that may also be due to an external cause. For example, when a condition, such as a myocardial infarction, is specifically stated as due to or precipitated by strenuous activity, such as shoveling snow, then external cause codes should be reported to identify the activity, place and external cause status. As was discussed previously, separate reporting of external cause codes is not necessary for poisoning, adverse effects, or underdosing of drugs and other substances (T36-T50), or for toxic effect of nonmedicinal substances (T51-T65), since the external cause is captured in a combination code from Chapter 19.

External Cause Coding and Third Party Payer Requirements

While not all third party payers require reporting of external cause codes, they are a valuable source of information to public health departments and other state agencies regarding the causes of death, injury, poisoning and adverse effects. In fact, more than half of all states have mandated that hospitals collect external cause data using statewide hospital discharge data systems. Another third of all states routinely collect external cause data even though it is not mandated. There are also 15 states that have mandated statewide hospital emergency department data systems requiring collection of external cause data.

These codes provide a framework for systematically collecting patient health-related information on the external cause of death, injury, poisoning and adverse effects. These codes define the manner of the death or injury, the mechanism, the place of occurrence of the event, the activity, and the status of the person at the time death or injury occurred. Manner refers to whether the cause of death or injury was unintentional/accidental, self-inflicted, assault, or undetermined. Mechanism describes how the injury occurred such as a motor vehicle accident, fall, contact with a sharp object or power tool, or being caught between moving objects. Place identifies where the injury occurred, such as a personal residence, playground, street, or place of employment. Activity indicates the activity of the person at the time the injury occurred such as swimming, running, bathing, or cooking. External cause status is used to indicate the status of the person at the time death or injury occurred such as work done for pay, military activity, or volunteer activity.

7th Characters

Most external cause codes require a 7th character to identify the episode of care. The 7th characters used in Chapter 20 are A, D and S. These external cause codes have the same definitions as they do for most injury codes found in Chapter 19. Initial encounter is defined as the period when the patient is receiving active treatment for the injury, poisoning, or other consequences of an external cause and is reported with 7th character 'A'. Subsequent encounters are identified with 7th character 'D'. This is an encounter after the active phase of treatment and when the patient is receiving routine care for the injury or poisoning during the period of healing or recovery. Sequela is identified by 7th character 'S' which is assigned for complications or conditions that arise as a direct result of an injury.

Chapter Guidelines

As with other chapter guidelines, the guidelines for Chapter 20 External Causes of Morbidity are provided so that there is standardization in the assignment of these codes. External cause codes are always secondary codes, and these codes can be used in any health care setting. An overview of the guidelines is provided here. For the complete guidelines related to external causes, the Official Guidelines for the Code Set should be consulted.

The general external cause coding guidelines relate to all external cause codes including those that describe the cause, the intent, the place of occurrence, the activity of the patient, and the patient's status at the time of the injury. External cause codes may be used with any code in ranges A00.0-T88.9 or Z00-Z99 when the health condition is due to an external cause. The most common health conditions related to external causes are those for injuries in categories S00-T88. It is appropriate to assign external cause codes to infections and diseases in categories A00-R99 and Z00-Z99 that are the result of an external cause, such as a heart attack resulting from strenuous activity.

External cause codes are assigned for the entire length of treatment for the condition resulting from the external cause. The appropriate 7th character must be assigned to identify the encounter as the initial encounter, subsequent encounter, or sequela. For conditions due to an external cause, the full range of external cause codes are used to completely describe the cause, intent, place of occurrence, activity of patient at time of event, and patient's status. No external cause code is required if the external cause and intent are captured by a code from another chapter. For example, codes for poisoning, adverse effect and underdosing of drugs, medicaments, and biological substances in categories T36-T50 and toxic effects of substances chiefly nonmedicinal as to source in categories T51-T65 capture both the external cause and the intent.

When applicable, place of occurrence (Y92), activity (Y93), and external cause status (Y99) codes are sequenced after the main external cause codes. Regardless of the number of external cause codes assigned, there is generally only one place of occurrence code, one activity code, and one external cause status code assigned. However, if a new injury should occur during hospitalization, it is allowable in such rare instances to assign an additional place of occurrence code. Codes from these categories are only assigned at the initial encounter for treatment so these codes do not make use of 7th characters. If the place, activity, or external cause status is not documented, no code is assigned. These codes do not apply to poisonings, adverse effects, misadventures, or sequela.

If the intent (accident, self-harm, assault) of the cause of an injury or other condition is unknown or unspecified, code the intent as accidental. All transport accident categories assume accidental intent. A code for undetermined intent is assigned only when the documentation in the medical record specifies that the intent cannot be determined.

The external cause of sequelae are reported using the code for the external cause with the 7th character extension 'S' for sequela. An external cause code is assigned for any condition described as a late effect or sequela resulting from a previous injury.

Chapter 21 – Factors Influencing Health Status and Contact with Health Services (Z00-Z99)

The codes for factors influencing health and contact with health services represent reasons for encounters. These codes are located in Chapter 21 and the initial alpha character is Z so they are referred to as Z-codes. While code descriptions in Chapter 21, such as Z00.110 Health examination of newborn under 8 days old may appear to be a description of a service or procedure, codes in this chapter are not procedure codes. These codes represent the reason for the encounter, service, or visit. The procedure must be reported with the appropriate procedure code.

Chapter Guidelines

There are extensive chapter-specific coding guidelines for factors influencing health status and contact with health services. The guidelines identify broad categories of Z-codes, such as status Z-codes and history Z-codes. Each of these broad categories contains categories and subcategories of Z-codes for similar types of patient visits/encounters with similar reporting rules. Z-codes may be used in any health care setting and most Z-codes may be either a principal/first-listed or secondary code depending on the circumstances of the encounter. However, certain Z-codes, such as Z02 Encounter for administrative examination, may only be used as a first-listed or principal diagnosis. An overview of the guidelines for the broad categories of Z-codes is provided here. Consult the Official Guidelines for the complete guidelines for Chapter 21.

Contact/Exposure – There are two categories of contact/exposure codes which may be reported as either a first-listed or secondary diagnosis although they are more commonly reported as a secondary diagnosis. Category Z20 indicates contact with, and suspected exposure to communicable diseases. These codes are reported for patients who do not show signs or symptoms of a disease but are suspected to have been exposed to it either by a close personal contact with an infected individual or by currently being in or having been in an area where the disease is epidemic. Category Z77 indicates contact with or suspected exposure to substances that are known to be hazardous to health. Code Z77.22 Exposure to tobacco smoke (second hand smoke) is included in this category.

Inoculations and Vaccinations – Inoculations and vaccinations may also be either the first-listed or a secondary diagnosis. There is a single code Z23 Encounter for immunization for reporting inoculations and vaccinations. A procedure code is required to capture the administration of the immunization of vaccination and to identify the specific immunization/vaccination provided.

Status – Status codes indicate that a patient is either a carrier of a disease or has the sequelae or residual of a past disease or condition. Codes for the presence of prosthetic or mechanical devices resulting from past treatment are categorized as status codes. Status codes should not be confused with history codes which indicate that a patient no longer has the condition. Status codes are not used with diagnosis codes that provide the same information as the status code. For example, code Z94.1 Heart transplant status should not be used with a code from subcategory T86.2- Complications of heart transplant because codes in subcategory T86.2- already identify the patient as a heart transplant recipient.

History (of) – There are two types of history Z-codes, personal and family. Personal history codes explain a patient's past medical condition that no longer exists and is not receiving any treatment, but that has the potential for recurrence, and therefore may require continued monitoring. Family history codes are for use when a patient has a family member who has had a particular disease that causes the patient to be at higher risk of also contracting the disease.

Screening – Screening is testing for disease or disease precursors in seemingly well individuals so that early detection and treatment can be provided for those who test positive for the disease (e.g. screening mammogram). The testing of a person to rule out or confirm a suspected diagnosis because the patient has some sign or symptom is a diagnostic examination not a screening and a sign or symptoms code is used to explain the reason for the visit.

Observation – There are three observation categories (Z03-Z05) for use in very limited circumstances when a person is being observed for a suspected condition that has been ruled out. The observation codes are to be used as principal diagnosis only. The only exception to this is when the principal diagnosis is required to be a code from category Z38, Liveborn infants according to place of birth and type of delivery. Then a code from category Z05, Encounter for observation and evaluation of newborn for suspected diseases and conditions ruled out, is sequenced after the Z38 code. Additional codes may be used in addition to the observation code, but only if they are unrelated to the suspected condition being observed.

Aftercare – Aftercare visit codes cover situations when the initial treatment of a disease has been performed and the patient requires continued care during the healing or recovery phase, or for the long-term consequences of the disease. Aftercare for injuries is not reported with Z-codes. The injury code is reported with the appropriate 7th character for subsequent care. Aftercare Z-codes/categories include Z42-Z49 and Z51. Z51 includes other aftercare and medical care.

Follow-up – The follow-up Z-codes are used to explain continuing surveillance following completed treatment of a disease, condition, or injury. They imply that the condition has been fully treated and no longer exists. Do not confuse follow-up codes with aftercare codes or injury codes with 7th character 'S'. Follow-up Z-codes/categories include: Z08-Z09 and Z39.

Donor – Codes in category Z52 Donors of organs and tissues are used for living individuals who are donating blood or other body tissue. These codes are only for individuals donating for other individuals, not for self-donations. The only exception to this rule is blood donation. There are codes for autologous blood donation in subcategory Z52.01-. Codes in category Z52 are not used to identify cadaveric donations.

Counseling – Counseling Z-codes are used when a patient or family member receives assistance in the aftermath of an illness or injury or when support is required in coping with family or social problems. They are not used in conjunction with a diagnosis code when the counseling component of care is considered integral to standard treatment. Counseling Z-codes/categories include: Z30.0-, Z31.5, Z31.6-, Z32.2-Z32.3, Z69-Z71, and Z76.81.

Encounters for Obstetrical and Reproductive Services – Routine prenatal visits and postpartum care are reported with Z-codes. Codes in category Z34 Encounter for supervision of normal pregnancy are always the first-listed diagnosis and are not to be used with any other code from the OB chapter. Codes in category Z3A Weeks of gestation may be assigned to provide additional information about the pregnancy. Codes in category Z37 Outcome of delivery should be included on all maternal delivery records. Outcome of delivery codes are always secondary codes and are never used on the newborn record. Examples of other conditions reported with Z-codes include family planning, and procreative management and counseling. Codes in category Z3A, Weeks of gestation, may be assigned to provide additional information about the pregnancy. Category Z3A codes should not be assigned for pregnancies with abortive outcomes (categories O00-O08), elective termination of pregnancy (code Z33.32), nor for postpartum conditions, as category Z3A is not applicable to these conditions. The date of the admission should be used to determine weeks of gestation for inpatient admissions that encompass more than one gestational week.

Newborns and Infants – There are a limited number of Z-codes for newborns and infants. Category Z38 Liveborn infants according to place of birth and type of delivery is always the principle diagnosis on the birth record. Subcategory Z00.11- Newborn health examination reports routine examination of the newborn. A 6th character is required that identifies the age of the newborn as under 8 days old (0) or 8-28 days old (1).

Routine and Administrative Examinations – An example of a routine examination is a general check-up. An example of an examination for administrative purposes is a pre-employment physical. These Z-codes are not to be used if the examination is for diagnosis of a suspected condition or for treatment purposes. In such cases the diagnosis code is used. During a routine exam, should a diagnosis or condition be discovered, it should be coded as an additional code. Some of the codes for routine health examinations distinguish between "with" and "without" abnormal findings. An examination with abnormal findings refers to a condition/diagnosis that is newly identified or a change in severity of a chronic condition (such as uncontrolled hypertension, or an acute exacerbation of chronic obstructive pulmonary disease) during a routine physical examination. Code assignment depends on the information that is known at the time the encounter is being coded. For example, if no abnormal findings were found during the examination, but the encounter is being coded before the test results are back, it is acceptable to assign the code for "without abnormal findings" diagnosis. When assigning a code for "with abnormal findings," additional codes should be assigned to identify the specific abnormal findings. Z-codes/categories for routine and administrative examinations include: Z00-Z02 (except Z02.9) and Z32.0-.

Miscellaneous Z-Codes – The miscellaneous Z-codes capture a number of other health care encounters that do not fall into one of the other categories. Certain of these codes identify the reason for the encounter; others are for use as additional codes that provide useful information on circumstances that may affect a patient's care and treatment. Miscellaneous Z-codes/categories are as follows: Z28 (except Z28.3), Z29, Z40-Z41 (except Z41.9) Z53, Z55-Z60, Z62-Z65, Z72-Z75 (except Z74.01 and only when the documentation specifies that the patient has an associated problem), Z76.0, Z76.3, Z76.5, Z91.1-, Z91.83, Z91.84-, and Z91.89.

Chapter 22 – Codes for Special Purposes (U00-U85)

This chapter is for the provisional assignment of new diseases of uncertain etiology or emergency use. Specifically, codes U00-U49 are to be used by WHO for the provisional assignment of new diseases of uncertain etiology or emergency use. Included in Chapter 22 are three codes:

- U07.0 Vaping-related disorder
- U07.1 COVID-19
- U09.9 COVID-19

U07.0 Vaping Related Disorder

The purpose of U07.0 is for coding encounters related to E-cigarette, or vaping, product use. This code has been implemented in response to the recent occurrences of vaping-related disorders. E-cigarettes work by heating a liquid in a pod or cartridge into an aerosol that is inhaled. Base ingredients, such as glycerol (vegetable glycerin) and propylene glycol create the vapor when heated. Other additives like nicotine, artificial flavorings, THC (tetrahydrocannabinol) or CBD (cannabinoid) oil, and vitamin E acetate are combined with the base liquid.

E-cigarette or vaping product use associated lung injury (EVALI) is the name given by the CDC to the dangerous lung disease linked to vaping. Symptoms include cough, shortness of breath, acute respiratory distress, chest pain, fever, stomach pain, diarrhea, nausea, vomiting, and weight loss. Damaging lung effects can be so severe as to stop the lungs from functioning.

Coding Guidance for U07.0

For patients documented with E-cigarette or vaping product use associated lung injury (EVALI), or acute lung injury, without further documentation identifying a specific condition [e.g., pneumonitis, bronchitis], assign only code U07.0. Per tabular instructions, when assigning U07.0, use additional code(s) to identify manifestations, such as:

- abdominal pain (R10.84)
- acute respiratory distress syndrome (J80)
- diarrhea (R19.7)
- drug-induced interstitial lung disorder (J70.4)
- lipoid pneumonia (J69.1)
- weight loss (R63.4)

Lung-related Complications – For patients presenting with lung conditions related to vaping, assign code U07.0 as the principal diagnosis. Assign additional codes for other specified respiratory manifestations, such as:

- J68.0 Bronchitis and pneumonitis due to chemicals, gases, fumes and vapors
- J69.1 Pneumonitis due to inhalation of oils and essences
- J80 Acute respiratory distress syndrome
- J82.8- Pulmonary eosinophilia, not elsewhere classified
- J84.114 Acute interstitial pneumonitis
- J96.0- Acute respiratory failure

Associated respiratory signs and symptoms due to vaping, such as cough, shortness of breath, etc., are not coded separately, when a definitive diagnosis has been established. However, it would be appropriate to code separately any gastrointestinal symptoms, such as diarrhea and abdominal pain.

Poisoning and Toxicity – Acute nicotine exposure can be toxic. Children and adults have been poisoned by swallowing, breathing, or even absorbing e-cigarette liquid through their skin or eyes. For these patients, assign code T65.291- Toxic effect of other nicotine and tobacco, accidental (unintentional). For a patient with acute tetrahydrocannabinol (THC) toxicity, assign code T40.711 Poisoning by cannabis, accidental (unintentional) or code T40.721 Poisoning by synthetic cannabinoids, accidental (unintentional).

Substance Use, Abuse, and Dependence – For patients with documented substance use, abuse, or dependence, additional codes identifying the substance(s) used should be assigned. When the provider documentation refers to use, abuse, and dependence of the same substance (e.g. nicotine, cannabis, etc.) together or interchangeably, only one code should be assigned to identify the pattern of use based on coding guidelines:

- If both use and abuse are documented, assign only the code for abuse
- If both abuse and dependence are documented, assign only the code for dependence
- If use, abuse and dependence are all documented, assign only the code for dependence
- If both use and dependence are documented, assign only the code for dependence

Assign as many codes as appropriate to identify each substance documented. Examples:

- F12.--- Cannabis related disorders
- F17.--- Nicotine related disorders

For vaping of nicotine with dependence, assign code F17.29- Nicotine dependence, other tobacco products since electronic nicotine delivery systems (ENDS) are non-combustible tobacco products.

U07.1 COVID-19

The purpose of U07.1 is for coding encounters related to infections due to SARS-CoV-2, the newly discovered strain of coronavirus emerging in December of 2019 causing the disease responsible for the recent pandemic. The disease it causes is named "coronavirus disease 2019", abbreviated as COVID-19. The disease causes respiratory illness with flu-like symptoms that range from mild to severe illness and death. Severe cases require hospitalization and ventilator assistance. Most patients will recover with supportive care.

Symptoms may appear 2-14 days after exposure and include cough, fever, shortness of breath, or difficulty breathing in serious cases. Older persons and those with an existing medical condition such as heart or lung disease, cancer, or diabetes are at greater risk for developing more serious illness. Emergency warning signs for COVID-19 infection that require immediate medical attention include trouble breathing; continual pain or pressure in the chest; a newly altered mental state such as confusion or the inability to be aroused; and a bluish tint to the lips or face.

Coding Guidance for U07.1

Code only a confirmed diagnosis of the 2019 novel coronavirus disease (COVID-19) as documented by the provider or documentation of a positive COVID-19 test result. For a confirmed diagnosis, assign code U07.1 COVID-19. This is an exception to the hospital inpatient guideline Section II, H. In this context, "confirmation" does not require documentation of a positive test result for COVID-19; the provider's documentation that the individual has COVID-19 is sufficient. If the provider documents "suspected," "possible," "probable," or "inconclusive" COVID-19, do not assign code U07.1. Instead, code the signs and symptoms reported.

Acute Respiratory Illnesses Due to COVID-19 – When the reason for the encounter/admission is a respiratory manifestation of COVID-19, assign U07.1 as the principal or first-listed diagnosis and assign code(s) for the respiratory manifestation(s) as additional diagnoses. The following conditions are examples of common respiratory manifestations of COVID-19:

- Pneumonia: Assign codes U07.1 COVID-19 and J12.82 Pneumonia due to coronavirus disease 2019.
- Acute bronchitis: Assign codes U07.1 and J20.8 Acute bronchitis due to other specified organisms. Note: Bronchitis not otherwise specified (NOS) due to COVID-19 should be coded using code U07.1 and J40 Bronchitis, not specified as acute or chronic.
- Lower respiratory infection: If the COVID-19 is documented as being associated with a lower respiratory infection, not otherwise specified (NOS), or an acute respiratory infection, NOS, assign codes U07.1 and J22 Unspecified acute lower respiratory infection. If the COVID-19 is documented as being associated with a respiratory infection, NOS, assign codes U07.1 and J98.8 Other specified respiratory disorders.

- Acute respiratory distress syndrome (ARDS) due to COVID 19: Assign codes U07.1 and J80 Acute respiratory distress syndrome.
- Acute respiratory failure due to COVID 19: Assign codes U07.1 and J96.0- Acute respiratory failure.

Note: When the reason for the encounter/admission is a non-respiratory manifestation (e.g., viral enteritis) of COVID-19, assign code U07.1 COVID-19 as the principal diagnosis and assign the appropriate code(s) for the non-respiratory manifestation(s) as additional diagnoses.

When COVID-19 meets the definition of principal diagnosis, code U07.1 COVID-19, should be sequenced first, followed by the appropriate codes for associated manifestations, except when another guideline requires that certain codes be sequenced first, such as for obstetric, sepsis, or transplant complications. (*See Section I.C.1.d. Sepsis, Severe Sepsis, and Septic Shock for a COVID-19 infection that progresses to sepsis. See Section I.C.19.g.3.a. Transplant complications other than kidney for a COVID-19 infection in a lung transplant patient.*)

Pregnancy, Childbirth, and Puerperium – When COVID-19 is the reason for the admission or encounter, assign code O98.5- Other viral diseases complicating pregnancy, childbirth and the puerperium, as the principal diagnosis, and code U07.1 COVID-19 along with the appropriate code(s) for any associated manifestation(s) as additional diagnoses. Codes from Chapter 15 always take sequencing priority. (*See Section I.C.15.s. for COVID-19 infection in pregnancy, childbirth, and the puerperium.*)

Newborns – For a newborn that tests positive for COVID-19, assign code U07.1 COVID-19, and the appropriate codes for any associated manifestation(s) in neonates/newborns in the absence of documentation indicating a specific type of transmission. For a newborn that tests positive for COVID-19 and the provider documents the condition was contracted in utero or during the birth process, assign codes P35.8 Other congenital viral diseases, and U07.1 COVID-19. When coding the birth episode in a newborn record, the appropriate code from category Z38 Liveborn infants according to place of birth and type of delivery, should be assigned as the principal diagnosis. (*See Section I.C.16.h. for COVID-19 infection in newborn.*)

Exposure – For asymptomatic individuals with actual or suspected exposure to COVID-19, assign code Z20.822 Contact with and (suspected) exposure to COVID-19. For symptomatic individuals with actual or suspected exposure to COVID-19 and the infection has been ruled out, or test results are inconclusive or unknown, assign code Z20.822 Contact with and (suspected) exposure to COVID-19. (*See Section I.C.21.c.1, Contact/Exposure, for additional guidance regarding the use of category Z20 codes.*)

Screening – During the COVID-19 pandemic, a screening code is generally not appropriate. For encounters for COVID-19 testing, including preoperative testing, code as exposure to COVID-19.

Note: Coding guidance will be updated as new information concerning the pandemic status becomes available.

Signs and Symptoms without Definifitive Diagnosis – For patients who have any signs/symptoms associated with COVID-19, but a definitive diagnosis has not be confirmed, assign the appropriate codes for each of the presenting signs and symptoms, such as:

- R05.1 Acute cough or R05.9 Cough, unspecified
- R06.02 Shortness of breath
- R50.9 Fever, unspecified

If a patient with signs/symptoms associated with COVID-19 also has an actual or suspected contact with or exposure to COVID-19, assign Z20.822.

Asymptomatic Individuals Testing Positive – For patients who are asymptomatic and test positive for COVID-19, assign U07.1. Although the individual is asymptomatic, the person has tested positive and is considered to have the COVID-19 infection.

Personal History – For patients with a history of COVID-19, assign code Z86.16 Personal history of COVID-19.

Follow-Up Visits – For individuals who previously had COVID-19, without residual symptom(s) or condition(s) and are being seen for a follow-up evaluation, when COVID-19 test results are negative, assign codes Z09 Encounter for follow-up examination after completed treatment for conditions other than malignant neoplasm and Z86.16 Personal history of COVID-19.

Encounter for Antibody Testing – For antibody testing that is not being performed to confirm a current COVID-19 infection, nor as a follow-up test after resolution of a previous COVID-19 infection, assign code Z01.84 Encounter for antibody response examination.

Multisystem Inflammatory Syndrome – For individuals with multisystem inflammatory syndrome (MIS) and COVID-19, assign code U07.1 COVID-19 as the principal diagnosis and code M35.81 Multisystem inflammatory syndrome, as an additional diagnosis.

If an individual with a history of COVID-19 develops MIS, assign codes M35.81 Multisystem inflammatory syndrome and U09.9 Post COVID-19 condition, unspecified.

Assign additional code(s) for an associated complications of MIS.

Post COVID-19 Condition – For sequela of a COVID-19 infection, or associated symptoms/conditions that develop following a previous COVID-19 infection, assign a code(s) for the specific symptoms/conditions related to the previous COVID-19 infection, if known, and code U09.9 Post COVID-19 condition, unspecified. Do not use code U09.9 for manifestations of an active (current) COVID-19 infection.

If a patient has a condition(s) associated with a previous COVID-19 infection and develops a new active (current) COVID-19 infection, code U09.9 may be assigned together with code U07.1 to identify that the patient also has a condition(s) associated with a previous COVID-19 infection. Code(s) for the specific condition(s) associated with the previous COVID-19 infection and code(s) for manifestation(s) of the new active (current) COVID-19 infection should also be assigned.

Introduction to ICD-10-PCS

ICD-10-PCS is a procedure coding system used to report inpatient procedures beginning October 1, 2015. As inpatient procedures associated with changing technology and medical advances are developed, the structure of ICD-10-PCS allows them to be easily incorporated as unique codes. This is possible because during the development phase, four attributes were identified as key components for the structure of the coding system – completeness, expandability, multiaxial, and standardized terminology. These components are defined as follows:

Completeness

Completeness refers to the ability to assign a unique code for all substantially different procedures, including unique codes for procedures that can be performed using different approaches.

Expandability

Expandability means the ability to add new unique codes to the coding system in the section and body system where they should reside.

Multiaxial

Multiaxial signifies the ability to assign codes using independent characters around each individual axis or component of the procedure. For example, if a new surgical approach is used for one of the root operations on a specific body part, a value for the new surgical approach can be added to the approach character without a need to add or change other code characters.

Standardized Terminology

ICD-10-PCS includes definitions of the terminology used. While the meaning of specific words varies in common usage, ICD-10-PCS does not include multiple meanings for the same term, and each term is assigned a specific meaning. For example, the term "excision" is defined in most medical dictionaries as surgical removal of part or all of a structure or organ. However, in ICD-10-PCS excision is defined as "cutting out or off, without replacement, a portion of a body part." If all of a body part is surgically removed without replacement, the procedure is defined as 'resection' in ICD-10-PCS.

General Development Principles

In the development of ICD-10-PCS, several general principles were followed:

Diagnostic Information is Not Included in Procedure Description

When procedures are performed for specific diseases or disorders, the disease or disorder is not contained in the procedure code. There are no codes for procedures exclusive to aneurysms, cleft lip, strictures, neoplasms, hernias, etc. The diagnosis codes, not the procedure codes, specify the disease or disorder.

Limited Use of Not Elsewhere Classified (NEC) Option

Because all significant components of a procedure are specified, there is generally no need for an NEC code option. However, limited NEC options are incorporated into ICD-10-PCS where necessary. For example, new devices are frequently developed, and therefore it is necessary to provide an "Other Device" option for use until the new device can be explicitly added to the coding system.

Level of Specificity

All procedures currently performed can be specified in ICD-10-PCS. The frequency with which a procedure is performed was not a consideration in the development of the system. Rather, a unique code is available for variations of a procedure that can be performed.

ICD-10-PCS Structure

ICD-10-PCS has a seven character alphanumeric code structure. Each character contains up to 34 possible values. Each value represents a specific option for the general character definition (e.g., stomach is one of the values for the body part character). The ten digits 0-9 and the 24 letters A-H, J-N and P-Z may be used in each character. The letters O and I are not used in order to avoid confusion with the digits 0 and 1.

Procedures are divided into sections that identify the general type of procedure (e.g., medical and surgical, obstetrics, imaging). The first character of the procedure code always specifies the section. The sections are shown in Table 1.

Table 1: ICD-10-PCS Sections

0	Medical and Surgical
1	Obstetrics
2	Placement
3	Administration
4	Measurement and Monitoring
5	Extracorporeal or Systemic Assistance and Performance
6	Extracorporeal or Systemic Therapies
7	Osteopathic
8	Other Procedures
9	Chiropractic
B	Imaging
C	Nuclear Medicine
D	Radiation Therapy
F	Physical Rehabilitation and Diagnostic Audiology
G	Mental Health
H	Substance Abuse Treatment
X	New Technology

The second through seventh characters mean the same thing within each section, but may mean different things in other sections. In all sections, the third character specifies the general type of procedure performed, or root operation (e.g., resection, transfusion, fluoroscopy), while the other characters give additional information such as the body part and approach. In ICD-10-PCS, the term "procedure" refers to the complete specification of the seven characters.

ICD-10-PCS for Ophthalmology

Ophthalmology procedures are reported with codes from the Medical and Surgical Eye section 080-08X.

ICD-10-PCS Format

The ICD-10-PCS is made up of three separate parts:

- Tables
- Index

The Index allows codes to be located by an alphabetic lookup. The index entry refers to a specific location in the Tables. The Tables must be used in order to construct a complete and valid code.

Tables in ICD-10-PCS

Each page in the Tables is composed of rows that specify the valid combinations of code values. *Table 2* is an excerpt from the ICD-10-PCS tables. In the system, the upper portion of each table specifies the values for the first three characters of the codes in that table. In the administration section, the first three characters are the section, the body system and the root operation.

In ICD-10-PCS, the values 3E0 specify the section Administration (3), the body system Physiological Systems/Anatomical Region (E), and the root operation Introduction (0). As shown in Table 2, the root operation (i.e., introduction) is accompanied by its definition. The lower portion of the table specifies all the valid combinations of the remaining characters four through seven. The four columns in the table specify the last four characters. In the administration section they are labeled Body System, Approach, Substance and Qualifier, respectively. Each row in the table specifies the valid combination of values for characters four through seven. The Tables contain only those combinations of values that result in a valid procedure code.

Table 2: Excerpt from the ICD-10-PCS tables

3 Administration **E Physiological Systems/Anatomical Regions** **0 Introduction: Putting in or on a therapeutic, diagnostic, nutritional, physiological, or prophylactic substance except blood or blood products**			
Character 4	**Character 5**	**Character 6**	**Character 7**
T Peripheral Nerves and Plexi X Cranial Nerves	3 Percutaneous	3 Anti-inflammatory B Anesthetic Agent T Destructive Agent	Z No Qualifier

There are 6 code options for the table above:

3E0T33Z Introduction (injection) anti-inflammatory peripheral nerves and plexi

3E0T3BZ Introduction (injection) local anesthetic peripheral nerves and plexi

3E0T3TZ Introduction (injection) destructive agent peripheral nerves and plexi

3E0X33Z Introduction (injection) anti-inflammatory peripheral cranial nerves

3E0X3BZ Introduction (injection) local anesthetic peripheral nerves and plexi

3E0X3TZ Introduction (injection) destructive agent cranial nerves

ICD-10-CM/PCS Coding

ICD-10-CM Anatomy and Physiology

Eye and Adnexa

Chapter Objectives

After studying this chapter, you should be able to:

- Describe the functions of the following:
  - Eyelid
  - Lacrimal System
  - Orbit
  - Conjunctiva
  - Sclera
  - Cornea
  - Iris
  - Ciliary Body
  - Lens
  - Choroid
  - Retina
  - Vitreous Body
  - Globe
  - Optic Nerve and Visual Pathways
  - Ocular Muscles
- Explain how the optic nerve and visual pathways impact the eyes and their relationship to the nervous system
- Identify infectious diseases of the eye and ocular adnexa
- Identify neoplasms of the eye and ocular adnexa
- Identify other diseases and conditions of the eyes, such as:
  - Cataracts
  - Glaucoma
  - Visual disturbances
  - Blindness
- Identify newborn conditions
- Define congenital anomalies and the impact they have on other organs and body functions
- Describe a variety of diseases and disease processes affecting the eye and ocular adnexa
- Identify how these diseases and disease processes affect and alter eye and ocular adnexa function
- Assign ICD-10-CM to a variety of diseases, injuries, and other conditions affecting the eyes and ocular adnexa

Overview

The eyes are the most complex of the four special sense organs. They are composed of structures that are specifically related to vision as well as accessory structures. The eyeball, optic nerve, and brain are the structures related to vision. Accessory structures include the eyebrows, eyelids, ocular muscles, and lacrimal glands. The cells of the eye that are responsible for vision are typically activated by a stimulus, such as light, in the external environment. When the light is detected, electrical impulses are sent to the visual center and other parts of the brain. In addition to allowing light perception, the eye performs other tasks such as color differentiation and depth perception.

The human eye is divided into three layers: the fibrous tunic, vascular tunic, and retina. These layers perform specific functions and are in turn subdivided into regions or portions that perform even more specific functions.

Fibrous Tunic

The fibrous tunic is also referred to as the sclerotic coat. This is the external layer of the eye. It is divided into two parts, the sclera, also called the white of the eye, and the anterior cornea. Because the fibrous tunic is exposed to the external environment, it is tougher than all other parts of the eye and provides protection to the internal eye.

The sclera includes:

- Episcleral layers
- Schlemm's canal
- Trabecular meshwork

The cornea contains:

- The limbus
- The following layers:
  - Epithelial layer
  - Bowman's layer
  - Stroma layer
  - Descemet's layer
  - Endothelium

Vascular Tunic

The vascular tunic is also referred to as the uvea or choroid coat. This is the middle layer of the eye that is pigmented with melanin. As its name implies this layer provides the eye with its blood supply. It also forms the iris and aides with vision by reducing the reflection of stray light within the eye. Structures contained in the vascular tunic include:

- Choroid
  - Capillary lamina of choroids
  - Bruch's membrane
  - Sattler's layer
- Ciliary body
  - Ciliary processes
  - Ciliary muscle
- Iris
  - Stroma
  - Pupil
  - Iris dilator muscle
  - Iris sphincter muscle

Retina

The retina is the inner layer of the eye, which is composed primarily of nervous tissue. Its primary function is image formation. It is composed of a nervous tissue layer and a pigmented layer. It contains:

- Cells
- Photoreceptor cells – rods, cones, horizontal
- Bipolar cells
- Retinal ganglion cells
- Layers
- Rods and cones
- Retinal pigment epithelium
- Other
- Macula
- Foveola
- Fovea

Eye Segments, Globe and Ocular Adnexa

In addition to the layers of the eye, the eye is divided into anterior and posterior segments. The terms anterior segment and posterior segment are often used by ophthalmologists and are found in coding references. The segments denote specific areas of the eye and include the structures contained in those areas. The structures contained in each segment are listed here and will be described in more detail in the next section. The term globe refers to the entire eyeball excluding the ocular adnexa and includes all the structures that make up the anterior and posterior segments. The ocular adnexa are accessory structures of the eye.

Anterior Segment

The anterior segment includes the following structures:

- Cornea
- Anterior Chamber
- Anterior Sclera
- Iris
- Ciliary Body
- Posterior Chamber
- Lens

The anterior segment also contains the aqueous humor which is the fluid contained in the anterior and posterior chambers.

Posterior Segment

The posterior segment is the segment of the eye behind the iris and includes the following:

- Vitreous body
- Vitreous humor
- Retina
- Choroid
- Posterior Sclera

Ocular Adnexa

The ocular adnexa include the following:

- Extraocular muscles
- Eyelids
- Lacrimal System
- Orbit
- Optic Nerve and Pathways

Eye Anatomy and Function

Conjunctiva

The conjunctiva is a clear, moist mucous membrane, made up of non-keratinizing squamous epithelium. It covers the sclera (the white part of the eye) and lines the inside of the eyelids. It assists in lubricating the eye by producing mucus and tears along with the lacrimal system and also serves to prevent foreign objects and microbes from penetrating into deeper structures of the eye. The part of the conjunctiva that coats the inner aspect of the eyelids is the palpebral conjunctiva; the covering on the outer surface of the eye is the ocular or bulbar conjunctiva.

Sclera

The sclera is the white part of the eye that is the opaque, protective, outer layer, which maintains the shape of the globe. It offers resistance to internal and external forces, provides an attachment for extraocular muscle insertions and is continuous with the dura mater and the cornea.

The sclera contains the following layers:

- Episcleral layer
- Stroma
- Lamina fusca
- Endothelium

Cornea

The cornea is a transparent fibrous coat that covers the front of the eye, including the iris, pupil and anterior chamber. It works with the lens to refract light, accounting for around two-thirds of the eye's optical power. Light is admitted through the cornea to the interior of the eye and light rays are bent so they can be brought to a fixed focus. The lacrimal glands, also called tear glands, keep the surface of the cornea moist and free of foreign bodies, such as dust. The cornea contains five layers:

1. Corneal epithelial layer
2. Bowman's layer
3. Corneal stroma layer
4. Descemet's membrane layer
5. Corneal endothelium layer

Corneal Epithelium Layer

The corneal epithelium layer is a thin multi-cellular tissue layer that is fast growing and easily regenerates. It is made up of non-keratinized stratified squamous epithelium and covers the front of the cornea. It contains several layers of cells, in which the top, exposed layer sheds constantly and the basal layer regenerates cells continuously.

Bowman's Layer

The Bowman's layer (also known as the anterior limiting membrane) is a condensed layer of collagen, which protects the corneal stroma. This durable layer consists of irregular collagen fibers (a type of stroma that assists in maintaining its shape) and lies in front of the corneal epithelium and stroma in the cornea. If the Bowman's membrane is damaged, scarring may occur.

Corneal Stroma Layer

The corneal stroma is a transparent, thick middle layer, containing regularly-arranged collagen fibers along with intermittently distributed interconnected keratocytes that lend to the general repair and maintenance of cells in the cornea.

Descemet's Membrane Layer

The Descemet's membrane layer, also known as the posterior limiting membrane, is a thin, acellular membranous layer that lies between the corneal proper substance and the corneal endothelium. It is the basement layer of the endothelium and is composed of collagen that differs from the stromal layer. Descemet's layer acts as a protective layer against infection and injuries and is easily regenerated after injury.

Corneal Endothelium

The corneal endothelium is a single layer of simple squamous mitochondria-rich cells that are responsible for regulating fluid and solute substance transport between the aqueous and corneal stromal compartments. It sits in aqueous humor and the cells do not regenerate. They stretch to compensate for dead cells, which reduce the overall cell density of the endothelium. It has an impact on fluid regulation that maintains the cornea in a slightly dehydrated state, which is required for optical transparency. If the endothelium cannot manage fluid balance, stromal swelling occurs due to excess fluids and loss of transparency will occur.

Schlemm's Canal and Trabecular Meshwork

Schlemm's canal (also known as the scleral venous sinus) is an endothelium-lined tube in the eye that collects aqueous humor from the anterior chamber and then delivers it to the bloodstream through the anterior ciliary veins.

The inside of the tube is lined with trabecular meshwork, which manages the outflow resistance of the aqueous humor. The trabecular meshwork is positioned at the base of the cornea near the ciliary body and drains the aqueous humor from the eye through the anterior chamber.

Choroid

The choroid is part of the vascular tunic. It is a highly vascular structure composed of capillaries and small arteries and veins that include connective tissue. It lies between the sclera and retina. It provides oxygen and other nutrients to the outer layers of the retina, and together with the ciliary body and the iris, it forms the uveal tract.

The choroid contains melanin (darkly colored pigment), which helps limit uncontrolled reflection within the eye that could result in the perception of mixed-up images.

Ciliary Body

The ciliary body is circumferential tissue composed of ciliary muscle and processes. The striated smooth muscle of the ciliary body controls accommodation, the process by which the eye changes optical power to maintain a clear image (focus) on an object as the distance changes. It also regulates the flow of aqueous humor into Schlemm's canal.

The ciliary body is coated by a double layer of ciliary epithelium, which produces the aqueous humor. The transparent inner layer covers the vitreous body and is continuous from the neural tissue of the retina. The outer layer is greatly pigmented, continuous with the retinal pigment epithelium, and comprises the cells of the dilator muscle in the iris.

Iris

The iris is the colored part of the eye, responsible for controlling the size and diameter of the pupil and the amount of light reaching the retina. For example, when the pupil is larger, more light enters and when it is smaller less light enters. The iris divides the area between the lens and the cornea into an anterior and posterior chamber. The iris consists of two layers: stroma (a fibrovascular tissue) and pigmented epithelial cells. The high pigment content blocks light from passing through the iris to the retina. It is attached to the sclera and the anterior ciliary body; both together are known as the anterior uvea. In front of the iris is the trabecular meshwork where the aqueous humor constantly drains out of the eye. This is the primary location where intraocular pressure is regulated and failure to control intraocular pressure can lead to disease, such as glaucoma. The iris, along with the anterior ciliary body, provides a smaller, secondary passageway for aqueous humor to drain from the eye.

Retina

The retina is a light-sensitive tissue lining that covers approximately 65% of the back inner surface of the eye. Rod and cone photosensitive cells, which are present in the retina, convert light energy into signals that are carried to the brain by the optic nerve. The macula lutea is located in the center of the retina. The macula is the region of the retina that provides the clearest and most distinct vision. Located in the middle of the macula is a small dimple, named the fovea or fovea centralis. It is the center of the eye's sharpest vision and has the most color perception. Conditions that affect the macula, such as macular degeneration, impair central vision affecting the sharpness of an image.

There are two distinct visual systems in the eye: Photopic and scotopic vision. Photopic vision is more sensitive to light, not color sensitive and is made up of rod cells. Scotopic vision is less sensitive to light, color sensitive and is made up of cone cells.

The single type of rod cell supports vision when light is low. These cells are cylindrical in shape and are located on the outer edges of the retina. They are mainly used in peripheral vision and because they require less light to function are also responsible for night vision.

There are three types of cone cells, each of which absorb light from a different portion of the light spectrum. They include:

- 1) Cones that absorb long-wavelength light (reds)
- 2) Cones that absorb middle-wavelength light (greens)
- 3) Cones that absorb short-wavelength light (blues)

Cone cells are a specialized type of neuron (nerve cell) that are responsible for color perception and visual acuity. They function best in bright light and are less sensitive to the light than rod cells. They also allow for the perception of color in finer detail and for faster changes in images than rod cells. The macula, a smaller, central area located in the retina contains the cone cells.

Rod and cone cells have a synaptic terminal, a bulb at the end of an axon (part of a neuron) in which neurotransmitter molecules are stored and released. (For more information on the nervous system, see Chapter 6). The synaptic terminal generates a synapse with another neuron, such as a bipolar cell. Bipolar cells synapse with either rods or cones, but not with both, which indicates they are designated to either one respectively. They transmit signals from the photoreceptors or the horizontal cells and pass these signals on to the ganglion cells (also called the retinal ganglion cell [RGC] found in the ganglion cell layer of the retina. Retinal ganglion cells collectively transmit visual information to the thalamus, hypothalamus and the mesencephalon (also called the midbrain), which are parts of the brain). Retinal ganglion cells all have a long axon that extends to the brain. These axons form the optic nerve, optic chiasm and optic tract, in addition to the retinohypothalamic tract, and contribute to circadian rhythms (sleep cycles) and papillary light reflex (resizing of the pupil).

The retinal ganglion cells are always active, even in the dark. They generate action potentials (a nerve action) and information is conducted back to brain via the optic nerve.

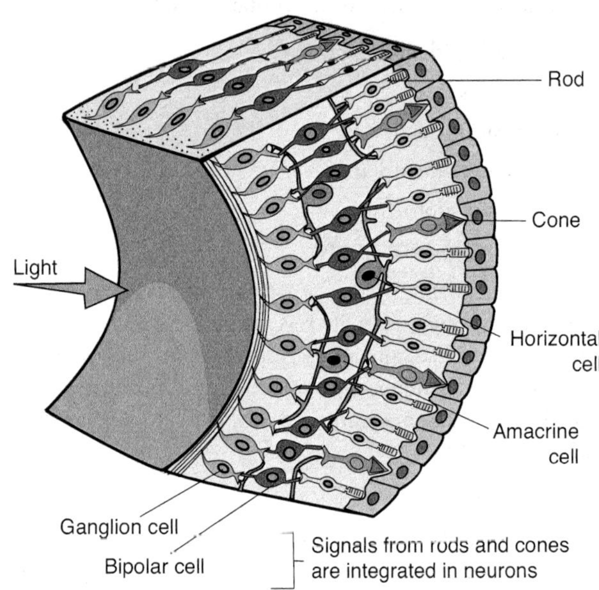

Anterior Chamber

The anterior chamber is a space in the eye filled with aqueous humor and lies between the iris and the cornea's endothelium.

Aqueous Humor

Secreted into the posterior chamber by the non-pigmented epithelium of the ciliary body, the aqueous humor flows through the pupil into the anterior chamber through a narrow cleft between the front of the lens and the back of the iris, through Schlemm's canal and into the anterior ciliary veins.

Its main function is to provide optical power to the cornea, but it also maintains intraocular pressure, shapes the globe, provides nutrients to the avascular optical tissue (e.g., lens, anterior vitreous), carries away waste products from the avascular tissue, and plays a minor role in defense against pathogens.

Posterior Chamber

This chamber is the space behind the iris and in front of the lens and holds aqueous humor for later transport to the anterior chamber.

Lens

The lens is just in front of the iris and is held in place by zonules (ring of fibrous strands), which extend from a circle of muscles. When the lens is relaxed, the lens is flattened (increased diameter); when contracted, the lens becomes more spherical (decreased diameter). This is called curvature of the lens and it enables the eye to adjust its focus between near and far objects.

The size of the pupil's opening is variable and is controlled by the autonomic nervous system. In dim light (or when danger is threatened), the pupil opens wide, allowing more light into the eye. In bright light, the pupil reduces in size and closes down. This reduces the amount of light that enters into the eye but also improves the formation of images.

Eyelids

The eyelids are folds of skin above and below the eye and are made up of skin, tarsal plates, epicanthic folds, meibomian glands, and the palpebral fissure. The eyelids open using the levator palpebrae muscle, either voluntarily or involuntarily, and serve to protect the eye from dust, foreign debris, and to spread tears and other secretions on the eye surface to keep it moist, even when asleep. Also, the blink reflex and eyelashes protect the eyes from foreign bodies.

There are two tarsal plates (tarsi) that are thick, elongated plates of dense connective tissue found in each eyelid. They are directly adjacent to the lid margins and contribute to form and support.

The epicanthic fold (epicanthus) is located on the upper eyelid, from the nasal bone to the inferior side of the eyebrow, and covers the inner corner (medial canthus) of the eye.

The meibomian glands (tarsal glands) are sebaceous glands at the rim of the eyelids inside the tarsal plates. They are responsible for the supply of sebum, an oily substance that prevents evaporation of tear film of the eye, which stops tears spilling onto the cheek. They also make the lids airtight when they are closed and block tear fluid, trapping tears between the oiled edge of the eyelid and the eyeball. There are approximately 50 glands on the upper eyelids and 25 glands on the lower eyelids.

The ciliary glands are tiny sweat glands arranged in rows close to the free margins of the eyelids. The small, narrow openings of the glands lie near the eyelash attachments.

The palpebral fissure is the separation between the upper and lower eyelids.

Globe

The globe of the eye (bulbus oculi) is the eyeball without its appendages (e.g., ocular muscle, optic nerve). It consists of a wall enclosing a cavity filled with fluid. It is surrounded by the socket (orbit) and covered externally by the eyelids.

Lacrimal System

The lacrimal system contains structures for tear production and drainage. It consists of the lacrimal glands, lake, canaliculi, puncta and sac and nasolacrimal duct.

The lacrimal gland secretes tears and with its excretory ducts moves the fluid to the surface of the eye providing both normal amounts on the surface of the eye and extra amounts for tears when the eye is irritated and during crying. The lacrimal lake is a tear pool located in the lower conjunctival cul-de-sac. It drains into the opening of the tear drainage system. The tiny openings on the inner part of each eyelid that tears drain through are the lacrimal puncta. Through the holes, the puncta connect and send tears through the lacrimal canaliculi. The lacrimal canaliculi (ducts) are narrow channels in each eyelid that drain tears from the lacrimal lake to the lacrimal sac. From the lacrimal sac, the nasolacrimal ducts carry tears into the nasal cavity.

Lacrimal system anatomy

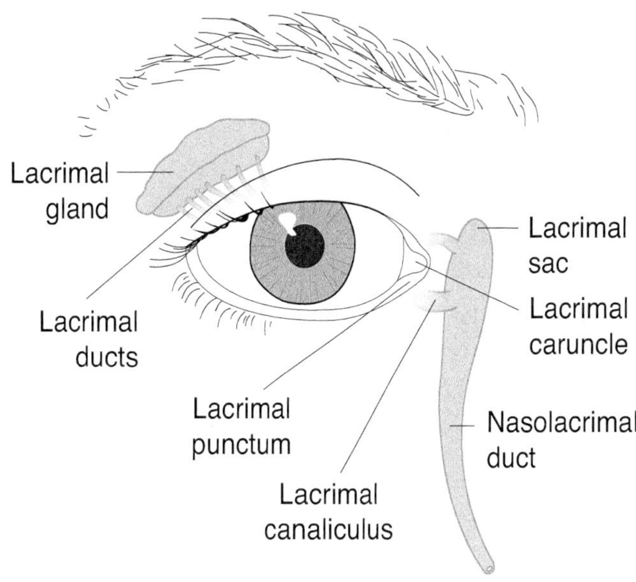

Orbit

The orbit is the socket in the skull in which the eye and its appendages are located. The orbit may mean the bone or the contents of the orbit.

Vitreous Body

The vitreous body—also referred to as vitreous humour (British), vitreous humor (US) or just the vitreous—is the transparent, colorless, gel that fills the space between the lens and the retina. It is produced by specific retinal cells and is of similar composition to the cornea. With very little solid matter, it holds the eye taut. Unlike the aqueous humor, this gel does not get replenished.

The vitreous assists in keeping the retina in place by pressing against the choroids and adhering to the retina in three areas: around the anterior border of the retina, in the macula (tiny spot in the retina), and at the optic nerve.

Optic Nerve and Visual Pathways

The optic nerve, also referred to as cranial nerve (CN) II, transmits visual information from the retina to the brain. It is considered to be a part of the central nervous system and is made up of three meningeal layers: dura, arachnoid, and pia mater. The layers contain retinal ganglion cell axons.

The optic nerve leaves the orbit through the optic canal towards the optic chiasm where it crosses with fibers from the temporal visual fields of both eyes. Most of the axons of the optic nerve terminate in the lateral geniculate nucleus (primary processing center for visual information), which is found inside the thalamus of the brain. The remaining axons terminate in the pretectal nucleus, which is responsible for reflexive eye movements, and the suprachiasmatic nucleus, which is responsible for sleep-wake cycle regulation.

Extraocular Muscles

The extraocular ocular muscles consist of six small, but very strong muscles that are responsible for eye movement. These six muscles turn or rotate the eye about the vertical, horizontal, and antero-posterior axes. Each of the six extraocular muscles is responsible for movement of the center of the eye, which is the pupil, in a specific direction or directions. The muscles and muscle movements are as follows:

Medial rectus: Moves the center of the eye inward toward the nose, also referred to as adduction.

Lateral rectus: Moves the center of the eye outward away from the nose, also referred to as abduction.

Superior rectus: Moves the center of the eye in three directions including:

- Upward movement, also referred to as elevation
- Assists with rotation of the eye inward, also referred to as intorsion
- Assists with movement of the eye inward toward the nose also referred to as adduction

Inferior rectus: Moves the center of the eye in three directions including:

- Downward movement, also referred to as depression
- Assists with rotation of the eye outward away from the nose, also referred to as extortion
- Assists with movement of the eye inward toward the nose, also referred to as adduction

Superior oblique: Moves the center of the eye in three directions including:

- Rotates the top of the eye inward toward the nose, also referred to as intorsion
- Assists with movement of the eye downward, also referred to as depression
- Assists with movement of the eye outward away from the nose, also referred to a extorsion

Inferior oblique: Moves the center of the eye in three directions including:

- Rotates the top of the eye away from the nose, also referred to as extorsion
- Assists with movement of the eye upward, also referred to as elevation
- Assists with movement of the eye outward, also referred to as abduction

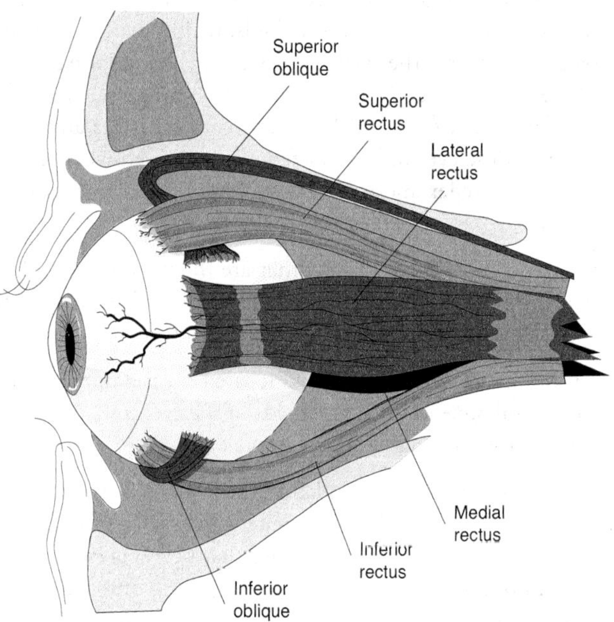

The extraocular muscles are contained within the orbit and, with the exception of the inferior oblique, form a cone around the eye. The apex of the cone is located at the posterior aspect of the orbit with the base of the cone being formed at the attachment of each muscle at the midline of the globe. The apex of the cone is formed by a tendinous ring-like structure called the annulus of Zinn. The optic nerve and ophthalmic artery and vein exit the eye through the annulus of Zinn.

The superior and inferior oblique muscles differ in configuration from other eye muscles. The superior oblique, although part of the cone, must pass through another ring-like tendon called the trochlea at the nasal portion of the orbit before attaching to the posterior aspect (apex) of the cone. The trochlea acts as a pulley for the superior oblique muscle. The inferior oblique does not form part of the cone. It arises from the lacrimal fossa in the nasal portion bony orbit and attaches to the inferior aspect of the eye.

Movement of the eyes is complex because in order to look in a specific direction the muscles of one eye must coordinate with the other. For example in order to look up and to the right, the lateral rectus and superior rectus of the right eye must coordinate with the medial rectus and superior rectus of the left eye. Any lack of coordination or weakness of a specific extraocular muscle can prevent the eyes from moving together which causes vision impairment.

ICD-10-CM Eye and Adnexa Coding Guidelines

In the general guidelines, there is an instruction related to the use of combination codes. ICD-10 has expanded the use of these types of to include additional coding scenarios related to eye and adnexa coding. For example only one code is required to identify diabetic retinopathy, with or without macular edema (E08.3-).

Chapter 7: Diseases of the Eye and Adnexa (H00-H59)
1. Glaucoma b. Assigning Glaucoma Codes Assign as many codes from category H40, Glaucoma, as needed to identify the type of glaucoma, the affected eye, and the glaucoma stage. Assign as many codes from category H40, Glaucoma, as needed to identify the type of glaucoma, the affected eye, and the glaucoma stage.
3. Bilateral glaucoma with same type and stage When a patient has bilateral glaucoma and both eyes are documented as being the same type and stage, and there is a code for bilateral glaucoma, report only the code for the type of glaucoma, bilateral, with the seventh character for the stage. When a patient has bilateral glaucoma and both eyes are documented as being the same type and stage, report as many codes as needed for the type of glaucoma with the appropriate seventh character for the stage And laterality.
4. Bilateral glaucoma stage with different types or stages When a patient has bilateral glaucoma and each eye is documented as having a different type or stage, and the classification distinguishes laterality, assign the appropriate code for each eye rather than the code for bilateral glaucoma. When a patient has bilateral glaucoma and each eye is documented as having a different type, and the classification does not distinguish laterality (i.e. subcategories H40.10, H40.11 and H40.20), assign one code for each type of glaucoma with the appropriate seventh character for the stage. When a patient has bilateral glaucoma and each eye is documented as having the same type, but different stage, and the classification does not distinguish laterality (i.e. subcategories H40.10, H40.11 and H40.20), assign a code for the type of glaucoma for each eye with the seventh character for the specific glaucoma stage documented for each eye.
5. Patient admitted with glaucoma and stage evolves during the admission If a patient is admitted with glaucoma and the stage progresses during the admission, assign the code for highest stage documented.
6. Indeterminate stage glaucoma Assignment of the seventh character "4" for "indeterminate stage" should be based on the clinical documentation. The seventh character "4" is used for glaucomas whose stage cannot be clinically determined. This seventh character should not be confused with the seventh character "0," unspecified, which should be assigned when there is no documentation regarding the stage of the glaucoma.

Documentation Elements of Eye and Adnexa

Key documentation elements for the eye and adnexa include the following:

- Laterality, meaning the side of the body affected, must be documented as right, left, or bilateral for most diseases and conditions located in this section.

Diseases, Disorders, Injuries and Other Conditions of Eye and Adnexa

This section of the chapter looks at a variety of diseases, disorders, injuries, and other conditions involving the eye and adnexa. The information presented in the anatomy and physiology section is expanded here to provide a better understanding regarding the part of the eye or adnexa affected and how these conditions affect function. Specific information is provided for more commonly encountered conditions involving the eye and adnexa.

Following the discussion of the various diseases, disease processes, disorders, injuries, and conditions, some diagnostic statements are provided with examples of coding scenarios. The coding practice is followed by questions to help reinforce the student's knowledge of anatomy, physiology, and coding concepts. Answers to the coding questions can be found by reviewing the text or referring to the coding book.

Answers to all coding practice questions are also provided at the end of the chapter.

Section 1 – Infectious Diseases of the Eye

Eye infections often involve the conjunctiva. Conjunctival infections may also involve other structures in conjunction with the conjunctiva, such as the cornea. In some cases other structures of the eye, such as the retina or iris or the entire eye are involved. When the entire eye is involved, it is called panophthalmitis. Only a few eye infections are reported with codes from *Chapter 1 – Certain Infectious and Parasitic Diseases*. The vast majority of eye infections are reported with codes from *Chapter 7 – Diseases of the Eye and Ocular Adnexa*. Two eye infections that are reported with codes from Chapter 1 are viral conjunctivitis and cytomegalovirus retinitis.

Bacterial Conjunctivitis

There are a number of different types of bacterial conjunctivitis, but the most common are pyogenic (pus-producing) bacteria that cause irritation and grittiness and/or a scratchy feeling and a yellowish or grey stringy, opaque mucopurulent discharge. This discharge causes the eyelids to stick together and crusting to occur around the eye and the surrounding skin. The eye is very red, and on microscopy, there are many white cells and desquamated epithelial cells in the tear duct along the eyelid margin. The more acute pyogenic infections can be painful.

Some bacteria do not cause exudates (discharge) or much redness. Instead there is a gritty and/or scratchy sensation in the eye, similar to having a foreign body in the eye. The tarsal conjunctiva is very red but the inflammation is typically milder than with other types of infections. As with viral conjunctivitis, the inflammation may spread from one eye to the other. Chronic giant papillary conjunctivitis is one type that is common among contact lens wearers.

Follicular Conjunctivitis

Follicular conjunctivitis is identified by lymphoid follicles in the conjunctival stroma. The lymphoid follicles are elevated, having germinal centers that have responded to an infectious agent.

Follicular conjunctival changes are most often associated with viral infections such as adenoviruses and herpes simplex, but may also be associated with chlamydia.

Viral Conjunctivitis

Commonly known as 'pink eye', viral conjunctivitis is typically associated with an infection of the throat or upper respiratory tract or a common cold. An adenovirus is the most common causative agent. Symptoms include tearing and itching, and if it begins in one eye, it may easily be spread to the other eye.

Viral Keratoconjunctivitis

This type of infection impacts both the cornea and the conjunctiva.

Cytomegalovirus (CMV) Retinitis

Caused by the herpes-group of viruses, most people are exposed to CMV during the course of their lifetime, but typically only those with a weakened immune system become ill with the infection, such as patients with:

- AIDS
- Organ transplant
- Bone marrow transplant
- Drugs that suppress the immune system
- Chemotherapy

Some patients with CMV have symptoms of blind spots, blurred vision and other vision problems, and floaters, although many are asymptomatic. The infection usually begins in one eye and eventually spreads to the other eye. If left untreated, progressive damage to the retina may lead to blindness in less than a year. Blindness may also occur if the virus becomes resistant to drug treatment or the patient's immune system further deteriorates. Patients with CMV are at risk of developing retinal detachment and systemic CMV infection may also occur.

Section 1 Coding Practice

Condition	ICD-10-CM
Acute conjunctivitis due to chlamydia	A74.0
Keratoconjunctivitis due to adenovirus type 8	B30.0
Conjunctivitis due to adenovirus	B30.1
Encounter for treatment of bilateral disseminated CMV retinitis in a patient with AIDS	H30.103, B25.8, B20

Section 1 Questions

What are some types of conjunctivitis that are reported with a single code from *Chapter 1 – Certain Infectious and Parasitic Diseases*?

____

____

If the inflammation involves both the conjunctiva and the cornea how is the condition reported?

____

____

What needs to be documented in order to appropriately choose a code to represent unspecified disseminated chorioretinal inflammation?

____

____

See end of chapter for Coding Practice answers.

Section 2 – Neoplasms of the Eye

All parts of the eye may be affected by neoplasms, which may be primary (e.g., rhabdomyosarcoma, retinoblastoma), secondary (metastatic) or benign (e.g., dermoid cyst).

Eyelid Tumors

One of the most common eyelid tumors is basal cell carcinoma. It affects the skin and is slow-growing. It can appear as a skin growth or bump that is pearly, white or light pink, flesh-colored or brown, or as a skin sore that bleeds easily, does not heal, and/or oozes or crusts over, appears scar-like without an injury, has irregular blood vessels in or around the spot, and/or it is sunken in the middle.

Other types of tumors of the eyelid include:

- Squamous carcinoma
- Malignant melanoma

Squamous Carcinoma

Nodular squamous conjunctival carcinoma is a form of squamous carcinoma. It is a nodular type of carcinoma that grows rapidly and is invasive. This type usually extends beneath the conjunctival epithelium, thus has the potential to be metastatic. There may be corkscrew-shaped blood vessels on the surface of the eye.

Melanoma

Melanomas begin in the melanocytes which are cells that product melanin, the pigment responsible for variations in skin color. Melanoma can also develop in other parts of the eye such as the choroid, conjunctiva, lacrimal gland, and retina because these sites also contain melanin-producing cells.

Two main types of melanoma are:

- Lentigo maligna melanoma (LMM) lesions are flat and tan with irregular borders and become increasingly mottled as they grow. This type spreads slowly, stays in the superficial layers and does not metastasize.
- Nodular melanoma (NM) lesions are slightly elevated, blue-black, and resemble blood blisters. This type grows rapidly and is normally fully invasive into other parts of the body.

Intraocular Tumors

The most common primary malignant intraocular tumor in adults is uveal melanoma. This type may occur in the choroid, iris, and ciliary body (ciliary body melanoma). Another type of common cancer is intraocular lymphoma. It is a subtype of primary nervous system lymphoma.

The most common malignant neoplasm of the eye in children is retinoblastoma. It develops rapidly in the cells of the retina and may occur in one or both eyes. Other symptoms are strabismus, white or yellow glow in the pupil, decreasing or loss of vision, and at times, the eye(s) can be painful and red.

Orbital Dermoid Cysts

An orbital dermal cyst is a mass of histologically normal tissue in an abnormal location. These cysts typically form at a suture juncture, most commonly at the fronto-zygomatic suture. Cysts at this site may have pressure effects on the eye muscles and optic nerve, causing diplopia and loss of vision.

Nevus

Benign by definition, nevi are circumscribed malformations not due to external causes and are composed of melanocytes. These types of tumors should be checked on a regular basis to ensure that the nevus has not turned into melanoma.

Giant Choroidal Nevi

Giant choroidal nevi is often confused with melanoma but the characteristics are different and include retinal pigment epithelium atrophy, retinal pigment epithelium hyperplasia, drusen (tiny or white accumulations of extracellular material that build up in the Bruch's membrane of the eye – normal in advancing age), and fibrous metaplasia.

Section 2 Coding Practice

Condition	ICD-10-CM
Eyelid melanoma, left eye	C43.12
Primary lacrimal gland malignancy, left side	C69.52
Primary conjunctiva malignancy, right eye	C69.01
Orbital dermoid cyst, right eye	D31.61
Giant choroidal nevi, left eye	D31.32

Section 2 Questions

Does laterality of the eye make a difference in code selection for neoplasms?

____

____

What term is looked up in the Alphabetic Index for orbital dermoid cyst?

____

____

See end of chapter for Coding Practice answers.

Section 3 – Eyelid Disorders

Entropion and Ectropion

An **entropion** is a turning inward of the eyelid so that the eyelashes rub against the surface of the eye. Typically only the lower eyelids are affected. This can irritate the eye and in severe cases may cause corneal abrasion, ulcer, or scarring. Entropions may be acquired or congenital. Acquired entropions occur most often in the elderly and are caused by spasm or weakening of the muscles of the eyelid. If the condition is due to muscle spasm the turning inward is typically intermittent. Depending on the severity of the problem it may be treated with artificial tears or lubricants. When the condition is due to weakening of the muscles, surgery is required to correct the position of the eyelid.

An **ectropion** is a turning outward of the eyelid, leaving the inner aspect of the eyelid exposed and prone to irritation. All or just a portion of the eyelid may be affected. The condition occurs primarily in the elderly and is due to an weakening of the eyelid muscles. Surgery is required to correct the condition.

Both entropions and ectropions are classified by type as:

- Senile – Age-related entropion
- Mechanical – Caused by fat pad herniation or eyelid lesion
- Spastic – Arising from contracture and spasm orbicularis oculi muscle
- Cicatricial – Caused by scarring of the palpebral conjunctiva

Blepharoptosis and Blepharochalasis

Blepharoptosis, also referred to as ptosis, is a drooping of the eyelid such that the upper eyelid margin partially covers the eye when the eyes are wide open. Ptosis can obstruct the superior visual field. Ptosis is caused by weakening of malfunction of the upper eyelid elevator muscles. These muscles include the levator palpebrae superioris and its aponeurosis and the Mueller muscle. Ptosis is subclassified as:

- Mechanical – Occurs when the weight of the eyelid is too heavy for the eyelid muscles to lift
- Myogenic – Occurs when there is some type of underlying muscle disorder
- Paralytic/Neurogenic – Occurs when there some type of nerve disorder

Ptosis of eyelid

(Drooping of the eyelid)

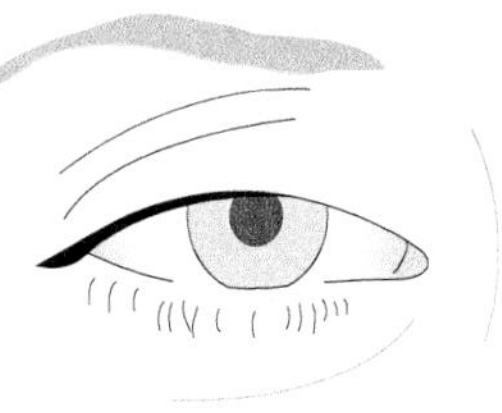

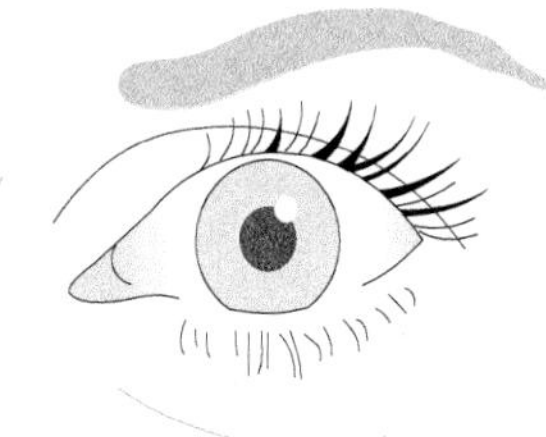

ICD-10-CM Anatomy & Physiology

Blepharochalasis is a rare condition characterized by recurrent episodes of edema of the upper eyelids that causes thinning, stretching and sagging of the skin of the eyelids. The lower eyelids are rarely involved. Episodes of swelling usually begin in adolescence or early adulthood but decrease in frequency and severity with age. During the active stage of the disease there is swelling of one or both eyelids, thinning of the eyelid skin, blepharoptosis or other eyelid malposition. Once the active phase has resolved, sequelae may include:

- Severe thinning of eyelid skin to the point where the iris may be visible through the skin.
- Fine wrinkling of eyelid skin, also referred to as cigarette-paper skin
- Stretched, redundant eyelid skin that may cause visual obstruction
- Subcutaneous dilated capillaries (telangiectasia)
- Pigmentary skin changes also called bronze deposits
- Blepharoptosis with levator aponeurosis dehiscence
- Eyelid malposition including ectropion or entropion
- Acquired horizontal narrowing of the eyelid (blepharophimosis) due to canthal tendon dehiscence
- Medial fat pad atrophy with pseudoepicanthal folds
- Orbital fat prolapse
- Lacrimal gland prolapse

Chalazion

When the meibomian gland (tiny oil gland in the eye) duct is blocked, a chalazion (also called a meibomian cyst) develops. Symptoms include eyelid tenderness or pain, increased tearing, and sensitivity to light. If the meibomian gland becomes infected it is called a hordeolum.

Blepharitis

Blepharitis is an inflammation of the eyelash follicles, along the edge of the eyelid. It is typically caused by seborrheic dermatitis (inflammatory skin condition), rosacea, bacteria, or a combination of these conditions. Other less common causes may be allergies or lice.

In blepharitis, excess oil is produced by the glands of the eyelid. Too much oil causes the normal bacteria on the skin to overgrow. The eyelids get red and irritated, causing skin flakes (scales) to cling to the base of the eyelashes and get crust-infested. Also, they become reddened, itchy, swollen, and burn. Blinking the eye may cause a granular or gritty sensation (e.g., foreign body sensation) and a loss of eyelashes may occur. Blepharitis may be related to repeated styes and chalazia.

There are two main types of blepharitis:

- **Anterior blepharitis** – affecting the outside front of the eyelid where the eyelashes attach
- **Posterior blepharitis** – associated with dysfunction of the meibomian glands of the eyelids

Both types of blepharitis typically occur at the same time, but in different degrees of severity.

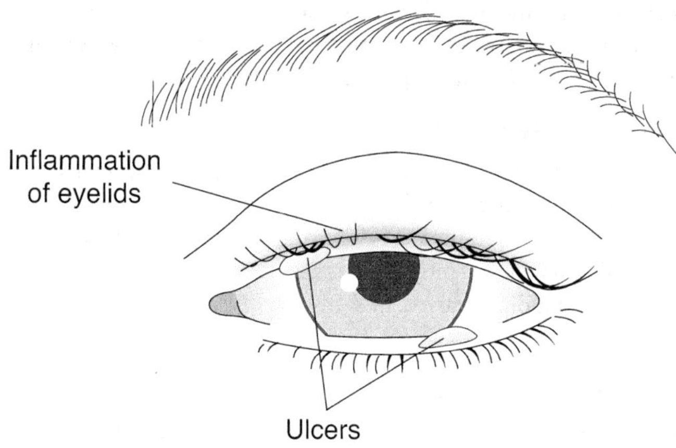

Hordeolum

A hordeolum is a common disorder of the eyelid generally caused by an acute infection, usually staphylococcal. The infection can involve either the meibomian glands, in which case it is known as an internal hordeola or in can involve the glands of Zeis in which case it is called a stye or external hordeola.

Section 3 Coding Practice

Condition	ICD-10-CM
Blepharitis, lower left eyelid	H01.005
Chalazion, right upper eyelid	H00.11
Infected meibomian gland left lower eyelid	H00.025
Senile ectropion left lower lid	H02.135
Neurogenic ptosis right upper lid	H02.431

Section 3 Questions

Why is an internal hordeolum code reported for an infected meibomian gland that is not specified as internal?

In addition to laterality, what else needs to be documented in the medical record to choose the appropriate code for ectropion?

See end of chapter for Coding Practice answers.

Section 4 – Lacrimal System

Conditions affecting the lacrimal system may affect the lacrimal gland, ducts, punctum, canaliculi, sac or nasolacrimal duct. Some common conditions include dacryoadenitis, dacryocystitis, and stenosis or obstruction of the lacrimal passages.

Dacryoadenitis

An inflammation of the tear-producing lacrimal gland, dacryoadenitis, is usually caused by bacteria or a virus, which includes mumps, Epstein-Barr virus, staphylococcus, and gonococcus. Noninfectious chronic dacryoadenitis is typically caused by sarcoidosis, thyroid eye disease, or orbital pseudotumors.

Symptoms include swelling of the outer portion of the upper lid with redness and tenderness, pain, excess tearing and/or discharge and swelling of the lymph nodes by the ear.

Dacryocystitis

This is an inflammation of the lacrimal sac. The lacrimal sac collects tears from the eye and the tears then drain through the nasolacrimal duct. The sac is connected to both the conjunctiva and the nasal mucosa. Bacteria can migrate from either of these sites causing an inflammatory response. Dacryocystitis may be acute, chronic or congenital.

Stenosis and Obstruction Lacrimal Passages

The lacrimal drainage system, which includes the punctum, canaliculi, sac, and nasolacrimal duct may become obstructed or stenosed. This causes a condition called epiphora which is an overflow of tears. Abnormalities in drainage of tears may be due to lacrimal pump malfunction or due to an anatomical obstruction and may be congenital or acquired.

Section 4 Coding Practice

Condition	ICD-10-CM
Chronic dacryoadenitis, right gland	H04.021
Chronic dacryocystitis affecting both eyes	H04.413
Obstruction of right nasolacrimal duct by dacryolith	H04.511
Bilateral obstruction nasolacrimal ducts, newborn	H04.533
Epiphora, left lacrimal gland	H04.202

Section 4 Questions

Is chronic enlargement of the lacrimal gland reported with the same code as chronic dacryoadenitis?

Are the codes for dacryocystitis specific to the lacrimal sac?

Is code H04.533 reported for congenital nasolacrimal duct obstruction?

The codes for epiphora are nonspecific. What additional information is required to assign a more specific code?

See end of chapter for Coding Practice answers.

Section 5 – Conjunctiva

One of the most common conditions affecting the conjunctiva is conjunctivitis. Infectious conjunctivitis has already been covered, but other types including allergic and chemical are discussed here. Other common conditions that affect the conjunctiva include pterygium, adhesions and scars, hemorrhage and vascular disorders.

Conjunctivitis

Conjunctivitis is an inflammation of the conjunctiva that results in redness and irritation of the conjunctiva. There are different types of noninfectious conjunctivitis, including allergic and chemical.

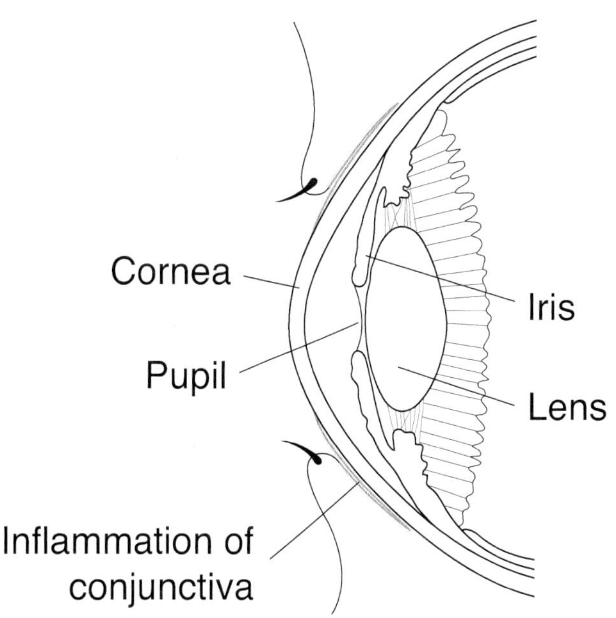

Allergic Conjunctivitis

Allergic conjunctivitis is a reaction to an external factor, such as animals or weeds, with itching, eye swelling, and edema of the conjunctiva. Increased production of tears and redness may also occur. Mast cells release histamine and other substances and blood vessels are stimulated causing dilation, irritation of nerve endings and increased secretion of tears. Atopic (acute attack caused by allergen) and vernal (seasonal allergens) are forms of allergic conjunctivitis.

Chemical Conjunctivitis

Also known as irritant or toxic conjunctivitis, chemical conjunctivitis may be severely painful. There is very little or no discharge or itching. The primary symptom is marked redness.

Depending on the type of chemical in the eye, very little of the eye may be affected with a splash injury and the inflammation maybe present only in the conjunctival sac. With caustic alkalis, necrosis of the conjunctiva may occur and a white eye is apparent (due to vascular closure), followed by the sloughing of dead epithelium.

Pterygium

A pterygium is an abnormal overgrowth of fibrovascular tissue that is continuous with the conjunctival tissue and extends into the cornea. The overgrowth of tissue may occur on either side of the eye but is more common on the nasal side. When a pterygium is present on both sides of the eye (nasal and temporal), it is called a double pterygium. Pterygia vary in size from small, slow-growing lesions that do not cause vision deficits to large rapidly growing lesions that distort the cornea causing irregular astigmatism. Amyloid is a protein that is deposited in some tissues as part of some disease processes. An amyloid pterygium is one with deposition of amyloid proteins in the growth. A central pterygium is one that extends over the center of the cornea. Peripheral pterygia are those that do not extend into the center of the cornea.

Section 5 Coding Practice

Condition	ICD-10-CM
Acute atopic conjunctivitis, bilateral	H10.13
Acute conjunctivitis due to cleaning solution splashed in both eyes	T52.91XA, H10.213
Acute conjunctivitis, left eye	H10.32
Simple conjunctivitis, right eye	H10.422

Section 5 Questions

For chemical or toxic conjunctivitis, does the episode of care need to be documented in the medical record before choosing a code?

____

____

Are two codes assigned for acute and chronic conjunctivitis occurring together?

____

____

See end of chapter for Coding Practice answers.

Section 6 – Sclera, Cornea, Iris, and Ciliary Body

The sclera, cornea, iris and ciliary body are structures in the anterior chamber of the eye. Conditions affecting the sclera include scleritis, episcleritis, and staphyloma. The cornea is subject to inflammatory conditions that such as corneal ulcer, keratitis, and keratoconjunctivitis; corneal neovascularization; corneal scars, opacities, pigmentations, and deposits as well as other conditions. Conditions affecting the iris and ciliary body include inflammatory conditions such as iritis, iridocyclitis, or cyclitis, cysts, and adhesions of the iris and ciliary body.

Scleritis and Episcleritis

Scleritis is an inflammation of the sclera. There are a number of different types. Anterior scleritis is inflammation of the sclera adjacent to the cornea. Brawny scleritis is a gelatinous-appearing inflammation surrounding the cornea that sometimes also involves the periphery of the cornea. Posterior scleritis is an inflammation of the sclera adjacent to the optic nerve that may extend into the retina and choroid.

Episcleritis is an inflammation of the thin layer of tissue that lies between conjunctiva and sclera. It is typically a mild, self-limiting condition localized to the superficial episcleral vascular network. There are two types of episcleritis, simple and nodular. Simple episcleritis, also referred to as episcleritis periodica fugax, is characterized by intermittent periods of diffuse moderate-to-severe inflammation occurring at 1 to 3 month periods. The episodes usually last 7-10 days. Nodular episcleritis is characterized by localized areas of inflammation of the episcleral tissues.

Staphyloma

A staphyloma is a bulging of the sclera or cornea containing uveal tissue. An anterior staphyloma is a bulging near the anterior pole of the eyeball. An equatorial staphyloma occurs near the area where the vortex veins exit. A posticum staphyloma is one near the posterior pole of the eyeball that is caused by degenerative changes in severe myopia.

Keratoconjunctivitis and Keratitis

Inflammation of the cornea may occur without involvement of the conjunctiva in which case it is referred to as keratitis or it may occur with inflammation of the conjunctiva in which case it is referred to a keratoconjunctivitis.

Keratoconjunctivitis

Inflammation of the cornea and conjunctiva is subdivided by type and/or cause which include:

Exposure keratoconjunctivitis – Inflammation caused by irritation of the cornea and conjunctiva due to the inability to completely close the eyelids.

Keratoconjunctivitis sicca – This type of inflammation is caused by insufficient tear production.

Neurotropic keratoconjunctivitis – This is an inflammation that occurs following administration of local anesthetic to the cornea and conjunctiva.

Phlyctenular keratoconjunctivitis – Inflammation with formation of small red nodules of lymphoid tissue near the corneoscleral limbus.

Vernal keratoconjunctivitis – This is a chronic inflammation that typically affects both eyes. It is often seasonal in nature occurring during warm weather. The bulbar form affects both the conjunctiva and cornea and is characterized by sensitivity to light, intense itching, and the presence of gelatinous nodules adjacent to the corneoscleral limbus.

Keratitis

Keratitis is an inflammation of the cornea in which intense pain and some impaired vision is experienced. Keratitis is typically subdivided into superficial keratitis and deep keratitis. Superficial keratitis involves the superficial layers of the cornea and typically does not cause corneal scarring. In contrast, deep keratitis, also referred to as keratitis profunda, involves the corneal stroma which is the connective tissue of the cornea. Types of superficial keratitis include:

Filamentary keratitis – Keratitis with twisted filaments of mucoid material on the surface of the cornea.

Photokeratitis (exposure keratitis) – Painful, inflamed cornea that develops due to over-exposure to ultraviolet lights.

Punctate keratitis – Inflammation that occurs with the death of cells on the surface of the cornea, which causes fiber-like deposits to form.

Types of deep keratitis include:

Diffuse interstitial keratitis – Diffuse inflammation of the corneal stroma that may be accompanied by neovascularization.

Sclerosing keratitis – Inflammation of the cornea and sclera with opacification of the corneal stroma.

Keratitis is commonly caused by bacteria (e.g., Staphylococcus aureus; improper contact care; extended contact wearing), viruses (e.g., herpes simplex (cold sores) secondary to an upper respiratory infection), exposure to ultraviolet lights or other intense lights, vitamin A deficiency, foreign bodies or chemicals in the eye, and allergens.

Symptoms of keratitis are painful and watery eyes, blurred vision, sensitivity to light, and vasculature, and for herpes simplex keratitis, a small white spot is apparent on the cornea.

Corneal Ulcers

A corneal ulcer is an open sore on the cornea, involving disruption of its epithelial layer with involvement of the corneal stroma.

Corneal ulcers are frequently caused by an infection in the eye due to:

- bacteria – e.g., improper contact lens care, extended contact lens wearing
- viruses – e.g., herpes simplex (cold sores), varicella (chicken pox, shingles)
- fungi – e.g., improper contact lens care, overuse of eye drops containing steroids
- a protozoan – e.g., Acanthamoeba

Other less common causes are:

- scratches (abrasions) – e.g., caused by trauma, chemical burns
- foreign bodies
- inadequate eye closure – e.g., Bell's palsy
- severely dry eyes – leaves eyes without germ-fighting tears
- severely allergic eyes

Symptoms of corneal ulcers are red eye, pain, foreign body sensation, tearing, pus or thick discharge from the eye, blurry vision, swollen eyelids, and/or a white or gray round spot on the cornea that is visible.

Corneal Neovascularization

The normal, healthy cornea is transparent and avascular, that is it does not contain blood vessels. However, when the cornea becomes diseased or injured, new blood vessels may grow into the cornea from the limbus. Conditions that can cause neovascularization include infection, immunological conditions, traumatic injury, corrosion burn, and even contact lenses. These conditions cause oxygen deprivation of the cornea. The body tries to compensate for the reduced amount of oxygen reaching the cornea by creating new blood vessels. Neovascularization may not produce any symptoms or individuals may experience eye pain, excessive tearing, light sensitivity, redness, intolerance to contact lenses, and decreased vision.

Iritis, Iridocyclitis, and Cyclitis

These inflammatory conditions may be acute or chronic. Acute conditions are classified as primary, recurrent, secondary infectious or noninfectious, and inflammation associated with hypopyon which is a condition in which there is an accumulation of pus in the anterior chamber of the eye. One type of chronic iridocyclitis is called lens-induced which is associated with the presence of an intraocular lens.

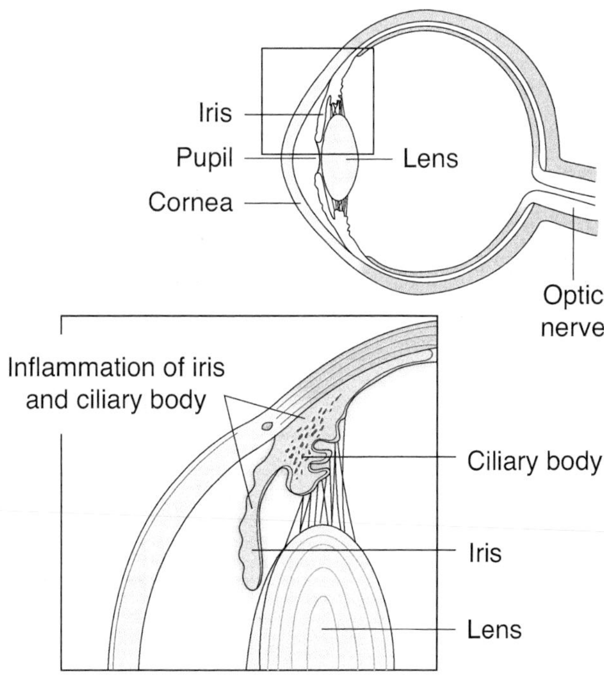

Cysts

Cysts may form in the iris or ciliary body. The most common type is a neuroepithelial iris cyst located at the root of the iris. Most cysts are located behind the iris and cause no symptoms. They are found on ophthalmological examination and typically appear as a bulge in the iris stroma. While most cysts do not require treatment, the physician must do further diagnostic studies to ensure that the bulge is not due to a tumor that would require removal. Other types of cysts that would require treatment are exudative and parasitic cysts. A definitive diagnosis can usually be made using an ultrasound study of the eye.

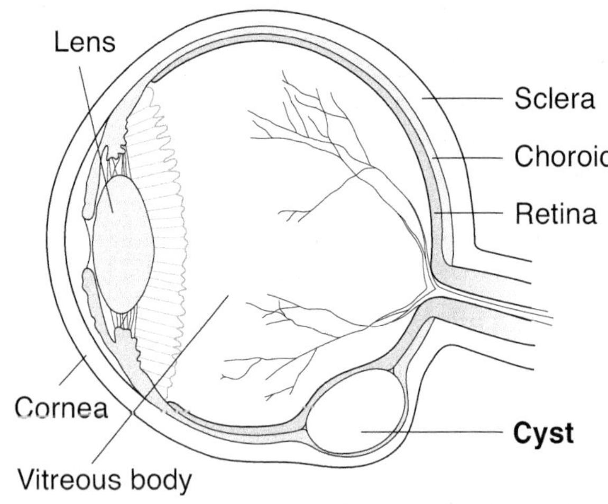

Synechiae and Goniosynechiae

Synechiae is another term for adhesion. Anterior synechiae are adhesions of the iris to the cornea. Posterior synechiae are adhesions of the iris to the lens capsule, and goniosynechiae are adhesions of the iris to the posterior surface of the cornea at the angle of the anterior chamber. Synechiae typically result from an infection or other disease process of the eye such as glaucoma or cataracts, or they may be a complication

Section 6 Coding Practice

Condition	ICD-10-CM
Filamentary keratitis, right eye	H16.121
Photokeratitis, left eye	H16.132
Punctate keratitis, right eye	H16.141
Superficial keratitis, left eye	H16.102
Central corneal ulcer, left eye	H16.012
Nodular episcleritis, right eye	H15.121
Bilateral vernal conjunctivitis with limbar and corneal involvement	H16.263
Corneal ghost vessels, right eye	H16.411
Chronic iridocyclitis, left eye	H20.12
Miotic pupillary, right eye	H21.271

Section 6 Questions

What type of keratitis in the coding practice above is not listed as a term under keratitis in the Alphabetic Index?

Does the type or site of the corneal ulcer affect code selection?

Are two codes required to report vernal conjunctivitis with limbar and corneal involvement?

What type of condition are corneal ghost vessels?

There is an excludes note for posterior cyclitis under H20.1- Chronic iridocyclitis. Does this mean that posterior cyclitis cannot be reported with chronic iridocyclitis?

Why is a neuroepithelial cyst reported with the code for idiopathic cyst?

See end of chapter for Coding Practice answers.

Section 7 – Lens

The lens of the eye is primarily affected by a single very common condition, cataracts. Other less common conditions that affect the lens include congenital or acquired aphakia which is the absence of the lens and dislocation of the lens a condition usually resulting from trauma to the eye.

Cataracts

In cataracts, there is partial or complete clouding on or in the lens or lens capsule of the eye, which may obscure vision. There are many different types of cataracts, ranging from infantile to senile.

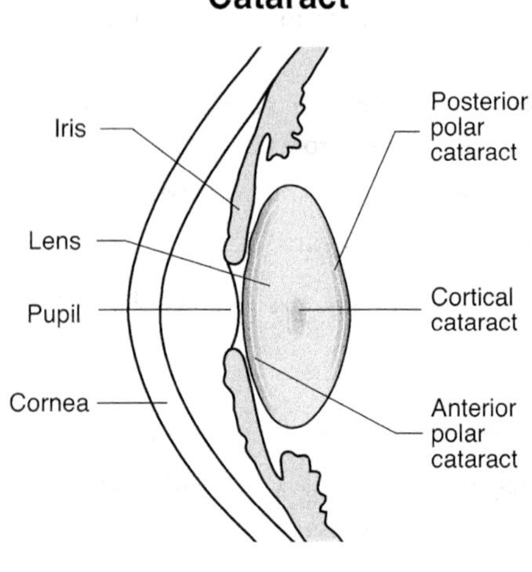

Infantile and Juvenile Cataracts

Infantile and juvenile cataracts occur early in life. Often the term infantile cataract is used interchangeably with congenital cataract. However, for disease classification purposes, the two are not the same. Congenital cataracts are present at birth, but may not be diagnosed until later in life. Infantile cataracts present early in life, but are not present at birth. Symptoms of infantile cataracts are nystagmus (unusual rapid eye movements) and, if cataracts are present in both eyes, failure of the infant to show visual awareness of what is around him.

Diseases and conditions that may cause or are associated with congenital cataracts include:

- Chondrodysplasia syndrome
- Conradi syndrome
- Down syndrome
- Ectodermal dysplasia
- Galactosemia
- Lowe syndrome
- Pierre-Robin syndrome
- Trisomy 13

Cataracts with Neovascularization

Neovascularization of the iris, termed rubeosis, is an abnormal blood vessel growth in the front of the eye. Many patients who have diabetes or an occluded vein are more susceptible to neovascularization and eventually, cataracts. The formation of the abnormal vessels can obstruct the drainage of aqueous fluid from the front of the eye, causing eye pressure to become elevated. This typically leads to neovascular glaucoma.

Cataracts in Inflammatory Disorders and Degenerative Diseases

Cataracts can be caused by an underlying inflammatory disorder, such as choroiditis, or a degenerative disease, such as degenerative myopia.

Drug-Induced Cataract

A drug-induced cataract is defined as one that has been induced by exposure to a drug, such as oral, topical, or inhaled steroids, or others that have been associated with cataracts to a lesser degree, including the long-term use of statins and phenothiazines.

Section 7 Coding Practice

Condition	ICD-10-CM
Anterior, subcapsular polar infantile cataract, left eye	H26.042
Congenital cataract	Q12.0
Infant & juvenile nuclear cataract, left eye	H26.032
Cataracts with neovascularization, right eye	H26.211
Cataract in chronic choroiditis, left eye	H26.222, H30.92
Myotonic cataract	G71.19, H28
Diabetic cataract, right eye	E11.36
Corticosteroid-induced cataract, right and left eyes	H26.33 ,T38.0X5S

Section 7 Questions

Presenile is not included in the code description for category H26. How is a presenile cataract coded?

____

____

How are cataracts that are secondary to inflammatory or degenerative disorders reported?

____

____

When reporting cataracts that are secondary to inflammatory or degenerative disorders, the associated disorder is also reported? How is the cataract code sequenced?

____

____

Why is the diabetic cataract in the coding practice reported with a code for type II diabetes when the diabetes is not identified as type II?

____

____

Is it a requirement to indicate the drug or toxin when coding a drug induced cataract?

____

____

See end of chapter for Coding Practice answers.

Section 8 – Choroid and Retina

Section 8a – Retinal Detachments

In retinal detachments, the retina is pulled or lifted away from its normal position. It may be a result of a retinal break, hole or tear, caused by injury or trauma, or occur in patients who are predisposed for this condition, such as ones with severe myopia (near-sightedness), after cataract surgery, and/or patients with proliferative diabetic retinopathy. If not treated immediately, this disorder can cause permanent vision loss.

Retinal breaks may occur when the vitreous gel separates from its attachments to the retina, typically in the peripheral parts of the retina. The separation sometimes exerts traction on the retina, and if the retina is weak, it will tear. The vitreous gel then can seep through the tear and build up behind the retina, which can cause the retina to separate from its point of attachment, resulting in detachment.

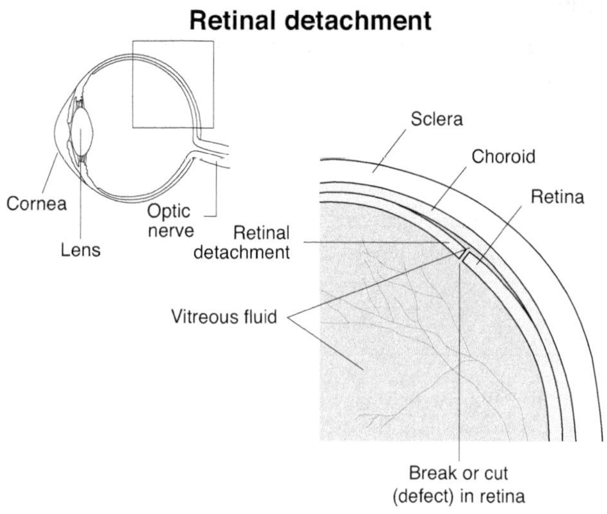

There are three main types of retinal detachments:

1. **Rhegmatogenous retinal detachment** – occurs due to a break, hole or tear in the retina that allows vitreous gel to pass from the vitreous space into the subretinal space between the sensory retina and the retinal pigment epithelium.
2. **Exudative, serous or secondary retinal detachment** – occurs due to inflammation, injury or vascular abnormalities that results in fluid accumulating underneath the retina without the presence of a hole, tear or break.
3. **Tractional retinal detachment** – occurs when fibrovascular tissue, caused by inflammation, injury or neovascularization, pulls the sensory retina from the retina pigment epithelium.

Section 8a Coding Practice

Condition	ICD-10-CM
Retinal detachment, right eye, with single break	H33.011
Horseshoe tear of left retina	H33.312
Total retinal detachment, right eye	H33.051
Subtotal retinal detachment, right eye	H33.8

Section 8a Questions

Is the term "partial" used in the descriptor of retinal detachments?

Is a horseshoe tear a type of retinal detachment? If not, how is it categorized?

Why is a subtotal retinal detachment reported with an "other specified" code?

See end of chapter for Coding Practice answers.

Section 8b – Macular Degeneration

One of the more common diseases of the macula is macular degeneration. Macular degeneration may be an acquired or hereditary eye disease. Age-related macular degeneration (ARMD) is an acquired type and the leading cause of blindness in the elderly. Hereditary types are seen in children and teenagers and are much less common than ARMD. Hereditary forms include Best's disease, Stargardt's disease, Sorsby's disease as well as others.

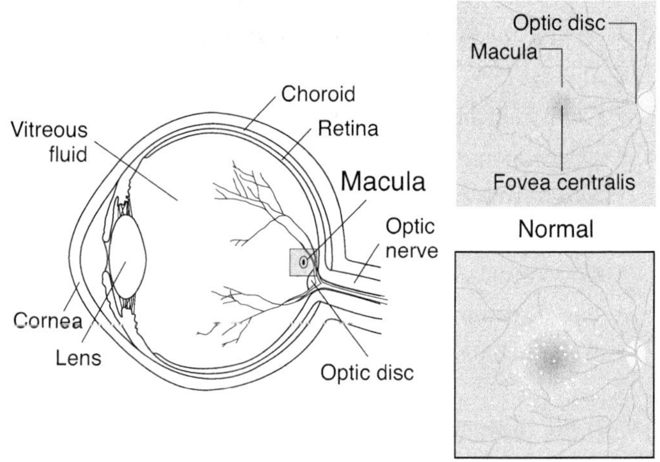

ARMD

There are two types of ARMD, dry and wet. Dry macular degeneration is due to thinning of the layers of the macular which causes gradual vision loss with tiny fragile blood vessels under the macula. Wet macular degeneration results when the tiny fragile blood vessels rupture causing hemorrhage. Blood and fluid that accumulates in the macula causes scarring and damage and vision loss may be rapid. Damaged macular tissue cannot be repaired. The first symptom of macular degeneration is usually blurred vision followed by distorted vision as more macular tissue is destroyed. For example, straight lines appear crooked. Eventually a small area of central vision may be completely destroyed. As damage to the macula progresses complete loss of central vision occurs; however, peripheral vision remains intact.

Hereditary Macular Degeneration

Best's disease, also referred to as vitelliform macular dystrophy, is an autosomal dominant disorder that typically presents in childhood. Examination of the eyes reveals macular lesions with a yellow or orange yolk-like appearance.

Stargardt's disease, also referred to as fundus flavimaculatus, is the most common form of inherited juvenile macular degeneration. It is an autosomal recessive disorder that results in a severe form of macular degeneration with characteristics similar to ARMD.

Sorsby's disease, also referred to as Sorsby's fundus dystrophy, is a rare inherited type of macular degeneration. Vision loss usually begins between ages 30 to 40. Individuals with this type of macular disease develop new choroidal blood vessels that can rupture causing wet macular degeneration similar to that seen in ARMD.

Section 8b Coding Practice

Condition	ICD-10-CM
Bilateral age-related wet macular degeneration, w/inactive scar	H35.32X3
Congenital macular degeneration	H35.53
Cystoid macular degeneration, left eye	H35.352

Section 8b Questions

What main term is congenital macular degeneration listed under in the Alphabetic Index?

What is the medical term for wet macular degeneration?

Which diagnosis above requires documentation of laterality to assign the most specific code?

See end of chapter for Coding Practice answers.

Section 9 – Glaucoma

Glaucoma is actually a group of diseases of the eyes characterized by damage of the optic nerve. The optic nerve damage is usually, but not always, caused by a dangerous increase in intraocular pressure (IOP), leading to progressive, irreversible loss of vision. This nerve damage entails loss of retinal ganglion cells in a pattern and is considered a type of optic neuropathy, which can lead to permanent damage to the optic nerve, loss of peripheral vision, and eventually, blindness.

There are many types of glaucoma, some that are chronic and some that are acute and require immediate and urgent care. Two of the more common forms of glaucoma are:

- Open-angle glaucoma
- Closed-angle glaucoma

Open-Angle Glaucoma

This type of glaucoma is chronic and tends to progress more slowly than closed angle glaucoma. There is an imbalance in the production and drainage of aqueous humor in the anterior chamber. Either too much is produced by the ciliary body or the trabecular meshwork in the anterior chamber is blocked and intraocular pressure increases. In most cases, the patient does not become symptomatic before the disease has progressed to a point where it is irreversible. Included in this type is primary open-angle glaucoma (POAG) which is the most common form of glaucoma.

Open-angle glaucoma

An increase in fluid pressure in the eye resulting from the outflow of ocular fluid being blocked

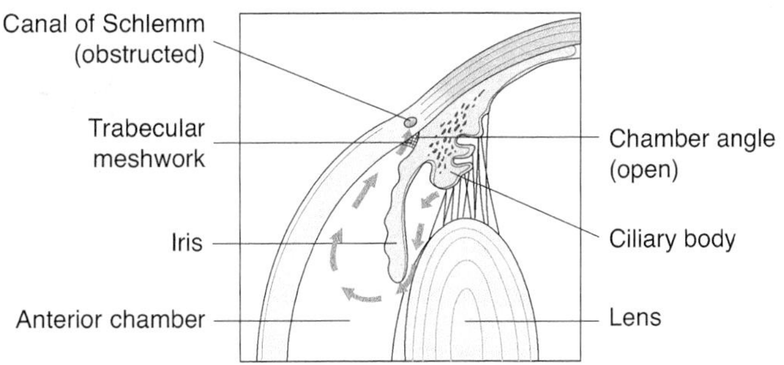

Normal-Tension Glaucoma

This type is an open-angle glaucoma, also called normal-pressure glaucoma, low-tension glaucoma or low-pressure glaucoma. Similar to POAG, normal-tension glaucoma may cause optic nerve damage and visual field loss, but the IOP remains in the normal range. Pain typically does not occur and permanent damage is not noticed until symptoms such as tunnel vision arise.

Closed-Angle Glaucoma

Closed angle glaucoma may appear rather quickly and is often painful. Symptoms include blurry vision, halos around lights, intense eye pain, dilated pupils, nausea and vomiting. This may be caught more quickly, before permanent damage of the optic nerve occurs. Narrow-angle glaucoma is included in the subcategory closed angle, also called angle-closure glaucoma.

Infantile Glaucoma

Infantile glaucoma, also known as congenital glaucoma, is present at birth, and is almost always diagnosed before the age of one. Most infants with this type of glaucoma are either born with narrow angle or with a defect in the drainage system of the eye.

Glaucoma described as childhood, infantile, juvenile, or congenital are all reported as congenital glaucoma with a code from *Chapter 17 – Congenital Malformations, Deformations, and Chromosomal Abnormalities*

Phacolytic Glaucoma

In phacolytic glaucoma, there is leakage of lens protein from a mature cataract into the aqueous fluid, blocking fluid outflow and causing pressure buildup.

Glaucoma Associated with Other Eye Conditions

Other diseases or conditions of the eye may cause glaucoma, such as chamber angle, iris, and other anterior segment anomalies. Others causes include vascular disorders, tumors, and cysts.

Secondary Glaucoma

Secondary glaucoma may develop in the presence of an eye infection, eye inflammation, tumor, enlarged cataract, or eye injury. In addition, secondary glaucoma is seen in advanced cases of cataracts or diabetes and may also be caused by drugs, such as steroids.

Pseudoexfoliative Glaucoma

This secondary type of glaucoma is where a flaky material peels off the outer layer of the lens within the eye. The material gathers in the angle between the cornea and the iris and may clog the drainage system of the eye, causing eye pressure to rise.

Section 9 Coding Practice

Condition	ICD-10-CM
Open-angle mild glaucoma, unspecified, right eye	H40.10X0
Primary mild open-angle glaucoma, right eye	H40.11X1
Acute angle-closure glaucoma, left eye	H40.212
Chronic severe angle-closure glaucoma, left eye	H40.2223
Intermittent angle-closure glaucoma, left eye	H40.232
Residual stage of angle-closure glaucoma, left eye	H40.242
Childhood glaucoma, right eye	Q15.0
Secondary vascular glaucoma, right eye	H40.89
Moderate pseudoexfoliation glaucoma, left eye	H40.1422
Corticosteroid-induced glaucoma, glaucomatous stage, right eye	H40.61X0 T38.0X5S
Corticosteroid-induced glaucoma, residual stage, right eye	H40.61X0 T38.0X5S

Section 9 Questions

When coding unspecified or primary open-angle glaucoma, does laterality affect code selection?

What are some examples of different types of primary angle-closure glaucoma?

Does Glaucoma associated with vascular disorders have a specific code.

Can steroid-induced glaucoma be reported with a single code?

See end of chapter for Coding Practice answers.

Section 10 – Vitreous Body and Globe

Conditions that affect the vitreous body include prolapse, hemorrhage, opacities, and degeneration. Conditions affecting the globe affect multiple structures of the eye, such as inflammation, degenerative conditions, and retained foreign bodies.

Vitreous Hemorrhage

The vitreous of the eye is normally a clear jelly-like fluid that fills the cavity behind the lens. A number of conditions can cause hemorrhage or bleeding into this cavity which is referred to as a vitreous hemorrhage. Vitreous hemorrhage causes a sudden loss of vision caused by blood blocking light perception which must be transmitted through the vitreous to the retina. Vitreous hemorrhage is associated with an aneurysm of a blood vessel in the eye, trauma, retinal tear, retinal detachment, neovascularization, as well as other conditions.

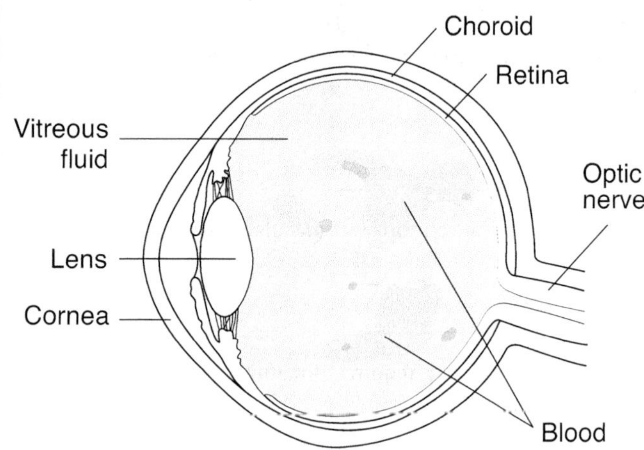

Endophthalmitis

Endophthalmitis is an inflammatory condition within the intraocular cavities affecting the aqueous or vitreous humor. It is typically caused by bacteria, fungi, or other microorganisms or may be a complication of eye surgery, such as when there is a part of the natural lens that is retained in the eye following cataract surgery. Symptoms include pain, swelling of the eyelids, redness, and decreased vision.

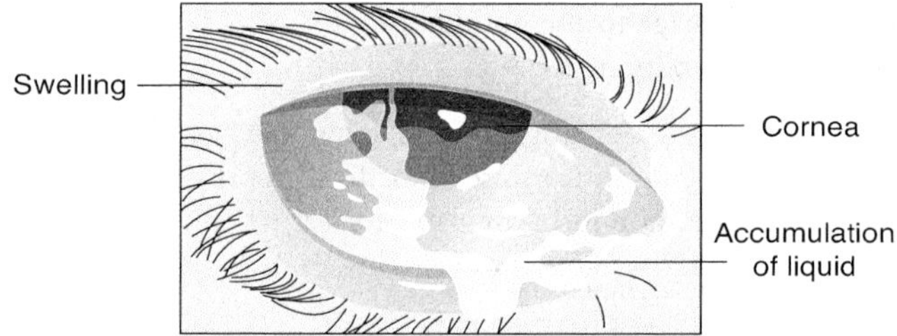

There are two types of endophthalmitis:

1. **Endogenous** (metastatic) results from the spread of organisms from a distant source of infection. This type occurs when there is a direct assault of an infection (e.g., septic emboli) or by changes in the vascular epithelium caused by substrates (substance on which an enzyme reacts) released during infection and intraocular tissue destruction occurs.
2. **Exogenous** results from a complication of ocular surgery (e.g., cataract, glaucoma, retinal), foreign bodies within the eyeball, and/or blunt or penetrating ocular trauma.

For both types of endophthalmitis, symptoms include white nodules that may occur on the lens capsule, iris, retina, or choroids. It may progress to inflammation of all ocular tissues with purulent exudate of the entire globe, and may spread to the orbital soft tissue.

Section 10 Coding Practice

Condition	ICD-10-CM
Purulent endophthalmitis, unspecified, right eye	H44.001
Acute endophthalmitis, right eye	H44.001
Chronic endophthalmitis, right eye	H44.001
Vitreous hemorrhage, left eye	H43.12

Section 10 Questions

Does ICD-10-CM differentiate between acute, chronic, and unspecified endophthalmitis?

How should subacute endophthalmitis be coded?

How is vitreous hemorrhage reported?

See end of chapter for Coding Practice answers.

Section 11 – Ocular Muscles

Conditions affecting the ocular muscles include strabismus, other disorders of binocular movement, and disorders of refraction and accommodation.

Strabismus

Strabismus is a condition where the eyes are not parallel and not aligned with one another. For example, one of the eyes turns or wanders in or out, or up or down. It usually involves lack of coordination between the extraocular muscles that prevent the gaze of each eye coming to the same point in space preventing binocular vision and affecting depth perception. If left untreated, strabismus may lead to amblyopia, which is described in the section visual disturbances. Forms of strabismus include:

Esotropia – Characterized by a turning inward of one or both eyes, also referred to as cross-eye. There is double vision, the eyes are not aligned in the same direction, there are uncoordinated eye movements, and/or there is visual loss in one eye without the ability to see in 3-D. Paralysis of the lateral rectus muscle causes an abnormal inward deviation of one eye.

Esotropia

A type of strabismus in which one or both eyes turn inwards

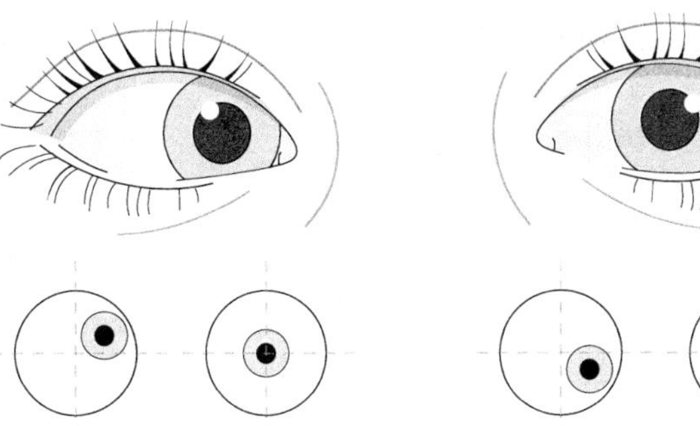

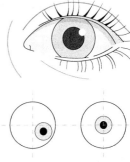

Esotropia with A pattern: eye deviates upwards and inwards

Esotropia with V pattern: eye deviates downwards and inwards

Exotropia – The eye is turned out. Exotropia most often occurs in children beginning between the ages of 2 and 4, but may occur at any age. It may be intermittent initially, occurring when the child is daydreaming, tired, or ill, but usually becomes more frequent if left untreated. Failure to treat exotropia can lead to permanently impaired vision.

Exotropia

A type of strabismus in which one or both eyes turn outwards

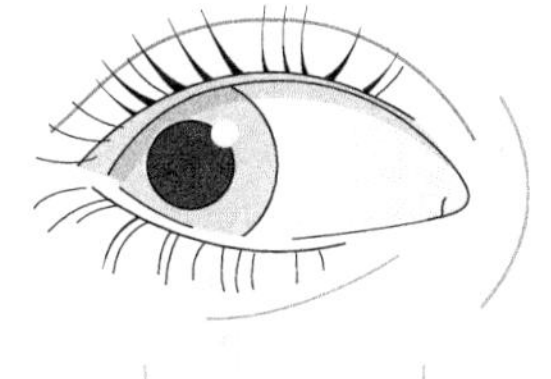

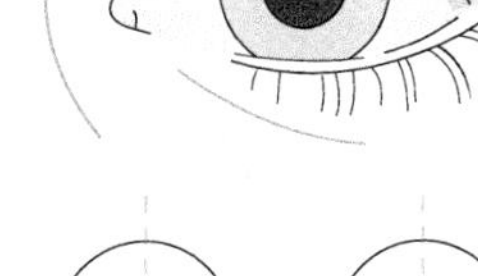

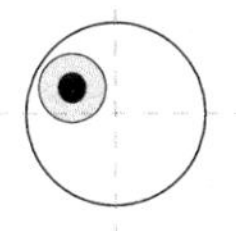

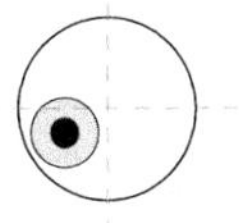

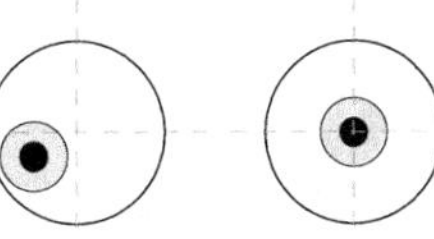

Exotropia with V pattern: eye deviates upwards and outwards

Exotropia with A pattern: eye deviates downwards and outwards

There are different types of esotropia and exotropia, which include:

- **Monocular** – affecting only one eye.
- **Alternating** – fixation alternates between the right and left eye so that at one moment the right eye fixates and the left eye turns inward, and the next, the left eye fixates and the right turns inward.

- **Intermittent** – This type is not always present; it may be visible when looking at close objects or when looking at distant objects and not close ones. Most intermittent types are accommodative, where an attempt is made to focus the eyes, but they converge, activating the accommodation reflex. With this condition, a loss of binocular control is possible.

Section 11 Coding Practice

Condition	ICD-10-CM
Alternating esotropia	H50.05
Alternating exotropia, A pattern	H50.16
Intermittent exotropia	H50.30

Section 11 Questions

How is strabismus classified?

What types of conditions are included under disorders of binocular movement?

See end of chapter for Coding Practice answers.

Section 12 – Disorders of Refraction and Accommodation

Myopia

Myopia, also called nearsightedness, is when the eyeball is too long or the lens is too spherical. Any distant images are brought to a focus in front of the retina and are quickly out of focus before the light hits the retina. Images that are nearby are seen much more clearly. Concave lenses of eyeglasses correct this problem by causing the light rays to separate and go in a different direction before they enter the eye.

Hypermetropia

Hypermetropia, also called farsightedness, is when the eyeball is too short or the lens has flattened out or is inflexible. The light rays that are entering the eye (especially close objects) will not be brought into focus by the time they reach the retina. It can be corrected with eyeglasses with convex lenses or contact lenses.

Section 12 Coding Practice

Condition	ICD-10-CM
Myopia, bilateral	H52.13
Hypermetropia, left eye	H52.02
Astigmatism, right eye	H52.201

Section 12 Questions

Does laterality affect the code selection for refraction disorders?

See end of chapter for Coding Practice answers.

Section 13 – Visual Disturbances

There are many different types of visual disturbances. They are typically symptoms of other disorders, such as:

- Vascular disease
- Neurological diseases and conditions
- Muscular disorders
- Cancer
- Trauma
- Diabetes
- Congenital conditions

Amblyopia

Amblyopia, also known as 'lazy eye', is loss of vision in an eye which is otherwise healthy. It may be caused by other disorders, such as strabismus, refractive disorders or injury. Eyesight in one eye does not develop normally during early childhood and the eye that is affected adjusts to avoid double vision, with the child preferring the better eye. Other causes of amblyopia may be nearsightedness, farsightedness, or astigmatism because one eye is out of focus.

Blurred Vision

Blurred vision refers to a loss of sharpness of vision and the inability to see small details. This may be caused by many things, such as an eye disease or injury, aging or a condition like diabetes.

Diplopia

Diplopia (double vision) causes a patient to see two objects instead of one. The most common reasons for diplopia are:

- Physiological change in the lens, conjunctiva, or retinal surface. Typically involves only one eye and is not corrected by covering the opposite eye.
- Inability of the brain to overlay images with both eyes. Usually involving both eyes and is corrected when one eye is covered. This condition is more often congenital, and/or can be nerve-related (e.g., multiple sclerosis, cranial nerve disorders) or muscle-related, caused by misaligned eyes.

Scotomas (Blind Spots)

Scotomas or scotomata, also referred to as blind spots, are areas in the field of vision that have been partially altered. A scotoma results in an area of partially diminished or entirely deteriorated visual acuity, surrounded by a normal field of vision. Everybody has a scotoma in their field of vision in an area where photoreceptors do not exist, although, underlying diseases, such as multiple sclerosis or vascular blockages in the eye, may cause more extensive scotomas.

A few different types are:

- **Annular scotoma** (ring) – A circular area of depressed vision that involves a fixation point.
- **Paracentral scotoma** – A blind spot that is adjacent to the fixation point.
- **Scintillating scotoma** – A localized area of diminished vision edged by shimmering colored lights. This is the visual aura that typically precedes a migraine headache.

Section 13 Coding Practice

Condition	ICD-10-CM
Blurred vision, left eye	H53.8
Diplopia, both eyes	H53.2
Ring scotoma, left eye	H53.452
Paracentral scotoma, right eye	H53.411
Scintillating scotoma, right eye	H53.121

Section 13 Questions

How is blurred vision reported?

The code for scintillating scotoma is not found under in the subcategory H53.4- Visual field defects with other types of scotomas. Where is scintillating scotoma listed and why?

Many conditions listed under visual disturbances can be symptoms of another condition. Explain how symptoms are coded using outpatient coding guidelines.

See end of chapter for Coding Practice answers.

Section 14 – Visual Impairment and Blindness

When a person is lacking in visual perception due to physiological or neurological factors, they are considered to have a form of visual impairment or blindness. There are different methods of classifying these conditions, from mild or moderate visual impairment to functional or total blindness.

Visual Impairment

Visual impairment is any chronic visual deficit that impairs everyday functioning and is not correctable by eyeglasses or contact lenses. There may be residual vision and light perception with the ability to tell dark from light and the direction of the light source.

Total Blindness

Total blindness is the complete lack of form and there is no visual light perception.

Legal Blindness

The World Health Organization (WHO) and the United States of America (USA) differ in their definitions of 'legal blindness'. The WHO identifies legal blindness as visual impairment on a 'Profound' to 'Total' level and the USA starts the definition earlier, with legal blindness starting one level earlier, at the 'Severe Visual Impairment' level.

Classification		Levels of Visual Impairment	Additional descriptors which may be encountered
"legal"	WHO	Visual acuity and/or visual field limitation (whichever is worse)	
	(Near-) Normal Vision	**Range of Normal Vision** 20/10 20/13 20/16 20/20 20/25 2.0 1.6 1.25 1.0 0.8	
	(Near-) Normal Vision	**Near-Normal Vision** 20/30 20/40 20/50 20/60 0.7 0.6 0.5 0.4 0.3	
	Low Vision	**Moderate Visual Impairment** 20/70 20/80 20/100 20/125 20/160 0.25 0.20 0.16 0.12	Moderate low vision
Legal Blindness (USA) both eyes	Low Vision	**Severe Visual Impairment** 20/200 20/250 20/320 20/400 0.10 0.08 0.06 0.05 Visual field: 20 degrees or less	Severe low vision, "Legal" blindness
Legal Blindness (USA) both eyes	Blindness (WHO) one or both eyes	**Profound Visual Impairment** 20/500 20/630 20/800 20/1000 0.04 0.03 0.025 0.02 Count fingers at: less than 3m (10 ft.) Visual field: 10 degrees or less	Profound low vision, Moderate blindness
Legal Blindness (USA) both eyes	Blindness (WHO) one or both eyes	**Near-Total Visual Impairment** Visual acuity: less than 0.02 (20/1000) Count fingers at: 1m (3ft.) or less Hand movements: 5m (15ft.) or less Light projection, light perception Visual field: 5 degrees or less	Severe blindness, Near-total blindness
Legal Blindness (USA) both eyes	Blindness (WHO) one or both eyes	**Total Visual Impairment** No light perception (NLP)	Total blindness

Visual acuity refers to best achievable acuity with correction.
Non-listed Snellen fractions may be classified by converting to the nearest decimal equivalent, e.g. 10/200 = .05, 6/30 = .20.
CF (count fingers) without designation of distance, may be classified to profound impairment.
HM (hand motion) without designation of distance, may be classified to near-total impairment.
Visual field measurements refer to the largest field diameter for a 1/100 white test object.

The table below gives a classification of severity of visual impairment recommended by a WHO Study Group on the Prevention of Blindness, Geneva, 6-10 November 1972.'

The term "low vision" in category H54 comprises categories 1 and 2 of the table. The term "blindness" compromises categories 3, 4 and 5, and the term "unqualified visual loss" is described with category 9.

If the extent of the visual field is taken into account, patients with a field no greater than 10 but greater than 5 around central fixation should be placed in category 3 and patients with a field no greater than 5 around central fixation should be placed in category 4, even if the central acuity is not impaired.

Category of visual impairment		Visual acuity with best possible correction	
		Maximum less than:	Minimum equal to or better than:
Low Vision (WHO)	1	6/18 3/10 (0.3) 20/70	6/60 1/10 (0.1) 20/200
	2	6/60 1/10 (0.1) 20/200	3/60 1/20 (0.05) 20/400
Blindness (WHO)	3	3/60 1/20 (0.05) 20/400	1/60 (finger counting at 1 meter) 1/50 (0.02) 5/300 (20/1200)
	4	1/60 (finger counting at 1 meter) 1/50 (0.02) 5/300	Light perception
	5	No light perception	
	9	Undetermined or unspecified	

Section 14 Coding Practice

Condition	ICD-10-CM
Bilateral blindness, no light perception, both eyes	H54.0X55
Left eye blindness , no light perception, right eye, low vision category 2	H54.1225

Section 14 Questions

How is visual impairment identified and reported?

See end of chapter for Coding Practice answers.

Section 15 – Other Disorders

There are two categories in the other disorders block of codes, nystagmus and other irregular eye movements and intraoperative and postoperative complications.

Nystagmus

Nystagmus is abnormal eye movement that usually results in blurred vision. There are a variety of types of nystagmus and the type of abnormal eye movement depends on the underlying cause.

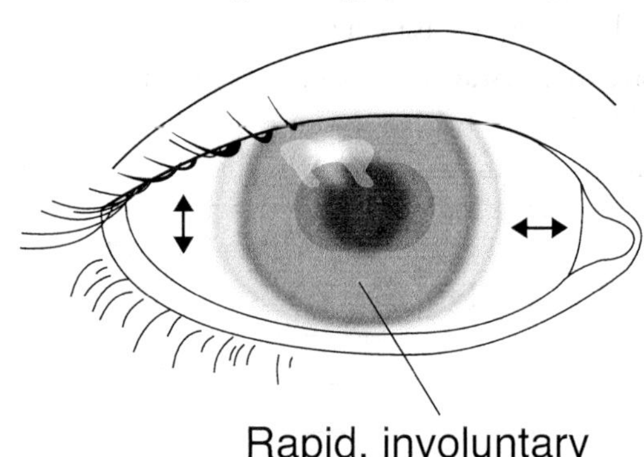

Horizontal nystagmus is a jerking movement that goes side to side. This condition is often associated with poor vision although by itself is not the cause.

Vertical nystagmus refers to up and down movement of the eye and typically indicates a problem with the central nervous system.

Childhood nystagmus is typically associated with eye defects, such as retinal disorders, although most are familial and not a symptom of a disease process. In adults, nystagmus can be a symptom of an underlying disease, such as multiple sclerosis or head trauma.

Intraoperative and Postoperative Complications

There are a number of intraoperative and postoperative complications that can affect the eye and ocular adnexa. As with all types of surgery there is always a possibility of intraoperative or postoperative hemorrhage or hematoma of the eye and surrounding structures and accidental puncture or laceration. Keratopathy and lens fragments are postoperative complications specific to cataract surgery. Chorioretinal scarring is a complication specific to surgery for retinal detachment.

Keratopathy Following Cataract Surgery

This complication may also be referred to as bullous aphakic keratopathy if the lens has been removed but not replaced with an intraocular lens implant or bullous pseudophakic keratopathy if an intraocular lens implant is present. In some individuals surgical trauma from the cataract extraction damages the corneal endothelium causing corneal edema and subepithelial bulla formation on the surface of the cornea. Bulla are fluid filled blisters. When the endothelial cells are damaged, the remaining cells rearrange themselves to cover the posterior corneal surface. The remaining endothelial cells become irregularly shaped and enlarged. The endothelium becomes unable to act as a pump to the cornea and the stroma begins to swell. The cornea thickens and folds are seen in the Descemet membrane.

Lens Fragments Following Cataract Surgery

If all lens material is not retrieved during cataract surgery, it is retained and may cause other complications, such as corneal edema or uveitis.

Chorioretinal Scarring Following Detachment Surgery

Chorioretinal scarring is a condition that is associated with surgical repair retinal detachment although it has other causes not related to surgical procedures such as infection and inflammation of the retina. Chorioretinal scarring is of concern because it can cause vision deficits.

Section 15 Coding Practice

Condition	ICD-10-CM
Bullous aphakic keratopathy of right eye, previous cataract surgery	H59.011
Retained cataracts fragments in left eye, following cataract surgery	H59.022
Right eye hemorrhage following cataract surgery	H59.311
Chorioretinal scars, right eye, after retinal detachment surgery	H59.811
Nystagmus, both eyes	H55.00

Section 15 Questions

From what section should postoperative complications related to eye surgery be coded?

What are some differences between coding intraoperative and postoperative complications related to eye surgery?

See end of chapter for Coding Practice answers.

Section 16 –Newborn and Congenital Conditions

Conditions affecting the eyes that originate during the perinatal period are limited in number. Retinopathy of prematurity is one condition and another relatively rare condition is birth trauma to the eye. However, there are a number of congenital conditions of the eye. Some conditions such as ptosis, ectropion, entropion, cataracts, and glaucoma were discussed previously because these conditions may be acquired, that is they may occur later in birth, or they may be present at birth in which case they are considered to be congenital malformations. A congenital condition not previously discussed is coloboma.

Coloboma

A coloboma is a congenital malformation in which part of the eye does not form due to failure of fusion of an embryonic feature called the intraocular fissure. The malformation is present at birth and may affect the various parts of the eye such as the eyelid, lens, iris, retina (including the macula), choroids, uvea, or optic disk. This causes a gap between those structures of the eye that fail to close up completely before a child is born.

The effect on eyesight is dependent on the size of the gap and can be mild or more severe. For example, if a small part of the eyelid is missing, vision may be normal, whereas if a large part of the optic nerve is missing, vision may be poor or a major portion of the visual field may be missing. Other conditions associated with a coloboma are microphthalmia (congenital deformity resulting in abnormally small eyes), glaucoma, nystagmus, scotoma, strabismus, eye surgery, or eye trauma.

Symptoms may include blurred vision, decreased visual acuity, and/or ghost or shadowy images.

Other specific types of coloboma with specific causes and/or symptoms are:

- **Lens** – A piece of lens is absent. The lens will usually appear with a notch.
- **Retina** (macula) – The center of the retina does not develop normally. Normal eye development is interrupted following inflammation of the retina in utero.
- **Optic disc** – The optic disc is slightly or largely hollowed out.

Retinopathy of Prematurity

Retinopathy of prematurity (ROP) is abnormal blood vessel development in the retina of a premature infant. There are five stages of ROP:

- Stage 1: Mild abnormal blood vessel growth
- Stage 2: Moderate abnormal blood vessel growth
- Stage 3: Severe abnormal blood vessel growth
- Stage 4: Severe abnormal blood vessel growth with partially detached retina
- Stage 5: Severe abnormal blood vessel growth with total retinal detachment

Symptoms of severe ROP are abnormal eye movements, crossed eyes, severe nearsightedness, and leukocoria (white shaded pupils).

Section 16 Coding Practice

Condition	ICD-10-CM
Lens coloboma, right eye	Q12.2
Retinal coloboma, right eye	Q14.1
Coloboma of optic disc, right eye	Q14.2
Retinopathy of prematurity, stage 3, right eye	H35.141

Section 16 Questions

From what chapter are colobomas coded?

Does laterality matter when coding colobomas?

If the site of the coloboma is not specified, how is it coded?

What additional documentation is needed when coding retinopathy of prematurity?

See end of chapter for Coding Practice answers.

Section 17 – Eye Injuries

Traumatic injuries of the eye and ocular adnexa are listed under injuries to the head in ICD-10-CM. Injuries may be superficial involving primarily the eyelid and periocular area or more severe injuries of the eye, ocular adnexa or orbit. Superficial injuries of the eyelid and periocular area include abrasion, foreign body, and insect bites. Injuries to deeper structures include eyelid and ocular laceration with or without foreign bodies, conjunctival and corneal abrasion, contusion of the eyeball and orbit, and avulsion of the eye. Some of the more common traumatic injuries are discussed below.

Eye Abrasions

An eye abrasion is wearing away of the layer of the eye (e.g., cornea, conjunctiva) as a result of applied friction force.

Foreign Bodies

Foreign bodies can enter the eyes at any time. Some are superficial and exit through the normal production of tears. If a foreign body is trapped under the eyelid, it may cause an abrasion on the conjunctiva and/or cornea, or remain there and require manual extraction. In more serious cases, the foreign body results in intraocular penetration because of electrical tools or a type of explosion. This type of injury typically requires manual extraction.

Eyelid and Ocular Lacerations

Lacerations of the eyelid can be minor, where the lid margin or the tarsal plate is not affected, or major, affecting the medial portion of the lower or upper eyelid and possibly the lacrimal canaliculus.

Some ocular lacerations can be superficial affecting only the conjunctiva, sclera, or only the front layers of the cornea. Others can penetrate the eyeball, have a foreign body, and have eye tissue prolapse or loss of intraocular tissue, and may be considered a rupture of the eyeball. These lacerations can seriously damage the eye structures that are necessary for vision and are predisposed to infection.

Ocular Burns

There are two types of burns of the eyes, thermal and corrosive. Burns that come from a heat source (excluding the sun) such as fire, electricity, or radiation are thermal burns. Burns caused by chemical are considered corrosive burns.

Chemical (Corrosive) Eye Injuries

Chemical burns (corrosion) of the eye can be defined as tissue damage in the eye or a serious decrease in vision due to exposure to a chemical or irritant. Mild chemicals or irritants disrupt or damage only the surface cells of the corneal epithelium and only a short time is required to repair these cells. If the chemical or irritant is stronger, it can go deeper into the next layer of the cornea, the stroma, which may cause irreversible damage or even deeper, into the corneal endothelial cell, possibly causing cataracts and/or glaucoma. There are three main categories of chemical burns:

Irritants – These typically have a normal pH and cause more irritation to the eye than damage, such as pepper spray.

Alkali burns – This chemical penetrates the surface of the eye and can cause severe injury to structures of the eye, such as the cornea and the lens. Examples of these are ammonia, lye, and lime, which are included in cleaning products, drain cleaners, and oven cleaners.

Acid burns – Usually less severe than an alkali burn, this chemical does not penetrate the eye as easily as alkali, but there are exceptions, such as hydrofluoric acid. This chemical usually only damages the front of the eye, but can cause damage to other layers resulting in blindness. Examples of acidic chemicals are acetic acid and sulfuric acid, found in vinegar, fingernail polish, and automobile batteries.

Section 17 Coding Practice

Condition	ICD-10-CM
Conjunctival abrasion, w/o foreign body, left eye, initial visit	S05.02XA
Corneal laceration with retained metal piece, right eye, initial visit	S05.51XA
Burn in left eye due to campfire, follow-up visit (aftercare)	T26.42XD
Ammonia in right eye affecting cornea, initial visit	T26.61XA

Section 17 Questions

For injuries, what additional documentation is needed to make the correct code selection?

What is the difference between thermal burns and corrosion burns?

Are there Official Coding Guidelines that should be followed when coding burns?

See end of chapter for Coding Practice answers.

Quiz — Eye and Ocular Adnexa

1. Which of the following is not one of the layers of the cornea?
   a. Bowman's layer
   b. Choroidal layer
   c. Descemet's membrane layer
   d. Endothelial layer

2. Identify in what part of the eye the rod and cone cells are located.
   a. Ciliary body
   b. Lens
   c. Retina
   d. Trabecular meshwork

3. Which of these is not a part of the lacrimal system?
   a. Nasolacrimal duct
   b. Lacrimal sac
   c. Lacrimal lake
   d. Nasal puncta

4. The vitreous helps to:
   a. Provide optical power to the cornea
   b. Assist in keeping the retina in place
   c. Maintain the supply of the sebum, an oily substance that prevents evaporation of tear film of the eye
   d. Supply the eye with moisture

5. Presenile cataracts are coded to:
   a. H26.0-
   b. H25.2-
   c. H25.81-
   d. H25.1-

6. Which one of the following types of glaucoma is identified by code H40.89 Other specified glaucoma?
   a. Childhood glaucoma
   b. Chamber-angle anomaly glaucoma
   c. Secondary vascular glaucoma
   d. Glaucoma associated with anomalies of the iris

7. Which of the following statements is true about melanomas?
   a. Melanoma starts in melanocytes.
   b. It is a mass of histologically normal tissue in an abnormal location.
   c. Includes retinal pigment epithelium atrophy, retinal pigment epithelium hyperplasia and drusens.
   d. There may be corkscrew-shaped blood vessels on the surface of the eye.

8. A coloboma should be coded from which section:
   a. Neoplasm section – C and D codes
   b. Infectious Disease section – A Codes
   c. Eye and Adnexa Section – H Codes
   d. Congenital Malformations and Deformations – Q Codes

9. Amblyopia is also called:
   a. Myopia
   b. Traumatic limitation
   c. Lazy eye
   d. Strabismus

10. Which are the three causes of corrosive burns?
    a. Radiation, sunburn, irritant
    b. Irritant, alkali, acid
    c. Fire burn, non-alkaline, radiation
    d. Oxidizer, electricity, acid

See next page for answers.

Quiz Answers — Eye and Ocular Adnexa

1. Which of the following is not one of the layers of the cornea?

   b. Choroidal layer

2. Identify in what part of the eye the rod and cone cells are located.

   c. Retina

3. Which of these is not a part of the lacrimal system?

   No selection. All are part of the lacrimal system.

4. The vitreous helps to:

   b. Assist in keeping the retina in place

5. Presenile cataracts are coded to:

   a. H26.0-

6. Which one of the following types of glaucoma is identified by code H40.89 Other specified glaucoma?

   c. Secondary vascular glaucoma

7. Which of the following statements is true about melanomas?

   a. Melanoma starts in melanocytes.

8. A coloboma should be coded from which section:

   d. Congenital Malformations and Deformations – Q Codes

9. Amblyopia is also called:

   c. Lazy eye

10. Which are the three causes of corrosive burns?

    b. Irritant, alkali, acid

Coding Practice Answers

Section 1 Coding Practice

Question: What are some types of conjunctivitis that are reported with a single code from *Chapter 1 – Certain Infectious and Parasitic Diseases*?

Answer: Conjunctivitis due to Acanthamoeba, adenovirus, Chlamydia, Cocksackievirus, diphtheria, enterovirus type 70, filariasis, gonococci, herpes simplex and zoster, other infectious disease NEC, meningococci, mucocutaneous leishmaniasis, and syphilis.

Question: If the inflammation involves both the conjunctiva and the cornea how is the condition reported?

Answer: It is reported with a code for keratoconjunctivitis.

Question: What needs to be documented in order to appropriately choose a code to represent unspecified disseminated chorioretinal inflammation?

Answer: H30.103 provides the additional information that the condition is bilateral affecting both eyes.

Section 2 Coding Practice

Question: Does laterality of the eye make a difference in code selection for neoplasms?

Answer: Yes. Laterality must be documented to allow assignment of a neoplasm code at the highest level of specificity.

Question: What main term is referenced in the Alphabetic Index to identify the correct code for orbital dermoid cyst?

Answer: Under the main term Cyst, dermoid, there is not a specific code for orbital, but there is an instruction to see Neoplasm, benign, by site.

Section 3 Coding Practice

Question: Why is an internal hordeolum code reported for an infected meibomian gland that is not specified as internal?

Answer: The meibomian glands are on the internal aspect of the eyelid and an infected meibomian gland is called a hordeolum.

Question: In addition to laterality, what else needs to be documented in the medical record to choose the appropriate code for ectropion?

Answer: Not only are ectropion codes specific to both sides (left or right), documentation needs to indicate if the upper or lower lids are affected

Section 4 Coding Practice

Question: Is chronic enlargement of the lacrimal gland reported with the same code as chronic dacryoadenitis?

Answer: No., there are specific codes for chronic enlargement of the lacrimal gland.

Question: Are the codes for dacryocystitis specific to the lacrimal sac?

Answer: No. The code for dacryocystitis is used for inflammation of the lacrimal sac and nasolacrimal duct. There is a separate code for reporting inflammation of the lacrimal canaliculi.

Question: Is code H04.533 reported for congenital nasolacrimal duct obstruction?

Answer: No. Congenital nasolacrimal duct obstruction is reported with code Q10.5.

Question: The codes for epiphora. What additional information is required to assign a more specific code?

Answer: In addition to documenting the cause as excess lacrimation or insufficient drainage, laterality must be specified as right, left or bilateral.

Section 5 Coding Practice

Question: For chemical or toxic conjunctivitis, does the episode of care need to be documented in the medical record before choosing a code?

Answer: The episode does not need to be specifically documented. However, if the chemical causes a corrosion or burn (T26.-), the episode of care needs to be documented to determine if it was an initial (A) or subsequent (D) visit or a sequela (S).

Question: Are two codes assigned for acute and chronic conjunctivitis occurring together?

Answer: Yes. When a patient with chronic conjunctivitis develops an acute conjunctivitis and both conditions are treated, two codes are required, one identifying the specific type of acute conjunctivitis and one for the chronic condition.

Section 6 Coding Practice

Question: What type of keratitis in the coding practice above is not listed as a term under keratitis in the Alphabetic Index?

Answer: Photokeratitis. There is a 'see' instruction for photokeratitis that is found under Keratitis, superficial, due to light.

Question: Does the type or site of the corneal ulcer affect code selection?

Answer: Yes. Code H16.002 is assigned for an unspecified corneal ulcer. To assign a more specific code, the corneal ulcer must be described as one of the following types: central, ring, marginal, Mooren's, mycotic, perforated, or with hypopyon.

Question: Are two codes required to report vernal conjunctivitis with limbar and corneal involvement?

Answer: No. A combination code is available to indicate that the limbar and corneal are involved.

Question: What type of condition are corneal ghost vessels?

Answer: This is a type of corneal neovascularization.

Question: There is an excludes note for posterior cyclitis under H20.1- Chronic iridocyclitis. Does this mean that posterior cyclitis cannot be reported with chronic iridocyclitis?

Answer: No. In this case there is an Excludes2 note which states that posterior cyclitis is not reported under subcategory H20.1. However, it is possible for the patient to have both conditions, in which case, both the code for chronic iridocyclitis and the code for posterior cyclitis would be reported.

Question: Why is a neuroepithelial cyst reported with the code for idiopathic cyst?

Answer: In the Alphabetic Index there is not a specific designation for neuroepithelial cyst, so the code listed for Cyst, iris H21.30- is used. This is the code for idiopathic cyst of the iris, ciliary body, or anterior chamber.

Section 7 Coding Practice

Question: Presenile is not included in the code description for category H26. How is presenile cataract coded?

Answer: Even though the term presenile is not included in the code description, in the Alphabetic Index, Cataract, presenile, is listed as the same codes as those described as infantile and juvenile cataracts.

Question: How are these cataracts that are secondary to inflammatory or degenerative disorders reports?

Answer: Cataracts occurring with inflammatory or degenerative disorders are reported codes from category H26.22-, Cataract secondary to ocular disorders (degenerative) (inflammatory).

Question: When reporting cataracts that are secondary to inflammatory or degenerative disorders, the associated disorder is also reported. How is the cataract code sequenced?

Answer: The coding instruction is to code also the associated ocular condition so the ocular disorder does not necessarily need to be coded first.

Question: Why is the diabetic cataract in the coding practice reported with a code for type II diabetes when the diabetes is not identified as type II?

Answer: Type II diabetes includes diabetes NOS.

Question: Is it a requirement to indicate the drug or toxin when coding a drug induced cataract?

Answer: Yes, two codes are also required. The cataract code is reported first and the adverse effect code for the glucocorticoid is reported second.

Section 8a Coding Practice

Question: Is the term 'partial' used in the descriptor of retinal detachments?

Answer: No. Partial retinal detachment is reported with the code for other retinal detachments (H33.8).

Question: Is a horseshoe tear a type of retinal detachment? If not, how it is categorized?

Answer: No. A horseshoe tear is a type of retinal break without detachment.

Question: Why is a subtotal retinal detachment reported with an 'other specified' code?

Answer: There is not a specific code for subtotal retinal detachment so it is reported with an 'other specified' code.

Section 8b Coding Practice

Question: What main term is congenital macular degeneration listed under in the Alphabetic Index?

Answer: Dystrophy, retina

Question: What is the medical term for wet macular degeneration?

Answer: Exudative. It is defined as any fluid that filters from the circulatory system into lesions or areas of inflammation.

Question: Which macular degeneration diagnosis above requires documentation of laterality to assign the most specific code?

Answer: Both cystoid and exudative age related macular degeneration require documentation of laterality.

Section 9 Coding Practice

Question: When coding unspecified or primary open-angle glaucoma, does laterality affect code selection?

Answer: Yes. Unspecified and primary open-angle glaucoma codes are identified by which eye is affected.

Question: What are some examples of different types of primary angle-closure glaucoma?

Answer: Acute, chronic, intermittent or residual stage.

Question: Does glaucoma associated with vascular disorders have a specific code

Answer: No. Glaucoma associated with an unspecified vascular disorder is reported with H40.89 Other specified glaucoma. If the vascular is more specifically identified as being due to retinal vein occlusion, code H40.5- would be reported with a second code H34.81- Central retinal vein occlusion.

Question: Can steroid-induced glaucoma be reported with a single code?

Answer: No. The code identifies the glaucoma secondary to drugs, but does not identify the stage and a second code is required to capture the adverse effect of corticosteroids.

Section 10 Coding Practice

Question: Does ICD-10-CM differentiate between acute, chronic, and unspecified endophthalmitis?

Answer: No. There is not a distinction between acute, chronic and unspecified.

Question: How should subacute endophthalmitis be coded?

Answer: Subacute endophthalmitis is reported with the same codes (H44.001-H44.009) as acute, chronic, or unspecified endophthalmitis.

Question: How is vitreous hemorrhage reported?

Answer: Vitreous hemorrhage is reported with codes for Disorders of the Vitreous Body and Globe (H43-H44).

Section 11 Coding Practice

Question: How is strabismus classified?

Answer: There are two categories, paralytic strabismus (H49) and other strabismus (H50). Other strabismus includes esotropia, exotropia, vertical strabismus, intermittent heterotopia, heterophoria, and mechanical strabismus.

Question: What types of conditions are included under disorders of binocular movement?

Answer: Palsy of conjugate gaze, convergence insufficiency and excess, and internuclear ophthalmoplegia.

Section 12 Coding Practice

Question: Does laterality affect the code selection for refraction disorders?

Answer: Laterality is included for most conditions. Diseases of the eyes and ocular adnexa are organized by disorders. Refraction disorders are grouped under the coding block that includes disorders of ocular muscles and binocular movement.

Section 13 Coding Practice

Question: How is blurred vision reported?

Answer: No. Code H53.8 reports other visual disturbances.

Question: The code for scintillating scotoma is not found under in the subcategory H53.4- Visual field defects with other types of scotomas. Where is scintillating scotoma listed and why?

Answer: It is listed under the subcategory H53.1- Subjective visual disturbances, and is considered a type of transient visual loss.

Question: Many conditions listed under visual disturbances can be symptoms of another condition. Explain how symptoms are coded using outpatient coding guidelines.

Answer: If the condition has not been confirmed by the physician, a symptom or sign is reported rather than the code for the condition. If symptoms are listed along with a confirmed condition, only the condition is coded.

Section 14 Coding Practice

Question: How is visual impairment identified and reported?

Answer: The level of visual impairment is defined by the category listed in the table and is specifically identified in the code. Blindness is reported for visual impairment categories 3, 4, and 5. Low vision is reported for categories 1 or 2. Unqualified visual loss is reported for category 9 which is for undetermined or unspecified visual acuity. Additionally, the level of visual impairment is reported based upon the category of visual loss, if any, in each eye.

Section 15 Coding Practice

Question: From what section should postoperative complications related to eye surgery be coded?

Answer: Most postoperative complications related to eye surgery are found at the end of *Chapter 7 – Diseases of the Eye and Ocular Adnexa* under category H59. Mechanical complications of intraocular lenses and prosthetic devices, implants and grafts are exceptions, which are found in *Chapter 19 – Injury, Poisoning and Certain Other Consequences of External Causes.*

Question: What are some differences between coding intraoperative and postoperative complications related to eye surgery?

Answer: The complication must be identified as affecting the right, left, or both eyes. Hemorrhage and hematoma must be designated as intraoperative or postoperative and for intraoperative hemorrhages the condition must be designated as due to an ophthalmic procedure or due to a procedure on another site.

Section 16 Coding Practice

Question: From what chapter are colobomas coded?

Answer: Colobomas are a congenital malformation of the part of the eye so they are coded from *Chapter 17 – Congenital Malformations, Deformations, and Chromosomal Abnormalities.*

Question: Does laterality matter when coding colobomas?

Answer: No.

Question: If the site of the coloboma is not specified, how is it coded?

Answer: Coloboma NOS is coded as a coloboma of the iris.

Question: What additional documentation is needed when coding retinopathy of prematurity?

Answer: Laterality must be documented to assign a code to the highest level of specificity.

Section 17 Coding Practice

Question: For injuries, what additional documentation is needed to make the correct code selection?

Answer: Episode of care must be designated.

Question: What is the difference between thermal burns and corrosion burns?

Answer: Thermal burns are any type of burn occurring from a heat source excluding sunburns. Corrosion burns are due to chemicals.

Question: Are there Official Coding Guidelines that should be followed when coding burns?

Answer: Yes. The guidelines for burn coding are listed in Section I.C.19.d of the Official Coding Guidelines.

ICD-10-CM Documentation

Introduction

The codes for diseases of the eye are located in Chapter 7 Diseases of the Eye and Adnexa (H00-H59).

The chapter begins with instructions to assign an external cause code following the code for the eye condition to identify the cause of the eye condition when applicable. Along with codes for diseases of the eye, are also codes for diseases and conditions affecting the adnexa, or the structures surrounding the eye, such as the tear (lacrimal) ducts and glands, the extraocular muscles, and the eyelids.

Coding diseases of the eye and adnexa can be difficult due to the complex anatomic structures of the ocular system. Provider documentation specifying the affected site is required in detail as body sites are very specific and require documentation of laterality for paired body parts and of upper versus lower sites as in right upper eyelid or right lower eyelid.

Documentation of the evaluation and treatment of eye disorders can be difficult to understand because ophthalmology has a distinctive language. Most ophthalmic terminology such as amblyopia, glaucoma, chalazion, and pterygium are derived from Greek and Latin words. For example, ophthalmologic medical record documentation often indicates "O.S." and "O.D." O.S. is an abbreviation for "oculus sinister," Latin for "left eye" and O.D. is an abbreviation for "oculus dexter," Latin for "right eye."

To help understand the coding and documentation requirements for diseases of the eye and adnexa the code blocks in ICD-10-CM are displayed in the following table.

ICD-10-CM Blocks	
H00-H05	Disorders of eyelid, lacrimal system and orbit
H10-H11	Disorders of conjunctiva
H15-H22	Disorders of sclera, cornea, iris and ciliary body
H25-H28	Disorders of lens
H30-H36	Disorders of choroid and retina
H40-H42	Glaucoma
H43-H44	Disorders of vitreous body and globe
H46-H47	Disorders of optic nerve and visual pathways
H49-H52	Disorders of ocular muscles, binocular movement, accommodation and refraction
H53-H54	Visual disturbances and blindness
H55-H57	Other disorders of eye and adnexa
H59	Intraoperative and postprocedural complications and disorders of eye and adnexa, not elsewhere classified

There is also a code block to classify all intraoperative and post procedural complications of treatment for eye and adnexal disorders.

Exclusions

There are no Excludes1 notes, but there are a number of Excludes2 notes, which are listed in the table below.

ICD-10-CM Excludes1	ICD-10-CM Excludes2
None	Certain conditions originating in the perinatal period (P04-P96) Certain infectious and parasitic diseases (A00-B99) Complications of pregnancy, childbirth and the puerperium (O00-O9A) Congenital malformations, deformations, and chromosomal abnormalities (Q00-Q99) Diabetes mellitus related eye conditions (E08.3-, E09.3-, E10.3-, E11.3-, E13.3-) Endocrine, nutritional and metabolic diseases (E00-E88) injury (trauma) of eye and orbit (S05.-) Injury, poisoning and certain other consequences of external causes (S00-T88) Neoplasms (C00-D49) Symptoms, signs and abnormal clinical and laboratory findings, not elsewhere classified (R00-R94) Syphilis related eye disorders (A50.01, A50.3-, A51.43, A52.71)

As can be seen in the exclusions table, several diseases coded to other chapters have associated eye manifestations, such as eye disorders associated with infectious diseases (Chapter 1) and diabetes (Chapter 4). ICD-10-CM contains many combination codes for conditions and common symptoms or manifestations. Most notably, there are combination codes for diabetes mellitus with eye conditions (E08.3-, E09.3-, E10.3-, E11.3-, E13.3-) such as diabetic retinopathy.

Besides diabetes related conditions and eye disorders associated with infectious and parasitic diseases, other disorders of the eye and adnexa are classified in different chapters, such as conditions associated with a neoplastic process, conditions originating in the perinatal period (P04-P96), complications of pregnancy, childbirth and the puerperium (O00-O9A) and congenital malformations, deformations, and chromosomal abnormalities (Q00-Q99). Conditions resulting from injury or trauma to the eye and orbit (S05.-) are classified in Chapter 19 - Injury, Poisoning and Certain Other Consequences of External Causes (S00-T88).

Reclassification of Codes into New Code Categories

In addition to reclassifying the entire section of codes, the restructuring of categories and reorganization of codes have resulted in different classifications of certain diseases and disorders in ICD-10-CM compared to the previous system. Certain diseases have been reclassified to different chapters or sections. For example, codes for postoperative complications affecting the eyes have been classified together in a separate code block in Chapter 7 and a distinction is made between intraoperative complications and postprocedural disorders.

Chapter Guidelines

Coding and sequencing guidelines for diseases of the eye and adnexa and complications due to the treatment of these conditions are found in the coding conventions, the general coding guidelines, and the chapter-specific coding guidelines. Close attention to the instructions in the Tabular List and Alphabetic Index is also needed in order to assign the most specific code possible.

There are specific guidelines addressing assignment of glaucoma codes. For example, when a patient is admitted with glaucoma and the stage evolves during the admission, coding guidelines direct the user to assign the code for the highest stage documented. Another example involves assignment of the code for "indeterminate" stage glaucoma, guidelines state that code assignment is based on the clinical documentation. Glaucoma codes are combination codes and the seventh character "4" is assigned to the code for indeterminate stage glaucoma cases whose stage cannot be clinically determined. Coding guidelines caution the user not to confuse the indeterminate stage with unspecified stage. The unspecified stage code is assigned only when there is no documentation regarding the stage of the glaucoma.

Codes identify the type of glaucoma, the affected eye, and the glaucoma stage in a single combination code. Laterality is a component of for choosing codes There are guidelines for coding bilateral glaucoma For bilateral glaucoma where both eyes are documented as the same type and stage, a single code for the type of glaucoma, bilateral, is reported with the seventh character identifying the stage. When bilateral glaucoma is documented and each eye is documented as having a different type or stage two codes are assigned rather than the code for bilateral glaucoma. Each code identifies the type of glaucoma, appropriate seventh character for the stage, and laterality (right, left).

General Documentation Requirements

Documentation requirements depend on the particular disease or disorder affecting the eye or the surrounding adnexa. Some of the general documentation requirements are discussed here, but greater detail for some of the more common diseases of the eye and adnexa will be provided in the next section.

In general, basic medical record documentation requirements include the severity or status of the disease (e.g., acute or chronic), as well as the site, etiology, and any secondary disease process. The provider's confirmation of any diagnosis found in laboratory or other diagnostic test reports must be documented for code assignment. Provider documentation should clearly specify any cause-and-effect relationship between medical treatment and an eye disorder. Documentation in the medical record should specify whether a complication occurred intraoperatively or postoperatively, such as intraoperative versus postoperative hemorrhage.

ICD-10-CM has included greater specificity regarding the type and cause of eye disorders which must be documented in the medical record. Many codes also require more specific documentation of the site such as upper or lower eyelid and laterality (right, left, bilateral).

In addition to these general documentation requirements, there are specific diseases and disorders that require greater detail in documentation to ensure optimal code assignment.

Code-Specific Documentation Requirements

In this section code categories, subcategories, and subclassifications for some of the more frequently reported diseases of the eye and adnexa are reviewed. The focus is on conditions with additional and more specific clinical documentation requirements. Although not all codes with significant documentation requirements are discussed, this section will provide a representative sample of the type of additional documentation needed for diseases of the eye and adnexa. The section is organized by the code category, subcategory, or subclassification depending on whether the documentation affects only a single code or an entire subcategory or category.

Conjunctivitis

Conjunctivitis is inflammation of the conjunctiva, which is the thin, clear membrane lining the inner surface of the eyelid and the outer surface of the eye. Inflammation may be caused by bacteria, viruses, allergens, or chemicals. Chronic allergic conjunctivitis is a prolonged allergic reaction to an allergen.

Giant papillary conjunctivitis is one of the most common complications of wearing contact lenses and has its own specific code. In giant papillary conjunctivitis, the inner surface of the eyelids becomes irritated and inflamed, and large bumps or papillae occur on the underside of the eyelid. The inflammation of the palpebral conjunctiva in giant papillary conjunctivitis results from repeated contact with and irritation of the conjunctiva, or as an allergic reaction to protein deposits on the surface of the contact lens.

Giant papillary conjunctivitis is not a true allergic reaction but rather is usually associated with hypersensitivity reactions. Hay fever or other associated allergies may play a role in the onset and the severity of the signs and symptoms, so provider documentation of any associated allergy is essential for accurate code assignment. As with other allergic diseases, a chronic condition can also develop and may be associated with an increased risk for the development of cataracts and glaucoma. Clear, complete documentation of the patient's condition is needed in order to assign the most accurate diagnosis code.

The signs and symptoms of giant papillary conjunctivitis include discomfort and a reduced tolerance to contact lens wear, conjunctival redness and edema, itching, mucous discharge, photophobia, and may include blurred vision. A diagnosis of giant papillary conjunctivitis can usually be confirmed using slit lamp biomicroscopy after ruling out other possible causes with similar presentation, such as seasonal and perennial allergic conjunctivitis or chlamydial conjunctivitis. Other types of chronic conjunctivitis must be differentiated in the medical record documentation as well, such as chronic follicular conjunctivitis, vernal conjunctivitis, parasitic conjunctivitis, or other chronic allergic conjunctivitis.

There is a separate code used to report other chronic allergic conjunctivitis (H10.45) when there is not a more specific code for the documented type of chronic conjunctivitis.

ICD-10-CM Coding and Documentation Requirements

Identify type:

- Chronic giant papillary conjunctivitis
- Other specified chronic allergic conjunctivitis

For chronic giant papillary conjunctivitis identify laterality:

- Right eye
- Left eye
- Bilateral
- Unspecified

ICD-10-CM Code/Documentation	
H10.411	Chronic giant papillary conjunctivitis, right eye
H10.412	Chronic giant papillary conjunctivitis, left eye
H10.413	Chronic giant papillary conjunctivitis, bilateral
H10.419	Chronic giant papillary conjunctivitis, unspecified

Documentation and Coding Example

Patient is a 19-year-old Caucasian female who presents to ophthalmologist with a 2 year history of itchy, burning, irritated eyes. Patient has worn contact lenses for five years and started to notice problems after one year of lens wear. She reported her symptoms numerous times to her optometrist and was told she had "dry eyes" and to use wetting drops. She saw a new optometrist 4 months ago who thought her problems were allergy related and prescribed Pataday eye drops and changed her to a daily wear contact lens. Patient attends college in another state and would not be able to follow up with her new optometrist so she was advised to see an eye doctor near her school if her symptoms did not improve in 2-3 months. Patient states she has used the Pataday drops daily and also uses Blink brand lubrication drops during the day and Sustane brand at night. She is unable to tolerate contact lenses for more than 2-3 hours and has rarely worn them in the past 3 months. On examination, this is an attractive, articulate young woman who has applied light makeup to enhance her face and eyes. She does admit to not being fastidious about removing her makeup every night. She states she does have seasonal allergies treated with Claritin and she takes vitamins and Chinese herbs prescribed by her acupuncturist. On examination, there is no evidence of blepharitis, conjunctival redness or inflammation. Corneas of both eyes are mildly pitted. Inverting the lid to look at the inner surface of her eyelids is extremely painful but even a quick look confirms that the surface is rough and red with raised papillae on **both the upper and lower lids bilaterally**. She is prescribed Lotemax Eye drops BID x 6 weeks and is to add Restasis eye drops BID beginning 2 weeks after starting the Lotemax. Patient is advised to refrain from contact lens use as much as possible. RTC in 3 months. She is advised to return sooner if her symptoms worsen or have not improved in 3-4 weeks.

Diagnosis: **Chronic giant papillary conjunctivitis secondary to contact lens use.**

ICD-10-CM Diagnosis Code(s)

H10.413 Chronic giant papillary conjunctivitis, bilateral

Coding Note(s)

There are several subcategory codes for different types of chronic conjunctivitis, in addition to the codes for chronic giant papillary conjunctivitis that also identify the affected eye.

Cataract

A senile cataract, now more commonly referred to as age-related cataract, is a disorder of the lens of the eye characterized by gradual, progressive thickening of the lens which becomes cloudy and eventually leads to vision impairment. Other forms of cataract exist including those that affect infants and children, those caused by trauma, drug-induced cataracts, and cataracts caused by underlying disease of the eye so careful review of the medical record documentation is required to ensure that the most appropriate code is selected.

The term age-related cataract has replaced senile cataract, and age-related cataracts are classified in category H25 and the condition is further differentiated by other characteristics of the cataract. For example, there are specific codes for the most common types of senile cataracts which include nuclear cataract, cortical cataract, and posterior subcapsular cataract as well as for less common types. As with all paired organs, cataract codes include laterality and must be specified as right, left, or bilateral. Additionally, there have been some terminology changes. For example, the term hypermature cataract has been replaced with the term morgagnian-type cataract which is classified in subcategory H25.2. Furthermore, some conditions that previously had a specific code are now reported using code H25.89 Other age-related cataract. For example, there is no longer a specific code for total or mature cataract, so in the absence of other more specific documentation code H25.89 is assigned.

Coding and Documentation Requirements

Identify type of age-related cataract:

- Combined forms
- Incipient
  - Anterior subcapsular polar
  - Cortical
  - Posterior subcapsular polar
  - Other incipient type

- Morgagnian type
- Nuclear
- Other specified type
- Unspecified type

Identify laterality:

- Right
- Left
- Bilateral
- Unspecified

ICD-10-CM Code/Documentation	
H25.011	Cortical age-related cataract, right eye
H25.012	Cortical age-related cataract, left eye
H25.013	Cortical age-related cataract, bilateral
H25.019	Cortical age-related cataract, unspecified
H25.031	Anterior subcapsular polar age-related cataract, right eye
H25.032	Anterior subcapsular polar age-related cataract, left eye
H25.033	Anterior subcapsular polar age-related cataract, bilateral
H25.039	Anterior subcapsular polar age-related cataract, unspecified
H25.041	Posterior subcapsular polar age-related cataract, right eye
H25.042	Posterior subcapsular polar age-related cataract, left eye
H25.043	Posterior subcapsular polar age-related cataract, bilateral
H25.049	Posterior subcapsular polar age-related cataract, unspecified

Documentation and Coding Example

Seventy-three-year-old Caucasian female presents for eye exam after noticing some loss of sharpness in her distance vision. She states the change in distance vision is mild but she is concerned about it. She does not drive or watch TV, but she does knit and read and these activities have not been impaired. On examination, this is a very petite, athletic appearing septuagenarian. She states she always keeps her skin covered and wears a brimmed hat while out of doors but has never worn sunglasses. Conjunctiva are clear, without redness or excess tearing. PERRLA. Cranial nerves are grossly intact, eye muscle movement is normal. There are no areas of scotoma. Color vision intact. Autorefraction of distance vision showed 20/40 OD and 20/50 OS. Acuity tested manually confirms these results and with refraction she is easily corrected to 20/15 OU. Near vision is excellent without evidence of astigmatism. Proparacaine eye gtts instilled and tonometry shows OD pressure of 13 mm Hg and OS pressure of 15 mm Hg. Mydriacyl 1% gtts instilled and slit lamp exam shows normal optic nerve and macula OU and **nuclear cataracts bilaterally**. The cataract OD is a LOC III NO2/NC2 and the cataract OS is slightly more opaque at a LOC III NO3/NC3.

Impression: **Bilateral nuclear cataracts in early stages.**

Plan: Dispense glasses to correct myopia. She is advised to wear sunglasses when out of doors. Follow up in 3 months. If changes are minimal she can be followed at 6 month intervals. Her diet was reviewed and she eats ample fresh fruits and vegetables, no processed foods, and healthy fats and protein sources. She is advised she can take a supplemental multivitamin/mineral if she wishes and that she should look for one that contains Lutein, Zeaxanthin and Omega-3 FA.

ICD-10-CM Diagnosis Code(s)

H25.13	Age-related nuclear cataract, bilateral
H52.13	Myopia, bilateral

Coding Note(s)

The outdated terminology of 'nuclear sclerosis' has been updated in ICD-10-CM, where the same condition is now classified as 'age-related nuclear cataract.' ICD-10-CM also captures laterality with specific codes for left, right, and bilateral cataracts.

Choroidal Degeneration/Dystrophies

The choroid is a tissue layer made up of blood vessels and connective tissue located between the sclera and retina. It supplies nutrients to the inner parts of the eye. Choroidal degeneration refers to disorders that present with progressive loss of cellular or tissue function resulting in structural changes in the choroid. Choroidal degeneration can occur as part of age-related macular degeneration. Provider documentation of any associated disease process is needed for optimal code assignment.

Careful review of the documentation is necessary when coding choroidal degeneration, atrophy, or dystrophy of the choroid. Atrophy refers to the anatomic changes from the loss of cells and tissue due to cell death and dystrophy refers to acquired cell or tissue degeneration as a result of a genetic defect or mutation. Previously there was a specific code for dystrophies primarily involving Bruch's membrane of the eye and specific codes for choroidal degeneration (sclerosis) unspecified, senile atrophy of the choroid, diffuse secondary atrophy of the choroid, and angioid streaks of the choroid (There is no longer a specific code for dystrophies involving Bruch's membrane. This condition is reported with the same codes as those for unspecified choroidal degeneration (H31.10-), age-related choroidal atrophy (H31.11-), or diffuse secondary atrophy of the choroid (H31.12-) depending on the physician's documentation.

Angioid streaks of choroid are no longer classified with codes for choroidal degenerations. This condition has been moved to subcategory H35.3 Degeneration of macula and posterior pole and is reported with code H35.33 Angioid streaks of macula. Laterality is not a component of the classification of angioid streaks of the macula so there is only a single code to report this condition.

It should also be noted that disease terminology has been updated to reflect current medical knowledge. For example, senile choroidal atrophy is the same as age-related choroidal atrophy The Alphabetic Index entry for Atrophy, choroid, senile will direct the coder to age-related choroidal atrophy.

Coding and Documentation Requirements

Identify condition:

- Choroidal degeneration (sclerosis) or atrophy
  - Age-related choroidal atrophy
  - Diffuse secondary atrophy of choroid
  - Unspecified choroidal degeneration

- Angioid streaks of macula (choroid)

Identify laterality for choroidal degeneration/atrophy:

- Right eye
- Left eye
- Bilateral
- Unspecified

ICD-10-CM Code/Documentation					
Choroidal Degeneration					
Degeneration unspecified		Age-related atrophy		Diffuse secondary atrophy	
H31.101	right eye	H31.111	right eye	H31.121	right eye
H31.102	left eye	H31.112	left eye	H31.122	left eye
H31.103	bilateral	H31.113	bilateral	H31.123	bilateral
H31.109	unspecified	H31.119	unspecified	H31.129	unspecified

Documentation and Coding Example

Seventy-nine-year-old Caucasian female presents to Ophthalmology clinic with her caregiver for continued monitoring of eye disease. Patient is well known to this practice, having been treated for **senile degenerative choroidal atrophy and retinal neovascularization in both eyes** for many years. She is a well-respected artist and a valued philanthropist in the community. She walks into the examination room on the arm of her caregiver but once settled into the chair she appears quite at ease and in control of her surroundings. Visual field acuity is significant for loss centrally in both eyes but she has fairly wide peripheral fields bilaterally. Intraocular pressure is normal in both eyes. She has been previously treated with intravitreal injections of Avastin and that seems to have controlled **neovascularization in her retinas**. Today we perform rapid sequence fluorescein angiography and optical coherence tomography. Both tests show hyperfluorescence dye leakage from retinal neovascularization but her disease appears stable at the present time. RTC in 3 months for recheck.

Diagnosis: **Bilateral age-related degenerative choroidal atrophy and retinal neovascularization.**

ICD-10-CM Diagnosis Code(s)

H31.113 Age-related choroidal atrophy, bilateral

H35.053 Retinal neovascularization, unspecified, bilateral

Coding Note(s)

In the Alphabetic Index, under the main term Atrophy, and subterms choroid and senile, the coder is referred to code H31.11- Age-related choroidal atrophy. An additional code is reported for retinal neovascularization because it is not an inherent part of the disease process for age-related choroidal atrophy.

Glaucoma

Glaucoma is a group of eye disorders characterized by elevated intraocular pressure that can cause optic nerve damage. There are a number of different types of glaucoma. The most common is a chronic condition called open angle glaucoma that develops painlessly over time. Another type, acute angle closure glaucoma, is a painful condition that develops quickly and must be treated emergently if vision is to be spared in one or both eyes. Congenital glaucoma is a type that is present at birth and usually results from abnormal eye development. Secondary glaucoma is caused by another condition such as trauma, eye disease, systemic illness, or as a side effect of medications, such as corticosteroids.

There is a great deal of variability in the care and resource utilization among glaucoma patients, so diagnosis codes that reflect disease severity allow for better management and treatment outcomes. Increased specificity of glaucoma codes was integrated to identify the stages of glaucoma. Codes reflect staging of glaucoma into mild, moderate, and severe disease based on the provider's documentation of the visual field in the patient's worse eye. There are also codes for indeterminate stage glaucoma and unspecified glaucoma stage. In order to code the patient's condition to the highest level of specificity, both the specific type and stage of glaucoma must be documented.

Glaucoma codes are located in two categories. Category H40 Glaucoma is specific to type, laterality, and stage. A 7th character is appended to capture the stage. The available 7th characters for reporting the stage are as follows:

0 – Stage unspecified
1 – Mild stage
2 – Moderate stage
3 – Severe stage
4 – Indeterminate stage

Three character category code H42 is used for Glaucoma in diseases classified elsewhere, has no additional qualifiers, and is reported secondary to the underlying condition, such as amyloidosis, aniridia, Lowe's syndrome, Rieger's anomaly, or other specified metabolic disorder.

ICD-10-CM Coding and Documentation Requirements

Identify type:

- Glaucoma in diseases classified elsewhere
  - Code first underlying condition such as:
    - » amyloidosis (E85.-)
    - » aniridia (Q13.1)
    - » glaucoma (in) diabetes mellitus (E08.39, E09.39, E10.39, E13.39)
    - » Lowe's syndrome (E72.03)
    - » Rieger's anomaly (Q13.81)
    - » specific metabolic disorder (E70-88)
- Glaucoma suspect
  - Anatomical narrow angle (primary angle closure suspect)
  - Open angle with borderline findings
    - » High risk
    - » Low risk
  - Ocular hypertension
  - Preglaucoma
  - Primary angle closure without glaucoma damage
  - Steroid responder
- Open-angle glaucoma
  - Capsular glaucoma with pseudoexfoliation of lens
  - Chronic simple glaucoma

  - Low-tension glaucoma
  - Pigmentary glaucoma
  - Primary open-angle glaucoma
  - Residual stage of open-angle glaucoma
  - Unspecified open angle glaucoma
- Primary angle-closure glaucoma
  - Acute angle-closure glaucoma (attack) (crisis)
  - Chronic (primary) angle-closure glaucoma
  - Intermittent angle-closure glaucoma
  - Residual stage of angle-closure glaucoma
  - Unspecified
- Secondary glaucoma (due to)
  - Drugs
  - Eye inflammation
  - Eye trauma
  - Other eye disorders
- Other specified type of glaucoma
  - Aqueous misdirection (malignant glaucoma)
  - Hypersecretion glaucoma
  - With increased episcleral venous pressure
  - Other specified type
- Unspecified type
- Identify laterality:
- Right eye
- Left eye
- Bilateral
- Unspecified
- Identify stage using the appropriate 7th character:
  - 0 – Stage unspecified
  - 1 – Mild stage
  - 2 – Moderate stage
  - 3 – Severe stage
  - 4 – Indeterminate stage

Note: Stage is not required for conditions listed under glaucoma suspect, residual stage, acute or intermittent angle-closure glaucoma, other specified types of glaucoma (aqueous misdirection, hypersecretion, glaucoma with increased episcleral venous pressure), unspecified glaucoma, or glaucoma in diseases classified elsewhere.

Use an additional code for adverse effect, if applicable, to identify the drug (T36-T50 with fifth or sixth character 5) in cases of glaucoma secondary to drugs.

Code also the underlying condition for glaucoma secondary to eye trauma, eye inflammation, and other eye disorders.

ICD-10-CM Code/Documentation	
A 7th character is required to identify the stage on the common glaucoma codes listed below	
H40.111	Primary open-angle glaucoma, right eye
H40.112	Primary open-angle glaucoma, left eye
H40.113	Primary open-angle glaucoma, bilateral
H40.119	Primary open-angle glaucoma, unspecified
H40.211	Acute angle-closure glaucoma, right eye
H40.212	Acute angle-closure glaucoma, left eye
H40.213	Acute angle-closure glaucoma, bilateral
H40.219	Acute angle-closure glaucoma, unspecified

Documentation and Coding Example

Patient is a 45-year-old African-American male who presents to the office today for ongoing care of glaucoma. This gentleman was diagnosed two years ago with **angle-closure glaucoma bilaterally.** Eye pressure was initially difficult to control and his **left eye progressed fairly rapidly to moderate disease. Clinically, the stage of disease in his right eye was difficult to determine, however both eyes appeared to be stabilized** at his exam six months ago using Cosopt eye drops bilaterally BID. Patient states he is having no side effects from the medication. On examination, his visual field perception is unchanged in both eyes with only minimal visual loss in the outer periphery of the right but circumferential in the left. Visual acuity is also unchanged on the right at 20/100 but slightly improved on the left at 20/200. His current glasses prescription for distance and reading is working fine for him. Right eye pressure is 22 mmHG, left is 23 mmHG. Slit lamp exam shows no unusual tissue growth and smooth conjunctiva and corneas bilaterally. Gonioscopy exam shows adequate fluid drainage in both eyes. Scanning laser polarimetry and optical coherence tomography is performed and compared to previous studies. Disease is stable at this time. Treatment options discussed with patient. He is not experiencing any side effects from the medication and he has good insurance coverage so it is not a financial burden to obtain the prescriptions each month. Patient has some anxiety about surgery on his eyes and as long as the medication is working, he prefers not to do any other type of treatment at this time. RTC in 6 months, sooner if symptoms arise.

Diagnosis: **Bilateral chronic angle-closure glaucoma.**

ICD-10-CM Diagnosis Code(s)

H40.2222 Chronic angle-closure glaucoma, left eye, moderate stage

H40.2214 Chronic angle-closure glaucoma, right eye, indeterminate stage

Coding Note(s)

When a patient has bilateral glaucoma and each eye is documented as having a different type or stage, and the classification distinguishes laterality, assign the appropriate code for each eye rather than the code for bilateral glaucoma. The seventh code character "2" is assigned to identify moderate stage glaucoma in the left eye and the seventh character "4" is assigned to the glaucoma code for the right eye because the stage cannot be clinically determined. The seventh character "4" is used for glaucomas whose stage cannot be clinically determined, and should not be confused with the seventh character "0," unspecified, which should be assigned when there is no documentation regarding the stage of the glaucoma.

Pterygium

A pterygium is a benign growth or thickening of the conjunctiva that grows onto the cornea. As it grows, the pterygium may become red and irritated and may cause visual disturbances. Pterygium is typically associated with ultraviolet light exposure but chronic conjunctival inflammation can cause localized amyloidosis.

There are a number of specific types of pterygiums identified in ICD-10-CM including a subcategory for amyloid pterygium (H11.01) which previously was reported with an unspecified code. Amyloid is a protein that gets deposited in the body organs and tissues where it may accumulate as in amyloid deposits on the conjunctiva.

ICD-10-CM Coding and Documentation Requirements

Identify type:

- Amyloid pterygium
- Central pterygium
- Double pterygium
- Peripheral pterygium
    - Progressive
    - Stationary
- Recurrent (same indent as peripheral)
- Unspecified pterygium

Identify laterality:

- Right eye
- Left eye
- Bilateral
- Unspecified

ICD-10-CM Code/Documentation	
H11.001	Unspecified pterygium of right eye
H11.002	Unspecified pterygium of left eye
H11.003	Unspecified pterygium of eye, bilateral
H11.009	Unspecified pterygium of eye, unspecified
H11.011	Amyloid pterygium of right eye
H11.012	Amyloid pterygium of left eye
H11.013	Amyloid pterygium of eye, bilateral
H11.019	Amyloid pterygium of eye, unspecified
H11.021	Central pterygium of right eye
H11.022	Central pterygium of left eye
H11.023	Central pterygium of eye, bilateral
H11.029	Central pterygium of unspecified eye
H11.031	Double pterygium of right eye
H11.032	Double pterygium of left eye
H11.033	Double pterygium of eye, bilateral
H11.039	Double pterygium of unspecified eye
H11.041	Peripheral pterygium, stationary, of right eye
H11.042	Peripheral pterygium, stationary, of left eye
H11.043	Peripheral pterygium, stationary, of eye, bilateral
H11.049	Peripheral pterygium, stationary, of unspecified eye
H11.051	Peripheral pterygium, stationary, of right eye
H11.052	Peripheral pterygium, progressive, of left eye
H11.053	Peripheral pterygium, progressive, of eye, bilateral
H11.059	Peripheral pterygium, progressive, of unspecified eye
H11.061	Recurrent pterygium of right eye
H11.062	Recurrent pterygium of left eye
H11.063	Recurrent pterygium of eye, bilateral
H11.069	Recurrent pterygium of unspecified eye

Documentation and Coding Example

This 34-year-old Caucasian male is self-referred to Ophthalmology with concerns about excessive tearing and patchy white growths in his eyes with occasional blurred vision in the left eye. Patient teaches physical education at the local high school and is an avid outdoorsman. He snowboards in winter, plays golf at least 9 months of the year, enjoys water sports on the local lake in the summer. He always wears sunglasses and/or a hat outside. He denies eye pain other than mild irritation relieved by OTC eye drops. On examination, visual acuity is 20/20, near and far. The eyes bilaterally have mild redness of the conjunctiva with no evidence of blepharitis. A small white patch is noted in the **upper inner edge of the right cornea** and a larger patch in the **lower outer edge of the left cornea.** Slit lamp exam confirms that they are located right on the edge of the cornea, slightly raised and contain a network of small blood vessels. **The characteristics are typical of amyloid pterygium.** Lesion on right eye is approximately 3mm x 4 mm and left eye measures 7mm x 9 mm. Corneal topography and photography is performed to document size and shape. Patient is counseled that these are usually benign growths but it would be wise to remove the lesion on the left because it is starting to affect vision. Patient is in agreement with that plan and is referred for surgical consultation.

Diagnosis:

Amyloid pterygium, right eye, 3mm x 4 mm.

Amyloid pterygium left eye, 7mm x 9 mm.

ICD-10-CM Diagnosis Code(s)

H11.013 Amyloid pterygium of eye, bilateral

Coding Note(s)

ICD-10-CM includes specific subcategories for the different types of pterygium. These codes further specify the affected eye as right, left, or bilateral.

Summary

Best practices in documentation of disorders of the eye and adnexa require more detailed information on the diagnosis and treatment of these conditions. In addition to general documentation requirements such as the severity or status of the disease, the affected site, the etiology, and any secondary disease process, there are specific diseases and disorders that require greater detail in medical record documentation to ensure optimal code assignment.

ICD-10-CM includes greater specificity regarding the type and the cause of eye disorders which must be documented in the medical record. Many codes require more specific documentation of the site including right, left, or bilateral and upper or lower eyelid.

Understanding new, updated, and more specific coding terminology will be needed in addition to more detailed documentation of the patient's condition. Some aspects of coding diseases of the eye and adnexa are improved in ICD-10-CM with the addition of a number of combination codes that identify both the disorder and the common manifestation.

Resources

Documentation checklists are available in Appendix B for the following condition(s):

- Cataract
- Conjunctivitis
- Diabetes Mellitus
- Glaucoma

Eye and Adnexa Quiz

1. Where are the combination codes for diabetes mellitus with eye conditions classified in ICD-10-CM?
   a. Chapter 1 - Certain infectious and parasitic diseases (A00-B99)
   b. Chapter 4 - Endocrine, nutritional and metabolic diseases (E00-E89)
   c. Chapter 7 - Diseases of the Eye and Adnexa (H00-H59)
   d. Chapter 18 - Symptoms, signs and abnormal clinical and laboratory findings, not elsewhere classified (R00-R99)
2. Which of the following disorders of the eye and adnexa are NOT classified in ICD-10-CM Chapter 7 Diseases of the Eye and Adnexa (H00-H59)?
   a. Conditions associated with a neoplastic process
   b. Complications of pregnancy, childbirth and the puerperium
   c. Conditions resulting from injury or trauma to the eye and orbit
   d. All of the above
3. Which of the following statements is true regarding coding of glaucoma?
   a. Dual codes are required to report the type and stage of glaucoma
   b. A combination code can be used to report the type and stage of glaucoma
   c. Laterality needs to be documented in the medical record
   d. Both B and D
4. How is a diagnosis of senile choroidal atrophy classified in?
   a. Age-related choroidal atrophy
   b. Choroidal degeneration or sclerosis
   c. Diffuse secondary atrophy of choroid
   d. All of the above
5. How are postprocedural complications of eye and adnexa classified?
   a. In Chapter 19 Injury, poisoning and certain other consequences of external causes (S00-T88)
   b. In Chapter 20 External causes of morbidity (V00-Y99)
   c. In Chapter 21 Factors influencing health status and contact with health services
   d. In Chapter 7 in a separate code block at the end of the chapter
6. The physician documents the patient's diagnosis as bilateral glaucoma but there is no documentation regarding determination of the stage of the glaucoma. What 7th character glaucoma stage is assigned in this case?
   a. 0
   b. 1
   c. 4
   d. None, the provider must be queried for documentation of the glaucoma stage
7. The physician documents bilateral glaucoma and documents each eye as having a different type or stage. How is this coded?
   a. One code is assigned for each type of glaucoma but only the 7th character for the highest glaucoma stage is assigned.
   b. The code for each eye is assigned for each type of glaucoma with the appropriate 7th character for the stage.
   c. The code for bilateral glaucoma is assigned with the 7th character for the highest glaucoma stage
   d. The code for bilateral glaucoma is assigned twice with the 7th character for Residual stage glaucoma
8. How is glaucoma associated with ocular trauma coded?
   a. With a code from Chapter 7 Diseases of the eye and adnexa (H00-H59)
   b. With a code from Chapter 19 Injury, poisoning and certain other consequences of external causes (S00-T88)
   c. With a code from Chapter 20 External causes of morbidity (V00-Y99)
   d. With a code from Chapter 21 Factors influencing health status and contact with health services
9. A patient was admitted with moderate stage glaucoma but during the admission, the stage progresses to severe glaucoma. What is the principal diagnosis?
   a. The code for the stage documented on discharge
   b. The code for the stage documented on admission
   c. The code for the highest glaucoma stage is documented
   d. The code for the indeterminate stage
10. The physician has documented that the patient has bilateral choroidal degeneration due to Bruch's membrane dystrophy. How is this coded?
   a. There are no codes for choroidal degeneration due to Bruch's membrane dystrophy so the physician must be queried.
   b. With code H31.8 Other specified disorders of the choroid
   c. With code H31.103 Choroidal degeneration, unspecified, bilateral
   d. With code H31.123 Diffuse secondary atrophy of choroid, bilateral

See next page for answers and rationales.

Eye and Adnexa Quiz Answers and Rationales

1. Where are the combination codes for diabetes mellitus with eye conditions classified in ICD-10-CM?

   b. Chapter 4 - Endocrine, nutritional and metabolic diseases (E00-E89)

   Rationale: According to the Excludes2 note at the beginning of Chapter 7 of ICD-10-CM, diabetes mellitus related eye conditions are coded to E08.3-, E09.3-, E10.3-, E11.3-, and E13.3-, classified in Chapter 4.

2. Which of the following disorders of the eye and adnexa are NOT classified in ICD-10-CM Chapter 7 Diseases of the Eye and Adnexa (H00-H59)?

   d. All of the above

   Rationale: All of the listed conditions are included in the list of excluded conditions at the beginning of Chapter 7.

3. Which of the following statements is true regarding coding of glaucoma?

   d. Both B and D

   Rationale: ICD-10-CM Tabular List includes combination codes that identify the type, stage and laterality of glaucoma. The ICD-10-CM guidelines for coding glaucoma provide additional direction.

4. How is a diagnosis of senile choroidal atrophy classified?

   a. Age-related choroidal atrophy

   Rationale: The Index entry for atrophy of the choroid, senile directs the coder to age-related choroidal atrophy.

5. How are postprocedural complications of eye and adnexa classified?

   d. In Chapter 7 in a separate code block at the end of the chapter

   Rationale: ICD-10-CM has a separate code block at the end of Chapter 7 (H59) to classify all intraoperative and postprocedural complications from treatment of eye and adnexa disorders together.

6. The physician documents the patient's diagnosis as bilateral glaucoma but there is no documentation regarding determination of the stage of the glaucoma. What 7th character glaucoma stage is assigned in this case?

   a. 0

   Rationale: The glaucoma codes in the Tabular List of ICD-10-CM include an instructional note directing the user to assign one of the listed 7th characters to the code to designate the stage of glaucoma. According to the ICD-10-CM Official Guidelines for Coding and Reporting Section I.C.7.a.5 the seventh character "0," unspecified, should be assigned when there is no documentation regarding the stage of the glaucoma.

7. The physician documents bilateral glaucoma and documents each eye as having a different type or stage. How is this coded?

   b. The code for each eye is assigned for each type of glaucoma with the appropriate 7th character for the stage.

   Rationale: According to the ICD-10-CM Official Guidelines for Coding and Reporting Section I.C.7.a.3, assign a code for the type of glaucoma for each eye with the seventh character for the specific glaucoma stage documented for each eye.

8. How is glaucoma associated with ocular trauma coded?

   a. With a code from Chapter 7 Diseases of the eye and adnexa (H00-H59)

   Rationale: In ICD-10-CM, glaucoma secondary to eye trauma is coded to H40.30-H40.33 based on the affected eye(s) with a 7th character of 0-4 to identify the glaucoma stage. An additional code is assigned also to identify the underlying condition.

9. A patient was admitted with moderate stage glaucoma but during the admission, the stage progresses to severe glaucoma. What is the principal diagnosis?

   c. The code for the highest glaucoma stage is documented

   Rationale: According to Section I.C.7.a.4 of the ICD-10-CM Official Guidelines for Coding and Reporting, when a patient is admitted with glaucoma and the stage evolves during the admission, assign the code for highest stage documented.

10. The physician has documented that the patient has bilateral choroidal degeneration due to Bruch's membrane dystrophy. How is this coded?

    c. With code H31.103 Choroidal degeneration, unspecified, bilateral

    Rationale: There is no entry in the alphabetic index for Dystrophy, Bruch's membrane. However, the physician has specified that the patient has choroidal degeneration due to Bruch's dystrophy. Searching the Alphabetic Index under the entry Degeneration, Bruch's membrane, the instruction is given to see degeneration, choroid and when that term is located, the code provided is H31.10-. The 6th character 3 is added to identify the condition as bilateral.

CPT® Procedural Coding

Introduction

Current Procedural Terminology (CPT®) codes are published by the American Medical Association (AMA). The purpose of this coding system is to provide a uniform language for reporting services provided to patients.

A CPT Category I code is a five-digit numeric code used to describe medical, surgical, radiological, laboratory, anesthesiology, and evaluation and management (E/M) services performed by physicians, and other health care providers or entities. There are over 8,000 CPT codes ranging from 00100 through 99607. Beginning in 2002, the AMA added Category III (emerging technology) codes. In 2004, the AMA introduced Category II (supplemental tracking) codes. Both Category II and III codes are five-digit alphanumeric codes.

The entire family of procedure codes acceptable to Medicare is referred to as HCPCS, which is an acronym for:

H Healthcare

C Common

P Procedure

C Coding

S System

This family is comprised of two distinct parts or levels: Level I and Level II.

HCPCS Level I Codes (CPT)

HCPCS Level I codes consist of the five-digit codes listed in the *CPT®* codebook published by the American Medical Association. These are the most frequently used codes to report services and procedures, since the codebook mainly consists of physician procedures. The codes are updated annually, and the new codes for the upcoming year are available at the end of the preceding year for use on January 1.

HCPCS Level II Codes

HCPCS Level II codes consist of five-digit alphanumeric codes utilizing letters A-V, and were developed specifically by the Centers for Medicare & Medicaid Services (CMS) to report services and supplies not found in Level I. HCPCS Level II is a standardized coding system that is used primarily to identify products; supplies; drugs and biologicals; durable medical equipment, prosthetics, orthotics, and supplies (DMEPOS); quality reporting measures; some physician and non-physician provider services; and other services, such as ambulance services. HCPCS Level II codes are recognized by Medicare and many other third-party payers.

The CPT Codebook

This coding reference book, which is updated annually, is organized into nine sections, sixteen appendices, and an alphabetic index. There are specific guidelines listed in the CPT codebook at the beginning of each section. These guidelines indicate interpretations and appropriate reporting of codes contained in that particular section. The guidelines should be reviewed prior to using any code in that section. The sections include:

- **Introduction and Illustrated Anatomical and Procedural Review** — Contains basic instructions for using the CPT codebook and reviews basic medical terminology and anatomy with additional information, references, and illustrations.
- **Evaluation and Management** — Provides the codes and guidelines for reporting patient evaluation and management services, most of which are face-to-face with the provider and based on established or new patient status. The codes are broadly grouped into place of service, such as office, hospital, outpatient or ambulatory surgical center, emergency department, nursing home or other residential facility and/or type of service, such as observation, consultations, critical care, newborn care, and preventive care.
- **Anesthesia** — Provides guidelines, codes, and modifiers for reporting services involving the administration of anesthesia for different types of procedures and on various locations of the body.
- **Surgery** — Identifies surgical procedures performed across all specialties and body systems. The procedure normally includes the necessary, related services in the surgical package without being stated as part of the code description.
- **Radiology** — Lists codes for diagnostic imaging, ultrasound, radiological guidance, radiation oncology, and nuclear medicine. Procedures in this section include X-ray, fluoroscopy, computed tomography, magnetic resonance imaging, angiography, lymphangiography, mammography, radiological supervision and interpretation for therapeutic transcatheter procedures, bone studies, radiation treatment and planning for cancer, brachytherapy, and radiopharmaceutical procedures.
- **Pathology and Laboratory** — Contains codes for reporting procedures and services processed in a laboratory facility. Tests include organ or disease panels, drug assays, urinalysis, chemistry profiles, microorganism identification, immunoassays, pathological examination of surgical samples, and reproductive-related procedures.
- **Medicine** — Identifies procedures that usually do not require operating room services. The medicine codes provided in this section cover a wide spectrum of specialties and include

both diagnostic and therapeutic procedures. This section includes procedures, such as neuromuscular testing, cardiac catheterization, acupuncture, dialysis, chemotherapy, vaccine administration, and psychiatric services.

- **Category II Codes** — List supplemental, optional tracking codes composed of four digits and the letter F. These codes are intended to reduce the need for record abstraction and chart review and facilitate data collection by those seeking to measure quality of patient care.
- **Category III Codes** — Provides temporary codes composed of four digits and the letter T, established for reporting and tracking data for emerging technology, services, and procedures. When a Category III code is available, it must be used rather than reporting an unlisted code. These codes may or may not be assigned a Category I code at a future date.

The appendices include:

- **Appendix A – Modifiers** — Lists all the applicable modifiers for the CPT codes to identify when a service or procedure was altered by a specific circumstance or to provide additional information about the procedure performed. This includes anesthesia physical status modifiers, CPT Level I modifiers approved for ambulatory surgical centers and hospital outpatient departments, Category II modifiers, and Level II HCPCS National modifiers.
- **Appendix B – Summary of Additions, Deletions, and Revisions** — Shows the current year's changes that were made to the codes.
- **Appendix C – Clinical Examples** — Gives real-life clinical scenarios and examples of patient evaluation and management encounters to help medical offices in reporting services provided to the patient.
- **Appendix D – Summary of CPT Add-on Codes** — Lists in numerical sequence all the codes designated in CPT as add-on codes. The add-on codes are only to be assigned in addition to the principal procedure and never stand alone. Add-on codes are also not subject to modifier 51 rules. These codes are additionally identified with a ✚ symbol.
- **Appendix E – Summary of CPT Codes Exempt from Modifier 51** — Lists in numerical sequence all the CPT codes designated as exempt from the use of modifier 51 that have not been identified as add-on procedures or services. These codes are additionally identified with a ⊘ symbol.
- **Appendix F – Summary of CPT Codes Exempt from Modifier 63** — Lists in numerical sequence all the CPT codes designated as exempt from the use of modifier 63. These codes are additionally identified with a parenthetical instruction.
- **Appendix G – Summary of CPT Codes That Include Moderate (Conscious) Sedation** — Summary of CPT codes that include moderate (conscious) sedation (formerly Appendix G) has been removed from the CPT code set. The codes that were previously included were revised to remove the moderate (conscious) sedation symbol. For guidance on reporting codes formerly listed in Appendix G, refer to the guidelines for codes 99151-99153 and 99155-99157.
- **Appendix H – Alphabetical Clinical Topics Listing** — The Alphabetical Clinical Topics Listing (formerly Appendix H) has been removed from the CPT codebook. Since performance measures are subject to change each year, the alphabetic index to performance measures is now maintained on the AMA website at www.ama-assn.org/go/cpt. The online version will continue to provide measures in table format listed alphabetically by the disease or condition and crosswalked to the Category II codes used to report the quality measure.
- **Appendix I – Genetic Testing Code Modifiers** — The list of Genetic Testing Code Modifiers (formerly Appendix I) has been removed from the CPT code set. The addition of hundreds of molecular pathology codes resulted in the deletion of the stacking codes to which these modifiers applied. For the most current updates for molecular pathology coding in the CPT code set, see the AMA CPT website at www.ama-assn.org/go/cpt.
- **Appendix J – Electrodiagnostic Medicine Listing of Sensory, Motor, and Mixed Nerves** — Assigns each sensory, motor, and mixed nerve with its proper nerve conduction study code in order to improve accurate reporting of codes 95907-95913.
- **Appendix K – Product Pending FDA Approval** — Identifies vaccines that have already been assigned Category I codes that are still awaiting FDA approval. These are identified with the symbol ⚡.
- **Appendix L – Vascular Families** — Outlines the tree of vascular families and identifies first-, second-, and third-order branches, assuming the beginning point is the aorta, vena cava, pulmonary artery, or portal vein.
- **Appendix M – Renumbered CPT Codes – Citations Crosswalk** — This listing identifies codes that were deleted and renumbered from 2007 to 2009, and their crosswalk to current year code(s).
- **Appendix N – Summary of Resequenced CPT Codes** — This list identifies codes that do not appear in numeric sequence. Instead of deleting and renumbering existing codes that need to be moved, the existing codes are now being moved to the correct location without being renumbered. Resequenced codes are relocated to appear with codes for the appropriate code concept. The CPT codebook lists the code in numeric sequence without the code description. Instead, a parenthetical note is listed referencing the range of codes in which the resequenced code appears. The resequenced code is identified with a # symbol, and the full code description is listed for the resequenced code.
- **Appendix O – Multianalyte Assays with Algorithmic Analyses** — This list identifies codes for Multianalyte Assays with Algorithmic Analyses (MAAA) procedures that utilize multiple results derived from various types of assays (e.g., molecular pathology assays, non-nucleic acid based assays) that are typically unique to a single clinical laboratory or manufacturer.
- **Appendix P – CPT Codes That May Be Used For Synchronous Telemedicine Services** — This appendix first appeared in 2017 to list codes that may be used for

reporting real-time telemedicine services when appended by modifier 95. These procedures include interactive electronic communication using audio-visual telecommunications equipment. These are identified with the ★ symbol.

- **Appendix Q – Severe Acute Respiratory Syndrome Coronavirus 2 (SARS-CoV-2) (coronavirus disease [COVID-19]) Vaccines** — This appendix is new to the CPT 2022 code set. The table in Appendix Q links the COVID-19 vaccine product codes (91300, 91301, 91302, 91303, 91304) to their associated immunization administration codes (0001A, 0002A, 0011A, 0012A, 0021A, 0022A, 0031A, 0041A, 0042A), manufacturer name, vaccine name(s), 10- and 11-digit National Drug Code (NDC) Labeler Product ID, and interval between doses. These codes are also located in the **Medicine** section of the CPT code set.
- **Appendix R – Digital Medicine—Services Taxonomy** — This appendix is new to the CPT 2022 code set. Appendix R is a listing of digital medicine services described in the CPT code set. The digital medicine–services taxonomy table in this appendix classifies CPT codes that are related to digital medicine services into discrete categories of clinician-to-patient services (eg, visit), clinician-to-clinician services (eg, consultation), patient-monitoring services, and digital diagnostic services.

Locating a CPT Code

Once familiar with the CPT codebook, identifying appropriate codes becomes less of a task. The numbers at the top of each page are for easy reference and give the range of codes located on that particular page.

Most sections list the sequence of codes in the following order:

- Top to bottom of body (head to toe)
- Central to peripheral in some subsections (i.e., cardiovascular and nervous system codes)
- Outside to inside of body (incision/excision)

There are two ways to locate a code in the CPT codebook:

- By anatomical site (numerically)
- The Index (alphabetically)

A code can be located simply by knowing the site or body system. For example, if a patient had an EKG performed in the emergency department, the user should try to locate a code through the Index. Alternatively, the coder could rationalize that a medicine service was performed to monitor the patient's heart which is part of the cardiovascular system. Since those medicine codes are found in the 93000 series of codes, the coder could then look in this section of the CPT codebook to locate the appropriate code.

The Index is organized by main terms, shown in bold typeface. There are four primary classes of main entries:

- Procedure or service – e.g., Cardiac Catheterization, Angioplasty
- Organ or other anatomic site – e.g., Heart, Chest, Abdomen
- Condition – e.g., Angina, Myocardial Infarction
- Synonyms, eponyms, and abbreviations – EKG, EMG, DXA

The main term is divided into specific sub-terms that help in selecting the appropriate code.

Whenever more than one code applies to a given index entry, a code range is listed. If two or more nonsequential codes apply, they will be separated by a comma. For example:

Electrocardiography

Evaluation … 0178T-0180T, 93000, 93010, 93660

If more than one sequential code applies, they will be separated by a hyphen. For example:

Office and/or Other Outpatient Services

Established patient … 99211-99215

A cross reference provides instructions to the user on where to look when entries are listed under another heading.

See directs the user to refer to the term listed. This is used primarily for synonyms, eponyms, and abbreviations, such as:

Ear Canal
See Auditory Canal

The alphabetic index is not a substitute for the main text of CPT. The user must always refer to the main text to ensure that the code selection is accurate and not assign any codes from the index entry alone.

CPT Symbols

In addition to understanding the layout of CPT and knowing how to reference the book, the user must also understand symbols and their meanings.

● Indicates a new code has been added to the edition the coder is referencing. For example:

● 0474T Insertion of anterior segment aqueous drainage device, with creation of intraocular reservoir, internal approach, into the supraciliary space

▲ Indicates the code number is the same, but the definition or description has changed since the last edition. For example:

▲ 67101 Repair of retinal detachment, including drainage of subretinal fluid when performed; cryotherapy

; Indicates a selection of suffixes that append to the main portion (prefix) of the code. For example:

96372 Therapeutic, prophylactic, or diagnostic injection (specify substance or drug); subcutaneous or intramuscular

96373 Therapeutic, prophylactic, or diagnostic injection (specify substance or drug); intra-arterial

96374 Therapeutic, prophylactic, or diagnostic injection (specify substance or drug); intravenous push single or initial substance/drug

⊘ Identifies codes that are exempt from the use of modifier 51, but have not been designated as add-on procedures/services.

⊘ 31500 Intubation, endotracheal, emergency procedure

Note: For more information on modifier 51, see the Modifier chapter.

★ Identifies telemedicine codes.

★ 90832 Psychotherapy, 30 minutes with patient

⁄⁄ Identifies codes that have been created for vaccines that are pending FDA approval (at the time of the publication of that year's CPT codebook).

⁄⁄ 90739 Hepatitis B vaccine (HepB), adult dosage, 2 dose schedule, for intramuscular use

Add-on Codes

Add-on procedures or services are ones that are performed in addition to the primary procedure/service. In the CPT codebook, a ✚ indicates a CPT add-on code.

99291 Critical care, evaluation and management of the critically ill or critically injured patient; first 30-74 minutes

✚99292 each additional 30 minutes (List separately in addition to code for primary service)

The add-on procedure is performed on the same day by the same provider that performed the primary procedure/service. These codes should never be reported alone and should not be reported with modifier 51.

Modifiers

Modifiers consist of two numeric or alphanumeric digits appended to a code to indicate when a service or procedure that still fits the code description was altered by a specific circumstance or when additional information about the procedure performed needs to be provided.

Unlisted Procedure or Service

The procedure performed may not always be found with a designated code assignment in the CPT codebook. Unlisted procedure codes are provided in every section to be used in these cases. An accompanying operative report or other visit documentation is required when reporting unlisted codes in order for the payer to identify what the procedure entailed and determine its eligibility for reimbursement. An unlisted procedure code should not be used when a Category III code best describes the procedure performed.

Surgical Package

The concept of a global fee for surgical procedures is a long-established concept under which a single fee is billed that pays for all necessary services normally furnished by the surgeon before, during, and after the procedure. Since the fee schedule is based on uniform national relative values, it is necessary to have a uniform national definition of global surgery to assure that equivalent payment is made for the same amount of work and resources.

The following items are included in the global package reimbursement:

- Local anesthesia, digital block, or topical anesthesia
- After the decision for surgery is made, one E/M service one day before or the day of surgery
- Postoperative care that occurs directly after the procedure
- Examining the patient in the recovery area
- Any postoperative care occurring during the designated postoperative period

To assist in this uniform implementation, the CPT Editorial Panel created five modifiers (24, 25, 59, 78, and 79) to identify a service or procedure furnished during a global period that is not a part of the global surgery fee, such as a service unrelated to the condition requiring surgery or for treating the underlying condition and not for normal recovery from the surgery. Use of these modifiers allows such services to be reported in addition to the global fee.

Category II Codes

The Category II section of CPT contains a set of supplemental tracking codes that can be used for performance measurement. This section of codes was implemented in 2004 to facilitate data collection about the quality of care rendered for specific conditions. These codes report certain services and test results that support nationally established performance measures with evidence of contributing to increased quality patient care. It is not required for providers to report these codes; the use of these codes is optional.

Category II codes consist of five-digit alphanumeric codes that end in an F, and the following categories are included in this code set:

- Composite Codes
- Patient Management
- Patient History
- Physical Examination
- Diagnostic/Screening Processes or Results
- Therapeutic, Preventive, or Other Interventions
- Follow-up or Other Outcomes
- Patient Safety
- Structural Measures
- Nonmeasure Code Listing

Category III Codes

Category III codes are temporary codes that identify emerging technologies, services, and procedures and allow for data collection to determine clinical efficacy, utilization, and outcomes. They are alphanumeric codes that consist of four numbers, followed by the letter T.

A Category III code should be reported instead of an unlisted code whenever it accurately describes the procedure that was performed. These temporary codes may or may not be assigned a Category I CPT code in the future.

2022 Ophthalmology CPT Codes and Crosswalks

The 2022 Ophthalmology CPT codes and crosswalks begin following the Surgery Guidelines section. Each code includes official CPT descriptions, official CPT Guidelines, Plain English Descriptions (PED), ICD-10-CM crosswalks, and Medicare-related information including: RVUs, Modifiers, and CCI edits (also known as NCCI).

Note: This Ophthalmology coding book is not intended to replace the AMA's CPT codebook. Use this book in conjunction with the official AMA 2022 CPT codebook.

Surgery Guidelines

Guidelines to direct general reporting of services are presented in the **Introduction**. Some of the commonalities are repeated here for the convenience of those referring to this section on **Surgery**. Other definitions and items unique to Surgery are also listed.

Services

Services rendered in the office, home, or hospital, consultations, and other medical services are listed in the **Evaluation and Management Services** section (99202-99499) beginning on page 19.* "Special Services, Procedures, and Reports" (99000-99082) are listed in the **Medicine** section.

CPT Surgical Package Definition

By their very nature, the services to any patient are variable. The CPT codes that represent a readily identifiable surgical procedure thereby include, on a procedure-by-procedure basis, a variety of services. In defining the specific services "included" in a given CPT surgical code, the following services related to the surgery when furnished by the physician or other qualified health care professional who performs the surgery are included in addition to the operation per se:

- Evaluation and Management (E/M) service(s) subsequent to the decision for surgery on the day before and/or day of surgery (including history and physical)
- Local infiltration, metacarpal/metatarsal/digital block or topical anesthesia
- Immediate postoperative care, including dictating operative notes, talking with the family and other physicians or other qualified health care professionals
- Writing orders
- Evaluating the patient in the postanesthesia recovery area
- Typical postoperative follow-up care

Follow-Up Care for Diagnostic Procedures

Follow-up care for diagnostic procedures (eg, endoscopy, arthroscopy, injection procedures for radiography) includes only that care related to recovery from the diagnostic procedure itself. Care of the condition for which the diagnostic procedure was performed or of other concomitant conditions is not included and may be listed separately.

Follow-Up Care for Therapeutic Surgical Procedures

Follow-up care for therapeutic surgical procedures includes only that care which is usually a part of the surgical service. Complications, exacerbations, recurrence, or the presence of other diseases or injuries requiring additional services should be separately reported.

Supplied Materials

Supplies and materials (eg, sterile trays/drugs), over and above those usually included with the procedure(s) rendered are reported separately. List drugs, trays, supplies, and materials provided. Identify as 99070 or specific supply code.

Reporting More Than One Procedure/Service

When more than one procedure/service is performed on the same date, same session or during a post-operative period (subject to the "surgical package" concept), several CPT modifiers may apply (see Appendix A* for definition).

Separate Procedure

Some of the procedures or services listed in the CPT codebook that are commonly carried out as an integral component of a total service or procedure have been identified by the inclusion of the term "separate procedure." The codes designated as "separate procedure" should not be reported in addition to the code for the total procedure or service of which it is considered an integral component.

However, when a procedure or service that is designated as a "separate procedure" is carried out independently or considered to be unrelated or distinct from other procedures/services provided at that time, it may be reported by itself, or in addition to other procedures/services by appending modifier 59 to the specific "separate procedure" code to indicate that the procedure is not considered to be a component of another procedure, but is a distinct, independent procedure. This may represent a different session, different procedure or surgery, different site or organ system, separate incision/excision, separate lesion, or separate injury (or area of injury in extensive injuries).

Unlisted Service or Procedure

A service or procedure may be provided that is not listed in this edition of the CPT codebook. When reporting such a service, the appropriate "Unlisted Procedure" code may be used to indicate the service, identifying it by "Special Report" as discussed in the section below. The "Unlisted Procedures" and accompanying codes for **Surgery** are as follows:

15999	Unlisted procedure, excision pressure ulcer
17999	Unlisted procedure, skin, mucous membrane and subcutaneous tissue
19499	Unlisted procedure, breast
20999	Unlisted procedure, musculoskeletal system, general
21089	Unlisted maxillofacial prosthetic procedure
21299	Unlisted craniofacial and maxillofacial procedure
21499	Unlisted musculoskeletal procedure, head
21899	Unlisted procedure, neck or thorax
22899	Unlisted procedure, spine
22999	Unlisted procedure, abdomen, musculoskeletal system
23929	Unlisted procedure, shoulder
24999	Unlisted procedure, humerus or elbow
25999	Unlisted procedure, forearm or wrist
26989	Unlisted procedure, hands or fingers
27299	Unlisted procedure, pelvis or hip joint
27599	Unlisted procedure, femur or knee
27899	Unlisted procedure, leg or ankle
28899	Unlisted procedure, foot or toes
29799	Unlisted procedure, casting or strapping
29999	Unlisted procedure, arthroscopy
30999	Unlisted procedure, nose
31299	Unlisted procedure, accessory sinuses
31599	Unlisted procedure, larynx
31899	Unlisted procedure, trachea, bronchi
32999	Unlisted procedure, lungs and pleura
33999	Unlisted procedure, cardiac surgery
36299	Unlisted procedure, vascular injection
37501	Unlisted vascular endoscopy procedure
37799	Unlisted procedure, vascular surgery
38129	Unlisted laparoscopy procedure, spleen
38589	Unlisted laparoscopy procedure, lymphatic system
38999	Unlisted procedure, hemic or lymphatic system
39499	Unlisted procedure, mediastinum
39599	Unlisted procedure, diaphragm
40799	Unlisted procedure, lips
40899	Unlisted procedure, vestibule of mouth
41599	Unlisted procedure, tongue, floor of mouth
41899	Unlisted procedure, dentoalveolar structures
42299	Unlisted procedure, palate, uvula
42699	Unlisted procedure, salivary glands or ducts
42999	Unlisted procedure, pharynx, adenoids, or tonsils
43289	Unlisted laparoscopy procedure, esophagus
43499	Unlisted procedure, esophagus
43659	Unlisted laparoscopy procedure, stomach
43999	Unlisted procedure, stomach
44238	Unlisted laparoscopy procedure, intestine (except rectum)
44799	Unlisted procedure, small intestine
44899	Unlisted procedure, Meckel's diverticulum and the mesentery
44979	Unlisted laparoscopy procedure, appendix
45399	Unlisted procedure, colon
45499	Unlisted laparoscopy procedure, rectum
45999	Unlisted procedure, rectum
46999	Unlisted procedure, anus
47379	Unlisted laparoscopic procedure, liver
47399	Unlisted procedure, liver
47579	Unlisted laparoscopy procedure, biliary tract
47999	Unlisted procedure, biliary tract
48999	Unlisted procedure, pancreas
49329	Unlisted laparoscopy procedure, abdomen, peritoneum and omentum
49659	Unlisted laparoscopy procedure, hernioplasty, herniorrhaphy, herniotomy
49999	Unlisted procedure, abdomen, peritoneum and omentum
50549	Unlisted laparoscopy procedure, renal
50949	Unlisted laparoscopy procedure, ureter
51999	Unlisted laparoscopy procedure, bladder
53899	Unlisted procedure, urinary system
54699	Unlisted laparoscopy procedure, testis
55559	Unlisted laparoscopy procedure, spermatic cord
55899	Unlisted procedure, male genital system
58578	Unlisted laparoscopy procedure, uterus
58579	Unlisted hysteroscopy procedure, uterus
58679	Unlisted laparoscopy procedure, oviduct, ovary
58999	Unlisted procedure, female genital system (nonobstetrical)

* Pages in this section refer to the AMA *CPT® 2022 Professional Edition.*

59897	Unlisted fetal invasive procedure, including ultrasound guidance, when performed
59898	Unlisted laparoscopy procedure, maternity care and delivery
59899	Unlisted procedure, maternity care and delivery
60659	Unlisted laparoscopy procedure, endocrine system
60699	Unlisted procedure, endocrine system
64999	Unlisted procedure, nervous system
66999	Unlisted procedure, anterior segment of eye
67299	Unlisted procedure, posterior segment
67399	Unlisted procedure, extraocular muscle
67599	Unlisted procedure, orbit
67999	Unlisted procedure, eyelids
68399	Unlisted procedure, conjunctiva
68899	Unlisted procedure, lacrimal system
69399	Unlisted procedure, external ear
69799	Unlisted procedure, middle ear
69949	Unlisted procedure, inner ear
69979	Unlisted procedure, temporal bone, middle fossa approach

Special Report

A service that is rarely provided, unusual, variable, or new may require a special report. Pertinent information should include an adequate definition or description of the nature, extent, and need for the procedure, and the time, effort, and equipment necessary to provide the service.

Imaging Guidance

When imaging guidance or imaging supervision and interpretation is included in a surgical procedure, guidelines for image documentation and report, included in the guidelines for Radiology (Including Nuclear Medicine and Diagnostic Ultrasound), will apply. Imaging guidance should not be reported for use of a nonimaging-guided tracking or localizing system (eg, radar signals, electromagnetic signals). Imaging guidance should only be reported when an imaging modality (eg, radiography, fluoroscopy, ultrasonography, magnetic resonance imaging, computed tomography, or nuclear medicine) is used and is appropriately documented.

Surgical Destruction

Surgical destruction is a part of a surgical procedure and different methods of destruction are not ordinarily listed separately unless the technique substantially alters the standard management of a problem or condition. Exceptions under special circumstances are provided for by separate code numbers.

▶Foreign Body/Implant Definition◀

▶An object intentionally placed by a physician or other qualified health care professional for any purpose (eg, diagnostic or therapeutic) is considered an implant. An object that is unintentionally placed (eg, trauma or ingestion) is considered a foreign body. If an implant (or part thereof) has moved from its original position or is structurally broken and no longer serves its intended purpose or presents a hazard to the patient, it qualifies as a foreign body for coding purposes, unless CPT coding instructions direct otherwise or a specific CPT code exists to describe the removal of that broken/moved implant.◀

Surgical Procedures on the Musculoskeletal System

Cast and strapping procedures appear at the end of this section.

The services listed below include the application and removal of the first cast or traction device only. Subsequent replacement of cast and/or traction device may require an additional listing.

Definitions

The terms "closed treatment," "open treatment," and "percutaneous skeletal fixation" have been carefully chosen to accurately reflect current orthopaedic procedural treatments.

Closed treatment specifically means that the fracture site is not surgically opened (exposed to the external environment and directly visualized). This terminology is used to describe procedures that treat fractures by three methods: (1) without manipulation; (2) with manipulation; or (3) with or without traction.

Open treatment is used when the fractured bone is either: (1) surgically opened (exposed to the external environment) and the fracture (bone ends) visualized and internal fixation may be used; or (2) the fractured bone is opened remote from the fracture site in order to insert an intramedullary nail across the fracture site (the fracture site is not opened and visualized).

Percutaneous skeletal fixation describes fracture treatment which is neither open nor closed. In this procedure, the fracture fragments are not visualized, but fixation (eg, pins) is placed across the fracture site, usually under X-ray imaging.

The type of fracture (eg, open, compound, closed) does not have any coding correlation with the type of treatment (eg, closed, open, or percutaneous) provided.

The codes for treatment of fractures and joint injuries (dislocations) are categorized by the type of manipulation (reduction) and stabilization (fixation or immobilization). These codes can apply to either open (compound) or closed fractures or joint injuries.

Skeletal traction is the application of a force (distracting or traction force) to a limb segment through a wire, pin, screw, or clamp that is attached (eg, penetrates) to bone.

Skin traction is the application of a force (longitudinal) to a limb using felt or strapping applied directly to skin only.

External fixation is the usage of skeletal pins plus an attaching mechanism/device used for temporary or definitive treatment of acute or chronic bony deformity.

Codes for obtaining autogenous bone grafts, cartilage, tendon, fascia lata grafts or other tissues through separate incisions are to be used only when the graft is not already listed as part of the basic procedure.

Re-reduction of a fracture and/or dislocation performed by the primary physician or other qualified health care professional may be identified by the addition of modifier 76 to the usual procedure number to indicate "Repeat Procedure or Service by Same Physician or Other Qualified Health Care Professional." (See Appendix A* guidelines.)

Codes for external fixation are to be used only when external fixation is not already listed as part of the basic procedure.

All codes for suction irrigation have been deleted. To report, list only the primary surgical procedure performed (eg, sequestrectomy, deep incision).

Manipulation is used throughout the musculoskeletal fracture and dislocation subsections to specifically mean the attempted reduction or restoration of a fracture or joint dislocation to its normal anatomic alignment by the application of manually applied forces.

Excision of subcutaneous soft connective tissue tumors (including simple or intermediate repair) involves the simple or marginal resection of tumors confined to subcutaneous tissue below the skin but above the deep fascia. These tumors are usually benign and are resected without removing a significant amount of surrounding normal tissue. Code selection is based on the location and size of the tumor. Code selection is determined by measuring the greatest diameter of the tumor plus that margin required for complete excision of the tumor. The margins refer to the most narrow margin required to adequately excise the tumor, based on the physician's judgment. The measurement of the tumor plus margin is made at the time of the excision. Appreciable vessel exploration and/or neuroplasty should be reported separately. Extensive undermining or other techniques to close a defect created by skin excision may require a complex repair which should be reported separately. Dissection or elevation of tissue planes to permit resection of the tumor is included in the excision. For excision of benign lesions of cutaneous origin (eg, sebaceous cyst), see 11400-11446.

Excision of fascial or subfascial soft tissue tumors (including simple or intermediate repair) involves the resection of tumors confined to the tissue within or below the deep fascia, but not involving the bone. These tumors are usually benign, are often intramuscular, and are resected without removing a significant amount of surrounding normal tissue. Code selection is based on size and location of the tumor. Code selection is determined by measuring the greatest diameter of the tumor plus that margin required for complete excision of the tumor. The margins refer to the most narrow margin required to adequately excise the tumor, based on individual judgment. The measurement of the tumor plus margin is made at the time of the excision. Appreciable vessel exploration and/or neuroplasty should be reported separately. Extensive undermining or other techniques to close a defect created by skin excision may require a complex repair which should be reported separately. Dissection or elevation of tissue planes to permit resection of the tumor is included in the excision.

Digital (ie, fingers and toes) subfascial tumors are defined as those tumors involving the tendons, tendon sheaths, or joints of the digit. Tumors which simply abut but do not breach the tendon, tendon sheath, or joint capsule are considered subcutaneous soft tissue tumors.

Radical resection of soft connective tissue tumors (including simple or intermediate repair) involves the resection of the tumor with wide margins of normal tissue. Appreciable vessel exploration and/or neuroplasty repair or reconstruction (eg, adjacent tissue transfer[s], flap[s]) should be reported separately. Extensive undermining or other techniques to close a defect created by skin excision may require a complex repair which should be

* Pages in this section refer to the AMA *CPT® 2022 Professional Edition.*

reported separately. Dissection or elevation of tissue planes to permit resection of the tumor is included in the excision. Although these tumors may be confined to a specific layer (eg, subcutaneous, subfascial), radical resection may involve removal of tissue from one or more layers. Radical resection of soft tissue tumors is most commonly used for malignant connective tissue tumors or very aggressive benign connective tissue tumors. Code selection is based on size and location of the tumor. Code selection is determined by measuring the greatest diameter of the tumor plus that margin required for complete excision of the tumor. The margins refer to the most narrow margin required to adequately excise the tumor, based on individual judgment. The measurement of the tumor plus margin is made at the time of the excision. For radical resection of tumor(s) of cutaneous origin (eg, melanoma), see 11600-11646.

Radical resection of bone tumors (including simple or intermediate repair) involves the resection of the tumor with wide margins of normal tissue. Appreciable vessel exploration and/or neuroplasty and complex bone repair or reconstruction (eg, adjacent tissue transfer[s], flap[s]) should be reported separately. Extensive undermining or other techniques to close a defect created by skin excision may require a complex repair which should be reported separately. Dissection or elevation of tissue planes to permit resection of the tumor is included in the excision. It may require removal of the entire bone if tumor growth is extensive (eg, clavicle). Radical resection of bone tumors is usually performed for malignant tumors or very aggressive benign tumors. If surrounding soft tissue is removed during these procedures, the radical resection of soft tissue tumor codes should not be reported separately. Code selection is based solely on the location of the tumor, **not** on the size of the tumor or whether the tumor is benign or malignant, primary or metastatic.

15820-15821

15820 Blepharoplasty, lower eyelid
15821 Blepharoplasty, lower eyelid; with extensive herniated fat pad

AMA Coding Guideline

Surgical Repair (Closure) Procedures on the Integumentary System

Use the codes in this section to designate wound closure utilizing sutures, staples, or tissue adhesives (eg, 2-cyanoacrylate), either singly or in combination with each other, or in combination with adhesive strips. Chemical cauterization, electrocauterization, or wound closure utilizing adhesive strips as the sole repair material are included in the appropriate E/M code.

Definitions

The repair of wounds may be classified as Simple, Intermediate, or Complex.

Simple repair is used when the wound is superficial (eg, involving primarily epidermis or dermis, or subcutaneous tissues without significant involvement of deeper structures) and requires simple one-layer closure. Hemostasis and local or topical anesthesia, when performed, are not reported separately.

Intermediate repair includes the repair of wounds that, in addition to the above, require layered closure of one or more of the deeper layers of subcutaneous tissue and superficial (non-muscle) fascia, in addition to the skin (epidermal and dermal) closure. It includes limited undermining (defined as a distance less than the maximum width of the defect, measured perpendicular to the closure line, along at least one entire edge of the defect). Single-layer closure of heavily contaminated wounds that have required extensive cleaning or removal of particulate matter also constitutes intermediate repair.

Complex repair includes the repair of wounds that, in addition to the requirements for intermediate repair, require at least one of the following: exposure of bone, cartilage, tendon, or named neurovascular structure; debridement of wound edges (eg, traumatic lacerations or avulsions); extensive undermining (defined as a distance greater than or equal to the maximum width of the defect, measured perpendicular to the closure line along at least one entire edge of the defect); involvement of free margins of helical rim, vermilion border, or nostril rim; placement of retention sutures. Necessary preparation includes creation of a limited defect for repairs or the debridement of complicated lacerations or avulsions. Complex repair does not include excision of benign (11400-11446) or malignant (11600-11646) lesions, excisional preparation of a wound bed (15002-15005) or debridement of an open fracture or open dislocation.

Instructions for listing services at time of wound repair:

1. The repaired wound(s) should be measured and recorded in centimeters, whether curved, angular, or stellate.

2. When multiple wounds are repaired, add together the lengths of those in the same classification (see above) and from all anatomic sites that are grouped together into the same code descriptor. For example, add together the lengths of intermediate repairs to the trunk and extremities. Do not add lengths of repairs from different groupings of anatomic sites (eg, face and extremities). Also, do not add together lengths of different classifications (eg, intermediate and complex repairs).

When more than one classification of wounds is repaired, list the more complicated as the primary procedure and the less complicated as the secondary procedure, using modifier 59.

3. Decontamination and/or debridement: Debridement is considered a separate procedure only when gross contamination requires prolonged cleansing, when appreciable amounts of devitalized or contaminated tissue are removed, or when debridement is carried out separately without immediate primary closure.

4. Involvement of nerves, blood vessels and tendons: Report under appropriate system (Nervous, Cardiovascular, Musculoskeletal) for repair of these structures. The repair of these associated wounds is included in the primary procedure unless it qualifies as a complex repair, in which case modifier 59 applies.

Simple ligation of vessels in an open wound is considered as part of any wound closure.

Simple "exploration" of nerves, blood vessels or tendons exposed in an open wound is also considered part of the essential treatment of the wound and is not a separate procedure unless appreciable dissection is required. If the wound requires enlargement, extension of dissection (to determine penetration), debridement, removal of foreign body(s), ligation or coagulation of minor subcutaneous and/or muscular blood vessel(s) of the subcutaneous tissue, muscle fascia, and/or muscle, not requiring thoracotomy or laparotomy, use codes 20100-20103, as appropriate.

AMA Coding Notes

Surgical Repair (Closure) Procedures on the Integumentary System

(For extensive debridement of soft tissue and/or bone, not associated with open fracture(s) and/or dislocation(s) resulting from penetrating and/or blunt trauma, see 11042-11047.)

(For extensive debridement of subcutaneous tissue, muscle fascia, muscle, and/or bone associated with open fracture(s) and/or dislocation(s), see 11010-11012.)

AMA *CPT® Assistant* ▯

15820: Feb 04: 11, May 04: 12, Feb 05: 16
15821: Feb 04: 11, May 04: 12, Feb 05: 16

Plain English Description

In 15820, loose or redundant skin of the lower eyelid just below the lashes is grasped, pulled taught, and trimmed away. If the musculature needs support, a stitch may be placed through the tendon at the lateral aspect of the eyelid and secured to the periosteum of the orbital rim. A running suture is placed to close the skin and repair the eyelid. In 15821, an incision is made in the conjunctiva of the lower lid and the underlying fat pad is exposed. The tendon on the lateral aspect of the eyelid is exposed and severed as needed to allow better exposure of the underlying fat pad. The herniated fat pad is dissected free of surrounding tissue. The fat may be removed, or more commonly, a subperiosteal tunnel is created at the medial aspect of the lower lid conjunctiva. The fat is transposed and positioned in the tear trough over the cheekbone. Loose sutures are placed through the skin to secure the fat pad in its new location. The lateral aspect of the eyelid is then incised and a wedge of eyelid is excised to allow tightening of the lower lid. A new tendon is fashioned and attached to the periosteum of the orbital rim using a single suture. Loose or redundant skin just below the lashes is grasped, pulled taught, and trimmed away. A running suture is placed to close the skin.

Blepharoplasty, lower eyelid

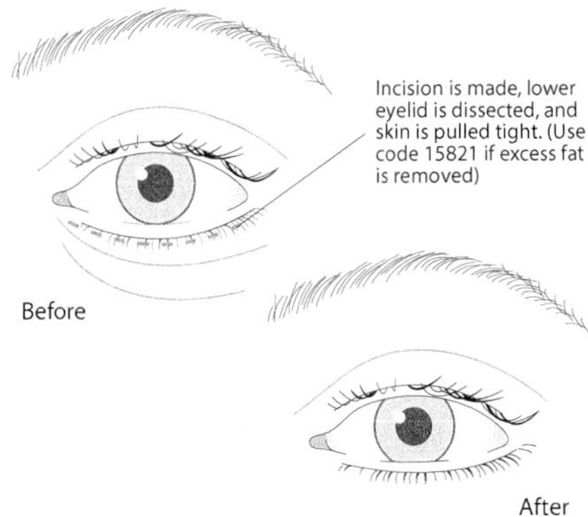
Incision is made, lower eyelid is dissected, and skin is pulled tight. (Use code 15821 if excess fat is removed)
Before
After

ICD-10-CM Diagnostic Codes

⇄	H02.32	Blepharochalasis right lower eyelid
⇄	H02.35	Blepharochalasis left lower eyelid
⇄	H02.832	Dermatochalasis of right lower eyelid
⇄	H02.835	Dermatochalasis of left lower eyelid
	Q10.3	Other congenital malformations of eyelid

CCI Edits

Refer to Appendix A for CCI edits.

Facility RVUs

Code	Work	PE Facility	MP	Total Facility
15820	6.27	8.31	0.47	15.05
15821	6.84	8.63	0.68	16.15

Non-facility RVUs

Code	Work	PE Non-Facility	MP	Total Non-Facility
15820	6.27	10.25	0.47	16.99
15821	6.84	10.76	0.68	18.28

Modifiers (PAR)

Code	Mod 50	Mod 51	Mod 62	Mod 66	Mod 80
15820	1	2	0	0	0
15821	1	2	0	0	0

Global Period

Code	Days
15820	090
15821	090

15822-15823

15822 Blepharoplasty, upper eyelid

15823 Blepharoplasty, upper eyelid; with excessive skin weighting down lid

(For bilateral blepharoplasty, add modifier 50)

AMA Coding Guideline

Surgical Repair (Closure) Procedures on the Integumentary System

Use the codes in this section to designate wound closure utilizing sutures, staples, or tissue adhesives (eg, 2-cyanoacrylate), either singly or in combination with each other, or in combination with adhesive strips. Chemical cauterization, electrocauterization, or wound closure utilizing adhesive strips as the sole repair material are included in the appropriate E/M code.

Definitions

The repair of wounds may be classified as Simple, Intermediate, or Complex.

Simple repair is used when the wound is superficial (eg, involving primarily epidermis or dermis, or subcutaneous tissues without significant involvement of deeper structures) and requires simple one-layer closure. Hemostasis and local or topical anesthesia, when performed, are not reported separately.

Intermediate repair includes the repair of wounds that, in addition to the above, require layered closure of one or more of the deeper layers of subcutaneous tissue and superficial (non-muscle) fascia, in addition to the skin (epidermal and dermal) closure. It includes limited undermining (defined as a distance less than the maximum width of the defect, measured perpendicular to the closure line, along at least one entire edge of the defect). Single-layer closure of heavily contaminated wounds that have required extensive cleaning or removal of particulate matter also constitutes intermediate repair.

Complex repair includes the repair of wounds that, in addition to the requirements for intermediate repair, require at least one of the following: exposure of bone, cartilage, tendon, or named neurovascular structure; debridement of wound edges (eg, traumatic lacerations or avulsions); extensive undermining (defined as a distance greater than or equal to the maximum width of the defect, measured perpendicular to the closure line along at least one entire edge of the defect); involvement of free margins of helical rim, vermilion border, or nostril rim; placement of retention sutures. Necessary preparation includes creation of a limited defect for repairs or the debridement of complicated lacerations or avulsions. Complex repair does not include excision of benign (11400-11446) or malignant (11600-11646) lesions, excisional preparation of a wound bed (15002-15005) or debridement of an open fracture or open dislocation.

Instructions for listing services at time of wound repair:

1. The repaired wound(s) should be measured and recorded in centimeters, whether curved, angular, or stellate.

2. When multiple wounds are repaired, add together the lengths of those in the same classification (see above) and from all anatomic sites that are grouped together into the same code descriptor. For example, add together the lengths of intermediate repairs to the trunk and extremities. Do not add lengths of repairs from different groupings of anatomic sites (eg, face and extremities). Also, do not add together lengths of different classifications (eg, intermediate and complex repairs).

When more than one classification of wounds is repaired, list the more complicated as the primary procedure and the less complicated as the secondary procedure, using modifier 59.

3. Decontamination and/or debridement: Debridement is considered a separate procedure only when gross contamination requires prolonged cleansing, when appreciable amounts of devitalized or contaminated tissue are removed, or when debridement is carried out separately without immediate primary closure.

4. Involvement of nerves, blood vessels and tendons: Report under appropriate system (Nervous, Cardiovascular, Musculoskeletal) for repair of these structures. The repair of these associated wounds is included in the primary procedure unless it qualifies as a complex repair, in which case modifier 59 applies.

Simple ligation of vessels in an open wound is considered as part of any wound closure.

Simple "exploration" of nerves, blood vessels or tendons exposed in an open wound is also considered part of the essential treatment of the wound and is not a separate procedure unless appreciable dissection is required. If the wound requires enlargement, extension of dissection (to determine penetration), debridement, removal of foreign body(s), ligation or coagulation of minor subcutaneous and/or muscular blood vessel(s) of the subcutaneous tissue, muscle fascia, and/or muscle, not requiring thoracotomy or laparotomy, use codes 20100-20103, as appropriate.

AMA Coding Notes

Surgical Repair (Closure) Procedures on the Integumentary System

(For extensive debridement of soft tissue and/or bone, not associated with open fracture(s) and/or dislocation(s) resulting from penetrating and/or blunt trauma, see 11042-11047.)

(For extensive debridement of subcutaneous tissue, muscle fascia, muscle, and/or bone associated with open fracture(s) and/or dislocation(s), see 11010-11012.)

AMA *CPT® Assistant* ▯

15822: Feb 04: 11, May 04: 12, Feb 05: 16

15823: Sep 00: 7, Feb 04: 11, May 04: 12, Feb 05: 16, Aug 11: 8, Mar 21: 11

Plain English Description

Upper eyelid blepharoplasty is used to modify or reconstruct a droopy eyelid by removing excess skin, muscle, and/or fat. Blepharoplasty may be indicated for functional problems including dermatochalasis, blepharoptosis, pseudoptosis, and ptosis or for cosmetic reasons. The skin is marked along the natural creases of the eyelid and the surgical area is infiltrated with local anesthetic. Using a steel blade, laser, or radiofrequency instruments, the skin is incised along the marked lines and the excess skin is removed. Using cautery, all or part of the orbicularis muscle underlying the skin may be removed. The orbital septum is then identified and incised just below its attachment to the arcus marginalis to expose the preaponeurotic fat. Using gentle pressure on the globe, the creamy yellow-white fat from the medial section is identified along with the darker yellow fat from the central section. Additional anesthetic may be injected into the fat capsules, which are then incised and the fat pads trimmed to contour the eyelid. The lateral orbital rim is examined for the lacrimal gland, which may require suturing to the orbital rim to prevent postoperative fullness in the lateral aspect of the lid. Alteration of the eyelid crease can be accomplished using supratarsal fixation sutures to create adherence between the skin and underlying tissue. The subcutaneous tissue at the lower aspect of the eyelid crease incision is attached to the levator aponeurosis just above the tarsus, or a mattress suture is placed through the skin, orbicularis oculi, levator aponeurosis, and conjunctiva then back out and through those same structures on the opposite side of the incision. Once adequate contouring and hemostasis have been established, the skin incisions are closed with sutures or tissue adhesive. Code 15822 includes upper lid blepharoplasty for conditions that reduce the upper and outer aspects of the peripheral visual field. Code 15823 includes excessive skin that weighs down the lid, obscuring the superior visual field in addition to the peripheral visual field.

Blepharoplasty, upper eyelid

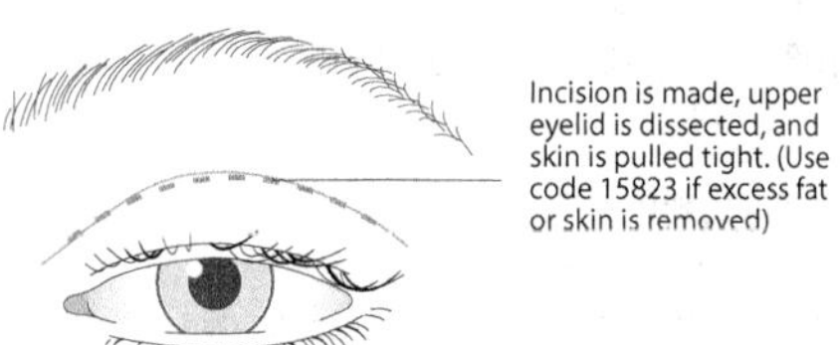
Incision is made, upper eyelid is dissected, and skin is pulled tight. (Use code 15823 if excess fat or skin is removed)
Before

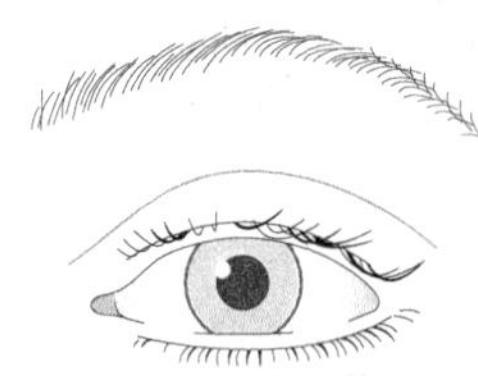
After

ICD-10-CM Diagnostic Codes

⇄	H02.031	Senile entropion of right upper eyelid
⇄	H02.034	Senile entropion of left upper eyelid
⇄	H02.31	Blepharochalasis right upper eyelid
⇄	H02.34	Blepharochalasis left upper eyelid
⇄	H02.401	Unspecified ptosis of right eyelid
⇄	H02.402	Unspecified ptosis of left eyelid
⇄	H02.403	Unspecified ptosis of bilateral eyelids
⇄	H02.411	Mechanical ptosis of right eyelid
⇄	H02.412	Mechanical ptosis of left eyelid
⇄	H02.413	Mechanical ptosis of bilateral eyelids
⇄	H02.421	Myogenic ptosis of right eyelid
⇄	H02.422	Myogenic ptosis of left eyelid
⇄	H02.423	Myogenic ptosis of bilateral eyelids
⇄	H02.431	Paralytic ptosis of right eyelid
⇄	H02.432	Paralytic ptosis of left eyelid
⇄	H02.433	Paralytic ptosis of bilateral eyelids
⇄	H02.831	Dermatochalasis of right upper eyelid
⇄	H02.834	Dermatochalasis of left upper eyelid
	H53.8	Other visual disturbances
	H53.9	Unspecified visual disturbance
	H54.7	Unspecified visual loss
	Q10.0	Congenital ptosis
	Q10.3	Other congenital malformations of eyelid

CCI Edits

Refer to Appendix A for CCI edits.

Facility RVUs ▯

Code	Work	PE Facility	MP	Total Facility
15822	4.62	6.60	0.54	11.76
15823	6.81	8.71	0.60	16.12

Non-facility RVUs ▯

Code	Work	PE Non-Facility	MP	Total Non-Facility
15822	4.62	8.51	0.54	13.67
15823	6.81	10.86	0.60	18.27

Modifiers (PAR) ▯

Code	Mod 50	Mod 51	Mod 62	Mod 66	Mod 80
15822	1	2	0	0	1
15823	1	2	0	0	1

Global Period

Code	Days
15822	090
15823	090

21385

21385 Open treatment of orbital floor blowout fracture; transantral approach (Caldwell-Luc type operation)

AMA Coding Guideline

Surgical Procedures on the Head

Skull, facial bones, and temporomandibular joint.

Please see the Surgery Guidelines section for the following guidelines:

- *Surgical Procedures on the Musculoskeletal System*

AMA Coding Notes

Fracture and/or Dislocation Procedures on the Head

(For operative repair of skull fracture, see 62000-62010)

(To report closed treatment of skull fracture, use the appropriate Evaluation and Management code)

Plain English Description

Open repair of an orbital floor blowout fracture using a transantral approach (Caldwell-Luc procedure) is performed to restore anatomic and functional defects of the globe. Orbital fractures are a common injury sustained with mid-facial trauma and may include extraocular muscle entrapment with impairment of eye movement in addition to aesthetic facial deformity. The upper lip is retracted to expose the gingivobuccal sulcus and a horizontal incision is made superior to the sulcus creating a wide mucosal band. Using a periosteal elevator, the periosteum and overlying soft tissue are elevated from the underlying maxillary bone to the infraorbital foramen. The maxillary sinus is entered via an antral window (Caldwell-Luc antrostomy) and the bone fragment is preserved. The maxillary sinus is visualized and the herniated orbital contents are removed or repositioned back into the orbit. The fracture is reduced and an implant may be inserted if a bony deficit is present. The sinus cavity is checked for hemostasis, the antral wall bone fragment is replaced, and the incision is closed with sutures.

Open treatment of orbital floor blowout fracture; transantral approach

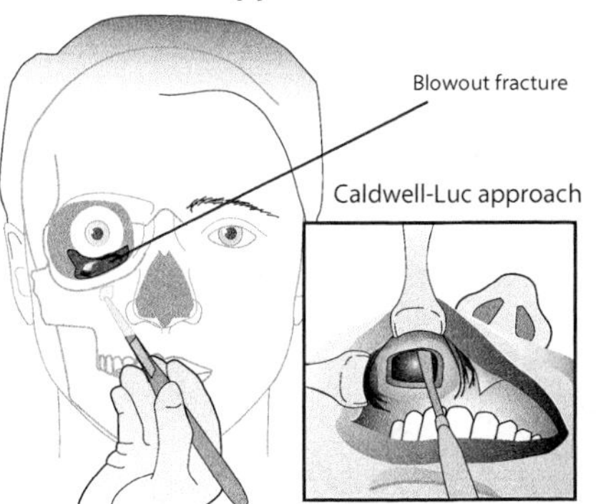

ICD-10-CM Diagnostic Codes

❼⇄	S02.31	Fracture of orbital floor, right side
❼⇄	S02.32	Fracture of orbital floor, left side

ICD-10-CM Coding Notes

For codes requiring a 7th character extension, refer to your ICD-10-CM book. Review the character descriptions and coding guidelines for proper selection. For some procedures, only certain characters will apply.

CCI Edits

Refer to Appendix A for CCI edits.

Facility RVUs ▯

Code	Work	PE Facility	MP	Total Facility
21385	9.57	10.46	1.75	21.78

Non-facility RVUs ▯

Code	Work	PE Non-Facility	MP	Total Non-Facility
21385	9.57	10.46	1.75	21.78

Modifiers (PAR) ▯

Code	Mod 50	Mod 51	Mod 62	Mod 66	Mod 80
21385	1	2	1	0	2

Global Period

Code	Days
21385	090

21386

21386 Open treatment of orbital floor blowout fracture; periorbital approach

AMA Coding Guideline

Surgical Procedures on the Head

Skull, facial bones, and temporomandibular joint.

Please see the Surgery Guidelines section for the following guidelines:

- *Surgical Procedures on the Musculoskeletal System*

AMA Coding Notes

Fracture and/or Dislocation Procedures on the Head

(For operative repair of skull fracture, see 62000-62010)

(To report closed treatment of skull fracture, use the appropriate Evaluation and Management code)

Plain English Description

Open repair of an orbital floor blowout fracture using a periorbital approach is performed to restore anatomic and functional defects of the globe. Orbital fractures are a common injury sustained with mid-facial trauma and may include extraocular muscle entrapment with impairment of eye movement in addition to aesthetic facial deformity. The conjunctiva is incised across the length of the lower eyelid just below the base of the tarsus. Traction sutures are placed and the conjunctiva is pulled superiorly to cover the cornea. The plane between the orbital septum and orbicularis muscle is bluntly dissected to the orbital rim. The periosteum is opened and elevated off the orbital floor. The herniated orbital tissue is removed or repositioned back into the orbit and the fracture is reduced. The surgical area is checked for hemostasis, the traction sutures are cut, the conjunctiva is repositioned, and the incision is closed with sutures.

Open treatment of orbital floor blowout fracture; periorbital approach

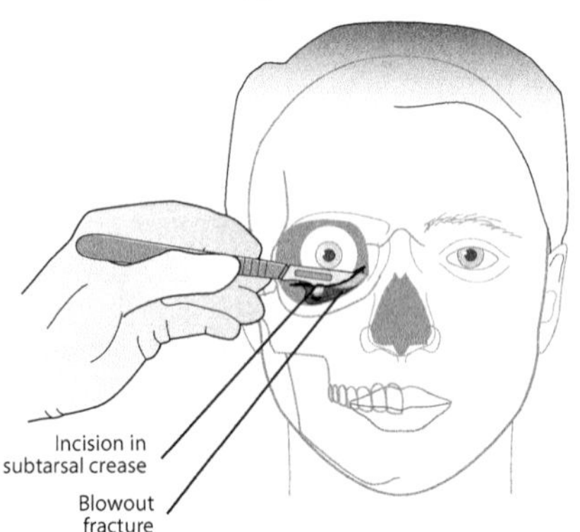

ICD-10-CM Diagnostic Codes

➐⇄	S02.31	Fracture of orbital floor, right side
➐⇄	S02.32	Fracture of orbital floor, left side

ICD-10-CM Coding Notes

For codes requiring a 7th character extension, refer to your ICD-10-CM book. Review the character descriptions and coding guidelines for proper selection. For some procedures, only certain characters will apply.

CCI Edits

Refer to Appendix A for CCI edits.

Facility RVUs ▢

Code	Work	PE Facility	MP	Total Facility
21386	9.57	9.16	1.75	20.48

Non-facility RVUs ▢

Code	Work	PE Non-Facility	MP	Total Non-Facility
21386	9.57	9.16	1.75	20.48

Modifiers (PAR) ▢

Code	Mod 50	Mod 51	Mod 62	Mod 66	Mod 80
21386	1	2	0	0	2

Global Period

Code	Days
21386	090

21387

21387 Open treatment of orbital floor blowout fracture; combined approach

AMA Coding Guideline

Surgical Procedures on the Head

Skull, facial bones, and temporomandibular joint.

Please see the Surgery Guidelines section for the following guidelines:

- *Surgical Procedures on the Musculoskeletal System*

AMA Coding Notes

Fracture and/or Dislocation Procedures on the Head

(For operative repair of skull fracture, see 62000-62010)

(To report closed treatment of skull fracture, use the appropriate Evaluation and Management code)

Plain English Description

Open repair of an orbital floor blowout fracture using a combined (transconjunctival with lateral canthotomy) approach is performed to restore anatomic and functional defects of the globe. Orbital fractures are a common injury sustained with mid-facial trauma and may include extraocular muscle entrapment with impairment of eye movement in addition to aesthetic facial deformity. Traction sutures are placed in the lower eyelid. A pointed scissor inserted horizontally at the outer lid angle is used to make an incision along the palpebral fissure through the skin, orbicularis oculi muscle, and conjuctiva. The lateral canthal tendon fibers that fan superficially are then transected and the lower lid is everted using the previously placed traction sutures. The lateral canthal tendon is transected using scissors to entirely free the lower eyelid. The conjunctiva is then incised across the length of the lower eyelid just below the base of the tarsus. Traction sutures are placed, and the conjunctiva is pulled superiorly to cover the cornea. The plane between the orbital septum and orbicularis muscle is bluntly dissected to the orbital rim. The periosteum is opened and elevated off the orbital floor. The herniated orbital tissue is removed or repositioned back into the orbit and the fracture is reduced. The surgical area is checked for hemostasis. Sutures are placed into the transected edges of the inferior and superior lateral canthal tendon and provisionally tightened. The traction sutures positioning the conjunctiva superiorly are cut and the conjunctiva is repositioned. The ends of lateral canthal tendon sutures are brought out of the conjunctival incision and that incision is then closed with sutures. The canthal suture is tightened bringing the lower eyelid back to its original position. The lateral canthotomy subcutaneous tissue is closed with sutures followed by closure of the skin incision.

Open treatment of orbital floor blowout fracture; combined approach

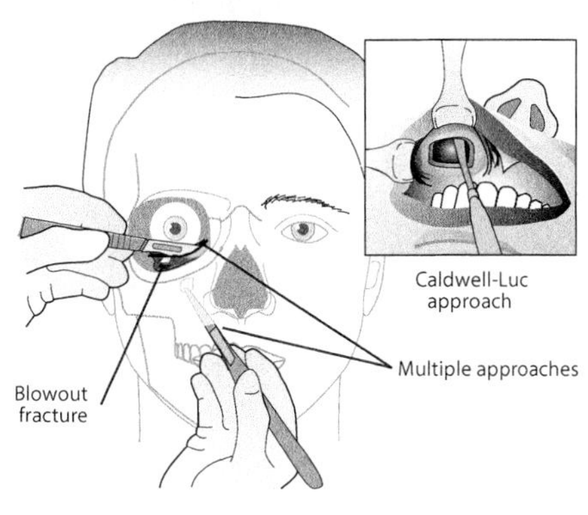

ICD-10-CM Diagnostic Codes

➐⇄	S02.31	Fracture of orbital floor, right side
➐⇄	S02.32	Fracture of orbital floor, left side

ICD-10-CM Coding Notes

For codes requiring a 7th character extension, refer to your ICD-10-CM book. Review the character descriptions and coding guidelines for proper selection. For some procedures, only certain characters will apply.

CCI Edits

Refer to Appendix A for CCI edits.

Facility RVUs ☐

Code	Work	PE Facility	MP	Total Facility
21387	10.11	10.77	1.84	22.72

Non-facility RVUs ☐

Code	Work	PE Non-Facility	MP	Total Non-Facility
21387	10.11	10.77	1.84	22.72

Modifiers (PAR) ☐

Code	Mod 50	Mod 51	Mod 62	Mod 66	Mod 80
21387	1	2	0	0	2

Global Period

Code	Days
21387	090

21390

21390 Open treatment of orbital floor blowout fracture; periorbital approach, with alloplastic or other implant

AMA Coding Guideline

Surgical Procedures on the Head

Skull, facial bones, and temporomandibular joint.

Please see the Surgery Guidelines section for the following guidelines:

- *Surgical Procedures on the Musculoskeletal System*

AMA Coding Notes

Fracture and/or Dislocation Procedures on the Head

(For operative repair of skull fracture, see 62000-62010)

(To report closed treatment of skull fracture, use the appropriate Evaluation and Management code)

AMA *CPT® Assistant* ▯

21390: Dec 20: 11

Plain English Description

Open repair of an orbital floor blowout fracture using a periorbital approach and alloplastic or other implant is performed to restore anatomic and functional defects of the globe. Orbital fractures are a common injury sustained with mid-facial trauma and may include extraocular muscle entrapment with impairment of eye movement in addition to aesthetic facial deformity. The conjunctiva is incised across the length of the lower eyelid just below the base of the tarsus. Traction sutures are placed and the conjunctiva is pulled superiorly to cover the cornea. The plane between the orbital septum and orbicularis muscle is bluntly dissected to the orbital rim. The periosteum is opened and elevated off the orbital floor. The herniated orbital tissue is removed or repositioned back into the orbit. The fracture is reduced and an orbital implant comprised of porous polyethylene, silicone, Teflon, Supramid, titanium mesh, bioresorbable copolymer plates, or Vicryl mesh is inserted to fill the bony deficit. The surgical area is checked for hemostasis, the traction sutures are cut, the conjunctiva is repositioned, and the incision is closed with sutures.

Open treatment of orbital floor blowout fracture; periorbital approach with alloplastic or other implant

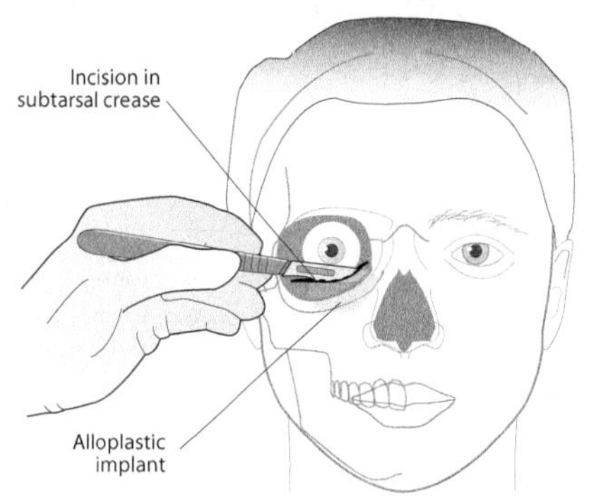

ICD-10-CM Diagnostic Codes

❼⇄	S02.31	Fracture of orbital floor, right side
❼⇄	S02.32	Fracture of orbital floor, left side

ICD-10-CM Coding Notes

For codes requiring a 7th character extension, refer to your ICD-10-CM book. Review the character descriptions and coding guidelines for proper selection. For some procedures, only certain characters will apply.

CCI Edits

Refer to Appendix A for CCI edits.

Facility RVUs ▯

Code	Work	PE Facility	MP	Total Facility
21390	11.23	10.99	1.48	23.70

Non-facility RVUs ▯

Code	Work	PE Non-Facility	MP	Total Non-Facility
21390	11.23	10.99	1.48	23.70

Modifiers (PAR) ▯

Code	Mod 50	Mod 51	Mod 62	Mod 66	Mod 80
21390	1	2	1	0	2

Global Period

Code	Days
21390	090

21395

21395 Open treatment of orbital floor blowout fracture; periorbital approach with bone graft (includes obtaining graft)

AMA Coding Guideline

Surgical Procedures on the Head

Skull, facial bones, and temporomandibular joint.

Please see the Surgery Guidelines section for the following guidelines:

- *Surgical Procedures on the Musculoskeletal System*

AMA Coding Notes

Fracture and/or Dislocation Procedures on the Head

(For operative repair of skull fracture, see 62000-62010)

(To report closed treatment of skull fracture, use the appropriate Evaluation and Management code)

Plain English Description

Open repair of an orbital floor blowout fracture using a periorbital approach with a bone graft is performed to restore anatomic and functional defects of the globe. Orbital fractures are a common injury sustained with mid-facial trauma and may include extraocular muscle entrapment with impairment of eye movement in addition to aesthetic facial deformity. The conjunctiva is incised across the length of the lower eyelid just below the base of the tarsus. Traction sutures are placed and the conjunctiva is pulled superiorly to cover the cornea. The plane between the orbital septum and orbicularis muscle is bluntly dissected to the orbital rim. The periosteum is opened and elevated off the orbital floor. The herniated orbital tissue is removed or repositioned back into the orbit. The fracture is reduced and an autogenous bone graft harvested from the maxillary wall, calvaria, iliac crest, rib, or fibula and shaped to match the contour of the bony deficit is inserted into the orbital space. The surgical area is checked for hemostasis, the traction sutures are cut, the conjunctiva is repositioned, and the incision is closed with sutures.

Open treatment of orbital floor blowout fracture; periorbital approach with bone graft

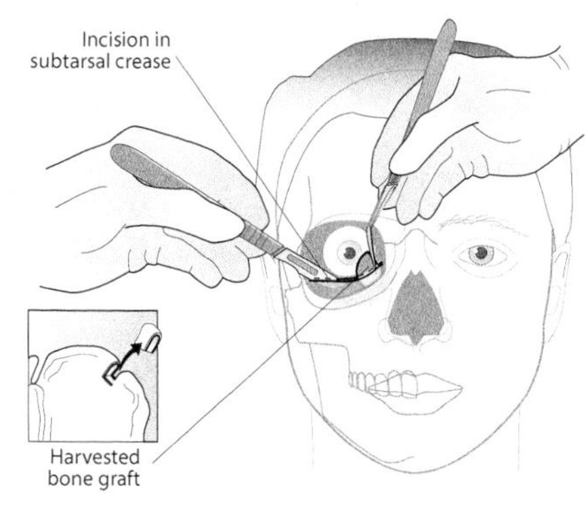

ICD-10-CM Diagnostic Codes

➐⇄	S02.31	Fracture of orbital floor, right side
➐⇄	S02.32	Fracture of orbital floor, left side

ICD-10-CM Coding Notes

For codes requiring a 7th character extension, refer to your ICD-10-CM book. Review the character descriptions and coding guidelines for proper selection. For some procedures, only certain characters will apply.

CCI Edits

Refer to Appendix A for CCI edits.

Facility RVUs ☐

Code	Work	PE Facility	MP	Total Facility
21395	14.70	12.52	2.69	29.91

Non-facility RVUs ☐

Code	Work	PE Non-Facility	MP	Total Non-Facility
21395	14.70	12.52	2.69	29.91

Modifiers (PAR) ☐

Code	Mod 50	Mod 51	Mod 62	Mod 66	Mod 80
21395	1	2	1	0	2

Global Period

Code	Days
21395	090

21400-21401

21400 Closed treatment of fracture of orbit, except blowout; without manipulation

21401 Closed treatment of fracture of orbit, except blowout; with manipulation

AMA Coding Guideline

Surgical Procedures on the Head

Skull, facial bones, and temporomandibular joint.

Please see the Surgery Guidelines section for the following guidelines:

- *Surgical Procedures on the Musculoskeletal System*

AMA Coding Notes

Fracture and/or Dislocation Procedures on the Head

(For operative repair of skull fracture, see 62000-62010)

(To report closed treatment of skull fracture, use the appropriate Evaluation and Management code)

Plain English Description

Closed treatment of a fracture of the orbit other than an orbital floor (blowout) fracture is performed Separately reportable radiographs are obtained to confirm the fracture. In 21400, a nondisplaced fracture of the orbit is evaluated. A neurovascular exam is performed to ensure that nerves and blood vessels at the site of injury are intact. No manipulation of fracture fragments is required. In 21401, a minimally displaced fracture of the orbit is evaluated. The displaced fracture fragments are manually reduced (manipulated) or a hook/screw is used to manipulate the fragments back to correct anatomic alignment. Separately reportable radiographs are obtained to confirm anatomic reduction.

Closed treatment of fracture of orbit, except blowout

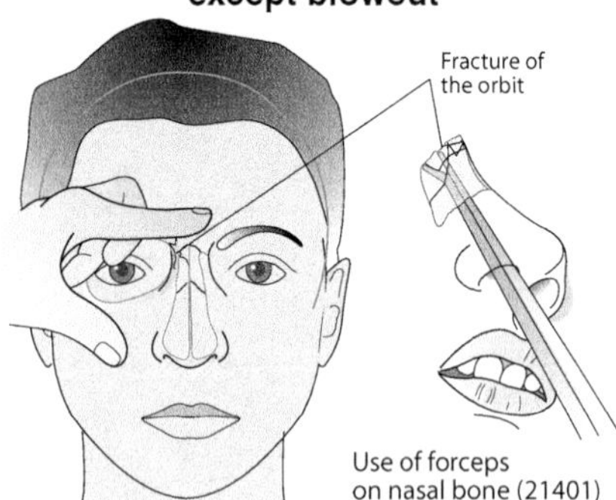

Without manipulation (21400); with manipulation (21401)

ICD-10-CM Diagnostic Codes

➐⇄	S02.121	Fracture of orbital roof, right side
➐⇄	S02.122	Fracture of orbital roof, left side
➐⇄	S02.831	Fracture of medial orbital wall, right side
➐⇄	S02.832	Fracture of medial orbital wall, left side
➐⇄	S02.841	Fracture of lateral orbital wall, right side
➐⇄	S02.842	Fracture of lateral orbital wall, left side
➐	S02.85	Fracture of orbit, unspecified

ICD-10-CM Coding Notes

For codes requiring a 7th character extension, refer to your ICD-10-CM book. Review the character descriptions and coding guidelines for proper selection. For some procedures, only certain characters will apply.

CCI Edits

Refer to Appendix A for CCI edits.

Facility RVUs ▯

Code	Work	PE Facility	MP	Total Facility
21400	1.50	3.13	0.25	4.88
21401	3.68	5.34	0.67	9.69

Non-facility RVUs ▯

Code	Work	PE Non-Facility	MP	Total Non-Facility
21400	1.50	4.52	0.25	6.27
21401	3.68	10.87	0.67	15.22

Modifiers (PAR) ▯

Code	Mod 50	Mod 51	Mod 62	Mod 66	Mod 80
21400	1	2	0	0	0
21401	1	2	0	0	2

Global Period

Code	Days
21400	090
21401	090

21406

21406 Open treatment of fracture of orbit, except blowout; without implant

AMA Coding Guideline

Surgical Procedures on the Head

Skull, facial bones, and temporomandibular joint.

Please see the Surgery Guidelines section for the following guidelines:

- *Surgical Procedures on the Musculoskeletal System*

AMA Coding Notes

Fracture and/or Dislocation Procedures on the Head

(For operative repair of skull fracture, see 62000-62010)

(To report closed treatment of skull fracture, use the appropriate Evaluation and Management code)

AMA *CPT® Assistant* ▢

21406: Dec 20: 11

Plain English Description

Open repair of a non-blowout orbital fracture, without implant is performed to restore the orbit to its natural shape. The natural skin creases are evaluated and incision lines are marked. A temporary tarsorrhaphy may be performed to protect the cornea by placing a mattress suture through the edges of the upper and lower eyelids to close the lids over the eye. The ends of the suture are grasped with a clamp and traction is applied upwards. The skin is incised along the marked lines to visualize the underlying orbicular muscle. The incision is extended subcutaneously over the pretarsal portion of the orbicularis oculi muscle to create a skin flap the full length of the incision. A dissection plane between the orbicularis oculi muscle and the septum orbitale is then created and suborbicular undermining of the muscle is performed using a slit-like lateral incision over the bony orbital rim. The suborbicular dissection plane is opened, leaving the orbital septum intact. The suborbicular pocket is extended downward over the whole lower palpebral region and the upper portion of the pocket below the tarsus is then opened. The remaining layer of the orbicularis oculi muscle is separated just below the lower border of the tarsus to create a skin muscle flap congruent with the lower eyelid. The eyelid and flap is retracted inferiorly over the anterior edge of the infraorbital rim and a periosteal elevator is employed to strip the periosteum from the bone. The intraorbital nerve is identified and preserved before continuing dissection along the upper facial surface of the anterior maxilla. The borders of the fracture are identified and orbital soft tissue that has herniated through any bony deficit is reduced. The fracture may be repaired with hardware, if indicated. The periosteum is then redraped over the bony surface and secured.

Open treatment of fracture of orbit, except blowout; without implant

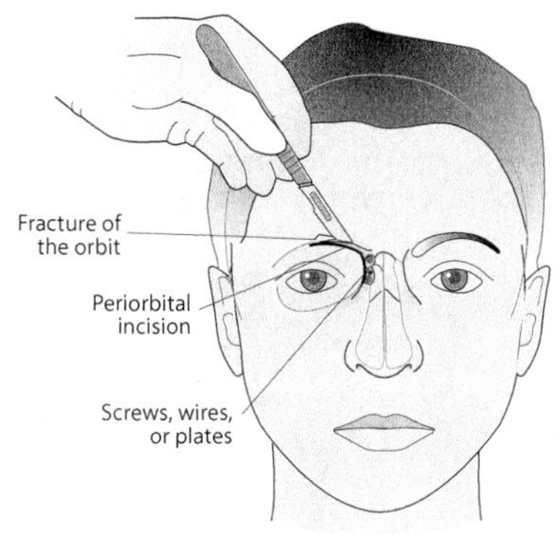

ICD-10-CM Diagnostic Codes

❼⇄	S02.121	Fracture of orbital roof, right side
❼⇄	S02.122	Fracture of orbital roof, left side
❼⇄	S02.831	Fracture of medial orbital wall, right side
❼⇄	S02.832	Fracture of medial orbital wall, left side
❼⇄	S02.841	Fracture of lateral orbital wall, right side
❼⇄	S02.842	Fracture of lateral orbital wall, left side
❼	S02.85	Fracture of orbit, unspecified

ICD-10-CM Coding Notes

For codes requiring a 7th character extension, refer to your ICD-10-CM book. Review the character descriptions and coding guidelines for proper selection. For some procedures, only certain characters will apply.

CCI Edits

Refer to Appendix A for CCI edits.

Facility RVUs ▢

Code	Work	PE Facility	MP	Total Facility
21406	7.42	8.54	1.36	17.32

Non-facility RVUs ▢

Code	Work	PE Non-Facility	MP	Total Non-Facility
21406	7.42	8.54	1.36	17.32

Modifiers (PAR) ▢

Code	Mod 50	Mod 51	Mod 62	Mod 66	Mod 80
21406	1	2	1	0	2

Global Period

Code	Days
21406	090

21407

21407 Open treatment of fracture of orbit, except blowout; with implant

AMA Coding Guideline

Surgical Procedures on the Head

Skull, facial bones, and temporomandibular joint.

Please see the Surgery Guidelines section for the following guidelines:

- *Surgical Procedures on the Musculoskeletal System*

AMA Coding Notes

Fracture and/or Dislocation Procedures on the Head

(For operative repair of skull fracture, see 62000-62010)

(To report closed treatment of skull fracture, use the appropriate Evaluation and Management code)

AMA *CPT® Assistant* ▢

21407: Dec 20: 11

Plain English Description

Open repair of a non-blowout orbital fracture, with implant is performed to restore the orbit to its natural shape. The natural skin creases are evaluated and incision lines are marked. A temporary tarsorrhaphy may be performed to protect the cornea by placing a mattress suture through the edges of the upper and lower eyelids to close the lids over the eye. The ends of the suture are grasped with a clamp and traction is applied upwards. The skin is incised along the marked lines to visualize the underlying orbicular muscle. The incision is extended subcutaneously over the pretarsal portion of the orbicularis oculi muscle to create a skin flap the full length of the incision. A dissection plane between the orbicularis oculi muscle and the septum orbitale is then created and suborbicular undermining of the muscle is performed using a slit-like lateral incision over the bony orbital rim. The suborbicular dissection plane is opened, leaving the orbital septum intact. The suborbicular pocket is extended downward over the whole lower palpebral region and the upper portion of the pocket below the tarsus is then opened. The remaining layer of the orbicularis oculi muscle is separated just below the lower border of the tarsus to create a skin muscle flap congruent with the lower eyelid. The eyelid and flap is retracted inferiorly over the anterior edge of the infraorbital rim and a periosteal elevator is employed to strip the periosteum from the bone. The intraorbital nerve is identified and preserved before continuing dissection along the upper facial surface of the anterior maxilla. The borders of the fracture are identified and orbital soft tissue that has herniated through any bony deficit is reduced. The fracture is reduced and an orbital implant (porous polyethylene, silicone, Teflon, Supramid, titanium mesh, bioresorbable copolymer plates) is inserted into the remaining bony deficit to prevent orbital soft tissue from prolapsing and restore the natural contour and volume of the orbit. The periosteum is then redraped over the implant and bony surface and secured with sutures.

Open treatment of fracture of orbit, except blowout; with implant

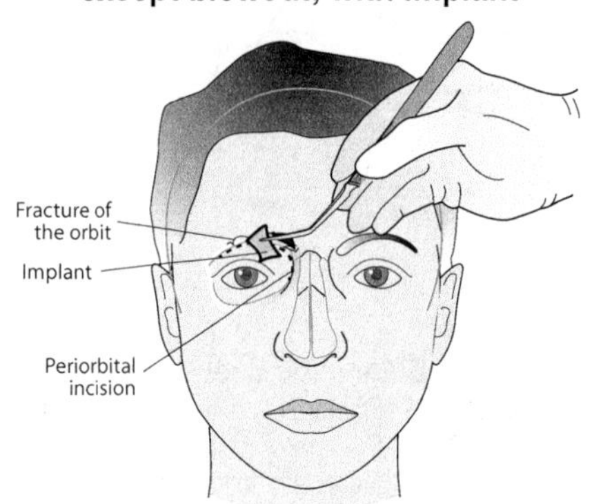

ICD-10-CM Diagnostic Codes

➐⇄	S02.121	Fracture of orbital roof, right side
➐⇄	S02.122	Fracture of orbital roof, left side
➐⇄	S02.831	Fracture of medial orbital wall, right side
➐⇄	S02.832	Fracture of medial orbital wall, left side
➐⇄	S02.841	Fracture of lateral orbital wall, right side
➐⇄	S02.842	Fracture of lateral orbital wall, left side
➐	S02.85	Fracture of orbit, unspecified

ICD-10-CM Coding Notes

For codes requiring a 7th character extension, refer to your ICD-10-CM book. Review the character descriptions and coding guidelines for proper selection. For some procedures, only certain characters will apply.

CCI Edits

Refer to Appendix A for CCI edits.

Facility RVUs ▢

Code	Work	PE Facility	MP	Total Facility
21407	9.02	8.81	1.12	18.95

Non-facility RVUs ▢

Code	Work	PE Non-Facility	MP	Total Non-Facility
21407	9.02	8.81	1.12	18.95

Modifiers (PAR) ▢

Code	Mod 50	Mod 51	Mod 62	Mod 66	Mod 80
21407	1	2	1	0	2

Global Period

Code	Days
21407	090

21408

21408 Open treatment of fracture of orbit, except blowout; with bone grafting (includes obtaining graft)

AMA Coding Guideline

Surgical Procedures on the Head

Skull, facial bones, and temporomandibular joint.

Please see the Surgery Guidelines section for the following guidelines:

- *Surgical Procedures on the Musculoskeletal System*

AMA Coding Notes

Fracture and/or Dislocation Procedures on the Head

(For operative repair of skull fracture, see 62000-62010)

(To report closed treatment of skull fracture, use the appropriate Evaluation and Management code)

Plain English Description

Open repair of a non-blowout orbital fracture, with bone grafting is performed to restore the orbit to its natural shape. The natural skin creases are evaluated and incision lines are marked. A temporary tarsorrhaphy may be performed to protect the cornea by placing a mattress suture through the edges of the upper and lower eyelids to close the lids over the eye. The ends of the suture are grasped with a clamp and traction is applied upwards. The skin is incised along the marked lines to visualize the underlying orbicular muscle. The incision is extended subcutaneously over the pretarsal portion of the orbicularis oculi muscle to create a skin flap the full length of the incision. A dissection plane between the orbicularis oculi muscle and the septum orbitale is then created and suborbicular undermining of the muscle is performed using a slit-like lateral incision over the bony orbital rim. The suborbicular dissection plane is opened, leaving the orbital septum intact. The suborbicular pocket is extended downward over the whole lower palpebral region and the upper portion of the pocket below the tarsus is then opened. The remaining layer of the orbicularis oculi muscle is separated just below the lower border of the tarsus to create a skin muscle flap congruent with the lower eyelid. The eyelid and flap is retracted inferiorly over the anterior edge of the infraorbital rim and a periosteal elevator is employed to strip the periosteum from the bone. The intraorbital nerve is identified and preserved before continuing dissection along the upper facial surface of the anterior maxilla. The borders of the fracture are identified and orbital soft tissue that has herniated through any bony deficit is reduced. The fracture is reduced and an autogenous bone graft harvested from the maxillary wall, calvaria, iliac crest, rib, or fibula and shaped to match the contour of the bony deficit is then inserted to prevent orbital soft tissue from prolapsing and restore the natural contour and volume of the orbit. The periosteum is then redraped over the grafted bony surface and secured with sutures.

Open treatment of fracture of orbit, except blowout; with bone grafting (includes obtaining graft)

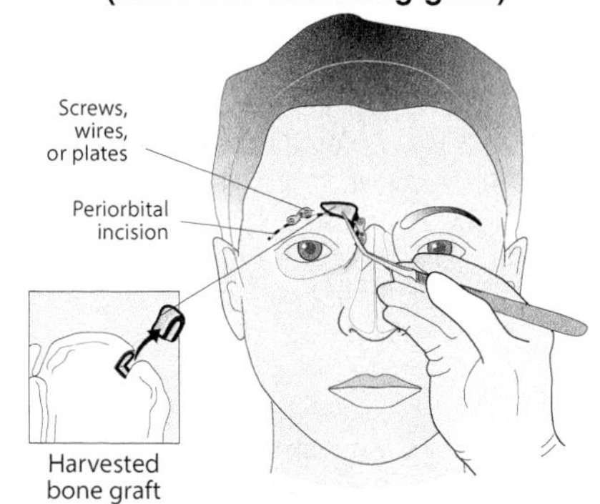

ICD-10-CM Diagnostic Codes

❼⇄	S02.121	Fracture of orbital roof, right side
❼⇄	S02.122	Fracture of orbital roof, left side
❼⇄	S02.831	Fracture of medial orbital wall, right side
❼⇄	S02.832	Fracture of medial orbital wall, left side
❼⇄	S02.841	Fracture of lateral orbital wall, right side
❼⇄	S02.842	Fracture of lateral orbital wall, left side
❼	S02.85	Fracture of orbit, unspecified

ICD-10-CM Coding Notes

For codes requiring a 7th character extension, refer to your ICD-10-CM book. Review the character descriptions and coding guidelines for proper selection. For some procedures, only certain characters will apply.

CCI Edits

Refer to Appendix A for CCI edits.

Facility RVUs ▯

Code	Work	PE Facility	MP	Total Facility
21408	12.78	11.64	2.33	26.75

Non-facility RVUs ▯

Code	Work	PE Non-Facility	MP	Total Non-Facility
21408	12.78	11.64	2.33	26.75

Modifiers (PAR) ▯

Code	Mod 50	Mod 51	Mod 62	Mod 66	Mod 80
21408	1	2	2	0	2

Global Period

Code	Days
21408	090

CPT® Procedural Coding

65091-65093

65091 Evisceration of ocular contents; without implant

65093 Evisceration of ocular contents; with implant

AMA Coding Notes

Surgical Procedures on the Eye and Ocular Adnexa

(For diagnostic and treatment ophthalmological services, see Medicine, Ophthalmology, and 92002 et seq)

(Do not report code 69990 in addition to codes 65091-68850)

Plain English Description

Evisceration of the eye is performed to treat eye infections that are unresponsive to antibiotics and for pain control or to improve the appearance in a blind eye. The cornea is excised and the ocular contents exposed. An ocular curette is then inserted into the space between the uveal tract and sclera. The ocular contents including the retina, uveal tract, vitreous and lens are then scraped away from the scleral shell. Bleeding from the vortex veins and central retinal artery is controlled with electrocautery and/or pressure. The scleral shell is carefully inspected and a swab used to remove any remaining uveal tissue. In 65091, evisceration is performed without placement of an implant. In 65093, an appropriately sized implant is inserted into the scleral shell. The sclera is then closed over the anterior surface of the implant in a layered fashion to prevent contraction of the sclera and extrusion of the implant.

Evisceration of ocular contents; with/without implant

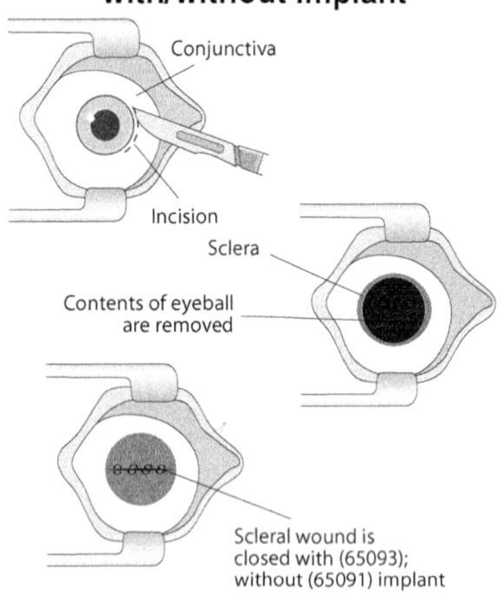

Conjunctiva
Incision
Sclera
Contents of eyeball are removed
Scleral wound is closed with (65093); without (65091) implant

ICD-10-CM Diagnostic Codes

	Code	Description
	A18.53	Tuberculous chorioretinitis
	A18.54	Tuberculous iridocyclitis
	B95.62	Methicillin resistant Staphylococcus aureus infection as the cause of diseases classified elsewhere
	D03.8	Melanoma in situ of other sites
⇄	D09.21	Carcinoma in situ of right eye
⇄	D09.22	Carcinoma in situ of left eye
⇄	D31.21	Benign neoplasm of right retina
⇄	D31.22	Benign neoplasm of left retina
⇄	D31.31	Benign neoplasm of right choroid
⇄	D31.32	Benign neoplasm of left choroid
⇄	D31.41	Benign neoplasm of right ciliary body
⇄	D31.42	Benign neoplasm of left ciliary body
⇄	H16.061	Mycotic corneal ulcer, right eye
⇄	H16.062	Mycotic corneal ulcer, left eye
⇄	H16.071	Perforated corneal ulcer, right eye
⇄	H16.072	Perforated corneal ulcer, left eye
⇄	H21.331	Parasitic cyst of iris, ciliary body or anterior chamber, right eye
⇄	H21.332	Parasitic cyst of iris, ciliary body or anterior chamber, left eye
⇄	H33.121	Parasitic cyst of retina, right eye
⇄	H33.122	Parasitic cyst of retina, left eye
⇄	H40.31X3	Glaucoma secondary to eye trauma, right eye, severe stage
⇄	H40.32X3	Glaucoma secondary to eye trauma, left eye, severe stage
⇄	H40.33X3	Glaucoma secondary to eye trauma, bilateral, severe stage
⇄	H40.41X3	Glaucoma secondary to eye inflammation, right eye, severe stage
⇄	H40.42X3	Glaucoma secondary to eye inflammation, left eye, severe stage
⇄	H40.43X3	Glaucoma secondary to eye inflammation, bilateral, severe stage
⇄	H40.51X3	Glaucoma secondary to other eye disorders, right eye, severe stage
⇄	H40.52X3	Glaucoma secondary to other eye disorders, left eye, severe stage
⇄	H40.53X3	Glaucoma secondary to other eye disorders, bilateral, severe stage
⇄	H44.001	Unspecified purulent endophthalmitis, right eye
⇄	H44.002	Unspecified purulent endophthalmitis, left eye
⇄	H44.003	Unspecified purulent endophthalmitis, bilateral
⇄	H44.011	Panophthalmitis (acute), right eye
⇄	H44.012	Panophthalmitis (acute), left eye
⇄	H44.013	Panophthalmitis (acute), bilateral
⇄	H44.021	Vitreous abscess (chronic), right eye
⇄	H44.022	Vitreous abscess (chronic), left eye
⇄	H44.023	Vitreous abscess (chronic), bilateral
⇄	H44.111	Panuveitis, right eye
⇄	H44.112	Panuveitis, left eye
⇄	H44.113	Panuveitis, bilateral
⇄	H44.121	Parasitic endophthalmitis, unspecified, right eye
⇄	H44.122	Parasitic endophthalmitis, unspecified, left eye
⇄	H44.123	Parasitic endophthalmitis, unspecified, bilateral
	H44.19	Other endophthalmitis
⇄	H57.11	Ocular pain, right eye
⇄	H57.12	Ocular pain, left eye
❼⇄	S05.21	Ocular laceration and rupture with prolapse or loss of intraocular tissue, right eye
❼⇄	S05.22	Ocular laceration and rupture with prolapse or loss of intraocular tissue, left eye
❼⇄	S05.51	Penetrating wound with foreign body of right eyeball
❼⇄	S05.52	Penetrating wound with foreign body of left eyeball
❼⇄	S05.61	Penetrating wound without foreign body of right eyeball
❼⇄	S05.62	Penetrating wound without foreign body of left eyeball
❼⇄	S05.8X1	Other injuries of right eye and orbit
❼⇄	S05.8X2	Other injuries of left eye and orbit

ICD-10-CM Coding Notes

For codes requiring a 7th character extension, refer to your ICD-10-CM book. Review the character descriptions and coding guidelines for proper selection. For some procedures, only certain characters will apply.

CCI Edits

Refer to Appendix A for CCI edits.

Facility RVUs ▯

Code	Work	PE Facility	MP	Total Facility
65091	7.26	14.34	0.56	22.16
65093	7.04	14.38	0.56	21.98

Non-facility RVUs ▯

Code	Work	PE Non-Facility	MP	Total Non-Facility
65091	7.26	14.34	0.56	22.16
65093	7.04	14.38	0.56	21.98

Modifiers (PAR) ▯

Code	Mod 50	Mod 51	Mod 62	Mod 66	Mod 80
65091	1	2	1	0	0
65093	1	2	1	0	1

Global Period

Code	Days
65091	090
65093	090

65101-65105

65101 Enucleation of eye; without implant

65103 Enucleation of eye; with implant, muscles not attached to implant

65105 Enucleation of eye; with implant, muscles attached to implant

(For conjunctivoplasty after enucleation, see 68320 et seq)

AMA Coding Notes

Surgical Procedures on the Eye and Ocular Adnexa

(For diagnostic and treatment ophthalmological services, see Medicine, Ophthalmology, and 92002 et seq)

(Do not report code 69990 in addition to codes 65091-68850)

Plain English Description

Enucleation of the eye is performed to treat tumors of the eye such as intraocular melanoma or retinoblastoma and for severe trauma to the eye. The globe is measured and the length of the optic nerve determined. The globe is illuminated and a dissecting microscope used to help visualize orbital structures and identify the extent of the lesion or trauma. A limbal incision is made around the conjunctiva and Tenon's capsule. The extraocular muscles are exposed and divided. The optic nerve is located and divided. The globe is removed. In 65101, an enucleation is performed without placement of an implant. In 65103, an appropriately sized implant is placed in the muscle cone without attachment to extraocular muscles. In 65105, an implant is placed in the muscle cone and the extraocular muscles are sutured to the implant.

Enucleation of eye with/without implant

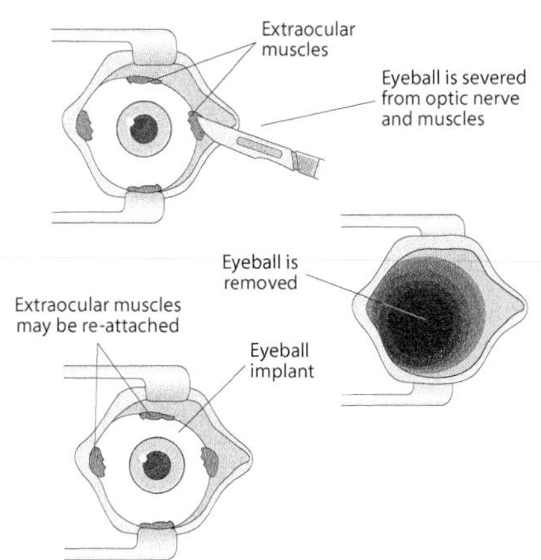

Procedure is completed without implant (65101); with implant, muscles not attached (65103); attached (65105)

ICD-10-CM Diagnostic Codes

	Code	Description
⇄	C69.01	Malignant neoplasm of right conjunctiva
⇄	C69.02	Malignant neoplasm of left conjunctiva
⇄	C69.11	Malignant neoplasm of right cornea
⇄	C69.12	Malignant neoplasm of left cornea
⇄	C69.21	Malignant neoplasm of right retina
⇄	C69.22	Malignant neoplasm of left retina
⇄	C69.31	Malignant neoplasm of right choroid
⇄	C69.32	Malignant neoplasm of left choroid
⇄	C69.41	Malignant neoplasm of right ciliary body
⇄	C69.42	Malignant neoplasm of left ciliary body
⇄	D09.22	Carcinoma in situ of left eye
⇄	D31.21	Benign neoplasm of right retina
⇄	D31.22	Benign neoplasm of left retina
⇄	D31.31	Benign neoplasm of right choroid
⇄	D31.32	Benign neoplasm of left choroid
⇄	H44.521	Atrophy of globe, right eye
⇄	H44.522	Atrophy of globe, left eye
⇄	H57.11	Ocular pain, right eye
⇄	H57.12	Ocular pain, left eye
	Q11.2	Microphthalmos
❼⇄	S05.21	Ocular laceration and rupture with prolapse or loss of intraocular tissue, right eye
❼⇄	S05.22	Ocular laceration and rupture with prolapse or loss of intraocular tissue, left eye
❼⇄	S05.51	Penetrating wound with foreign body of right eyeball
❼⇄	S05.52	Penetrating wound with foreign body of left eyeball
❼⇄	S05.61	Penetrating wound without foreign body of right eyeball
❼⇄	S05.62	Penetrating wound without foreign body of left eyeball
❼⇄	S05.71	Avulsion of right eye
❼⇄	S05.72	Avulsion of left eye
❼⇄	S05.8X1	Other injuries of right eye and orbit
❼⇄	S05.8X2	Other injuries of left eye and orbit
❼⇄	T26.21	Burn with resulting rupture and destruction of right eyeball
❼⇄	T26.22	Burn with resulting rupture and destruction of left eyeball
❼⇄	T26.71	Corrosion with resulting rupture and destruction of right eyeball
❼⇄	T26.72	Corrosion with resulting rupture and destruction of left eyeball

ICD-10-CM Coding Notes

For codes requiring a 7th character extension, refer to your ICD-10-CM book. Review the character descriptions and coding guidelines for proper selection. For some procedures, only certain characters will apply.

CCI Edits

Refer to Appendix A for CCI edits.

Facility RVUs ▯

Code	Work	PE Facility	MP	Total Facility
65101	8.30	16.33	0.64	25.27
65103	8.84	16.53	0.67	26.04
65105	9.93	17.60	0.77	28.30

Non-facility RVUs ▯

Code	Work	PE Non-Facility	MP	Total Non-Facility
65101	8.30	16.33	0.64	25.27
65103	8.84	16.53	0.67	26.04
65105	9.93	17.60	0.77	28.30

Modifiers (PAR) ▯

Code	Mod 50	Mod 51	Mod 62	Mod 66	Mod 80
65101	1	2	0	0	1
65103	1	2	1	0	1
65105	1	2	1	0	2

Global Period

Code	Days
65101	090
65103	090
65105	090

65110-65114

65110 Exenteration of orbit (does not include skin graft), removal of orbital contents; only

65112 Exenteration of orbit (does not include skin graft), removal of orbital contents; with therapeutic removal of bone

65114 Exenteration of orbit (does not include skin graft), removal of orbital contents; with muscle or myocutaneous flap

(For skin graft to orbit (split skin), see 15120, 15121; free, full thickness, see 15260, 15261)

(For eyelid repair involving more than skin, see 67930 et seq)

AMA Coding Notes

Surgical Procedures on the Eye and Ocular Adnexa

(For diagnostic and treatment ophthalmological services, see Medicine, Ophthalmology, and 92002 et seq)

(Do not report code 69990 in addition to codes 65091-68850)

Plain English Description

Exenteration is performed primarily for orbital tumors or intraocular tumors that extend into the orbit or extraorbital structures, such as the eyelids or bone surrounding the eye. If the eyelid anatomy is free of disease, full thickness incisions are made through the entire eyelid just above the upper lash line and just below the loser lash line. If only the skin of the eyelid is preserved, the skin is incised just above the upper lash line and just below the lower lash line. The skin of the eyelid is dissected from underlying subcutaneous tissue and both superiorly and inferiorly to the level of the orbital rim. If the eyelids are completely removed full-thickness incisions are made through the skin and soft tissue along the orbital rim. The periosteum of the orbital rim is then dissected off of underlying bone in a circular fashion until the entire the globe and orbital contents have been completely freed. The entire globe and orbital contents are then removed. Underlying bony structures are inspected for evidence of tumor extension. If tumor is present in the bones of the orbits is, boney tissue is excised as well. If the entire eyelids or skin of the eyelids have been preserved, the eyelids are closed in layers. If the eyelids have been completely excised separately reportable skin grafts may be used to close the defect. Use 65110 when no bone is removed and the defect can be closed without the use of muscle or myocutaneous flaps. Use 65112 when bone is removed. Use 65114 when muscle or myocutaneous flap is used to close the surgical defect. A free muscle or myocutaneous flap is developed taking care to preserve blood supply to the flap. Commonly used free muscle flaps include the abdominis rectus or latissimus dorsi muscles. The free flap is trimmed to the desired size and shape. Blood vessels in the free flap are sutured to blood vessels surrounding the eye. The edges of the flap are secured with sutures.

ICD-10-CM Diagnostic Codes

	C41.0	Malignant neoplasm of bones of skull and face
⇄	C43.111	Malignant melanoma of right upper eyelid, including canthus
⇄	C43.112	Malignant melanoma of right lower eyelid, including canthus
⇄	C43.121	Malignant melanoma of left upper eyelid, including canthus
⇄	C43.122	Malignant melanoma of left lower eyelid, including canthus
⇄	C69.01	Malignant neoplasm of right conjunctiva
⇄	C69.11	Malignant neoplasm of right cornea
⇄	C69.21	Malignant neoplasm of right retina
⇄	C69.31	Malignant neoplasm of right choroid
⇄	C69.41	Malignant neoplasm of right ciliary body
⇄	C69.51	Malignant neoplasm of right lacrimal gland and duct
⇄	C69.61	Malignant neoplasm of right orbit
⇄	C69.81	Malignant neoplasm of overlapping sites of right eye and adnexa
⇄	D09.21	Carcinoma in situ of right eye

CCI Edits

Refer to Appendix A for CCI edits.

Facility RVUs □

Code	Work	PE Facility	MP	Total Facility
65110	15.70	22.00	1.20	38.90
65112	18.51	24.56	1.41	44.48
65114	19.65	25.27	1.51	46.43

Non-facility RVUs □

Code	Work	PE Non-Facility	MP	Total Non-Facility
65110	15.70	22.00	1.20	38.90
65112	18.51	24.56	1.41	44.48
65114	19.65	25.27	1.51	46.43

Modifiers (PAR) □

Code	Mod 50	Mod 51	Mod 62	Mod 66	Mod 80
65110	1	2	1	0	2
65112	1	2	1	0	2
65114	1	2	1	0	2

Global Period

Code	Days
65110	090
65112	090
65114	090

65125

65125 Modification of ocular implant with placement or replacement of pegs (eg, drilling receptacle for prosthesis appendage) (separate procedure)

AMA Coding Guideline

Secondary Implant(s) Procedures on the Eyeball

An ocular implant is an implant inside muscular cone; an orbital implant is an implant outside muscular cone.

AMA Coding Notes

Surgical Procedures on the Eye and Ocular Adnexa

(For diagnostic and treatment ophthalmological services, see Medicine, Ophthalmology, and 92002 et seq)

(Do not report code 69990 in addition to codes 65091-68850)

Plain English Description

The ocular implant is removed in a separately reportable procedure. The ocular implant is then modified to improve the fit in the eye socket. Pegs are removed as needed and new holes drilled for repositioning of the pegs. Additional pegs may be placed to better secure the implant within the eye socket.

Modification of ocular implant

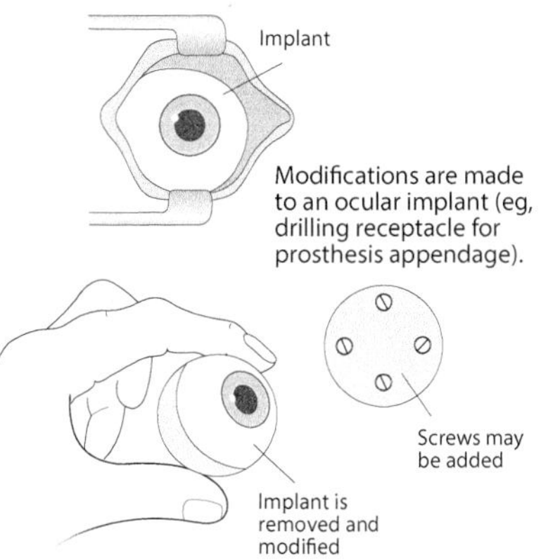

ICD-10-CM Diagnostic Codes

➐⇄	T85.310	Breakdown (mechanical) of prosthetic orbit of right eye
➐⇄	T85.311	Breakdown (mechanical) of prosthetic orbit of left eye
➐⇄	T85.318	Breakdown (mechanical) of other ocular prosthetic devices, implants and grafts
➐⇄	T85.320	Displacement of prosthetic orbit of right eye
➐⇄	T85.321	Displacement of prosthetic orbit of left eye
➐⇄	T85.328	Displacement of other ocular prosthetic devices, implants and grafts
➐⇄	T85.390	Other mechanical complication of prosthetic orbit of right eye
➐⇄	T85.391	Other mechanical complication of prosthetic orbit of left eye
➐⇄	T85.398	Other mechanical complication of other ocular prosthetic devices, implants and grafts
➐	T85.79	Infection and inflammatory reaction due to other internal prosthetic devices, implants and grafts
⇄	Z44.21	Encounter for fitting and adjustment of artificial right eye
⇄	Z44.22	Encounter for fitting and adjustment of artificial left eye
	Z85.840	Personal history of malignant neoplasm of eye
	Z87.828	Personal history of other (healed) physical injury and trauma
	Z90.01	Acquired absence of eye
	Z97.0	Presence of artificial eye

ICD-10-CM Coding Notes

For codes requiring a 7th character extension, refer to your ICD-10-CM book. Review the character descriptions and coding guidelines for proper selection. For some procedures, only certain characters will apply.

CCI Edits

Refer to Appendix A for CCI edits.

Facility RVUs ▯

Code	Work	PE Facility	MP	Total Facility
65125	3.27	4.97	0.25	8.49

Non-facility RVUs ▯

Code	Work	PE Non-Facility	MP	Total Non-Facility
65125	3.27	9.98	0.25	13.50

Modifiers (PAR) ▯

Code	Mod 50	Mod 51	Mod 62	Mod 66	Mod 80
65125	1	2	1	0	1

Global Period

Code	Days
65125	090

65130

65130 Insertion of ocular implant secondary; after evisceration, in scleral shell

AMA Coding Guideline

Secondary Implant(s) Procedures on the Eyeball

An ocular implant is an implant inside muscular cone; an orbital implant is an implant outside muscular cone.

AMA Coding Notes

Surgical Procedures on the Eye and Ocular Adnexa

(For diagnostic and treatment ophthalmological services, see Medicine, Ophthalmology, and 92002 et seq)

(Do not report code 69990 in addition to codes 65091-68850)

Plain English Description

If the remaining scleral shell has been closed, it is opened. An appropriately sized implant is selected and placed in the sclera shell. The sclera is then closed over the anterior surface of the implant in a layered fashion to prevent contraction of the sclera and extrusion of the implant.

Insertion of ocular implant

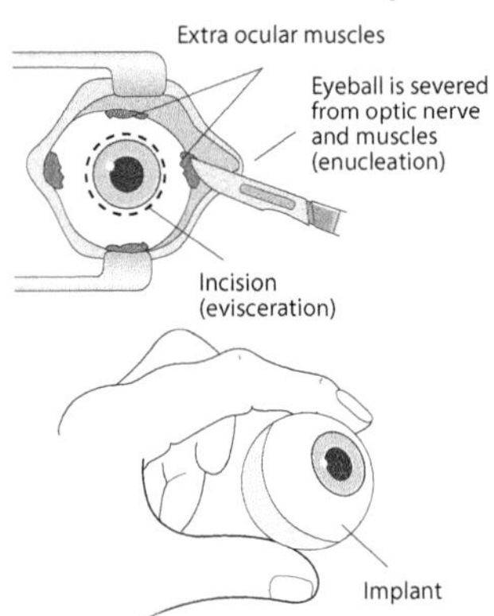

Post evisceration scleral shell implant (65130)

ICD-10-CM Diagnostic Codes

⇄	Z44.22	Encounter for fitting and adjustment of artificial left eye
	Z85.840	Personal history of malignant neoplasm of eye
	Z87.828	Personal history of other (healed) physical injury and trauma
	Z90.01	Acquired absence of eye
	Z97.0	Presence of artificial eye

CCI Edits

Refer to Appendix A for CCI edits.

Facility RVUs ▯

Code	Work	PE Facility	MP	Total Facility
65130	8.42	16.28	0.65	25.35

Non-facility RVUs ▯

Code	Work	PE Non-Facility	MP	Total Non-Facility
65130	8.42	16.28	0.65	25.35

Modifiers (PAR) ▯

Code	Mod 50	Mod 51	Mod 62	Mod 66	Mod 80
65130	1	2	1	0	1

Global Period

Code	Days
65130	090

65135-65140

65135 Insertion of ocular implant secondary; after enucleation, muscles not attached to implant

65140 Insertion of ocular implant secondary; after enucleation, muscles attached to implant

AMA Coding Guideline

Secondary Implant(s) Procedures on the Eyeball

An ocular implant is an implant inside muscular cone; an orbital implant is an implant outside muscular cone.

AMA Coding Notes

Surgical Procedures on the Eye and Ocular Adnexa

(For diagnostic and treatment ophthalmological services, see Medicine, Ophthalmology, and 92002 et seq)

(Do not report code 69990 in addition to codes 65091-68850)

Plain English Description

If the eyelid has been closed with sutures it is opened and the muscle cone inspected. An appropriately sized ocular implant is selected and placed in the muscle cone. In 65135, the implant is not attached to the extraocular muscles. Ocular implants are composed of porous material, such as mesh or biosynthetic material. Surrounding tissue will eventually grow into the porous implant and secure it within the muscle cone. In 65140, the muscles are secured to the implant with sutures. The sutures can be easily placed through the porous implant material. The eye muscle tissue will eventually grow into the implant.

Insertion of ocular implant

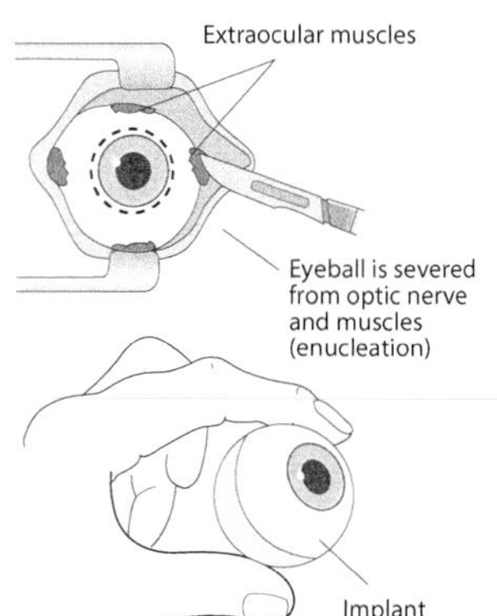

Post enucleation implant without (65135); with (65140) muscle attachment

ICD-10-CM Diagnostic Codes

⇄	Z44.21	Encounter for fitting and adjustment of artificial right eye
⇄	Z44.22	Encounter for fitting and adjustment of artificial left eye
	Z85.840	Personal history of malignant neoplasm of eye
	Z87.828	Personal history of other (healed) physical injury and trauma
	Z90.01	Acquired absence of eye
	Z97.0	Presence of artificial eye

CCI Edits

Refer to Appendix A for CCI edits.

Facility RVUs

Code	Work	PE Facility	MP	Total Facility
65135	8.60	16.39	0.65	25.64
65140	9.46	17.34	0.73	27.53

Non-facility RVUs

Code	Work	PE Non-Facility	MP	Total Non-Facility
65135	8.60	16.39	0.65	25.64
65140	9.46	17.34	0.73	27.53

Modifiers (PAR)

Code	Mod 50	Mod 51	Mod 62	Mod 66	Mod 80
65135	1	2	0	0	1
65140	1	2	0	0	1

Global Period

Code	Days
65135	090
65140	090

65150-65155

65150 Reinsertion of ocular implant; with or without conjunctival graft

65155 Reinsertion of ocular implant; with use of foreign material for reinforcement and/or attachment of muscles to implant

AMA Coding Guideline

Secondary Implant(s) Procedures on the Eyeball

An ocular implant is an implant inside muscular cone; an orbital implant is an implant outside muscular cone.

AMA Coding Notes

Surgical Procedures on the Eye and Ocular Adnexa

(For diagnostic and treatment ophthalmological services, see Medicine, Ophthalmology, and 92002 et seq)

(Do not report code 69990 in addition to codes 65091-68850)

Plain English Description

The scleral shell or muscle cone is exposed. The ocular implant is then reinserted in the scleral shell or muscle cone. In 65150, if the patient has had a previous evisceration procedure, the sclera is closed over the anterior surface of the implant in a layered fashion to prevent contraction of the sclera and extrusion of the implant. Alternatively, a conjunctival graft may be used to secure and/or cover the implant. If the patient has had an enucleation procedure, a conjunctival graft may be fashioned and used to secure and/or completely cover the implant. In 65155, synthetic material such as pegs or mesh is used to secure the implant and attach extraocular muscles.

Reinsertion of ocular implant with/without conjunctival graft

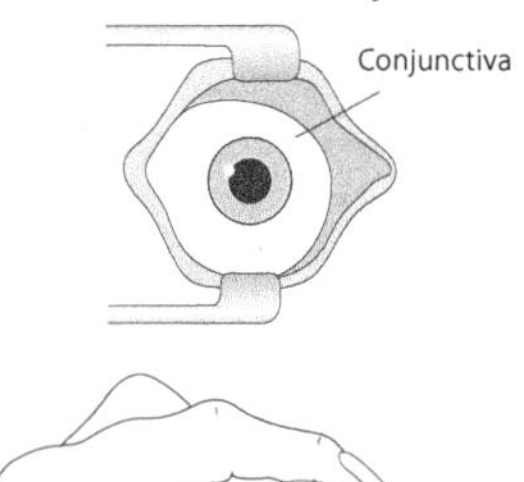

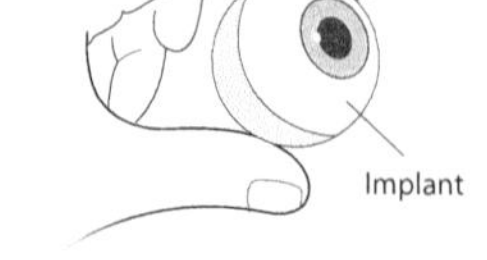

Reinsertion with/without conjuctival graft (65150); with use of foreign material for reinforcement/attachment of muscles to implant (65155)

ICD-10-CM Diagnostic Codes

⇄	H57.11	Ocular pain, right eye
⇄	H57.12	Ocular pain, left eye
⇄	H57.13	Ocular pain, bilateral
❼⇄	T85.310	Breakdown (mechanical) of prosthetic orbit of right eye
❼⇄	T85.311	Breakdown (mechanical) of prosthetic orbit of left eye
❼⇄	T85.318	Breakdown (mechanical) of other ocular prosthetic devices, implants and grafts
❼⇄	T85.320	Displacement of prosthetic orbit of right eye
❼⇄	T85.321	Displacement of prosthetic orbit of left eye
❼⇄	T85.328	Displacement of other ocular prosthetic devices, implants and grafts
❼⇄	T85.390	Other mechanical complication of prosthetic orbit of right eye
❼⇄	T85.391	Other mechanical complication of prosthetic orbit of left eye
❼⇄	T85.398	Other mechanical complication of other ocular prosthetic devices, implants and grafts
❼	T85.79	Infection and inflammatory reaction due to other internal prosthetic devices, implants and grafts
⇄	Z44.21	Encounter for fitting and adjustment of artificial right eye
	Z85.840	Personal history of malignant neoplasm of eye
	Z87.828	Personal history of other (healed) physical injury and trauma
	Z90.01	Acquired absence of eye
	Z97.0	Presence of artificial eye

ICD-10-CM Coding Notes

For codes requiring a 7th character extension, refer to your ICD-10-CM book. Review the character descriptions and coding guidelines for proper selection. For some procedures, only certain characters will apply.

CCI Edits

Refer to Appendix A for CCI edits.

Facility RVUs ▢

Code	Work	PE Facility	MP	Total Facility
65150	6.43	14.01	0.50	20.94
65155	10.10	17.72	0.77	28.59

Non-facility RVUs ▢

Code	Work	PE Non-Facility	MP	Total Non-Facility
65150	6.43	14.01	0.50	20.94
65155	10.10	17.72	0.77	28.59

Modifiers (PAR) ▢

Code	Mod 50	Mod 51	Mod 62	Mod 66	Mod 80
65150	1	2	0	0	0
65155	1	2	0	0	1

Global Period

Code	Days
65150	090
65155	090

65175

65175 Removal of ocular implant

(For orbital implant (implant outside muscle cone) insertion, use 67550; removal, use 67560)

AMA Coding Guideline

Secondary Implant(s) Procedures on the Eyeball

An ocular implant is an implant inside muscular cone; an orbital implant is an implant outside muscular cone.

AMA Coding Notes

Surgical Procedures on the Eye and Ocular Adnexa

(For diagnostic and treatment ophthalmological services, see Medicine, Ophthalmology, and 92002 et seq)

(Do not report code 69990 in addition to codes 65091-68850)

Plain English Description

The ocular implant is exposed. If the patient has had a previous evisceration procedure, the scleral shell that has been secured over the anterior aspect of the implant is opened. The ocular implant is then dissected free of sclera and removed. If the patient has had a previous enucleation procedure, any overlying tissue or synthetic grafts are removed. The ocular implant is then dissected free of surrounding tissue and removed.

Removal of ocular implant

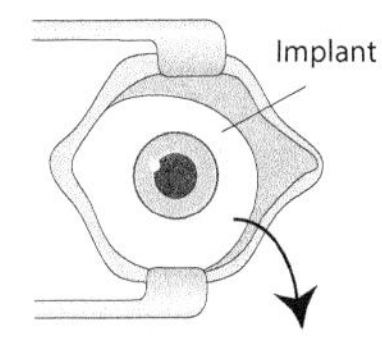

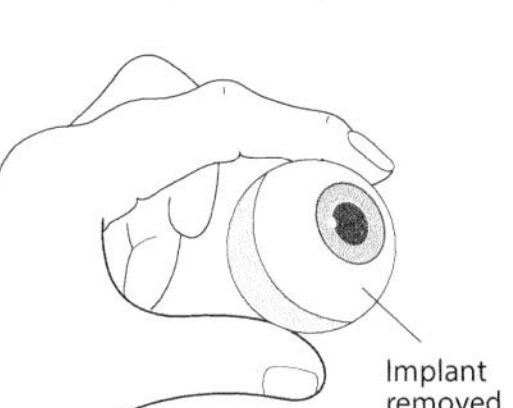

An implant from enucleated/eviscerated eye is removed.

ICD-10-CM Diagnostic Codes

	H05.00	Unspecified acute inflammation of orbit
⇄	H05.011	Cellulitis of right orbit
⇄	H05.012	Cellulitis of left orbit
⇄	H05.021	Osteomyelitis of right orbit
⇄	H05.022	Osteomyelitis of left orbit
⇄	H05.031	Periostitis of right orbit
⇄	H05.032	Periostitis of left orbit
⇄	H05.111	Granuloma of right orbit
⇄	H05.112	Granuloma of left orbit
⇄	H05.351	Exostosis of right orbit
⇄	H05.352	Exostosis of left orbit
⇄	H57.11	Ocular pain, right eye
⇄	H57.12	Ocular pain, left eye
❼⇄	T85.310	Breakdown (mechanical) of prosthetic orbit of right eye
❼⇄	T85.311	Breakdown (mechanical) of prosthetic orbit of left eye
❼⇄	T85.318	Breakdown (mechanical) of other ocular prosthetic devices, implants and grafts
❼⇄	T85.320	Displacement of prosthetic orbit of right eye
❼⇄	T85.321	Displacement of prosthetic orbit of left eye
❼⇄	T85.328	Displacement of other ocular prosthetic devices, implants and grafts
❼⇄	T85.390	Other mechanical complication of prosthetic orbit of right eye
❼⇄	T85.391	Other mechanical complication of prosthetic orbit of left eye
❼⇄	T85.398	Other mechanical complication of other ocular prosthetic devices, implants and grafts
⇄	Z44.21	Encounter for fitting and adjustment of artificial right eye
⇄	Z44.22	Encounter for fitting and adjustment of artificial left eye
	Z85.840	Personal history of malignant neoplasm of eye
	Z87.828	Personal history of other (healed) physical injury and trauma
	Z90.01	Acquired absence of eye
	Z97.0	Presence of artificial eye

ICD-10-CM Coding Notes

For codes requiring a 7th character extension, refer to your ICD-10-CM book. Review the character descriptions and coding guidelines for proper selection. For some procedures, only certain characters will apply.

CCI Edits

Refer to Appendix A for CCI edits.

Facility RVUs ▢

Code	Work	PE Facility	MP	Total Facility
65175	7.40	15.22	0.57	23.19

Non-facility RVUs ▢

Code	Work	PE Non-Facility	MP	Total Non-Facility
65175	7.40	15.22	0.57	23.19

Modifiers (PAR) ▢

Code	Mod 50	Mod 51	Mod 62	Mod 66	Mod 80
65175	1	2	1	0	1

Global Period

Code	Days
65175	090

65205-65210

65205 Removal of foreign body, external eye; conjunctival superficial

65210 Removal of foreign body, external eye; conjunctival embedded (includes concretions), subconjunctival, or scleral nonperforating

AMA Coding Notes

Removal of Foreign Body Procedures on the Eyeball

(For removal of implanted material: ocular implant, use 65175; anterior segment implant, use 65920; posterior segment implant, use 67120; orbital implant, use 67560)

(For diagnostic x-ray for foreign body, use 70030)

(For diagnostic echography for foreign body, use 76529)

(For removal of foreign body from orbit: frontal approach, use 67413; lateral approach, use 67430)

(For removal of foreign body from eyelid, embedded, use 67938)

(For removal of foreign body from lacrimal system, use 68530)

Surgical Procedures on the Eye and Ocular Adnexa

(For diagnostic and treatment ophthalmological services, see Medicine, Ophthalmology, and 92002 et seq)

(Do not report code 69990 in addition to codes 65091-68850)

AMA *CPT® Assistant*

65205: Mar 05: 17, Oct 13: 19

Plain English Description

A foreign body is removed from the conjunctiva, subconjunctiva, or sclera. The conjunctiva is the mucous membrane covering the anterior surface of the eyeball (bulbar conjunctiva) and the posterior surface of the eyelid (palpebral conjunctiva). The subconjunctiva is the tissue immediately below the conjunctiva. The sclera, also referred to as the white of the eye, is the fibrous layer that forms the outer envelope of the eye. The eye is examined and the foreign body identified. Anesthetic eye drops are applied as needed. In 65205, a superficial conjunctival foreign body is removed using saline irrigation or a cotton swab. In 65210, an embedded foreign body is removed from the conjunctiva, subconjunctiva, or sclera using a cotton-tipped swab or forceps. The eye is copiously irrigated with saline solution following removal of the foreign body.

Removal of foreign body, external eye

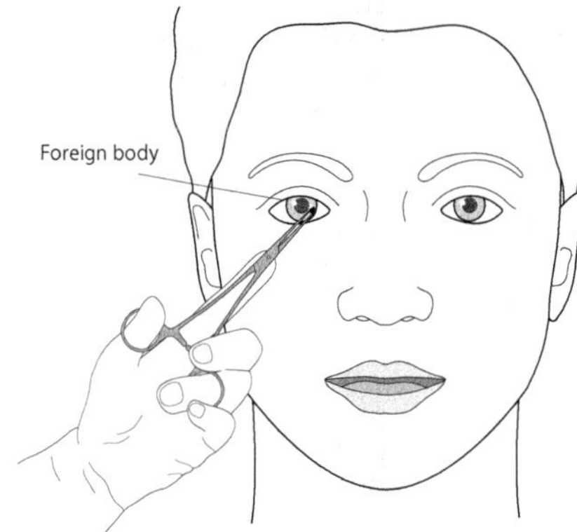

The physician removes a foreign body from the outer covering of the eye.

ICD-10-CM Diagnostic Codes

⇄	H11.121	Conjunctival concretions, right eye
⇄	H11.122	Conjunctival concretions, left eye
⇄	H11.123	Conjunctival concretions, bilateral
➐⇄	T15.11	Foreign body in conjunctival sac, right eye
➐⇄	T15.12	Foreign body in conjunctival sac, left eye
➐⇄	T15.81	Foreign body in other and multiple parts of external eye, right eye
➐⇄	T15.82	Foreign body in other and multiple parts of external eye, left eye
➐⇄	T15.91	Foreign body on external eye, part unspecified, right eye
➐⇄	T15.92	Foreign body on external eye, part unspecified, left eye
	Z18.10	Retained metal fragments, unspecified
	Z18.11	Retained magnetic metal fragments
	Z18.12	Retained nonmagnetic metal fragments
	Z18.2	Retained plastic fragments
	Z18.33	Retained wood fragments
	Z18.39	Other retained organic fragments
	Z18.81	Retained glass fragments
	Z18.83	Retained stone or crystalline fragments
	Z18.89	Other specified retained foreign body fragments
	Z18.9	Retained foreign body fragments, unspecified material

ICD-10-CM Coding Notes

For codes requiring a 7th character extension, refer to your ICD-10-CM book. Review the character descriptions and coding guidelines for proper selection. For some procedures, only certain characters will apply.

CCI Edits

Refer to Appendix A for CCI edits.

Facility RVUs

Code	Work	PE Facility	MP	Total Facility
65205	0.49	0.32	0.04	0.85
65210	0.61	0.40	0.04	1.05

Non-facility RVUs

Code	Work	PE Non-Facility	MP	Total Non-Facility
65205	0.49	0.32	0.04	0.85
65210	0.61	0.49	0.04	1.14

Modifiers (PAR)

Code	Mod 50	Mod 51	Mod 62	Mod 66	Mod 80
65205	1	2	0	0	1
65210	1	2	0	0	1

Global Period

Code	Days
65205	000
65210	000

65220-65222

65220 Removal of foreign body, external eye; corneal, without slit lamp

65222 Removal of foreign body, external eye; corneal, with slit lamp

(For repair of corneal laceration with foreign body, use 65275)

AMA Coding Notes

Removal of Foreign Body Procedures on the Eyeball

(For removal of implanted material: ocular implant, use 65175; anterior segment implant, use 65920; posterior segment implant, use 67120; orbital implant, use 67560)

(For diagnostic x-ray for foreign body, use 70030)

(For diagnostic echography for foreign body, use 76529)

(For removal of foreign body from orbit: frontal approach, use 67413; lateral approach, use 67430)

(For removal of foreign body from eyelid, embedded, use 67938)

(For removal of foreign body from lacrimal system, use 68530)

Surgical Procedures on the Eye and Ocular Adnexa

(For diagnostic and treatment ophthalmological services, see Medicine, Ophthalmology, and 92002 et seq)

(Do not report code 69990 in addition to codes 65091-68850)

Plain English Description

A foreign body is removed from the cornea. The cornea is the transparent tissue that covers the anterior aspect of the eye. The cornea refracts light helping the eye to focus. Anesthetic drops are instilled into the eye. The physician checks visual acuity and performs a funduscopy to locate the foreign body. A slit lamp, which is an instrument used to illuminate and provide a magnified, three-dimensional view of the eye, may be also be used. A superficial corneal foreign body may be removed with a moistened cotton swab. An embedded foreign body is removed under magnification with an ophthalmic spud or needle. If a metallic foreign body has left a rust ring, the rust impregnated corneal tissue is removed using a corneal burr. The eye is flushed with saline solution to remove any foreign body fragments. The corneal defect caused by the foreign body is treated like a corneal abrasion using antibiotic ointment and an eye patch. Use 65220 if the foreign body is removed without a slit lamp and 65222 if a slit lamp is used.

Removal of foreign body, external eye; corneal

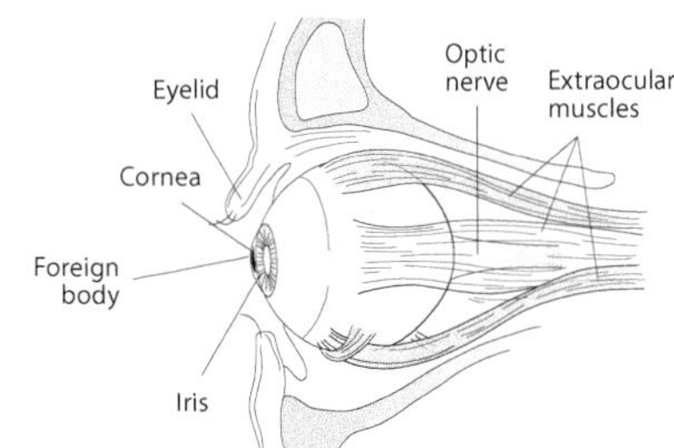

A foreign body is removed from the cornea of the eye with (65222); without (65220) slit lamp.

ICD-10-CM Diagnostic Codes

⑦⇄	T15.01	Foreign body in cornea, right eye
⑦⇄	T15.02	Foreign body in cornea, left eye
⑦⇄	T15.81	Foreign body in other and multiple parts of external eye, right eye
⑦⇄	T15.82	Foreign body in other and multiple parts of external eye, left eye
⑦⇄	T15.91	Foreign body on external eye, part unspecified, right eye
⑦⇄	T15.92	Foreign body on external eye, part unspecified, left eye
	Z18.10	Retained metal fragments, unspecified
	Z18.11	Retained magnetic metal fragments
	Z18.12	Retained nonmagnetic metal fragments
	Z18.2	Retained plastic fragments
	Z18.33	Retained wood fragments
	Z18.39	Other retained organic fragments
	Z18.81	Retained glass fragments
	Z18.83	Retained stone or crystalline fragments
	Z18.89	Other specified retained foreign body fragments
	Z18.9	Retained foreign body fragments, unspecified material

ICD-10-CM Coding Notes

For codes requiring a 7th character extension, refer to your ICD-10-CM book. Review the character descriptions and coding guidelines for proper selection. For some procedures, only certain characters will apply.

CCI Edits

Refer to Appendix A for CCI edits.

Facility RVUs ▯

Code	Work	PE Facility	MP	Total Facility
65220	0.71	0.40	0.09	1.20
65222	0.84	0.57	0.05	1.46

Non-facility RVUs ▯

Code	Work	PE Non-Facility	MP	Total Non-Facility
65220	0.71	0.97	0.09	1.77
65222	0.84	1.09	0.05	1.98

Modifiers (PAR) ▯

Code	Mod 50	Mod 51	Mod 62	Mod 66	Mod 80
65220	1	2	0	0	1
65222	1	2	0	0	1

Global Period

Code	Days
65220	000
65222	000

CPT® Procedural Coding

65235

65235 Removal of foreign body, intraocular; from anterior chamber of eye or lens

(For removal of implanted material from anterior segment, use 65920)

AMA Coding Notes

Removal of Foreign Body Procedures on the Eyeball

(For removal of implanted material: ocular implant, use 65175; anterior segment implant, use 65920; posterior segment implant, use 67120; orbital implant, use 67560)

(For diagnostic x-ray for foreign body, use 70030)

(For diagnostic echography for foreign body, use 76529)

(For removal of foreign body from orbit: frontal approach, use 67413; lateral approach, use 67430)

(For removal of foreign body from eyelid, embedded, use 67938)

(For removal of foreign body from lacrimal system, use 68530)

Surgical Procedures on the Eye and Ocular Adnexa

(For diagnostic and treatment ophthalmological services, see Medicine, Ophthalmology, and 92002 et seq)

(Do not report code 69990 in addition to codes 65091-68850)

Plain English Description

The anterior chamber lies behind the cornea and in front of the iris and lens. The anterior chamber is filled with a clear watery fluid called aqueous humor. The injury to the eye is inspected and the location of the intraocular foreign body determined to be in the anterior chamber or lens without penetration into deeper structures of the eye. The site of entry is located and the wound enlarged as needed. Alternatively, a separate incision may be made to provide access to the foreign body. A metallic foreign body is removed using a magnet. A non-metallic foreign body is removed using forceps. The wound is closed with sutures as needed.

Removal of foreign body, intraocular; from anterior chamber of eye lens

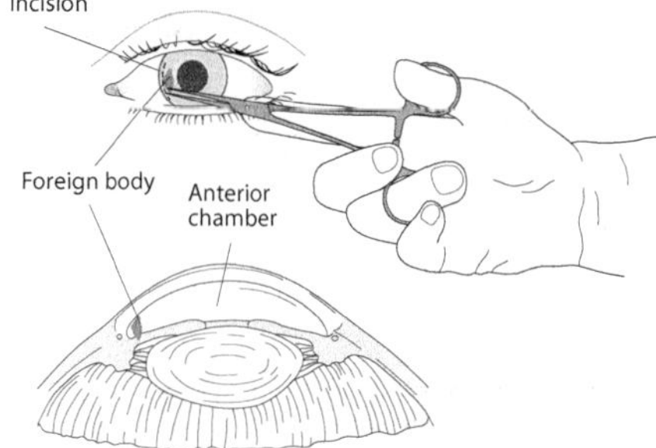

Through an incision, intraocular forceps are used to remove a foreign body from the anterior chamber of the eye lens.

ICD-10-CM Diagnostic Codes

⇄	H44.611	Retained (old) magnetic foreign body in anterior chamber, right eye
⇄	H44.612	Retained (old) magnetic foreign body in anterior chamber, left eye
⇄	H44.613	Retained (old) magnetic foreign body in anterior chamber, bilateral
⇄	H44.631	Retained (old) magnetic foreign body in lens, right eye
⇄	H44.632	Retained (old) magnetic foreign body in lens, left eye
⇄	H44.633	Retained (old) magnetic foreign body in lens, bilateral
⇄	H44.691	Retained (old) intraocular foreign body, magnetic, in other or multiple sites, right eye
⇄	H44.692	Retained (old) intraocular foreign body, magnetic, in other or multiple sites, left eye
⇄	H44.693	Retained (old) intraocular foreign body, magnetic, in other or multiple sites, bilateral
⇄	H44.711	Retained (nonmagnetic) (old) foreign body in anterior chamber, right eye
⇄	H44.712	Retained (nonmagnetic) (old) foreign body in anterior chamber, left eye
⇄	H44.713	Retained (nonmagnetic) (old) foreign body in anterior chamber, bilateral
⇄	H44.731	Retained (nonmagnetic) (old) foreign body in lens, right eye
⇄	H44.732	Retained (nonmagnetic) (old) foreign body in lens, left eye
⇄	H44.733	Retained (nonmagnetic) (old) foreign body in lens, bilateral
⇄	H44.791	Retained (old) intraocular foreign body, nonmagnetic, in other or multiple sites, right eye
⇄	H44.792	Retained (old) intraocular foreign body, nonmagnetic, in other or multiple sites, left eye
⇄	H44.793	Retained (old) intraocular foreign body, nonmagnetic, in other or multiple sites, bilateral
⇄	H59.021	Cataract (lens) fragments in eye following cataract surgery, right eye
⇄	H59.022	Cataract (lens) fragments in eye following cataract surgery, left eye
⇄	H59.023	Cataract (lens) fragments in eye following cataract surgery, bilateral
❼⇄	S05.51	Penetrating wound with foreign body of right eyeball
❼⇄	S05.52	Penetrating wound with foreign body of left eyeball
	Z18.10	Retained metal fragments, unspecified
	Z18.11	Retained magnetic metal fragments
	Z18.12	Retained nonmagnetic metal fragments
	Z18.2	Retained plastic fragments
	Z18.33	Retained wood fragments
	Z18.39	Other retained organic fragments
	Z18.81	Retained glass fragments
	Z18.83	Retained stone or crystalline fragments
	Z18.89	Other specified retained foreign body fragments
	Z18.9	Retained foreign body fragments, unspecified material

ICD-10-CM Coding Notes

For codes requiring a 7th character extension, refer to your ICD-10-CM book. Review the character descriptions and coding guidelines for proper selection. For some procedures, only certain characters will apply.

CCI Edits

Refer to Appendix A for CCI edits.

Facility RVUs ▯

Code	Work	PE Facility	MP	Total Facility
65235	9.01	11.54	0.70	21.25

Non-facility RVUs ▯

Code	Work	PE Non-Facility	MP	Total Non-Facility
65235	9.01	11.54	0.70	21.25

Modifiers (PAR) ▯

Code	Mod 50	Mod 51	Mod 62	Mod 66	Mod 80
65235	1	2	0	0	0

Global Period

Code	Days
65235	090

● New ▲ Revised ✚ Add On ⊘Modifier 51 Exempt ★Telemedicine ▯ CPT QuickRef ⁄FDA Pending ⇄ Laterality ❼ Seventh Character ♂Male ♀Female

65260-65265

65260 Removal of foreign body, intraocular; from posterior segment, magnetic extraction, anterior or posterior route

65265 Removal of foreign body, intraocular; from posterior segment, nonmagnetic extraction

(For removal of implanted material from posterior segment, use 67120)

AMA Coding Notes

Removal of Foreign Body Procedures on the Eyeball

(For removal of implanted material: ocular implant, use 65175; anterior segment implant, use 65920; posterior segment implant, use 67120; orbital implant, use 67560)

(For diagnostic x-ray for foreign body, use 70030)

(For diagnostic echography for foreign body, use 76529)

(For removal of foreign body from orbit: frontal approach, use 67413; lateral approach, use 67430)

(For removal of foreign body from eyelid, embedded, use 67938)

(For removal of foreign body from lacrimal system, use 68530)

Surgical Procedures on the Eye and Ocular Adnexa

(For diagnostic and treatment ophthalmological services, see Medicine, Ophthalmology, and 92002 et seq)

(Do not report code 69990 in addition to codes 65091-68850)

Plain English Description

The posterior segment of the eye is a large cavity that lies between the lens and the retina. It is filled vitreous humor, a soft jelly-like substance. The injury to the eye is inspected and the location of the intraocular foreign body determined to be in the posterior segment. The site of entry is located and the wound enlarged as needed. Alternatively, a separate incision may be made to provide access to the foreign body. Use 65260 for a metallic foreign body that is removed using a magnet and 65265 for a non-metallic foreign body that is removed using forceps or other technique. The wound is closed with sutures as needed.

Removal of foreign body, intraocular from posterior segment

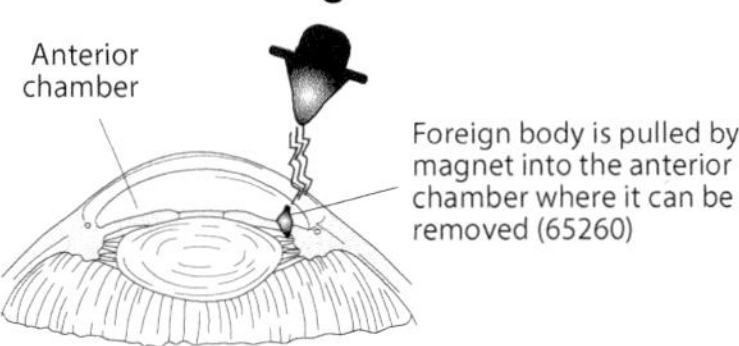
Anterior chamber
Foreign body is pulled by magnet into the anterior chamber where it can be removed (65260)

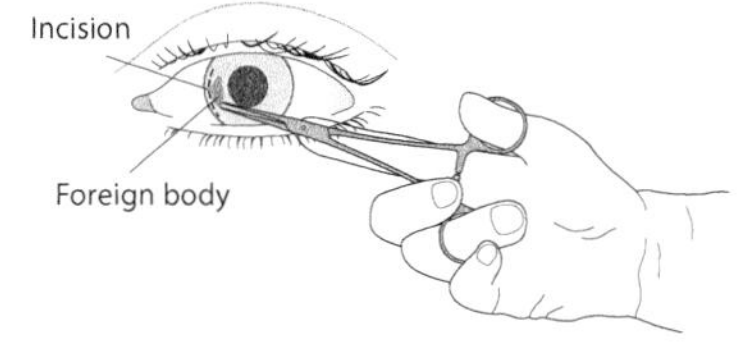
Incision
Foreign body

Through an incision, intraocular forceps are used to remove a foreign body from the posterior segment (65265).

ICD-10-CM Diagnostic Codes

⇄	H44.601	Unspecified retained (old) intraocular foreign body, magnetic, right eye
⇄	H44.602	Unspecified retained (old) intraocular foreign body, magnetic, left eye
⇄	H44.603	Unspecified retained (old) intraocular foreign body, magnetic, bilateral
⇄	H44.641	Retained (old) magnetic foreign body in posterior wall of globe, right eye
⇄	H44.642	Retained (old) magnetic foreign body in posterior wall of globe, left eye
⇄	H44.643	Retained (old) magnetic foreign body in posterior wall of globe, bilateral
⇄	H44.651	Retained (old) magnetic foreign body in vitreous body, right eye
⇄	H44.652	Retained (old) magnetic foreign body in vitreous body, left eye
⇄	H44.653	Retained (old) magnetic foreign body in vitreous body, bilateral
⇄	H44.691	Retained (old) intraocular foreign body, magnetic, in other or multiple sites, right eye
⇄	H44.692	Retained (old) intraocular foreign body, magnetic, in other or multiple sites, left eye
⇄	H44.693	Retained (old) intraocular foreign body, magnetic, in other or multiple sites, bilateral
⇄	H44.701	Unspecified retained (old) intraocular foreign body, nonmagnetic, right eye
⇄	H44.702	Unspecified retained (old) intraocular foreign body, nonmagnetic, left eye
⇄	H44.703	Unspecified retained (old) intraocular foreign body, nonmagnetic, bilateral
⇄	H44.741	Retained (nonmagnetic) (old) foreign body in posterior wall of globe, right eye
⇄	H44.742	Retained (nonmagnetic) (old) foreign body in posterior wall of globe, left eye
⇄	H44.743	Retained (nonmagnetic) (old) foreign body in posterior wall of globe, bilateral
⇄	H44.751	Retained (nonmagnetic) (old) foreign body in vitreous body, right eye
⇄	H44.752	Retained (nonmagnetic) (old) foreign body in vitreous body, left eye
⇄	H44.753	Retained (nonmagnetic) (old) foreign body in vitreous body, bilateral
⇄	H44.791	Retained (old) intraocular foreign body, nonmagnetic, in other or multiple sites, right eye
⇄	H44.792	Retained (old) intraocular foreign body, nonmagnetic, in other or multiple sites, left eye
⇄	H44.793	Retained (old) intraocular foreign body, nonmagnetic, in other or multiple sites, bilateral
❼⇄	S05.51	Penetrating wound with foreign body of right eyeball
❼⇄	S05.52	Penetrating wound with foreign body of left eyeball
	Z18.10	Retained metal fragments, unspecified
	Z18.11	Retained magnetic metal fragments
	Z18.12	Retained nonmagnetic metal fragments
	Z18.2	Retained plastic fragments
	Z18.33	Retained wood fragments
	Z18.39	Other retained organic fragments
	Z18.81	Retained glass fragments
	Z18.83	Retained stone or crystalline fragments
	Z18.89	Other specified retained foreign body fragments
	Z18.9	Retained foreign body fragments, unspecified material

ICD-10-CM Coding Notes

For codes requiring a 7th character extension, refer to your ICD-10-CM book. Review the character descriptions and coding guidelines for proper selection. For some procedures, only certain characters will apply.

CCI Edits

Refer to Appendix A for CCI edits.

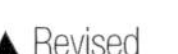
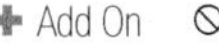

Facility RVUs

Code	Work	PE Facility	MP	Total Facility
65260	12.54	15.08	0.96	28.58
65265	14.34	16.73	1.10	32.17

Non-facility RVUs

Code	Work	PE Non-Facility	MP	Total Non-Facility
65260	12.54	15.08	0.96	28.58
65265	14.34	16.73	1.10	32.17

Modifiers (PAR)

Code	Mod 50	Mod 51	Mod 62	Mod 66	Mod 80
65260	1	2	0	0	2
65265	1	2	1	0	2

Global Period

Code	Days
65260	090
65265	090

65270

65270 Repair of laceration; conjunctiva, with or without nonperforating laceration sclera, direct closure

AMA Coding Notes

Repair of Laceration Procedures on the Eyeball

(For fracture of orbit, see 21385 et seq)

(For repair of wound of eyelid, skin, linear, simple, see 12011-12018; intermediate, layered closure, see 12051-12057; linear, complex, see 13151-13160; other, see 67930, 67935)

(For repair of wound of lacrimal system, use 68700)

(For repair of operative wound, use 66250)

Surgical Procedures on the Eye and Ocular Adnexa

(For diagnostic and treatment ophthalmological services, see Medicine, Ophthalmology, and 92002 et seq)

(Do not report code 69990 in addition to codes 65091-68850)

AMA *CPT® Assistant* ☐

65270: Aug 12: 9

Plain English Description

The conjunctiva is a transparent mucous membrane that covers the sclera (white of the eye) and the inner surface of the eyelids. Local anesthetic is administered. The eye is carefully examined and the injury determined to be limited to the conjunctiva. A partial thickness laceration of the sclera may also be present; however, there is no penetration of the globe. The edges of the laceration are debrided as needed. If the sclera is lacerated, it is closed first with absorbable suture material followed by direct repair of the conjunctival laceration.

Repair of laceration; conjunctiva

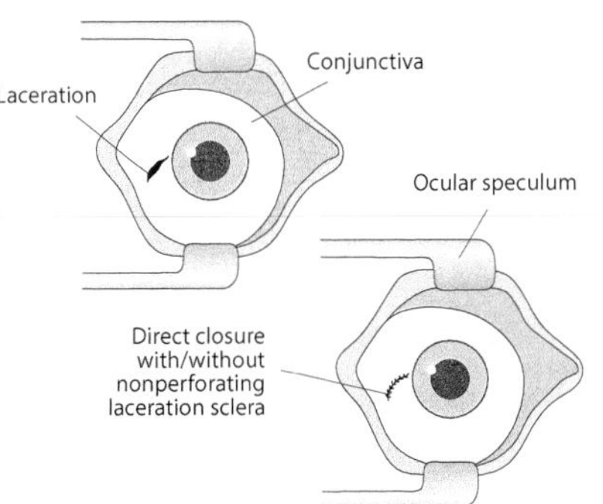

ICD-10-CM Diagnostic Codes

❼⇄	S05.01	Injury of conjunctiva and corneal abrasion without foreign body, right eye
❼⇄	S05.02	Injury of conjunctiva and corneal abrasion without foreign body, left eye
❼⇄	S05.31	Ocular laceration without prolapse or loss of intraocular tissue, right eye
❼⇄	S05.32	Ocular laceration without prolapse or loss of intraocular tissue, left eye
❼⇄	S05.8X1	Other injuries of right eye and orbit
❼⇄	S05.8X2	Other injuries of left eye and orbit

ICD-10-CM Coding Notes

For codes requiring a 7th character extension, refer to your ICD-10-CM book. Review the character descriptions and coding guidelines for proper selection. For some procedures, only certain characters will apply.

CCI Edits

Refer to Appendix A for CCI edits.

Facility RVUs ☐

Code	Work	PE Facility	MP	Total Facility
65270	1.95	1.98	0.14	4.07

Non-facility RVUs ☐

Code	Work	PE Non-Facility	MP	Total Non-Facility
65270	1.95	6.40	0.14	8.49

Modifiers (PAR) ☐

Code	Mod 50	Mod 51	Mod 62	Mod 66	Mod 80
65270	1	2	0	0	0

Global Period

Code	Days
65270	010

65272-65273

65272 Repair of laceration; conjunctiva, by mobilization and rearrangement, without hospitalization

65273 Repair of laceration; conjunctiva, by mobilization and rearrangement, with hospitalization

AMA Coding Notes

Repair of Laceration Procedures on the Eyeball

(For fracture of orbit, see 21385 et seq)

(For repair of wound of eyelid, skin, linear, simple, see 12011-12018; intermediate, layered closure, see 12051-12057; linear, complex, see 13151-13160; other, see 67930, 67935)

(For repair of wound of lacrimal system, use 68700)

(For repair of operative wound, use 66250)

Surgical Procedures on the Eye and Ocular Adnexa

(For diagnostic and treatment ophthalmological services, see Medicine, Ophthalmology, and 92002 et seq)

(Do not report code 69990 in addition to codes 65091-68850)

Plain English Description

The conjunctiva is a transparent mucous membrane that covers the sclera (white of the eye) and the inner surface of the eyelids. Local anesthetic is administered. The eye is carefully examined to ensure that there is no injury to the globe. The edges of the laceration are debrided as needed. The conjunctiva is mobilized and rearranged to relieve tension on the edges of the laceration. A flap may be developed to ensure adequate coverage of the defect. The defect is repaired using absorbable sutures. Use 65272 when the injury does not require hospitalization and 65273 when hospitalization is required.

Repair of laceration; conjunctiva

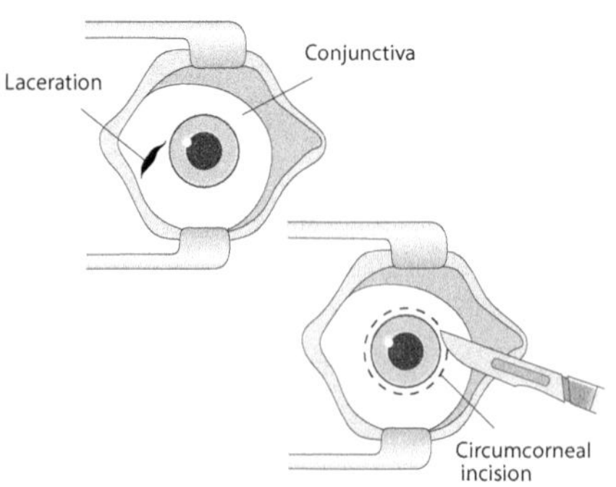

Extensive laceration conjunctiva, by mobilization/rearrangement without (65272); with (65273) hospitalization

ICD-10-CM Diagnostic Codes

❼⇄	S05.01	Injury of conjunctiva and corneal abrasion without foreign body, right eye
❼⇄	S05.02	Injury of conjunctiva and corneal abrasion without foreign body, left eye
❼⇄	S05.31	Ocular laceration without prolapse or loss of intraocular tissue, right eye
❼⇄	S05.32	Ocular laceration without prolapse or loss of intraocular tissue, left eye
❼⇄	S05.8X1	Other injuries of right eye and orbit
❼⇄	S05.8X2	Other injuries of left eye and orbit

ICD-10-CM Coding Notes

For codes requiring a 7th character extension, refer to your ICD-10-CM book. Review the character descriptions and coding guidelines for proper selection. For some procedures, only certain characters will apply.

CCI Edits

Refer to Appendix A for CCI edits.

Facility RVUs ☐

Code	Work	PE Facility	MP	Total Facility
65272	4.62	5.28	0.35	10.25
65273	5.16	5.46	0.40	11.02

Non-facility RVUs ☐

Code	Work	PE Non-Facility	MP	Total Non-Facility
65272	4.62	10.65	0.35	15.62
65273	5.16	5.46	0.40	11.02

Modifiers (PAR) ☐

Code	Mod 50	Mod 51	Mod 62	Mod 66	Mod 80
65272	1	2	0	0	1
65273	1	2	1	0	1

Global Period

Code	Days
65272	090
65273	090

65275

65275 Repair of laceration; cornea, nonperforating, with or without removal foreign body

AMA Coding Notes

Repair of Laceration Procedures on the Eyeball

(For fracture of orbit, see 21385 et seq)

(For repair of wound of eyelid, skin, linear, simple, see 12011-12018; intermediate, layered closure, see 12051-12057; linear, complex, see 13151-13160; other, see 67930, 67935)

(For repair of wound of lacrimal system, use 68700)

(For repair of operative wound, use 66250)

Surgical Procedures on the Eye and Ocular Adnexa

(For diagnostic and treatment ophthalmological services, see Medicine, Ophthalmology, and 92002 et seq)

(Do not report code 69990 in addition to codes 65091-68850)

Plain English Description

The cornea is a clear dome of tissue located at the front of the eye. It covers and protects the uvea, a three layer (iris, ciliary body, choroid) pigmented area that encircles the black pupil. A non-perforating laceration does not violate the globe (fluid-filled cavity behind the cornea and sclera). The eye is irrigated to remove foreign bodies and dirt and examined using a slit lamp (ophthalmic microscope). A Seidel test using fluorescein dye may be performed. The laceration is sutured using tight, longer sutures at the periphery of the laceration to compress and flatten the area and steepen the center of the cornea followed by shorter, appositional sutures in the central cornea. Antibiotic and/or steroid ophthalmic drops may be instilled and the eye is patched.

Repair of laceration; cornea with/without foreign body removal

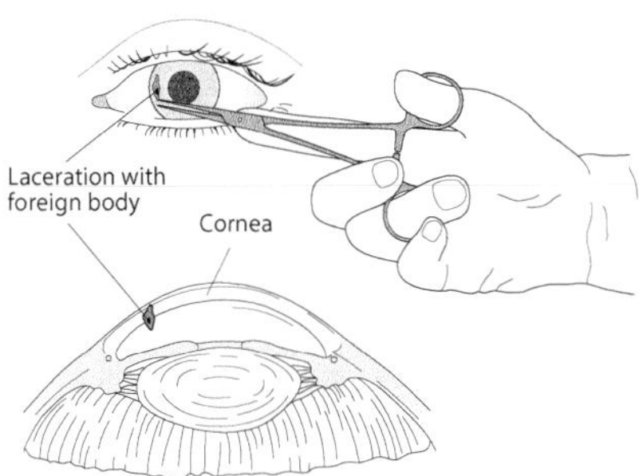

After removing any foreign body, a laceration of the cornea is repaired.

ICD-10-CM Diagnostic Codes

➐⇄	S05.01	Injury of conjunctiva and corneal abrasion without foreign body, right eye
➐⇄	S05.02	Injury of conjunctiva and corneal abrasion without foreign body, left eye
➐⇄	S05.31	Ocular laceration without prolapse or loss of intraocular tissue, right eye
➐⇄	S05.32	Ocular laceration without prolapse or loss of intraocular tissue, left eye
➐⇄	S05.8X1	Other injuries of right eye and orbit
➐⇄	S05.8X2	Other injuries of left eye and orbit
➐⇄	T15.01	Foreign body in cornea, right eye
➐⇄	T15.02	Foreign body in cornea, left eye

ICD-10-CM Coding Notes

For codes requiring a 7th character extension, refer to your ICD-10-CM book. Review the character descriptions and coding guidelines for proper selection. For some procedures, only certain characters will apply.

CCI Edits

Refer to Appendix A for CCI edits.

Facility RVUs ▢

Code	Work	PE Facility	MP	Total Facility
65275	6.29	6.60	0.50	13.39

Non-facility RVUs ▢

Code	Work	PE Non-Facility	MP	Total Non-Facility
65275	6.29	10.49	0.50	17.28

Modifiers (PAR) ▢

Code	Mod 50	Mod 51	Mod 62	Mod 66	Mod 80
65275	1	2	0	0	0

Global Period

Code	Days
65275	090

CPT® Procedural Coding

65280

65280 Repair of laceration; cornea and/or sclera, perforating, not involving uveal tissue

AMA Coding Notes

Repair of Laceration Procedures on the Eyeball

(For fracture of orbit, see 21385 et seq)

(For repair of wound of eyelid, skin, linear, simple, see 12011-12018; intermediate, layered closure, see 12051-12057; linear, complex, see 13151-13160; other, see 67930, 67935)

(For repair of wound of lacrimal system, use 68700)

(For repair of operative wound, use 66250)

Surgical Procedures on the Eye and Ocular Adnexa

(For diagnostic and treatment ophthalmological services, see Medicine, Ophthalmology, and 92002 et seq)

(Do not report code 69990 in addition to codes 65091-68850)

AMA *CPT® Assistant*

65280: Aug 12: 9

Plain English Description

The sclera is the opaque, white, outer layer of the eye made up of fibrous tissue and collagen. It extends from the cornea at the front of the eye to the optic nerve at the back of the eye. A thin transparent membrane called the conjunctiva covers the sclera at the front of the eye. The cornea is a clear dome of tissue also located at the front of the eye. It covers and protects the uvea, a three layer (iris, ciliary body, choroid) pigmented area that encircles the black pupil. The margin of the cornea and sclera is called the limbus. A perforating laceration, also called a full thickness laceration, of the cornea and/or sclera is repaired. The eye is irrigated to remove foreign bodies and dirt and examined using a slit lamp (ophthalmic microscope). A Seidel test using fluorescein dye may be performed. Using fine nylon suture, the first stitch is placed at the limbus to approximate the wound. Next, the corneal wound is sutured, followed by the sclera. The conjunctiva is closed with fine nylon suture. Antibiotic and/or steroid ophthalmic drops may be instilled and the eye is patched.

Repair of laceration; cornea/sclera, perforating

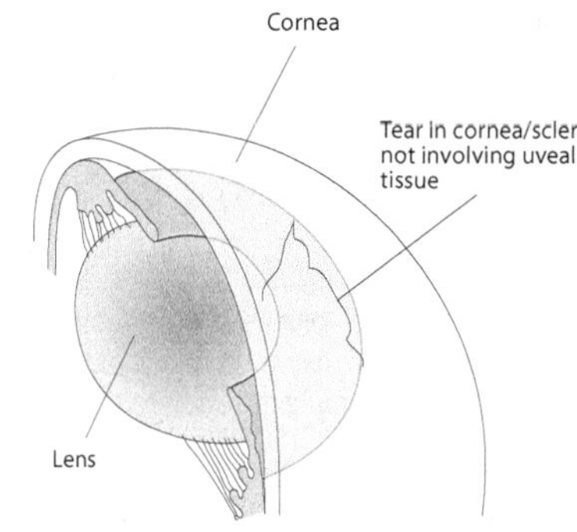

ICD-10-CM Diagnostic Codes

➐⇄	S05.31	Ocular laceration without prolapse or loss of intraocular tissue, right eye
➐⇄	S05.32	Ocular laceration without prolapse or loss of intraocular tissue, left eye
➐⇄	S05.51	Penetrating wound with foreign body of right eyeball
➐⇄	S05.52	Penetrating wound with foreign body of left eyeball
➐⇄	S05.61	Penetrating wound without foreign body of right eyeball
➐⇄	S05.62	Penetrating wound without foreign body of left eyeball
➐⇄	S05.8X1	Other injuries of right eye and orbit
➐⇄	S05.8X2	Other injuries of left eye and orbit
➐⇄	T15.01	Foreign body in cornea, right eye
➐⇄	T15.02	Foreign body in cornea, left eye
➐⇄	T15.81	Foreign body in other and multiple parts of external eye, right eye
➐⇄	T15.82	Foreign body in other and multiple parts of external eye, left eye

ICD-10-CM Coding Notes

For codes requiring a 7th character extension, refer to your ICD-10-CM book. Review the character descriptions and coding guidelines for proper selection. For some procedures, only certain characters will apply.

CCI Edits

Refer to Appendix A for CCI edits.

Facility RVUs

Code	Work	PE Facility	MP	Total Facility
65280	9.10	9.63	0.70	19.43

Non-facility RVUs

Code	Work	PE Non-Facility	MP	Total Non-Facility
65280	9.10	9.63	0.70	19.43

Modifiers (PAR)

Code	Mod 50	Mod 51	Mod 62	Mod 66	Mod 80
65280	1	2	0	0	0

Global Period

Code	Days
65280	090

65285

65285 Repair of laceration; cornea and/or sclera, perforating, with reposition or resection of uveal tissue

(65280 and 65285 are not used for repair of a surgical wound)

AMA Coding Notes

Repair of Laceration Procedures on the Eyeball

(For fracture of orbit, see 21385 et seq)

(For repair of wound of eyelid, skin, linear, simple, see 12011-12018; intermediate, layered closure, see 12051-12057; linear, complex, see 13151-13160; other, see 67930, 67935)

(For repair of wound of lacrimal system, use 68700)

(For repair of operative wound, use 66250)

Surgical Procedures on the Eye and Ocular Adnexa

(For diagnostic and treatment ophthalmological services, see Medicine, Ophthalmology, and 92002 et seq)

(Do not report code 69990 in addition to codes 65091-68850)

AMA *CPT® Assistant* ▯

65285: Aug 12: 9

Plain English Description

Repair of a perforating corneal and/or scleral laceration with reposition or resection of uveal tissue is accomplished using conventional sutures. The goal of treatment is to ensure a watertight globe, reestablish original eye anatomy, and restore or preserve visual function. The corneal component is approached first. Vitreous or lens fragments are cut flush with the cornea. A limbal incision is made and working through that incision, uveal or retinal fragments are repositioned with a sweeping technique. The uveal surface and wound are checked for epithelial tissue, which is carefully peeled off if it is present. The corneal laceration is then closed. The anterior and posterior edges of the cornea are opposed using long tight sutures at the periphery and shorter, wider, central sutures preserving the natural curvature of the structure and avoiding entrapment of the iris. The scleral laceration is addressed next. Using gentle peritomy, the conjunctiva adjacent to the laceration is carefully dissected to explore the wound. Vitreous tissue that has prolapsed is excised, viable uveal/retinal tissue is repositioned and the sclera is closed with sutures. A deeply penetrating scleral wound can be left alone to heal. A paracentesis may be created and sterile water injected through it to fill the anterior chamber and check the globe for a watertight seal. At the end of the surgical procedure, antibiotics may be injected directly into the conjunctiva or other areas of the eye, and the eye is covered with a sterile dressing and eye shield.

Repair of laceration; cornea/sclera, perforating

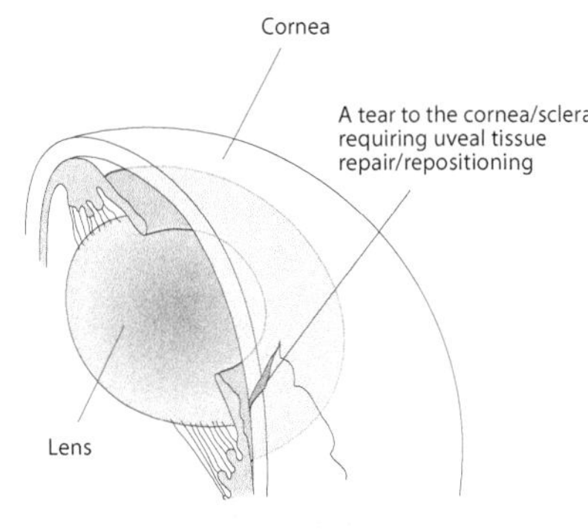

ICD-10-CM Diagnostic Codes

	Code	Description
⑦⇄	S05.31	Ocular laceration without prolapse or loss of intraocular tissue, right eye
⑦⇄	S05.32	Ocular laceration without prolapse or loss of intraocular tissue, left eye
⑦⇄	S05.51	Penetrating wound with foreign body of right eyeball
⑦⇄	S05.52	Penetrating wound with foreign body of left eyeball
⑦⇄	S05.61	Penetrating wound without foreign body of right eyeball
⑦⇄	S05.62	Penetrating wound without foreign body of left eyeball
⑦⇄	S05.8X1	Other injuries of right eye and orbit
⑦⇄	S05.8X2	Other injuries of left eye and orbit
⑦⇄	T15.01	Foreign body in cornea, right eye
⑦⇄	T15.02	Foreign body in cornea, left eye
⑦⇄	T15.81	Foreign body in other and multiple parts of external eye, right eye
⑦⇄	T15.82	Foreign body in other and multiple parts of external eye, left eye

ICD-10-CM Coding Notes

For codes requiring a 7th character extension, refer to your ICD-10-CM book. Review the character descriptions and coding guidelines for proper selection. For some procedures, only certain characters will apply.

CCI Edits

Refer to Appendix A for CCI edits.

Facility RVUs ▯

Code	Work	PE Facility	MP	Total Facility
65285	15.36	15.47	1.20	32.03

Non-facility RVUs ▯

Code	Work	PE Non-Facility	MP	Total Non-Facility
65285	15.36	15.47	1.20	32.03

Modifiers (PAR) ▯

Code	Mod 50	Mod 51	Mod 62	Mod 66	Mod 80
65285	1	2	0	0	1

Global Period

Code	Days
65285	090

65286

65286 Repair of laceration; application of tissue glue, wounds of cornea and/or sclera

(Repair of laceration includes use of conjunctival flap and restoration of anterior chamber, by air or saline injection when indicated)

(For repair of iris or ciliary body, use 66680)

AMA Coding Notes

Repair of Laceration Procedures on the Eyeball

(For fracture of orbit, see 21385 et seq)

(For repair of wound of eyelid, skin, linear, simple, see 12011-12018; intermediate, layered closure, see 12051-12057; linear, complex, see 13151-13160; other, see 67930, 67935)

(For repair of wound of lacrimal system, use 68700)

(For repair of operative wound, use 66250)

Surgical Procedures on the Eye and Ocular Adnexa

(For diagnostic and treatment ophthalmological services, see Medicine, Ophthalmology, and 92002 et seq)

(Do not report code 69990 in addition to codes 65091-68850)

AMA *CPT® Assistant* ▯

65286: May 99: 11, Apr 09: 5

Plain English Description

Repair of a superficial corneal and/or scleral laceration may be accomplished using an application of liquid tissue adhesive (fibrin, chondroitin, isobutyl cyanoacrylate) and a bandage contact lens. The goal of treatment is to ensure a watertight globe, reestablish original eye anatomy, and restore or preserve visual function. The eye is irrigated and the wound is carefully examined under a slit lamp or operating microscope. The edges of the laceration are manually approximated and liquid tissue adhesive is brushed over the wound. The liquid undergoes a chemical reaction when it comes in contact with moisture and polymerizes to bind the epithelium together and allow healing to take place in the underlying tissue. A bandage contact lens may be applied over the liquid tissue adhesive. The lens provides pressure patching over a large surface area to protect the eye from the mechanical trauma of lid closure and helps to relieve pain.

Repair of laceration; cornea/sclera application of tissue glue

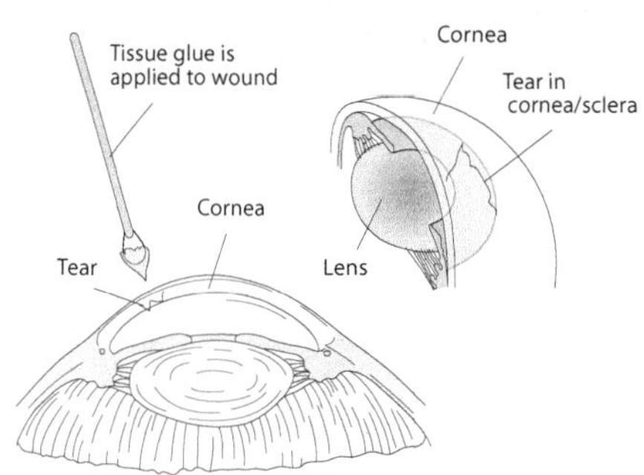

ICD-10-CM Diagnostic Codes

❼⇄	S05.01	Injury of conjunctiva and corneal abrasion without foreign body, right eye
❼⇄	S05.02	Injury of conjunctiva and corneal abrasion without foreign body, left eye
❼⇄	S05.31	Ocular laceration without prolapse or loss of intraocular tissue, right eye
❼⇄	S05.32	Ocular laceration without prolapse or loss of intraocular tissue, left eye
❼⇄	S05.51	Penetrating wound with foreign body of right eyeball
❼⇄	S05.52	Penetrating wound with foreign body of left eyeball
❼⇄	S05.61	Penetrating wound without foreign body of right eyeball
❼⇄	S05.62	Penetrating wound without foreign body of left eyeball
❼⇄	S05.8X1	Other injuries of right eye and orbit
❼⇄	S05.8X2	Other injuries of left eye and orbit
❼⇄	T15.01	Foreign body in cornea, right eye
❼⇄	T15.02	Foreign body in cornea, left eye

ICD-10-CM Coding Notes

For codes requiring a 7th character extension, refer to your ICD-10-CM book. Review the character descriptions and coding guidelines for proper selection. For some procedures, only certain characters will apply.

CCI Edits

Refer to Appendix A for CCI edits.

Facility RVUs ▯

Code	Work	PE Facility	MP	Total Facility
65286	6.63	7.23	0.51	14.37

Non-facility RVUs ▯

Code	Work	PE Non-Facility	MP	Total Non-Facility
65286	6.63	13.47	0.51	20.61

Modifiers (PAR) ▯

Code	Mod 50	Mod 51	Mod 62	Mod 66	Mod 80
65286	1	2	0	0	1

Global Period

Code	Days
65286	090

65290

65290 Repair of wound, extraocular muscle, tendon and/or Tenon's capsule

AMA Coding Notes

Repair of Laceration Procedures on the Eyeball

(For fracture of orbit, see 21385 et seq)

(For repair of wound of eyelid, skin, linear, simple, see 12011-12018; intermediate, layered closure, see 12051-12057; linear, complex, see 13151-13160; other, see 67930, 67935)

(For repair of wound of lacrimal system, use 68700)

(For repair of operative wound, use 66250)

Surgical Procedures on the Eye and Ocular Adnexa

(For diagnostic and treatment ophthalmological services, see Medicine, Ophthalmology, and 92002 et seq)

(Do not report code 69990 in addition to codes 65091-68850)

Plain English Description

Repair of a wound, extraocular muscle, tendon and/or Tenon's capsule is accomplished using conventional sutures. The eye is carefully examined under slit lamp or operating microscope to evaluate the wound and damage to eye structures. The eyeball is suspended in the orbit enveloped inside of Tenon's capsule, a fibrous tissue that covers the eyeball from the entrance of the optic nerve to the corneal limbus and attaches firmly to the conjunctiva. Three paired extraocular muscles—the horizontal rectus, vertical rectus, and oblique muscles are attached to the sclera/globe by broad thin tendons. A wound to the eye surface on the cornea or sclera may disrupt the integrity of muscle(s), tendon(s) and/or Tenon's capsule. The ends of a transected muscle or tendon are located, reapproximated, and repaired using suture. Tenon's capsule is carefully dissected to expose foreign bodies and trapped tissue and is then closed with sutures. At the end of the surgical procedure, antibiotics may be injected directly into the conjunctiva or other areas of the eye and the eye is covered with a sterile dressing and eye shield.

Repair of wound, extraocular muscle, tendon/Tenon's capsule

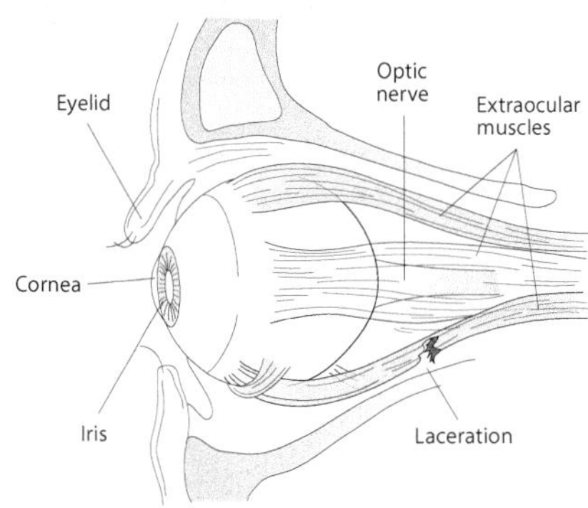

A deep laceration of the extraocular muscle, tendon/Tenon's capsule is repaired.

ICD-10-CM Diagnostic Codes

❼⇄	S01.101	Unspecified open wound of right eyelid and periocular area
❼⇄	S01.102	Unspecified open wound of left eyelid and periocular area
❼⇄	S01.111	Laceration without foreign body of right eyelid and periocular area
❼⇄	S01.112	Laceration without foreign body of left eyelid and periocular area
❼⇄	S01.121	Laceration with foreign body of right eyelid and periocular area
❼⇄	S01.122	Laceration with foreign body of left eyelid and periocular area
❼⇄	S01.131	Puncture wound without foreign body of right eyelid and periocular area
❼⇄	S01.132	Puncture wound without foreign body of left eyelid and periocular area
❼⇄	S01.141	Puncture wound with foreign body of right eyelid and periocular area
❼⇄	S01.142	Puncture wound with foreign body of left eyelid and periocular area
❼⇄	S01.151	Open bite of right eyelid and periocular area
❼⇄	S01.152	Open bite of left eyelid and periocular area
❼⇄	S05.41	Penetrating wound of orbit with or without foreign body, right eye
❼⇄	S05.42	Penetrating wound of orbit with or without foreign body, left eye

ICD-10-CM Coding Notes

For codes requiring a 7th character extension, refer to your ICD-10-CM book. Review the character descriptions and coding guidelines for proper selection. For some procedures, only certain characters will apply.

CCI Edits

Refer to Appendix A for CCI edits.

Facility RVUs ☐

Code	Work	PE Facility	MP	Total Facility
65290	6.53	7.17	0.50	14.20

Non-facility RVUs ☐

Code	Work	PE Non-Facility	MP	Total Non-Facility
65290	6.53	7.17	0.50	14.20

Modifiers (PAR) ☐

Code	Mod 50	Mod 51	Mod 62	Mod 66	Mod 80
65290	1	2	1	0	1

Global Period

Code	Days
65290	090

65400

65400 Excision of lesion, cornea (keratectomy, lamellar, partial), except pterygium

AMA Coding Notes

Surgical Procedures on the Eye and Ocular Adnexa

(For diagnostic and treatment ophthalmological services, see Medicine, Ophthalmology, and 92002 et seq)

(Do not report code 69990 in addition to codes 65091-68850)

Plain English Description

Corneal lesions that require excision can include dystrophic, degenerative, and hypertrophic or scar tissue. Using a slit lamp or operating microscope, the lesion is visualized. Surface epithelial cells are gently debrided from the cornea using blunt forceps, spatula, or sponge to delineate the margins of the lesion and expose the deeper corneal epithelium and subepithelial fibrous and fibrovascular tissue. Blunt or sharp dissection of the deeper lesion is then carried out and the surface of the cornea may be polished using a diamond burr. A bandage contact lens is inserted at the conclusion of the procedure to facilitate healing and regeneration of corneal epithelial cells from limbic stem cells.

Excision of lesion, cornea (keratectomy, lamellar, partial), except pterygium

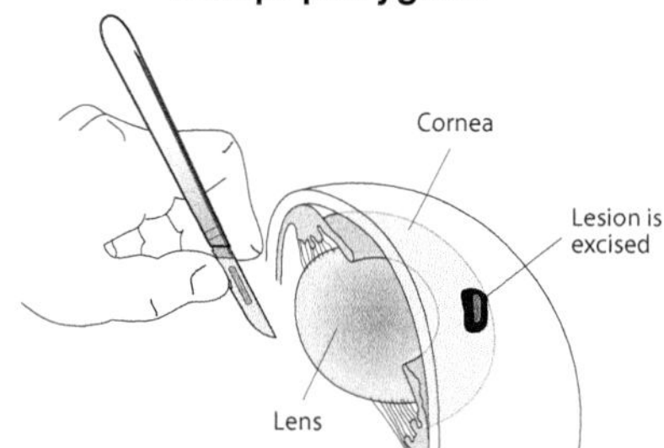

ICD-10-CM Diagnostic Codes

⇄	D09.21	Carcinoma in situ of right eye
⇄	D09.22	Carcinoma in situ of left eye
⇄	D31.11	Benign neoplasm of right cornea
⇄	D31.12	Benign neoplasm of left cornea
	D48.7	Neoplasm of uncertain behavior of other specified sites
⇄	H17.01	Adherent leukoma, right eye
⇄	H17.02	Adherent leukoma, left eye
⇄	H17.03	Adherent leukoma, bilateral
⇄	H17.11	Central corneal opacity, right eye
⇄	H17.12	Central corneal opacity, left eye
⇄	H17.13	Central corneal opacity, bilateral
	H17.89	Other corneal scars and opacities
⇄	H18.011	Anterior corneal pigmentations, right eye
⇄	H18.012	Anterior corneal pigmentations, left eye
⇄	H18.022	Argentous corneal deposits, left eye
⇄	H18.032	Corneal deposits in metabolic disorders, left eye
⇄	H18.052	Posterior corneal pigmentations, left eye
⇄	H18.062	Stromal corneal pigmentations, left eye
⇄	H18.422	Band keratopathy, left eye
⇄	H18.452	Nodular corneal degeneration, left eye
⇄	H18.511	Endothelial corneal dystrophy, right eye
⇄	H18.512	Endothelial corneal dystrophy, left eye
⇄	H18.513	Endothelial corneal dystrophy, bilateral
⇄	H18.591	Other hereditary corneal dystrophies, right eye
⇄	H18.592	Other hereditary corneal dystrophies, left eye
⇄	H18.593	Other hereditary corneal dystrophies, bilateral
⇄	H18.832	Recurrent erosion of cornea, left eye
⇄	H18.892	Other specified disorders of cornea, left eye
⇄	H25.12	Age-related nuclear cataract, left eye

CCI Edits

Refer to Appendix A for CCI edits.

Pub 100

65400: Pub 100-03, 1, 80.7-80.71

Facility RVUs ▢

Code	Work	PE Facility	MP	Total Facility
65400	7.50	9.37	0.57	17.44

Non-facility RVUs ▢

Code	Work	PE Non-Facility	MP	Total Non-Facility
65400	7.50	12.15	0.57	20.22

Modifiers (PAR) ▢

Code	Mod 50	Mod 51	Mod 62	Mod 66	Mod 80
65400	1	2	0	0	1

Global Period

Code	Days
65400	090

65410

65410 Biopsy of cornea

AMA Coding Notes

Surgical Procedures on the Eye and Ocular Adnexa

(For diagnostic and treatment ophthalmological services, see Medicine, Ophthalmology, and 92002 et seq)

(Do not report code 69990 in addition to codes 65091-68850)

Plain English Description

A surgical blade or aspiration cutter is used to obtain a tissue sample from the cornea or from a corneal lesion. A small incision is made over the area to be biopsied. If a surgical blade is used, a small amount of tissue is excised from the cornea or corneal lesion. If an aspiration cutter is used, a probe is introduced through the incision. Tissue samples are obtained and submitted for pathology examination.

Biopsy of cornea

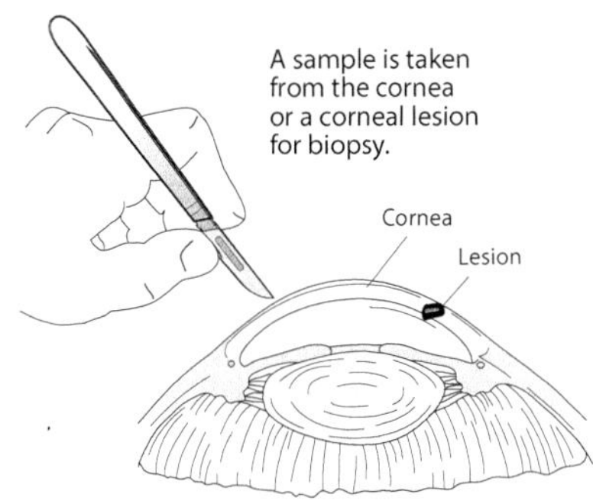
A sample is taken from the cornea or a corneal lesion for biopsy.
Cornea
Lesion

ICD-10-CM Diagnostic Codes

	Code	Description
	A18.51	Tuberculous episcleritis
	A18.52	Tuberculous keratitis
	A18.53	Tuberculous chorioretinitis
	A18.54	Tuberculous iridocyclitis
	A18.59	Other tuberculosis of eye
	B48.8	Other specified mycoses
	B60.10	Acanthamebiasis, unspecified
	B60.11	Meningoencephalitis due to Acanthamoeba (culbertsoni)
	B60.12	Conjunctivitis due to Acanthamoeba
	B60.13	Keratoconjunctivitis due to Acanthamoeba
	B60.19	Other acanthamebic disease
	B60.2	Naegleriasis
⇄	C69.11	Malignant neoplasm of right cornea
	C79.32	Secondary malignant neoplasm of cerebral meninges
⇄	D09.21	Carcinoma in situ of right eye
⇄	D31.11	Benign neoplasm of right cornea
⇄	H16.011	Central corneal ulcer, right eye
⇄	H16.031	Corneal ulcer with hypopyon, right eye
⇄	H16.041	Marginal corneal ulcer, right eye
⇄	H16.061	Mycotic corneal ulcer, right eye
⇄	H16.071	Perforated corneal ulcer, right eye
⇄	H16.301	Unspecified interstitial keratitis, right eye
⇄	H16.311	Corneal abscess, right eye
⇄	H16.321	Diffuse interstitial keratitis, right eye
⇄	H16.331	Sclerosing keratitis, right eye
⇄	H17.01	Adherent leukoma, right eye
	H17.89	Other corneal scars and opacities
⇄	H18.001	Unspecified corneal deposit, right eye
⇄	H18.011	Anterior corneal pigmentations, right eye
⇄	H18.021	Argentous corneal deposits, right eye
⇄	H18.031	Corneal deposits in metabolic disorders, right eye
⇄	H18.041	Kayser-Fleischer ring, right eye
⇄	H18.051	Posterior corneal pigmentations, right eye
⇄	H18.061	Stromal corneal pigmentations, right eye
⇄	H18.421	Band keratopathy, right eye
⇄	H18.451	Nodular corneal degeneration, right eye
⇄	H18.461	Peripheral corneal degeneration, right eye
	H18.49	Other corneal degeneration
⇄	H18.721	Corneal staphyloma, right eye
⇄	H18.791	Other corneal deformities, right eye
⇄	H18.831	Recurrent erosion of cornea, right eye
⇄	H18.891	Other specified disorders of cornea, right eye
	M35.01	Sjögren syndrome with keratoconjunctivitis

CCI Edits

Refer to Appendix A for CCI edits.

Facility RVUs

Code	Work	PE Facility	MP	Total Facility
65410	1.47	1.36	0.11	2.94

Non-facility RVUs

Code	Work	PE Non-Facility	MP	Total Non-Facility
65410	1.47	2.60	0.11	4.18

Modifiers (PAR)

Code	Mod 50	Mod 51	Mod 62	Mod 66	Mod 80
65410	1	2	0	0	0

Global Period

Code	Days
65410	000

65420-65426

65420 Excision or transposition of pterygium; without graft

65426 Excision or transposition of pterygium; with graft

AMA Coding Notes

Surgical Procedures on the Eye and Ocular Adnexa

(For diagnostic and treatment ophthalmological services, see Medicine, Ophthalmology, and 92002 et seq)

(Do not report code 69990 in addition to codes 65091-68850)

AMA *CPT® Assistant* ▯

65420: Dec 07: 13

65426: May 18: 11

Plain English Description

The physician performs an excision or transposition of a pterygium without the use of a graft, also referred to as a simple excision or bare sclera technique. A pterygium is a raised, triangular growth of conjunctiva at the corner of the eye that extends into the sclera and may also invade the cornea. If the pterygium extends into the central cornea, it is removed surgically. The pterygium is dissected free of underlying sclera and corneal tissue and a simple excision performed. The sclera is left open to heal. In 65426, the pterygium is removed and the scleral defect repaired using a graft. The pterygium is dissected down to the level of the Tenon's capsule and the fibrous tissue forming the pterygium is removed. An autograft, such as a free conjunctival graft, is then harvested from under the eyelid of the patient and used to repair the defect. Alternatively, an allograft, such as an amniotic membrane graft obtained from a tissue bank, may be used. The graft is sutured onto the conjunctiva or secured using fibrin tissue glue.

Excision or transposition of pterygium

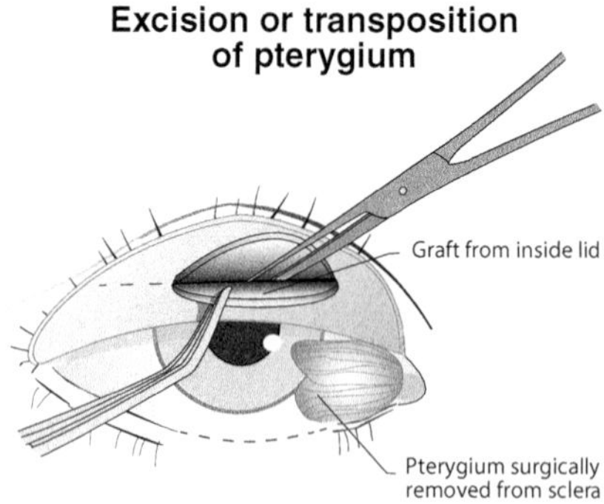

Without graft (65420); with graft (65426)

ICD-10-CM Diagnostic Codes

⇄	H11.011	Amyloid pterygium of right eye
⇄	H11.012	Amyloid pterygium of left eye
⇄	H11.013	Amyloid pterygium of eye, bilateral
⇄	H11.021	Central pterygium of right eye
⇄	H11.022	Central pterygium of left eye
⇄	H11.023	Central pterygium of eye, bilateral
⇄	H11.031	Double pterygium of right eye
⇄	H11.032	Double pterygium of left eye
⇄	H11.033	Double pterygium of eye, bilateral
⇄	H11.041	Peripheral pterygium, stationary, right eye
⇄	H11.042	Peripheral pterygium, stationary, left eye
⇄	H11.043	Peripheral pterygium, stationary, bilateral
⇄	H11.051	Peripheral pterygium, progressive, right eye
⇄	H11.052	Peripheral pterygium, progressive, left eye
⇄	H11.053	Peripheral pterygium, progressive, bilateral
⇄	H11.061	Recurrent pterygium of right eye
⇄	H11.062	Recurrent pterygium of left eye
⇄	H11.063	Recurrent pterygium of eye, bilateral
⇄	H11.151	Pinguecula, right eye
⇄	H11.152	Pinguecula, left eye
⇄	H11.153	Pinguecula, bilateral
⇄	H11.811	Pseudopterygium of conjunctiva, right eye
⇄	H11.812	Pseudopterygium of conjunctiva, left eye
⇄	H11.813	Pseudopterygium of conjunctiva, bilateral

CCI Edits

Refer to Appendix A for CCI edits.

Facility RVUs ▯

Code	Work	PE Facility	MP	Total Facility
65420	4.36	6.28	0.34	10.98
65426	6.05	7.32	0.45	13.82

Non-facility RVUs ▯

Code	Work	PE Non-Facility	MP	Total Non-Facility
65420	4.36	11.24	0.34	15.94
65426	6.05	13.27	0.45	19.77

Modifiers (PAR) ▯

Code	Mod 50	Mod 51	Mod 62	Mod 66	Mod 80
65420	1	2	0	0	1
65426	1	2	0	0	1

Global Period

Code	Days
65420	090
65426	090

65430

65430 Scraping of cornea, diagnostic, for smear and/or culture

AMA Coding Notes

Surgical Procedures on the Eye and Ocular Adnexa

(For diagnostic and treatment ophthalmological services, see Medicine, Ophthalmology, and 92002 et seq)

(Do not report code 69990 in addition to codes 65091-68850)

Plain English Description

The eye is examined with the help of a slit lamp, magnifiers, loupe, or operating microscope. Eye drops are instilled to numb the eye. The cornea or corneal lesion is then scraped using a sterile Kimura spatula or surgical blade. If the tissue sample is obtained from a corneal lesion, samples are obtained from the base and sides of the lesion. The tissue sample is applied to one or more prepared glass slides and separately reportable microscopic examination is performed.

Scraping of cornea, diagnostic, for smear/culture

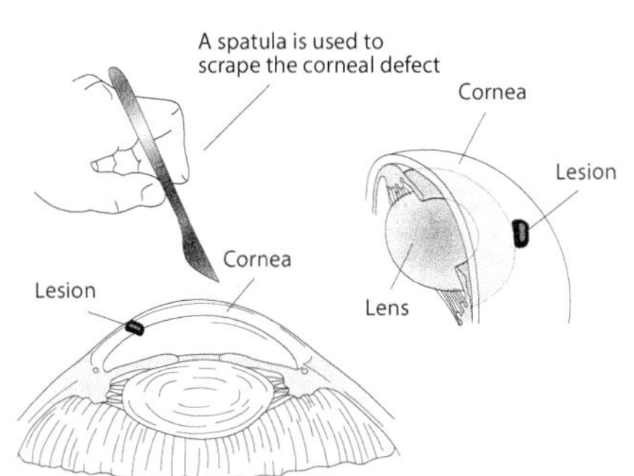

ICD-10-CM Diagnostic Codes

	A18.50	Tuberculosis of eye, unspecified
	A18.52	Tuberculous keratitis
	A18.59	Other tuberculosis of eye
	A50.31	Late congenital syphilitic interstitial keratitis
	A54.33	Gonococcal keratitis
	B00.52	Herpesviral keratitis
	B02.30	Zoster ocular disease, unspecified
	B02.31	Zoster conjunctivitis
	B02.33	Zoster keratitis
	B02.34	Zoster scleritis
	B02.39	Other herpes zoster eye disease
	B30.0	Keratoconjunctivitis due to adenovirus
	B48.8	Other specified mycoses
	B60.10	Acanthamebiasis, unspecified
	B60.11	Meningoencephalitis due to Acanthamoeba (culbertsoni)
	B60.12	Conjunctivitis due to Acanthamoeba
	B60.13	Keratoconjunctivitis due to Acanthamoeba
	B60.19	Other acanthamebic disease
	B60.2	Naegleriasis
⇄	H04.122	Dry eye syndrome of left lacrimal gland
⇄	H16.011	Central corneal ulcer, right eye
⇄	H16.021	Ring corneal ulcer, right eye
⇄	H16.031	Corneal ulcer with hypopyon, right eye
⇄	H16.041	Marginal corneal ulcer, right eye
⇄	H16.051	Mooren's corneal ulcer, right eye
⇄	H16.061	Mycotic corneal ulcer, right eye
⇄	H16.071	Perforated corneal ulcer, right eye
⇄	H16.111	Macular keratitis, right eye
⇄	H16.121	Filamentary keratitis, right eye
⇄	H16.122	Filamentary keratitis, left eye
⇄	H16.141	Punctate keratitis, right eye
⇄	H16.221	Keratoconjunctivitis sicca, not specified as Sjögren's, right eye
⇄	H16.251	Phlyctenular keratoconjunctivitis, right eye
⇄	H16.291	Other keratoconjunctivitis, right eye
⇄	H16.321	Diffuse interstitial keratitis, right eye
⇄	H16.331	Sclerosing keratitis, right eye
⇄	H16.391	Other interstitial and deep keratitis, right eye
	H16.8	Other keratitis
⇄	H17.11	Central corneal opacity, right eye
	H17.89	Other corneal scars and opacities
	H17.9	Unspecified corneal scar and opacity
⇄	H18.001	Unspecified corneal deposit, right eye
	M35.01	Sjögren syndrome with keratoconjunctivitis

CCI Edits

Refer to Appendix A for CCI edits.

Facility RVUs ▢

Code	Work	PE Facility	MP	Total Facility
65430	1.47	1.35	0.11	2.93

Non-facility RVUs ▢

Code	Work	PE Non-Facility	MP	Total Non-Facility
65430	1.47	1.77	0.11	3.35

Modifiers (PAR) ▢

Code	Mod 50	Mod 51	Mod 62	Mod 66	Mod 80
65430	1	2	0	0	1

Global Period

Code	Days
65430	000

65435-65436

65435 Removal of corneal epithelium; with or without chemocauterization (abrasion, curettage)

(Do not report 65435 in conjunction with 0402T)

65436 Removal of corneal epithelium; with application of chelating agent (eg, EDTA)

AMA Coding Notes

Surgical Procedures on the Eye and Ocular Adnexa

(For diagnostic and treatment ophthalmological services, see Medicine, Ophthalmology, and 92002 et seq)

(Do not report code 69990 in addition to codes 65091-68850)

AMA *CPT® Assistant* ▢

65435: Feb 16: 12

Plain English Description

The physician removes the corneal epithelium with or without the use of chemocauterization using abrasion or curettage. The procedure is performed to remove a diseased, eroded, damaged, or dystrophied layer of epithelium from the cornea of the eye. The soft epithelial layer of the cornea is removed using a brushing or scraping instrument. The surface epithelium is separated and removed from the underlying and harder Bowman's layer. A chemical may then be applied to cauterize the newly exposed underlying tissue. In 65436, the corneal epithelium is removed and a chelating agent such as ethylenediaminetetraacetic acid (EDTA) applied. The epithelium is removed with a sponge or blade. The chelating agent is then applied using surgical sponges or a reservoir such as a corneal trephine or well. Additional scraping may be performed to remove calcifications or deposits from the Bowman's layer following application of the chelating agent.

Removal of corneal epithelium

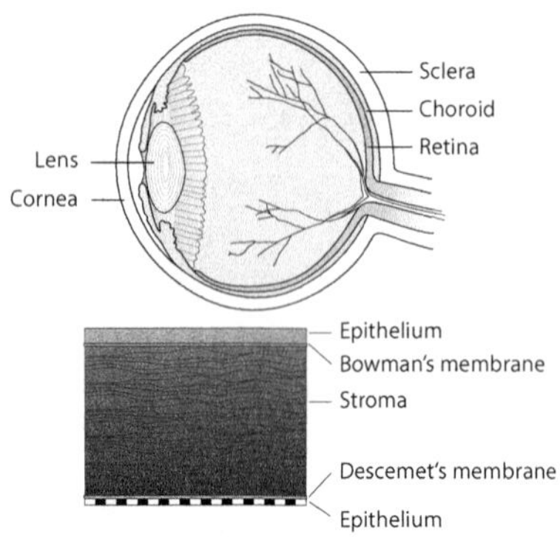

The outer layer of the cornea is removed, with/without chemocauterization (65435); with application of chelating agent (65436).

ICD-10-CM Diagnostic Codes

	B00.52	Herpesviral keratitis
	B02.30	Zoster ocular disease, unspecified
	B02.34	Zoster scleritis
	B02.39	Other herpes zoster eye disease
⇄	H04.122	Dry eye syndrome of left lacrimal gland
⇄	H16.002	Unspecified corneal ulcer, left eye
⇄	H16.122	Filamentary keratitis, left eye
	H17.89	Other corneal scars and opacities
	H17.9	Unspecified corneal scar and opacity
⇄	H18.312	Folds and rupture in Bowman's membrane, left eye
	H18.40	Unspecified corneal degeneration
⇄	H18.412	Arcus senilis, left eye
⇄	H18.422	Band keratopathy, left eye
	H18.43	Other calcerous corneal degeneration
⇄	H18.442	Keratomalacia, left eye
⇄	H18.452	Nodular corneal degeneration, left eye
⇄	H18.462	Peripheral corneal degeneration, left eye
	H18.49	Other corneal degeneration
⇄	H18.501	Unspecified hereditary corneal dystrophies, right eye
⇄	H18.502	Unspecified hereditary corneal dystrophies, left eye
⇄	H18.503	Unspecified hereditary corneal dystrophies, bilateral
⇄	H18.511	Endothelial corneal dystrophy, right eye
⇄	H18.512	Endothelial corneal dystrophy, left eye
⇄	H18.513	Endothelial corneal dystrophy, bilateral
⇄	H18.521	Epithelial (juvenile) corneal dystrophy, right eye
⇄	H18.522	Epithelial (juvenile) corneal dystrophy, left eye
⇄	H18.523	Epithelial (juvenile) corneal dystrophy, bilateral
⇄	H18.531	Granular corneal dystrophy, right eye
⇄	H18.532	Granular corneal dystrophy, left eye
⇄	H18.533	Granular corneal dystrophy, bilateral
⇄	H18.591	Other hereditary corneal dystrophies, right eye
⇄	H18.592	Other hereditary corneal dystrophies, left eye
⇄	H18.593	Other hereditary corneal dystrophies, bilateral
⇄	H18.832	Recurrent erosion of cornea, left eye
⇄	H57.12	Ocular pain, left eye
❼⇄	S05.02	Injury of conjunctiva and corneal abrasion without foreign body, left eye
❼⇄	T15.02	Foreign body in cornea, left eye
❼⇄	T26.12	Burn of cornea and conjunctival sac, left eye
❼⇄	T26.62	Corrosion of cornea and conjunctival sac, left eye

ICD-10-CM Coding Notes

For codes requiring a 7th character extension, refer to your ICD-10-CM book. Review the character descriptions and coding guidelines for proper selection. For some procedures, only certain characters will apply.

CCI Edits

Refer to Appendix A for CCI edits.

Facility RVUs ▢

Code	Work	PE Facility	MP	Total Facility
65435	0.92	1.00	0.08	2.00
65436	4.82	5.49	0.37	10.68

Non-facility RVUs ▢

Code	Work	PE Non-Facility	MP	Total Non-Facility
65435	0.92	1.40	0.08	2.40
65436	4.82	6.06	0.37	11.25

Modifiers (PAR) ▢

Code	Mod 50	Mod 51	Mod 62	Mod 66	Mod 80
65435	1	2	0	0	1
65436	1	2	0	0	1

Global Period

Code	Days
65435	000
65436	090

65450

65450 Destruction of lesion of cornea by cryotherapy, photocoagulation or thermocauterization

AMA Coding Notes

Surgical Procedures on the Eye and Ocular Adnexa

(For diagnostic and treatment ophthalmological services, see Medicine, Ophthalmology, and 92002 et seq)

(Do not report code 69990 in addition to codes 65091-68850)

Plain English Description

Eye drops are instilled to numb the eye. Cryotherapy involves applying a freezing probe directly to the lesion. The extreme cold destroys the lesion. Photocoagulation is performed using a laser. The laser beam is fired at the cornea and destroys the lesion. Thermocauterization is performed by touching the lesion with a heat probe to destroy it by burning.

Destruction of lesion of cornea by cryotherapy/photocoagulation/ thermocauterization

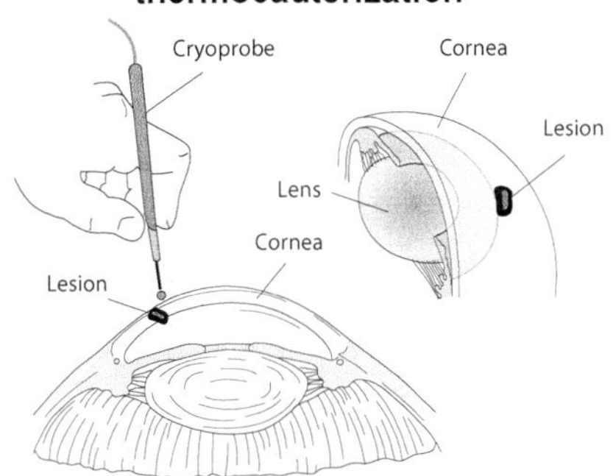

ICD-10-CM Diagnostic Codes

⇄ C69.12 Malignant neoplasm of left cornea
⇄ C69.92 Malignant neoplasm of unspecified site of left eye
⇄ D09.21 Carcinoma in situ of right eye
⇄ D31.12 Benign neoplasm of left cornea
⇄ D31.92 Benign neoplasm of unspecified part of left eye
D48.7 Neoplasm of uncertain behavior of other specified sites
D49.89 Neoplasm of unspecified behavior of other specified sites
⇄ H18.531 Granular corneal dystrophy, right eye
⇄ H18.532 Granular corneal dystrophy, left eye
⇄ H18.533 Granular corneal dystrophy, bilateral
⇄ H18.551 Macular corneal dystrophy, right eye
⇄ H18.552 Macular corneal dystrophy, left eye
⇄ H18.553 Macular corneal dystrophy, bilateral
⇄ H18.591 Other hereditary corneal dystrophies, right eye
⇄ H18.592 Other hereditary corneal dystrophies, left eye
⇄ H18.593 Other hereditary corneal dystrophies, bilateral
⇄ H18.792 Other corneal deformities, left eye
⇄ H18.832 Recurrent erosion of cornea, left eye

CCI Edits

Refer to Appendix A for CCI edits.

Facility RVUs ▯

Code	Work	PE Facility	MP	Total Facility
65450	3.47	5.58	0.25	9.30

Non-facility RVUs ▯

Code	Work	PE Non-Facility	MP	Total Non-Facility
65450	3.47	5.81	0.25	9.53

Modifiers (PAR) ▯

Code	Mod 50	Mod 51	Mod 62	Mod 66	Mod 80
65450	1	2	0	0	1

Global Period

Code	Days
65450	090

65600

65600 Multiple punctures of anterior cornea (eg, for corneal erosion, tattoo)

AMA Coding Notes

Surgical Procedures on the Eye and Ocular Adnexa

(For diagnostic and treatment ophthalmological services, see Medicine, Ophthalmology, and 92002 et seq)

(Do not report code 69990 in addition to codes 65091-68850)

Plain English Description

Multiple punctures of the anterior cornea are performed to treat recurrent corneal erosion or a disfiguring corneal scar. Eye drops are instilled to numb the eye. To treat corneal erosion, a 23- to 25-gauge bent needle is used to puncture the anterior corneal stroma. The small puncture wounds in the cornea promote healing of the erosion by causing intentional scarring of the cornea. Alternatively, puncturing of the anterior cornea may be performed to treat a disfiguring corneal scar following surgery or other trauma. Multiple punctures are performed as described above and an ink stain is applied until the desired cosmetic effect is attained.

Multiple punctures of anterior cornea (eg, for corneal erosion, tattoo)

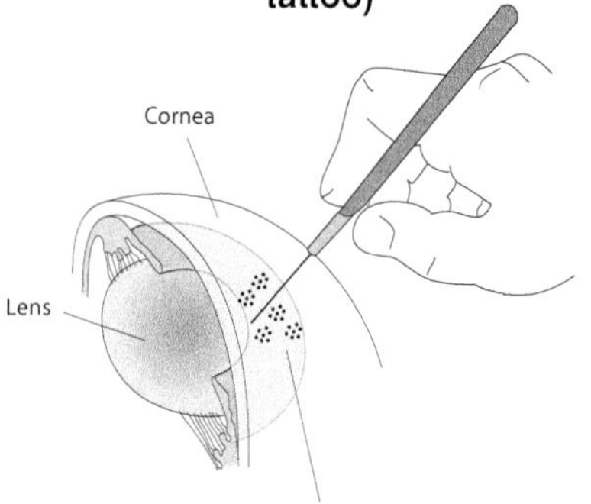
Cornea
Lens
Fine needle is used to make hundreds of tiny holes in the epithelium

ICD-10-CM Diagnostic Codes

	Code	Description
	H17.89	Other corneal scars and opacities
⇄	H18.12	Bullous keratopathy, left eye
⇄	H18.412	Arcus senilis, left eye
⇄	H18.422	Band keratopathy, left eye
	H18.43	Other calcerous corneal degeneration
⇄	H18.442	Keratomalacia, left eye
⇄	H18.452	Nodular corneal degeneration, left eye
⇄	H18.462	Peripheral corneal degeneration, left eye
	H18.49	Other corneal degeneration
⇄	H18.511	Endothelial corneal dystrophy, right eye
⇄	H18.512	Endothelial corneal dystrophy, left eye
⇄	H18.513	Endothelial corneal dystrophy, bilateral
⇄	H18.591	Other hereditary corneal dystrophies, right eye
⇄	H18.592	Other hereditary corneal dystrophies, left eye
⇄	H18.593	Other hereditary corneal dystrophies, bilateral
⇄	H18.792	Other corneal deformities, left eye
⇄	H18.832	Recurrent erosion of cornea, left eye
⇄	H18.892	Other specified disorders of cornea, left eye
	H53.71	Glare sensitivity
	H53.72	Impaired contrast sensitivity
	H53.8	Other visual disturbances
❼⇄	S05.02	Injury of conjunctiva and corneal abrasion without foreign body, left eye

ICD-10-CM Coding Notes

For codes requiring a 7th character extension, refer to your ICD-10-CM book. Review the character descriptions and coding guidelines for proper selection. For some procedures, only certain characters will apply.

CCI Edits

Refer to Appendix A for CCI edits.

Facility RVUs ▯

Code	Work	PE Facility	MP	Total Facility
65600	4.20	5.30	0.32	9.82

Non-facility RVUs ▯

Code	Work	PE Non-Facility	MP	Total Non-Facility
65600	4.20	8.35	0.32	12.87

Modifiers (PAR) ▯

Code	Mod 50	Mod 51	Mod 62	Mod 66	Mod 80
65600	1	2	0	0	1

Global Period

Code	Days
65600	090

65710

65710 Keratoplasty (corneal transplant); anterior lamellar

AMA Coding Guideline

Keratoplasty Procedures on the Cornea

Corneal transplant includes use of fresh or preserved grafts. The preparation of donor material is included for penetrating or anterior lamellar keratoplasty, but reported separately for endothelial keratoplasty. Do not report 65710-65757 in conjunction with 92025.

AMA Coding Notes

Keratoplasty Procedures on the Cornea

(Keratoplasty excludes refractive keratoplasty procedures, 65760, 65765, and 65767)

Surgical Procedures on the Eye and Ocular Adnexa

(For diagnostic and treatment ophthalmological services, see Medicine, Ophthalmology, and 92002 et seq)

(Do not report code 69990 in addition to codes 65091-68850)

AMA *CPT® Assistant* ☐

65710: Oct 02: 8, Apr 09: 5, Dec 09: 13, Aug 12: 15

Plain English Description

Anterior lamellar keratoplasty is performed to replace the diseased, or scarred, partial thickness portion of the anterior cornea selectively, leaving the rest of the healthy cornea undisturbed. The anterior corneal surface is trephined to a depth of 400 micrometers. A 25-gauge bent needle attached to a syringe is inserted with the bevel downward into the corneal stroma, through the trephine cut. Air is then injected to form a big bubble and to detach the deep stromal layers from Descemet's membrane and facilitate lamellar dissection. The anterior stromal disc is then removed with a rounded blade. The anterior chamber is entered and aqueous humor is partially released before a miotic agent is injected. A bubble test is performed to see if the big bubble is properly formed by injecting a small amount of air into the anterior chamber. If it stays within the periphery, pushed by the convex shape of the detached Descemet's membrane, the big bubble has formed in the cornea. A small, oblique incision is made in the corneal stromal surface to collapse the big bubble. The small bubble in the anterior chamber migrates to the central area. Viscoelastic material is then used to fill the space between Descemet's membrane and the detached stroma and to separate the tissue. Microscissors are used to excise the remaining deep corneal stroma and expose the smooth membrane surface. The donor cornea is trephined, stripped of its Descemet's membrane and epithelium, placed into host cornea bed, and sutured into place.

Keratoplasty (corneal transplant); anterior lamellar

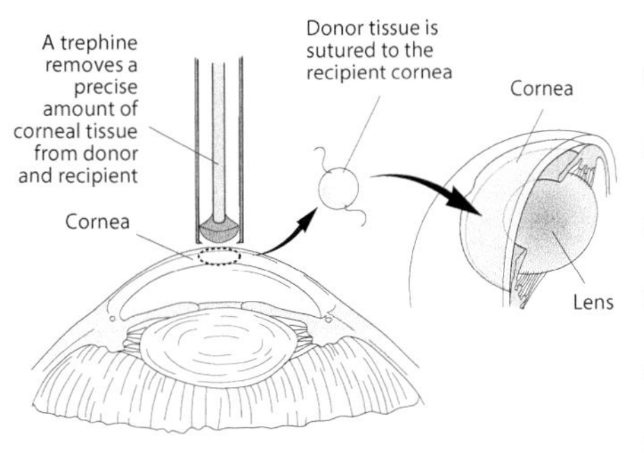
A trephine removes a precise amount of corneal tissue from donor and recipient
Donor tissue is sutured to the recipient cornea
Cornea
Cornea
Lens

ICD-10-CM Diagnostic Codes

	Code	Description
⇄	H11.231	Symblepharon, right eye
⇄	H11.232	Symblepharon, left eye
⇄	H11.233	Symblepharon, bilateral
⇄	H16.001	Unspecified corneal ulcer, right eye
⇄	H16.002	Unspecified corneal ulcer, left eye
⇄	H16.003	Unspecified corneal ulcer, bilateral
⇄	H16.011	Central corneal ulcer, right eye
⇄	H16.012	Central corneal ulcer, left eye
⇄	H16.013	Central corneal ulcer, bilateral
⇄	H16.041	Marginal corneal ulcer, right eye
⇄	H16.042	Marginal corneal ulcer, left eye
⇄	H16.043	Marginal corneal ulcer, bilateral
⇄	H17.11	Central corneal opacity, right eye
⇄	H17.12	Central corneal opacity, left eye
⇄	H17.13	Central corneal opacity, bilateral
⇄	H17.811	Minor opacity of cornea, right eye
⇄	H17.812	Minor opacity of cornea, left eye
⇄	H17.813	Minor opacity of cornea, bilateral
	H17.89	Other corneal scars and opacities
	H17.9	Unspecified corneal scar and opacity
⇄	H18.11	Bullous keratopathy, right eye
⇄	H18.12	Bullous keratopathy, left eye
⇄	H18.13	Bullous keratopathy, bilateral
⇄	H18.211	Corneal edema secondary to contact lens, right eye
⇄	H18.212	Corneal edema secondary to contact lens, left eye
⇄	H18.213	Corneal edema secondary to contact lens, bilateral
⇄	H18.221	Idiopathic corneal edema, right eye
⇄	H18.222	Idiopathic corneal edema, left eye
⇄	H18.223	Idiopathic corneal edema, bilateral
⇄	H18.231	Secondary corneal edema, right eye
⇄	H18.232	Secondary corneal edema, left eye
⇄	H18.233	Secondary corneal edema, bilateral
⇄	H18.421	Band keratopathy, right eye
⇄	H18.422	Band keratopathy, left eye
⇄	H18.423	Band keratopathy, bilateral
⇄	H18.441	Keratomalacia, right eye
⇄	H18.442	Keratomalacia, left eye
⇄	H18.443	Keratomalacia, bilateral
⇄	H18.451	Nodular corneal degeneration, right eye
⇄	H18.452	Nodular corneal degeneration, left eye
⇄	H18.453	Nodular corneal degeneration, bilateral
⇄	H18.461	Peripheral corneal degeneration, right eye
⇄	H18.462	Peripheral corneal degeneration, left eye
⇄	H18.463	Peripheral corneal degeneration, bilateral
	H18.49	Other corneal degeneration
⇄	H18.511	Endothelial corneal dystrophy, right eye
⇄	H18.512	Endothelial corneal dystrophy, left eye
⇄	H18.513	Endothelial corneal dystrophy, bilateral
⇄	H18.521	Epithelial (juvenile) corneal dystrophy, right eye
⇄	H18.522	Epithelial (juvenile) corneal dystrophy, left eye
⇄	H18.523	Epithelial (juvenile) corneal dystrophy, bilateral
⇄	H18.531	Granular corneal dystrophy, right eye
⇄	H18.532	Granular corneal dystrophy, left eye
⇄	H18.533	Granular corneal dystrophy, bilateral
⇄	H18.541	Lattice corneal dystrophy, right eye
⇄	H18.542	Lattice corneal dystrophy, left eye
⇄	H18.543	Lattice corneal dystrophy, bilateral
⇄	H18.551	Macular corneal dystrophy, right eye
⇄	H18.552	Macular corneal dystrophy, left eye
⇄	H18.553	Macular corneal dystrophy, bilateral
⇄	H18.591	Other hereditary corneal dystrophies, right eye
⇄	H18.592	Other hereditary corneal dystrophies, left eye
⇄	H18.593	Other hereditary corneal dystrophies, bilateral
⇄	H18.611	Keratoconus, stable, right eye
⇄	H18.612	Keratoconus, stable, left eye
⇄	H18.613	Keratoconus, stable, bilateral
⇄	H18.711	Corneal ectasia, right eye
⇄	H18.712	Corneal ectasia, left eye
⇄	H18.713	Corneal ectasia, bilateral
⇄	H18.721	Corneal staphyloma, right eye
⇄	H18.722	Corneal staphyloma, left eye
⇄	H18.723	Corneal staphyloma, bilateral
⇄	H18.731	Descemetocele, right eye
⇄	H18.732	Descemetocele, left eye
⇄	H18.733	Descemetocele, bilateral
⇄	H18.791	Other corneal deformities, right eye
⇄	H18.792	Other corneal deformities, left eye
⇄	H18.793	Other corneal deformities, bilateral
⇄	H18.831	Recurrent erosion of cornea, right eye
⇄	H18.832	Recurrent erosion of cornea, left eye
⇄	H18.833	Recurrent erosion of cornea, bilateral
❼⇄	T85.310	Breakdown (mechanical) of prosthetic orbit of right eye
❼⇄	T85.311	Breakdown (mechanical) of prosthetic orbit of left eye
❼⇄	T85.318	Breakdown (mechanical) of other ocular prosthetic devices, implants and grafts
❼⇄	T85.320	Displacement of prosthetic orbit of right eye
❼⇄	T85.321	Displacement of prosthetic orbit of left eye

● New ▲ Revised ✚ Add On ⊘Modifier 51 Exempt ★Telemedicine ☐ CPT QuickRef ⁄⁄FDA Pending ⇄ Laterality ❼ Seventh Character ♂Male ♀Female

➐⇄	T85.328	Displacement of other ocular prosthetic devices, implants and grafts
➐⇄	T85.390	Other mechanical complication of prosthetic orbit of right eye
➐⇄	T85.391	Other mechanical complication of prosthetic orbit of left eye
➐⇄	T85.398	Other mechanical complication of other ocular prosthetic devices, implants and grafts
⇄	T86.8401	Corneal transplant rejection, right eye
⇄	T86.8402	Corneal transplant rejection, left eye
⇄	T86.8403	Corneal transplant rejection, bilateral
⇄	T86.8411	Corneal transplant failure, right eye
⇄	T86.8412	Corneal transplant failure, left eye
⇄	T86.8413	Corneal transplant failure, bilateral
⇄	T86.8481	Other complications of corneal transplant, right eye
⇄	T86.8482	Other complications of corneal transplant, left eye
⇄	T86.8483	Other complications of corneal transplant, bilateral
	Z94.7	Corneal transplant status

ICD-10-CM Coding Notes

For codes requiring a 7th character extension, refer to your ICD-10-CM book. Review the character descriptions and coding guidelines for proper selection. For some procedures, only certain characters will apply.

CCI Edits

Refer to Appendix A for CCI edits.

Facility RVUs ▯

Code	Work	PE Facility	MP	Total Facility
65710	14.45	17.67	1.10	33.22

Non-facility RVUs ▯

Code	Work	PE Non-Facility	MP	Total Non-Facility
65710	14.45	17.67	1.10	33.22

Modifiers (PAR) ▯

Code	Mod 50	Mod 51	Mod 62	Mod 66	Mod 80
65710	1	2	1	0	2

Global Period

Code	Days
65710	090

65730

65730 Keratoplasty (corneal transplant); penetrating (except in aphakia or pseudophakia)

AMA Coding Guideline

Keratoplasty Procedures on the Cornea

Corneal transplant includes use of fresh or preserved grafts. The preparation of donor material is included for penetrating or anterior lamellar keratoplasty, but reported separately for endothelial keratoplasty. Do not report 65710-65757 in conjunction with 92025.

AMA Coding Notes

Keratoplasty Procedures on the Cornea

(Keratoplasty excludes refractive keratoplasty procedures, 65760, 65765, and 65767)

Surgical Procedures on the Eye and Ocular Adnexa

(For diagnostic and treatment ophthalmological services, see Medicine, Ophthalmology, and 92002 et seq)

(Do not report code 69990 in addition to codes 65091-68850)

AMA *CPT® Assistant* ▯

65730: Oct 02: 8, Feb 06: 1, Apr 09: 5, Dec 09: 13, Aug 12: 15

Plain English Description

This is a full-thickness corneal transplant procedure that may be performed for conditions such as viral keratitis, keratoconus, and Fuchs' endothelial dystrophy, bullous keratopathy, or corneal scarring and dystrophy due to trauma or keratitis. The patient's eyes are miosed before the surgery to prevent damage to the lens and avoid causing cataract. The recipient cornea is trephined with a manual, motorized, or vacuum trephine. In order to avoid rapid decompression of the eye, only a partial-thickness trephination cut is made first, followed by a full-thickness cut to remove damaged cornea. The size of the graft is decided, and the donor corneoscleral graft button is cut with the epithelial side up in a concave setting until it is 0.5 mm larger than the recipient bed. The donor button is fitted and stitched into place using radially interrupted sutures placed at 12, 3, 6, and 9 o'clock positions, or with a single continuous running suture. The volume in the anterior chamber is recreated with a balanced salt solution injection.

Keratoplasty (corneal transplant); penetrating (except in aphakia/pseudophakia)

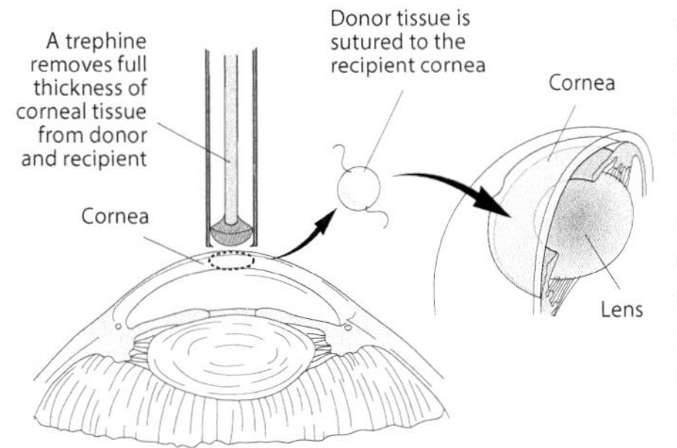

ICD-10-CM Diagnostic Codes

	B00.50	Herpesviral ocular disease, unspecified
	B00.52	Herpesviral keratitis
	B02.33	Zoster keratitis
	B94.0	Sequelae of trachoma
	E50.6	Vitamin A deficiency with xerophthalmic scars of cornea
⇄	H16.011	Central corneal ulcer, right eye
⇄	H16.012	Central corneal ulcer, left eye
⇄	H16.013	Central corneal ulcer, bilateral
⇄	H16.031	Corneal ulcer with hypopyon, right eye
⇄	H16.032	Corneal ulcer with hypopyon, left eye
⇄	H16.033	Corneal ulcer with hypopyon, bilateral
⇄	H16.041	Marginal corneal ulcer, right eye
⇄	H16.042	Marginal corneal ulcer, left eye
⇄	H16.043	Marginal corneal ulcer, bilateral
⇄	H16.051	Mooren's corneal ulcer, right eye
⇄	H16.052	Mooren's corneal ulcer, left eye
⇄	H16.053	Mooren's corneal ulcer, bilateral
⇄	H16.061	Mycotic corneal ulcer, right eye
⇄	H16.062	Mycotic corneal ulcer, left eye
⇄	H16.063	Mycotic corneal ulcer, bilateral
⇄	H16.071	Perforated corneal ulcer, right eye
⇄	H16.072	Perforated corneal ulcer, left eye
⇄	H16.073	Perforated corneal ulcer, bilateral
⇄	H17.01	Adherent leukoma, right eye
⇄	H17.02	Adherent leukoma, left eye
⇄	H17.03	Adherent leukoma, bilateral
⇄	H17.11	Central corneal opacity, right eye
⇄	H17.12	Central corneal opacity, left eye
⇄	H17.13	Central corneal opacity, bilateral
⇄	H17.811	Minor opacity of cornea, right eye
⇄	H17.812	Minor opacity of cornea, left eye
⇄	H17.813	Minor opacity of cornea, bilateral
⇄	H17.821	Peripheral opacity of cornea, right eye
⇄	H17.822	Peripheral opacity of cornea, left eye
⇄	H17.823	Peripheral opacity of cornea, bilateral
	H17.89	Other corneal scars and opacities
⇄	H18.11	Bullous keratopathy, right eye
⇄	H18.12	Bullous keratopathy, left eye
⇄	H18.13	Bullous keratopathy, bilateral
	H18.20	Unspecified corneal edema
⇄	H18.211	Corneal edema secondary to contact lens, right eye
⇄	H18.212	Corneal edema secondary to contact lens, left eye
⇄	H18.213	Corneal edema secondary to contact lens, bilateral
⇄	H18.221	Idiopathic corneal edema, right eye
⇄	H18.222	Idiopathic corneal edema, left eye
⇄	H18.223	Idiopathic corneal edema, bilateral
⇄	H18.231	Secondary corneal edema, right eye
⇄	H18.232	Secondary corneal edema, left eye
⇄	H18.233	Secondary corneal edema, bilateral
⇄	H18.421	Band keratopathy, right eye
⇄	H18.422	Band keratopathy, left eye
⇄	H18.423	Band keratopathy, bilateral
	H18.43	Other calcerous corneal degeneration
⇄	H18.441	Keratomalacia, right eye
⇄	H18.442	Keratomalacia, left eye
⇄	H18.443	Keratomalacia, bilateral
⇄	H18.451	Nodular corneal degeneration, right eye
⇄	H18.452	Nodular corneal degeneration, left eye
⇄	H18.453	Nodular corneal degeneration, bilateral
⇄	H18.461	Peripheral corneal degeneration, right eye
⇄	H18.462	Peripheral corneal degeneration, left eye
⇄	H18.463	Peripheral corneal degeneration, bilateral
	H18.49	Other corneal degeneration
⇄	H18.511	Endothelial corneal dystrophy, right eye
⇄	H18.512	Endothelial corneal dystrophy, left eye
⇄	H18.513	Endothelial corneal dystrophy, bilateral
⇄	H18.521	Epithelial (juvenile) corneal dystrophy, right eye
⇄	H18.522	Epithelial (juvenile) corneal dystrophy, left eye
⇄	H18.523	Epithelial (juvenile) corneal dystrophy, bilateral
⇄	H18.531	Granular corneal dystrophy, right eye
⇄	H18.532	Granular corneal dystrophy, left eye
⇄	H18.533	Granular corneal dystrophy, bilateral
⇄	H18.541	Lattice corneal dystrophy, right eye
⇄	H18.542	Lattice corneal dystrophy, left eye
⇄	H18.543	Lattice corneal dystrophy, bilateral
⇄	H18.551	Macular corneal dystrophy, right eye
⇄	H18.552	Macular corneal dystrophy, left eye
⇄	H18.553	Macular corneal dystrophy, bilateral
⇄	H18.591	Other hereditary corneal dystrophies, right eye
⇄	H18.592	Other hereditary corneal dystrophies, left eye
⇄	H18.593	Other hereditary corneal dystrophies, bilateral
⇄	H18.602	Keratoconus, unspecified, left eye
⇄	H18.612	Keratoconus, stable, left eye
⇄	H18.622	Keratoconus, unstable, left eye
⇄	H18.831	Recurrent erosion of cornea, right eye

⇄	H18.832	Recurrent erosion of cornea, left eye
⇄	H18.833	Recurrent erosion of cornea, bilateral
❼⇄	T26.61	Corrosion of cornea and conjunctival sac, right eye
❼⇄	T26.62	Corrosion of cornea and conjunctival sac, left eye
❼⇄	T85.310	Breakdown (mechanical) of prosthetic orbit of right eye
❼⇄	T85.311	Breakdown (mechanical) of prosthetic orbit of left eye
❼⇄	T85.318	Breakdown (mechanical) of other ocular prosthetic devices, implants and grafts
❼⇄	T85.320	Displacement of prosthetic orbit of right eye
❼⇄	T85.321	Displacement of prosthetic orbit of left eye
❼⇄	T85.328	Displacement of other ocular prosthetic devices, implants and grafts
❼⇄	T85.390	Other mechanical complication of prosthetic orbit of right eye
❼⇄	T85.391	Other mechanical complication of prosthetic orbit of left eye
❼⇄	T85.398	Other mechanical complication of other ocular prosthetic devices, implants and grafts
⇄	T86.8401	Corneal transplant rejection, right eye
⇄	T86.8402	Corneal transplant rejection, left eye
⇄	T86.8403	Corneal transplant rejection, bilateral
⇄	T86.8411	Corneal transplant failure, right eye
⇄	T86.8412	Corneal transplant failure, left eye
⇄	T86.8413	Corneal transplant failure, bilateral
⇄	T86.8481	Other complications of corneal transplant, right eye
⇄	T86.8482	Other complications of corneal transplant, left eye
⇄	T86.8483	Other complications of corneal transplant, bilateral

ICD-10-CM Coding Notes

For codes requiring a 7th character extension, refer to your ICD-10-CM book. Review the character descriptions and coding guidelines for proper selection. For some procedures, only certain characters will apply.

CCI Edits

Refer to Appendix A for CCI edits.

Facility RVUs ▯

Code	Work	PE Facility	MP	Total Facility
65730	16.35	18.80	1.26	36.41

Non-facility RVUs ▯

Code	Work	PE Non-Facility	MP	Total Non-Facility
65730	16.35	18.80	1.26	36.41

Modifiers (PAR) ▯

Code	Mod 50	Mod 51	Mod 62	Mod 66	Mod 80
65730	1	2	1	0	2

Global Period

Code	Days
65730	090

65750-65755

65750 Keratoplasty (corneal transplant); penetrating (in aphakia)

65755 Keratoplasty (corneal transplant); penetrating (in pseudophakia)

AMA Coding Guideline

Keratoplasty Procedures on the Cornea

Corneal transplant includes use of fresh or preserved grafts. The preparation of donor material is included for penetrating or anterior lamellar keratoplasty, but reported separately for endothelial keratoplasty. Do not report 65710-65757 in conjunction with 92025.

AMA Coding Notes

Keratoplasty Procedures on the Cornea

(Keratoplasty excludes refractive keratoplasty procedures, 65760, 65765, and 65767)

Surgical Procedures on the Eye and Ocular Adnexa

(For diagnostic and treatment ophthalmological services, see Medicine, Ophthalmology, and 92002 et seq)

(Do not report code 69990 in addition to codes 65091-68850)

AMA *CPT® Assistant*

65750: Oct 02: 8, Apr 09: 5, Dec 09: 13, Aug 12: 15

65755: Winter 90: 8, Oct 02: 9, Apr 09: 5, Dec 09: 13, Aug 12: 15

Plain English Description

Keratoplasty is a procedure used to improve visual acuity by replacing diseased or damaged corneal tissue with clear, healthy tissue from a donor. Using an operating microscope to visualize the eye, a trephine is used to remove a circular section of the patient's cornea. The anterior chamber is filled with viscoelastic fluid and a similar circle cut from the donor tissue is placed epithelial side down on the recipient eye and sutured in place. Antibiotic eye drops may be instilled, and the eye is covered with a patch and/or shield. Code 65750 includes penetrating keratoplasty for corneal edema following cataract extraction. Code 65755 includes penetrating keratoplasty with the presence of a pseudophakia intraocular lens.

Keratoplasty (corneal transplant); penetrating (in aphakia)

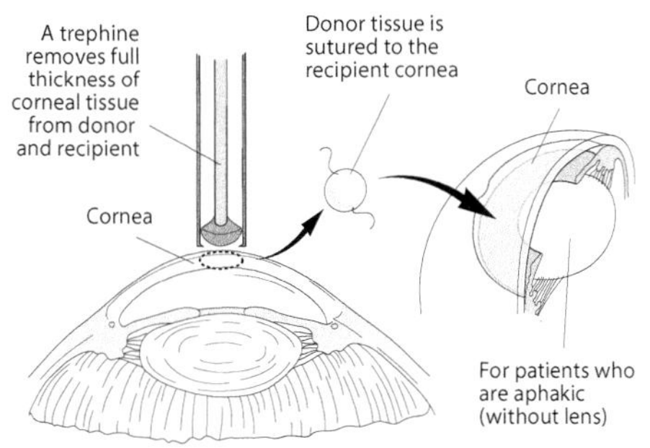

ICD-10-CM Diagnostic Codes

	B60.13	Keratoconjunctivitis due to Acanthamoeba
	E50.6	Vitamin A deficiency with xerophthalmic scars of cornea
⇄	H16.071	Perforated corneal ulcer, right eye
⇄	H16.072	Perforated corneal ulcer, left eye
⇄	H16.073	Perforated corneal ulcer, bilateral
⇄	H16.441	Deep vascularization of cornea, right eye
⇄	H16.442	Deep vascularization of cornea, left eye
⇄	H16.443	Deep vascularization of cornea, bilateral
	H16.8	Other keratitis
⇄	H17.01	Adherent leukoma, right eye
⇄	H17.02	Adherent leukoma, left eye
⇄	H17.03	Adherent leukoma, bilateral
⇄	H17.11	Central corneal opacity, right eye
⇄	H17.12	Central corneal opacity, left eye
⇄	H17.13	Central corneal opacity, bilateral
⇄	H17.821	Peripheral opacity of cornea, right eye
⇄	H17.822	Peripheral opacity of cornea, left eye
⇄	H17.823	Peripheral opacity of cornea, bilateral
	H17.89	Other corneal scars and opacities
	H17.9	Unspecified corneal scar and opacity
⇄	H18.011	Anterior corneal pigmentations, right eye
⇄	H18.012	Anterior corneal pigmentations, left eye
⇄	H18.013	Anterior corneal pigmentations, bilateral
⇄	H18.021	Argentous corneal deposits, right eye
⇄	H18.022	Argentous corneal deposits, left eye
⇄	H18.023	Argentous corneal deposits, bilateral
⇄	H18.11	Bullous keratopathy, right eye
⇄	H18.12	Bullous keratopathy, left eye
⇄	H18.13	Bullous keratopathy, bilateral
⇄	H18.231	Secondary corneal edema, right eye
⇄	H18.232	Secondary corneal edema, left eye
⇄	H18.233	Secondary corneal edema, bilateral
⇄	H18.311	Folds and rupture in Bowman's membrane, right eye
⇄	H18.312	Folds and rupture in Bowman's membrane, left eye
⇄	H18.313	Folds and rupture in Bowman's membrane, bilateral
⇄	H18.451	Nodular corneal degeneration, right eye
⇄	H18.452	Nodular corneal degeneration, left eye
⇄	H18.453	Nodular corneal degeneration, bilateral
⇄	H18.511	Endothelial corneal dystrophy, right eye
⇄	H18.512	Endothelial corneal dystrophy, left eye
⇄	H18.513	Endothelial corneal dystrophy, bilateral
⇄	H18.531	Granular corneal dystrophy, right eye
⇄	H18.532	Granular corneal dystrophy, left eye
⇄	H18.533	Granular corneal dystrophy, bilateral
⇄	H18.601	Keratoconus, unspecified, right eye
⇄	H18.602	Keratoconus, unspecified, left eye
⇄	H18.603	Keratoconus, unspecified, bilateral
⇄	H18.621	Keratoconus, unstable, right eye
⇄	H18.622	Keratoconus, unstable, left eye
⇄	H18.623	Keratoconus, unstable, bilateral
⇄	H21.511	Anterior synechiae (iris), right eye
⇄	H21.512	Anterior synechiae (iris), left eye
⇄	H21.513	Anterior synechiae (iris), bilateral
⇄	H27.01	Aphakia, right eye
⇄	H27.02	Aphakia, left eye
⇄	H27.03	Aphakia, bilateral
⇄	H43.01	Vitreous prolapse, right eye
⇄	H43.02	Vitreous prolapse, left eye
⇄	H43.03	Vitreous prolapse, bilateral
⇄	H59.021	Cataract (lens) fragments in eye following cataract surgery, right eye
⇄	H59.022	Cataract (lens) fragments in eye following cataract surgery, left eye
⇄	H59.023	Cataract (lens) fragments in eye following cataract surgery, bilateral
	Q12.3	Congenital aphakia
	Q13.4	Other congenital corneal malformations
❼⇄	S05.21	Ocular laceration and rupture with prolapse or loss of intraocular tissue, right eye
❼⇄	S05.22	Ocular laceration and rupture with prolapse or loss of intraocular tissue, left eye
❼⇄	S05.31	Ocular laceration without prolapse or loss of intraocular tissue, right eye
❼⇄	S05.32	Ocular laceration without prolapse or loss of intraocular tissue, left eye
❼⇄	S05.51	Penetrating wound with foreign body of right eyeball
❼⇄	S05.52	Penetrating wound with foreign body of left eyeball
❼⇄	S05.8X1	Other injuries of right eye and orbit
❼⇄	S05.8X2	Other injuries of left eye and orbit
❼⇄	T26.61	Corrosion of cornea and conjunctival sac, right eye
❼⇄	T26.62	Corrosion of cornea and conjunctival sac, left eye

❼	T85.21	Breakdown (mechanical) of intraocular lens
❼	T85.22	Displacement of intraocular lens
❼	T85.29	Other mechanical complication of intraocular lens
❼	T85.79	Infection and inflammatory reaction due to other internal prosthetic devices, implants and grafts
❼	T85.848	Pain due to other internal prosthetic devices, implants and grafts
❼	T85.898	Other specified complication of other internal prosthetic devices, implants and grafts
⇄	T86.8421	Corneal transplant infection, right eye
⇄	T86.8422	Corneal transplant infection, left eye
⇄	T86.8423	Corneal transplant infection, bilateral
⇄	T86.8481	Other complications of corneal transplant, right eye
⇄	T86.8482	Other complications of corneal transplant, left eye
⇄	T86.8483	Other complications of corneal transplant, bilateral
	Z96.1	Presence of intraocular lens

ICD-10-CM Coding Notes

For codes requiring a 7th character extension, refer to your ICD-10-CM book. Review the character descriptions and coding guidelines for proper selection. For some procedures, only certain characters will apply.

CCI Edits

Refer to Appendix A for CCI edits.

Facility RVUs ☐

Code	Work	PE Facility	MP	Total Facility
65750	16.90	18.51	1.29	36.70
65755	16.79	18.45	1.29	36.53

Non-facility RVUs ☐

Code	Work	PE Non-Facility	MP	Total Non-Facility
65750	16.90	18.51	1.29	36.70
65755	16.79	18.45	1.29	36.53

Modifiers (PAR) ☐

Code	Mod 50	Mod 51	Mod 62	Mod 66	Mod 80
65750	1	2	1	0	2
65755	1	2	1	0	2

Global Period

Code	Days
65750	090
65755	090

65756

65756 Keratoplasty (corneal transplant); endothelial

AMA Coding Guideline

Keratoplasty Procedures on the Cornea

Corneal transplant includes use of fresh or preserved grafts. The preparation of donor material is included for penetrating or anterior lamellar keratoplasty, but reported separately for endothelial keratoplasty. Do not report 65710-65757 in conjunction with 92025.

AMA Coding Notes

Keratoplasty Procedures on the Cornea

(Keratoplasty excludes refractive keratoplasty procedures, 65760, 65765, and 65767)

Surgical Procedures on the Eye and Ocular Adnexa

(For diagnostic and treatment ophthalmological services, see Medicine, Ophthalmology, and 92002 et seq)

(Do not report code 69990 in addition to codes 65091-68850)

Plain English Description

There are two techniques commonly used: deep lamellar endothelial keratoplasty (DLEK) and Descemet's stripping endothelial keratoplasty (DSEK). Endothelial keratoplasty is used to treat endothelial dysfunction, which includes conditions such as Fuchs' dystrophy, pseudophakic bullous keratopathy (PBK), aphakic bullous keratopathy (ABK), and posterior polymorphous dystrophy (PPMD). The conjunctival tissue is incised around the whole circumference of the cornea (peritomy) using scissors and forceps. A 5 mm scleral tunnel is created beginning 1.5 mm from the limbus. Paracentesis is performed on each side of the scleral tunnel. The anterior chamber is filled with viscoelastic (Healon). If DLEK technique is used, the posterior corneal stroma is dissected away. A keratome is used to enter the anterior chamber and the posterior cornea is removed by scissor dissection. The Healon is removed from the anterior chamber by irrigation and aspiration. A temporary suture is placed in the sclera tunnel. The prepared donor lenticle is folded and grasped with forceps. The temporary suture in the sclera tunnel is removed and the donor lenticle is placed into the anterior chamber. The sclera tunnel is closed and the lenticle is unfolded by infiltrating air into the anterior chamber. The lenticle is tucked into place using hooks; the anterior chamber is filled with balanced saline solution; and the conjunctiva is closed. If DSEK technique is used, the Descemet's membrane is first scored with a Sinskey hook and then stripped using a hook, strippers, or an irrigation/aspiration device. The edge is roughened and the prepared lenticle is folded and placed in the anterior chamber. The sclera tunnel is closed and the lenticle is unfolded and positioned by infiltrating air into the anterior chamber. Fluid is massaged out of the interface. The pupil is dilated and the conjunctiva is closed.

Keratoplasty (corneal transplant); endothelial

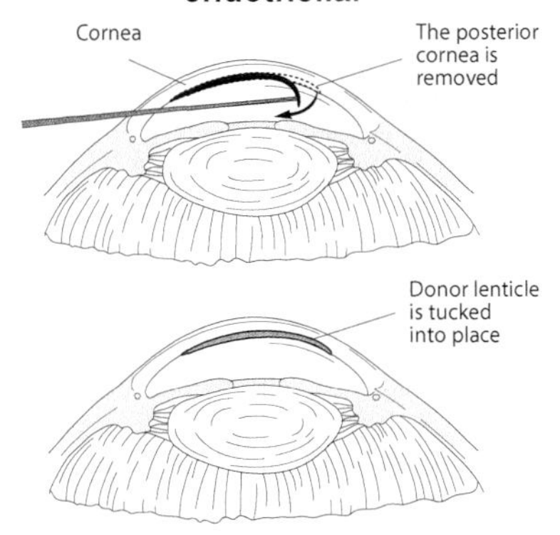
Cornea
The posterior cornea is removed
Donor lenticle is tucked into place

ICD-10-CM Diagnostic Codes

	Code	Description
⇄	H18.12	Bullous keratopathy, left eye
⇄	H18.511	Endothelial corneal dystrophy, right eye
⇄	H18.512	Endothelial corneal dystrophy, left eye
⇄	H18.513	Endothelial corneal dystrophy, bilateral
⇄	H18.591	Other hereditary corneal dystrophies, right eye
⇄	H18.592	Other hereditary corneal dystrophies, left eye
⇄	H18.593	Other hereditary corneal dystrophies, bilateral

CCI Edits

Refer to Appendix A for CCI edits.

Facility RVUs ▢

Code	Work	PE Facility	MP	Total Facility
65756	16.84	15.93	1.29	34.06

Non-facility RVUs ▢

Code	Work	PE Non-Facility	MP	Total Non-Facility
65756	16.84	15.93	1.29	34.06

Modifiers (PAR) ▢

Code	Mod 50	Mod 51	Mod 62	Mod 66	Mod 80
65756	1	2	1	0	2

Global Period

Code	Days
65756	090

65757

+ 65757 Backbench preparation of corneal endothelial allograft prior to transplantation (List separately in addition to code for primary procedure)

(Use 65757 in conjunction with 65756)

AMA Coding Guideline

Keratoplasty Procedures on the Cornea

Corneal transplant includes use of fresh or preserved grafts. The preparation of donor material is included for penetrating or anterior lamellar keratoplasty, but reported separately for endothelial keratoplasty. Do not report 65710-65757 in conjunction with 92025.

AMA Coding Notes

Keratoplasty Procedures on the Cornea

(Keratoplasty excludes refractive keratoplasty procedures, 65760, 65765, and 65767)

Surgical Procedures on the Eye and Ocular Adnexa

(For diagnostic and treatment ophthalmological services, see Medicine, Ophthalmology, and 92002 et seq)

(Do not report code 69990 in addition to codes 65091-68850)

AMA *CPT® Assistant*

65757: Aug 14: 15

Plain English Description

The physician prepares a corneal endothelial allograft in a backbench (back table) procedure prior to transplantation. The donor tissue may be prepared using a microkeratome in an automated technique or it may be prepared manually without the use of a microkeratome. Using an automated microkeratome system, the artificial anterior chamber is filled with preservation solution. The donor tissue endothelium is coated with a thin layer of Healon and placed in the artificial anterior chamber. The artificial chamber is pressurized and the epithelial cells are wiped from the surface of the cornea. The horizontal meridian of the donor tissue is marked so that it can be properly oriented during transplantation. The microkeratome head is mounted on the guide ring, positioned for resection, and then passed over the donor cornea. A free cap of anterior tissue is resected and held above the blade on the microkeratome head. The residual stromal bed is dried using sponges and the diameter and smoothness of the cut is evaluated. The anterior tissue cap is placed back in position using the previously placed reference marks. The exact center of the anterior tissue cap is marked and maintained in position until it adheres to the stromal bed. Alternatively, the donor tissue may be prepared without the use of a microkeratome. The donor tissue is placed in the artificial anterior chamber as described above. A diamond knife is set to the proper depth and a curved incision is made in the peripheral donor limbal area next to the edge of the metal cap of the artificial anterior chamber. Deeper stromal tissue is cut using a crescent blade until the desired plane has been reached. Dissectors are then used to continue all the way to the limbus of the donor tissue. A second manual technique uses a suction trephine placed on the surface of the donor tissue with suction applied. Trephination is carried down to the desired depth. The trephine is removed and the cut inspected to ensure it is of the proper depth. The donor tissue is now dismounted from the artificial anterior chamber and removed from the post, taking care not to damage the endothelium. The donor sclera is irrigated above and below the endothelial surface to remove any residual Healon. The donor tissue is placed on a standard punch trephine block, taking care to properly position the tissue using the previously placed central ink mark. The donor tissue is folded along the horizontal meridian prior to transplantation. The physician now proceeds with the separately reportable endothelial corneal transplant procedure.

Backbench preparation of corneal endothelial allograft

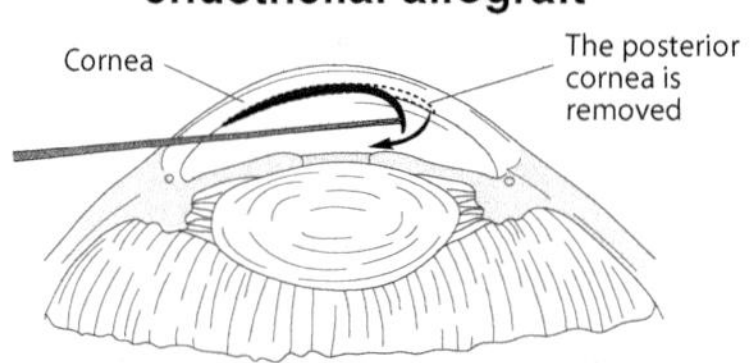
Cornea
The posterior cornea is removed

Using one of several techniques, the physician prepares a corneal endothelial allograft in a backbench procedure prior to transplantation.

ICD-10-CM Diagnostic Codes

See Primary Procedure code for crosswalks.

CCI Edits

Refer to Appendix A for CCI edits.

Facility RVUs

Code	Work	PE Facility	MP	Total Facility
65757	0.00	0.00	0.00	0.00

Non-facility RVUs

Code	Work	PE Non-Facility	MP	Total Non-Facility
65757	0.00	0.00	0.00	0.00

Modifiers (PAR)

Code	Mod 50	Mod 51	Mod 62	Mod 66	Mod 80
65757	0	0	0	0	0

Global Period

Code	Days
65757	ZZZ

65760

65760 Keratomileusis

AMA Coding Guideline

Other Procedures on the Cornea

Do not report 65760-65771 in conjunction with 92025.

AMA Coding Notes

Surgical Procedures on the Eye and Ocular Adnexa

(For diagnostic and treatment ophthalmological services, see Medicine, Ophthalmology, and 92002 et seq)

(Do not report code 69990 in addition to codes 65091-68850)

AMA *CPT® Assistant*

65760: Oct 02: 9

Plain English Description

Keratomileusis is a type of keratoplasty in which the cornea is surgically reshaped to the desired curvature and sutured back in place to correct a refractive error and improve visual acuity. Using an operating microscope to visualize the eye, the anterior lamella is peeled back and a section of corneal tissue is removed and frozen. The posterior surface of the corneal tissue is reshaped using a lathe, laser, or knife blade, and the tissue is sutured back into place. At the conclusion of the procedure, the eye may be covered with a patch or shield.

Keratomileusis

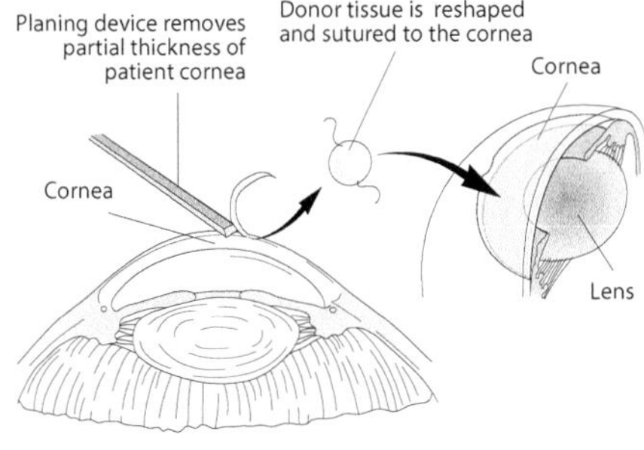
Planing device removes partial thickness of patient cornea
Donor tissue is reshaped and sutured to the cornea
Cornea
Cornea
Lens

ICD-10-CM Diagnostic Codes

⇄	C69.11	Malignant neoplasm of right cornea
⇄	C69.12	Malignant neoplasm of left cornea
⇄	D31.11	Benign neoplasm of right cornea
⇄	D31.12	Benign neoplasm of left cornea
⇄	H18.791	Other corneal deformities, right eye
⇄	H18.821	Corneal disorder due to contact lens, right eye
⇄	H18.831	Recurrent erosion of cornea, right eye
⇄	H18.832	Recurrent erosion of cornea, left eye
⇄	H52.11	Myopia, right eye
	H52.6	Other disorders of refraction
	Q13.3	Congenital corneal opacity
	Q13.4	Other congenital corneal malformations

CCI Edits

Refer to Appendix A for CCI edits.

Pub 100

65760: Pub 100-03, 1, 80.7-80.71

Facility RVUs

Code	Work	PE Facility	MP	Total Facility
65760	0.00	0.00	0.00	0.00

Non-facility RVUs

Code	Work	PE Non-Facility	MP	Total Non-Facility
65760	0.00	0.00	0.00	0.00

Modifiers (PAR)

Code	Mod 50	Mod 51	Mod 62	Mod 66	Mod 80
65760	9	9	9	9	9

Global Period

Code	Days
65760	XXX

65765

65765 Keratophakia

AMA Coding Guideline

Other Procedures on the Cornea

Do not report 65760-65771 in conjunction with 92025.

AMA Coding Notes

Surgical Procedures on the Eye and Ocular Adnexa

(For diagnostic and treatment ophthalmological services, see Medicine, Ophthalmology, and 92002 et seq)

(Do not report code 69990 in addition to codes 65091-68850)

AMA *CPT® Assistant* ▢

65765: Oct 02: 10

Plain English Description

Keratophakia is a type of keratoplasty in which a piece of frozen donor cornea is shaped to the desired curvature and inserted between layers of the recipient cornea to correct a refractive error and improve visual acuity in patients with aphakia, myopia, presbyopia, and stigmatism. Using an operating microscope to visualize the eye, the anterior lamella is peeled back and an implant of donor corneal tissue that has been reshaped to the correct curvature for the patient, or an intraocular lens, is placed deep within the corneal stroma and sutured in place. At the conclusion of the procedure, the eye may be covered with a patch or shield.

Keratophakia

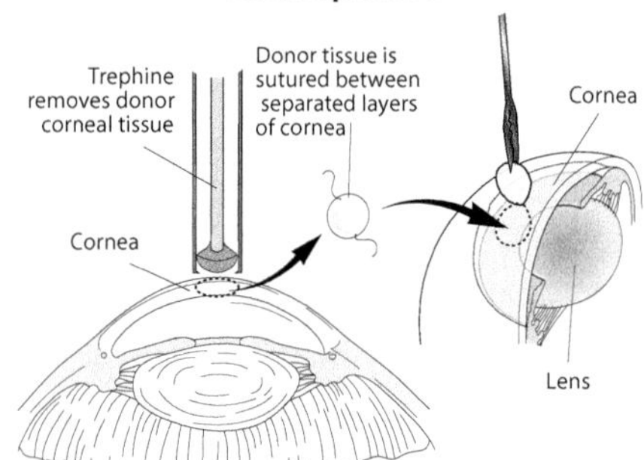

ICD-10-CM Diagnostic Codes

⇄	H18.12	Bullous keratopathy, left eye
⇄	H18.212	Corneal edema secondary to contact lens, left eye
⇄	H18.222	Idiopathic corneal edema, left eye
⇄	H18.232	Secondary corneal edema, left eye
⇄	H18.511	Endothelial corneal dystrophy, right eye
⇄	H18.512	Endothelial corneal dystrophy, left eye
⇄	H18.513	Endothelial corneal dystrophy, bilateral
⇄	H52.02	Hypermetropia, left eye
⇄	H52.12	Myopia, left eye
	H52.4	Presbyopia
	H52.6	Other disorders of refraction
	H52.7	Unspecified disorder of refraction
	Q15.0	Congenital glaucoma

CCI Edits

Refer to Appendix A for CCI edits.

Pub 100

65765: Pub 100-03, 1, 80.7-80.71

Facility RVUs ▢

Code	Work	PE Facility	MP	Total Facility
65765	0.00	0.00	0.00	0.00

Non-facility RVUs ▢

Code	Work	PE Non-Facility	MP	Total Non-Facility
65765	0.00	0.00	0.00	0.00

Modifiers (PAR) ▢

Code	Mod 50	Mod 51	Mod 62	Mod 66	Mod 80
65765	9	9	9	9	9

Global Period

Code	Days
65765	XXX

65767

65767 Epikeratoplasty

AMA Coding Guideline

Other Procedures on the Cornea

Do not report 65760-65771 in conjunction with 92025.

AMA Coding Notes

Surgical Procedures on the Eye and Ocular Adnexa

(For diagnostic and treatment ophthalmological services, see Medicine, Ophthalmology, and 92002 et seq)

(Do not report code 69990 in addition to codes 65091-68850)

AMA *CPT® Assistant* ☐

65767: Winter 90: 8, Oct 02: 10

Plain English Description

The corneal epithelium in the damaged or thinned region of the cornea is removed. Donor corneal tissue that has been reshaped and freeze dried is obtained and is used to fill the corneal defect in the recipient. The corneal graft is secured with sutures. The eyelids may be temporarily sutured closed to allow the patient's corneal tissue to grow into and over the surface of the graft. Usually within 4-5 days the corneal epithelium has healed and the eyelid sutures are removed. The patient continues to use eye drops or ointment until the graft is completely stabilized by the overgrowth of new corneal epithelium, which usually takes 2-3 months.

Epikeratoplasty

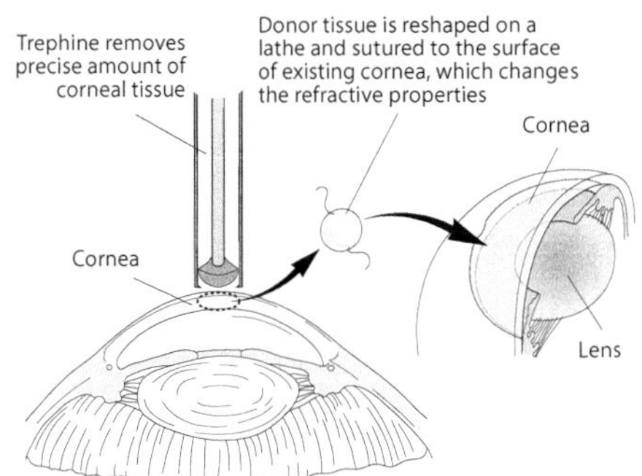
Trephine removes precise amount of corneal tissue
Donor tissue is reshaped on a lathe and sutured to the surface of existing cornea, which changes the refractive properties
Cornea
Cornea
Lens

ICD-10-CM Diagnostic Codes

⇄	H18.11	Bullous keratopathy, right eye
⇄	H18.12	Bullous keratopathy, left eye
⇄	H18.13	Bullous keratopathy, bilateral
⇄	H18.211	Corneal edema secondary to contact lens, right eye
⇄	H18.212	Corneal edema secondary to contact lens, left eye
⇄	H18.213	Corneal edema secondary to contact lens, bilateral
⇄	H18.221	Idiopathic corneal edema, right eye
⇄	H18.222	Idiopathic corneal edema, left eye
⇄	H18.223	Idiopathic corneal edema, bilateral
⇄	H18.231	Secondary corneal edema, right eye
⇄	H18.232	Secondary corneal edema, left eye
⇄	H18.233	Secondary corneal edema, bilateral
⇄	H52.11	Myopia, right eye
⇄	H52.12	Myopia, left eye
⇄	H52.13	Myopia, bilateral
	H52.6	Other disorders of refraction
	Q15.0	Congenital glaucoma
❼⇄	T85.310	Breakdown (mechanical) of prosthetic orbit of right eye
❼⇄	T85.311	Breakdown (mechanical) of prosthetic orbit of left eye
❼⇄	T85.318	Breakdown (mechanical) of other ocular prosthetic devices, implants and grafts
❼⇄	T85.320	Displacement of prosthetic orbit of right eye
❼⇄	T85.321	Displacement of prosthetic orbit of left eye
❼⇄	T85.328	Displacement of other ocular prosthetic devices, implants and grafts
❼⇄	T85.390	Other mechanical complication of prosthetic orbit of right eye
❼⇄	T85.391	Other mechanical complication of prosthetic orbit of left eye
❼⇄	T85.398	Other mechanical complication of other ocular prosthetic devices, implants and grafts
⇄	T86.8401	Corneal transplant rejection, right eye
⇄	T86.8402	Corneal transplant rejection, left eye
⇄	T86.8403	Corneal transplant rejection, bilateral
⇄	T86.8411	Corneal transplant failure, right eye
⇄	T86.8412	Corneal transplant failure, left eye
⇄	T86.8413	Corneal transplant failure, bilateral
⇄	T86.8481	Other complications of corneal transplant, right eye
⇄	T86.8482	Other complications of corneal transplant, left eye
⇄	T86.8483	Other complications of corneal transplant, bilateral

ICD-10-CM Coding Notes

For codes requiring a 7th character extension, refer to your ICD-10-CM book. Review the character descriptions and coding guidelines for proper selection. For some procedures, only certain characters will apply.

CCI Edits

Refer to Appendix A for CCI edits.

Facility RVUs ☐

Code	Work	PE Facility	MP	Total Facility
65767	0.00	0.00	0.00	0.00

Non-facility RVUs ☐

Code	Work	PE Non-Facility	MP	Total Non-Facility
65767	0.00	0.00	0.00	0.00

Modifiers (PAR) ☐

Code	Mod 50	Mod 51	Mod 62	Mod 66	Mod 80
65767	9	9	9	9	9

Global Period

Code	Days
65767	XXX

65770

65770 Keratoprosthesis

AMA Coding Guideline

Other Procedures on the Cornea

Do not report 65760-65771 in conjunction with 92025.

AMA Coding Notes

Surgical Procedures on the Eye and Ocular Adnexa

(For diagnostic and treatment ophthalmological services, see Medicine, Ophthalmology, and 92002 et seq)

(Do not report code 69990 in addition to codes 65091-68850)

AMA *CPT® Assistant* ▢

65770: Oct 02: 10

Plain English Description

A keratoprosthesis is a synthetic substitute used to replace the cornea, usually due to human donor corneal transplant failure or when a donor transplant is not likely to succeed. The synthetic corneal transplant consists of a clear plastic prosthetic graft that takes the place of the cornea. The prosthesis is sutured into human donor tissue that is then sutured to the patient's damaged cornea. Once the keratoprosthesis is properly positioned and secured with sutures a soft contact lens is placed over the eye and must be worn continuously (24 hours a day) every day.

Keratoprosthesis

Tube positioned in the cornea

A tube is inserted from outside the eye into the cornea to restore vision

Cornea

ICD-10-CM Diagnostic Codes

	H17.89	Other corneal scars and opacities
⇄	H18.11	Bullous keratopathy, right eye
⇄	H18.12	Bullous keratopathy, left eye
⇄	H18.13	Bullous keratopathy, bilateral
⇄	H18.231	Secondary corneal edema, right eye
⇄	H18.232	Secondary corneal edema, left eye
⇄	H18.233	Secondary corneal edema, bilateral
⇄	H18.511	Endothelial corneal dystrophy, right eye
⇄	H18.512	Endothelial corneal dystrophy, left eye
⇄	H18.513	Endothelial corneal dystrophy, bilateral
⇄	H18.531	Granular corneal dystrophy, right eye
⇄	H18.532	Granular corneal dystrophy, left eye
⇄	H18.533	Granular corneal dystrophy, bilateral
⇄	H18.541	Lattice corneal dystrophy, right eye
⇄	H18.542	Lattice corneal dystrophy, left eye
⇄	H18.543	Lattice corneal dystrophy, bilateral
⇄	H18.551	Macular corneal dystrophy, right eye
⇄	H18.552	Macular corneal dystrophy, left eye
⇄	H18.553	Macular corneal dystrophy, bilateral
	L12.8	Other pemphigoid
➐⇄	S05.21	Ocular laceration and rupture with prolapse or loss of intraocular tissue, right eye
➐⇄	S05.22	Ocular laceration and rupture with prolapse or loss of intraocular tissue, left eye
➐⇄	T26.11	Burn of cornea and conjunctival sac, right eye
➐⇄	T26.12	Burn of cornea and conjunctival sac, left eye
➐⇄	T26.61	Corrosion of cornea and conjunctival sac, right eye
➐⇄	T26.62	Corrosion of cornea and conjunctival sac, left eye
➐⇄	T85.310	Breakdown (mechanical) of prosthetic orbit of right eye
➐⇄	T85.311	Breakdown (mechanical) of prosthetic orbit of left eye
➐⇄	T85.318	Breakdown (mechanical) of other ocular prosthetic devices, implants and grafts
➐⇄	T85.320	Displacement of prosthetic orbit of right eye
➐⇄	T85.321	Displacement of prosthetic orbit of left eye
➐⇄	T85.328	Displacement of other ocular prosthetic devices, implants and grafts
➐⇄	T85.390	Other mechanical complication of prosthetic orbit of right eye
➐⇄	T85.391	Other mechanical complication of prosthetic orbit of left eye
➐⇄	T85.398	Other mechanical complication of other ocular prosthetic devices, implants and grafts
➐	T85.79	Infection and inflammatory reaction due to other internal prosthetic devices, implants and grafts
➐	T85.848	Pain due to other internal prosthetic devices, implants and grafts
➐	T85.898	Other specified complication of other internal prosthetic devices, implants and grafts
⇄	T86.8401	Corneal transplant rejection, right eye
⇄	T86.8402	Corneal transplant rejection, left eye
⇄	T86.8403	Corneal transplant rejection, bilateral
⇄	T86.8411	Corneal transplant failure, right eye
⇄	T86.8412	Corneal transplant failure, left eye
⇄	T86.8413	Corneal transplant failure, bilateral
⇄	T86.8421	Corneal transplant infection, right eye
⇄	T86.8422	Corneal transplant infection, left eye
⇄	T86.8423	Corneal transplant infection, bilateral
⇄	T86.8481	Other complications of corneal transplant, right eye
⇄	T86.8482	Other complications of corneal transplant, left eye
⇄	T86.8483	Other complications of corneal transplant, bilateral
	Z94.7	Corneal transplant status

ICD-10-CM Coding Notes

For codes requiring a 7th character extension, refer to your ICD-10-CM book. Review the character descriptions and coding guidelines for proper selection. For some procedures, only certain characters will apply.

CCI Edits

Refer to Appendix A for CCI edits.

Facility RVUs ▢

Code	Work	PE Facility	MP	Total Facility
65770	19.74	19.55	1.52	40.81

Non-facility RVUs ▢

Code	Work	PE Non-Facility	MP	Total Non-Facility
65770	19.74	19.55	1.52	40.81

Modifiers (PAR) ▢

Code	Mod 50	Mod 51	Mod 62	Mod 66	Mod 80
65770	1	2	0	0	2

Global Period

Code	Days
65770	090

65771

65771 Radial keratotomy

AMA Coding Guideline

Other Procedures on the Cornea

Do not report 65760-65771 in conjunction with 92025.

AMA Coding Notes

Surgical Procedures on the Eye and Ocular Adnexa

(For diagnostic and treatment ophthalmological services, see Medicine, Ophthalmology, and 92002 et seq)

(Do not report code 69990 in addition to codes 65091-68850)

AMA *CPT® Assistant* ☐

65771: Winter 90: 8, Oct 02: 10

Plain English Description

Radial keratotomy is performed to correct nearsightedness. This procedure is no longer commonly performed having been replaced with photorefractive keratectomy (PRK), laser in situ keratomileusis (LASIK), or epi-LASIK. The eye is first mapped using a slit lamp and markings placed. The number and location of incisions is determined based on the severity of the patient's nearsightedness. The patient is then positioned supine and the eye is prepared and draped. A topical anesthetic is applied to the eye. The cornea is irrigated with saline and a viscolubricant eye solution may be instilled. The globe of the eye is secured using a suction device or forceps. Incisions are then made in the cornea from the center of the cornea to the outer edge using a diamond blade that has been precisely calibrated to achieve the necessary depth of incision. As incisions are made, the cornea relaxes and flattens bringing the central aspect of the cornea closer to the retina, which in turn corrects nearsightedness. Upon completion of the procedure the eye may be covered with soft bandage or patch or a contact lens bandage may be applied.

Radial keratotomy

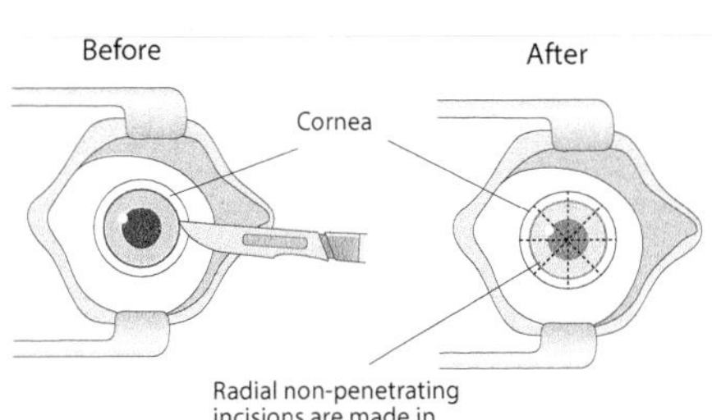
Before
After
Cornea
Radial non-penetrating incisions are made in the cornea

ICD-10-CM Diagnostic Codes

⇄ H44.2A1 Degenerative myopia with choroidal neovascularization, right eye
⇄ H44.2A2 Degenerative myopia with choroidal neovascularization, left eye
⇄ H44.2A3 Degenerative myopia with choroidal neovascularization, bilateral eye
⇄ H44.2B1 Degenerative myopia with macular hole, right eye
⇄ H44.2B2 Degenerative myopia with macular hole, left eye
⇄ H44.2B3 Degenerative myopia with macular hole, bilateral eye
⇄ H44.2C1 Degenerative myopia with retinal detachment, right eye
⇄ H44.2C2 Degenerative myopia with retinal detachment, left eye
⇄ H44.2C3 Degenerative myopia with retinal detachment, bilateral eye
⇄ H44.2D1 Degenerative myopia with foveoschisis, right eye
⇄ H44.2D2 Degenerative myopia with foveoschisis, left eye
⇄ H44.2D3 Degenerative myopia with foveoschisis, bilateral eye
⇄ H44.2E1 Degenerative myopia with other maculopathy, right eye
⇄ H44.2E2 Degenerative myopia with other maculopathy, left eye
⇄ H44.2E3 Degenerative myopia with other maculopathy, bilateral eye
⇄ H52.11 Myopia, right eye

CCI Edits

Refer to Appendix A for CCI edits.

Pub 100

65771: Pub 100-03, 1, 80.7-80.71

Facility RVUs ☐

Code	Work	PE Facility	MP	Total Facility
65771	0.00	0.00	0.00	0.00

Non-facility RVUs ☐

Code	Work	PE Non-Facility	MP	Total Non-Facility
65771	0.00	0.00	0.00	0.00

Modifiers (PAR) ☐

Code	Mod 50	Mod 51	Mod 62	Mod 66	Mod 80
65771	9	9	9	9	9

Global Period

Code	Days
65771	XXX

65772

65772 Corneal relaxing incision for correction of surgically induced astigmatism

AMA Coding Guideline

Other Procedures on the Cornea

Do not report 65760-65771 in conjunction with 92025.

AMA Coding Notes

Surgical Procedures on the Eye and Ocular Adnexa

(For diagnostic and treatment ophthalmological services, see Medicine, Ophthalmology, and 92002 et seq)

(Do not report code 69990 in addition to codes 65091-68850)

AMA *CPT® Assistant* ▢

65772: Oct 02: 10, 12

Plain English Description

Astigmatism occurs when the naturally spherical (round) cornea takes on an oval configuration. This change in shape causes vision to become less sharp (blurry). Surgically induced astigmatism may occur following cataract removal or refractive procedures such as LASIK. A low degree of astigmatism can be corrected using peripheral corneal relaxing incisions (PCRI) or limbal relaxing incisions (LRI). The eye is first mapped using a slit lamp and markings placed. The patient is then positioned supine and the eye is prepared and draped. The cornea is anesthetized using a topical anesthetic. The cornea is irrigated with saline and a viscolubricant eye solution may be instilled. The globe of the eye is secured using a suction device or forceps and a diamond knife is used to incise the previously marked areas around the axis of the cornea. These small incisions allow the cornea to return to a more natural, spherical shape and vision to be sharper or clearer. At the conclusion of the procedure a corneal contact lens bandage may be placed, antibiotic eye drops are instilled and the eye is then patched.

Corneal relaxing incision

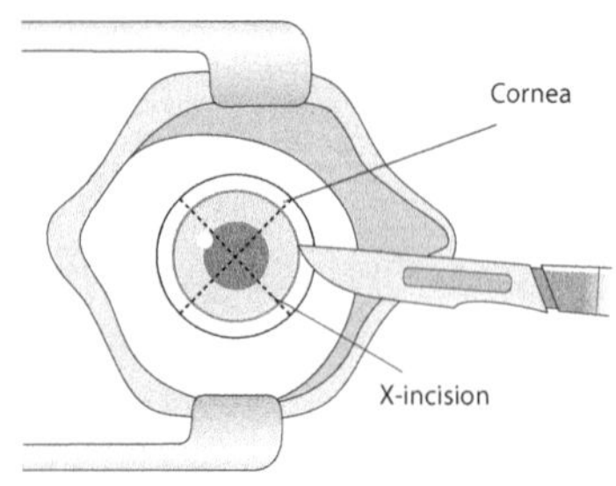

Incisions are made in the cornea to correct a surgically induced astigmatism.

ICD-10-CM Diagnostic Codes

⇄	H52.211	Irregular astigmatism, right eye
⇄	H52.212	Irregular astigmatism, left eye
⇄	H52.213	Irregular astigmatism, bilateral
⇄	H52.221	Regular astigmatism, right eye
⇄	H52.222	Regular astigmatism, left eye
⇄	H52.223	Regular astigmatism, bilateral
❼	T81.89	Other complications of procedures, not elsewhere classified
❼⇄	T85.310	Breakdown (mechanical) of prosthetic orbit of right eye
❼⇄	T85.311	Breakdown (mechanical) of prosthetic orbit of left eye
❼⇄	T85.318	Breakdown (mechanical) of other ocular prosthetic devices, implants and grafts
❼⇄	T85.320	Displacement of prosthetic orbit of right eye
❼⇄	T85.321	Displacement of prosthetic orbit of left eye
❼⇄	T85.328	Displacement of other ocular prosthetic devices, implants and grafts
❼⇄	T85.390	Other mechanical complication of prosthetic orbit of right eye
❼⇄	T85.391	Other mechanical complication of prosthetic orbit of left eye
❼⇄	T85.398	Other mechanical complication of other ocular prosthetic devices, implants and grafts
⇄	T86.8401	Corneal transplant rejection, right eye
⇄	T86.8402	Corneal transplant rejection, left eye
⇄	T86.8403	Corneal transplant rejection, bilateral
⇄	T86.8411	Corneal transplant failure, right eye
⇄	T86.8412	Corneal transplant failure, left eye
⇄	T86.8413	Corneal transplant failure, bilateral
	Z94.7	Corneal transplant status
	Z96.1	Presence of intraocular lens
	Z98.83	Filtering (vitreous) bleb after glaucoma surgery status

ICD-10-CM Coding Notes

For codes requiring a 7th character extension, refer to your ICD-10-CM book. Review the character descriptions and coding guidelines for proper selection. For some procedures, only certain characters will apply.

CCI Edits

Refer to Appendix A for CCI edits.

Facility RVUs ▢

Code	Work	PE Facility	MP	Total Facility
65772	5.09	6.22	0.39	11.70

Non-facility RVUs ▢

Code	Work	PE Non-Facility	MP	Total Non-Facility
65772	5.09	7.84	0.39	13.32

Modifiers (PAR) ▢

Code	Mod 50	Mod 51	Mod 62	Mod 66	Mod 80
65772	1	2	0	0	1

Global Period

Code	Days
65772	090

65775

65775 Corneal wedge resection for correction of surgically induced astigmatism

(For fitting of contact lens for treatment of disease, see 92071, 92072)

(For unlisted procedures on cornea, use 66999)

AMA Coding Guideline

Other Procedures on the Cornea

Do not report 65760-65771 in conjunction with 92025.

AMA Coding Notes

Surgical Procedures on the Eye and Ocular Adnexa

(For diagnostic and treatment ophthalmological services, see Medicine, Ophthalmology, and 92002 et seq)

(Do not report code 69990 in addition to codes 65091-68850)

AMA *CPT® Assistant* ▢

65775: Oct 02: 10, 12, Aug 12: 9

Plain English Description

Astigmatism occurs when the naturally spherical (round) cornea takes on an oval configuration. This change in shape causes vision to become less sharp (blurry). Surgically induced astigmatism may occur following cataract removal or refractive procedures such as LASIK. A high degree of astigmatism is usually corrected using corneal wedge resection. The eye is first mapped using a slit lamp and markings placed. The patient is then positioned supine and the eye is prepared and draped. The cornea is anesthetized using a topical anesthetic. The cornea is irrigated with saline and a viscolubricant eye solution may be instilled. The globe of the eye is secured using a suction device or forceps and a diamond knife is used to incise the previously marked area of the cornea. A sliver of corneal tissue is excised and the wound closed with 10-0 nylon. The removal of small section of tissue allows the cornea to return to a more natural, spherical shape and vision to be sharper or clearer. At the conclusion of the procedure a corneal contact lens bandage may be applied, antibiotic eye drops are instilled and the eye is then patched.

Corneal relaxing incision

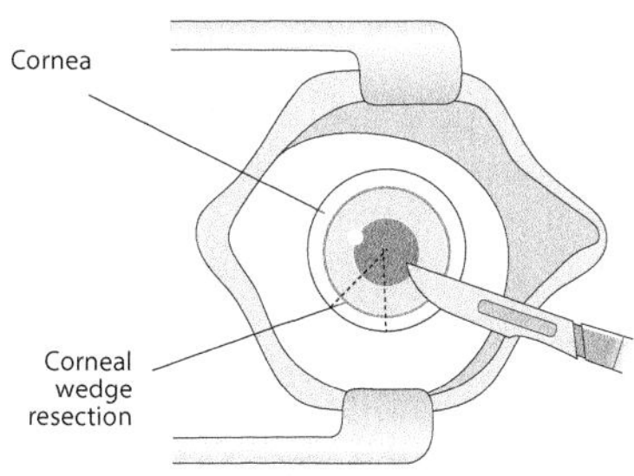

Incisions are made in the cornea to correct surgically induced astigmatism.

ICD-10-CM Diagnostic Codes

⇄	H52.211	Irregular astigmatism, right eye
⇄	H52.212	Irregular astigmatism, left eye
⇄	H52.213	Irregular astigmatism, bilateral
⇄	H52.221	Regular astigmatism, right eye
⇄	H52.222	Regular astigmatism, left eye
⇄	H52.223	Regular astigmatism, bilateral
➐	T81.89	Other complications of procedures, not elsewhere classified
⇄	T86.8411	Corneal transplant failure, right eye
⇄	T86.8412	Corneal transplant failure, left eye
⇄	T86.8413	Corneal transplant failure, bilateral
	Z94.7	Corneal transplant status
	Z96.1	Presence of intraocular lens
	Z98.83	Filtering (vitreous) bleb after glaucoma surgery status

ICD-10-CM Coding Notes

For codes requiring a 7th character extension, refer to your ICD-10-CM book. Review the character descriptions and coding guidelines for proper selection. For some procedures, only certain characters will apply.

CCI Edits

Refer to Appendix A for CCI edits.

Facility RVUs ▢

Code	Work	PE Facility	MP	Total Facility
65775	6.91	9.26	0.54	16.71

Non-facility RVUs ▢

Code	Work	PE Non-Facility	MP	Total Non-Facility
65775	6.91	9.26	0.54	16.71

Modifiers (PAR) ▢

Code	Mod 50	Mod 51	Mod 62	Mod 66	Mod 80
65775	1	2	0	0	1

Global Period

Code	Days
65775	090

65778-65779

65778 Placement of amniotic membrane on the ocular surface; without sutures

65779 Placement of amniotic membrane on the ocular surface; single layer, sutured

(Do not report 65778, 65779 in conjunction with 65430, 65435, 65780)

(For placement of amniotic membrane using tissue glue, use 66999)

AMA Coding Guideline

Other Procedures on the Cornea

Do not report 65760-65771 in conjunction with 92025.

AMA Coding Notes

Surgical Procedures on the Eye and Ocular Adnexa

(For diagnostic and treatment ophthalmological services, see Medicine, Ophthalmology, and 92002 et seq)

(Do not report code 69990 in addition to codes 65091-68850)

AMA *CPT® Assistant* ▢

65778: May 14: 5, Feb 18: 11

65779: May 14: 5, Feb 18: 11

Plain English Description

Amniotic membrane, previously harvested from placental tissue and dried, is placed on the ocular surface of the eye to promote wound healing. The eye is irrigated with normal saline and antibiotic drops are used as needed for 24-48 hours before applying the amniotic membrane. Anesthetic eye drops and/or facial nerve block is used to anesthetize the eye. An eye speculum is applied to the eye to keep it open. In 65778, a self-retaining amniotic membrane graft is applied. This method of graft placement may also be referred to as spreading or sutureless. A dried piece of amniotic membrane approximately the size of the conjunctival sac is obtained from the tissue bank. A circular opening is cut into the membrane so that uninvolved portions of the cornea are not covered. Covering the entire cornea can result in temporary hazy vision in the affected eye. The amniotic membrane is then spread over the wound as well as the healthy conjunctiva. The membrane is spread from the upper fornix with the patient looking down and then over the lower fornix with the patient looking up. The eye speculum is removed. Liquid paraffin is used to seal the eye closed and both eyes are bandaged closed for 24-48 hours to allow the amniotic membrane to be absorbed. In 65779, the amniotic membrane is sutured over the wound. A dried piece of amniotic membrane conforming to the size and shape of the wound is obtained from the tissue bank. A suture is passed through each corner of the membrane graft. The graft is placed over the wound and the previously placed membrane sutures are passed through the conjunctiva to secure the graft to the eye. The speculum is removed, liquid paraffin is used to seal the eye closed, and both eyes are bandaged closed for 24-48 hours. The sutures are removed three days after the membrane placement.

Placement of amniotic membrane on the ocular surface

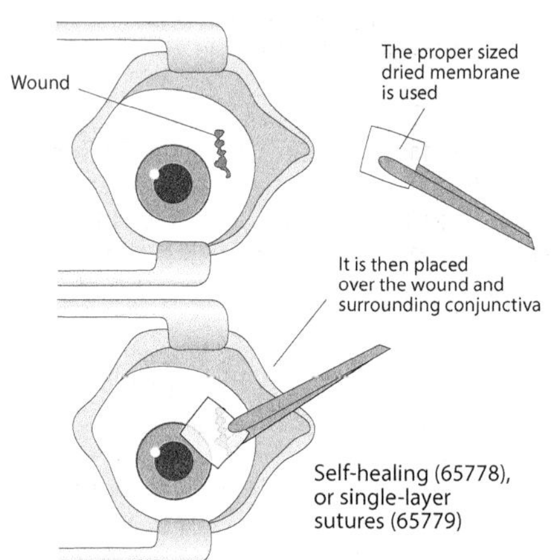

ICD-10-CM Diagnostic Codes

⇄	H11.012	Amyloid pterygium of left eye
⇄	H11.022	Central pterygium of left eye
⇄	H11.032	Double pterygium of left eye
⇄	H11.042	Peripheral pterygium, stationary, left eye
⇄	H11.052	Peripheral pterygium, progressive, left eye
⇄	H11.062	Recurrent pterygium of left eye
⇄	H11.152	Pinguecula, left eye
⇄	H11.242	Scarring of conjunctiva, left eye
⇄	H16.012	Central corneal ulcer, left eye
⇄	H16.022	Ring corneal ulcer, left eye
⇄	H16.032	Corneal ulcer with hypopyon, left eye
⇄	H16.042	Marginal corneal ulcer, left eye
⇄	H16.052	Mooren's corneal ulcer, left eye
⇄	H16.062	Mycotic corneal ulcer, left eye
⇄	H16.072	Perforated corneal ulcer, left eye
	H17.89	Other corneal scars and opacities
⇄	H18.521	Epithelial (juvenile) corneal dystrophy, right eye
⇄	H18.522	Epithelial (juvenile) corneal dystrophy, left eye
⇄	H18.523	Epithelial (juvenile) corneal dystrophy, bilateral
⇄	H18.832	Recurrent erosion of cornea, left eye
	L51.1	Stevens-Johnson syndrome
	L51.3	Stevens-Johnson syndrome-toxic epidermal necrolysis overlap syndrome
❼⇄	T26.12	Burn of cornea and conjunctival sac, left eye
❼⇄	T26.32	Burns of other specified parts of left eye and adnexa
❼⇄	T26.42	Burn of left eye and adnexa, part unspecified
❼⇄	T26.62	Corrosion of cornea and conjunctival sac, left eye
❼⇄	T26.82	Corrosions of other specified parts of left eye and adnexa
❼⇄	T26.92	Corrosion of left eye and adnexa, part unspecified

ICD-10-CM Coding Notes

For codes requiring a 7th character extension, refer to your ICD-10-CM book. Review the character descriptions and coding guidelines for proper selection. For some procedures, only certain characters will apply.

CCI Edits

Refer to Appendix A for CCI edits.

Facility RVUs ▢

Code	Work	PE Facility	MP	Total Facility
65778	1.00	0.50	0.05	1.55
65779	2.50	1.60	0.20	4.30

Non-facility RVUs ▢

Code	Work	PE Non-Facility	MP	Total Non-Facility
65778	1.00	39.77	0.05	40.82
65779	2.50	32.68	0.20	35.38

Modifiers (PAR) ▢

Code	Mod 50	Mod 51	Mod 62	Mod 66	Mod 80
65778	1	2	0	0	0
65779	1	2	0	0	0

Global Period

Code	Days
65778	000
65779	000

65780

65780 Ocular surface reconstruction; amniotic membrane transplantation, multiple layers

(For placement of amniotic membrane without reconstruction using no sutures or single layer suture technique, see 65778, 65779)

AMA Coding Guideline

Other Procedures on the Cornea

Do not report 65760-65771 in conjunction with 92025.

AMA Coding Notes

Surgical Procedures on the Eye and Ocular Adnexa

(For diagnostic and treatment ophthalmological services, see Medicine, Ophthalmology, and 92002 et seq)

(Do not report code 69990 in addition to codes 65091-68850)

AMA *CPT® Assistant*

65780: May 04: 10, Jun 09: 9, May 14: 5, Feb 18: 11

Plain English Description

This procedure is performed to treat damage to the ocular surface caused by injury or a disease process. When the repair is performed by amniotic membrane reconstruction, the physician may use an inlay or overlay technique or for deeper defects the amniotic membrane may be used as a filler to repair the ocular surface. Amniotic membrane grafts act as a basement membrane over which epithelialization takes place. The amniotic membrane graft is obtained from the tissue bank and prepared for transplant. The corneal epithelium is debrided as needed. The graft material is trimmed to the size of the corneal defect. Using an inlay technique, the graft is carefully placed in the defect taking care not to extend the graft edges beyond the defect. The graft is secured with interrupted sutures. Using an overlay technique, the entire corneal surface including the limbus is covered with the amniotic membrane graft. The overlay graft protects the underlying damaged epithelium while at the same time allowing oxygen and moisture to reach it, which promotes regeneration of the epithelium and healing of the cornea. Deeper defects may require amniotic membrane filler graft, which is a multilayered amniotic membrane graft. Once the multilayered graft has been placed in the defect and secured with sutures, it may be covered with an inlay or overlay graft.

Ocular surface reconstruction

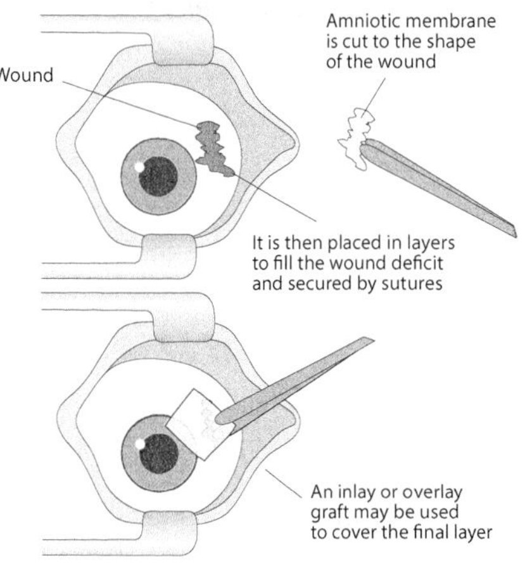

Wound
Amniotic membrane is cut to the shape of the wound
It is then placed in layers to fill the wound deficit and secured by sutures
An inlay or overlay graft may be used to cover the final layer

ICD-10-CM Diagnostic Codes

⇄	D31.11	Benign neoplasm of right cornea
⇄	H11.011	Amyloid pterygium of right eye
⇄	H11.021	Central pterygium of right eye
⇄	H11.031	Double pterygium of right eye
⇄	H11.041	Peripheral pterygium, stationary, right eye
⇄	H11.051	Peripheral pterygium, progressive, right eye
⇄	H11.061	Recurrent pterygium of right eye
⇄	H11.121	Conjunctival concretions, right eye
⇄	H11.141	Conjunctival xerosis, unspecified, right eye
⇄	H11.231	Symblepharon, right eye
⇄	H11.811	Pseudopterygium of conjunctiva, right eye
⇄	H11.821	Conjunctivochalasis, right eye
⇄	H16.021	Ring corneal ulcer, right eye
⇄	H16.031	Corneal ulcer with hypopyon, right eye
⇄	H16.041	Marginal corneal ulcer, right eye
⇄	H16.061	Mycotic corneal ulcer, right eye
⇄	H16.071	Perforated corneal ulcer, right eye
⇄	H16.211	Exposure keratoconjunctivitis, right eye
⇄	H16.231	Neurotrophic keratoconjunctivitis, right eye
	H17.89	Other corneal scars and opacities
⇄	H18.11	Bullous keratopathy, right eye
⇄	H18.211	Corneal edema secondary to contact lens, right eye
⇄	H18.411	Arcus senilis, right eye
⇄	H18.421	Band keratopathy, right eye
⇄	H18.441	Keratomalacia, right eye
⇄	H18.461	Peripheral corneal degeneration, right eye
⇄	H18.511	Endothelial corneal dystrophy, right eye
⇄	H18.512	Endothelial corneal dystrophy, left eye
⇄	H18.513	Endothelial corneal dystrophy, bilateral
⇄	H18.531	Granular corneal dystrophy, right eye
⇄	H18.532	Granular corneal dystrophy, left eye
⇄	H18.533	Granular corneal dystrophy, bilateral
⇄	H18.541	Lattice corneal dystrophy, right eye
⇄	H18.542	Lattice corneal dystrophy, left eye
⇄	H18.543	Lattice corneal dystrophy, bilateral
⇄	H18.551	Macular corneal dystrophy, right eye
⇄	H18.552	Macular corneal dystrophy, left eye
⇄	H18.553	Macular corneal dystrophy, bilateral
⇄	H18.591	Other hereditary corneal dystrophies, right eye
⇄	H18.592	Other hereditary corneal dystrophies, left eye
⇄	H18.593	Other hereditary corneal dystrophies, bilateral
⇄	H18.821	Corneal disorder due to contact lens, right eye
⇄	H18.831	Recurrent erosion of cornea, right eye
	L51.1	Stevens-Johnson syndrome
	L51.3	Stevens-Johnson syndrome-toxic epidermal necrolysis overlap syndrome
	M35.01	Sjögren syndrome with keratoconjunctivitis
❼⇄	T26.11	Burn of cornea and conjunctival sac, right eye
❼⇄	T26.61	Corrosion of cornea and conjunctival sac, right eye

ICD-10-CM Coding Notes

For codes requiring a 7th character extension, refer to your ICD-10-CM book. Review the character descriptions and coding guidelines for proper selection. For some procedures, only certain characters will apply.

CCI Edits

Refer to Appendix A for CCI edits.

Facility RVUs

Code	Work	PE Facility	MP	Total Facility
65780	7.81	10.96	0.60	19.37

Non-facility RVUs

Code	Work	PE Non-Facility	MP	Total Non-Facility
65780	7.81	10.96	0.60	19.37

Modifiers (PAR)

Code	Mod 50	Mod 51	Mod 62	Mod 66	Mod 80
65780	1	2	1	0	1

Global Period

Code	Days
65780	090

65781

65781 Ocular surface reconstruction; limbal stem cell allograft (eg, cadaveric or living donor)

AMA Coding Guideline

Other Procedures on the Cornea

Do not report 65760-65771 in conjunction with 92025.

AMA Coding Notes

Surgical Procedures on the Eye and Ocular Adnexa

(For diagnostic and treatment ophthalmological services, see Medicine, Ophthalmology, and 92002 et seq)

(Do not report code 69990 in addition to codes 65091-68850)

AMA *CPT® Assistant* ▯

65781: May 04: 10

Plain English Description

This procedure is performed to treat damage to the cornea caused by injury or a disease process. Limbal stem cell allograft is performed only on patients with severe damage to the ocular surface causing inability of the eye to heal itself. Limbal stem cells arise from the white outer coating of eyeball, also referred to as the limbus. The limbal stem cells give rise to corneal epithelial cells, which form the outermost layer of the cornea and act as a protective barrier to germs and other contaminants. If a live donor allograft is used, the limbal cells are harvested in a strip from the eye of the donor in a separately reportable procedure. Alternatively, previously harvested limbal stem cells from a cadaver may be used. In the patient receiving the transplant, the corneal epithelium is debrided to remove the damaged epithelial stem cells and the transplant bed is prepared for the allograft. The conjunctiva is resected and the sclera exposed to a point 4-5 mm beyond the limbus. The limbal stem cell allograft is then placed in the prepared transplant bed and secured with sutures. Antibiotic and corticosteroid ointments are applied to the surgical wound. The eye is patched and covered with an eye shield.

Ocular reconstruction, limbal stem cell allograft

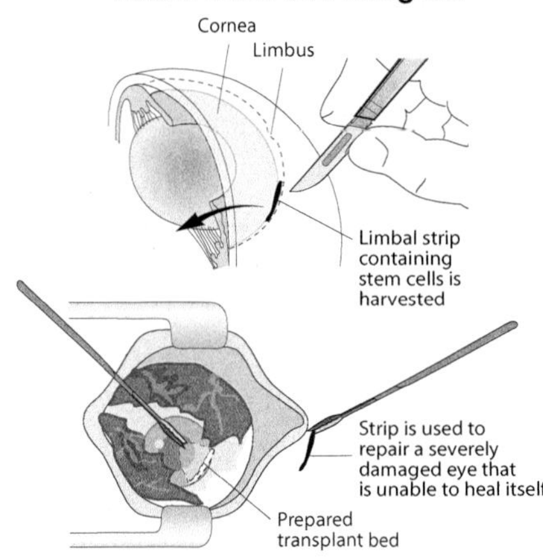
Cornea
Limbus
Limbal strip containing stem cells is harvested
Strip is used to repair a severely damaged eye that is unable to heal itself
Prepared transplant bed

ICD-10-CM Diagnostic Codes

⇄ D31.02 Benign neoplasm of left conjunctiva
⇄ H11.012 Amyloid pterygium of left eye
⇄ H11.022 Central pterygium of left eye
⇄ H11.032 Double pterygium of left eye
⇄ H11.042 Peripheral pterygium, stationary, left eye
⇄ H11.052 Peripheral pterygium, progressive, left eye
⇄ H11.062 Recurrent pterygium of left eye
⇄ H11.812 Pseudopterygium of conjunctiva, left eye
⇄ H18.412 Arcus senilis, left eye
⇄ H18.422 Band keratopathy, left eye
H18.43 Other calcerous corneal degeneration
⇄ H18.442 Keratomalacia, left eye
⇄ H18.511 Endothelial corneal dystrophy, right eye
⇄ H18.512 Endothelial corneal dystrophy, left eye
⇄ H18.513 Endothelial corneal dystrophy, bilateral
⇄ H18.521 Epithelial (juvenile) corneal dystrophy, right eye
⇄ H18.522 Epithelial (juvenile) corneal dystrophy, left eye
⇄ H18.523 Epithelial (juvenile) corneal dystrophy, bilateral
⇄ H18.531 Granular corneal dystrophy, right eye
⇄ H18.532 Granular corneal dystrophy, left eye
⇄ H18.533 Granular corneal dystrophy, bilateral
⇄ H18.541 Lattice corneal dystrophy, right eye
⇄ H18.542 Lattice corneal dystrophy, left eye
⇄ H18.543 Lattice corneal dystrophy, bilateral
⇄ H18.551 Macular corneal dystrophy, right eye
⇄ H18.552 Macular corneal dystrophy, left eye
⇄ H18.553 Macular corneal dystrophy, bilateral
⇄ H18.591 Other hereditary corneal dystrophies, right eye
⇄ H18.592 Other hereditary corneal dystrophies, left eye
⇄ H18.593 Other hereditary corneal dystrophies, bilateral
⇄ H18.822 Corneal disorder due to contact lens, left eye
⇄ H18.832 Recurrent erosion of cornea, left eye
L51.1 Stevens-Johnson syndrome
L51.3 Stevens-Johnson syndrome-toxic epidermal necrolysis overlap syndrome
❼⇄ T26.12 Burn of cornea and conjunctival sac, left eye
❼⇄ T26.62 Corrosion of cornea and conjunctival sac, left eye

ICD-10-CM Coding Notes

For codes requiring a 7th character extension, refer to your ICD-10-CM book. Review the character descriptions and coding guidelines for proper selection. For some procedures, only certain characters will apply.

CCI Edits

Refer to Appendix A for CCI edits.

Facility RVUs ▯

Code	Work	PE Facility	MP	Total Facility
65781	18.14	18.84	1.40	38.38

Non-facility RVUs ▯

Code	Work	PE Non-Facility	MP	Total Non-Facility
65781	18.14	18.84	1.40	38.38

Modifiers (PAR) ▯

Code	Mod 50	Mod 51	Mod 62	Mod 66	Mod 80
65781	1	2	1	0	2

Global Period

Code	Days
65781	090

65782

65782 Ocular surface reconstruction; limbal conjunctival autograft (includes obtaining graft)

(For harvesting conjunctival allograft, living donor, use 68371)

AMA Coding Guideline

Other Procedures on the Cornea

Do not report 65760-65771 in conjunction with 92025.

AMA Coding Notes

Surgical Procedures on the Eye and Ocular Adnexa

(For diagnostic and treatment ophthalmological services, see Medicine, Ophthalmology, and 92002 et seq)

(Do not report code 69990 in addition to codes 65091-68850)

AMA *CPT® Assistant* ▯

65782: Feb 04: 11, May 04: 10, Feb 05: 15-16

Plain English Description

This procedure is performed to treat damage to the cornea caused by injury or a disease process. Limbal conjunctival autograft is performed only on patients with severe damage to the ocular surface causing inability of the eye to heal itself. The limbus is the white outer coating of the eyeball. The limbus contains stem cells that give rise to corneal epithelial cells, which form the outermost layer of the cornea and act as a protective barrier to germs and other contaminants. If only one eye is damaged the physician obtains a graft from the patient's healthy eye. The limbal conjunctival autograft is harvested in a strip from the healthy eye. The corneal epithelium of the damaged eye is debrided to remove the damaged epithelial stem cells and the transplant bed is prepared for the allograft. The conjunctiva is resected and the sclera exposed to a point 4-5 mm beyond the limbus. The limbal conjunctival autograft is then placed in the prepared transplant bed and secured with sutures. Antibiotic and corticosteroid ointments are applied to the surgical wound. The eye is patched and covered with an eye shield.

Ocular reconstruction, limbal conjunctival autograft

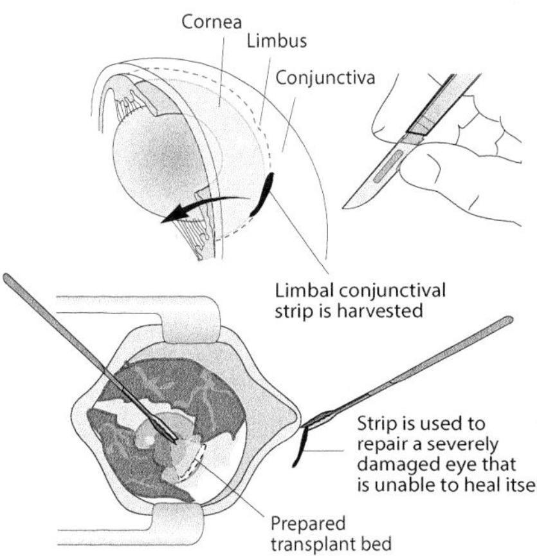
Cornea
Limbus
Conjunctiva
Limbal conjunctival strip is harvested
Strip is used to repair a severely damaged eye that is unable to heal itself
Prepared transplant bed

ICD-10-CM Diagnostic Codes

	Code	Description
⇄	H11.011	Amyloid pterygium of right eye
⇄	H11.021	Central pterygium of right eye
⇄	H11.031	Double pterygium of right eye
⇄	H11.041	Peripheral pterygium, stationary, right eye
⇄	H11.051	Peripheral pterygium, progressive, right eye
⇄	H11.061	Recurrent pterygium of right eye
⇄	H11.811	Pseudopterygium of conjunctiva, right eye
⇄	H16.011	Central corneal ulcer, right eye
⇄	H16.021	Ring corneal ulcer, right eye
⇄	H16.031	Corneal ulcer with hypopyon, right eye
⇄	H16.041	Marginal corneal ulcer, right eye
⇄	H16.051	Mooren's corneal ulcer, right eye
⇄	H16.061	Mycotic corneal ulcer, right eye
⇄	H16.071	Perforated corneal ulcer, right eye
⇄	H16.231	Neurotrophic keratoconjunctivitis, right eye
⇄	H17.821	Peripheral opacity of cornea, right eye
⇄	H18.41	Arcus senilis
⇄	H18.421	Band keratopathy, right eye
	H18.43	Other calcerous corneal degeneration
⇄	H18.441	Keratomalacia, right eye
⇄	H18.451	Nodular corneal degeneration, right eye
⇄	H18.461	Peripheral corneal degeneration, right eye
	H18.49	Other corneal degeneration
⇄	H18.511	Endothelial corneal dystrophy, right eye
⇄	H18.512	Endothelial corneal dystrophy, left eye
⇄	H18.513	Endothelial corneal dystrophy, bilateral
⇄	H18.521	Epithelial (juvenile) corneal dystrophy, right eye
⇄	H18.522	Epithelial (juvenile) corneal dystrophy, left eye
⇄	H18.523	Epithelial (juvenile) corneal dystrophy, bilateral
⇄	H18.531	Granular corneal dystrophy, right eye
⇄	H18.532	Granular corneal dystrophy, left eye
⇄	H18.533	Granular corneal dystrophy, bilateral
⇄	H18.541	Lattice corneal dystrophy, right eye
⇄	H18.542	Lattice corneal dystrophy, left eye
⇄	H18.543	Lattice corneal dystrophy, bilateral
⇄	H18.551	Macular corneal dystrophy, right eye
⇄	H18.552	Macular corneal dystrophy, left eye
⇄	H18.553	Macular corneal dystrophy, bilateral
⇄	H18.591	Other hereditary corneal dystrophies, right eye
⇄	H18.592	Other hereditary corneal dystrophies, left eye
⇄	H18.593	Other hereditary corneal dystrophies, bilateral
⇄	H18.821	Corneal disorder due to contact lens, right eye
⇄	H18.831	Recurrent erosion of cornea, right eye
	L51.1	Stevens-Johnson syndrome
	L51.3	Stevens-Johnson syndrome-toxic epidermal necrolysis overlap syndrome
❼⇄	T26.11	Burn of cornea and conjunctival sac, right eye
❼⇄	T26.31	Burns of other specified parts of right eye and adnexa
❼⇄	T26.61	Corrosion of cornea and conjunctival sac, right eye
❼⇄	T26.81	Corrosions of other specified parts of right eye and adnexa

ICD-10-CM Coding Notes

For codes requiring a 7th character extension, refer to your ICD-10-CM book. Review the character descriptions and coding guidelines for proper selection. For some procedures, only certain characters will apply.

CCI Edits

Refer to Appendix A for CCI edits.

Facility RVUs ▯

Code	Work	PE Facility	MP	Total Facility
65782	15.43	16.53	1.18	33.14

Non-facility RVUs ▯

Code	Work	PE Non-Facility	MP	Total Non-Facility
65782	15.43	16.53	1.18	33.14

Modifiers (PAR) ▯

Code	Mod 50	Mod 51	Mod 62	Mod 66	Mod 80
65782	1	2	1	0	1

Global Period

Code	Days
65782	090

65785

65785 Implantation of intrastromal corneal ring segments

AMA Coding Guideline

Other Procedures on the Cornea

Do not report 65760-65771 in conjunction with 92025.

AMA Coding Notes

Surgical Procedures on the Eye and Ocular Adnexa

(For diagnostic and treatment ophthalmological services, see Medicine, Ophthalmology, and 92002 et seq)

(Do not report code 69990 in addition to codes 65091-68850)

Plain English Description

Intrastromal corneal ring segments are micro-thin, flexible, crescent-shaped plastic inserts made of polymethylmethacrylate in a range of thicknesses that can be implanted into the periphery of the cornea to improve visual acuity. A small incision is made in the cornea and channels are created with a laser or special dissecting device. One or two corneal ring implant segments are then placed within each channel, selecting the appropriate thicknesses for the degree of correction needed. The implants flatten the curvature of the anterior cornea and physically alter its shape, which affects the refraction in the eye and improves vision. Intrastromal corneal ring segments are used to correct myopia and astigmatism, most often in patients who have undergone refractive laser surgery and have associated corneal ectasia or keratoconus.

Intrastromal corneal ring transplant

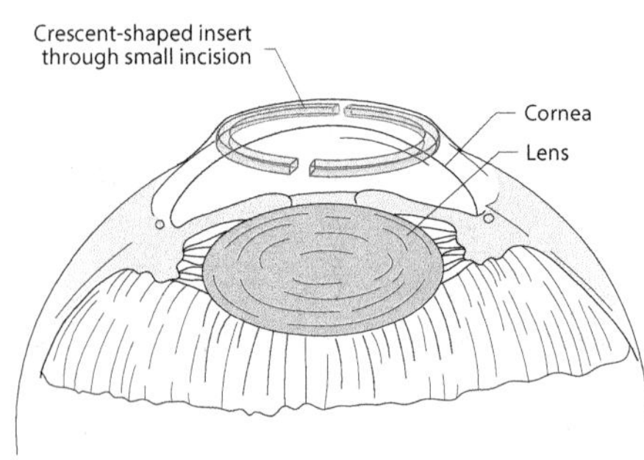

ICD-10-CM Diagnostic Codes

	Code	Description
⇄	H18.601	Keratoconus, unspecified, right eye
⇄	H18.611	Keratoconus, stable, right eye
⇄	H18.621	Keratoconus, unstable, right eye
⇄	H44.21	Degenerative myopia, right eye
⇄	H44.2A1	Degenerative myopia with choroidal neovascularization, right eye
⇄	H44.2A2	Degenerative myopia with choroidal neovascularization, left eye
⇄	H44.2A3	Degenerative myopia with choroidal neovascularization, bilateral eye
⇄	H44.2B1	Degenerative myopia with macular hole, right eye
⇄	H44.2B2	Degenerative myopia with macular hole, left eye
⇄	H44.2B3	Degenerative myopia with macular hole, bilateral eye
⇄	H44.2C1	Degenerative myopia with retinal detachment, right eye
⇄	H44.2C2	Degenerative myopia with retinal detachment, left eye
⇄	H44.2C3	Degenerative myopia with retinal detachment, bilateral eye
⇄	H44.2D1	Degenerative myopia with foveoschisis, right eye
⇄	H44.2D2	Degenerative myopia with foveoschisis, left eye
⇄	H44.2D3	Degenerative myopia with foveoschisis, bilateral eye
⇄	H44.2E1	Degenerative myopia with other maculopathy, right eye
⇄	H44.2E2	Degenerative myopia with other maculopathy, left eye
⇄	H44.2E3	Degenerative myopia with other maculopathy, bilateral eye
⇄	H52.11	Myopia, right eye
⇄	H52.211	Irregular astigmatism, right eye
⇄	H52.221	Regular astigmatism, right eye
	Q13.4	Other congenital corneal malformations

CCI Edits

Refer to Appendix A for CCI edits.

Facility RVUs ▢

Code	Work	PE Facility	MP	Total Facility
65785	5.39	7.01	0.41	12.81

Non-facility RVUs ▢

Code	Work	PE Non-Facility	MP	Total Non-Facility
65785	5.39	59.95	0.41	65.75

Modifiers (PAR) ▢

Code	Mod 50	Mod 51	Mod 62	Mod 66	Mod 80
65785	1	2	1	0	1

Global Period

Code	Days
65785	090

65800

65800 Paracentesis of anterior chamber of eye (separate procedure); with removal of aqueous

AMA Coding Notes

Surgical Procedures on the Eye and Ocular Adnexa

(For diagnostic and treatment ophthalmological services, see Medicine, Ophthalmology, and 92002 et seq)

(Do not report code 69990 in addition to codes 65091-68850)

AMA *CPT® Assistant* ◻

65800: Nov 12: 10

Plain English Description

Removal of aqueous from the anterior chamber of the eye may be performed as a diagnostic or therapeutic procedure. Diagnostic removal of aqueous is performed for a condition such as uveitis to diagnose infectious organisms. Therapeutic removal of aqueous may be performed to lower intraocular pressure. Eye drops are instilled to numb the eye. The patient is positioned at the slit lamp. A needle attached to a syringe or an aqueous pipette is inserted at the paralimbal aspect of the cornea above and parallel to the iris. If a needle and syringe is used, the plunger is pulled and aqueous is aspirated into the syringe. If an aqueous pipette is used, the suction-infusion bulb that was compressed at the time of insertion in order to create a vacuum is released and aqueous is aspirated.

Paracentesis of anterior chamber of eye diagnostic

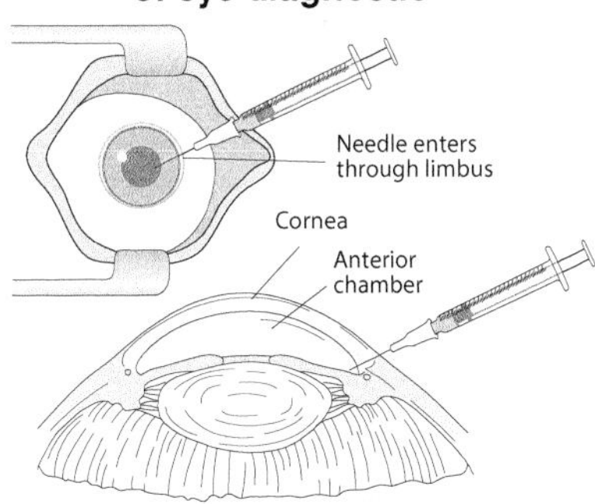

A needle is inserted into the anterior chamber for diagnostic (65800) purposes.

ICD-10-CM Diagnostic Codes

⇄	H20.042	Secondary noninfectious iridocyclitis, left eye
⇄	H20.052	Hypopyon, left eye
⇄	H25.11	Age-related nuclear cataract, right eye
➐⇄	H35.321	Exudative age-related macular degeneration, right eye
➐⇄	H35.322	Exudative age-related macular degeneration, left eye
➐⇄	H35.323	Exudative age-related macular degeneration, bilateral
⇄	H35.352	Cystoid macular degeneration, left eye
	H35.81	Retinal edema
⇄	H40.061	Primary angle closure without glaucoma damage, right eye
⇄	H40.062	Primary angle closure without glaucoma damage, left eye
⇄	H40.063	Primary angle closure without glaucoma damage, bilateral
⇄	H40.211	Acute angle-closure glaucoma, right eye
⇄	H40.212	Acute angle-closure glaucoma, left eye
⇄	H40.213	Acute angle-closure glaucoma, bilateral
➐⇄	H40.31	Glaucoma secondary to eye trauma, right eye
➐⇄	H40.41	Glaucoma secondary to eye inflammation, right eye
➐⇄	H40.51	Glaucoma secondary to other eye disorders, right eye
⇄	H40.831	Aqueous misdirection, right eye

ICD-10-CM Coding Notes

For codes requiring a 7th character extension, refer to your ICD-10-CM book. Review the character descriptions and coding guidelines for proper selection. For some procedures, only certain characters will apply.

CCI Edits

Refer to Appendix A for CCI edits.

Facility RVUs ◻

Code	Work	PE Facility	MP	Total Facility
65800	1.53	0.94	0.11	2.58

Non-facility RVUs ◻

Code	Work	PE Non-Facility	MP	Total Non-Facility
65800	1.53	1.83	0.11	3.47

Modifiers (PAR) ◻

Code	Mod 50	Mod 51	Mod 62	Mod 66	Mod 80
65800	1	2	0	0	1

Global Period

Code	Days
65800	000

65810

65810 Paracentesis of anterior chamber of eye (separate procedure); with removal of vitreous and/or discission of anterior hyaloid membrane, with or without air injection

AMA Coding Notes

Surgical Procedures on the Eye and Ocular Adnexa

(For diagnostic and treatment ophthalmological services, see Medicine, Ophthalmology, and 92002 et seq)

(Do not report code 69990 in addition to codes 65091-68850)

AMA *CPT® Assistant* ▯

65810: Nov 12: 10

Plain English Description

The physician repairs a condition in which the aqueous fluid in the front chamber of the eye pushes forward between the cornea and the lens. The physician may remove some of the fluid and/or remove part of the membrane that separates the fluid from the rest of the eye. The physician may also inject air into the eye to equalize the pressure in the eye.

Paracentesis of anterior chamber of eye with removal of vitreous/discission of hyaloid membrane, with/without air injection

A laser may be used to destroy hyaloid membrane.

ICD-10-CM Diagnostic Codes

E08.311 Diabetes mellitus due to underlying condition with unspecified diabetic retinopathy with macular edema

E08.319 Diabetes mellitus due to underlying condition with unspecified diabetic retinopathy without macular edema

⑦⇄ E08.321 Diabetes mellitus due to underlying condition with mild nonproliferative diabetic retinopathy with macular edema

⑦⇄ E08.329 Diabetes mellitus due to underlying condition with mild nonproliferative diabetic retinopathy without macular edema

⑦⇄ E08.331 Diabetes mellitus due to underlying condition with moderate nonproliferative diabetic retinopathy with macular edema

⑦⇄ E08.339 Diabetes mellitus due to underlying condition with moderate nonproliferative diabetic retinopathy without macular edema

⑦⇄ E08.341 Diabetes mellitus due to underlying condition with severe nonproliferative diabetic retinopathy with macular edema

⑦⇄ E08.349 Diabetes mellitus due to underlying condition with severe nonproliferative diabetic retinopathy without macular edema

⑦⇄ E08.351 Diabetes mellitus due to underlying condition with proliferative diabetic retinopathy with macular edema

⑦⇄ E08.352 Diabetes mellitus due to underlying condition with proliferative diabetic retinopathy with traction retinal detachment involving the macula

⑦⇄ E08.353 Diabetes mellitus due to underlying condition with proliferative diabetic retinopathy with traction retinal detachment not involving the macula

⑦⇄ E08.354 Diabetes mellitus due to underlying condition with proliferative diabetic retinopathy with combined traction retinal detachment and rhegmatogenous retinal detachment

⑦⇄ E08.355 Diabetes mellitus due to underlying condition with stable proliferative diabetic retinopathy

⑦⇄ E08.359 Diabetes mellitus due to underlying condition with proliferative diabetic retinopathy without macular edema

E08.36 Diabetes mellitus due to underlying condition with diabetic cataract

⑦⇄ E08.37 Diabetes mellitus due to underlying condition with diabetic macular edema, resolved following treatment

E08.39 Diabetes mellitus due to underlying condition with other diabetic ophthalmic complication

E09.311 Drug or chemical induced diabetes mellitus with unspecified diabetic retinopathy with macular edema

E09.319 Drug or chemical induced diabetes mellitus with unspecified diabetic retinopathy without macular edema

⑦⇄ E09.321 Drug or chemical induced diabetes mellitus with mild nonproliferative diabetic retinopathy with macular edema

⑦⇄ E09.329 Drug or chemical induced diabetes mellitus with mild nonproliferative diabetic retinopathy without macular edema

⑦⇄ E09.331 Drug or chemical induced diabetes mellitus with moderate nonproliferative diabetic retinopathy with macular edema

⑦⇄ E09.339 Drug or chemical induced diabetes mellitus with moderate nonproliferative diabetic retinopathy without macular edema

⑦⇄ E09.341 Drug or chemical induced diabetes mellitus with severe nonproliferative diabetic retinopathy with macular edema

⑦⇄ E09.349 Drug or chemical induced diabetes mellitus with severe nonproliferative diabetic retinopathy without macular edema

⑦⇄ E09.351 Drug or chemical induced diabetes mellitus with proliferative diabetic retinopathy with macular edema

⑦⇄ E09.352 Drug or chemical induced diabetes mellitus with proliferative diabetic retinopathy with traction retinal detachment involving the macula

⑦⇄ E09.354 Drug or chemical induced diabetes mellitus with proliferative diabetic retinopathy with combined traction retinal detachment and rhegmatogenous retinal detachment

⑦⇄ E09.355 Drug or chemical induced diabetes mellitus with stable proliferative diabetic retinopathy

⑦⇄ E09.359 Drug or chemical induced diabetes mellitus with proliferative diabetic retinopathy without macular edema

E09.36 Drug or chemical induced diabetes mellitus with diabetic cataract

⑦⇄ E09.37 Drug or chemical induced diabetes mellitus with diabetic macular edema, resolved following treatment

E09.39 Drug or chemical induced diabetes mellitus with other diabetic ophthalmic complication

E09.65 Drug or chemical induced diabetes mellitus with hyperglycemia

E10.31 Type 1 diabetes mellitus with unspecified diabetic retinopathy

E10.311 Type 1 diabetes mellitus with unspecified diabetic retinopathy with macular edema

E10.319 Type 1 diabetes mellitus with unspecified diabetic retinopathy without macular edema

⑦⇄ E10.321 Type 1 diabetes mellitus with mild nonproliferative diabetic retinopathy with macular edema

⑦⇄ E10.329 Type 1 diabetes mellitus with mild nonproliferative diabetic retinopathy without macular edema

⑦⇄ E10.331 Type 1 diabetes mellitus with moderate nonproliferative diabetic retinopathy with macular edema

⑦⇄ E10.339 Type 1 diabetes mellitus with moderate nonproliferative diabetic retinopathy without macular edema

⑦⇄ E10.341 Type 1 diabetes mellitus with severe nonproliferative diabetic retinopathy with macular edema

⑦⇄ E10.349 Type 1 diabetes mellitus with severe nonproliferative diabetic retinopathy without macular edema

➐⇄	E10.351	Type 1 diabetes mellitus with proliferative diabetic retinopathy with macular edema
➐⇄	E10.352	Type 1 diabetes mellitus with proliferative diabetic retinopathy with traction retinal detachment involving the macula
➐⇄	E10.353	Type 1 diabetes mellitus with proliferative diabetic retinopathy with traction retinal detachment not involving the macula
➐⇄	E10.354	Type 1 diabetes mellitus with proliferative diabetic retinopathy with combined traction retinal detachment and rhegmatogenous retinal detachment
➐⇄	E10.355	Type 1 diabetes mellitus with stable proliferative diabetic retinopathy
➐⇄	E10.359	Type 1 diabetes mellitus with proliferative diabetic retinopathy without macular edema
	E10.36	Type 1 diabetes mellitus with diabetic cataract
➐⇄	E10.37	Type 1 diabetes mellitus with diabetic macular edema, resolved following treatment
	E10.39	Type 1 diabetes mellitus with other diabetic ophthalmic complication
	E11.311	Type 2 diabetes mellitus with unspecified diabetic retinopathy with macular edema
	E11.319	Type 2 diabetes mellitus with unspecified diabetic retinopathy without macular edema
➐⇄	E11.321	Type 2 diabetes mellitus with mild nonproliferative diabetic retinopathy with macular edema
➐⇄	E11.329	Type 2 diabetes mellitus with mild nonproliferative diabetic retinopathy without macular edema
➐⇄	E11.331	Type 2 diabetes mellitus with moderate nonproliferative diabetic retinopathy with macular edema
➐⇄	E11.339	Type 2 diabetes mellitus with moderate nonproliferative diabetic retinopathy without macular edema
➐⇄	E11.341	Type 2 diabetes mellitus with severe nonproliferative diabetic retinopathy with macular edema
➐⇄	E11.349	Type 2 diabetes mellitus with severe nonproliferative diabetic retinopathy without macular edema
➐⇄	E11.351	Type 2 diabetes mellitus with proliferative diabetic retinopathy with macular edema
➐⇄	E11.352	Type 2 diabetes mellitus with proliferative diabetic retinopathy with traction retinal detachment involving the macula
➐⇄	E11.353	Type 2 diabetes mellitus with proliferative diabetic retinopathy with traction retinal detachment not involving the macula
➐⇄	E11.354	Type 2 diabetes mellitus with proliferative diabetic retinopathy with combined traction retinal detachment and rhegmatogenous retinal detachment
➐⇄	E11.355	Type 2 diabetes mellitus with stable proliferative diabetic retinopathy
➐⇄	E11.359	Type 2 diabetes mellitus with proliferative diabetic retinopathy without macular edema
	E11.36	Type 2 diabetes mellitus with diabetic cataract
➐⇄	E11.37	Type 2 diabetes mellitus with diabetic macular edema, resolved following treatment
	E11.39	Type 2 diabetes mellitus with other diabetic ophthalmic complication
	E13.311	Other specified diabetes mellitus with unspecified diabetic retinopathy with macular edema
	E13.319	Other specified diabetes mellitus with unspecified diabetic retinopathy without macular edema
➐⇄	E13.351	Other specified diabetes mellitus with proliferative diabetic retinopathy with macular edema
➐⇄	E13.359	Other specified diabetes mellitus with proliferative diabetic retinopathy without macular edema
⇄	H43.0	Vitreous prolapse
⇄	H43.1	Vitreous hemorrhage
⇄	H43.81	Vitreous degeneration
	H43.89	Other disorders of vitreous body
⇄	H44.001	Unspecified purulent endophthalmitis, right eye
⇄	H44.011	Panophthalmitis (acute), right eye
⇄	H44.021	Vitreous abscess (chronic), right eye

ICD-10-CM Coding Notes

For codes requiring a 7th character extension, refer to your ICD-10-CM book. Review the character descriptions and coding guidelines for proper selection. For some procedures, only certain characters will apply.

CCI Edits

Refer to Appendix A for CCI edits.

Facility RVUs ▯

Code	Work	PE Facility	MP	Total Facility
65810	5.82	7.17	0.43	13.42

Non-facility RVUs ▯

Code	Work	PE Non-Facility	MP	Total Non-Facility
65810	5.82	7.17	0.43	13.42

Modifiers (PAR) ▯

Code	Mod 50	Mod 51	Mod 62	Mod 66	Mod 80
65810	1	2	0	0	1

Global Period

Code	Days
65810	090

65815

65815 Paracentesis of anterior chamber of eye (separate procedure); with removal of blood, with or without irrigation and/or air injection

(For injection, see 66020-66030)

(For removal of blood clot, use 65930)

AMA Coding Notes

Surgical Procedures on the Eye and Ocular Adnexa

(For diagnostic and treatment ophthalmological services, see Medicine, Ophthalmology, and 92002 et seq)

(Do not report code 69990 in addition to codes 65091-68850)

AMA *CPT® Assistant*

65815: Nov 12: 10

Plain English Description

This procedure is performed to treat hyphema, which is a collection of blood in the anterior chamber of the eye, usually resulting from trauma. Eye drops are instilled to numb the eye. Two paracentesis sites are created using a knife blade. A needle or cannula is inserted into one of the sites and loose blood is irrigated from the eye with balanced saline solution. Intraocular pressure is monitored during the procedure. If a blood clot is present and the removal of loose blood does not reduce the intraocular pressure, the paracentesis site may be enlarged slightly and the blood clot removed using irrigation and aspiration. Following the irrigation aspiration procedure, air may be injected into the eye to stabilize eye pressure.

Paracentesis of anterior chamber of eye with removal of blood, with/without air injection/irrigation

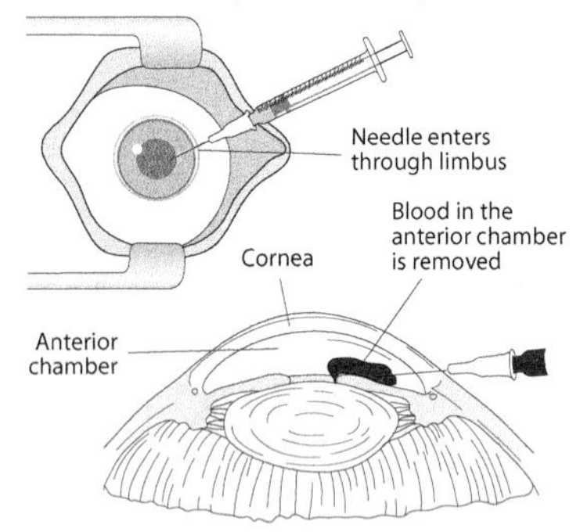
Needle enters through limbus
Blood in the anterior chamber is removed
Cornea
Anterior chamber

The physician may irrigate with saline to remove blood, then air may be injected to restore normal pressure.

ICD-10-CM Diagnostic Codes

	Code	Description
⇄	H21.0	Hyphema
❼⇄	S01.112	Laceration without foreign body of left eyelid and periocular area
❼⇄	S01.122	Laceration with foreign body of left eyelid and periocular area
❼⇄	S01.132	Puncture wound without foreign body of left eyelid and periocular area
❼⇄	S01.142	Puncture wound with foreign body of left eyelid and periocular area
❼⇄	S01.152	Open bite of left eyelid and periocular area
❼⇄	S05.12	Contusion of eyeball and orbital tissues, left eye
❼⇄	S05.22	Ocular laceration and rupture with prolapse or loss of intraocular tissue, left eye
❼⇄	S05.52	Penetrating wound with foreign body of left eyeball
❼⇄	S05.62	Penetrating wound without foreign body of left eyeball
❼⇄	S05.8X1	Other injuries of right eye and orbit
❼⇄	S05.8X2	Other injuries of left eye and orbit
❼	T81.32	Disruption of internal operation (surgical) wound, not elsewhere classified

ICD-10-CM Coding Notes

For codes requiring a 7th character extension, refer to your ICD-10-CM book. Review the character descriptions and coding guidelines for proper selection. For some procedures, only certain characters will apply.

CCI Edits

Refer to Appendix A for CCI edits.

Facility RVUs

Code	Work	PE Facility	MP	Total Facility
65815	6.00	7.33	0.44	13.77

Non-facility RVUs

Code	Work	PE Non-Facility	MP	Total Non-Facility
65815	6.00	12.49	0.44	18.93

Modifiers (PAR)

Code	Mod 50	Mod 51	Mod 62	Mod 66	Mod 80
65815	1	2	0	0	1

Global Period

Code	Days
65815	090

65820

65820 Goniotomy

(Do not report modifier 63 in conjunction with 65820)

(For use of ophthalmic endoscope with 65820, use 66990)

AMA Coding Notes

Surgical Procedures on the Eye and Ocular Adnexa

(For diagnostic and treatment ophthalmological services, see Medicine, Ophthalmology, and 92002 et seq)

(Do not report code 69990 in addition to codes 65091-68850)

AMA *CPT® Assistant* ▢

65820: Sep 05: 12, Jul 18: 3, Dec 18: 9, Sep 19: 11

Plain English Description

The physician performs a goniotomy, used to treat congenital glaucoma in children. Congenital glaucoma can cause developmental arrest of the iris and ciliary body, which may then lead to obstruction of the trabecular network, preventing drainage of aqueous fluid from the eye and causing increased intraocular pressure. Mitotic eye drops are administered to constrict the pupil. The eye is then stabilized using forceps or sutures. The cornea is punctured and a viscoelastic tube is placed in the anterior chamber through which fluid is introduced. A gonioscopy lens is placed on the eye and the anterior trabecular meshwork is incised using a needle or knife blade. The tubing is then removed; sterile saline is injected; and the corneal puncture site to the anterior chamber is closed.

Goniotomy

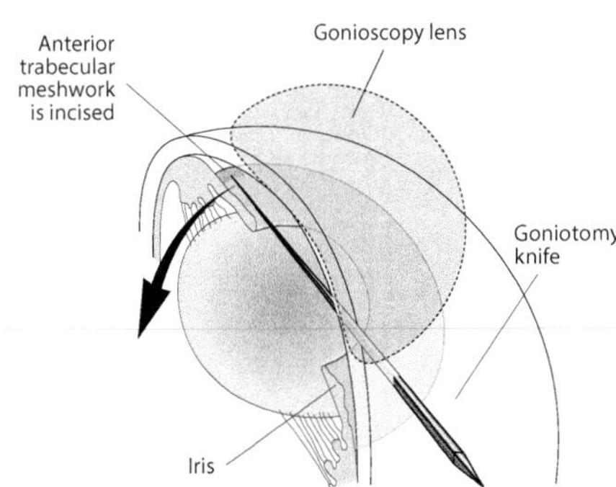

ICD-10-CM Diagnostic Codes

❼⇄	H40.111	Primary open-angle glaucoma, right eye
❼⇄	H40.112	Primary open-angle glaucoma, left eye
❼⇄	H40.113	Primary open-angle glaucoma, bilateral
❼⇄	H40.121	Low-tension glaucoma, right eye
❼⇄	H40.131	Pigmentary glaucoma, right eye
⇄	H40.151	Residual stage of open-angle glaucoma, right eye
⇄	H40.831	Aqueous misdirection, right eye
	H40.89	Other specified glaucoma
	H42	Glaucoma in diseases classified elsewhere
	Q13.4	Other congenital corneal malformations
	Q13.81	Rieger's anomaly
	Q13.9	Congenital malformation of anterior segment of eye, unspecified
	Q15.0	Congenital glaucoma
	Q85.00	Neurofibromatosis, unspecified
	Q85.01	Neurofibromatosis, type 1
	Q85.8	Other phakomatoses, not elsewhere classified
	Q85.9	Phakomatosis, unspecified

ICD-10-CM Coding Notes

For codes requiring a 7th character extension, refer to your ICD-10-CM book. Review the character descriptions and coding guidelines for proper selection. For some procedures, only certain characters will apply.

CCI Edits

Refer to Appendix A for CCI edits.

Facility RVUs ▢

Code	Work	PE Facility	MP	Total Facility
65820	8.91	14.63	0.68	24.22

Non-facility RVUs ▢

Code	Work	PE Non-Facility	MP	Total Non-Facility
65820	8.91	14.63	0.68	24.22

Modifiers (PAR) ▢

Code	Mod 50	Mod 51	Mod 62	Mod 66	Mod 80
65820	1	2	0	0	0

Global Period

Code	Days
65820	090

65850

65850 Trabeculotomy ab externo

AMA Coding Notes

Surgical Procedures on the Eye and Ocular Adnexa

(For diagnostic and treatment ophthalmological services, see Medicine, Ophthalmology, and 92002 et seq)

(Do not report code 69990 in addition to codes 65091-68850)

Plain English Description

This procedure is performed to treat congenital and open angle glaucoma. An ab externo approach involves opening the trabecular meshwork in front of Schlemm's canal. Mitotic eye drops are administered to constrict the pupil. A slit lamp and gonioscopy lens are used to guide the trabeculotome as it is introduced into Schlemm's canal. The trabeculotome is rotated as it is advanced into the anterior chamber and an opening is created in the trabecular meshwork to release intraocular pressure. The trabeculotome is removed.

Trabeculotomy ab externo

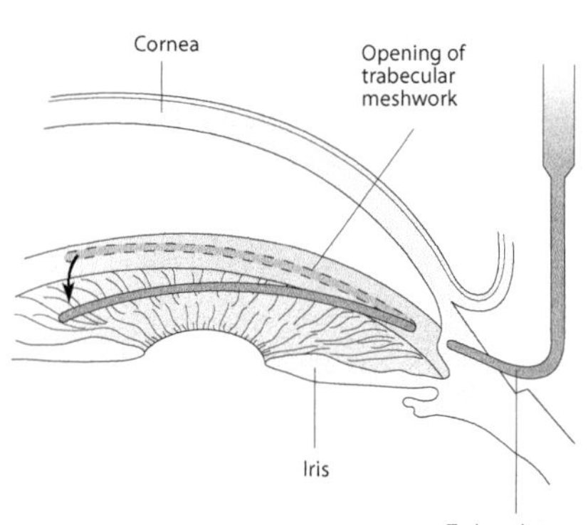

ICD-10-CM Diagnostic Codes

	Code	Description
⇄	H15.832	Staphyloma posticum, left eye
⇄	H15.842	Scleral ectasia, left eye
⇄	H15.852	Ring staphyloma, left eye
⇄	H25.12	Age-related nuclear cataract, left eye
⇄	H25.812	Combined forms of age-related cataract, left eye
⇄	H40.032	Anatomical narrow angle, left eye
❼	H40.10	Unspecified open-angle glaucoma
❼⇄	H40.111	Primary open-angle glaucoma, right eye
❼⇄	H40.112	Primary open-angle glaucoma, left eye
❼⇄	H40.113	Primary open-angle glaucoma, bilateral
❼⇄	H40.122	Low-tension glaucoma, left eye
❼⇄	H40.123	Low-tension glaucoma, bilateral
❼⇄	H40.142	Capsular glaucoma with pseudoexfoliation of lens, left eye
❼⇄	H40.222	Chronic angle-closure glaucoma, left eye
❼⇄	H40.32	Glaucoma secondary to eye trauma, left eye
❼⇄	H40.42	Glaucoma secondary to eye inflammation, left eye
❼⇄	H40.52	Glaucoma secondary to other eye disorders, left eye
❼⇄	H40.62	Glaucoma secondary to drugs, left eye
⇄	H40.832	Aqueous misdirection, left eye
	H40.89	Other specified glaucoma
⇄	H43.392	Other vitreous opacities, left eye
	Q13.4	Other congenital corneal malformations
	Q13.81	Rieger's anomaly
	Q15.0	Congenital glaucoma
	Q85.00	Neurofibromatosis, unspecified
	Q85.01	Neurofibromatosis, type 1
	Q85.8	Other phakomatoses, not elsewhere classified
	Q85.9	Phakomatosis, unspecified

ICD-10-CM Coding Notes

For codes requiring a 7th character extension, refer to your ICD-10-CM book. Review the character descriptions and coding guidelines for proper selection. For some procedures, only certain characters will apply.

CCI Edits

Refer to Appendix A for CCI edits.

Facility RVUs ▯

Code	Work	PE Facility	MP	Total Facility
65850	11.39	12.22	0.89	24.50

Non-facility RVUs ▯

Code	Work	PE Non-Facility	MP	Total Non-Facility
65850	11.39	12.22	0.89	24.50

Modifiers (PAR) ▯

Code	Mod 50	Mod 51	Mod 62	Mod 66	Mod 80
65850	1	2	1	0	1

Global Period

Code	Days
65850	090

65855

65855 Trabeculoplasty by laser surgery

(Do not report 65855 in conjunction with 65860, 65865, 65870, 65875, 65880)

(For trabeculectomy, use 66170)

AMA Coding Notes

Surgical Procedures on the Eye and Ocular Adnexa

(For diagnostic and treatment ophthalmological services, see Medicine, Ophthalmology, and 92002 et seq)

(Do not report code 69990 in addition to codes 65091-68850)

AMA *CPT® Assistant*

65855: Mar 98: 7, Mar 03: 23

Plain English Description

The procedure may also be referred to as argon laser trabeculoplasty (ALT) or selective laser trabeculoplasty (SLT). This procedure is performed for primary open angle glaucoma, pseudoexfoliation syndrome, and pigmentary dispersion syndrome. Eye drops are administered to constrict the pupil, decrease the amount of fluid in the eyes, and prevent elevation of eye pressure. A slit lamp and gonioscopy lens are used to guide the laser beam into the trabecular meshwork. The laser is activated and small burns are made in the trabecular meshwork. The treatment typically involves creating 40 to 80 burns over 180 degrees of trabecular meshwork.

Trabeculoplasty by laser surgery

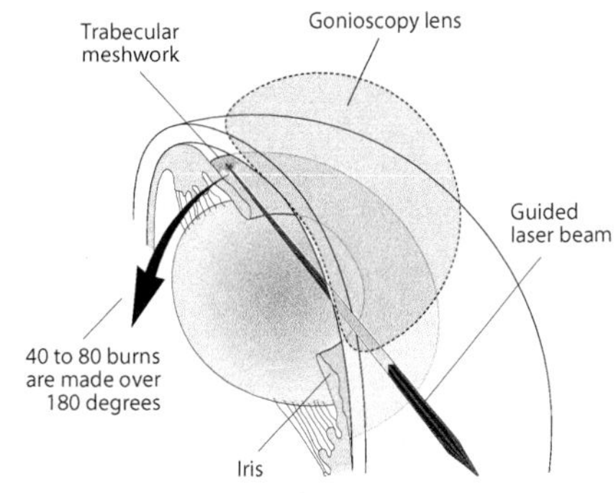

ICD-10-CM Diagnostic Codes

⇄ H18.041 Kayser-Fleischer ring, right eye
⇄ H21.231 Degeneration of iris (pigmentary), right eye
⇄ H25.11 Age-related nuclear cataract, right eye
H25.89 Other age-related cataract
⇄ H40.001 Preglaucoma, unspecified, right eye
⇄ H40.011 Open angle with borderline findings, low risk, right eye
⇄ H40.031 Anatomical narrow angle, right eye
⇄ H40.051 Ocular hypertension, right eye
❼ H40.10 Unspecified open-angle glaucoma
❼⇄ H40.111 Primary open-angle glaucoma, right eye
❼⇄ H40.112 Primary open-angle glaucoma, left eye
❼⇄ H40.113 Primary open-angle glaucoma, bilateral
❼⇄ H40.121 Low-tension glaucoma, right eye
❼⇄ H40.131 Pigmentary glaucoma, right eye
❼⇄ H40.141 Capsular glaucoma with pseudoexfoliation of lens, right eye
⇄ H40.152 Residual stage of open-angle glaucoma, left eye
❼⇄ H40.221 Chronic angle-closure glaucoma, right eye
❼⇄ H40.31 Glaucoma secondary to eye trauma, right eye
❼⇄ H40.41 Glaucoma secondary to eye inflammation, right eye
❼⇄ H40.51 Glaucoma secondary to other eye disorders, right eye
❼⇄ H40.61 Glaucoma secondary to drugs, right eye
⇄ H40.831 Aqueous misdirection, right eye

ICD-10-CM Coding Notes

For codes requiring a 7th character extension, refer to your ICD-10-CM book. Review the character descriptions and coding guidelines for proper selection. For some procedures, only certain characters will apply.

CCI Edits

Refer to Appendix A for CCI edits.

Pub 100

65855: Pub 100-03, 1, 140.5

Facility RVUs

Code	Work	PE Facility	MP	Total Facility
65855	3.00	2.71	0.23	5.94

Non-facility RVUs

Code	Work	PE Non-Facility	MP	Total Non-Facility
65855	3.00	3.95	0.23	7.18

Modifiers (PAR)

Code	Mod 50	Mod 51	Mod 62	Mod 66	Mod 80
65855	1	2	1	1	1

Global Period

Code	Days
65855	010

65860

65860 Severing adhesions of anterior segment, laser technique (separate procedure)

AMA Coding Notes

Surgical Procedures on the Eye and Ocular Adnexa

(For diagnostic and treatment ophthalmological services, see Medicine, Ophthalmology, and 92002 et seq)

(Do not report code 69990 in addition to codes 65091-68850)

Plain English Description

Adhesions in the anterior segment are severed using laser technique. Eye drops are administered to numb the eye. A slit lamp and gonioscopy lens are used to guide the laser beam. The laser is activated and scar tissue in the anterior segment is severed.

Severing adhesions of anterior segment, laser technique

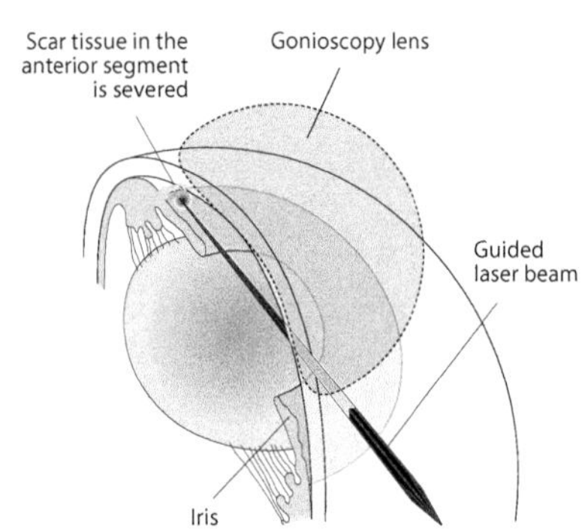

ICD-10-CM Diagnostic Codes

⇄	H16.012	Central corneal ulcer, left eye
⇄	H16.022	Ring corneal ulcer, left eye
⇄	H16.032	Corneal ulcer with hypopyon, left eye
⇄	H16.042	Marginal corneal ulcer, left eye
⇄	H16.052	Mooren's corneal ulcer, left eye
⇄	H16.062	Mycotic corneal ulcer, left eye
⇄	H16.072	Perforated corneal ulcer, left eye
⇄	H17.02	Adherent leukoma, left eye
⇄	H17.12	Central corneal opacity, left eye
⇄	H20.012	Primary iridocyclitis, left eye
⇄	H20.022	Recurrent acute iridocyclitis, left eye
⇄	H20.12	Chronic iridocyclitis, left eye
⇄	H26.492	Other secondary cataract, left eye
⇄	H35.352	Cystoid macular degeneration, left eye
❼⇄	H40.111	Primary open-angle glaucoma, right eye
❼⇄	H40.112	Primary open-angle glaucoma, left eye
❼⇄	H40.113	Primary open-angle glaucoma, bilateral
❼⇄	H40.122	Low-tension glaucoma, left eye
❼⇄	H40.132	Pigmentary glaucoma, left eye
❼⇄	H40.142	Capsular glaucoma with pseudoexfoliation of lens, left eye
❼⇄	H40.222	Chronic angle-closure glaucoma, left eye
❼⇄	H40.32	Glaucoma secondary to eye trauma, left eye
❼⇄	H40.42	Glaucoma secondary to eye inflammation, left eye
❼⇄	H40.52	Glaucoma secondary to other eye disorders, left eye
❼⇄	H40.62	Glaucoma secondary to drugs, left eye
⇄	H43.392	Other vitreous opacities, left eye
⇄	H44.412	Flat anterior chamber hypotony of left eye

ICD-10-CM Coding Notes

For codes requiring a 7th character extension, refer to your ICD-10-CM book. Review the character descriptions and coding guidelines for proper selection. For some procedures, only certain characters will apply.

CCI Edits

Refer to Appendix A for CCI edits.

Pub 100

65860: Pub 100-03, 1, 140.5

Facility RVUs ▯

Code	Work	PE Facility	MP	Total Facility
65860	3.59	3.31	0.27	7.17

Non-facility RVUs ▯

Code	Work	PE Non-Facility	MP	Total Non-Facility
65860	3.59	5.11	0.27	8.97

Modifiers (PAR) ▯

Code	Mod 50	Mod 51	Mod 62	Mod 66	Mod 80
65860	1	2	0	0	0

Global Period

Code	Days
65860	090

65865-65880

65865 Severing adhesions of anterior segment of eye, incisional technique (with or without injection of air or liquid) (separate procedure); goniosynechiae

(For trabeculoplasty by laser surgery, use 65855)

65870 Severing adhesions of anterior segment of eye, incisional technique (with or without injection of air or liquid) (separate procedure); anterior synechiae, except goniosynechiae

65875 Severing adhesions of anterior segment of eye, incisional technique (with or without injection of air or liquid) (separate procedure); posterior synechiae

(For use of ophthalmic endoscope with 65875, use 66990)

65880 Severing adhesions of anterior segment of eye, incisional technique (with or without injection of air or liquid) (separate procedure); corneovitreal adhesions

(For laser surgery, use 66821)

AMA Coding Notes

Surgical Procedures on the Eye and Ocular Adnexa

(For diagnostic and treatment ophthalmological services, see Medicine, Ophthalmology, and 92002 et seq)

(Do not report code 69990 in addition to codes 65091-68850)

AMA *CPT® Assistant* ▢

65875: Sep 05: 12

Plain English Description

Adhesions in the anterior segment are severed using an incisional technique with or without injection of air or liquid. In 65865, goniosynechiae are incised. Goniosynechiae are adhesions of the iris to the posterior surface of the cornea in the iridocorneal angle of the anterior chamber. Goniosynechiae are associated with angle closure glaucoma. An incision is made in the cornea and a needle or knife blade used to severe the adhesive tissue connecting the iris to the posterior surface of the cornea. Air or fluid may be injected to stabilize pressure in the eye if aqueous fluid is lost during the procedure. In 65870, adhesions between the iris and anterior segment structures other than the cornea are severed using a needle or knife blade. In 65875, posterior synechiae are severed using a needle or knife blade. Posterior synechiae are adhesions between the iris and lens capsule. In 65880, corneovitreal adhesions are severed using a needle or knife blade. Corneovitreal adhesions are adhesions between the cornea and vitreous matter filling the anterior segment.

Severing adhesions of anterior segment, incisional technique

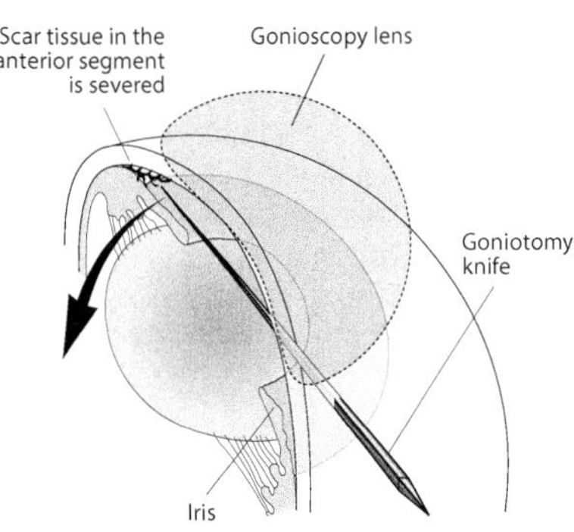

Gonio (65865); anterior (65870); posterior (65875); synechiae; corneovitreal (65880) adhesions

ICD-10-CM Diagnostic Codes

	Code	Description
⇄	H17.01	Adherent leukoma, right eye
⇄	H17.11	Central corneal opacity, right eye
	H17.89	Other corneal scars and opacities
⇄	H20.011	Primary iridocyclitis, right eye
⇄	H20.021	Recurrent acute iridocyclitis, right eye
⇄	H20.11	Chronic iridocyclitis, right eye
⇄	H21.511	Anterior synechiae (iris), right eye
⇄	H21.521	Goniosynechiae, right eye
⇄	H21.541	Posterior synechiae (iris), right eye
❼⇄	H40.111	Primary open-angle glaucoma, right eye
❼⇄	H40.112	Primary open-angle glaucoma, left eye
❼⇄	H40.113	Primary open-angle glaucoma, bilateral
❼⇄	H40.121	Low-tension glaucoma, right eye
❼⇄	H40.131	Pigmentary glaucoma, right eye
❼⇄	H40.141	Capsular glaucoma with pseudoexfoliation of lens, right eye
❼⇄	H40.221	Chronic angle-closure glaucoma, right eye
❼⇄	H40.31	Glaucoma secondary to eye trauma, right eye
❼⇄	H40.41	Glaucoma secondary to eye inflammation, right eye
❼⇄	H40.51	Glaucoma secondary to other eye disorders, right eye
❼⇄	H40.61	Glaucoma secondary to drugs, right eye
⇄	H44.411	Flat anterior chamber hypotony of right eye

ICD-10-CM Coding Notes

For codes requiring a 7th character extension, refer to your ICD-10-CM book. Review the character descriptions and coding guidelines for proper selection. For some procedures, only certain characters will apply.

CCI Edits

Refer to Appendix A for CCI edits.

Facility RVUs ▢

Code	Work	PE Facility	MP	Total Facility
65865	5.77	7.69	0.43	13.89
65870	7.39	9.32	0.57	17.28
65875	7.81	10.01	0.60	18.42
65880	8.36	10.35	0.65	19.36

Non-facility RVUs ▢

Code	Work	PE Non-Facility	MP	Total Non-Facility
65865	5.77	7.69	0.43	13.89
65870	7.39	9.32	0.57	17.28
65875	7.81	10.01	0.60	18.42
65880	8.36	10.35	0.65	19.36

Modifiers (PAR) ▢

Code	Mod 50	Mod 51	Mod 62	Mod 66	Mod 80
65865	1	2	1	0	1
65870	1	2	1	0	1
65875	1	2	1	0	1
65880	1	2	0	0	1

Global Period

Code	Days
65865	090
65870	090
65875	090
65880	090

65900

65900 Removal of epithelial downgrowth, anterior chamber of eye

AMA Coding Notes

Surgical Procedures on the Eye and Ocular Adnexa

(For diagnostic and treatment ophthalmological services, see Medicine, Ophthalmology, and 92002 et seq)

(Do not report code 69990 in addition to codes 65091-68850)

Plain English Description

Epithelial downgrowths (ingrowths) are a complication of surgical or nonsurgical trauma to the eye. The corneal or conjunctival epithelium gains access to the anterior (inner) chamber of the eye and grows on the back of the cornea, trabecular meshwork and/or anterior surface of the iris. The condition may also present as a fluid-filled cystic lesion or as free-floating epithelial cells. Symptoms can include pain, increased intraocular pressure (glaucoma) and inflammation. The eye is anesthetized using a topical ophthalmic anesthetic. Using an operative microscope or slit lamp the flap edge from the previous incision or traumatic wound is located and opened using a Sinskey hook or similar instrument. If the area of downgrowth is extensive a cyclodialysis spatula may be used to further elevate the flap. The stromal bed is scraped with a blade or knife and the flap replaced. Alternatively, epithelial tissue can be removed surgically using direct electrocautery or photocoagulation. If the downgrowth presents as a cystic lesion, cyst aspiration with cauterization, diathermy or injection of sclerosing agents or alcohol may be performed. Following removal of the downgrowths, the eye is irrigated, a corneal contact lens bandage may be placed followed by the instillation of antibiotic and/or steroid eye drops. The eye is then patched.

Removal of epithelial downgrowth, anterior chamber of eye

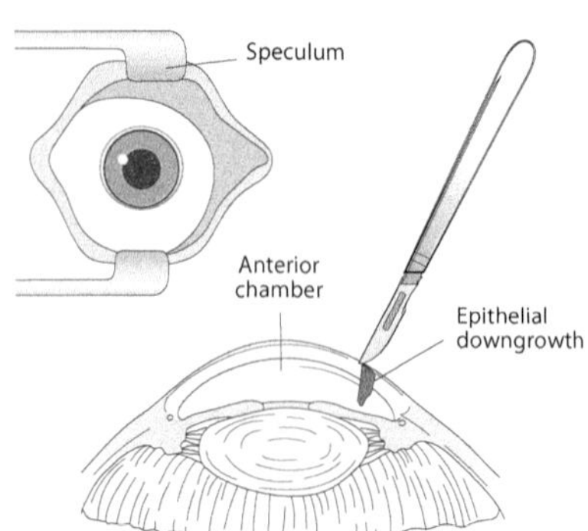

An improperly healing surgical wound to the cornea that has grown down into the anterior chamber is excised.

ICD-10-CM Diagnostic Codes

	Code	Description
⇄	H21.321	Implantation cysts of iris, ciliary body or anterior chamber, right eye
⇄	H21.322	Implantation cysts of iris, ciliary body or anterior chamber, left eye
⇄	H21.323	Implantation cysts of iris, ciliary body or anterior chamber, bilateral
❼	T85.21	Breakdown (mechanical) of intraocular lens
❼	T85.22	Displacement of intraocular lens
❼	T85.29	Other mechanical complication of intraocular lens
❼⇄	T85.310	Breakdown (mechanical) of prosthetic orbit of right eye
❼⇄	T85.311	Breakdown (mechanical) of prosthetic orbit of left eye
❼⇄	T85.318	Breakdown (mechanical) of other ocular prosthetic devices, implants and grafts
❼⇄	T85.320	Displacement of prosthetic orbit of right eye
❼⇄	T85.321	Displacement of prosthetic orbit of left eye
❼⇄	T85.328	Displacement of other ocular prosthetic devices, implants and grafts
❼⇄	T85.390	Other mechanical complication of prosthetic orbit of right eye
❼⇄	T85.391	Other mechanical complication of prosthetic orbit of left eye
❼⇄	T85.398	Other mechanical complication of other ocular prosthetic devices, implants and grafts
⇄	T86.8401	Corneal transplant rejection, right eye
⇄	T86.8402	Corneal transplant rejection, left eye
⇄	T86.8403	Corneal transplant rejection, bilateral
⇄	T86.8411	Corneal transplant failure, right eye
⇄	T86.8412	Corneal transplant failure, left eye
⇄	T86.8413	Corneal transplant failure, bilateral
⇄	T86.8481	Other complications of corneal transplant, right eye
⇄	T86.8482	Other complications of corneal transplant, left eye
⇄	T86.8483	Other complications of corneal transplant, bilateral

ICD-10-CM Coding Notes

For codes requiring a 7th character extension, refer to your ICD-10-CM book. Review the character descriptions and coding guidelines for proper selection. For some procedures, only certain characters will apply.

CCI Edits

Refer to Appendix A for CCI edits.

Facility RVUs ▯

Code	Work	PE Facility	MP	Total Facility
65900	12.51	15.41	0.96	28.88

Non-facility RVUs ▯

Code	Work	PE Non-Facility	MP	Total Non-Facility
65900	12.51	15.41	0.96	28.88

Modifiers (PAR) ▯

Code	Mod 50	Mod 51	Mod 62	Mod 66	Mod 80
65900	1	2	0	0	2

Global Period

Code	Days
65900	090

65920

65920 Removal of implanted material, anterior segment of eye

(For use of ophthalmic endoscope with 65920, use 66990)

AMA Coding Notes

Surgical Procedures on the Eye and Ocular Adnexa

(For diagnostic and treatment ophthalmological services, see Medicine, Ophthalmology, and 92002 et seq)

(Do not report code 69990 in addition to codes 65091-68850)

AMA *CPT® Assistant* ▯

65920: Sep 05: 12

Plain English Description

Material implants are manufactured objects placed into the eye during a surgical procedure and can include intraocular lenses and tube shunts. Removal of implanted material from the anterior chamber of the eye is performed under an operating microscope. A scleral incision is made close to the limbus to access the anterior chamber, a fluid-filled space directly behind the cornea and in front of the iris. The implanted material is located and any anchoring sutures are cut. The implanted material is then removed from the anterior chamber. Ocular pressure is checked and fluid is injected into the chamber if indicated. The scleral incision is closed with suture and the eye may be covered with a patch or shield.

Removal of implanted material, anterior segment of eye

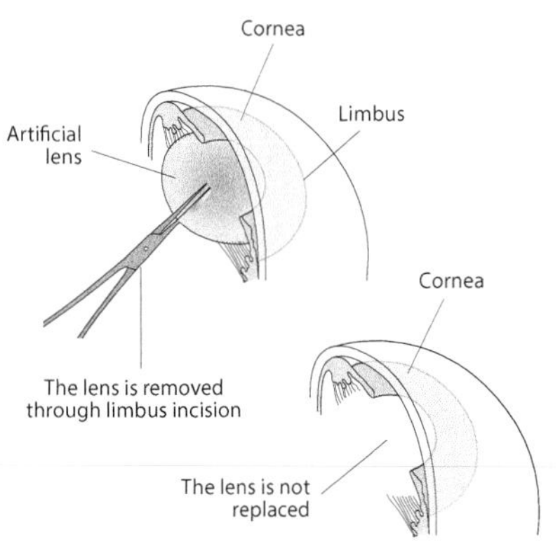

ICD-10-CM Diagnostic Codes

⇄	H18.11	Bullous keratopathy, right eye
⇄	H18.12	Bullous keratopathy, left eye
⇄	H18.13	Bullous keratopathy, bilateral
⇄	H20.21	Lens-induced iridocyclitis, right eye
⇄	H20.22	Lens-induced iridocyclitis, left eye
⇄	H20.23	Lens-induced iridocyclitis, bilateral
⇄	H27.121	Anterior dislocation of lens, right eye
⇄	H27.122	Anterior dislocation of lens, left eye
⇄	H27.123	Anterior dislocation of lens, bilateral
⇄	H40.041	Steroid responder, right eye
⇄	H40.042	Steroid responder, left eye
⇄	H40.043	Steroid responder, bilateral
❼	T85.21	Breakdown (mechanical) of intraocular lens
❼	T85.22	Displacement of intraocular lens
❼	T85.29	Other mechanical complication of intraocular lens
❼⇄	T85.310	Breakdown (mechanical) of prosthetic orbit of right eye
❼⇄	T85.311	Breakdown (mechanical) of prosthetic orbit of left eye
❼⇄	T85.318	Breakdown (mechanical) of other ocular prosthetic devices, implants and grafts
❼⇄	T85.320	Displacement of prosthetic orbit of right eye
❼⇄	T85.321	Displacement of prosthetic orbit of left eye
❼⇄	T85.328	Displacement of other ocular prosthetic devices, implants and grafts
❼⇄	T85.390	Other mechanical complication of prosthetic orbit of right eye
❼⇄	T85.391	Other mechanical complication of prosthetic orbit of left eye
❼⇄	T85.398	Other mechanical complication of other ocular prosthetic devices, implants and grafts
⇄	T86.8401	Corneal transplant rejection, right eye
⇄	T86.8402	Corneal transplant rejection, left eye
⇄	T86.8403	Corneal transplant rejection, bilateral
⇄	T86.8411	Corneal transplant failure, right eye
⇄	T86.8412	Corneal transplant failure, left eye
⇄	T86.8413	Corneal transplant failure, bilateral
⇄	T86.8421	Corneal transplant infection, right eye
⇄	T86.8422	Corneal transplant infection, left eye
⇄	T86.8423	Corneal transplant infection, bilateral
⇄	T86.8481	Other complications of corneal transplant, right eye
⇄	T86.8482	Other complications of corneal transplant, left eye
⇄	T86.8483	Other complications of corneal transplant, bilateral
	Z45.89	Encounter for adjustment and management of other implanted devices
	Z45.9	Encounter for adjustment and management of unspecified implanted device
	Z46.89	Encounter for fitting and adjustment of other specified devices

ICD-10-CM Coding Notes

For codes requiring a 7th character extension, refer to your ICD-10-CM book. Review the character descriptions and coding guidelines for proper selection. For some procedures, only certain characters will apply.

CCI Edits

Refer to Appendix A for CCI edits.

Facility RVUs ▯

Code	Work	PE Facility	MP	Total Facility
65920	9.99	12.22	0.77	22.98

Non-facility RVUs ▯

Code	Work	PE Non-Facility	MP	Total Non-Facility
65920	9.99	12.22	0.77	22.98

Modifiers (PAR) ▯

Code	Mod 50	Mod 51	Mod 62	Mod 66	Mod 80
65920	1	2	1	0	1

Global Period

Code	Days
65920	090

65930

65930 Removal of blood clot, anterior segment of eye

AMA Coding Notes

Surgical Procedures on the Eye and Ocular Adnexa

(For diagnostic and treatment ophthalmological services, see Medicine, Ophthalmology, and 92002 et seq)

(Do not report code 69990 in addition to codes 65091-68850)

Plain English Description

A blood clot or hyphema in the anterior segment of the eye may result from blunt or penetrating trauma to the exposed area of the eye, as a complication from intraocular surgery or spontaneously in the form of neovascularization in patients with diabetes mellitus, ischemic disease, cicatrix formation, ocular neoplasm or uveitis. Red blood cells suspend in the aqueous humor forming the clot, which then leads to inflammation, increased intraocular pressure and pain. Blood staining the cornea eventually leads to visual impairment if the clot is not removed. The patient is positioned supine and an operating microscopic put in place. An incision is made in the clear cornea using a diamond blade parallel to the plane of the iris. A 20-gauge Ocutome is attached to an infusion of balanced salt solution plus (BSS-Plus) and placed into the anterior chamber of the eye. The chamber is irrigated with this fluid to break up the clot and the fluid and blood are then aspirated using suction. An air bubble is placed into the chamber at the completion of the procedure and the incision in the cornea is closed with 10-0 suture. Antibiotic eye drops may be instilled and the eye is then patched.

Removal of blood clot, anterior segment of eye

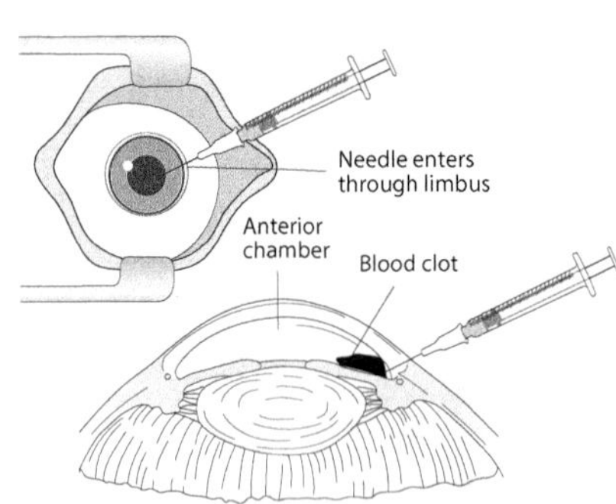

A needle is inserted into the anterior chamber to aspirate a blood clot between the iris and cornea.

ICD-10-CM Diagnostic Codes

⇄	H21.01	Hyphema, right eye
⇄	H21.02	Hyphema, left eye
⇄	H21.03	Hyphema, bilateral
⇄	H59.311	Postprocedural hemorrhage of right eye and adnexa following an ophthalmic procedure
⇄	H59.312	Postprocedural hemorrhage of left eye and adnexa following an ophthalmic procedure
⇄	H59.313	Postprocedural hemorrhage of eye and adnexa following an ophthalmic procedure, bilateral
⇄	H59.321	Postprocedural hemorrhage of right eye and adnexa following other procedure
⇄	H59.322	Postprocedural hemorrhage of left eye and adnexa following other procedure
⇄	H59.323	Postprocedural hemorrhage of eye and adnexa following other procedure, bilateral
❼⇄	S05.11	Contusion of eyeball and orbital tissues, right eye
❼⇄	S05.12	Contusion of eyeball and orbital tissues, left eye
❼⇄	S05.21	Ocular laceration and rupture with prolapse or loss of intraocular tissue, right eye
❼⇄	S05.22	Ocular laceration and rupture with prolapse or loss of intraocular tissue, left eye
❼⇄	S05.31	Ocular laceration without prolapse or loss of intraocular tissue, right eye
❼⇄	S05.32	Ocular laceration without prolapse or loss of intraocular tissue, left eye
❼⇄	S05.51	Penetrating wound with foreign body of right eyeball
❼⇄	S05.52	Penetrating wound with foreign body of left eyeball
❼⇄	S05.61	Penetrating wound without foreign body of right eyeball
❼⇄	S05.62	Penetrating wound without foreign body of left eyeball
❼⇄	S05.8X1	Other injuries of right eye and orbit
❼⇄	S05.8X2	Other injuries of left eye and orbit
⇄	T86.8481	Other complications of corneal transplant, right eye
⇄	T86.8482	Other complications of corneal transplant, left eye
⇄	T86.8483	Other complications of corneal transplant, bilateral

ICD-10-CM Coding Notes

For codes requiring a 7th character extension, refer to your ICD-10-CM book. Review the character descriptions and coding guidelines for proper selection. For some procedures, only certain characters will apply.

CCI Edits

Refer to Appendix A for CCI edits.

Facility RVUs ▯

Code	Work	PE Facility	MP	Total Facility
65930	8.39	9.61	0.65	18.65

Non-facility RVUs ▯

Code	Work	PE Non-Facility	MP	Total Non-Facility
65930	8.39	9.61	0.65	18.65

Modifiers (PAR) ▯

Code	Mod 50	Mod 51	Mod 62	Mod 66	Mod 80
65930	1	2	1	0	1

Global Period

Code	Days
65930	090

66020-66030

66020 Injection, anterior chamber of eye (separate procedure); air or liquid

66030 Injection, anterior chamber of eye (separate procedure); medication

(For unlisted procedures on anterior segment, use 66999)

AMA Coding Notes

Surgical Procedures on the Eye and Ocular Adnexa

(For diagnostic and treatment ophthalmological services, see Medicine, Ophthalmology, and 92002 et seq)

(Do not report code 69990 in addition to codes 65091-68850)

AMA *CPT® Assistant*

66020: Nov 12: 10

66030: Nov 12: 10

Plain English Description

The anterior chamber of the eye is the area behind the cornea and in front of the iris and lens that holds most of the clear, watery fluid called the aqueous humor. In 66020, air or liquid is injected into the anterior chamber. The patient is positioned supine with head and neck supported. A topical ophthalmic anesthetic is applied and the eye is then cleansed with antiseptic. An eyelid speculum is placed and the injection site is marked. A fine needle with attached syringe is inserted through the cornea and into the fluid-filled cavity behind it. Air or liquid is then injected into the cavity. The needle is withdrawn, antibiotic eye drops are instilled and the eye may be patched. In 66030, medication is injected into the anterior chamber using the same technique, also called an intracameral injection.

Injection anterior chamber of eye air/liquid/medication

Needle enters through limbus

Cornea

Anterior chamber

A needle is inserted into the anterior chamber to inject air/liquid (66020); medication (66030).

ICD-10-CM Diagnostic Codes

	Code	Description
	D49.89	Neoplasm of unspecified behavior of other specified sites
⇄	H18.11	Bullous keratopathy, right eye
⇄	H18.12	Bullous keratopathy, left eye
⇄	H18.13	Bullous keratopathy, bilateral
⇄	H18.331	Rupture in Descemet's membrane, right eye
⇄	H18.332	Rupture in Descemet's membrane, left eye
⇄	H18.333	Rupture in Descemet's membrane, bilateral
	H20.00	Unspecified acute and subacute iridocyclitis
⇄	H20.011	Primary iridocyclitis, right eye
⇄	H20.012	Primary iridocyclitis, left eye
⇄	H20.013	Primary iridocyclitis, bilateral
	H20.9	Unspecified iridocyclitis
⇄	H21.521	Goniosynechiae, right eye
⇄	H21.522	Goniosynechiae, left eye
⇄	H21.523	Goniosynechiae, bilateral
⇄	H25.041	Posterior subcapsular polar age-related cataract, right eye
⇄	H25.042	Posterior subcapsular polar age-related cataract, left eye
⇄	H25.043	Posterior subcapsular polar age-related cataract, bilateral
⇄	H25.11	Age-related nuclear cataract, right eye
⇄	H25.12	Age-related nuclear cataract, left eye
⇄	H25.13	Age-related nuclear cataract, bilateral
	H25.9	Unspecified age-related cataract
⇄	H33.21	Serous retinal detachment, right eye
⇄	H33.22	Serous retinal detachment, left eye
⇄	H33.23	Serous retinal detachment, bilateral
⇄	H33.41	Traction detachment of retina, right eye
⇄	H33.42	Traction detachment of retina, left eye
⇄	H33.43	Traction detachment of retina, bilateral
➐⇄	H35.321	Exudative age-related macular degeneration, right eye
➐⇄	H35.322	Exudative age-related macular degeneration, left eye
➐⇄	H35.323	Exudative age-related macular degeneration, bilateral
⇄	H35.341	Macular cyst, hole, or pseudohole, right eye
⇄	H35.342	Macular cyst, hole, or pseudohole, left eye
⇄	H35.343	Macular cyst, hole, or pseudohole, bilateral
⇄	H35.351	Cystoid macular degeneration, right eye
⇄	H35.352	Cystoid macular degeneration, left eye
⇄	H35.353	Cystoid macular degeneration, bilateral
⇄	H35.371	Puckering of macula, right eye
⇄	H35.372	Puckering of macula, left eye
⇄	H35.373	Puckering of macula, bilateral
⇄	H35.61	Retinal hemorrhage, right eye
⇄	H35.62	Retinal hemorrhage, left eye
⇄	H35.63	Retinal hemorrhage, bilateral
	H40.10X0	Unspecified open-angle glaucoma, stage unspecified
	H40.10X1	Unspecified open-angle glaucoma, mild stage
	H40.10X2	Unspecified open-angle glaucoma, moderate stage
	H40.10X3	Unspecified open-angle glaucoma, severe stage
	H40.10X4	Unspecified open-angle glaucoma, indeterminate stage
⇄	H40.1110	Primary open-angle glaucoma, right eye, stage unspecified
⇄	H40.1112	Primary open-angle glaucoma, right eye, moderate stage
⇄	H40.1113	Primary open-angle glaucoma, right eye, severe stage
⇄	H40.1114	Primary open-angle glaucoma, right eye, indeterminate stage
➐⇄	H40.112	Primary open-angle glaucoma, left eye
⇄	H40.1120	Primary open-angle glaucoma, left eye, stage unspecified
⇄	H40.1121	Primary open-angle glaucoma, left eye, mild stage
⇄	H40.1122	Primary open-angle glaucoma, left eye, moderate stage
⇄	H40.1123	Primary open-angle glaucoma, left eye, severe stage
⇄	H40.1124	Primary open-angle glaucoma, left eye, indeterminate stage
⇄	H40.1130	Primary open-angle glaucoma, bilateral, stage unspecified
⇄	H40.1131	Primary open-angle glaucoma, bilateral, mild stage
⇄	H40.1132	Primary open-angle glaucoma, bilateral, moderate stage
⇄	H40.1133	Primary open-angle glaucoma, bilateral, severe stage
⇄	H40.1134	Primary open-angle glaucoma, bilateral, indeterminate stage
➐⇄	H40.121	Low-tension glaucoma, right eye
➐⇄	H40.122	Low-tension glaucoma, left eye
➐⇄	H40.123	Low-tension glaucoma, bilateral
⇄	H40.831	Aqueous misdirection, right eye
⇄	H40.832	Aqueous misdirection, left eye
⇄	H40.833	Aqueous misdirection, bilateral
⇄	H43.11	Vitreous hemorrhage, right eye
⇄	H43.12	Vitreous hemorrhage, left eye
⇄	H43.13	Vitreous hemorrhage, bilateral
⇄	H44.001	Unspecified purulent endophthalmitis, right eye
⇄	H44.002	Unspecified purulent endophthalmitis, left eye
⇄	H44.003	Unspecified purulent endophthalmitis, bilateral
⇄	H44.2C1	Degenerative myopia with retinal detachment, right eye
⇄	H44.2C2	Degenerative myopia with retinal detachment, left eye
⇄	H44.2C3	Degenerative myopia with retinal detachment, bilateral eye
⇄	H44.411	Flat anterior chamber hypotony of right eye
⇄	H44.412	Flat anterior chamber hypotony of left eye
⇄	H44.413	Flat anterior chamber hypotony of eye, bilateral
⇄	H44.431	Hypotony of eye due to other ocular disorders, right eye
⇄	H44.432	Hypotony of eye due to other ocular disorders, left eye
⇄	H44.433	Hypotony of eye due to other ocular disorders, bilateral
	H59.40	Inflammation (infection) of postprocedural bleb, unspecified

	H59.41	Inflammation (infection) of postprocedural bleb, stage 1
	H59.42	Inflammation (infection) of postprocedural bleb, stage 2
	H59.43	Inflammation (infection) of postprocedural bleb, stage 3
⇄	T86.8421	Corneal transplant infection, right eye
⇄	T86.8422	Corneal transplant infection, left eye
⇄	T86.8423	Corneal transplant infection, bilateral
⇄	T86.8481	Other complications of corneal transplant, right eye
⇄	T86.8482	Other complications of corneal transplant, left eye
⇄	T86.8483	Other complications of corneal transplant, bilateral

ICD-10-CM Coding Notes

For codes requiring a 7th character extension, refer to your ICD-10-CM book. Review the character descriptions and coding guidelines for proper selection. For some procedures, only certain characters will apply.

CCI Edits

Refer to Appendix A for CCI edits.

Facility RVUs ▢

Code	Work	PE Facility	MP	Total Facility
66020	1.64	2.02	0.12	3.78
66030	1.30	1.81	0.10	3.21

Non-facility RVUs ▢

Code	Work	PE Non-Facility	MP	Total Non-Facility
66020	1.64	4.05	0.12	5.81
66030	1.30	3.85	0.10	5.25

Modifiers (PAR) ▢

Code	Mod 50	Mod 51	Mod 62	Mod 66	Mod 80
66020	1	2	0	0	1
66030	1	2	0	0	1

Global Period

Code	Days
66020	010
66030	010

66130

66130 Excision of lesion, sclera

AMA Coding Notes

Excision Procedures on the Anterior Sclera of the Eye

(For removal of intraocular foreign body, use 65235)

(For operations on posterior sclera, use 67250, 67255)

Surgical Procedures on the Eye and Ocular Adnexa

(For diagnostic and treatment ophthalmological services, see Medicine, Ophthalmology, and 92002 et seq)

(Do not report code 69990 in addition to codes 65091-68850)

Plain English Description

Lesions of the sclera are usually benign in nature. They can include pingueculae found most often in the open space between the eyelids and characterized by a yellowish color and slight elevation. Pigmented lesions that arise from melanocytes and non-melanocytes can be acquired or congenital. Scleral lesions may be removed for cosmetic reasons or when they become enlarged and cause discomfort. A topical ophthalmic anesthetic is applied and the eye is prepared with an antibacterial solution. An eyelid speculum is inserted and the lesion is excised. Separately reportable tissue grafting may be performed to repair the surgical defect resulting from the excision. At the conclusion of the procedure, the cytotoxic (anti-cancer) drug Mitomycin C may be applied briefly to reduce scarring and then flushed away.

Excision of lesion, sclera

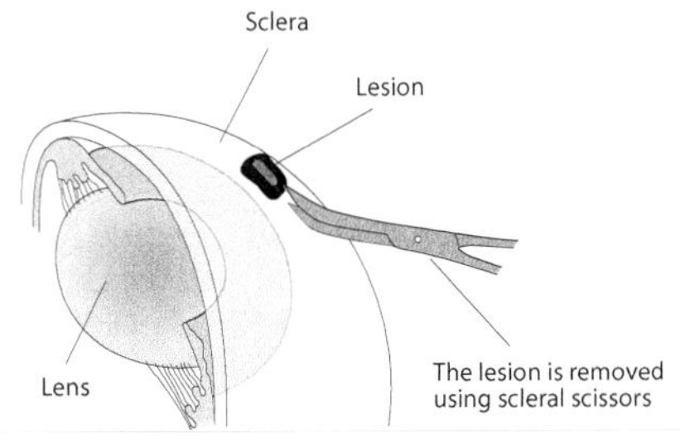

ICD-10-CM Diagnostic Codes

	Code	Description
⇄	C69.41	Malignant neoplasm of right ciliary body
⇄	C69.42	Malignant neoplasm of left ciliary body
	C79.49	Secondary malignant neoplasm of other parts of nervous system
⇄	D09.21	Carcinoma in situ of right eye
⇄	D09.22	Carcinoma in situ of left eye
⇄	D31.41	Benign neoplasm of right ciliary body
⇄	D31.42	Benign neoplasm of left ciliary body
	D48.7	Neoplasm of uncertain behavior of other specified sites
	D49.89	Neoplasm of unspecified behavior of other specified sites
⇄	H10.812	Pingueculitis, left eye
	H15.89	Other disorders of sclera
	H15.9	Unspecified disorder of sclera

CCI Edits

Refer to Appendix A for CCI edits.

Facility RVUs ☐

Code	Work	PE Facility	MP	Total Facility
66130	7.83	7.91	0.60	16.34

Non-facility RVUs ☐

Code	Work	PE Non-Facility	MP	Total Non-Facility
66130	7.83	12.33	0.60	20.76

Modifiers (PAR) ☐

Code	Mod 50	Mod 51	Mod 62	Mod 66	Mod 80
66130	1	2	0	0	0

Global Period

Code	Days
66130	090

66150

66150 Fistulization of sclera for glaucoma; trephination with iridectomy

AMA Coding Notes

Excision Procedures on the Anterior Sclera of the Eye

(For removal of intraocular foreign body, use 65235)

(For operations on posterior sclera, use 67250, 67255)

Surgical Procedures on the Eye and Ocular Adnexa

(For diagnostic and treatment ophthalmological services, see Medicine, Ophthalmology, and 92002 et seq)

(Do not report code 69990 in addition to codes 65091-68850)

AMA *CPT® Assistant* ▯

66150: Jul 18: 3

Plain English Description

Scleral fistulization to treat glaucoma is performed using trephination with iridectomy. The eye is visualized under an operating microscope and an incision is made in the conjunctiva near the limbus to expose the sclera. A flap is created in the sclera and a surgical instrument called a trephine is used to remove a small disc of tissue from the iris. The opening in the iris (iridectomy) allows fluid to flow between the anterior and posterior chambers of the eye, lowering the intraocular pressure. The scleral incision is closed with sutures followed by closure of the conjunctiva.

Fistulization of sclera for glaucoma

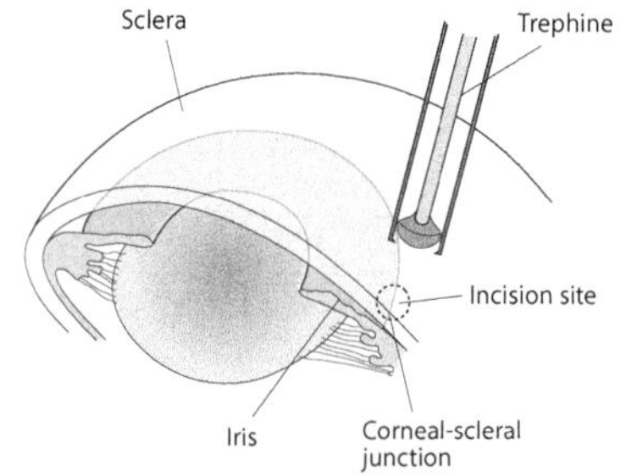

The physician creates a collection area to improve the flow of aqueous by trephination.

ICD-10-CM Diagnostic Codes

⇄	H40.021	Open angle with borderline findings, high risk, right eye
⇄	H40.061	Primary angle closure without glaucoma damage, right eye
❼⇄	H40.111	Primary open-angle glaucoma, right eye
❼⇄	H40.112	Primary open-angle glaucoma, left eye
❼⇄	H40.113	Primary open-angle glaucoma, bilateral
❼⇄	H40.121	Low-tension glaucoma, right eye
❼⇄	H40.131	Pigmentary glaucoma, right eye
❼⇄	H40.141	Capsular glaucoma with pseudoexfoliation of lens, right eye
⇄	H40.151	Residual stage of open-angle glaucoma, right eye
⇄	H40.211	Acute angle-closure glaucoma, right eye
❼⇄	H40.221	Chronic angle-closure glaucoma, right eye
⇄	H40.231	Intermittent angle-closure glaucoma, right eye
❼⇄	H40.31	Glaucoma secondary to eye trauma, right eye
❼⇄	H40.41	Glaucoma secondary to eye inflammation, right eye
❼⇄	H40.51	Glaucoma secondary to other eye disorders, right eye
❼⇄	H40.61	Glaucoma secondary to drugs, right eye
⇄	H40.831	Aqueous misdirection, right eye
	H40.89	Other specified glaucoma
	Q15.0	Congenital glaucoma

ICD-10-CM Coding Notes

For codes requiring a 7th character extension, refer to your ICD-10-CM book. Review the character descriptions and coding guidelines for proper selection. For some procedures, only certain characters will apply.

CCI Edits

Refer to Appendix A for CCI edits.

Facility RVUs ▯

Code	Work	PE Facility	MP	Total Facility
66150	10.53	14.11	0.79	25.43

Non-facility RVUs ▯

Code	Work	PE Non-Facility	MP	Total Non-Facility
66150	10.53	14.11	0.79	25.43

Modifiers (PAR) ▯

Code	Mod 50	Mod 51	Mod 62	Mod 66	Mod 80
66150	1	2	1	0	1

Global Period

Code	Days
66150	090

66155

66155 Fistulization of sclera for glaucoma; thermocauterization with iridectomy

AMA Coding Notes

Excision Procedures on the Anterior Sclera of the Eye

(For removal of intraocular foreign body, use 65235)

(For operations on posterior sclera, use 67250, 67255)

Surgical Procedures on the Eye and Ocular Adnexa

(For diagnostic and treatment ophthalmological services, see Medicine, Ophthalmology, and 92002 et seq)

(Do not report code 69990 in addition to codes 65091-68850)

AMA *CPT® Assistant* ☐

66155: Jul 18: 3

Plain English Description

Scleral fistulization to treat glaucoma is performed using thermocauterization with iridectomy. The eye is visualized under an operating microscope and an incision is made in the conjunctiva near the limbus to expose the sclera. An opening is created in the area of the pars plana of the ciliary body and a Fugo blade is used to dissolve tissue bands and create a small hole in the iris (iridectomy). The vascular ciliary body bleeds minimally when a Fugo blade is employed because it utilizes plasma energy around an ablation filament creating thermocauterization of the tissue as it cuts. The iridectomy allows fluid to drain from the posterior chamber into the subconjunctival lymphatics and lowers intraocular pressure. The scleral incision is closed with sutures followed by closure of the conjunctiva.

Fistulization of sclera for glaucoma

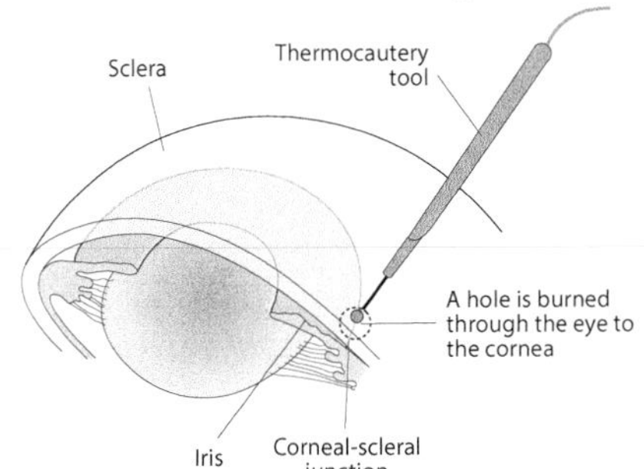

The physician creates a collection area to improve the flow of aqueous by thermocautery.

ICD-10-CM Diagnostic Codes

⇄	H40.022	Open angle with borderline findings, high risk, left eye
⇄	H40.062	Primary angle closure without glaucoma damage, left eye
❼⇄	H40.111	Primary open-angle glaucoma, right eye
❼⇄	H40.112	Primary open-angle glaucoma, left eye
❼⇄	H40.113	Primary open-angle glaucoma, bilateral
❼⇄	H40.122	Low-tension glaucoma, left eye
❼⇄	H40.132	Pigmentary glaucoma, left eye
❼⇄	H40.142	Capsular glaucoma with pseudoexfoliation of lens, left eye
⇄	H40.152	Residual stage of open-angle glaucoma, left eye
⇄	H40.212	Acute angle-closure glaucoma, left eye
❼⇄	H40.222	Chronic angle-closure glaucoma, left eye
⇄	H40.232	Intermittent angle-closure glaucoma, left eye
⇄	H40.242	Residual stage of angle-closure glaucoma, left eye
❼⇄	H40.32	Glaucoma secondary to eye trauma, left eye
❼⇄	H40.42	Glaucoma secondary to eye inflammation, left eye
❼⇄	H40.52	Glaucoma secondary to other eye disorders, left eye
❼⇄	H40.62	Glaucoma secondary to drugs, left eye
⇄	H40.832	Aqueous misdirection, left eye
	H40.89	Other specified glaucoma
	Q15.0	Congenital glaucoma

ICD-10-CM Coding Notes

For codes requiring a 7th character extension, refer to your ICD-10-CM book. Review the character descriptions and coding guidelines for proper selection. For some procedures, only certain characters will apply.

CCI Edits

Refer to Appendix A for CCI edits.

Facility RVUs ☐

Code	Work	PE Facility	MP	Total Facility
66155	10.52	14.11	0.79	25.42

Non-facility RVUs ☐

Code	Work	PE Non-Facility	MP	Total Non-Facility
66155	10.52	14.11	0.79	25.42

Modifiers (PAR) ☐

Code	Mod 50	Mod 51	Mod 62	Mod 66	Mod 80
66155	1	2	0	0	1

Global Period

Code	Days
66155	090

66160

66160 Fistulization of sclera for glaucoma; sclerectomy with punch or scissors, with iridectomy

AMA Coding Notes

Excision Procedures on the Anterior Sclera of the Eye

(For removal of intraocular foreign body, use 65235)

(For operations on posterior sclera, use 67250, 67255)

Surgical Procedures on the Eye and Ocular Adnexa

(For diagnostic and treatment ophthalmological services, see Medicine, Ophthalmology, and 92002 et seq)

(Do not report code 69990 in addition to codes 65091-68850)

AMA *CPT® Assistant* ▢

66160: Jul 18: 3

Plain English Description

Scleral fistulization to treat glaucoma is performed using sclerectomy with iridectomy. The eye is visualized under an operating microscope and an incision is made in the conjunctiva. The sclera is incised close to the limbus, and using a punch or scissors, a scleral lip is excised. The iris is opened with forceps to create a smooth, inverted iris flap (iridectomy) under the sclera. The iridectomy allows fluid to drain from the posterior chamber and lowers intraocular pressure. The scleral incision is closed with sutures followed by closure of the conjunctiva.

Fistulization of sclera for glaucoma; with punch or scissors, with iridectomy

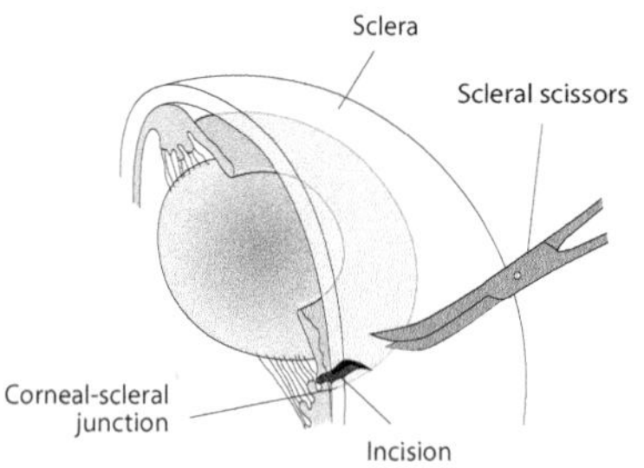

A portion of the iris and sclera are removed to create a fluid collection area in the anterior chamber.

ICD-10-CM Diagnostic Codes

⇄	H21.261	Iris atrophy (essential) (progressive), right eye
❼⇄	H40.141	Capsular glaucoma with pseudoexfoliation of lens, right eye
⇄	H40.211	Acute angle-closure glaucoma, right eye
❼⇄	H40.221	Chronic angle-closure glaucoma, right eye
⇄	H40.231	Intermittent angle-closure glaucoma, right eye
⇄	H40.241	Residual stage of angle-closure glaucoma, right eye
⇄	H40.831	Aqueous misdirection, right eye
	H40.89	Other specified glaucoma

ICD-10-CM Coding Notes

For codes requiring a 7th character extension, refer to your ICD-10-CM book. Review the character descriptions and coding guidelines for proper selection. For some procedures, only certain characters will apply.

CCI Edits

Refer to Appendix A for CCI edits.

Facility RVUs ▢

Code	Work	PE Facility	MP	Total Facility
66160	12.39	15.25	0.95	28.59

Non-facility RVUs ▢

Code	Work	PE Non-Facility	MP	Total Non-Facility
66160	12.39	15.25	0.95	28.59

Modifiers (PAR) ▢

Code	Mod 50	Mod 51	Mod 62	Mod 66	Mod 80
66160	1	2	1	0	1

Global Period

Code	Days
66160	090

66170-66172

66170 Fistulization of sclera for glaucoma; trabeculectomy ab externo in absence of previous surgery

(For trabeculotomy ab externo, use 65850)

(For repair of operative wound, use 66250)

66172 Fistulization of sclera for glaucoma; trabeculectomy ab externo with scarring from previous ocular surgery or trauma (includes injection of antifibrotic agents)

AMA Coding Notes

Excision Procedures on the Anterior Sclera of the Eye

(For removal of intraocular foreign body, use 65235)

(For operations on posterior sclera, use 67250, 67255)

Surgical Procedures on the Eye and Ocular Adnexa

(For diagnostic and treatment ophthalmological services, see Medicine, Ophthalmology, and 92002 et seq)

(Do not report code 69990 in addition to codes 65091-68850)

AMA *CPT® Assistant* ☐

66170: Jul 03: 4, Nov 03: 10, Dec 12: 14, Jul 18: 3, Dec 18: 9

66172: Jul 03: 4, Nov 03: 10, Dec 12: 14, Jul 18: 3, Dec 18: 10, Apr 19: 7

Plain English Description

The physician creates a new drainage tube for eye fluids through the fibrous covering of the eye. This is performed to treat a condition in which fluid drains from the front chamber of the eye slower than new fluid is produced. The physician removes some of the tissue connecting the iris to the fibrous membrane that surrounds the eye, leaving a passage for fluid to drain into the space between the fibrous membrane and the other structures of the eye. Code 66172 if this procedure is performed after a previous eye surgery to reduce scar tissue.

ICD-10-CM Diagnostic Codes

❼⇄	H40.111	Primary open-angle glaucoma, right eye
❼⇄	H40.112	Primary open-angle glaucoma, left eye
❼⇄	H40.113	Primary open-angle glaucoma, bilateral
❼⇄	H40.122	Low-tension glaucoma, left eye
❼⇄	H40.132	Pigmentary glaucoma, left eye
❼⇄	H40.142	Capsular glaucoma with pseudoexfoliation of lens, left eye
❼	H40.20	Unspecified primary angle-closure glaucoma
❼⇄	H40.222	Chronic angle-closure glaucoma, left eye
❼⇄	H40.52	Glaucoma secondary to other eye disorders, left eye

ICD-10-CM Coding Notes

For codes requiring a 7th character extension, refer to your ICD-10-CM book. Review the character descriptions and coding guidelines for proper selection. For some procedures, only certain characters will apply.

CCI Edits

Refer to Appendix A for CCI edits.

Facility RVUs ☐

Code	Work	PE Facility	MP	Total Facility
66170	13.94	16.66	1.07	31.67
66172	14.84	18.58	1.16	34.58

Non-facility RVUs ☐

Code	Work	PE Non-Facility	MP	Total Non-Facility
66170	13.94	16.66	1.07	31.67
66172	14.84	18.58	1.16	34.58

Modifiers (PAR) ☐

Code	Mod 50	Mod 51	Mod 62	Mod 66	Mod 80
66170	1	2	1	0	2
66172	1	2	1	0	2

Global Period

Code	Days
66170	090
66172	090

66174-66175

66174 Transluminal dilation of aqueous outflow canal; without retention of device or stent

(Do not report 66174 in conjunction with 65820)

66175 Transluminal dilation of aqueous outflow canal; with retention of device or stent

AMA Coding Notes

Excision Procedures on the Anterior Sclera of the Eye

(For removal of intraocular foreign body, use 65235)

(For operations on posterior sclera, use 67250, 67255)

Surgical Procedures on the Eye and Ocular Adnexa

(For diagnostic and treatment ophthalmological services, see Medicine, Ophthalmology, and 92002 et seq)

(Do not report code 69990 in addition to codes 65091-68850)

AMA *CPT® Assistant* ▢

66174: Dec 18: 9, Sep 19: 11

Plain English Description

Transluminal dilation of the aqueous outflow canal (Schlemm's canal) without retention is performed to treat open angle glaucoma. This procedure is also referred to as glaucoma canaloplasty or enhanced viscocanalostomy. The procedure reduces intraocular pressure (IOP) in patients with glaucoma by forcibly opening Schlemm's canal to restore natural drainage of fluid from the eye. A scleral flap is created. The canal is exposed and deroofed. The scleral flap may be extended to expose Descemet's membrane and a window (Descemet's window) is created. The canal is then intubated with a flexible hollow microcatheter with a lighted tip. The lighted tip illuminates the canal as the microcatheter is advanced. A viscoelastic, such as high viscosity sodium hyaluronate, is instilled to dilate the canal and facilitate advancement of the microcatheter. After it has been passed through the entire length of the canal, the microcatheter is withdrawn. The scleral flap is closed. Use 66174 when the procedure is performed without retention of a device or stent. Use 66175 when transluminal dilation of the aqueous outflow canal is performed with retention of a device or stent. The procedure is performed as described above except that a device, such as a suture, or a stent is left in the canal. After the microcannula has been passed through the entire length of the canal, either a flexible stent or a suture is advanced along the path of the microcannula through the full length of the canal as well. The flexible stent or suture is left in the canal and the microcannula is withdrawn. If a suture is used to permanently open the canal, the suture is tied off and left in place. The suture cinches and stretches the trabecular meshwork inward and opens the canal.

Transluminal dilation of aqueous outflow canal

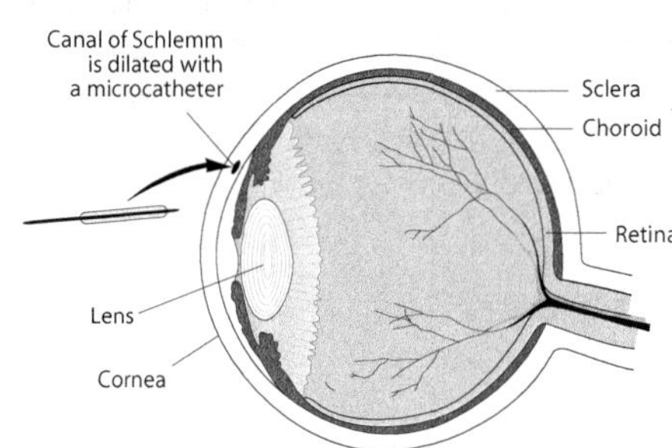

With (66174), or without (66175) retention of device or stent

ICD-10-CM Diagnostic Codes

⇄	H21.41	Pupillary membranes, right eye
⇄	H21.501	Unspecified adhesions of iris, right eye
⇄	H21.511	Anterior synechiae (iris), right eye
⇄	H21.521	Goniosynechiae, right eye
⇄	H21.541	Posterior synechiae (iris), right eye
⇄	H40.001	Preglaucoma, unspecified, right eye
⇄	H40.011	Open angle with borderline findings, low risk, right eye
⇄	H40.021	Open angle with borderline findings, high risk, right eye
⇄	H40.031	Anatomical narrow angle, right eye
⇄	H40.041	Steroid responder, right eye
❼	H40.10	Unspecified open-angle glaucoma
❼⇄	H40.111	Primary open-angle glaucoma, right eye
❼⇄	H40.112	Primary open-angle glaucoma, left eye
❼⇄	H40.113	Primary open-angle glaucoma, bilateral
❼⇄	H40.121	Low-tension glaucoma, right eye
❼⇄	H40.131	Pigmentary glaucoma, right eye
❼⇄	H40.141	Capsular glaucoma with pseudoexfoliation of lens, right eye
⇄	H40.151	Residual stage of open-angle glaucoma, right eye
❼	H40.20	Unspecified primary angle-closure glaucoma
⇄	H40.211	Acute angle-closure glaucoma, right eye
❼⇄	H40.221	Chronic angle-closure glaucoma, right eye
⇄	H40.231	Intermittent angle-closure glaucoma, right eye
⇄	H40.241	Residual stage of angle-closure glaucoma, right eye
❼⇄	H40.31	Glaucoma secondary to eye trauma, right eye
❼⇄	H40.51	Glaucoma secondary to other eye disorders, right eye
❼⇄	H40.61	Glaucoma secondary to drugs, right eye
⇄	H40.811	Glaucoma with increased episcleral venous pressure, right eye
⇄	H40.821	Hypersecretion glaucoma, right eye
⇄	H40.831	Aqueous misdirection, right eye
	H40.89	Other specified glaucoma
	H40.9	Unspecified glaucoma
	Q15.0	Congenital glaucoma

ICD-10-CM Coding Notes

For codes requiring a 7th character extension, refer to your ICD-10-CM book. Review the character descriptions and coding guidelines for proper selection. For some procedures, only certain characters will apply.

CCI Edits

Refer to Appendix A for CCI edits.

Facility RVUs ▢

Code	Work	PE Facility	MP	Total Facility
66174	7.62	13.77	0.60	21.99
66175	9.34	13.02	0.73	23.09

Non-facility RVUs ▢

Code	Work	PE Non-Facility	MP	Total Non-Facility
66174	7.62	13.77	0.60	21.99
66175	9.34	13.02	0.73	23.09

Modifiers (PAR) ▢

Code	Mod 50	Mod 51	Mod 62	Mod 66	Mod 80
66174	1	2	1	0	2
66175	1	2	1	0	2

Global Period

Code	Days
66174	090
66175	090

66179-66180

66179 Aqueous shunt to extraocular equatorial plate reservoir, external approach; without graft

66180 Aqueous shunt to extraocular equatorial plate reservoir, external approach; with graft

(Do not report 66180 in conjunction with 67255)

AMA Coding Notes

Surgical Procedures on the Eye and Ocular Adnexa

(For diagnostic and treatment ophthalmological services, see Medicine, Ophthalmology, and 92002 et seq)

(Do not report code 69990 in addition to codes 65091-68850)

AMA *CPT® Assistant* ▯

66179: Jan 15: 10, Jul 18: 3

66180: Winter 90: 8, Aug 03: 9, Sep 03: 2, Jun 12: 15, Jan 15: 10, Jul 18: 3

Plain English Description

Normal outflow of vitreous fluid begins at the aqueous humor and passes through the trabecular meshwork, enters Schlemm's canal (a space lined with endothelial cells) finally draining into the collector channel and the aqueous veins. An aqueous shunt to extraocular reservoir (Molteno, Schocket, Krupin-Denver) bypasses the trabecular meshwork and Schlemm's canal. The shunt is used to reduce intraocular pressure (IOP) when traditional medical (pharmacological) or surgical (trabeculectomy) therapy have failed. This procedure is most often implemented when increased intraocular pressure (IOP) is caused by iris swelling, abnormal vessel formation or iridocorneal endothelial (ICE) syndrome. With the patient supine and under general anesthesia, a small silicon tube is implanted into the anterior chamber of the eye allowing vitreous fluid to drain through the tube and collect in a tiny plate sutured on the anterior eye between the sclera and the conjunctiva (usually in the area of the upper eye lid). After collecting in the plate, the vitreous fluid is then absorbed by blood vessels on the surface of the anterior eye. In 66180, a scleral or corneal patch graft from donor tissue may be placed over the plate to keep it in position and reduce the incidence of conjunctival ulceration. At the conclusion of the procedure, the cytotoxic (anti-cancer) drug Mitomycin C may be applied briefly to reduce scarring and then flushed away. A contact lens bandage may be applied and antibiotic and/or steroid drops may be instilled. The eye is then patched.

Aqueous shunt to extraocular reservoir

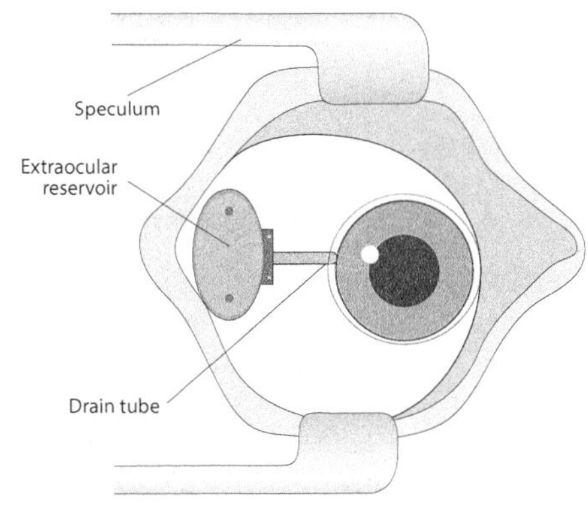

A tube which drains fluid from the eye to a reservoir outside the eye socket is placed.

ICD-10-CM Diagnostic Codes

	Code	Description
⇄	H20.12	Chronic iridocyclitis, left eye
⇄	H20.22	Lens-induced iridocyclitis, left eye
	H21.1	Other vascular disorders of iris and ciliary body
⇄	H21.322	Implantation cysts of iris, ciliary body or anterior chamber, left eye
⇄	H21.532	Iridodialysis, left eye
❼⇄	H40.111	Primary open-angle glaucoma, right eye
❼⇄	H40.112	Primary open-angle glaucoma, left eye
❼⇄	H40.113	Primary open-angle glaucoma, bilateral
❼⇄	H40.122	Low-tension glaucoma, left eye
❼⇄	H40.132	Pigmentary glaucoma, left eye
❼⇄	H40.142	Capsular glaucoma with pseudoexfoliation of lens, left eye
⇄	H40.152	Residual stage of open-angle glaucoma, left eye
❼⇄	H40.222	Chronic angle-closure glaucoma, left eye
❼⇄	H40.32	Glaucoma secondary to eye trauma, left eye
❼⇄	H40.42	Glaucoma secondary to eye inflammation, left eye
❼⇄	H40.52	Glaucoma secondary to other eye disorders, left eye
❼⇄	H40.62	Glaucoma secondary to drugs, left eye
	H40.89	Other specified glaucoma
⇄	H44.112	Panuveitis, left eye
	Q15.0	Congenital glaucoma

ICD-10-CM Coding Notes

For codes requiring a 7th character extension, refer to your ICD-10-CM book. Review the character descriptions and coding guidelines for proper selection. For some procedures, only certain characters will apply.

CCI Edits

Refer to Appendix A for CCI edits.

Facility RVUs ▯

Code	Work	PE Facility	MP	Total Facility
66179	14.00	16.23	1.07	31.30
66180	15.00	16.83	1.16	32.99

Non-facility RVUs ▯

Code	Work	PE Non-Facility	MP	Total Non-Facility
66179	14.00	16.23	1.07	31.30
66180	15.00	16.83	1.16	32.99

Modifiers (PAR) ▯

Code	Mod 50	Mod 51	Mod 62	Mod 66	Mod 80
66179	1	2	0	0	2
66180	1	2	0	0	2

Global Period

Code	Days
66179	090
66180	090

CPT® Procedural Coding

66183

66183 Insertion of anterior segment aqueous drainage device, without extraocular reservoir, external approach

AMA Coding Notes

Surgical Procedures on the Eye and Ocular Adnexa

(For diagnostic and treatment ophthalmological services, see Medicine, Ophthalmology, and 92002 et seq)

(Do not report code 69990 in addition to codes 65091-68850)

AMA *CPT® Assistant* ▢

66183: May 14: 5, Jul 18: 3

Plain English Description

Insertion of an anterior segment aqueous drainage device is used to treat chronic or progressive open angle glaucoma. Using an external approach, which may also be described as non-penetrating deep sclerectomy, the conjunctiva is incised and a scleral flap is created with the base of the flap located at the corneoscleral junction (limbus). An incision is made into the anterior chamber and aqueous flow is established. A miniature drainage device (shunt), about the size of a grain of rice, is implanted between the anterior chamber and under the scleral flap in order to facilitate drainage of aqueous humor from the anterior chamber to the space under the conjunctiva. The scleral flap is secured with sutures and the conjunctival incision is closed.

ICD-10-CM Diagnostic Codes

⇄	H20.051	Hypopyon, right eye
⇄	H20.12	Chronic iridocyclitis, left eye
⇄	H31.421	Serous choroidal detachment, right eye
❼⇄	H40.111	Primary open-angle glaucoma, right eye
❼⇄	H40.112	Primary open-angle glaucoma, left eye
❼⇄	H40.113	Primary open-angle glaucoma, bilateral
❼⇄	H40.121	Low-tension glaucoma, right eye
❼⇄	H40.122	Low-tension glaucoma, left eye
❼⇄	H40.131	Pigmentary glaucoma, right eye
❼⇄	H40.132	Pigmentary glaucoma, left eye
❼⇄	H40.141	Capsular glaucoma with pseudoexfoliation of lens, right eye
⇄	H40.152	Residual stage of open-angle glaucoma, left eye
❼⇄	H40.221	Chronic angle-closure glaucoma, right eye
❼⇄	H40.222	Chronic angle-closure glaucoma, left eye
❼⇄	H40.31	Glaucoma secondary to eye trauma, right eye
❼⇄	H40.41	Glaucoma secondary to eye inflammation, right eye
❼⇄	H40.51	Glaucoma secondary to other eye disorders, right eye
❼⇄	H40.61	Glaucoma secondary to drugs, right eye
⇄	H40.832	Aqueous misdirection, left eye
	H40.89	Other specified glaucoma
⇄	H44.412	Flat anterior chamber hypotony of left eye
⇄	H44.421	Hypotony of right eye due to ocular fistula
	Q15.0	Congenital glaucoma

ICD-10-CM Coding Notes

For codes requiring a 7th character extension, refer to your ICD-10-CM book. Review the character descriptions and coding guidelines for proper selection. For some procedures, only certain characters will apply.

CCI Edits

Refer to Appendix A for CCI edits.

Facility RVUs ▢

Code	Work	PE Facility	MP	Total Facility
66183	13.20	15.60	1.01	29.81

Non-facility RVUs ▢

Code	Work	PE Non-Facility	MP	Total Non-Facility
66183	13.20	15.60	1.01	29.81

Modifiers (PAR) ▢

Code	Mod 50	Mod 51	Mod 62	Mod 66	Mod 80
66183	1	2	0	0	2

Global Period

Code	Days
66183	090

66184-66185

66184 Revision of aqueous shunt to extraocular equatorial plate reservoir; without graft

66185 Revision of aqueous shunt to extraocular equatorial plate reservoir; with graft

(Do not report 66185 in conjunction with 67255)

(For removal of implanted shunt, use 67120)

AMA Coding Notes

Surgical Procedures on the Eye and Ocular Adnexa

(For diagnostic and treatment ophthalmological services, see Medicine, Ophthalmology, and 92002 et seq)

(Do not report code 69990 in addition to codes 65091-68850)

AMA *CPT® Assistant* ▯

66184: Jan 15: 10

66185: Winter 90: 8, Jan 15: 10

Plain English Description

A number of conditions may require revision of aqueous shunt to extraocular plate reservoir. With the sudden drop in intraocular pressure (IOP) from the newly created drainage system, the anterior chamber may decrease the amount of fluid it produces. This can be treated by priming the pump with a viscoelastic fluid to raise IOP in the anterior chamber and stimulate the production of vitreous humor. However, some conditions require revision of the shunt, including corneal damage, small cataracts, infection, and bleeding. The most common problem requiring revision of the aqueous shunt is the buildup of scar tissue at the posterior plate. An incision is made in the conjunctival tissue over the plate. The scar tissue is then removed. Once the scar tissue is removed, the conjunctival incision is sutured closed. In 66185, a scleral or corneal patch graft from donor tissue may be placed over the plate to keep it in position after the revision and reduce the incidence of conjunctival ulceration. At the conclusion of the procedure, the cytotoxic (anti-cancer) drug Mitomycin C may be applied briefly to reduce recurrence of scarring and then flushed away. A contact lens bandage may be applied and antibiotic and/or steroid drops may be instilled. The eye is then patched.

Revision of aqueous shunt to extraocular reservoir

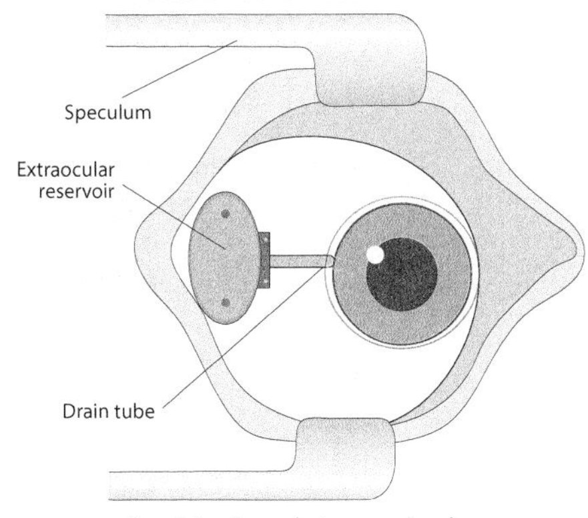

A revision is made to a previously placed aqueous shunt.

ICD-10-CM Diagnostic Codes

	Code	Description
⇄	H20.051	Hypopyon, right eye
⇄	H20.12	Chronic iridocyclitis, left eye
⇄	H31.421	Serous choroidal detachment, right eye
➐	H40.10	Unspecified open-angle glaucoma
➐⇄	H40.111	Primary open-angle glaucoma, right eye
➐⇄	H40.112	Primary open-angle glaucoma, left eye
➐⇄	H40.113	Primary open-angle glaucoma, bilateral
➐⇄	H40.121	Low-tension glaucoma, right eye
➐⇄	H40.122	Low-tension glaucoma, left eye
➐⇄	H40.131	Pigmentary glaucoma, right eye
➐⇄	H40.132	Pigmentary glaucoma, left eye
➐⇄	H40.141	Capsular glaucoma with pseudoexfoliation of lens, right eye
⇄	H40.151	Residual stage of open-angle glaucoma, right eye
➐	H40.20	Unspecified primary angle-closure glaucoma
➐⇄	H40.221	Chronic angle-closure glaucoma, right eye
➐⇄	H40.222	Chronic angle-closure glaucoma, left eye
➐⇄	H40.31	Glaucoma secondary to eye trauma, right eye
➐⇄	H40.41	Glaucoma secondary to eye inflammation, right eye
➐⇄	H40.51	Glaucoma secondary to other eye disorders, right eye
➐⇄	H40.61	Glaucoma secondary to drugs, right eye
⇄	H40.831	Aqueous misdirection, right eye
	H40.89	Other specified glaucoma
⇄	H44.412	Flat anterior chamber hypotony of left eye
⇄	H44.421	Hypotony of right eye due to ocular fistula
	Q15.0	Congenital glaucoma
➐	T85.618	Breakdown (mechanical) of other specified internal prosthetic devices, implants and grafts
➐	T85.638	Leakage of other specified internal prosthetic devices, implants and grafts
➐	T85.698	Other mechanical complication of other specified internal prosthetic devices, implants and grafts
➐	T85.79	Infection and inflammatory reaction due to other internal prosthetic devices, implants and grafts
➐	T85.898	Other specified complication of other internal prosthetic devices, implants and grafts

ICD-10-CM Coding Notes

For codes requiring a 7th character extension, refer to your ICD-10-CM book. Review the character descriptions and coding guidelines for proper selection. For some procedures, only certain characters will apply.

CCI Edits

Refer to Appendix A for CCI edits.

Facility RVUs ▯

Code	Work	PE Facility	MP	Total Facility
66184	9.58	12.62	0.73	22.93
66185	10.58	13.24	0.83	24.65

Non-facility RVUs ▯

Code	Work	PE Non-Facility	MP	Total Non-Facility
66184	9.58	12.62	0.73	22.93
66185	10.58	13.24	0.83	24.65

Modifiers (PAR) ▯

Code	Mod 50	Mod 51	Mod 62	Mod 66	Mod 80
66184	1	2	0	0	2
66185	1	2	0	0	2

Global Period

Code	Days
66184	090
66185	090

66225

66225 Repair of scleral staphyloma with graft

(For scleral reinforcement, see 67250, 67255)

AMA Coding Notes

Repair or Revision Procedures on the Anterior Sclera of the Eye

(For scleral procedures in retinal surgery, see 67101 et seq)

Surgical Procedures on the Eye and Ocular Adnexa

(For diagnostic and treatment ophthalmological services, see Medicine, Ophthalmology, and 92002 et seq)

(Do not report code 69990 in addition to codes 65091-68850)

Plain English Description

A staphyloma is a protrusion of uveal tissue through a weak area of the sclera or cornea. Staphylomas usually arise in an area that has been injured or weakened by disease or inflammation. There are five areas in which staphylomas are found. Anterior segment staphylomas involve the cornea and adjacent scleral tissue. Intercalary or limbal staphylomas are found at the margin where the cornea and sclera meet and often present with secondary angle closure glaucoma or corneal astigmatism. Ciliary staphylomas are located in an area lined with ciliary bodies approximately 2-3 mm from the limbus. Equatorial staphylomas are found in a region perforated by vortex veins. Posterior or macular staphylomas are located at the back of the eye and are diagnosed by ophthalmoscopy often after the patient presents with myopia. In 66225, the protruding tissue is excised and the weak region of the sclera is reinforced with a tissue graft, such as an allogenic fascial graft fixed with fibrin tissue glue.

Repair of scleral staphyloma

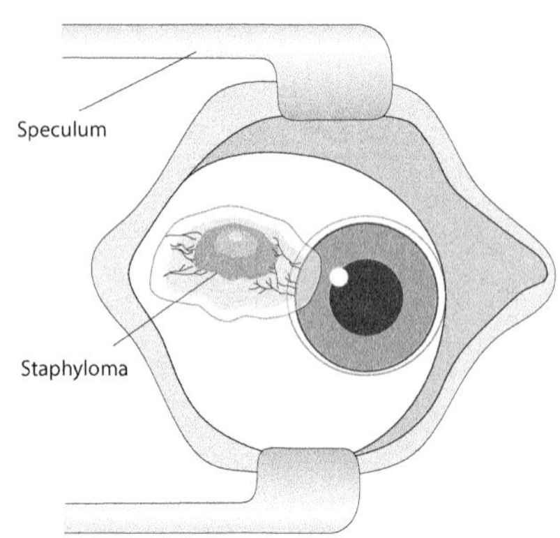

A scleral staphyloma is repaired with a graft.

ICD-10-CM Diagnostic Codes

	Code	Description
⇄	H15.011	Anterior scleritis, right eye
⇄	H15.012	Anterior scleritis, left eye
⇄	H15.013	Anterior scleritis, bilateral
⇄	H15.811	Equatorial staphyloma, right eye
⇄	H15.812	Equatorial staphyloma, left eye
⇄	H15.813	Equatorial staphyloma, bilateral
⇄	H15.821	Localized anterior staphyloma, right eye
⇄	H15.822	Localized anterior staphyloma, left eye
⇄	H15.823	Localized anterior staphyloma, bilateral
⇄	H15.841	Scleral ectasia, right eye
⇄	H15.842	Scleral ectasia, left eye
⇄	H15.843	Scleral ectasia, bilateral
⇄	H15.851	Ring staphyloma, right eye
⇄	H15.852	Ring staphyloma, left eye
⇄	H15.853	Ring staphyloma, bilateral
	H15.89	Other disorders of sclera
❼⇄	H40.51	Glaucoma secondary to other eye disorders, right eye
❼⇄	H40.52	Glaucoma secondary to other eye disorders, left eye
❼⇄	H40.53	Glaucoma secondary to other eye disorders, bilateral
⇄	H52.11	Myopia, right eye
⇄	H52.12	Myopia, left eye
⇄	H52.13	Myopia, bilateral
⇄	H52.211	Irregular astigmatism, right eye
⇄	H52.212	Irregular astigmatism, left eye
⇄	H52.213	Irregular astigmatism, bilateral
⇄	H52.221	Regular astigmatism, right eye
⇄	H52.222	Regular astigmatism, left eye
⇄	H52.223	Regular astigmatism, bilateral
⇄	S05.51XS	Penetrating wound with foreign body of right eyeball, sequela
⇄	S05.52XS	Penetrating wound with foreign body of left eyeball, sequela
⇄	S05.61XS	Penetrating wound without foreign body of right eyeball, sequela
⇄	S05.62XS	Penetrating wound without foreign body of left eyeball, sequela

ICD-10-CM Coding Notes

For codes requiring a 7th character extension, refer to your ICD-10-CM book. Review the character descriptions and coding guidelines for proper selection. For some procedures, only certain characters will apply.

CCI Edits

Refer to Appendix A for CCI edits.

Facility RVUs ▯

Code	Work	PE Facility	MP	Total Facility
66225	12.63	13.51	0.98	27.12

Non-facility RVUs ▯

Code	Work	PE Non-Facility	MP	Total Non-Facility
66225	12.63	13.51	0.98	27.12

Modifiers (PAR) ▯

Code	Mod 50	Mod 51	Mod 62	Mod 66	Mod 80
66225	1	2	1	0	1

Global Period

Code	Days
66225	090

66250

66250 Revision or repair of operative wound of anterior segment, any type, early or late, major or minor procedure

(For unlisted procedures on anterior sclera, use 66999)

AMA Coding Notes

Repair or Revision Procedures on the Anterior Sclera of the Eye

(For scleral procedures in retinal surgery, see 67101 et seq)

Surgical Procedures on the Eye and Ocular Adnexa

(For diagnostic and treatment ophthalmological services, see Medicine, Ophthalmology, and 92002 et seq)

(Do not report code 69990 in addition to codes 65091-68850)

AMA *CPT® Assistant* ▯

66250: Oct 10: 15, Dec 10: 15, Dec 18: 9

Plain English Description

The physician revises or repairs any type of wound to the front of the eye that resulted from surgery.

Revision or repair of operative wound of anterior segment, any type, early/late major/minor procedure

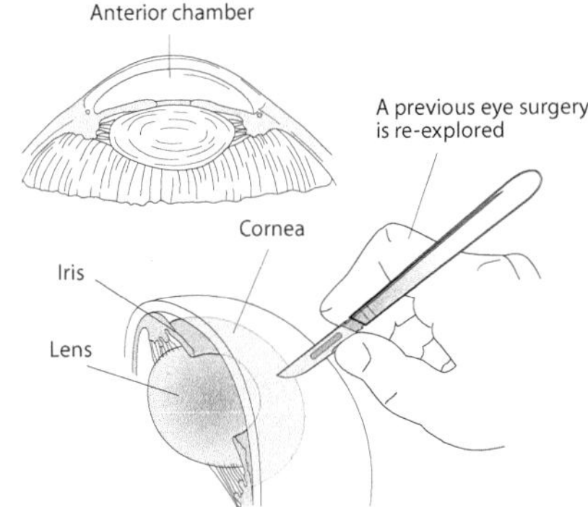

ICD-10-CM Diagnostic Codes

⇄	H59.011	Keratopathy (bullous aphakic) following cataract surgery, right eye
⇄	H59.012	Keratopathy (bullous aphakic) following cataract surgery, left eye
⇄	H59.013	Keratopathy (bullous aphakic) following cataract surgery, bilateral
⇄	H59.031	Cystoid macular edema following cataract surgery, right eye
⇄	H59.032	Cystoid macular edema following cataract surgery, left eye
⇄	H59.033	Cystoid macular edema following cataract surgery, bilateral
⇄	H59.091	Other disorders of the right eye following cataract surgery
⇄	H59.092	Other disorders of the left eye following cataract surgery
⇄	H59.093	Other disorders of the eye following cataract surgery, bilateral
⇄	H59.811	Chorioretinal scars after surgery for detachment, right eye
⇄	H59.812	Chorioretinal scars after surgery for detachment, left eye
⇄	H59.813	Chorioretinal scars after surgery for detachment, bilateral
❼	T81.31	Disruption of external operation (surgical) wound, not elsewhere classified
❼	T81.49	Infection following a procedure, other surgical site
❼	T81.82	Emphysema (subcutaneous) resulting from a procedure
❼⇄	T85.310	Breakdown (mechanical) of prosthetic orbit of right eye
❼⇄	T85.311	Breakdown (mechanical) of prosthetic orbit of left eye
❼⇄	T85.318	Breakdown (mechanical) of other ocular prosthetic devices, implants and grafts
❼⇄	T85.320	Displacement of prosthetic orbit of right eye
❼⇄	T85.321	Displacement of prosthetic orbit of left eye
❼⇄	T85.328	Displacement of other ocular prosthetic devices, implants and grafts
❼⇄	T85.390	Other mechanical complication of prosthetic orbit of right eye
❼⇄	T85.391	Other mechanical complication of prosthetic orbit of left eye
❼⇄	T85.398	Other mechanical complication of other ocular prosthetic devices, implants and grafts
⇄	T86.8401	Corneal transplant rejection, right eye
⇄	T86.8402	Corneal transplant rejection, left eye
⇄	T86.8403	Corneal transplant rejection, bilateral
⇄	T86.8411	Corneal transplant failure, right eye
⇄	T86.8412	Corneal transplant failure, left eye
⇄	T86.8413	Corneal transplant failure, bilateral
⇄	T86.8421	Corneal transplant infection, right eye
⇄	T86.8422	Corneal transplant infection, left eye
⇄	T86.8423	Corneal transplant infection, bilateral
⇄	T86.8481	Other complications of corneal transplant, right eye
⇄	T86.8482	Other complications of corneal transplant, left eye
⇄	T86.8483	Other complications of corneal transplant, bilateral
	Z94.7	Corneal transplant status
	Z98.83	Filtering (vitreous) bleb after glaucoma surgery status

ICD-10-CM Coding Notes

For codes requiring a 7th character extension, refer to your ICD-10-CM book. Review the character descriptions and coding guidelines for proper selection. For some procedures, only certain characters will apply.

CCI Edits

Refer to Appendix A for CCI edits.

Facility RVUs ▯

Code	Work	PE Facility	MP	Total Facility
66250	7.10	8.44	0.56	16.10

Non-facility RVUs ▯

Code	Work	PE Non-Facility	MP	Total Non-Facility
66250	7.10	14.54	0.56	22.20

Modifiers (PAR) ▯

Code	Mod 50	Mod 51	Mod 62	Mod 66	Mod 80
66250	1	2	0	0	1

Global Period

Code	Days
66250	090

66500-66505

66500 Iridotomy by stab incision (separate procedure); except transfixion

66505 Iridotomy by stab incision (separate procedure); with transfixion as for iris bombe

(For iridotomy by photocoagulation, use 66761)

AMA Coding Notes

Surgical Procedures on the Eye and Ocular Adnexa

(For diagnostic and treatment ophthalmological services, see Medicine, Ophthalmology, and 92002 et seq)

(Do not report code 69990 in addition to codes 65091-68850)

Plain English Description

Stab incision iridotomy with or without transfixion may be used to treat glaucoma, iris atrophy, papillary membrane adhesions, and aniridia. Using an operating microscope to visualize the eye, a stab incision is made through the conjunctiva and into the lamellar sclera. A superficial tunnel is then carefully dissected using a side-to-side technique up to the limbus. The dissection is extended into the lamellar cornea and the anterior chamber is entered horizontally. The blade is withdrawn in a single, smooth movement to open the tunnel. An ophthalmic viscoelastic fluid is injected through the tunnel and the globe is rotated downward allowing a membrane punch to slide along the tunnel and into the anterior chamber. The posterior lip of the corneal section is grasped and punched. To compromise the tunnel, additional punches may be taken in clear cornea and extended up to the limbus. The anterior chamber is then irrigated through the tunnel to remove excess viscoelastic fluid and monitor for leakage. The conjunctival incision is closed with sutures. Code 66505 includes iridotomy by stab incision with transfixion as for iris bombe, a condition in which there is apposition of the iris to the anterior chamber blocking the flow of aqueous fluid from the posterior chamber. The increased pressure in the posterior chamber causes anterior bowing, or bulging of the iris and obstruction of the trabecular meshwork. Transfixion restores communication between the anterior and posterior chamber, returning the iris to its normal position, while reducing tension.

Iridotomy by stab incision

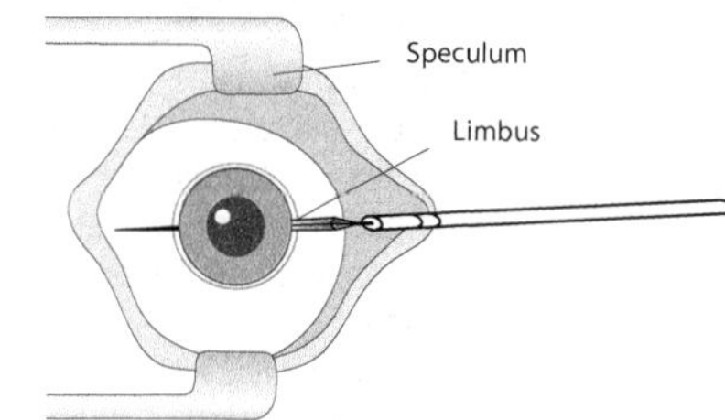

The physician slices through the iris to increase aqueous affected by pupillary block (66500); with transfixion as for iris bombe (66505).

ICD-10-CM Diagnostic Codes

	Code	Description
	A18.54	Tuberculous iridocyclitis
⇄	H20.012	Primary iridocyclitis, left eye
⇄	H20.022	Recurrent acute iridocyclitis, left eye
⇄	H20.032	Secondary infectious iridocyclitis, left eye
⇄	H20.042	Secondary noninfectious iridocyclitis, left eye
⇄	H20.052	Hypopyon, left eye
⇄	H20.12	Chronic iridocyclitis, left eye
⇄	H20.22	Lens-induced iridocyclitis, left eye
⇄	H20.812	Fuchs' heterochromic cyclitis, left eye
⇄	H20.822	Vogt-Koyanagi syndrome, left eye
⇄	H21.262	Iris atrophy (essential) (progressive), left eye
⇄	H21.42	Pupillary membranes, left eye
⇄	H40.212	Acute angle-closure glaucoma, left eye
❼⇄	H40.222	Chronic angle-closure glaucoma, left eye
⇄	H40.232	Intermittent angle-closure glaucoma, left eye
⇄	H40.242	Residual stage of angle-closure glaucoma, left eye
❼⇄	H40.41	Glaucoma secondary to eye inflammation, right eye
❼⇄	H40.51	Glaucoma secondary to other eye disorders, right eye
❼⇄	H40.52	Glaucoma secondary to other eye disorders, left eye
❼⇄	H40.53	Glaucoma secondary to other eye disorders, bilateral
⇄	H40.832	Aqueous misdirection, left eye
	H40.89	Other specified glaucoma
	Q13.1	Absence of iris

ICD-10-CM Coding Notes

For codes requiring a 7th character extension, refer to your ICD-10-CM book. Review the character descriptions and coding guidelines for proper selection. For some procedures, only certain characters will apply.

CCI Edits

Refer to Appendix A for CCI edits.

Facility RVUs ▯

Code	Work	PE Facility	MP	Total Facility
66500	3.83	7.49	0.29	11.61
66505	4.22	8.07	0.33	12.62

Non-facility RVUs ▯

Code	Work	PE Non-Facility	MP	Total Non-Facility
66500	3.83	7.49	0.29	11.61
66505	4.22	8.07	0.33	12.62

Modifiers (PAR) ▯

Code	Mod 50	Mod 51	Mod 62	Mod 66	Mod 80
66500	1	2	1	0	1
66505	1	2	0	0	1

Global Period

Code	Days
66500	090
66505	090

66600-66605

66600 Iridectomy, with corneoscleral or corneal section; for removal of lesion

66605 Iridectomy, with corneoscleral or corneal section; with cyclectomy

AMA Coding Notes

Surgical Procedures on the Eye and Ocular Adnexa

(For diagnostic and treatment ophthalmological services, see Medicine, Ophthalmology, and 92002 et seq)

(Do not report code 69990 in addition to codes 65091-68850)

AMA *CPT® Assistant* ▢

66600: Mar 21: 7

Plain English Description

The physician performs an iridectomy for removal of a lesion with a corneoscleral or corneal section. Iridectomy involves excising or removing a small, full thickness section of the iris. A local anesthetic is applied to the eye. An incision is made in the cornea or at the limbus of the sclera. The lesion on the iris is excised along with a margin of healthy tissue. In 66605, the physician performs an iridectomy with a cyclectomy. In this procedure the physician removes a portion of the ciliary body, which lies immediately behind the iris, along with a small full-thickness section of the iris. The ciliary body produces aqueous humor, the clear fluid that fills the front of the eye, and also controls accommodation by contracting and relaxing to allow the ability of the eye to focus on a close or distant object. Cyclectomy may be performed to remove a lesion on the ciliary body. A local anesthetic is applied to the eye. An incision is made in the cornea or at the limbus of the sclera. A section of iris is excised along with a portion of the underlying ciliary body.

Iridectomy, with corneoscleral or corneal section

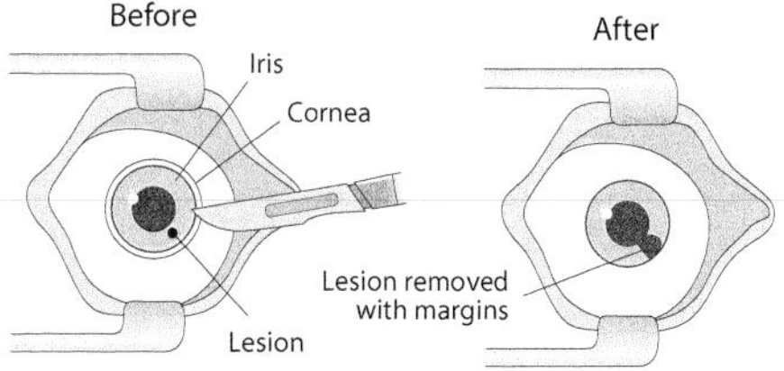

A full thickness section of the iris is removed for removal of lesion (66600); with cyclectomy (66605).

ICD-10-CM Diagnostic Codes

⇄	C69.41	Malignant neoplasm of right ciliary body
⇄	D09.21	Carcinoma in situ of right eye
⇄	D31.41	Benign neoplasm of right ciliary body
	D48.7	Neoplasm of uncertain behavior of other specified sites
⇄	H20.011	Primary iridocyclitis, right eye
⇄	H20.021	Recurrent acute iridocyclitis, right eye
⇄	H20.031	Secondary infectious iridocyclitis, right eye
⇄	H20.041	Secondary noninfectious iridocyclitis, right eye
⇄	H20.051	Hypopyon, right eye
⇄	H20.11	Chronic iridocyclitis, right eye
⇄	H20.21	Lens-induced iridocyclitis, right eye
⇄	H20.811	Fuchs' heterochromic cyclitis, right eye
⇄	H20.821	Vogt-Koyanagi syndrome, right eye
⇄	H21.261	Iris atrophy (essential) (progressive), right eye
⇄	H21.301	Idiopathic cysts of iris, ciliary body or anterior chamber, right eye
⇄	H21.311	Exudative cysts of iris or anterior chamber, right eye
⇄	H21.321	Implantation cysts of iris, ciliary body or anterior chamber, right eye
⇄	H21.41	Pupillary membranes, right eye
❼⇄	H40.41	Glaucoma secondary to eye inflammation, right eye

ICD-10-CM Coding Notes

For codes requiring a 7th character extension, refer to your ICD-10-CM book. Review the character descriptions and coding guidelines for proper selection. For some procedures, only certain characters will apply.

CCI Edits

Refer to Appendix A for CCI edits.

Facility RVUs ▢

Code	Work	PE Facility	MP	Total Facility
66600	10.12	15.71	0.77	26.60
66605	14.22	16.46	1.09	31.77

Non-facility RVUs ▢

Code	Work	PE Non-Facility	MP	Total Non-Facility
66600	10.12	15.71	0.77	26.60
66605	14.22	16.46	1.09	31.77

Modifiers (PAR) ▢

Code	Mod 50	Mod 51	Mod 62	Mod 66	Mod 80
66600	1	2	0	0	1
66605	1	2	0	0	1

Global Period

Code	Days
66600	090
66605	090

66625-66630

66625 Iridectomy, with corneoscleral or corneal section; peripheral for glaucoma (separate procedure)

66630 Iridectomy, with corneoscleral or corneal section; sector for glaucoma (separate procedure)

AMA Coding Notes

Surgical Procedures on the Eye and Ocular Adnexa

(For diagnostic and treatment ophthalmological services, see Medicine, Ophthalmology, and 92002 et seq)

(Do not report code 69990 in addition to codes 65091-68850)

Plain English Description

A portion of the iris is removed to treat glaucoma. Removing a portion of the iris allows fluid to drain from the anterior chamber to the posterior chamber, thereby reducing intraocular pressure (IOP). This procedure is typically performed for angle-closure glaucoma when laser iridotomy fails to achieve the necessary reduction in IOP. A topical anesthetic is applied to the eye. An incision is made in the cornea usually at the limbus where the cornea and sclera join. In 66625, a small full-thickness section of the iris is excised. In 66630, a larger full-thickness wedge-shaped section of the iris is excised. The corneal incision is typically not closed because it will close and heal on its own. Antibiotic drops may be applied along with a contact lens bandage and/or an eye patch.

Iridectomy, with corneoscleral/corneal section; sector for glaucoma

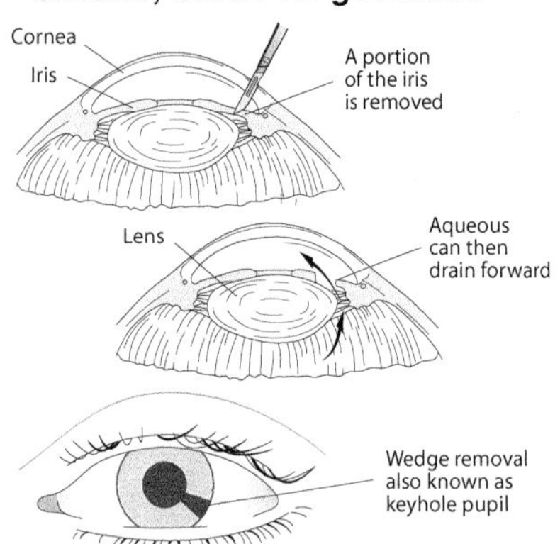

ICD-10-CM Diagnostic Codes

⇄	H40.062	Primary angle closure without glaucoma damage, left eye
❼⇄	H40.111	Primary open-angle glaucoma, right eye
❼⇄	H40.112	Primary open-angle glaucoma, left eye
❼⇄	H40.113	Primary open-angle glaucoma, bilateral
❼⇄	H40.122	Low-tension glaucoma, left eye
❼⇄	H40.132	Pigmentary glaucoma, left eye
❼⇄	H40.142	Capsular glaucoma with pseudoexfoliation of lens, left eye
⇄	H40.212	Acute angle-closure glaucoma, left eye
❼⇄	H40.222	Chronic angle-closure glaucoma, left eye
⇄	H40.232	Intermittent angle-closure glaucoma, left eye
⇄	H40.242	Residual stage of angle-closure glaucoma, left eye
❼⇄	H40.32	Glaucoma secondary to eye trauma, left eye
❼⇄	H40.42	Glaucoma secondary to eye inflammation, left eye
❼⇄	H40.52	Glaucoma secondary to other eye disorders, left eye
❼⇄	H40.61	Glaucoma secondary to drugs, right eye
❼⇄	H40.62	Glaucoma secondary to drugs, left eye
⇄	H40.832	Aqueous misdirection, left eye
	H40.89	Other specified glaucoma

ICD-10-CM Coding Notes

For codes requiring a 7th character extension, refer to your ICD-10-CM book. Review the character descriptions and coding guidelines for proper selection. For some procedures, only certain characters will apply.

CCI Edits

Refer to Appendix A for CCI edits.

Facility RVUs ▢

Code	Work	PE Facility	MP	Total Facility
66625	5.30	6.71	0.40	12.41
66630	7.28	8.56	0.56	16.40

Non-facility RVUs ▢

Code	Work	PE Non-Facility	MP	Total Non-Facility
66625	5.30	6.71	0.40	12.41
66630	7.28	8.56	0.56	16.40

Modifiers (PAR) ▢

Code	Mod 50	Mod 51	Mod 62	Mod 66	Mod 80
66625	1	2	0	0	1
66630	1	2	0	0	1

Global Period

Code	Days
66625	090
66630	090

66635

66635 Iridectomy, with corneoscleral or corneal section; optical (separate procedure)

(For coreoplasty by photocoagulation, use 66762)

AMA Coding Notes

Surgical Procedures on the Eye and Ocular Adnexa

(For diagnostic and treatment ophthalmological services, see Medicine, Ophthalmology, and 92002 et seq)

(Do not report code 69990 in addition to codes 65091-68850)

Plain English Description

The physician performs an optical iridectomy with corneoscleral or corneal section. Iridectomy involves excising or removing a small, full-thickness section of the iris. Optical iridectomy is performed to create an artificial pupil in the eye by removing a section of iris at the center of the eye. A local anesthetic is applied to the eye. An incision is made in the cornea or at the limbus of the sclera. Iris forceps or an iris hook is introduced through the corneal or limbal incision and the edge of the pupil is grasped. Iridectomy forceps are then introduced and the iris is grasped near the edge of the pupil and drawn out through the corneal or limbal incision. Iridectomy scissors are used to snip off a small fragment of iris. Excision of the iris continues in a radial fashion to form an artificial pupil at the center of the eye.

Iridectomy, with corneoscleral/corneal section; optical

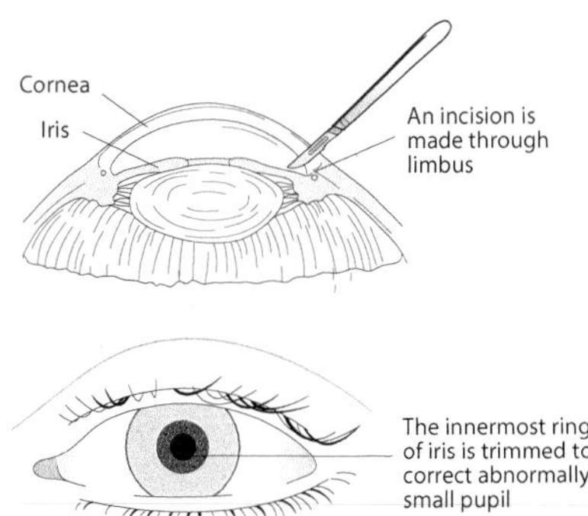
Cornea
Iris
An incision is made through limbus
The innermost ring of iris is trimmed to correct abnormally small pupil

ICD-10-CM Diagnostic Codes

⇄	H21.41	Pupillary membranes, right eye
⇄	H21.561	Pupillary abnormality, right eye
	H21.89	Other specified disorders of iris and ciliary body
	H22	Disorders of iris and ciliary body in diseases classified elsewhere
⇄	H31.401	Unspecified choroidal detachment, right eye
⇄	H31.411	Hemorrhagic choroidal detachment, right eye
⇄	H31.421	Serous choroidal detachment, right eye
⇄	H44.2A1	Degenerative myopia with choroidal neovascularization, right eye
⇄	H44.2A2	Degenerative myopia with choroidal neovascularization, left eye
⇄	H44.2A3	Degenerative myopia with choroidal neovascularization, bilateral eye

CCI Edits

Refer to Appendix A for CCI edits.

Facility RVUs

Code	Work	PE Facility	MP	Total Facility
66635	7.37	8.62	0.57	16.56

Non-facility RVUs

Code	Work	PE Non-Facility	MP	Total Non-Facility
66635	7.37	8.62	0.57	16.56

Modifiers (PAR)

Code	Mod 50	Mod 51	Mod 62	Mod 66	Mod 80
66635	1	2	0	0	1

Global Period

Code	Days
66635	090

66680

66680 Repair of iris, ciliary body (as for iridodialysis)

(For reposition or resection of uveal tissue with perforating wound of cornea or sclera, use 65285)

AMA Coding Notes

Surgical Procedures on the Eye and Ocular Adnexa

(For diagnostic and treatment ophthalmological services, see Medicine, Ophthalmology, and 92002 et seq)

(Do not report code 69990 in addition to codes 65091-68850)

AMA *CPT® Assistant* ▢

66680: Mar 21: 7

Plain English Description

An injury to the iris or ciliary body, such as one that results in iridodialysis, is repaired. Iridodialysis refers to separation of the iris root from the ciliary body or scleral spur. This results in an irregular D-shaped pupil. A miotic agent is used to constrict the pupil. A corneal incision is made and any synechiae are lysed to fully mobilization the iris leaflets. If the injury extends into the iris sphincter it is repaired first. The edges are carefully approximated to ensure a centrally located pupil. The remainder of the iris injury is repaired with sutures by passing the needle through a paracentesis tract in the anterior chamber and then through the iris. The needle passes through the proximal and distal leaflets of the iris and then out through the peripheral cornea. If iridodialysis has occurred the iris root is reattached to the ciliary body or scleral spur. The sutures are then tied and buried in the anterior chamber.

Repair of iris, ciliary body

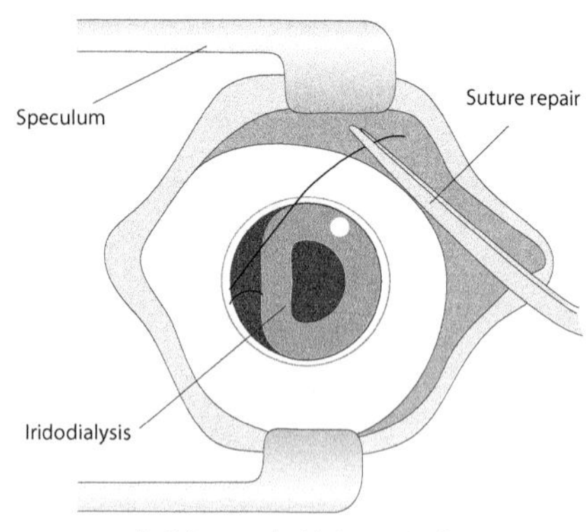

An injury to the iris is repaired.

ICD-10-CM Diagnostic Codes

⇄ H16.101 Unspecified superficial keratitis, right eye
⇄ H16.102 Unspecified superficial keratitis, left eye
⇄ H16.103 Unspecified superficial keratitis, bilateral
⇄ H18.11 Bullous keratopathy, right eye
⇄ H18.12 Bullous keratopathy, left eye
⇄ H18.13 Bullous keratopathy, bilateral
⇄ H21.211 Degeneration of chamber angle, right eye
⇄ H21.212 Degeneration of chamber angle, left eye
⇄ H21.213 Degeneration of chamber angle, bilateral
⇄ H21.221 Degeneration of ciliary body, right eye
⇄ H21.222 Degeneration of ciliary body, left eye
⇄ H21.223 Degeneration of ciliary body, bilateral
⇄ H21.231 Degeneration of iris (pigmentary), right eye
⇄ H21.232 Degeneration of iris (pigmentary), left eye
⇄ H21.233 Degeneration of iris (pigmentary), bilateral
⇄ H21.241 Degeneration of pupillary margin, right eye
⇄ H21.242 Degeneration of pupillary margin, left eye
⇄ H21.243 Degeneration of pupillary margin, bilateral
⇄ H21.251 Iridoschisis, right eye
⇄ H21.252 Iridoschisis, left eye
⇄ H21.253 Iridoschisis, bilateral
⇄ H21.261 Iris atrophy (essential) (progressive), right eye
⇄ H21.262 Iris atrophy (essential) (progressive), left eye
⇄ H21.263 Iris atrophy (essential) (progressive), bilateral
⇄ H21.271 Miotic pupillary cyst, right eye
⇄ H21.272 Miotic pupillary cyst, left eye
⇄ H21.273 Miotic pupillary cyst, bilateral
⇄ H21.502 Unspecified adhesions of iris, left eye
⇄ H21.511 Anterior synechiae (iris), right eye
⇄ H21.512 Anterior synechiae (iris), left eye
⇄ H21.513 Anterior synechiae (iris), bilateral
⇄ H21.531 Iridodialysis, right eye
⇄ H21.532 Iridodialysis, left eye
⇄ H21.533 Iridodialysis, bilateral
⇄ H21.541 Posterior synechiae (iris), right eye
⇄ H21.542 Posterior synechiae (iris), left eye
⇄ H21.543 Posterior synechiae (iris), bilateral
⇄ H21.561 Pupillary abnormality, right eye
⇄ H21.562 Pupillary abnormality, left eye
⇄ H21.563 Pupillary abnormality, bilateral
⇄ H27.01 Aphakia, right eye
⇄ H27.02 Aphakia, left eye
⇄ H27.03 Aphakia, bilateral
⇄ H43.01 Vitreous prolapse, right eye
⇄ H43.02 Vitreous prolapse, left eye
⇄ H43.03 Vitreous prolapse, bilateral
⇄ H43.311 Vitreous membranes and strands, right eye
⇄ H43.312 Vitreous membranes and strands, left eye
⇄ H43.313 Vitreous membranes and strands, bilateral
H57.00 Unspecified anomaly of pupillary function
H57.9 Unspecified disorder of eye and adnexa
❼⇄ S05.21 Ocular laceration and rupture with prolapse or loss of intraocular tissue, right eye
❼⇄ S05.22 Ocular laceration and rupture with prolapse or loss of intraocular tissue, left eye
❼ T85.21 Breakdown (mechanical) of intraocular lens
❼ T85.22 Displacement of intraocular lens
❼ T85.29 Other mechanical complication of intraocular lens
⇄ T86.8401 Corneal transplant rejection, right eye
⇄ T86.8402 Corneal transplant rejection, left eye
⇄ T86.8403 Corneal transplant rejection, bilateral
⇄ T86.8411 Corneal transplant failure, right eye
⇄ T86.8412 Corneal transplant failure, left eye
⇄ T86.8413 Corneal transplant failure, bilateral

ICD-10-CM Coding Notes

For codes requiring a 7th character extension, refer to your ICD-10-CM book. Review the character descriptions and coding guidelines for proper selection. For some procedures, only certain characters will apply.

CCI Edits

Refer to Appendix A for CCI edits.

Facility RVUs ▢

Code	Work	PE Facility	MP	Total Facility
66680	6.39	8.26	0.50	15.15

Non-facility RVUs ▢

Code	Work	PE Non-Facility	MP	Total Non-Facility
66680	6.39	8.26	0.50	15.15

Modifiers (PAR) ▢

Code	Mod 50	Mod 51	Mod 62	Mod 66	Mod 80
66680	1	2	1	0	1

Global Period

Code	Days
66680	090

● New ▲ Revised ✚ Add On ⊘Modifier 51 Exempt ★Telemedicine ▢ CPT QuickRef ⁄ FDA Pending ⇄ Laterality ❼ Seventh Character ♂Male ♀Female

66682

66682 Suture of iris, ciliary body (separate procedure) with retrieval of suture through small incision (eg, McCannel suture)

AMA Coding Notes

Surgical Procedures on the Eye and Ocular Adnexa

(For diagnostic and treatment ophthalmological services, see Medicine, Ophthalmology, and 92002 et seq)

(Do not report code 69990 in addition to codes 65091-68850)

AMA *CPT® Assistant*

66682: Mar 21: 7

Plain English Description

A small incision is made in the conjunctiva at the limbus adjacent to the site of injury in the iris and/or ciliary body. Suture material is threaded through the first needle. The needle is then inserted at a point 180 degrees from the site of the injury in the iris. The needle is passed through the cornea, anterior chamber, iris base, iris root and sclera exiting at the site of the injury. Several centimeters of suture are pulled through the wound. The suture material is left attached to the needle. The needle is then retracted back into the anterior chamber and a second pass is made through the iris root on the other side of the defect. The needle and suture material are again brought through the sclera a short distance from the first exit site. The two ends of the suture material are then tied over the sclera and the knot is buried. The conjunctival incision is closed. This type of suture repair may be referred to as a McCannel double arm suture.

Repair of iris, ciliary body with retrieval of suture through small incision (eg, McCannel suture)

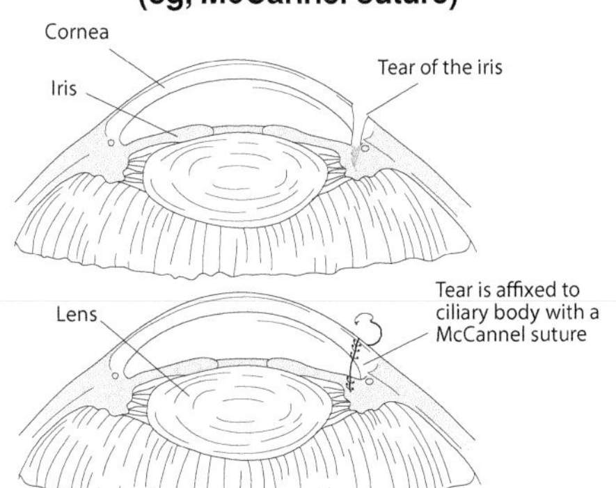
Cornea
Iris
Tear of the iris
Lens
Tear is affixed to ciliary body with a McCannel suture

ICD-10-CM Diagnostic Codes

- ⇄ H18.11 Bullous keratopathy, right eye
- ⇄ H21.211 Degeneration of chamber angle, right eye
- ⇄ H21.221 Degeneration of ciliary body, right eye
- ⇄ H21.231 Degeneration of iris (pigmentary), right eye
- ⇄ H21.241 Degeneration of pupillary margin, right eye
- ⇄ H21.261 Iris atrophy (essential) (progressive), right eye
- ⇄ H21.271 Miotic pupillary cyst, right eye
- ⇄ H21.531 Iridodialysis, right eye
- ⇄ H21.541 Posterior synechiae (iris), right eye
- ⇄ H21.561 Pupillary abnormality, right eye
- ⇄ H25.11 Age-related nuclear cataract, right eye
- ⇄ H26.031 Infantile and juvenile nuclear cataract, right eye
- ⇄ H27.01 Aphakia, right eye
- ⇄ H27.111 Subluxation of lens, right eye
- ⇄ H27.121 Anterior dislocation of lens, right eye
- ⇄ H27.131 Posterior dislocation of lens, right eye
- ⇄ H43.01 Vitreous prolapse, right eye
- ➐⇄ S05.01 Injury of conjunctiva and corneal abrasion without foreign body, right eye
- ➐⇄ S05.11 Contusion of eyeball and orbital tissues, right eye
- ➐⇄ S05.21 Ocular laceration and rupture with prolapse or loss of intraocular tissue, right eye
- ➐⇄ S05.51 Penetrating wound with foreign body of right eyeball
- ➐⇄ S05.61 Penetrating wound without foreign body of right eyeball
- ➐ T85.21 Breakdown (mechanical) of intraocular lens
- ➐ T85.22 Displacement of intraocular lens
- ➐ T85.29 Other mechanical complication of intraocular lens

ICD-10-CM Coding Notes

For codes requiring a 7th character extension, refer to your ICD-10-CM book. Review the character descriptions and coding guidelines for proper selection. For some procedures, only certain characters will apply.

CCI Edits

Refer to Appendix A for CCI edits.

Facility RVUs

Code	Work	PE Facility	MP	Total Facility
66682	7.33	13.11	0.57	21.01

Non-facility RVUs

Code	Work	PE Non-Facility	MP	Total Non-Facility
66682	7.33	13.11	0.57	21.01

Modifiers (PAR)

Code	Mod 50	Mod 51	Mod 62	Mod 66	Mod 80
66682	1	2	0	0	1

Global Period

Code	Days
66682	090

66700

66700 Ciliary body destruction; diathermy

AMA Coding Notes

Surgical Procedures on the Eye and Ocular Adnexa

(For diagnostic and treatment ophthalmological services, see Medicine, Ophthalmology, and 92002 et seq)

(Do not report code 69990 in addition to codes 65091-68850)

Plain English Description

The ciliary body is located just behind the iris. The two primary functions of the ciliary body include production of aqueous humor, which is the clear fluid that fills the anterior chamber, and accommodation, which changes the shape of the crystalline lens allowing the eye to focus on near or far objects. Destruction of the ciliary body is performed to treat glaucoma that has failed to respond to medication and other more conservative surgical procedures. Destruction of the ciliary body reduces inflow of aqueous to the anterior chamber thereby reducing intraocular pressure. A local periocular anesthetic is administered. A lid speculum is placed on the eye to hold the eyelids open. Diathermy, also referred to as electrodiathermy, uses an extra-ocular transcleral or transconjunctival approach. Alternatively, a scleral flap may be elevated to access the ciliary body. The ciliary body is destroyed using a heat probe.

Ciliary body destruction; diathermy

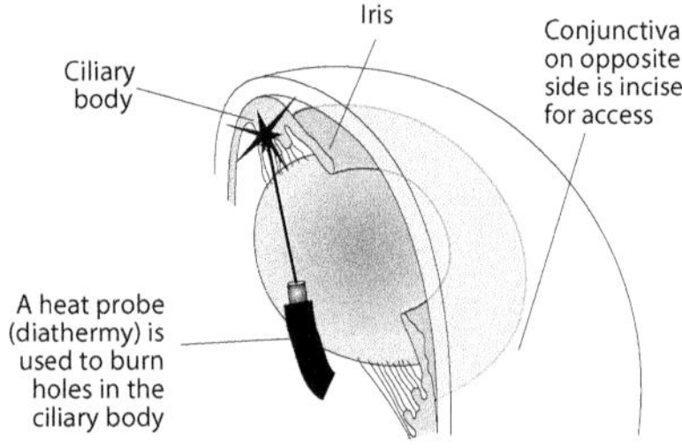

ICD-10-CM Diagnostic Codes

	Code	Description
⇄	H21.0	Hyphema
	H21.1	Other vascular disorders of iris and ciliary body
	H21.89	Other specified disorders of iris and ciliary body
	H22	Disorders of iris and ciliary body in diseases classified elsewhere
⇄	H40.022	Open angle with borderline findings, high risk, left eye
⇄	H40.062	Primary angle closure without glaucoma damage, left eye
❼⇄	H40.111	Primary open-angle glaucoma, right eye
❼⇄	H40.112	Primary open-angle glaucoma, left eye
❼⇄	H40.113	Primary open-angle glaucoma, bilateral
❼⇄	H40.122	Low-tension glaucoma, left eye
❼⇄	H40.132	Pigmentary glaucoma, left eye
❼⇄	H40.142	Capsular glaucoma with pseudoexfoliation of lens, left eye
⇄	H40.152	Residual stage of open-angle glaucoma, left eye
❼⇄	H40.222	Chronic angle-closure glaucoma, left eye
⇄	H40.242	Residual stage of angle-closure glaucoma, left eye
❼⇄	H40.32	Glaucoma secondary to eye trauma, left eye
❼⇄	H40.42	Glaucoma secondary to eye inflammation, left eye
❼⇄	H40.52	Glaucoma secondary to other eye disorders, left eye
❼⇄	H40.62	Glaucoma secondary to drugs, left eye
⇄	H40.822	Hypersecretion glaucoma, left eye
⇄	H40.832	Aqueous misdirection, left eye
	H40.89	Other specified glaucoma
	Q13.4	Other congenital corneal malformations
	Q13.81	Rieger's anomaly
	Q13.9	Congenital malformation of anterior segment of eye, unspecified
	Q15.0	Congenital glaucoma

ICD-10-CM Coding Notes

For codes requiring a 7th character extension, refer to your ICD-10-CM book. Review the character descriptions and coding guidelines for proper selection. For some procedures, only certain characters will apply.

CCI Edits

Refer to Appendix A for CCI edits.

Facility RVUs ▢

Code	Work	PE Facility	MP	Total Facility
66700	5.14	5.79	0.40	11.33

Non-facility RVUs ▢

Code	Work	PE Non-Facility	MP	Total Non-Facility
66700	5.14	7.64	0.40	13.18

Modifiers (PAR) ▢

Code	Mod 50	Mod 51	Mod 62	Mod 66	Mod 80
66700	1	2	0	0	0

Global Period

Code	Days
66700	090

66710-66711

66710 Ciliary body destruction; cyclophotocoagulation, transscleral

66711 Ciliary body destruction; cyclophotocoagulation, endoscopic, without concomitant removal of crystalline lens

(For endoscopic cyclophotocoagulation performed at same encounter as extracapsular cataract removal with intraocular lens insertion, see 66987, 66988)

(Do not report 66711 in conjunction with 66990)

AMA Coding Notes

Surgical Procedures on the Eye and Ocular Adnexa

(For diagnostic and treatment ophthalmological services, see Medicine, Ophthalmology, and 92002 et seq)

(Do not report code 69990 in addition to codes 65091-68850)

AMA *CPT® Assistant* ▯

66710: Mar 05: 20, Sep 05: 5

66711: Mar 05: 20, Sep 05: 5, 12, Dec 19: 6

Plain English Description

The ciliary body is located just behind the iris and produces aqueous humor, the clear fluid that fills the anterior chamber, as well as accommodation, which changes the shape of the crystalline lens allowing the eye to focus on near or far objects. Ciliary body destruction is performed to treat glaucoma that has failed to respond to medication or conservative outflow surgical procedures. Partial destruction of the ciliary body reduces inflow of aqueous to the anterior chamber thereby reducing intraocular pressure. For eyes with little visual potential, the ciliary body may be destroyed using cyclophotocoagulation via an extraocular transscleral approach (66710). A local periocular anesthetic is administered. A lid speculum is placed on the eye to hold the eyelids open. The laser probe is positioned over the ciliary body. No incisions are made. The laser energy travels through the sclera to the ciliary body and partially destroys it, although damage may be done to adjacent tissues. For eyes with more visual potential, endoscopic cyclophotocoagulation (ECP) is used (66711). Viscoelastic material is injected into the anterior chamber over the pupil and lens and under the iris to allow better visualization. Through a limbal or pars plana incision, a laser probe is inserted that emits pulsed, continuous wave energy to treat each ciliary process until it shrinks and turns white while viewing continuously on the monitor. The probe combines a laser diode emitting pulsed wave energy, a light source, a laser aiming beam, and video camera imaging. Up to 180 degrees of ciliary processes can be photocoagulated through one incision. Up to 360 degrees may be treated. A second incision may be made to allow access to another section of the ciliary body and the processes are destroyed in the same manner until a sufficient amount has been destroyed to reduce intraocular pressure with enough ciliary body preserved to allow some production of aqueous. The viscoelastic material is removed by irrigation and aspiration. A balanced saline solution is injected to replace the viscoelastic material. The incisions are checked for fluid leakage and repaired with sutures as needed.

Ciliary body destruction; cyclophotocoagulation

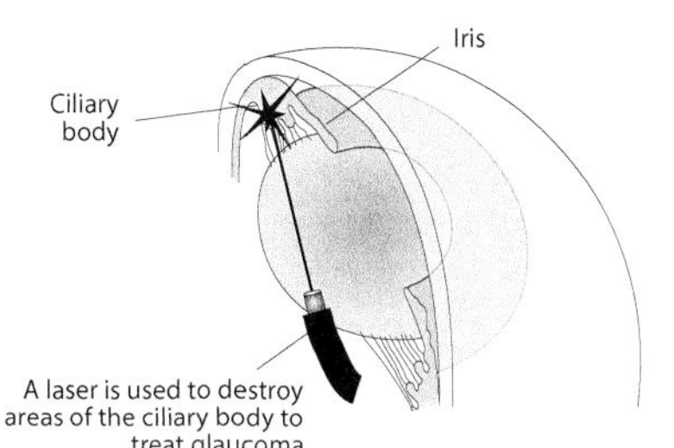

Transscleral (66710), or endoscopic (66711) approach

ICD-10-CM Diagnostic Codes

⇄	H21.01	Hyphema, right eye
⇄	H21.02	Hyphema, left eye
⇄	H21.03	Hyphema, bilateral
	H21.1	Other vascular disorders of iris and ciliary body
⇄	H21.541	Posterior synechiae (iris), right eye
⇄	H21.542	Posterior synechiae (iris), left eye
⇄	H21.543	Posterior synechiae (iris), bilateral
⇄	H40.021	Open angle with borderline findings, high risk, right eye
⇄	H40.022	Open angle with borderline findings, high risk, left eye
⇄	H40.023	Open angle with borderline findings, high risk, bilateral
⇄	H40.031	Anatomical narrow angle, right eye
⇄	H40.032	Anatomical narrow angle, left eye
⇄	H40.033	Anatomical narrow angle, bilateral
⇄	H40.061	Primary angle closure without glaucoma damage, right eye
⇄	H40.062	Primary angle closure without glaucoma damage, left eye
⇄	H40.063	Primary angle closure without glaucoma damage, bilateral
❼	H40.10	Unspecified open-angle glaucoma
❼⇄	H40.111	Primary open-angle glaucoma, right eye
❼⇄	H40.112	Primary open-angle glaucoma, left eye
❼⇄	H40.113	Primary open-angle glaucoma, bilateral
❼⇄	H40.121	Low-tension glaucoma, right eye
❼⇄	H40.122	Low-tension glaucoma, left eye
❼⇄	H40.123	Low-tension glaucoma, bilateral
❼⇄	H40.131	Pigmentary glaucoma, right eye
❼⇄	H40.132	Pigmentary glaucoma, left eye
❼⇄	H40.133	Pigmentary glaucoma, bilateral
❼⇄	H40.141	Capsular glaucoma with pseudoexfoliation of lens, right eye
❼⇄	H40.142	Capsular glaucoma with pseudoexfoliation of lens, left eye
❼⇄	H40.143	Capsular glaucoma with pseudoexfoliation of lens, bilateral
⇄	H40.151	Residual stage of open-angle glaucoma, right eye
⇄	H40.152	Residual stage of open-angle glaucoma, left eye
⇄	H40.153	Residual stage of open-angle glaucoma, bilateral
❼	H40.20	Unspecified primary angle-closure glaucoma
❼⇄	H40.221	Chronic angle-closure glaucoma, right eye
❼⇄	H40.222	Chronic angle-closure glaucoma, left eye
❼⇄	H40.223	Chronic angle-closure glaucoma, bilateral
⇄	H40.241	Residual stage of angle-closure glaucoma, right eye
⇄	H40.242	Residual stage of angle-closure glaucoma, left eye
⇄	H40.243	Residual stage of angle-closure glaucoma, bilateral
❼⇄	H40.31	Glaucoma secondary to eye trauma, right eye
❼⇄	H40.32	Glaucoma secondary to eye trauma, left eye
❼⇄	H40.33	Glaucoma secondary to eye trauma, bilateral
❼⇄	H40.41	Glaucoma secondary to eye inflammation, right eye
❼⇄	H40.42	Glaucoma secondary to eye inflammation, left eye
❼⇄	H40.43	Glaucoma secondary to eye inflammation, bilateral
❼⇄	H40.51	Glaucoma secondary to other eye disorders, right eye
❼⇄	H40.52	Glaucoma secondary to other eye disorders, left eye
❼⇄	H40.53	Glaucoma secondary to other eye disorders, bilateral
⇄	H40.821	Hypersecretion glaucoma, right eye
⇄	H40.822	Hypersecretion glaucoma, left eye
⇄	H40.823	Hypersecretion glaucoma, bilateral
⇄	H40.831	Aqueous misdirection, right eye
⇄	H40.832	Aqueous misdirection, left eye
⇄	H40.833	Aqueous misdirection, bilateral
	H40.89	Other specified glaucoma
	H50.51	Esophoria
	Q13.4	Other congenital corneal malformations
	Q13.81	Rieger's anomaly
	Q13.9	Congenital malformation of anterior segment of eye, unspecified
	Q15.0	Congenital glaucoma

ICD-10-CM Coding Notes

For codes requiring a 7th character extension, refer to your ICD-10-CM book. Review the character descriptions and coding guidelines for proper selection. For some procedures, only certain characters will apply.

CCI Edits

Refer to Appendix A for CCI edits.

Facility RVUs

Code	Work	PE Facility	MP	Total Facility
66710	5.14	5.79	0.40	11.33
66711	5.62	8.60	0.42	14.64

Non-facility RVUs

Code	Work	PE Non-Facility	MP	Total Non-Facility
66710	5.14	7.38	0.40	12.92
66711	5.62	8.60	0.42	14.64

Modifiers (PAR)

Code	Mod 50	Mod 51	Mod 62	Mod 66	Mod 80
66710	1	2	0	0	1
66711	1	3	0	0	1

Global Period

Code	Days
66710	090
66711	090

66720

66720 Ciliary body destruction; cryotherapy

AMA Coding Notes

Surgical Procedures on the Eye and Ocular Adnexa

(For diagnostic and treatment ophthalmological services, see Medicine, Ophthalmology, and 92002 et seq)

(Do not report code 69990 in addition to codes 65091-68850)

Plain English Description

The ciliary body is located just behind the iris. The two primary functions of the ciliary body include production of aqueous humor, which is the clear fluid that fills the anterior chamber, and accommodation, which changes the shape of the crystalline lens allowing the eye to focus on near or far objects. Destruction of the ciliary body is performed to treat glaucoma that has failed to respond to medication and other more conservative surgical procedures. Partial destruction of the ciliary body reduces inflow of aqueous to the anterior chamber thereby reducing intraocular pressure. A local periocular anesthetic is administered. A lid speculum is placed on the eye to hold the eyelids open. Cryotherapy nonselectively destroys ciliary body tissue. A cryoprobe is used to rapidly freeze part of the ciliary body. The tissue is then slowly thawed. The freeze-thaw cycle is repeated until the desired amount of ciliary body tissue has been destroyed.

Ciliary body destruction; cryotherapy

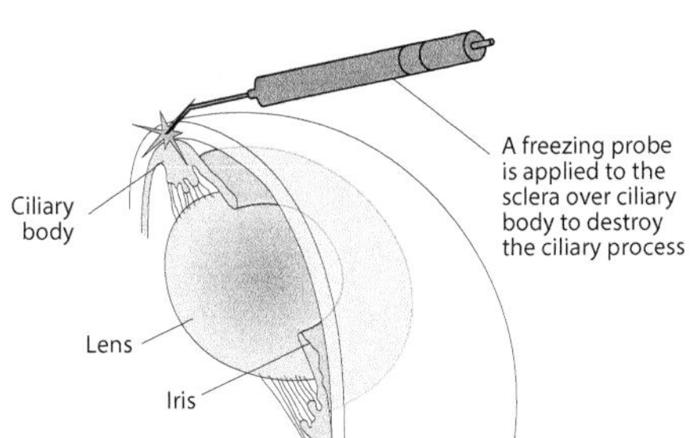
Ciliary body
Lens
Iris
A freezing probe is applied to the sclera over ciliary body to destroy the ciliary process

ICD-10-CM Diagnostic Codes

⇄	H21.01	Hyphema, right eye
	H21.1	Other vascular disorders of iris and ciliary body
⇄	H40.022	Open angle with borderline findings, high risk, left eye
⇄	H40.062	Primary angle closure without glaucoma damage, left eye
➐	H40.10	Unspecified open-angle glaucoma
➐⇄	H40.111	Primary open-angle glaucoma, right eye
➐⇄	H40.112	Primary open-angle glaucoma, left eye
➐⇄	H40.113	Primary open-angle glaucoma, bilateral
➐⇄	H40.122	Low-tension glaucoma, left eye
➐⇄	H40.132	Pigmentary glaucoma, left eye
➐⇄	H40.142	Capsular glaucoma with pseudoexfoliation of lens, left eye
⇄	H40.152	Residual stage of open-angle glaucoma, left eye
➐	H40.20	Unspecified primary angle-closure glaucoma
⇄	H40.212	Acute angle-closure glaucoma, left eye
➐⇄	H40.222	Chronic angle-closure glaucoma, left eye
⇄	H40.232	Intermittent angle-closure glaucoma, left eye
⇄	H40.242	Residual stage of angle-closure glaucoma, left eye
➐⇄	H40.32	Glaucoma secondary to eye trauma, left eye
➐⇄	H40.42	Glaucoma secondary to eye inflammation, left eye
➐⇄	H40.52	Glaucoma secondary to other eye disorders, left eye
➐⇄	H40.62	Glaucoma secondary to drugs, left eye
⇄	H40.822	Hypersecretion glaucoma, left eye
⇄	H40.832	Aqueous misdirection, left eye
	H40.89	Other specified glaucoma
	Q13.4	Other congenital corneal malformations
	Q13.81	Rieger's anomaly
	Q15.0	Congenital glaucoma

ICD-10-CM Coding Notes

For codes requiring a 7th character extension, refer to your ICD-10-CM book. Review the character descriptions and coding guidelines for proper selection. For some procedures, only certain characters will apply.

CCI Edits

Refer to Appendix A for CCI edits.

Facility RVUs ▯

Code	Work	PE Facility	MP	Total Facility
66720	4.75	6.74	0.37	11.86

Non-facility RVUs ▯

Code	Work	PE Non-Facility	MP	Total Non-Facility
66720	4.75	8.48	0.37	13.60

Modifiers (PAR) ▯

Code	Mod 50	Mod 51	Mod 62	Mod 66	Mod 80
66720	1	2	0	0	1

Global Period

Code	Days
66720	090

66740

66740 Ciliary body destruction; cyclodialysis

AMA Coding Notes

Surgical Procedures on the Eye and Ocular Adnexa

(For diagnostic and treatment ophthalmological services, see Medicine, Ophthalmology, and 92002 et seq)

(Do not report code 69990 in addition to codes 65091-68850)

Plain English Description

The ciliary body is located just behind the iris. The two primary functions of the ciliary body include the production of aqueous humor, which is the clear fluid that fills the anterior chamber, and accommodation, which changes the shape of the crystalline lens allowing the eye to focus on near or far objects. Destruction of the ciliary body is performed to treat glaucoma that has failed to respond to medication and other more conservative surgical procedures. A local periocular anesthetic is administered. A lid speculum is placed on the eye to hold the eyelids open. Cyclodialysis involves separating the ciliary body from the scleral spur. This creates a communication between the anterior chamber and suprachoroidal space that allows aqueous to flow out of the anterior chamber thereby reducing intraocular pressure.

Ciliary body destruction; cyclodialysis

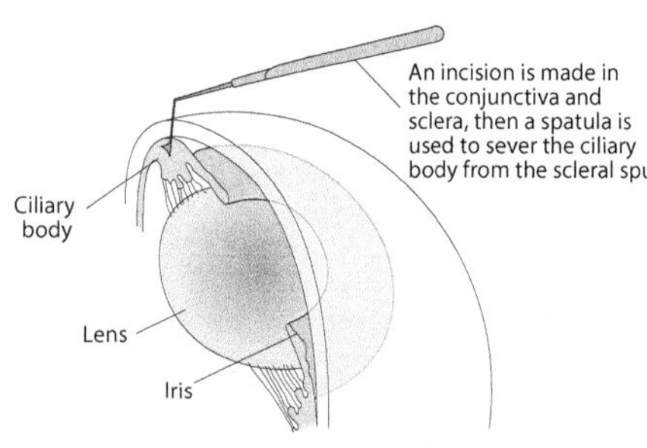
An incision is made in the conjunctiva and sclera, then a spatula is used to sever the ciliary body from the scleral spur
Ciliary body
Lens
Iris

ICD-10-CM Diagnostic Codes

⇄	H21.01	Hyphema, right eye
	H21.1	Other vascular disorders of iris and ciliary body
⇄	H40.021	Open angle with borderline findings, high risk, right eye
⇄	H40.061	Primary angle closure without glaucoma damage, right eye
❼	H40.10	Unspecified open-angle glaucoma
❼⇄	H40.111	Primary open-angle glaucoma, right eye
❼⇄	H40.112	Primary open-angle glaucoma, left eye
❼⇄	H40.113	Primary open-angle glaucoma, bilateral
❼⇄	H40.121	Low-tension glaucoma, right eye
❼⇄	H40.131	Pigmentary glaucoma, right eye
⇄	H40.151	Residual stage of open-angle glaucoma, right eye
⇄	H40.211	Acute angle-closure glaucoma, right eye
❼⇄	H40.221	Chronic angle-closure glaucoma, right eye
⇄	H40.231	Intermittent angle-closure glaucoma, right eye
⇄	H40.241	Residual stage of angle-closure glaucoma, right eye
❼⇄	H40.41	Glaucoma secondary to eye inflammation, right eye
❼⇄	H40.51	Glaucoma secondary to other eye disorders, right eye
⇄	H40.831	Aqueous misdirection, right eye
	H40.89	Other specified glaucoma
	Q13.4	Other congenital corneal malformations
	Q13.81	Rieger's anomaly
	Q13.9	Congenital malformation of anterior segment of eye, unspecified
	Q15.0	Congenital glaucoma

ICD-10-CM Coding Notes

For codes requiring a 7th character extension, refer to your ICD-10-CM book. Review the character descriptions and coding guidelines for proper selection. For some procedures, only certain characters will apply.

CCI Edits

Refer to Appendix A for CCI edits.

Facility RVUs ▯

Code	Work	PE Facility	MP	Total Facility
66740	5.14	5.79	0.40	11.33

Non-facility RVUs ▯

Code	Work	PE Non-Facility	MP	Total Non-Facility
66740	5.14	7.27	0.40	12.81

Modifiers (PAR) ▯

Code	Mod 50	Mod 51	Mod 62	Mod 66	Mod 80
66740	1	2	0	0	1

Global Period

Code	Days
66740	090

66761

66761 Iridotomy/iridectomy by laser surgery (eg, for glaucoma) (per session)

AMA Coding Notes

Surgical Procedures on the Eye and Ocular Adnexa

(For diagnostic and treatment ophthalmological services, see Medicine, Ophthalmology, and 92002 et seq)

(Do not report code 69990 in addition to codes 65091-68850)

AMA *CPT® Assistant* ▯

66761: Mar 98: 7

Plain English Description

Iridotomy or iridectomy is performed to treat closed angle glaucoma. An intraocular pressure lowering eye drop is administered one hour prior to surgery and again immediately prior to surgery. Eye drops are administered to constrict the pupil. The patient is seated at the laser and an iridotomy contact lens is placed on the upper part of the front of the eye to magnify the lens and improve accuracy of laser beam projection. The laser is aimed at the 11 o'clock or 1 o'clock position and laser pulses are applied to the iris until a hole is formed. Once the laser has completely penetrated the iris, aqueous fluid begins to flow out of the anterior chamber. Following the laser procedure, the anterior chamber angle is examined using a gonioscope to ensure that the hole is wide enough to allow drainage of aqueous and lower the intraocular pressure. Multiple sessions may be required to ensure adequate drainage of aqueous and each session is reported separately.

Iridectomy/iridotomy, by laser (eg, for glaucoma)

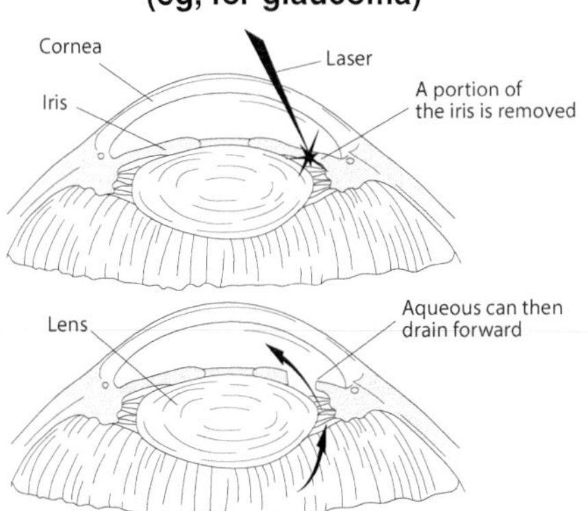

ICD-10-CM Diagnostic Codes

⇄	H40.022	Open angle with borderline findings, high risk, left eye
⇄	H40.062	Primary angle closure without glaucoma damage, left eye
❼⇄	H40.111	Primary open-angle glaucoma, right eye
❼⇄	H40.112	Primary open-angle glaucoma, left eye
❼⇄	H40.113	Primary open-angle glaucoma, bilateral
❼⇄	H40.122	Low-tension glaucoma, left eye
❼⇄	H40.132	Pigmentary glaucoma, left eye
❼⇄	H40.142	Capsular glaucoma with pseudoexfoliation of lens, left eye
⇄	H40.152	Residual stage of open-angle glaucoma, left eye
⇄	H40.212	Acute angle-closure glaucoma, left eye
❼⇄	H40.222	Chronic angle-closure glaucoma, left eye
⇄	H40.242	Residual stage of angle-closure glaucoma, left eye
❼⇄	H40.42	Glaucoma secondary to eye inflammation, left eye
❼⇄	H40.52	Glaucoma secondary to other eye disorders, left eye
⇄	H40.832	Aqueous misdirection, left eye
	H40.89	Other specified glaucoma
	H53.71	Glare sensitivity
	H53.72	Impaired contrast sensitivity
	H53.8	Other visual disturbances
	H53.9	Unspecified visual disturbance
⇄	H57.12	Ocular pain, left eye
	Q13.4	Other congenital corneal malformations
	Q13.81	Rieger's anomaly
	Q13.9	Congenital malformation of anterior segment of eye, unspecified
	Q15.0	Congenital glaucoma

ICD-10-CM Coding Notes

For codes requiring a 7th character extension, refer to your ICD-10-CM book. Review the character descriptions and coding guidelines for proper selection. For some procedures, only certain characters will apply.

CCI Edits

Refer to Appendix A for CCI edits.

Pub 100

66761: Pub 100-03, 1, 140.5

Facility RVUs ▯

Code	Work	PE Facility	MP	Total Facility
66761	3.00	3.62	0.23	6.85

Non-facility RVUs ▯

Code	Work	PE Non-Facility	MP	Total Non-Facility
66761	3.00	5.54	0.23	8.77

Modifiers (PAR) ▯

Code	Mod 50	Mod 51	Mod 62	Mod 66	Mod 80
66761	1	2	0	0	1

Global Period

Code	Days
66761	010

66762

66762 Iridoplasty by photocoagulation (1 or more sessions) (eg, for improvement of vision, for widening of anterior chamber angle)

AMA Coding Notes

Surgical Procedures on the Eye and Ocular Adnexa

(For diagnostic and treatment ophthalmological services, see Medicine, Ophthalmology, and 92002 et seq)

(Do not report code 69990 in addition to codes 65091-68850)

AMA *CPT® Assistant* ▢

66762: Mar 98: 7

Plain English Description

This procedure is performed to treat closed angle glaucoma and plateau iris. Eye drops are administered to constrict the pupil. The patient is seated at the laser and the physician carefully inspects the iris for areas of pigmentation at the periphery. Multiple laser burns are then placed around the periphery of the iris in the pigmented areas if possible. As the laser burns are placed the physician observes the iris, which will contract as tissue shrinks in response to the laser treatment. Twenty or more laser burns may be required to open the anterior chamber angle allowing better drainage of aqueous. Following the laser procedure, the anterior chamber angle is examined using a gonioscope to ensure that it wide enough to allow drainage of aqueous and lower intraocular pressure.

Iridoplasty by photocoagulation

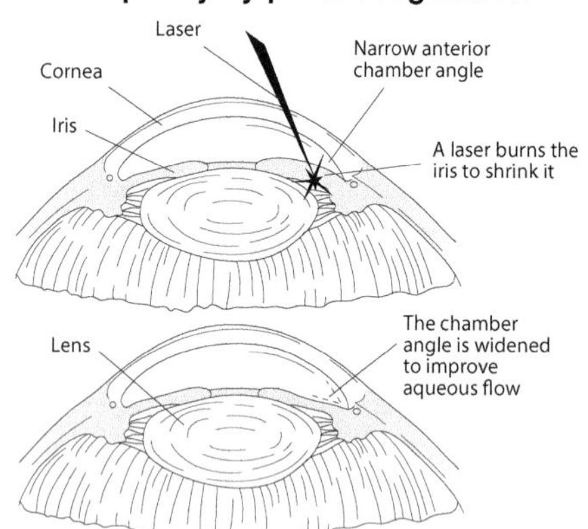

ICD-10-CM Diagnostic Codes

⇄ H18.221 Idiopathic corneal edema, right eye
⇄ H21.501 Unspecified adhesions of iris, right eye
⇄ H21.521 Goniosynechiae, right eye
⇄ H21.531 Iridodialysis, right eye
⇄ H21.551 Recession of chamber angle, right eye
⇄ H21.561 Pupillary abnormality, right eye
H21.82 Plateau iris syndrome (post-iridectomy) (postprocedural)
⇄ H40.011 Open angle with borderline findings, low risk, right eye
⇄ H40.031 Anatomical narrow angle, right eye
❼⇄ H40.111 Primary open-angle glaucoma, right eye
❼⇄ H40.112 Primary open-angle glaucoma, left eye
❼⇄ H40.113 Primary open-angle glaucoma, bilateral
❼⇄ H40.121 Low-tension glaucoma, right eye
❼⇄ H40.131 Pigmentary glaucoma, right eye
⇄ H40.151 Residual stage of open-angle glaucoma, right eye
⇄ H40.211 Acute angle-closure glaucoma, right eye
❼⇄ H40.221 Chronic angle-closure glaucoma, right eye
⇄ H40.231 Intermittent angle-closure glaucoma, right eye
⇄ H40.831 Aqueous misdirection, right eye
H57.03 Miosis
Q15.0 Congenital glaucoma

ICD-10-CM Coding Notes

For codes requiring a 7th character extension, refer to your ICD-10-CM book. Review the character descriptions and coding guidelines for proper selection. For some procedures, only certain characters will apply.

CCI Edits

Refer to Appendix A for CCI edits.

Facility RVUs ▢

Code	Work	PE Facility	MP	Total Facility
66762	5.38	6.49	0.41	12.28

Non-facility RVUs ▢

Code	Work	PE Non-Facility	MP	Total Non-Facility
66762	5.38	8.12	0.41	13.91

Modifiers (PAR) ▢

Code	Mod 50	Mod 51	Mod 62	Mod 66	Mod 80
66762	1	2	0	0	1

Global Period

Code	Days
66762	090

66770

66770 Destruction of cyst or lesion iris or ciliary body (nonexcisional procedure)

(For excision lesion iris, ciliary body, see 66600, 66605; for removal of epithelial downgrowth, use 65900)

(For unlisted procedures on iris, ciliary body, use 66999)

AMA Coding Notes

Surgical Procedures on the Eye and Ocular Adnexa

(For diagnostic and treatment ophthalmological services, see Medicine, Ophthalmology, and 92002 et seq)

(Do not report code 69990 in addition to codes 65091-68850)

Plain English Description

Cysts or lesions of the iris or ciliary body can be primary (no known cause) or secondary (following trauma). Asymptomatic cysts and lesions are usually found during a routine eye examination and require no treatment. Cysts or lesions that block the visual axis (pupil) can cause secondary glaucoma (increased intraocular pressure) and/or loss of visual acuity. The most common site of cysts or lesions is the pigmented iris epithelium from the central pupillary margin to the peripheral iris. Less commonly a cyst or lesion will arise from the stroma, which is lined with non-keratinized squamous epithelium. Infants and children are more likely to have cysts or lesions in the stromal area. Destruction of a cyst or lesion can be accomplished under local or general anesthesia. Cysts are usually treated by inserting a fine-gauge needle into the base, aspirating the fluid and replacing the volume with ethyl alcohol (ETOH) x 1 minute. The ETOH solution is then aspirated back out allowing the cyst to collapse. Cysts and lesions may also be treated using endodiathermy (heat), cryotherapy (cold) and laser photocoagulation.

Destruction of cyst/lesion iris or ciliary body

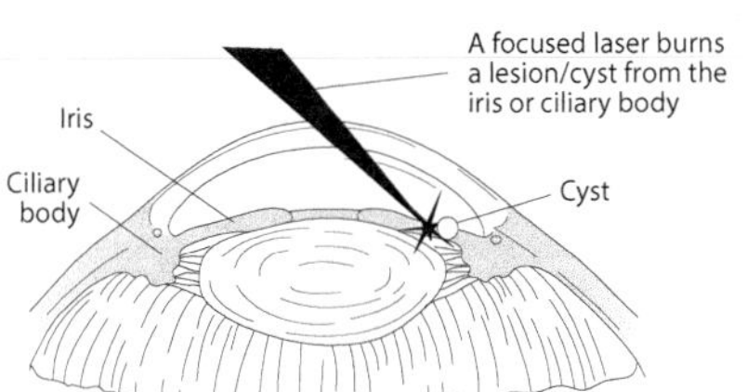
A focused laser burns a lesion/cyst from the iris or ciliary body
Iris
Ciliary body
Cyst

ICD-10-CM Diagnostic Codes

⇄	C69.92	Malignant neoplasm of unspecified site of left eye
⇄	D09.22	Carcinoma in situ of left eye
⇄	D31.52	Benign neoplasm of left lacrimal gland and duct
	D48.7	Neoplasm of uncertain behavior of other specified sites
	D49.89	Neoplasm of unspecified behavior of other specified sites
⇄	H21.272	Miotic pupillary cyst, left eye
⇄	H21.302	Idiopathic cysts of iris, ciliary body or anterior chamber, left eye
⇄	H21.312	Exudative cysts of iris or anterior chamber, left eye
⇄	H21.322	Implantation cysts of iris, ciliary body or anterior chamber, left eye
⇄	H21.352	Exudative cyst of pars plana, left eye
⇄	H21.502	Unspecified adhesions of iris, left eye

CCI Edits

Refer to Appendix A for CCI edits.

Facility RVUs ▢

Code	Work	PE Facility	MP	Total Facility
66770	6.13	7.31	0.45	13.89

Non-facility RVUs ▢

Code	Work	PE Non-Facility	MP	Total Non-Facility
66770	6.13	8.83	0.45	15.41

Modifiers (PAR) ▢

Code	Mod 50	Mod 51	Mod 62	Mod 66	Mod 80
66770	1	2	0	0	1

Global Period

Code	Days
66770	090

66820-66821

66820 Discission of secondary membranous cataract (opacified posterior lens capsule and/or anterior hyaloid); stab incision technique (Ziegler or Wheeler knife)

66821 Discission of secondary membranous cataract (opacified posterior lens capsule and/or anterior hyaloid); laser surgery (eg, YAG laser) (1 or more stages)

AMA Coding Notes

Surgical Procedures on the Eye and Ocular Adnexa

(For diagnostic and treatment ophthalmological services, see Medicine, Ophthalmology, and 92002 et seq)

(Do not report code 69990 in addition to codes 65091-68850)

Plain English Description

A secondary membranous cataract, also referred to as an after-cataract, is treated by discission using a stab incision technique (Ziegler or Wheeler knife). This procedure is performed when the remaining posterior portion of the lens capsule or the anterior hyaloid membrane that covers the anterior outer surface of the vitreous body in the posterior cavity of the eye becomes opacified or cloudy and impairs vision. This condition is sometimes referred to as posterior capsule opacification (PCO). A small surgical needle with a knife-like tip is inserted through the edge of the cornea and advanced into the posterior lens capsule and/or the anterior hyaloid membrane beneath the lens capsule. The posterior lens capsule and/or anterior hyaloid are incised using the small needle-knife and the secondary membranous cataract is opened providing an area of clear vision. In 66821, the secondary membranous cataract is opened by laser surgery in one or more stages. This procedure may also be referred to as a YAG laser capsulotomy. Eye drops may be used to dilate the pupil. A test shot is placed with the laser to mark the center of the pupil on the posterior capsule. Using a slit lamp microscope, the laser is aimed at the posterior capsule and fired in a pattern that opens the center to provide an area of clear vision. More than one session may be required to create an adequate sized opening in the center of the posterior lens.

Discission of secondary membranous cataract

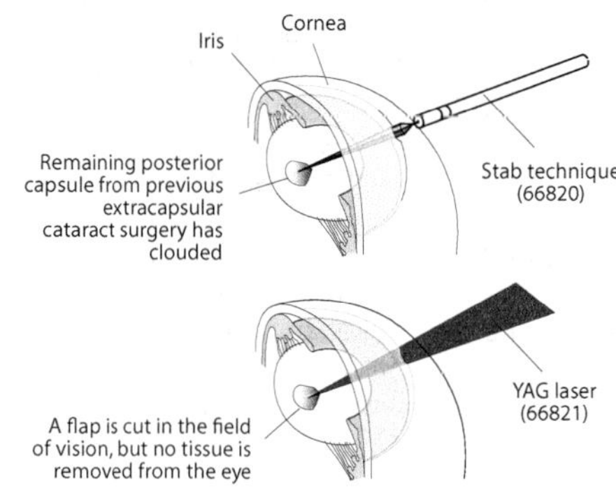
Iris
Cornea
Remaining posterior capsule from previous extracapsular cataract surgery has clouded
Stab technique (66820)
A flap is cut in the field of vision, but no tissue is removed from the eye
YAG laser (66821)

ICD-10-CM Diagnostic Codes

	Code	Description
	E10.311	Type 1 diabetes mellitus with unspecified diabetic retinopathy with macular edema
	E10.319	Type 1 diabetes mellitus with unspecified diabetic retinopathy without macular edema
➐⇄	E10.321	Type 1 diabetes mellitus with mild nonproliferative diabetic retinopathy with macular edema
➐⇄	E10.329	Type 1 diabetes mellitus with mild nonproliferative diabetic retinopathy without macular edema
➐⇄	E10.331	Type 1 diabetes mellitus with moderate nonproliferative diabetic retinopathy with macular edema
➐⇄	E10.339	Type 1 diabetes mellitus with moderate nonproliferative diabetic retinopathy without macular edema
➐⇄	E10.341	Type 1 diabetes mellitus with severe nonproliferative diabetic retinopathy with macular edema
➐⇄	E10.349	Type 1 diabetes mellitus with severe nonproliferative diabetic retinopathy without macular edema
➐⇄	E10.351	Type 1 diabetes mellitus with proliferative diabetic retinopathy with macular edema
➐⇄	E10.359	Type 1 diabetes mellitus with proliferative diabetic retinopathy without macular edema
	E10.36	Type 1 diabetes mellitus with diabetic cataract
	E10.39	Type 1 diabetes mellitus with other diabetic ophthalmic complication
	E10.65	Type 1 diabetes mellitus with hyperglycemia
	E11.311	Type 2 diabetes mellitus with unspecified diabetic retinopathy with macular edema
	E11.319	Type 2 diabetes mellitus with unspecified diabetic retinopathy without macular edema
➐⇄	E11.321	Type 2 diabetes mellitus with mild nonproliferative diabetic retinopathy with macular edema
➐⇄	E11.329	Type 2 diabetes mellitus with mild nonproliferative diabetic retinopathy without macular edema
➐⇄	E11.331	Type 2 diabetes mellitus with moderate nonproliferative diabetic retinopathy with macular edema
➐⇄	E11.339	Type 2 diabetes mellitus with moderate nonproliferative diabetic retinopathy without macular edema
➐⇄	E11.341	Type 2 diabetes mellitus with severe nonproliferative diabetic retinopathy with macular edema
➐⇄	E11.349	Type 2 diabetes mellitus with severe nonproliferative diabetic retinopathy without macular edema
➐⇄	E11.351	Type 2 diabetes mellitus with proliferative diabetic retinopathy with macular edema
➐⇄	E11.359	Type 2 diabetes mellitus with proliferative diabetic retinopathy without macular edema
	E11.36	Type 2 diabetes mellitus with diabetic cataract
	E11.39	Type 2 diabetes mellitus with other diabetic ophthalmic complication
	H17.89	Other corneal scars and opacities
⇄	H26.411	Soemmering's ring, right eye
⇄	H26.491	Other secondary cataract, right eye
➐	T85.21	Breakdown (mechanical) of intraocular lens
➐	T85.22	Displacement of intraocular lens
➐	T85.29	Other mechanical complication of intraocular lens
	Z96.1	Presence of intraocular lens

ICD-10-CM Coding Notes

For codes requiring a 7th character extension, refer to your ICD-10-CM book. Review the character descriptions and coding guidelines for proper selection. For some procedures, only certain characters will apply.

CCI Edits

Refer to Appendix A for CCI edits.

Pub 100

66820: Pub 100-03, 1, 10.1

66821: Pub 100-03, 1, 10.1, Pub 100-03, 1, 140.5

Facility RVUs

Code	Work	PE Facility	MP	Total Facility
66820	4.01	9.63	0.31	13.95
66821	3.42	5.37	0.25	9.04

Non-facility RVUs

Code	Work	PE Non-Facility	MP	Total Non-Facility
66820	4.01	9.63	0.31	13.95
66821	3.42	6.08	0.25	9.75

Modifiers (PAR)

Code	Mod 50	Mod 51	Mod 62	Mod 66	Mod 80
66820	1	2	0	0	1
66821	1	2	0	0	1

Global Period

Code	Days
66820	090
66821	090

66825

66825 Repositioning of intraocular lens prosthesis, requiring an incision (separate procedure)

AMA Coding Notes

Surgical Procedures on the Eye and Ocular Adnexa

(For diagnostic and treatment ophthalmological services, see Medicine, Ophthalmology, and 92002 et seq)

(Do not report code 69990 in addition to codes 65091-68850)

Plain English Description

An intraocular lens (IOL) prosthesis may require repositioning when a toric lens is off axis, a multifocal lens or sulcus-fixated lens in decentered, or a single-piece haptic lens escapes from the capsular bag. Using an operating microscope, a scleral incision is made and the IOL is located and elevated using a vitreoretinal pick or hook. The IOL is then grasped with forceps and brought to the posterior chamber. Using a Sinskey hook inserted either through the sclerotomy or a limbic stab incision, the IOL is rotated into place. If there is inadequate capsular support, transcleral sutures or iris sutures may be placed. The scleral incision is closed with sutures and a patch or shield is placed over the eye.

Repositioning of intraocular lens prosthesis, requiring an incision

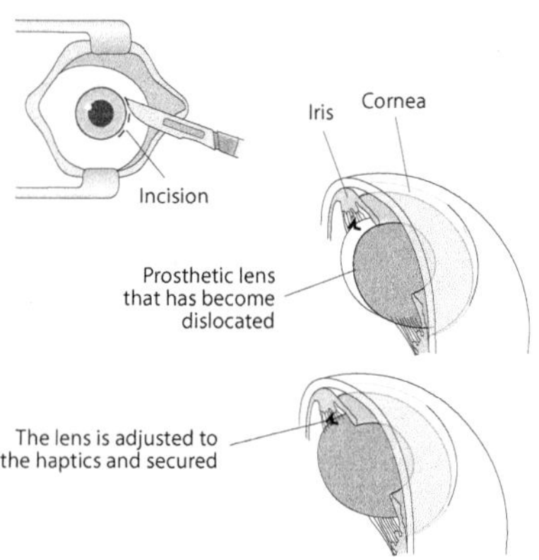

ICD-10-CM Diagnostic Codes

⇄	H21.512	Anterior synechiae (iris), left eye
⇄	H27.112	Subluxation of lens, left eye
⇄	H27.122	Anterior dislocation of lens, left eye
⇄	H27.132	Posterior dislocation of lens, left eye
➐	T85.21	Breakdown (mechanical) of intraocular lens
➐	T85.22	Displacement of intraocular lens
➐	T85.29	Other mechanical complication of intraocular lens
	Z96.1	Presence of intraocular lens
⇄	Z98.42	Cataract extraction status, left eye

ICD-10-CM Coding Notes

For codes requiring a 7th character extension, refer to your ICD-10-CM book. Review the character descriptions and coding guidelines for proper selection. For some procedures, only certain characters will apply.

CCI Edits

Refer to Appendix A for CCI edits.

Pub 100

66825: Pub 100-03, 1, 80.12

Facility RVUs ▢

Code	Work	PE Facility	MP	Total Facility
66825	9.01	14.80	0.70	24.51

Non-facility RVUs ▢

Code	Work	PE Non-Facility	MP	Total Non-Facility
66825	9.01	14.80	0.70	24.51

Modifiers (PAR) ▢

Code	Mod 50	Mod 51	Mod 62	Mod 66	Mod 80
66825	1	2	0	0	0

Global Period

Code	Days
66825	090

66830

66830 Removal of secondary membranous cataract (opacified posterior lens capsule and/or anterior hyaloid) with corneo-scleral section, with or without iridectomy (iridocapsulotomy, iridocapsulectomy)

AMA Coding Guideline

Removal of Lens Material Procedures of the Eye

Lateral canthotomy, iridectomy, iridotomy, anterior capsulotomy, posterior capsulotomy, the use of viscoelastic agents, enzymatic zonulysis, use of other pharmacologic agents, and subconjunctival or sub-tenon injections are included as part of the code for the extraction of lens.

AMA Coding Notes

Surgical Procedures on the Eye and Ocular Adnexa

(For diagnostic and treatment ophthalmological services, see Medicine, Ophthalmology, and 92002 et seq)

(Do not report code 69990 in addition to codes 65091-68850)

Plain English Description

Secondary membranous cataracts are a complication of cataract surgery. After a cataract is removed from the anterior chamber and replaced with an intraocular lens, epithelial and fibroblastic cells from the cataract may remain and proliferate on the anterior surface of the posterior capsule, forming a hazy membrane. The posterior capsule is incised and the tissue is separated and retracted. A vitreous cutter or needle/hook is used to manually remove the tissue. Access to the posterior capsule may require an incision through the iris and capsular membrane surrounding the lens of the eye (iridectomy, iridocapsulotomy, iridocapsulectomy). The pressure is checked in the anterior chamber and fluid may be injected to inflate the chamber to a normal intraocular pressure. The instruments are removed and the wound(s) are checked for fluid leakage. Sutures may be placed if required to close the incision.

Removal of secondary membranous cataract with/without iridectomy

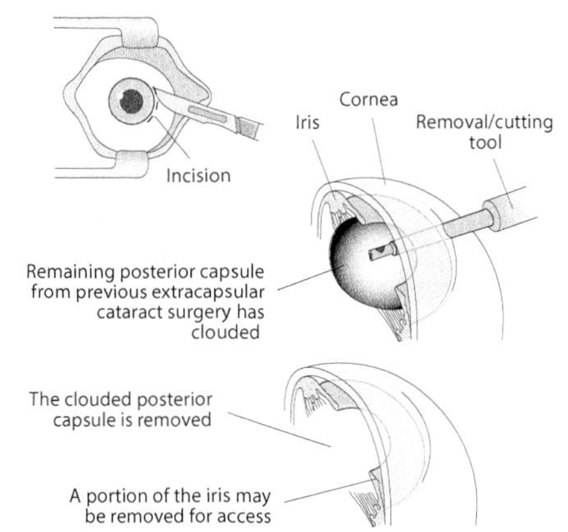

ICD-10-CM Diagnostic Codes

⇄	H26.411	Soemmering's ring, right eye
⇄	H26.491	Other secondary cataract, right eye
⇄	H59.021	Cataract (lens) fragments in eye following cataract surgery, right eye
	Z96.1	Presence of intraocular lens
⇄	Z98.41	Cataract extraction status, right eye

CCI Edits

Refer to Appendix A for CCI edits.

Pub 100

66830: Pub 100-03, 1, 10.1

Facility RVUs ☐

Code	Work	PE Facility	MP	Total Facility
66830	9.47	10.34	0.73	20.54

Non-facility RVUs ☐

Code	Work	PE Non-Facility	MP	Total Non-Facility
66830	9.47	10.34	0.73	20.54

Modifiers (PAR) ☐

Code	Mod 50	Mod 51	Mod 62	Mod 66	Mod 80
66830	1	2	0	0	1

Global Period

Code	Days
66830	090

66840

66840 Removal of lens material; aspiration technique, 1 or more stages

AMA Coding Guideline

Removal of Lens Material Procedures of the Eye

Lateral canthotomy, iridectomy, iridotomy, anterior capsulotomy, posterior capsulotomy, the use of viscoelastic agents, enzymatic zonulysis, use of other pharmacologic agents, and subconjunctival or sub-tenon injections are included as part of the code for the extraction of lens.

AMA Coding Notes

Surgical Procedures on the Eye and Ocular Adnexa

(For diagnostic and treatment ophthalmological services, see Medicine, Ophthalmology, and 92002 et seq)

(Do not report code 69990 in addition to codes 65091-68850)

AMA *CPT® Assistant* ▢

66840: Fall 92: 4, Jan 09: 7, Apr 09: 9, Sep 09: 5, Apr 16: 8, Jun 16: 6, Sep 16: 9

Plain English Description

To remove lens material by aspiration technique, the eye is visualized using an operating microscope and the anterior chamber is accessed with a needle or blade, creating one or more paracenteses. An irrigation and aspiration tool is inserted into the anterior chamber through the paracentesis and the lens material is gently pulled from the periphery to the pupillary center and aspirated. The pressure is checked in the anterior chamber and fluid may be injected to inflate the chamber to a normal intraocular pressure. The instruments are removed and the wound(s) is checked for fluid leakage. Sutures may be placed if required to close the incision(s).

Removal of lens material; aspiration technique, 1 or more stages

ICD-10-CM Diagnostic Codes

	E08.36	Diabetes mellitus due to underlying condition with diabetic cataract
	E09.36	Drug or chemical induced diabetes mellitus with diabetic cataract
	E10.311	Type 1 diabetes mellitus with unspecified diabetic retinopathy with macular edema
	E10.319	Type 1 diabetes mellitus with unspecified diabetic retinopathy without macular edema
❼⇄	E10.321	Type 1 diabetes mellitus with mild nonproliferative diabetic retinopathy with macular edema
❼⇄	E10.329	Type 1 diabetes mellitus with mild nonproliferative diabetic retinopathy without macular edema
❼⇄	E10.331	Type 1 diabetes mellitus with moderate nonproliferative diabetic retinopathy with macular edema
❼⇄	E10.339	Type 1 diabetes mellitus with moderate nonproliferative diabetic retinopathy without macular edema
❼⇄	E10.341	Type 1 diabetes mellitus with severe nonproliferative diabetic retinopathy with macular edema
❼⇄	E10.349	Type 1 diabetes mellitus with severe nonproliferative diabetic retinopathy without macular edema
❼⇄	E10.351	Type 1 diabetes mellitus with proliferative diabetic retinopathy with macular edema
❼⇄	E10.359	Type 1 diabetes mellitus with proliferative diabetic retinopathy without macular edema
	E10.36	Type 1 diabetes mellitus with diabetic cataract
	E10.39	Type 1 diabetes mellitus with other diabetic ophthalmic complication
	E11.311	Type 2 diabetes mellitus with unspecified diabetic retinopathy with macular edema
	E11.319	Type 2 diabetes mellitus with unspecified diabetic retinopathy without macular edema
❼⇄	E11.321	Type 2 diabetes mellitus with mild nonproliferative diabetic retinopathy with macular edema
❼⇄	E11.329	Type 2 diabetes mellitus with mild nonproliferative diabetic retinopathy without macular edema
❼⇄	E11.331	Type 2 diabetes mellitus with moderate nonproliferative diabetic retinopathy with macular edema
❼⇄	E11.339	Type 2 diabetes mellitus with moderate nonproliferative diabetic retinopathy without macular edema
❼⇄	E11.341	Type 2 diabetes mellitus with severe nonproliferative diabetic retinopathy with macular edema
❼⇄	E11.349	Type 2 diabetes mellitus with severe nonproliferative diabetic retinopathy without macular edema
❼⇄	E11.351	Type 2 diabetes mellitus with proliferative diabetic retinopathy with macular edema
❼⇄	E11.359	Type 2 diabetes mellitus with proliferative diabetic retinopathy without macular edema
	E11.36	Type 2 diabetes mellitus with diabetic cataract
	E11.39	Type 2 diabetes mellitus with other diabetic ophthalmic complication
	E13.36	Other specified diabetes mellitus with diabetic cataract
⇄	H20.22	Lens-induced iridocyclitis, left eye
⇄	H25.012	Cortical age-related cataract, left eye
⇄	H25.032	Anterior subcapsular polar age-related cataract, left eye
⇄	H25.042	Posterior subcapsular polar age-related cataract, left eye
⇄	H25.092	Other age-related incipient cataract, left eye
⇄	H25.12	Age-related nuclear cataract, left eye
⇄	H25.22	Age-related cataract, morgagnian type, left eye
⇄	H25.812	Combined forms of age-related cataract, left eye
	H25.89	Other age-related cataract
⇄	H26.012	Infantile and juvenile cortical, lamellar, or zonular cataract, left eye
⇄	H26.032	Infantile and juvenile nuclear cataract, left eye
⇄	H26.042	Anterior subcapsular polar infantile and juvenile cataract, left eye
⇄	H26.052	Posterior subcapsular polar infantile and juvenile cataract, left eye
⇄	H26.062	Combined forms of infantile and juvenile cataract, left eye
⇄	H27.112	Subluxation of lens, left eye
⇄	H43.02	Vitreous prolapse, left eye
	Z96.1	Presence of intraocular lens
⇄	Z98.42	Cataract extraction status, left eye

ICD-10-CM Coding Notes

For codes requiring a 7th character extension, refer to your ICD-10-CM book. Review the character descriptions and coding guidelines for proper selection. For some procedures, only certain characters will apply.

CCI Edits

Refer to Appendix A for CCI edits.

Facility RVUs ▢

Code	Work	PE Facility	MP	Total Facility
66840	9.18	10.16	0.72	20.06

Non-facility RVUs ▢

Code	Work	PE Non-Facility	MP	Total Non-Facility
66840	9.18	10.16	0.72	20.06

Modifiers (PAR) ▢

Code	Mod 50	Mod 51	Mod 62	Mod 66	Mod 80
66840	1	2	0	0	1

Global Period

Code	Days
66840	090

66850

66850 Removal of lens material; phacofragmentation technique (mechanical or ultrasonic) (eg, phacoemulsification), with aspiration

AMA Coding Guideline

Removal of Lens Material Procedures of the Eye

Lateral canthotomy, iridectomy, iridotomy, anterior capsulotomy, posterior capsulotomy, the use of viscoelastic agents, enzymatic zonulysis, use of other pharmacologic agents, and subconjunctival or sub-tenon injections are included as part of the code for the extraction of lens.

AMA Coding Notes

Surgical Procedures on the Eye and Ocular Adnexa

(For diagnostic and treatment ophthalmological services, see Medicine, Ophthalmology, and 92002 et seq)

(Do not report code 69990 in addition to codes 65091-68850)

AMA *CPT® Assistant* ☐

66850: Fall 92: 6, Jan 09: 7, Apr 09: 9, Sep 09: 5, Jun 16: 6

Plain English Description

To remove lens material by phacoemulsification aspiration technique, the eye is visualized using an operating microscope and the anterior chamber is accessed with a needle or blade, creating one or more paracenteses. A probe is inserted through the paracentesis into the anterior chamber and the lens material is broken up using ultrasound. The probe is removed and an irrigation and aspiration tool is inserted into the anterior chamber through the paracentesis. The fragmented pieces of lens material are gently pulled from the periphery to the pupillary center and aspirated. The pressure is checked in the anterior chamber and fluid may be injected to inflate the chamber to a normal intraocular pressure. The instruments are removed and the wound(s) are checked for fluid leakage. Sutures may be placed if required to close the incision(s).

Removal of lens material; phacofragmentation, mechanical/ ultrasonic, with aspiration

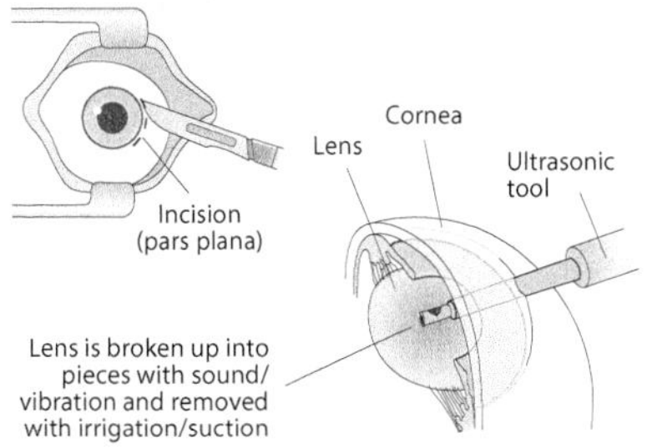
Cornea
Lens
Ultrasonic tool
Incision (pars plana)
Lens is broken up into pieces with sound/ vibration and removed with irrigation/suction

ICD-10-CM Diagnostic Codes

E08.36 Diabetes mellitus due to underlying condition with diabetic cataract
E09.36 Drug or chemical induced diabetes mellitus with diabetic cataract
E10.311 Type 1 diabetes mellitus with unspecified diabetic retinopathy with macular edema
E10.319 Type 1 diabetes mellitus with unspecified diabetic retinopathy without macular edema
➐⇄ E10.321 Type 1 diabetes mellitus with mild nonproliferative diabetic retinopathy with macular edema
➐⇄ E10.329 Type 1 diabetes mellitus with mild nonproliferative diabetic retinopathy without macular edema
➐⇄ E10.331 Type 1 diabetes mellitus with moderate nonproliferative diabetic retinopathy with macular edema
➐⇄ E10.339 Type 1 diabetes mellitus with moderate nonproliferative diabetic retinopathy without macular edema
➐⇄ E10.341 Type 1 diabetes mellitus with severe nonproliferative diabetic retinopathy with macular edema
➐⇄ E10.349 Type 1 diabetes mellitus with severe nonproliferative diabetic retinopathy without macular edema
➐⇄ E10.351 Type 1 diabetes mellitus with proliferative diabetic retinopathy with macular edema
➐⇄ E10.359 Type 1 diabetes mellitus with proliferative diabetic retinopathy without macular edema
E10.36 Type 1 diabetes mellitus with diabetic cataract
E10.39 Type 1 diabetes mellitus with other diabetic ophthalmic complication
E11.311 Type 2 diabetes mellitus with unspecified diabetic retinopathy with macular edema
E11.319 Type 2 diabetes mellitus with unspecified diabetic retinopathy without macular edema
➐⇄ E11.321 Type 2 diabetes mellitus with mild nonproliferative diabetic retinopathy with macular edema
➐⇄ E11.329 Type 2 diabetes mellitus with mild nonproliferative diabetic retinopathy without macular edema
➐⇄ E11.331 Type 2 diabetes mellitus with moderate nonproliferative diabetic retinopathy with macular edema
➐⇄ E11.339 Type 2 diabetes mellitus with moderate nonproliferative diabetic retinopathy without macular edema
➐⇄ E11.341 Type 2 diabetes mellitus with severe nonproliferative diabetic retinopathy with macular edema
➐⇄ E11.349 Type 2 diabetes mellitus with severe nonproliferative diabetic retinopathy without macular edema
➐⇄ E11.351 Type 2 diabetes mellitus with proliferative diabetic retinopathy with macular edema
➐⇄ E11.359 Type 2 diabetes mellitus with proliferative diabetic retinopathy without macular edema
E11.36 Type 2 diabetes mellitus with diabetic cataract
E11.39 Type 2 diabetes mellitus with other diabetic ophthalmic complication
E13.36 Other specified diabetes mellitus with diabetic cataract
⇄ H20.21 Lens-induced iridocyclitis, right eye
⇄ H25.011 Cortical age-related cataract, right eye
⇄ H25.031 Anterior subcapsular polar age-related cataract, right eye
⇄ H25.041 Posterior subcapsular polar age-related cataract, right eye
⇄ H25.091 Other age-related incipient cataract, right eye
⇄ H25.11 Age-related nuclear cataract, right eye
⇄ H25.21 Age-related cataract, morgagnian type, right eye
⇄ H25.811 Combined forms of age-related cataract, right eye
H25.89 Other age-related cataract
⇄ H26.001 Unspecified infantile and juvenile cataract, right eye
⇄ H26.011 Infantile and juvenile cortical, lamellar, or zonular cataract, right eye
⇄ H26.031 Infantile and juvenile nuclear cataract, right eye
⇄ H26.041 Anterior subcapsular polar infantile and juvenile cataract, right eye
⇄ H26.051 Posterior subcapsular polar infantile and juvenile cataract, right eye
⇄ H26.061 Combined forms of infantile and juvenile cataract, right eye
⇄ H27.111 Subluxation of lens, right eye
⇄ H27.131 Posterior dislocation of lens, right eye
⇄ H43.01 Vitreous prolapse, right eye
⇄ H43.11 Vitreous hemorrhage, right eye
Q12.0 Congenital cataract
Q12.2 Coloboma of lens
Q12.4 Spherophakia
Q12.8 Other congenital lens malformations
Q12.9 Congenital lens malformation, unspecified

ICD-10-CM Coding Notes

For codes requiring a 7th character extension, refer to your ICD-10-CM book. Review the character descriptions and coding guidelines for proper selection. For some procedures, only certain characters will apply.

CCI Edits

Refer to Appendix A for CCI edits.

Pub 100

66850: Pub 100-03, 1, 80.10

Facility RVUs

Code	Work	PE Facility	MP	Total Facility
66850	10.55	11.45	0.79	22.79

Non-facility RVUs

Code	Work	PE Non-Facility	MP	Total Non-Facility
66850	10.55	11.45	0.79	22.79

Modifiers (PAR)

Code	Mod 50	Mod 51	Mod 62	Mod 66	Mod 80
66850	1	2	0	0	1

Global Period

Code	Days
66850	090

66852

66852 Removal of lens material; pars plana approach, with or without vitrectomy

AMA Coding Guideline

Removal of Lens Material Procedures of the Eye

Lateral canthotomy, iridectomy, iridotomy, anterior capsulotomy, posterior capsulotomy, the use of viscoelastic agents, enzymatic zonulysis, use of other pharmacologic agents, and subconjunctival or sub-tenon injections are included as part of the code for the extraction of lens.

AMA Coding Notes

Surgical Procedures on the Eye and Ocular Adnexa

(For diagnostic and treatment ophthalmological services, see Medicine, Ophthalmology, and 92002 et seq)

(Do not report code 69990 in addition to codes 65091-68850)

AMA *CPT® Assistant* ☐

66852: Fall 92: 8, Jan 09: 7, Apr 09: 9, Sep 09: 5, Jun 16: 6

Plain English Description

To remove lens material using a pars plana approach, with or without vitrectomy, the eye is visualized using an operating microscope. The posterior segment is accessed through a pars plana incision, opening the conjunctiva and Tenon's layer to expose the sclera. Hemostasis is achieved with cautery; the sclera is marked at the inferotemporal quadrant; and two sutures are placed on either side of the mark. Using a microvitreoretinal (MVR) blade, the sclera is incised at the mark between the two sutures. An infusion line is inserted and secured with the sutures, then visualized with a light pipe. It may be necessary to make a second sclerotomy in the inferotemporal quadrant to position the infusion line correctly. Superior sclerotomies are then made using the MVR blade, and a light pipe and vitreo cutter are passed through into the posterior segment. The lens material is removed using irrigation and aspiration. Vitreous fluid (vitrectomy) may be removed with the lens material. The intraocular pressure is monitored and maintained to ensure that the eye stays formed during the irrigation and aspiration. Fluid may be injected to inflate the chamber to a normal intraocular pressure at the conclusion of the procedure. Instruments are removed, and the sclerotomies are closed with suture and checked for fluid leakage. The infusion line is removed and closed with the previously placed sutures, followed by closure of the conjunctiva.

Removal of lens material; pars plana approach, with or without vitrectomy

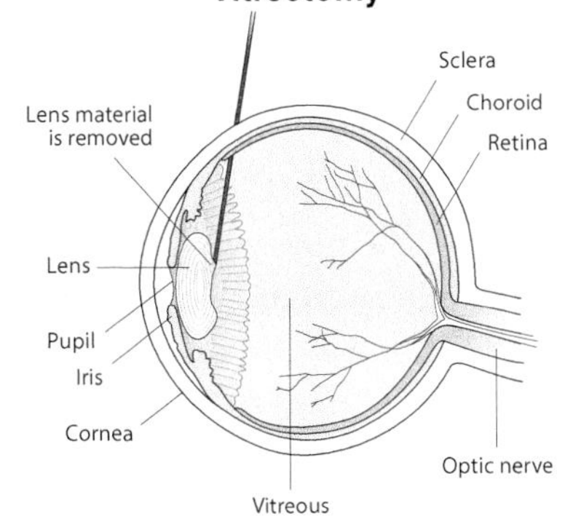

ICD-10-CM Diagnostic Codes

	E10.311	Type 1 diabetes mellitus with unspecified diabetic retinopathy with macular edema
	E10.319	Type 1 diabetes mellitus with unspecified diabetic retinopathy without macular edema
❼⇄	E10.321	Type 1 diabetes mellitus with mild nonproliferative diabetic retinopathy with macular edema
❼⇄	E10.329	Type 1 diabetes mellitus with mild nonproliferative diabetic retinopathy without macular edema
❼⇄	E10.331	Type 1 diabetes mellitus with moderate nonproliferative diabetic retinopathy with macular edema
❼⇄	E10.339	Type 1 diabetes mellitus with moderate nonproliferative diabetic retinopathy without macular edema
❼⇄	E10.341	Type 1 diabetes mellitus with severe nonproliferative diabetic retinopathy with macular edema
❼⇄	E10.349	Type 1 diabetes mellitus with severe nonproliferative diabetic retinopathy without macular edema
❼⇄	E10.351	Type 1 diabetes mellitus with proliferative diabetic retinopathy with macular edema
❼⇄	E10.359	Type 1 diabetes mellitus with proliferative diabetic retinopathy without macular edema
	E10.36	Type 1 diabetes mellitus with diabetic cataract
	E10.39	Type 1 diabetes mellitus with other diabetic ophthalmic complication
	E11.311	Type 2 diabetes mellitus with unspecified diabetic retinopathy with macular edema
	E11.319	Type 2 diabetes mellitus with unspecified diabetic retinopathy without macular edema
❼⇄	E11.321	Type 2 diabetes mellitus with mild nonproliferative diabetic retinopathy with macular edema
❼⇄	E11.329	Type 2 diabetes mellitus with mild nonproliferative diabetic retinopathy without macular edema
❼⇄	E11.331	Type 2 diabetes mellitus with moderate nonproliferative diabetic retinopathy with macular edema
❼⇄	E11.339	Type 2 diabetes mellitus with moderate nonproliferative diabetic retinopathy without macular edema
❼⇄	E11.341	Type 2 diabetes mellitus with severe nonproliferative diabetic retinopathy with macular edema
❼⇄	E11.349	Type 2 diabetes mellitus with severe nonproliferative diabetic retinopathy without macular edema
❼⇄	E11.351	Type 2 diabetes mellitus with proliferative diabetic retinopathy with macular edema
❼⇄	E11.359	Type 2 diabetes mellitus with proliferative diabetic retinopathy without macular edema
	E11.36	Type 2 diabetes mellitus with diabetic cataract
	E11.39	Type 2 diabetes mellitus with other diabetic ophthalmic complication
⇄	H25.012	Cortical age-related cataract, left eye
⇄	H25.032	Anterior subcapsular polar age-related cataract, left eye
⇄	H25.042	Posterior subcapsular polar age-related cataract, left eye
⇄	H25.092	Other age-related incipient cataract, left eye
⇄	H25.22	Age-related cataract, morgagnian type, left eye
⇄	H25.812	Combined forms of age-related cataract, left eye
	H25.89	Other age-related cataract
⇄	H26.002	Unspecified infantile and juvenile cataract, left eye
⇄	H26.012	Infantile and juvenile cortical, lamellar, or zonular cataract, left eye
⇄	H26.032	Infantile and juvenile nuclear cataract, left eye
⇄	H26.042	Anterior subcapsular polar infantile and juvenile cataract, left eye
⇄	H26.052	Posterior subcapsular polar infantile and juvenile cataract, left eye
⇄	H26.062	Combined forms of infantile and juvenile cataract, left eye
⇄	H26.102	Unspecified traumatic cataract, left eye
⇄	H26.112	Localized traumatic opacities, left eye
⇄	H26.132	Total traumatic cataract, left eye
⇄	H27.112	Subluxation of lens, left eye
⇄	H27.132	Posterior dislocation of lens, left eye
⇄	H43.12	Vitreous hemorrhage, left eye
⇄	H43.392	Other vitreous opacities, left eye
⇄	H59.022	Cataract (lens) fragments in eye following cataract surgery, left eye
⇄	Z98.42	Cataract extraction status, left eye

ICD-10-CM Coding Notes

For codes requiring a 7th character extension, refer to your ICD-10-CM book. Review the character descriptions and coding guidelines for proper selection. For some procedures, only certain characters will apply.

CCI Edits

Refer to Appendix A for CCI edits.

Pub 100

66852: Pub 100-03, 1, 80.11

Facility RVUs

Code	Work	PE Facility	MP	Total Facility
66852	11.41	11.98	0.89	24.28

Non-facility RVUs

Code	Work	PE Non-Facility	MP	Total Non-Facility
66852	11.41	11.98	0.89	24.28

Modifiers (PAR)

Code	Mod 50	Mod 51	Mod 62	Mod 66	Mod 80
66852	1	2	1	0	0

Global Period

Code	Days
66852	090

66920-66930

66920 Removal of lens material; intracapsular

66930 Removal of lens material; intracapsular, for dislocated lens

AMA Coding Guideline

Removal of Lens Material Procedures of the Eye

Lateral canthotomy, iridectomy, iridotomy, anterior capsulotomy, posterior capsulotomy, the use of viscoelastic agents, enzymatic zonulysis, use of other pharmacologic agents, and subconjunctival or sub-tenon injections are included as part of the code for the extraction of lens.

AMA Coding Notes

Surgical Procedures on the Eye and Ocular Adnexa

(For diagnostic and treatment ophthalmological services, see Medicine, Ophthalmology, and 92002 et seq)

(Do not report code 69990 in addition to codes 65091-68850)

AMA *CPT® Assistant* ▯

66920: Fall 92: 8, Sep 09: 5

66930: Fall 92: 8, Sep 09: 5

Plain English Description

An incision is made at the corneoscleral junction. The lens capsule is exposed. Medication is injected to dissolve the zonal fibers that hold the lens in place. A cryoprobe is inserted and the lens is frozen. The probe is withdrawn and the natural lens and lens capsule are removed. The surgical wound is repaired with sutures. Temporary sutures are placed through the upper and lower eyelids to keep the eye closed until the eye has healed. A soft bandage or patch may also be applied to the eye. Use 66920 when intracapsular removal of lens material is performed for a condition other than a dislocated lens. Use 66930 when the procedure is performed to remove a dislocated natural lens and lens capsule.

Removal of lens material; intracapsular

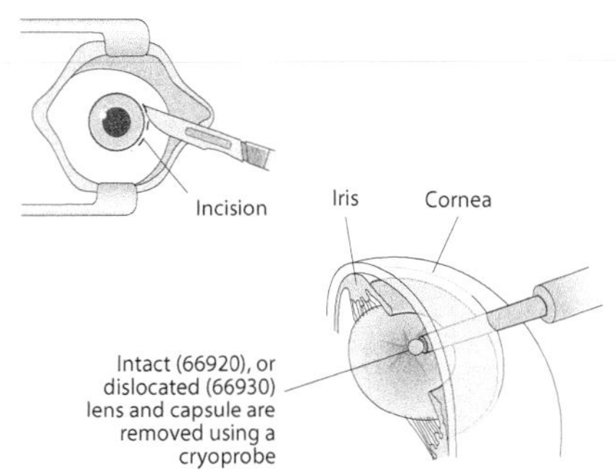
Incision
Iris
Cornea
Intact (66920), or dislocated (66930) lens and capsule are removed using a cryoprobe

ICD-10-CM Diagnostic Codes

	Code	Description
⇄	H20.11	Chronic iridocyclitis, right eye
⇄	H25.011	Cortical age-related cataract, right eye
⇄	H25.031	Anterior subcapsular polar age-related cataract, right eye
⇄	H25.041	Posterior subcapsular polar age-related cataract, right eye
⇄	H25.11	Age-related nuclear cataract, right eye
⇄	H25.21	Age-related cataract, morgagnian type, right eye
⇄	H25.811	Combined forms of age-related cataract, right eye
	H25.89	Other age-related cataract
⇄	H26.101	Unspecified traumatic cataract, right eye
⇄	H26.111	Localized traumatic opacities, right eye
⇄	H26.131	Total traumatic cataract, right eye
	H26.8	Other specified cataract
⇄	H27.111	Subluxation of lens, right eye
⇄	H27.121	Anterior dislocation of lens, right eye
⇄	H27.131	Posterior dislocation of lens, right eye
	H27.8	Other specified disorders of lens
⇄	H44.631	Retained (old) magnetic foreign body in lens, right eye
⇄	H44.731	Retained (nonmagnetic) (old) foreign body in lens, right eye
⇄	H59.021	Cataract (lens) fragments in eye following cataract surgery, right eye
❼⇄	S05.21	Ocular laceration and rupture with prolapse or loss of intraocular tissue, right eye
❼⇄	S05.31	Ocular laceration without prolapse or loss of intraocular tissue, right eye
❼⇄	S05.32	Ocular laceration without prolapse or loss of intraocular tissue, left eye
❼⇄	S05.51	Penetrating wound with foreign body of right eyeball
❼⇄	S05.61	Penetrating wound without foreign body of right eyeball
❼⇄	S05.8X1	Other injuries of right eye and orbit
❼⇄	S05.8X2	Other injuries of left eye and orbit

ICD-10-CM Coding Notes

For codes requiring a 7th character extension, refer to your ICD-10-CM book. Review the character descriptions and coding guidelines for proper selection. For some procedures, only certain characters will apply.

CCI Edits

Refer to Appendix A for CCI edits.

Facility RVUs ▯

Code	Work	PE Facility	MP	Total Facility
66920	10.13	10.75	0.77	21.65
66930	11.61	12.31	0.90	24.82

Non-facility RVUs ▯

Code	Work	PE Non-Facility	MP	Total Non-Facility
66920	10.13	10.75	0.77	21.65
66930	11.61	12.31	0.90	24.82

Modifiers (PAR) ▯

Code	Mod 50	Mod 51	Mod 62	Mod 66	Mod 80
66920	1	2	1	0	0
66930	1	2	0	0	0

Global Period

Code	Days
66920	090
66930	090

66940

66940 Removal of lens material; extracapsular (other than 66840, 66850, 66852)

(For removal of intralenticular foreign body without lens extraction, use 65235)

(For repair of operative wound, use 66250)

AMA Coding Guideline
Removal of Lens Material Procedures of the Eye

Lateral canthotomy, iridectomy, iridotomy, anterior capsulotomy, posterior capsulotomy, the use of viscoelastic agents, enzymatic zonulysis, use of other pharmacologic agents, and subconjunctival or sub-tenon injections are included as part of the code for the extraction of lens.

AMA Coding Notes
Surgical Procedures on the Eye and Ocular Adnexa

(For diagnostic and treatment ophthalmological services, see Medicine, Ophthalmology, and 92002 et seq)

(Do not report code 69990 in addition to codes 65091-68850)

AMA *CPT® Assistant* ▢

66940: Fall 92: 4, Jan 09: 7, Apr 09: 9, Sep 09: 5, Jun 16: 6

Plain English Description

To remove lens material using extracapsular technique, the eye is visualized using an operating microscope and an incision is made in the cornea close to the scleral border. A circular tear is made in the front of the lens capsule and the capsule is opened. Lens material is removed using instruments and/or suction, and the incision is closed with sutures.

Removal of lens material; extracapsular (other than 66840, 66850, 66852)

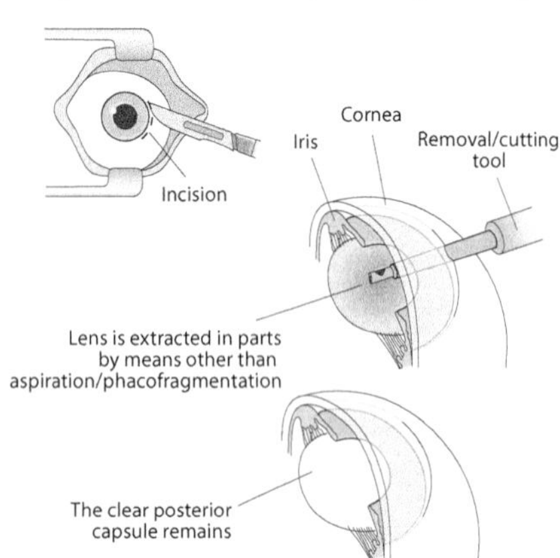
Cornea
Iris
Removal/cutting tool
Incision
Lens is extracted in parts by means other than aspiration/phacofragmentation
The clear posterior capsule remains

ICD-10-CM Diagnostic Codes

⇄ H25.012 Cortical age-related cataract, left eye
⇄ H25.032 Anterior subcapsular polar age-related cataract, left eye
⇄ H25.042 Posterior subcapsular polar age-related cataract, left eye
⇄ H25.092 Other age-related incipient cataract, left eye
⇄ H25.12 Age-related nuclear cataract, left eye
⇄ H25.812 Combined forms of age-related cataract, left eye
H25.89 Other age-related cataract
⇄ H26.002 Unspecified infantile and juvenile cataract, left eye
⇄ H26.012 Infantile and juvenile cortical, lamellar, or zonular cataract, left eye
⇄ H26.032 Infantile and juvenile nuclear cataract, left eye
⇄ H26.042 Anterior subcapsular polar infantile and juvenile cataract, left eye
⇄ H26.052 Posterior subcapsular polar infantile and juvenile cataract, left eye
⇄ H26.062 Combined forms of infantile and juvenile cataract, left eye
⇄ H26.102 Unspecified traumatic cataract, left eye
⇄ H26.112 Localized traumatic opacities, left eye
⇄ H26.132 Total traumatic cataract, left eye
H26.8 Other specified cataract
⇄ H27.122 Anterior dislocation of lens, left eye
⇄ H27.132 Posterior dislocation of lens, left eye

CCI Edits

Refer to Appendix A for CCI edits.

Facility RVUs ▢

Code	Work	PE Facility	MP	Total Facility
66940	10.37	11.55	0.79	22.71

Non-facility RVUs ▢

Code	Work	PE Non-Facility	MP	Total Non-Facility
66940	10.37	11.55	0.79	22.71

Modifiers (PAR) ▢

Code	Mod 50	Mod 51	Mod 62	Mod 66	Mod 80
66940	1	2	1	0	0

Global Period

Code	Days
66940	090

66982

66982 Extracapsular cataract removal with insertion of intraocular lens prosthesis (1-stage procedure), manual or mechanical technique (eg, irrigation and aspiration or phacoemulsification), complex, requiring devices or techniques not generally used in routine cataract surgery (eg, iris expansion device, suture support for intraocular lens, or primary posterior capsulorrhexis) or performed on patients in the amblyogenic developmental stage; without endoscopic cyclophotocoagulation

(For complex extracapsular cataract removal with concomitant endoscopic cyclophotocoagulation, use 66987)

(For complex extracapsular cataract removal with intraocular lens implant and concomitant intraocular aqueous drainage device by internal approach, use 66989)

(For insertion of ocular telescope prosthesis including removal of crystalline lens, use 0308T)

AMA Coding Notes

Surgical Procedures on the Eye and Ocular Adnexa

(For diagnostic and treatment ophthalmological services, see Medicine, Ophthalmology, and 92002 et seq)

(Do not report code 69990 in addition to codes 65091-68850)

AMA *CPT® Assistant* ▯

66982: Feb 01: 7, Nov 03: 10, Sep 09: 5, Mar 13: 6, Mar 16: 10, Dec 17: 14, Dec 18: 6, Dec 19: 6, Mar 21: 7

Plain English Description

Complex extracapsular cataract removal is performed with insertion of intraocular lens (IOL) prosthesis using manual or mechanical technique without endoscopic cyclophotocoagulation. A complex procedure uses devices or techniques not generally used in routine cataract surgery. This is necessary for children because primary posterior capsulotomy or capsulorrhexis is required for IOL insertion, the anterior capsule in children is more difficult to open, and the cortex is more difficult to remove due to lens adhesion. Complexity is also increased with certain conditions, such as uveitis, glaucoma, pseudoexfoliation syndrome, or Marfan syndrome. Patients with prior intraocular surgery or other trauma to the eye, or dense, hard, white cataracts may also require a more complex procedure. An incision is made in the corneoscleral junction (fornix) for insertion of the phacoemulsification device. A side port incision is made. An attempt is made to dilate the pupil. If unsuccessful, a spatula is inserted and posterior synechiae are lysed. Four incisions are made and an expansion device consisting of four hooks is inserted. The iris is retracted using the hooks. A circular tear is made in the anterior lens capsule, which is opened, and the phacoemulsification probe is inserted. The probe uses ultrasound to break up the cataract and remove the pieces by aspiration. Once the cataract has been removed, the softer cortex surrounding the cataract is removed by suction. Viscoelastic material is injected into the lens capsule to maintain its shape. In a child, the posterior capsule is also incised to facilitate insertion of the IOL. The IOL is inserted and the viscoelastic material is removed. The incisions are checked for water tightness. Subconjunctival injection of water or saline is performed to restore intraocular pressure and the eye is dressed.

Extracapsular cataract removal with insertion of intraocular lens prosthesis, manual/mechanical, complex

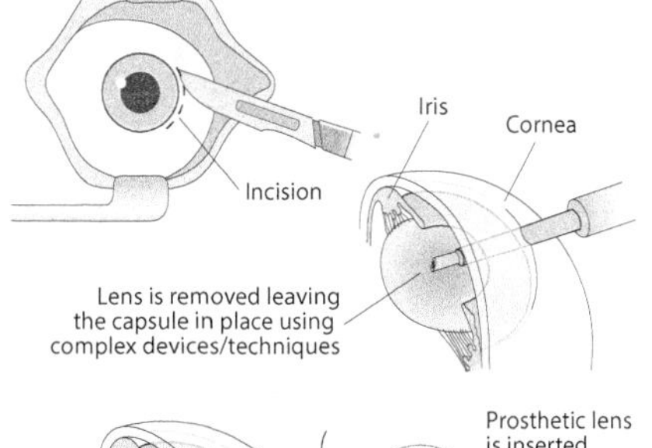
Iris
Cornea
Incision
Lens is removed leaving the capsule in place using complex devices/techniques
Prosthetic lens is inserted
Intraocular lens in anterior chamber

ICD-10-CM Diagnostic Codes

	Code	Description
⇄	H20.11	Chronic iridocyclitis, right eye
⇄	H20.12	Chronic iridocyclitis, left eye
⇄	H20.13	Chronic iridocyclitis, bilateral
⇄	H21.541	Posterior synechiae (iris), right eye
⇄	H21.542	Posterior synechiae (iris), left eye
⇄	H21.543	Posterior synechiae (iris), bilateral
⇄	H25.011	Cortical age-related cataract, right eye
⇄	H25.012	Cortical age-related cataract, left eye
⇄	H25.013	Cortical age-related cataract, bilateral
⇄	H25.041	Posterior subcapsular polar age-related cataract, right eye
⇄	H25.042	Posterior subcapsular polar age-related cataract, left eye
⇄	H25.043	Posterior subcapsular polar age-related cataract, bilateral
⇄	H25.11	Age-related nuclear cataract, right eye
⇄	H25.12	Age-related nuclear cataract, left eye
⇄	H25.13	Age-related nuclear cataract, bilateral
⇄	H25.21	Age-related cataract, morgagnian type, right eye
⇄	H25.22	Age-related cataract, morgagnian type, left eye
⇄	H25.23	Age-related cataract, morgagnian type, bilateral
⇄	H25.811	Combined forms of age-related cataract, right eye
⇄	H25.812	Combined forms of age-related cataract, left eye
⇄	H25.813	Combined forms of age-related cataract, bilateral
	H25.89	Other age-related cataract
⇄	H26.001	Unspecified infantile and juvenile cataract, right eye
⇄	H26.002	Unspecified infantile and juvenile cataract, left eye
⇄	H26.003	Unspecified infantile and juvenile cataract, bilateral
⇄	H26.031	Infantile and juvenile nuclear cataract, right eye
⇄	H26.032	Infantile and juvenile nuclear cataract, left eye
⇄	H26.033	Infantile and juvenile nuclear cataract, bilateral
⇄	H26.041	Anterior subcapsular polar infantile and juvenile cataract, right eye
⇄	H26.042	Anterior subcapsular polar infantile and juvenile cataract, left eye
⇄	H26.043	Anterior subcapsular polar infantile and juvenile cataract, bilateral
⇄	H26.051	Posterior subcapsular polar infantile and juvenile cataract, right eye
⇄	H26.052	Posterior subcapsular polar infantile and juvenile cataract, left eye
⇄	H26.053	Posterior subcapsular polar infantile and juvenile cataract, bilateral
⇄	H26.101	Unspecified traumatic cataract, right eye
⇄	H26.102	Unspecified traumatic cataract, left eye
⇄	H26.103	Unspecified traumatic cataract, bilateral
⇄	H26.111	Localized traumatic opacities, right eye
⇄	H26.112	Localized traumatic opacities, left eye
⇄	H26.113	Localized traumatic opacities, bilateral
⇄	H26.121	Partially resolved traumatic cataract, right eye
⇄	H26.122	Partially resolved traumatic cataract, left eye
⇄	H26.123	Partially resolved traumatic cataract, bilateral
⇄	H26.131	Total traumatic cataract, right eye
⇄	H26.132	Total traumatic cataract, left eye
⇄	H26.133	Total traumatic cataract, bilateral
	H26.20	Unspecified complicated cataract
⇄	H26.211	Cataract with neovascularization, right eye
⇄	H26.212	Cataract with neovascularization, left eye
⇄	H26.213	Cataract with neovascularization, bilateral

⇄ H26.221 Cataract secondary to ocular disorders (degenerative) (inflammatory), right eye
⇄ H26.222 Cataract secondary to ocular disorders (degenerative) (inflammatory), left eye
⇄ H26.223 Cataract secondary to ocular disorders (degenerative) (inflammatory), bilateral
⇄ H26.231 Glaucomatous flecks (subcapsular), right eye
⇄ H26.232 Glaucomatous flecks (subcapsular), left eye
⇄ H26.233 Glaucomatous flecks (subcapsular), bilateral
H26.8 Other specified cataract
⇄ H30.001 Unspecified focal chorioretinal inflammation, right eye
⇄ H30.002 Unspecified focal chorioretinal inflammation, left eye
⇄ H30.003 Unspecified focal chorioretinal inflammation, bilateral
⇄ H30.891 Other chorioretinal inflammations, right eye
⇄ H30.892 Other chorioretinal inflammations, left eye
⇄ H30.893 Other chorioretinal inflammations, bilateral
H35.52 Pigmentary retinal dystrophy
⇄ H40.1411 Capsular glaucoma with pseudoexfoliation of lens, right eye, mild stage
⇄ H40.1412 Capsular glaucoma with pseudoexfoliation of lens, right eye, moderate stage
⇄ H40.1413 Capsular glaucoma with pseudoexfoliation of lens, right eye, severe stage
⇄ H40.1414 Capsular glaucoma with pseudoexfoliation of lens, right eye, indeterminate stage
⇄ H40.1421 Capsular glaucoma with pseudoexfoliation of lens, left eye, mild stage
⇄ H40.1422 Capsular glaucoma with pseudoexfoliation of lens, left eye, moderate stage
⇄ H40.1423 Capsular glaucoma with pseudoexfoliation of lens, left eye, severe stage
⇄ H40.1424 Capsular glaucoma with pseudoexfoliation of lens, left eye, indeterminate stage
⇄ H40.1431 Capsular glaucoma with pseudoexfoliation of lens, bilateral, mild stage
⇄ H40.1432 Capsular glaucoma with pseudoexfoliation of lens, bilateral, moderate stage
⇄ H40.1433 Capsular glaucoma with pseudoexfoliation of lens, bilateral, severe stage
⇄ H40.1434 Capsular glaucoma with pseudoexfoliation of lens, bilateral, indeterminate stage
⇄ H40.51X1 Glaucoma secondary to other eye disorders, right eye, mild stage
⇄ H40.51X2 Glaucoma secondary to other eye disorders, right eye, moderate stage
⇄ H40.51X3 Glaucoma secondary to other eye disorders, right eye, severe stage
⇄ H40.51X4 Glaucoma secondary to other eye disorders, right eye, indeterminate stage
⇄ H40.52X1 Glaucoma secondary to other eye disorders, left eye, mild stage
⇄ H40.52X2 Glaucoma secondary to other eye disorders, left eye, moderate stage
⇄ H40.52X3 Glaucoma secondary to other eye disorders, left eye, severe stage
⇄ H40.52X4 Glaucoma secondary to other eye disorders, left eye, indeterminate stage
⇄ H40.53X1 Glaucoma secondary to other eye disorders, bilateral, mild stage
⇄ H40.53X2 Glaucoma secondary to other eye disorders, bilateral, moderate stage
⇄ H40.53X3 Glaucoma secondary to other eye disorders, bilateral, severe stage
⇄ H40.53X4 Glaucoma secondary to other eye disorders, bilateral, indeterminate stage
H40.89 Other specified glaucoma
⇄ H44.111 Panuveitis, right eye
⇄ H44.112 Panuveitis, left eye
⇄ H44.113 Panuveitis, bilateral
⇄ H44.21 Degenerative myopia, right eye
⇄ H44.22 Degenerative myopia, left eye
⇄ H44.23 Degenerative myopia, bilateral
⇄ H44.2A1 Degenerative myopia with choroidal neovascularization, right eye
⇄ H44.2A2 Degenerative myopia with choroidal neovascularization, left eye
⇄ H44.2A3 Degenerative myopia with choroidal neovascularization, bilateral eye
⇄ H44.2B1 Degenerative myopia with macular hole, right eye
⇄ H44.2B2 Degenerative myopia with macular hole, left eye
⇄ H44.2B3 Degenerative myopia with macular hole, bilateral eye
⇄ H44.2C1 Degenerative myopia with retinal detachment, right eye
⇄ H44.2C2 Degenerative myopia with retinal detachment, left eye
⇄ H44.2C3 Degenerative myopia with retinal detachment, bilateral eye
⇄ H44.2D1 Degenerative myopia with foveoschisis, right eye
⇄ H44.2D2 Degenerative myopia with foveoschisis, left eye
⇄ H44.2D3 Degenerative myopia with foveoschisis, bilateral eye
⇄ H44.2E1 Degenerative myopia with other maculopathy, right eye
⇄ H44.2E2 Degenerative myopia with other maculopathy, left eye
⇄ H44.2E3 Degenerative myopia with other maculopathy, bilateral eye
⇄ H44.311 Chalcosis, right eye
⇄ H44.312 Chalcosis, left eye
⇄ H44.313 Chalcosis, bilateral
Q12.0 Congenital cataract
Z96.1 Presence of intraocular lens
⇄ Z98.41 Cataract extraction status, right eye
⇄ Z98.42 Cataract extraction status, left eye

CCI Edits

Refer to Appendix A for CCI edits.

Pub 100

66982: Pub 100-03, 1, 10.1, Pub 100-03, 1, 80.10, Pub 100-03, 1, 80.12, Pub 100-04, 14, 40.3, Pub 100-04, 32, 120 120.4

Facility RVUs ▯

Code	Work	PE Facility	MP	Total Facility
66982	10.25	10.54	0.77	21.56

Non-facility RVUs ▯

Code	Work	PE Non-Facility	MP	Total Non-Facility
66982	10.25	10.54	0.77	21.56

Modifiers (PAR) ▯

Code	Mod 50	Mod 51	Mod 62	Mod 66	Mod 80
66982	1	2	0	0	1

Global Period

Code	Days
66982	090

66983

66983 Intracapsular cataract extraction with insertion of intraocular lens prosthesis (1 stage procedure)

(Do not report 66983 in conjunction with 0308T)

AMA Coding Notes

Surgical Procedures on the Eye and Ocular Adnexa

(For diagnostic and treatment ophthalmological services, see Medicine, Ophthalmology, and 92002 et seq)

(Do not report code 69990 in addition to codes 65091-68850)

AMA *CPT® Assistant*

66983: Fall 92: 5, 8, Nov 03: 10, Sep 09: 5, Mar 13: 6, Dec 19: 6, Mar 21: 7

Plain English Description

The physician performs an intracapsular cataract extraction (ICCE) with insertion of an intraocular lens (IOL) prosthesis. ICCE is rarely used today due to the development of more advanced extracapsular techniques. A large incision is made at the corneoscleral junction (fornix). The eye is injected with a substance that dissolves the zonular fibers that hold the lens in place. A cryoprobe is placed on the lens and liquid nitrogen is applied to freeze the lens. The probe is then withdrawn with the attached native lens. When the native lens is removed, the IOL is implanted in front of the iris. The eyelid is then sutured closed to allow the eye to heal.

Intracapsular cataract extraction with insertion of intraocular lens prosthesis

ICD-10-CM Diagnostic Codes

	E08.36	Diabetes mellitus due to underlying condition with diabetic cataract
	E09.36	Drug or chemical induced diabetes mellitus with diabetic cataract
	E10.311	Type 1 diabetes mellitus with unspecified diabetic retinopathy with macular edema
	E10.319	Type 1 diabetes mellitus with unspecified diabetic retinopathy without macular edema
❼⇄	E10.321	Type 1 diabetes mellitus with mild nonproliferative diabetic retinopathy with macular edema
❼⇄	E10.329	Type 1 diabetes mellitus with mild nonproliferative diabetic retinopathy without macular edema
❼⇄	E10.331	Type 1 diabetes mellitus with moderate nonproliferative diabetic retinopathy with macular edema
❼⇄	E10.339	Type 1 diabetes mellitus with moderate nonproliferative diabetic retinopathy without macular edema
❼⇄	E10.341	Type 1 diabetes mellitus with severe nonproliferative diabetic retinopathy with macular edema
❼⇄	E10.349	Type 1 diabetes mellitus with severe nonproliferative diabetic retinopathy without macular edema
❼⇄	E10.351	Type 1 diabetes mellitus with proliferative diabetic retinopathy with macular edema
❼⇄	E10.359	Type 1 diabetes mellitus with proliferative diabetic retinopathy without macular edema
	E10.36	Type 1 diabetes mellitus with diabetic cataract
	E10.39	Type 1 diabetes mellitus with other diabetic ophthalmic complication
	E11.311	Type 2 diabetes mellitus with unspecified diabetic retinopathy with macular edema
	E11.319	Type 2 diabetes mellitus with unspecified diabetic retinopathy without macular edema
❼⇄	E11.321	Type 2 diabetes mellitus with mild nonproliferative diabetic retinopathy with macular edema
❼⇄	E11.329	Type 2 diabetes mellitus with mild nonproliferative diabetic retinopathy without macular edema
❼⇄	E11.339	Type 2 diabetes mellitus with moderate nonproliferative diabetic retinopathy without macular edema
❼⇄	E11.341	Type 2 diabetes mellitus with severe nonproliferative diabetic retinopathy with macular edema
❼⇄	E11.349	Type 2 diabetes mellitus with severe nonproliferative diabetic retinopathy without macular edema
❼⇄	E11.351	Type 2 diabetes mellitus with proliferative diabetic retinopathy with macular edema
❼⇄	E11.359	Type 2 diabetes mellitus with proliferative diabetic retinopathy without macular edema
	E11.36	Type 2 diabetes mellitus with diabetic cataract
	E11.39	Type 2 diabetes mellitus with other diabetic ophthalmic complication
	E11.65	Type 2 diabetes mellitus with hyperglycemia
⇄	H25.012	Cortical age-related cataract, left eye
⇄	H25.032	Anterior subcapsular polar age-related cataract, left eye
⇄	H25.042	Posterior subcapsular polar age-related cataract, left eye
⇄	H25.092	Other age-related incipient cataract, left eye
⇄	H25.12	Age-related nuclear cataract, left eye
⇄	H25.22	Age-related cataract, morgagnian type, left eye
⇄	H25.812	Combined forms of age-related cataract, left eye
	H25.89	Other age-related cataract
⇄	H26.032	Infantile and juvenile nuclear cataract, left eye
⇄	H26.112	Localized traumatic opacities, left eye
⇄	H26.132	Total traumatic cataract, left eye
	H26.8	Other specified cataract
	Q12.0	Congenital cataract
	Z96.1	Presence of intraocular lens
⇄	Z98.42	Cataract extraction status, left eye

ICD-10-CM Coding Notes

For codes requiring a 7th character extension, refer to your ICD-10-CM book. Review the character descriptions and coding guidelines for proper selection. For some procedures, only certain characters will apply.

CCI Edits

Refer to Appendix A for CCI edits.

Pub 100

66983: Pub 100-03, 1, 10.1, Pub 100-03, 1, 80.12, Pub 100-04, 14, 40.3, Pub 100-04, 32, 120-120.4

Facility RVUs

Code	Work	PE Facility	MP	Total Facility
66983	0.00	0.00	0.00	0.00

Non-facility RVUs

Code	Work	PE Non-Facility	MP	Total Non-Facility
66983	0.00	0.00	0.00	0.00

Modifiers (PAR)

Code	Mod 50	Mod 51	Mod 62	Mod 66	Mod 80
66983	1	2	0	0	1

Global Period

Code	Days
66983	090

66984

66984 Extracapsular cataract removal with insertion of intraocular lens prosthesis (1 stage procedure), manual or mechanical technique (eg, irrigation and aspiration or phacoemulsification); without endoscopic cyclophotocoagulation

(For complex extracapsular cataract removal, use 66982)

(For extracapsular cataract removal with concomitant endoscopic cyclophotocoagulation, use 66988)

(For extracapsular cataract removal with concomitant intraocular aqueous drainage device by internal approach, use 66989)

(For insertion of ocular telescope prosthesis including removal of crystalline lens, use 0308T)

(For insertion of intraocular anterior segment drainage device into the trabecular meshwork without concomitant cataract removal with intraocular lens implant, use 0671T)

AMA Coding Notes

Surgical Procedures on the Eye and Ocular Adnexa

(For diagnostic and treatment ophthalmological services, see Medicine, Ophthalmology, and 92002 et seq)

(Do not report code 69990 in addition to codes 65091-68850)

AMA *CPT® Assistant* ▢

66984: Fall 92: 5, 8, Feb 01: 7, Nov 03: 10, Mar 05: 11, Sep 09: 5, Mar 13: 6, Dec 18: 6, Dec 19: 6, Dec 20: 13, Mar 21: 7

Plain English Description

Extracapsular cataract removal is performed with insertion of an intraocular lens (IOL) prosthesis to remove the cloudy membrane that has formed over the surface of the lens. An incision is made in the corneoscleral junction (fornix) for insertion of the phacoemulsification device. A side port incision is made and the pupil is dilated. A circular tear is made in the anterior lens capsule, which is opened, and the phacoemulsification probe is inserted. The device uses ultrasound to break up the cataract and aspirate the pieces for removal, or manual cutting and suction is used. A bubble of air is injected into the anterior chamber for protection of the cornea. The intraocular lens is placed into the eye and the incision may be closed with sutures. Water or saline is injected to re-establish intraocular pressure and the eye is dressed.

Extracapsular cataract removal with insertion of intraocular lens prosthesis

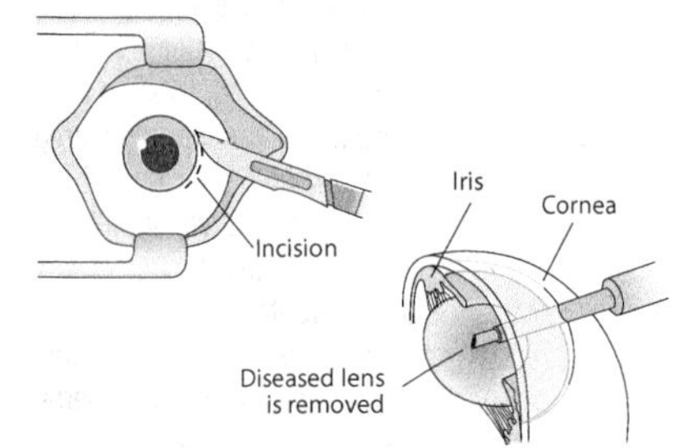

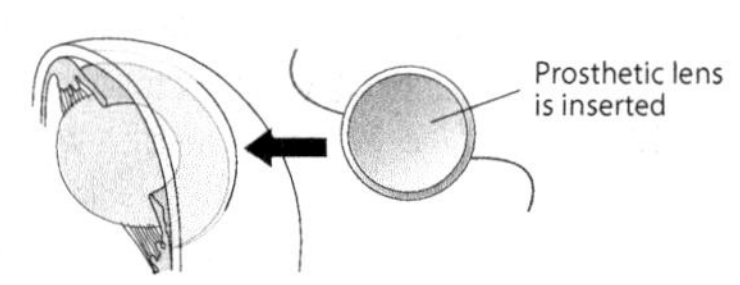

ICD-10-CM Diagnostic Codes

	Code	Description
	E10.36	Type 1 diabetes mellitus with diabetic cataract
	E11.36	Type 2 diabetes mellitus with diabetic cataract
⇄	H25.011	Cortical age-related cataract, right eye
⇄	H25.012	Cortical age-related cataract, left eye
⇄	H25.013	Cortical age-related cataract, bilateral
⇄	H25.031	Anterior subcapsular polar age-related cataract, right eye
⇄	H25.032	Anterior subcapsular polar age-related cataract, left eye
⇄	H25.033	Anterior subcapsular polar age-related cataract, bilateral
⇄	H25.041	Posterior subcapsular polar age-related cataract, right eye
⇄	H25.042	Posterior subcapsular polar age-related cataract, left eye
⇄	H25.043	Posterior subcapsular polar age-related cataract, bilateral
⇄	H25.091	Other age-related incipient cataract, right eye
⇄	H25.092	Other age-related incipient cataract, left eye
⇄	H25.093	Other age-related incipient cataract, bilateral
⇄	H25.11	Age-related nuclear cataract, right eye
⇄	H25.12	Age-related nuclear cataract, left eye
⇄	H25.13	Age-related nuclear cataract, bilateral
⇄	H25.21	Age-related cataract, morgagnian type, right eye
⇄	H25.22	Age-related cataract, morgagnian type, left eye
⇄	H25.23	Age-related cataract, morgagnian type, bilateral
⇄	H25.811	Combined forms of age-related cataract, right eye
⇄	H25.812	Combined forms of age-related cataract, left eye
⇄	H25.813	Combined forms of age-related cataract, bilateral
	H25.89	Other age-related cataract
⇄	H26.111	Localized traumatic opacities, right eye
⇄	H26.112	Localized traumatic opacities, left eye
⇄	H26.113	Localized traumatic opacities, bilateral
⇄	H26.131	Total traumatic cataract, right eye
⇄	H26.132	Total traumatic cataract, left eye
⇄	H26.133	Total traumatic cataract, bilateral
	H26.8	Other specified cataract
	H26.9	Unspecified cataract

CCI Edits

Refer to Appendix A for CCI edits.

Pub 100

66984: Pub 100-03, 1, 10.1, Pub 100-03, 1, 80.10, Pub 100-03, 1, 80.12, Pub 100-04, 14, 40.3, Pub 100-04, 32, 120-120.4

Facility RVUs ▢

Code	Work	PE Facility	MP	Total Facility
66984	7.35	7.83	0.56	15.74

Non-facility RVUs ▢

Code	Work	PE Non-Facility	MP	Total Non-Facility
66984	7.35	7.83	0.56	15.74

Modifiers (PAR) ▢

Code	Mod 50	Mod 51	Mod 62	Mod 66	Mod 80
66984	1	2	0	0	1

Global Period

Code	Days
66984	090

66985

66985 Insertion of intraocular lens prosthesis (secondary implant), not associated with concurrent cataract removal

(To code implant at time of concurrent cataract surgery, see 66982, 66983, 66984)

(To report supply of intraocular lens prosthesis, use 99070)

(For ultrasonic determination of intraocular lens power, use 76519)

(For removal of implanted material from anterior segment, use 65920)

(For secondary fixation (separate procedure), use 66682)

(For use of ophthalmic endoscope with 66985, use 66990)

AMA Coding Notes

Surgical Procedures on the Eye and Ocular Adnexa

(For diagnostic and treatment ophthalmological services, see Medicine, Ophthalmology, and 92002 et seq)

(Do not report code 69990 in addition to codes 65091-68850)

AMA *CPT® Assistant* ▯

66985: Sep 05: 12, Sep 09: 5, Dec 11: 16, Mar 13: 6, Mar 21: 7

Plain English Description

A secondary intraocular lens (IOL) prosthesis may be placed over an existing IOL implant ("piggybacked") to correct refractive errors following previous cataract surgery. The cornea is incised and viscoelastic material is injected into the anterior chamber to protect the corneal endothelium. The ciliary sulcus space is then distended with viscoelastic material, and the IOL mounted on an injector is placed into the eye. The lead haptic may be placed directly into the ciliary sulcus with the trailing haptic inserted into the eye and tucked behind the iris, or the entire lens can be delivered completely into the anterior chamber and both haptics secured under the iris. The viscoelastic material is removed from the eye and the corneal incision is closed with suture or stromal hydration.

Insertion of intraocular lens prosthesis, not associated with concurrent cataract removal

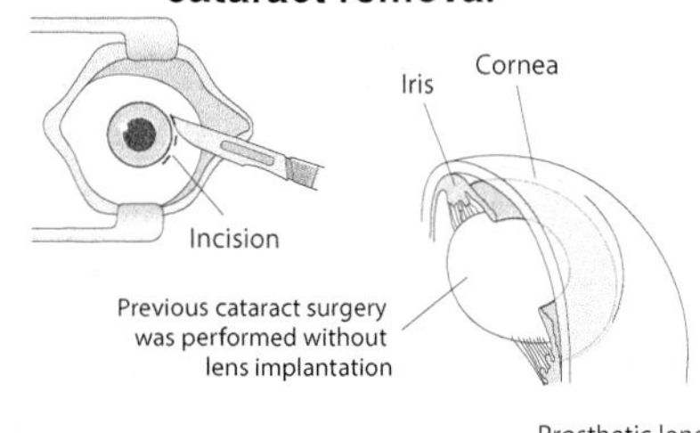

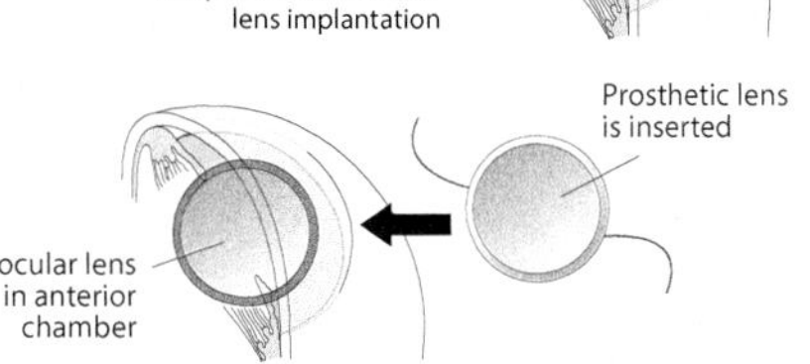

ICD-10-CM Diagnostic Codes

⇄	H25.11	Age-related nuclear cataract, right eye
⇄	H25.12	Age-related nuclear cataract, left eye
⇄	H25.13	Age-related nuclear cataract, bilateral
⇄	H27.01	Aphakia, right eye
⇄	H27.02	Aphakia, left eye
⇄	H27.03	Aphakia, bilateral
⇄	H27.111	Subluxation of lens, right eye
⇄	H27.112	Subluxation of lens, left eye
⇄	H27.113	Subluxation of lens, bilateral
⇄	H27.131	Posterior dislocation of lens, right eye
⇄	H27.132	Posterior dislocation of lens, left eye
⇄	H27.133	Posterior dislocation of lens, bilateral
⇄	H43.01	Vitreous prolapse, right eye
⇄	H43.02	Vitreous prolapse, left eye
⇄	H43.03	Vitreous prolapse, bilateral
⇄	H59.021	Cataract (lens) fragments in eye following cataract surgery, right eye
⇄	H59.022	Cataract (lens) fragments in eye following cataract surgery, left eye
⇄	H59.023	Cataract (lens) fragments in eye following cataract surgery, bilateral
❼	T85.21	Breakdown (mechanical) of intraocular lens
❼	T85.22	Displacement of intraocular lens
❼	T85.29	Other mechanical complication of intraocular lens
⇄	T86.8421	Corneal transplant infection, right eye
⇄	T86.8422	Corneal transplant infection, left eye
⇄	T86.8423	Corneal transplant infection, bilateral
⇄	T86.8481	Other complications of corneal transplant, right eye
⇄	T86.8482	Other complications of corneal transplant, left eye
⇄	T86.8483	Other complications of corneal transplant, bilateral
	Z96.1	Presence of intraocular lens
⇄	Z98.42	Cataract extraction status, left eye
	Z98.83	Filtering (vitreous) bleb after glaucoma surgery status

ICD-10-CM Coding Notes

For codes requiring a 7th character extension, refer to your ICD-10-CM book. Review the character descriptions and coding guidelines for proper selection. For some procedures, only certain characters will apply.

CCI Edits

Refer to Appendix A for CCI edits.

Pub 100

66985: Pub 100-03, 1, 10.1, Pub 100-03, 1, 80.12, Pub 100-04, 14, 40.3, Pub 100-04, 32, 120-120.4

Facility RVUs ▯

Code	Work	PE Facility	MP	Total Facility
66985	9.98	11.52	0.77	22.27

Non-facility RVUs ▯

Code	Work	PE Non-Facility	MP	Total Non-Facility
66985	9.98	11.52	0.77	22.27

Modifiers (PAR) ▯

Code	Mod 50	Mod 51	Mod 62	Mod 66	Mod 80
66985	1	2	1	0	1

Global Period

Code	Days
66985	090

66986

66986 Exchange of intraocular lens

(For use of ophthalmic endoscope with 66986, use 66990)

AMA Coding Notes

Surgical Procedures on the Eye and Ocular Adnexa

(For diagnostic and treatment ophthalmological services, see Medicine, Ophthalmology, and 92002 et seq)

(Do not report code 69990 in addition to codes 65091-68850)

AMA *CPT® Assistant* ▢

66986: Sep 05: 12, Mar 21: 7

Plain English Description

The exchange of a previously placed intraocular lens (IOL) may be required to correct refractive errors following cataract surgery. The cornea is incised to create a paracentesis, and the anterior chamber is inflated with viscoelastic. A capsulorrhexis needle is advanced and dispersive viscoelastic is injected to separate the anterior capsule from the IOL. A blunt spatula is then used to dissect the anterior capsule from the IOL. Viscoelastic is then injected under the IOL to dissect it from the posterior capsule and the IOL is lifted, injecting more dispersive viscoelastic as necessary. A second paracentesis may be required to access 360 degrees around the IOL and complete the dissection. The IOL is dialed out of the capsule and into the anterior chamber where it can be folded and removed or cut with scissors and removed in pieces. Using a lens injector, the exchange IOL may be inserted behind the first IOL, before it is removed or it can be inserted after removal of the first IOL. The viscoelastic is removed from the eye and the corneal incision(s) are closed with suture or stromal hydration.

Exchange intraocular lens

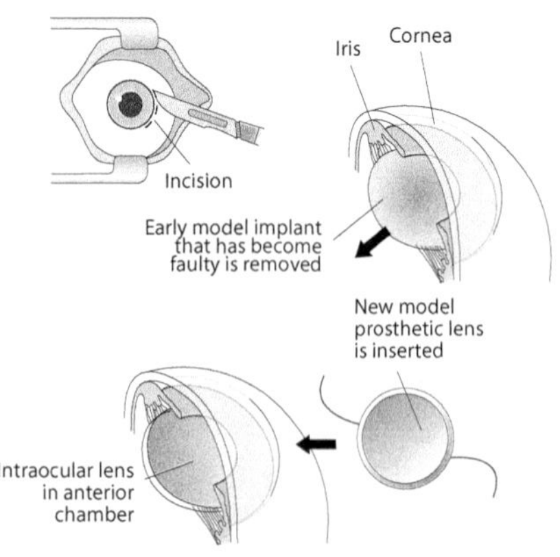
Iris
Cornea
Incision
Early model implant that has become faulty is removed
New model prosthetic lens is inserted
Intraocular lens in anterior chamber

ICD-10-CM Diagnostic Codes

⇄ H20.11 Chronic iridocyclitis, right eye
⇄ H25.11 Age-related nuclear cataract, right eye
⇄ H27.01 Aphakia, right eye
⇄ H27.111 Subluxation of lens, right eye
⇄ H27.121 Anterior dislocation of lens, right eye
⇄ H27.131 Posterior dislocation of lens, right eye
⇄ H43.01 Vitreous prolapse, right eye
⇄ H59.021 Cataract (lens) fragments in eye following cataract surgery, right eye
➐ T85.21 Breakdown (mechanical) of intraocular lens
➐ T85.22 Displacement of intraocular lens
➐ T85.29 Other mechanical complication of intraocular lens
Z96.1 Presence of intraocular lens
⇄ Z98.41 Cataract extraction status, right eye

ICD-10-CM Coding Notes

For codes requiring a 7th character extension, refer to your ICD-10-CM book. Review the character descriptions and coding guidelines for proper selection. For some procedures, only certain characters will apply.

CCI Edits

Refer to Appendix A for CCI edits.

Pub 100

66986: Pub 100-03, 1, 80.12, Pub 100-04, 14, 40.3, Pub 100-04, 32, 120-120.4

Facility RVUs ▢

Code	Work	PE Facility	MP	Total Facility
66986	12.26	12.93	0.95	26.14

Non-facility RVUs ▢

Code	Work	PE Non-Facility	MP	Total Non-Facility
66986	12.26	12.93	0.95	26.14

Modifiers (PAR) ▢

Code	Mod 50	Mod 51	Mod 62	Mod 66	Mod 80
66986	1	2	1	0	1

Global Period

Code	Days
66986	090

66987

66987 Extracapsular cataract removal with insertion of intraocular lens prosthesis (1-stage procedure), manual or mechanical technique (eg, irrigation and aspiration or phacoemulsification), complex, requiring devices or techniques not generally used in routine cataract surgery (eg, iris expansion device, suture support for intraocular lens, or primary posterior capsulorrhexis) or performed on patients in the amblyogenic developmental stage; with endoscopic cyclophotocoagulation

(For complex extracapsular cataract removal without endoscopic cyclophotocoagulation, use 66982)

(For insertion of ocular telescope prosthesis including removal of crystalline lens, use 0308T)

AMA Coding Notes

Surgical Procedures on the Eye and Ocular Adnexa

(For diagnostic and treatment ophthalmological services, see Medicine, Ophthalmology, and 92002 et seq)

(Do not report code 69990 in addition to codes 65091-68850)

AMA *CPT® Assistant* ▯

66987: Dec 19: 6

Plain English Description

Complex extracapsular cataract removal is performed with insertion of intraocular lens (IOL) prosthesis using manual or mechanical technique with endoscopic cyclophotocoagulation. A complex procedure uses devices or techniques not generally used in routine cataract surgery. This is necessary for children because primary posterior capsulotomy or capsulorrhexis is required for IOL insertion, the anterior capsule in children is more difficult to open, and the cortex is more difficult to remove due to lens adhesion. Complexity is also increased with certain conditions, such as uveitis, glaucoma, pseudoexfoliation syndrome, or Marfan syndrome. Patients with prior intraocular surgery or other trauma to the eye, or dense, hard, white cataracts may also require a more complex procedure.

An incision is made in the corneoscleral junction (fornix) for insertion of the phacoemulsification device. A side port incision is made. An attempt is made to dilate the pupil. If unsuccessful, a spatula is inserted and posterior synechiae are lysed. Four incisions are made and an expansion device consisting of four hooks is inserted. The iris is retracted using the hooks. A circular tear is made in the anterior lens capsule, which is opened, and the phacoemulsification probe is inserted. The probe uses ultrasound to break up the cataract and remove the pieces by aspiration. Once the cataract has been removed, the softer cortex surrounding the cataract is removed by suction. Viscoelastic material is injected into the lens capsule to maintain its shape. In a child, the posterior capsule is also incised to facilitate insertion of the IOL. Endoscopic cyclophotocoagulation (ECP) is performed with phacoemulsification cataract removal on glaucoma patients and may result in a reduced need for medication. A laser probe is inserted that emits pulsed, continuous wave energy to treat each ciliary process until it shrinks and turns white while viewing continuously on the monitor. The probe combines a laser diode emitting pulsed wave energy, a light source, a laser aiming beam, and video camera imaging. 180 to 360 degrees may be treated. The IOL is inserted and the viscoelastic material is removed. The incisions are checked for water tightness. Subconjunctival injection of water or saline is performed to restore intraocular pressure and the eye is dressed.

Extracapsular cataract removal with lens insertion, complex, with endoscopic cyclophotocoagulation

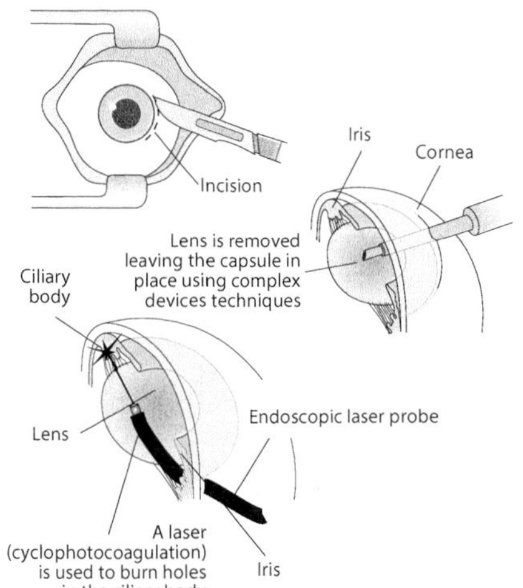

ICD-10-CM Diagnostic Codes

⇄	H20.11	Chronic iridocyclitis, right eye
⇄	H21.54	Posterior synechiae (iris)
⇄	H25.011	Cortical age-related cataract, right eye
⇄	H25.041	Posterior subcapsular polar age-related cataract, right eye
⇄	H25.11	Age-related nuclear cataract, right eye
⇄	H25.21	Age-related cataract, morgagnian type, right eye
⇄	H25.811	Combined forms of age-related cataract, right eye
	H25.89	Other age-related cataract
⇄	H26.001	Unspecified infantile and juvenile cataract, right eye
⇄	H26.031	Infantile and juvenile nuclear cataract, right eye
⇄	H26.041	Anterior subcapsular polar infantile and juvenile cataract, right eye
⇄	H26.051	Posterior subcapsular polar infantile and juvenile cataract, right eye
⇄	H26.101	Unspecified traumatic cataract, right eye
⇄	H26.11	Localized traumatic opacities
⇄	H26.121	Partially resolved traumatic cataract, right eye
⇄	H26.131	Total traumatic cataract, right eye
	H26.20	Unspecified complicated cataract
⇄	H26.221	Cataract secondary to ocular disorders (degenerative) (inflammatory), right eye
⇄	H26.231	Glaucomatous flecks (subcapsular), right eye
	H26.8	Other specified cataract
⇄	H30.001	Unspecified focal chorioretinal inflammation, right eye
⇄	H30.891	Other chorioretinal inflammations, right eye
	H35.52	Pigmentary retinal dystrophy
⇄	H40.021	Open angle with borderline findings, high risk, right eye
⇄	H40.022	Open angle with borderline findings, high risk, left eye
⇄	H40.023	Open angle with borderline findings, high risk, bilateral
⇄	H40.031	Anatomical narrow angle, right eye
⇄	H40.032	Anatomical narrow angle, left eye
⇄	H40.033	Anatomical narrow angle, bilateral
❼⇄	H40.111	Primary open-angle glaucoma, right eye
❼⇄	H40.112	Primary open-angle glaucoma, left eye
❼⇄	H40.113	Primary open-angle glaucoma, bilateral
❼⇄	H40.141	Capsular glaucoma with pseudoexfoliation of lens, right eye
❼⇄	H40.142	Capsular glaucoma with pseudoexfoliation of lens, left eye
❼⇄	H40.143	Capsular glaucoma with pseudoexfoliation of lens, bilateral
❼⇄	H40.51	Glaucoma secondary to other eye disorders, right eye
❼⇄	H40.52	Glaucoma secondary to other eye disorders, left eye
❼⇄	H40.53	Glaucoma secondary to other eye disorders, bilateral
	H40.89	Other specified glaucoma
⇄	H44.21	Degenerative myopia, right eye
⇄	H44.2A1	Degenerative myopia with choroidal neovascularization, right eye
⇄	H44.2A2	Degenerative myopia with choroidal neovascularization, left eye
⇄	H44.2A3	Degenerative myopia with choroidal neovascularization, bilateral eye
⇄	H44.2B1	Degenerative myopia with macular hole, right eye
⇄	H44.2B2	Degenerative myopia with macular hole, left eye
⇄	H44.2B3	Degenerative myopia with macular hole, bilateral eye
⇄	H44.2C1	Degenerative myopia with retinal detachment, right eye
⇄	H44.2C2	Degenerative myopia with retinal detachment, left eye

⇄	H44.2C3	Degenerative myopia with retinal detachment, bilateral eye
⇄	H44.2D1	Degenerative myopia with foveoschisis, right eye
⇄	H44.2D2	Degenerative myopia with foveoschisis, left eye
⇄	H44.2D3	Degenerative myopia with foveoschisis, bilateral eye
⇄	H44.2E1	Degenerative myopia with other maculopathy, right eye
⇄	H44.2E2	Degenerative myopia with other maculopathy, left eye
⇄	H44.2E3	Degenerative myopia with other maculopathy, bilateral eye
⇄	H44.311	Chalcosis, right eye
	Q12.0	Congenital cataract
	Z96.1	Presence of intraocular lens
⇄	Z98.41	Cataract extraction status, right eye

ICD-10-CM Coding Notes

For codes requiring a 7th character extension, refer to your ICD-10-CM book. Review the character descriptions and coding guidelines for proper selection. For some procedures, only certain characters will apply.

CCI Edits

Refer to Appendix A for CCI edits.

Facility RVUs ▯

Code	Work	PE Facility	MP	Total Facility
66987	0.00	0.00	0.00	0.00

Non-facility RVUs ▯

Code	Work	PE Non-Facility	MP	Total Non-Facility
66987	0.00	0.00	0.00	0.00

Modifiers (PAR) ▯

Code	Mod 50	Mod 51	Mod 62	Mod 66	Mod 80
66987	1	2	1	1	0

Global Period

Code	Days
66987	090

66988

66988 Extracapsular cataract removal with insertion of intraocular lens prosthesis (1 stage procedure), manual or mechanical technique (eg, irrigation and aspiration or phacoemulsification); with endoscopic cyclophotocoagulation

(For extracapsular cataract removal without endoscopic cyclophotocoagulation, use 66984)

(For complex extracapsular cataract removal with endoscopic cyclophotocoagulation, use 66987)

(For insertion of ocular telescope prosthesis, including removal of crystalline lens, use 0308T)

AMA Coding Notes

Surgical Procedures on the Eye and Ocular Adnexa

(For diagnostic and treatment ophthalmological services, see Medicine, Ophthalmology, and 92002 et seq)

(Do not report code 69990 in addition to codes 65091-68850)

AMA *CPT® Assistant* ☐

66988: Dec 19: 6

Plain English Description

Extracapsular cataract removal is performed with insertion of an intraocular lens (IOL) prosthesis and endoscopic cyclophotocoagulation (ECP). An incision is made in the corneoscleral junction (fornix) for insertion of the phacoemulsification device. A side port incision is made and the pupil is dilated. A circular tear is made in the anterior lens capsule, which is opened, and the phacoemulsification probe is inserted. The device uses ultrasound to break up the cataract and aspirate the pieces for removal, or manual cutting and suction is used. A bubble of air is injected into the anterior chamber for protection of the cornea. Endoscopic cyclophotocoagulation (ECP) is performed with phacoemulsification cataract removal on glaucoma patients and may result in a reduced need for medication. A laser probe is inserted that emits pulsed, continuous wave energy to treat each ciliary process until it shrinks and turns white while viewing continuously on the monitor. The probe combines a laser diode emitting pulsed wave energy, a light source, a laser aiming beam, and video camera imaging. 180 to 360 degrees may be treated. The IOL is inserted and the incisions are checked for water tightness. Subconjunctival injection of water or saline is performed to restore intraocular pressure and the eye is dressed.

Extracapsular cataract removal with lens insertion and endoscopic cyclophotocoagulation

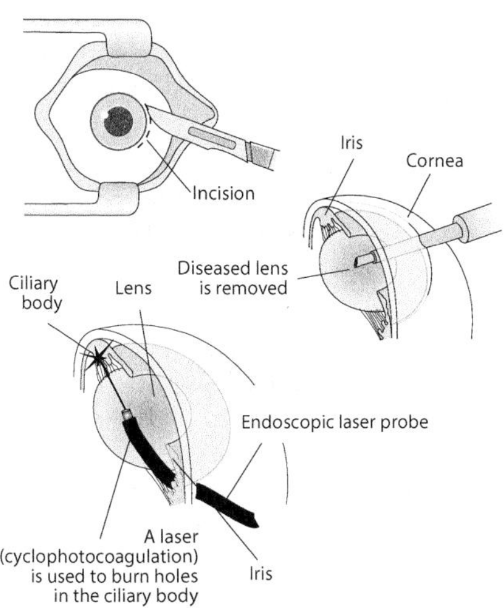

ICD-10-CM Diagnostic Codes

	E10.36	Type 1 diabetes mellitus with diabetic cataract
	E11.36	Type 2 diabetes mellitus with diabetic cataract
⇄	H25.011	Cortical age-related cataract, right eye
⇄	H25.031	Anterior subcapsular polar age-related cataract, right eye
⇄	H25.041	Posterior subcapsular polar age-related cataract, right eye
⇄	H25.091	Other age-related incipient cataract, right eye
⇄	H25.11	Age-related nuclear cataract, right eye
⇄	H25.21	Age-related cataract, morgagnian type, right eye
⇄	H25.812	Combined forms of age-related cataract, left eye
	H25.89	Other age-related cataract
⇄	H26.031	Infantile and juvenile nuclear cataract, right eye
⇄	H26.111	Localized traumatic opacities, right eye
⇄	H26.131	Total traumatic cataract, right eye
	H26.8	Other specified cataract
	H26.9	Unspecified cataract
⇄	H40.021	Open angle with borderline findings, high risk, right eye
⇄	H40.022	Open angle with borderline findings, high risk, left eye
⇄	H40.023	Open angle with borderline findings, high risk, bilateral
⇄	H40.031	Anatomical narrow angle, right eye
⇄	H40.032	Anatomical narrow angle, left eye
⇄	H40.033	Anatomical narrow angle, bilateral
➐	H40.10	Unspecified open-angle glaucoma
➐⇄	H40.111	Primary open-angle glaucoma, right eye
➐⇄	H40.112	Primary open-angle glaucoma, left eye
➐⇄	H40.113	Primary open-angle glaucoma, bilateral
➐⇄	H40.121	Low-tension glaucoma, right eye
➐⇄	H40.122	Low-tension glaucoma, left eye
➐⇄	H40.123	Low-tension glaucoma, bilateral
➐⇄	H40.141	Capsular glaucoma with pseudoexfoliation of lens, right eye
➐⇄	H40.142	Capsular glaucoma with pseudoexfoliation of lens, left eye
➐⇄	H40.143	Capsular glaucoma with pseudoexfoliation of lens, bilateral
➐⇄	H40.51	Glaucoma secondary to other eye disorders, right eye
➐⇄	H40.52	Glaucoma secondary to other eye disorders, left eye
➐⇄	H40.53	Glaucoma secondary to other eye disorders, bilateral

ICD-10-CM Coding Notes

For codes requiring a 7th character extension, refer to your ICD-10-CM book. Review the character descriptions and coding guidelines for proper selection. For some procedures, only certain characters will apply.

CCI Edits

Refer to Appendix A for CCI edits.

Facility RVUs ☐

Code	Work	PE Facility	MP	Total Facility
66988	0.00	0.00	0.00	0.00

Non-facility RVUs ☐

Code	Work	PE Non-Facility	MP	Total Non-Facility
66988	0.00	0.00	0.00	0.00

Modifiers (PAR) ☐

Code	Mod 50	Mod 51	Mod 62	Mod 66	Mod 80
66988	1	2	1	1	0

Global Period

Code	Days
66988	090

66989

- 66989 **Extracapsular cataract removal with insertion of intraocular lens prosthesis (1-stage procedure), manual or mechanical technique (eg, irrigation and aspiration or phacoemulsification), complex, requiring devices or techniques not generally used in routine cataract surgery (eg, iris expansion device, suture support for intraocular lens, or primary posterior capsulorrhexis) or performed on patients in the amblyogenic developmental stage; with insertion of intraocular (eg, trabecular meshwork, supraciliary, suprachoroidal) anterior segment aqueous drainage device, without extraocular reservoir, internal approach, one or more**

(For complex extracapsular cataract removal with intraocular lens implant without concomitant aqueous drainage device, use 66982)

(For insertion of intraocular anterior segment drainage device into the trabecular meshwork without concomitant cataract removal with intraocular lens implant, use 0671T)

AMA Coding Notes

Surgical Procedures on the Eye and Ocular Adnexa

(For diagnostic and treatment ophthalmological services, see Medicine, Ophthalmology, and 92002 et seq)

(Do not report code 69990 in addition to codes 65091-68850)

Plain English Description

Complex extracapsular cataract removal is performed with insertion of intraocular lens (IOL) prosthesis using manual or mechanical technique with the insertion of an intraocular anterior segment aqueous drainage device. A complex procedure uses devices or techniques not generally used in routine cataract surgery. This is necessary for children because primary posterior capsulotomy or capsulorrhexis is required for IOL insertion, the anterior capsule in children is more difficult to open, and the cortex is more difficult to remove due to lens adhesion. Complexity is also increased with certain conditions, such as uveitis, glaucoma, pseudoexfoliation syndrome or Marfan syndrome. Patients with prior intraocular surgery or other trauma to the eye, or dense, hard, white cataracts may also require a more complex procedure.
An incision is made in the corneoscleral junction (fornix) for insertion of the phacoemulsification device. A side port incision is made. An attempt is made to dilate the pupil. If unsuccessful, a spatula is inserted and posterior synechiae are lysed. Four incisions are made and an expansion device consisting of four hooks is inserted. The iris is retracted using the hooks. A circular tear is made in the anterior lens capsule, which is opened, and the phacoemulsification probe is inserted. The probe uses ultrasound to break up the cataract and remove the pieces by aspiration. Once the cataract has been removed, the softer cortex surrounding the cataract is removed by suction. Viscoelastic material is injected into the lens capsule to maintain its shape. In a child, the posterior capsule is also incised to facilitate insertion of the IOL. The IOL is inserted and the viscoelastic material is removed. An anterior segment aqueous drainage device without extraocular reservoir is also inserted to treat chronic or progressive open angle glaucoma. A magnification lens, such as a gonioscope, is used to place and position the drainage device (shunt) at the angle of the anterior chamber. The drainage device may traverse the sclera with the terminal end positioned in the suprachoroidal space, or end in the trabecular meshwork; alternatively, it may rest in the supraciliary space between the sclera and ciliary body to create a channel for aqueous fluid to flow out, reducing intraocular pressure. The incisions are checked for water tightness, and the eye is dressed.

ICD-10-CM Diagnostic Codes

	Code	Description
⇄	H20.11	Chronic iridocyclitis, right eye
⇄	H20.12	Chronic iridocyclitis, left eye
⇄	H20.13	Chronic iridocyclitis, bilateral
⇄	H21.541	Posterior synechiae (iris), right eye
⇄	H21.542	Posterior synechiae (iris), left eye
⇄	H21.543	Posterior synechiae (iris), bilateral
⇄	H25.011	Cortical age-related cataract, right eye
⇄	H25.012	Cortical age-related cataract, left eye
⇄	H25.013	Cortical age-related cataract, bilateral
⇄	H25.041	Posterior subcapsular polar age-related cataract, right eye
⇄	H25.042	Posterior subcapsular polar age-related cataract, left eye
⇄	H25.043	Posterior subcapsular polar age-related cataract, bilateral
⇄	H25.11	Age-related nuclear cataract, right eye
⇄	H25.12	Age-related nuclear cataract, left eye
⇄	H25.13	Age-related nuclear cataract, bilateral
⇄	H25.21	Age-related cataract, morgagnian type, right eye
⇄	H25.22	Age-related cataract, morgagnian type, left eye
⇄	H25.23	Age-related cataract, morgagnian type, bilateral
⇄	H25.811	Combined forms of age-related cataract, right eye
⇄	H25.812	Combined forms of age-related cataract, left eye
⇄	H25.813	Combined forms of age-related cataract, bilateral
	H25.89	Other age-related cataract
⇄	H26.001	Unspecified infantile and juvenile cataract, right eye
⇄	H26.002	Unspecified infantile and juvenile cataract, left eye
⇄	H26.003	Unspecified infantile and juvenile cataract, bilateral
⇄	H26.031	Infantile and juvenile nuclear cataract, right eye
⇄	H26.032	Infantile and juvenile nuclear cataract, left eye
⇄	H26.033	Infantile and juvenile nuclear cataract, bilateral
⇄	H26.041	Anterior subcapsular polar infantile and juvenile cataract, right eye
⇄	H26.042	Anterior subcapsular polar infantile and juvenile cataract, left eye
⇄	H26.043	Anterior subcapsular polar infantile and juvenile cataract, bilateral
⇄	H26.051	Posterior subcapsular polar infantile and juvenile cataract, right eye
⇄	H26.052	Posterior subcapsular polar infantile and juvenile cataract, left eye
⇄	H26.053	Posterior subcapsular polar infantile and juvenile cataract, bilateral
⇄	H26.101	Unspecified traumatic cataract, right eye
⇄	H26.102	Unspecified traumatic cataract, left eye
⇄	H26.103	Unspecified traumatic cataract, bilateral
⇄	H26.111	Localized traumatic opacities, right eye
⇄	H26.112	Localized traumatic opacities, left eye
⇄	H26.113	Localized traumatic opacities, bilateral
⇄	H26.121	Partially resolved traumatic cataract, right eye
⇄	H26.122	Partially resolved traumatic cataract, left eye
⇄	H26.123	Partially resolved traumatic cataract, bilateral
⇄	H26.131	Total traumatic cataract, right eye
⇄	H26.132	Total traumatic cataract, left eye
⇄	H26.133	Total traumatic cataract, bilateral
	H26.20	Unspecified complicated cataract
⇄	H26.211	Cataract with neovascularization, right eye
⇄	H26.212	Cataract with neovascularization, left eye
⇄	H26.213	Cataract with neovascularization, bilateral
⇄	H26.221	Cataract secondary to ocular disorders (degenerative) (inflammatory), right eye
⇄	H26.222	Cataract secondary to ocular disorders (degenerative) (inflammatory), left eye
⇄	H26.223	Cataract secondary to ocular disorders (degenerative) (inflammatory), bilateral
⇄	H26.231	Glaucomatous flecks (subcapsular), right eye

⇄ H26.232 Glaucomatous flecks (subcapsular), left eye
⇄ H26.233 Glaucomatous flecks (subcapsular), bilateral
H26.8 Other specified cataract
⇄ H30.001 Unspecified focal chorioretinal inflammation, right eye
⇄ H30.002 Unspecified focal chorioretinal inflammation, left eye
⇄ H30.003 Unspecified focal chorioretinal inflammation, bilateral
⇄ H30.891 Other chorioretinal inflammations, right eye
⇄ H30.892 Other chorioretinal inflammations, left eye
⇄ H30.893 Other chorioretinal inflammations, bilateral
H35.52 Pigmentary retinal dystrophy
⇄ H40.1111 Primary open-angle glaucoma, right eye, mild stage
⇄ H40.1112 Primary open-angle glaucoma, right eye, moderate stage
⇄ H40.1113 Primary open-angle glaucoma, right eye, severe stage
⇄ H40.1114 Primary open-angle glaucoma, right eye, indeterminate stage
⇄ H40.1121 Primary open-angle glaucoma, left eye, mild stage
⇄ H40.1122 Primary open-angle glaucoma, left eye, moderate stage
⇄ H40.1123 Primary open-angle glaucoma, left eye, severe stage
⇄ H40.1124 Primary open-angle glaucoma, left eye, indeterminate stage
⇄ H40.1131 Primary open-angle glaucoma, bilateral, mild stage
⇄ H40.1132 Primary open-angle glaucoma, bilateral, moderate stage
⇄ H40.1133 Primary open-angle glaucoma, bilateral, severe stage
⇄ H40.1134 Primary open-angle glaucoma, bilateral, indeterminate stage
⇄ H40.1411 Capsular glaucoma with pseudoexfoliation of lens, right eye, mild stage
⇄ H40.1412 Capsular glaucoma with pseudoexfoliation of lens, right eye, moderate stage
⇄ H40.1413 Capsular glaucoma with pseudoexfoliation of lens, right eye, severe stage
⇄ H40.1414 Capsular glaucoma with pseudoexfoliation of lens, right eye, indeterminate stage
⇄ H40.1421 Capsular glaucoma with pseudoexfoliation of lens, left eye, mild stage
⇄ H40.1422 Capsular glaucoma with pseudoexfoliation of lens, left eye, moderate stage
⇄ H40.1423 Capsular glaucoma with pseudoexfoliation of lens, left eye, severe stage
⇄ H40.1424 Capsular glaucoma with pseudoexfoliation of lens, left eye, indeterminate stage
⇄ H40.1431 Capsular glaucoma with pseudoexfoliation of lens, bilateral, mild stage
⇄ H40.1432 Capsular glaucoma with pseudoexfoliation of lens, bilateral, moderate stage
⇄ H40.1433 Capsular glaucoma with pseudoexfoliation of lens, bilateral, severe stage
⇄ H40.1434 Capsular glaucoma with pseudoexfoliation of lens, bilateral, indeterminate stage
⇄ H40.51X1 Glaucoma secondary to other eye disorders, right eye, mild stage
⇄ H40.51X2 Glaucoma secondary to other eye disorders, right eye, moderate stage
⇄ H40.51X3 Glaucoma secondary to other eye disorders, right eye, severe stage
⇄ H40.51X4 Glaucoma secondary to other eye disorders, right eye, indeterminate stage
⇄ H40.52X1 Glaucoma secondary to other eye disorders, left eye, mild stage
⇄ H40.52X2 Glaucoma secondary to other eye disorders, left eye, moderate stage
⇄ H40.52X3 Glaucoma secondary to other eye disorders, left eye, severe stage
⇄ H40.52X4 Glaucoma secondary to other eye disorders, left eye, indeterminate stage
⇄ H40.53X1 Glaucoma secondary to other eye disorders, bilateral, mild stage
⇄ H40.53X2 Glaucoma secondary to other eye disorders, bilateral, moderate stage
⇄ H40.53X3 Glaucoma secondary to other eye disorders, bilateral, severe stage
⇄ H40.53X4 Glaucoma secondary to other eye disorders, bilateral, indeterminate stage
H40.89 Other specified glaucoma
⇄ H44.111 Panuveitis, right eye
⇄ H44.112 Panuveitis, left eye
⇄ H44.113 Panuveitis, bilateral
⇄ H44.21 Degenerative myopia, right eye
⇄ H44.22 Degenerative myopia, left eye
⇄ H44.23 Degenerative myopia, bilateral
⇄ H44.2A1 Degenerative myopia with choroidal neovascularization, right eye
⇄ H44.2A2 Degenerative myopia with choroidal neovascularization, left eye
⇄ H44.2A3 Degenerative myopia with choroidal neovascularization, bilateral eye
⇄ H44.2B1 Degenerative myopia with macular hole, right eye
⇄ H44.2B2 Degenerative myopia with macular hole, left eye
⇄ H44.2B3 Degenerative myopia with macular hole, bilateral eye
⇄ H44.2C1 Degenerative myopia with retinal detachment, right eye
⇄ H44.2C2 Degenerative myopia with retinal detachment, left eye
⇄ H44.2C3 Degenerative myopia with retinal detachment, bilateral eye
⇄ H44.2D1 Degenerative myopia with foveoschisis, right eye
⇄ H44.2D2 Degenerative myopia with foveoschisis, left eye
⇄ H44.2D3 Degenerative myopia with foveoschisis, bilateral eye
⇄ H44.2E1 Degenerative myopia with other maculopathy, right eye
⇄ H44.2E2 Degenerative myopia with other maculopathy, left eye
⇄ H44.2E3 Degenerative myopia with other maculopathy, bilateral eye
⇄ H44.311 Chalcosis, right eye
⇄ H44.312 Chalcosis, left eye
⇄ H44.313 Chalcosis, bilateral
Q12.0 Congenital cataract
Z96.1 Presence of intraocular lens
⇄ Z98.41 Cataract extraction status, right eye
⇄ Z98.42 Cataract extraction status, left eye

CCI Edits

Refer to Appendix A for CCI edits.

Facility RVUs ▯

Code	Work	PE Facility	MP	Total Facility
66989	12.13	11.69	0.93	24.75

Non-facility RVUs ▯

Code	Work	PE Non-Facility	MP	Total Non-Facility
66989	12.13	11.69	0.93	24.75

Modifiers (PAR) ▯

Code	Mod 50	Mod 51	Mod 62	Mod 66	Mod 80
66989					

Global Period

Code	Days
66989	090

66990

+ 66990 Use of ophthalmic endoscope (List separately in addition to code for primary procedure)

(66990 may be used only with codes 65820, 65875, 65920, 66985, 66986, 67036, 67039, 67040, 67041, 67042, 67043, 67113)

AMA Coding Notes

Surgical Procedures on the Eye and Ocular Adnexa

(For diagnostic and treatment ophthalmological services, see Medicine, Ophthalmology, and 92002 et seq)

(Do not report code 69990 in addition to codes 65091-68850)

AMA *CPT® Assistant*

66990: Sep 05: 12, Oct 08: 3

Plain English Description

An ophthalmic endoscope provides better visualization of the anterior chamber, lens, and posterior segment than an operating microscope for certain types of procedures. Two stab incisions are made in the limbus. A cannula is inserted through one stab incision and viscoelastic material injected as needed to improve visualization. The endoscope is then inserted through the second stab incision and the surgical site carefully examined. Information obtained during the endoscopic exam is used to help plan the best surgical course for the patient. The physician then proceeds with the corrective procedure using endoscopic visualization as needed.

Ciliary body destruction; diathermy

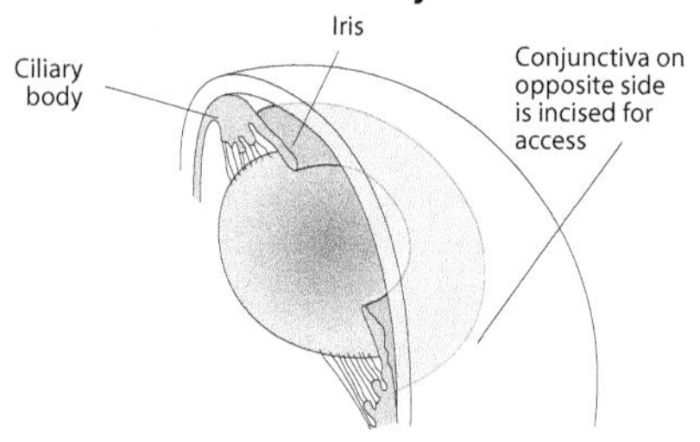

A heat probe (diathermy) is used to burn holes in the ciliary body.

ICD-10-CM Diagnostic Codes

See Primary Procedure code for crosswalks.

CCI Edits

Refer to Appendix A for CCI edits.

Facility RVUs

Code	Work	PE Facility	MP	Total Facility
66990	1.51	0.93	0.11	2.55

Non-facility RVUs

Code	Work	PE Non-Facility	MP	Total Non-Facility
66990	1.51	0.93	0.11	2.55

Modifiers (PAR)

Code	Mod 50	Mod 51	Mod 62	Mod 66	Mod 80
66990	0	0	0	0	1

Global Period

Code	Days
66990	ZZZ

66991

● **66991 Extracapsular cataract removal with insertion of intraocular lens prosthesis (1 stage procedure), manual or mechanical technique (eg, irrigation and aspiration or phacoemulsification); with insertion of intraocular (eg, trabecular meshwork, supraciliary, suprachoroidal) anterior segment aqueous drainage device, without extraocular reservoir, internal approach, one or more**

(For extracapsular cataract removal with intraocular lens implant without concomitant aqueous drainage device, use 66984)

(For insertion of intraocular anterior segment drainage device into the trabecular meshwork without concomitant cataract removal with intraocular lens implant, use 0671T)

AMA Coding Notes

Surgical Procedures on the Eye and Ocular Adnexa

(For diagnostic and treatment ophthalmological services, see Medicine, Ophthalmology, and 92002 et seq)

(Do not report code 69990 in addition to codes 65091-68850)

Plain English Description

Extracapsular cataract removal is performed with insertion of an intraocular lens (IOL) prosthesis to remove the cloudy membrane that has formed over the surface of the lens. An incision is made in the corneoscleral junction (fornix) for insertion of the phacoemulsification device. A side port incision is made and the pupil is dilated. A circular tear is made in the anterior lens capsule, which is opened, and the phacoemulsification probe is inserted. The device uses ultrasound to break up the cataract and aspirate the pieces for removal, or manual cutting and suction is used. A bubble of air is injected into the anterior chamber for protection of the cornea. The intraocular lens is placed into the eye, and an anterior segment aqueous drainage device without extraocular reservoir is also inserted to treat chronic or progressive open angle glaucoma. A magnification lens, such as a gonioscope, is used to place and position the shunt at the angle of the anterior chamber. The drainage device may traverse the sclera with the terminal end positioned in the suprachoroidal space, or end in the trabecular meshwork; alternatively, it may rest in the supraciliary space between the sclera and ciliary body to create a channel for aqueous fluid to flow out, reducing intraocular pressure. Incisions may be closed with sutures, and the eye is dressed.

ICD-10-CM Diagnostic Codes

	E10.36	Type 1 diabetes mellitus with diabetic cataract
	E11.36	Type 2 diabetes mellitus with diabetic cataract
⇄	H25.011	Cortical age-related cataract, right eye
⇄	H25.012	Cortical age-related cataract, left eye
⇄	H25.013	Cortical age-related cataract, bilateral
⇄	H25.031	Anterior subcapsular polar age-related cataract, right eye
⇄	H25.032	Anterior subcapsular polar age-related cataract, left eye
⇄	H25.033	Anterior subcapsular polar age-related cataract, bilateral
⇄	H25.041	Posterior subcapsular polar age-related cataract, right eye
⇄	H25.042	Posterior subcapsular polar age-related cataract, left eye
⇄	H25.043	Posterior subcapsular polar age-related cataract, bilateral
⇄	H25.091	Other age-related incipient cataract, right eye
⇄	H25.092	Other age-related incipient cataract, left eye
⇄	H25.093	Other age-related incipient cataract, bilateral
⇄	H25.11	Age-related nuclear cataract, right eye
⇄	H25.12	Age-related nuclear cataract, left eye
⇄	H25.13	Age-related nuclear cataract, bilateral
⇄	H25.21	Age-related cataract, morgagnian type, right eye
⇄	H25.22	Age-related cataract, morgagnian type, left eye
⇄	H25.23	Age-related cataract, morgagnian type, bilateral
⇄	H25.811	Combined forms of age-related cataract, right eye
⇄	H25.812	Combined forms of age-related cataract, left eye
⇄	H25.813	Combined forms of age-related cataract, bilateral
	H25.89	Other age-related cataract
⇄	H26.111	Localized traumatic opacities, right eye
⇄	H26.112	Localized traumatic opacities, left eye
⇄	H26.113	Localized traumatic opacities, bilateral
⇄	H26.131	Total traumatic cataract, right eye
⇄	H26.132	Total traumatic cataract, left eye
⇄	H26.133	Total traumatic cataract, bilateral
	H26.8	Other specified cataract
	H26.9	Unspecified cataract
⇄	H40.1111	Primary open-angle glaucoma, right eye, mild stage
⇄	H40.1112	Primary open-angle glaucoma, right eye, moderate stage
⇄	H40.1113	Primary open-angle glaucoma, right eye, severe stage
⇄	H40.1114	Primary open-angle glaucoma, right eye, indeterminate stage
⇄	H40.1121	Primary open-angle glaucoma, left eye, mild stage
⇄	H40.1122	Primary open-angle glaucoma, left eye, moderate stage
⇄	H40.1123	Primary open-angle glaucoma, left eye, severe stage
⇄	H40.1124	Primary open-angle glaucoma, left eye, indeterminate stage
⇄	H40.1131	Primary open-angle glaucoma, bilateral, mild stage
⇄	H40.1132	Primary open-angle glaucoma, bilateral, moderate stage
⇄	H40.1133	Primary open-angle glaucoma, bilateral, severe stage
⇄	H40.1134	Primary open-angle glaucoma, bilateral, indeterminate stage

CCI Edits

Refer to Appendix A for CCI edits.

Facility RVUs ▯

Code	Work	PE Facility	MP	Total Facility
66991	9.23	9.84	0.68	19.75

Non-facility RVUs ▯

Code	Work	PE Non-Facility	MP	Total Non-Facility
66991	9.23	9.84	0.68	19.75

Modifiers (PAR) ▯

Code	Mod 50	Mod 51	Mod 62	Mod 66	Mod 80
66991					

Global Period

Code	Days
66991	090

67005-67010

67005 Removal of vitreous, anterior approach (open sky technique or limbal incision); partial removal

67010 Removal of vitreous, anterior approach (open sky technique or limbal incision); subtotal removal with mechanical vitrectomy

(For removal of vitreous by paracentesis of anterior chamber, use 65810)

(For removal of corneovitreal adhesions, use 65880)

AMA Coding Notes

Surgical Procedures on the Eye and Ocular Adnexa

(For diagnostic and treatment ophthalmological services, see Medicine, Ophthalmology, and 92002 et seq)

(Do not report code 69990 in addition to codes 65091-68850)

AMA *CPT® Assistant* ▢

67005: Fall 92: 4

67010: Fall 92: 4

Plain English Description

Vitreous is a clear gel-like substance that fills the posterior chamber of the eye. An anterior approach requires either an open sky technique or a limbal incision. Using an open sky technique, an incision is made in the cornea. Alternatively, a curvilinear incision is made in the limbus, which is the edge of the cornea where the cornea joins the sclera. Vitreous removal has three components, cutting of vitreous strands, suction, and infusion of saline. In 67005, a needle or scissors is used for partial removal of the vitreous. In 67010, a mechanical device is used to remove the vitreous, such rotoextractors or a VISC device. This procedure may also involve severing of membranes and adhesions to achieve subtotal removal of the vitreous.

Removal of vitreous, anterior approach; partial, subtotal/mechanical

Sclera
Choroid
Retina
Lens
Cornea
Cornea/limbal approach
Vitreous is removed partial using a needle (67005); most/all using mechanical tool (67010)

ICD-10-CM Diagnostic Codes

- E08.311 Diabetes mellitus due to underlying condition with unspecified diabetic retinopathy with macular edema
- E08.319 Diabetes mellitus due to underlying condition with unspecified diabetic retinopathy without macular edema
- ❼⇄ E08.321 Diabetes mellitus due to underlying condition with mild nonproliferative diabetic retinopathy with macular edema
- ❼⇄ E08.329 Diabetes mellitus due to underlying condition with mild nonproliferative diabetic retinopathy without macular edema
- ❼⇄ E08.331 Diabetes mellitus due to underlying condition with moderate nonproliferative diabetic retinopathy with macular edema
- ❼⇄ E08.339 Diabetes mellitus due to underlying condition with moderate nonproliferative diabetic retinopathy without macular edema
- ❼⇄ E08.341 Diabetes mellitus due to underlying condition with severe nonproliferative diabetic retinopathy with macular edema
- ❼⇄ E08.349 Diabetes mellitus due to underlying condition with severe nonproliferative diabetic retinopathy without macular edema
- ❼⇄ E08.351 Diabetes mellitus due to underlying condition with proliferative diabetic retinopathy with macular edema
- ❼⇄ E08.352 Diabetes mellitus due to underlying condition with proliferative diabetic retinopathy with traction retinal detachment involving the macula
- ❼⇄ E08.353 Diabetes mellitus due to underlying condition with proliferative diabetic retinopathy with traction retinal detachment not involving the macula
- ❼⇄ E08.354 Diabetes mellitus due to underlying condition with proliferative diabetic retinopathy with combined traction retinal detachment and rhegmatogenous retinal detachment
- ❼⇄ E08.355 Diabetes mellitus due to underlying condition with stable proliferative diabetic retinopathy
- ❼⇄ E08.359 Diabetes mellitus due to underlying condition with proliferative diabetic retinopathy without macular edema
- E08.36 Diabetes mellitus due to underlying condition with diabetic cataract
- ❼⇄ E08.37 Diabetes mellitus due to underlying condition with diabetic macular edema, resolved following treatment
- E08.39 Diabetes mellitus due to underlying condition with other diabetic ophthalmic complication
- E08.65 Diabetes mellitus due to underlying condition with hyperglycemia
- E09.311 Drug or chemical induced diabetes mellitus with unspecified diabetic retinopathy with macular edema
- E09.319 Drug or chemical induced diabetes mellitus with unspecified diabetic retinopathy without macular edema
- ❼⇄ E09.321 Drug or chemical induced diabetes mellitus with mild nonproliferative diabetic retinopathy with macular edema
- ❼⇄ E09.329 Drug or chemical induced diabetes mellitus with mild nonproliferative diabetic retinopathy without macular edema
- ❼⇄ E09.331 Drug or chemical induced diabetes mellitus with moderate nonproliferative diabetic retinopathy with macular edema
- ❼⇄ E09.339 Drug or chemical induced diabetes mellitus with moderate nonproliferative diabetic retinopathy without macular edema
- ❼⇄ E09.341 Drug or chemical induced diabetes mellitus with severe nonproliferative diabetic retinopathy with macular edema
- ❼⇄ E09.349 Drug or chemical induced diabetes mellitus with severe nonproliferative diabetic retinopathy without macular edema
- ❼⇄ E09.351 Drug or chemical induced diabetes mellitus with proliferative diabetic retinopathy with macular edema
- ❼⇄ E09.352 Drug or chemical induced diabetes mellitus with proliferative diabetic retinopathy with traction retinal detachment involving the macula
- ❼⇄ E09.353 Drug or chemical induced diabetes mellitus with proliferative diabetic retinopathy with traction retinal detachment not involving the macula
- ❼⇄ E09.354 Drug or chemical induced diabetes mellitus with proliferative diabetic retinopathy with combined traction retinal detachment and rhegmatogenous retinal detachment
- ❼⇄ E09.355 Drug or chemical induced diabetes mellitus with stable proliferative diabetic retinopathy
- ❼⇄ E09.359 Drug or chemical induced diabetes mellitus with proliferative diabetic retinopathy without macular edema
- E09.36 Drug or chemical induced diabetes mellitus with diabetic cataract
- ❼⇄ E09.37 Drug or chemical induced diabetes mellitus with diabetic macular edema, resolved following treatment
- E09.39 Drug or chemical induced diabetes mellitus with other diabetic ophthalmic complication
- E09.65 Drug or chemical induced diabetes mellitus with hyperglycemia
- E10.311 Type 1 diabetes mellitus with unspecified diabetic retinopathy with macular edema
- E10.319 Type 1 diabetes mellitus with unspecified diabetic retinopathy without macular edema
- ❼⇄ E10.321 Type 1 diabetes mellitus with mild nonproliferative diabetic retinopathy with macular edema

● New ▲ Revised ✚ Add On ⊘Modifier 51 Exempt ★Telemedicine ▢ CPT QuickRef ⁄FDA Pending ⇄ Laterality ❼ Seventh Character ♂Male ♀Female

❼⇄	E10.329	Type 1 diabetes mellitus with mild nonproliferative diabetic retinopathy without macular edema
❼⇄	E10.331	Type 1 diabetes mellitus with moderate nonproliferative diabetic retinopathy with macular edema
❼⇄	E10.339	Type 1 diabetes mellitus with moderate nonproliferative diabetic retinopathy without macular edema
❼⇄	E10.341	Type 1 diabetes mellitus with severe nonproliferative diabetic retinopathy with macular edema
❼⇄	E10.349	Type 1 diabetes mellitus with severe nonproliferative diabetic retinopathy without macular edema
❼⇄	E10.351	Type 1 diabetes mellitus with proliferative diabetic retinopathy with macular edema
❼⇄	E10.352	Type 1 diabetes mellitus with proliferative diabetic retinopathy with traction retinal detachment involving the macula
❼⇄	E10.353	Type 1 diabetes mellitus with proliferative diabetic retinopathy with traction retinal detachment not involving the macula
❼⇄	E10.354	Type 1 diabetes mellitus with proliferative diabetic retinopathy with combined traction retinal detachment and rhegmatogenous retinal detachment
❼⇄	E10.355	Type 1 diabetes mellitus with stable proliferative diabetic retinopathy
	E10.36	Type 1 diabetes mellitus with diabetic cataract
❼⇄	E10.37	Type 1 diabetes mellitus with diabetic macular edema, resolved following treatment
	E10.39	Type 1 diabetes mellitus with other diabetic ophthalmic complication
	E10.65	Type 1 diabetes mellitus with hyperglycemia
	E11.311	Type 2 diabetes mellitus with unspecified diabetic retinopathy with macular edema
	E11.319	Type 2 diabetes mellitus with unspecified diabetic retinopathy without macular edema
❼⇄	E11.329	Type 2 diabetes mellitus with mild nonproliferative diabetic retinopathy without macular edema
❼⇄	E11.331	Type 2 diabetes mellitus with moderate nonproliferative diabetic retinopathy with macular edema
❼⇄	E11.339	Type 2 diabetes mellitus with moderate nonproliferative diabetic retinopathy without macular edema
❼⇄	E11.341	Type 2 diabetes mellitus with severe nonproliferative diabetic retinopathy with macular edema
❼⇄	E11.349	Type 2 diabetes mellitus with severe nonproliferative diabetic retinopathy without macular edema
❼⇄	E11.351	Type 2 diabetes mellitus with proliferative diabetic retinopathy with macular edema
❼⇄	E11.352	Type 2 diabetes mellitus with proliferative diabetic retinopathy with traction retinal detachment involving the macula
❼⇄	E11.353	Type 2 diabetes mellitus with proliferative diabetic retinopathy with traction retinal detachment not involving the macula
❼⇄	E11.354	Type 2 diabetes mellitus with proliferative diabetic retinopathy with combined traction retinal detachment and rhegmatogenous retinal detachment
❼⇄	E11.355	Type 2 diabetes mellitus with stable proliferative diabetic retinopathy
❼⇄	E11.359	Type 2 diabetes mellitus with proliferative diabetic retinopathy without macular edema
	E11.36	Type 2 diabetes mellitus with diabetic cataract
❼⇄	E11.37	Type 2 diabetes mellitus with diabetic macular edema, resolved following treatment
	E11.39	Type 2 diabetes mellitus with other diabetic ophthalmic complication
	E11.65	Type 2 diabetes mellitus with hyperglycemia
	E13.36	Other specified diabetes mellitus with diabetic cataract
⇄	H33.032	Retinal detachment with giant retinal tear, left eye
⇄	H33.052	Total retinal detachment, left eye
⇄	H33.42	Traction detachment of retina, left eye
⇄	H35.022	Exudative retinopathy, left eye
⇄	H35.102	Retinopathy of prematurity, unspecified, left eye
⇄	H35.22	Other non-diabetic proliferative retinopathy, left eye
❼⇄	H35.311	Nonexudative age-related macular degeneration, right eye
❼⇄	H35.312	Nonexudative age-related macular degeneration, left eye
❼⇄	H35.313	Nonexudative age-related macular degeneration, bilateral
	H44.19	Other endophthalmitis
⇄	H44.2C1	Degenerative myopia with retinal detachment, right eye
⇄	H44.2C2	Degenerative myopia with retinal detachment, left eye
⇄	H44.2C3	Degenerative myopia with retinal detachment, bilateral eye
❼	T85.21	Breakdown (mechanical) of intraocular lens
❼	T85.22	Displacement of intraocular lens
❼	T85.29	Other mechanical complication of intraocular lens

ICD-10-CM Coding Notes

For codes requiring a 7th character extension, refer to your ICD-10-CM book. Review the character descriptions and coding guidelines for proper selection. For some procedures, only certain characters will apply.

CCI Edits

Refer to Appendix A for CCI edits.

Pub 100

67010: Pub 100-03, 1, 80.11

Facility RVUs ▯

Code	Work	PE Facility	MP	Total Facility
67005	5.89	7.39	0.44	13.72
67010	7.06	8.11	0.55	15.72

Non-facility RVUs ▯

Code	Work	PE Non-Facility	MP	Total Non-Facility
67005	5.89	7.39	0.44	13.72
67010	7.06	8.11	0.55	15.72

Modifiers (PAR) ▯

Code	Mod 50	Mod 51	Mod 62	Mod 66	Mod 80
67005	1	2	1	0	1
67010	1	2	1	0	1

Global Period

Code	Days
67005	090
67010	090

67015

67015 Aspiration or release of vitreous, subretinal or choroidal fluid, pars plana approach (posterior sclerotomy)

AMA Coding Notes

Surgical Procedures on the Eye and Ocular Adnexa

(For diagnostic and treatment ophthalmological services, see Medicine, Ophthalmology, and 92002 et seq)

(Do not report code 69990 in addition to codes 65091-68850)

Plain English Description

Ocular fluid normally moves between the vitreous and the choroid through a membrane called the retinal pigment epithelium (RPE). The RPE actively pumps ions and water from the vitreous into the choroid without pooling. When there is an increase in inflow or a decrease in outflow, fluid may accumulate in the subretinal space, causing an increase in ocular pressure and placing the patient at risk for retinal detachment. Vitreous, subretinal, and/or choroidal fluid may be aspirated to relieve the intraocular pressure. Anesthetic drops are instilled and an antibacterial solution is used to wash the surface of the eye. An area in the pars plana is identified and marked. A small-gauge needle attached to an empty syringe is inserted through the marked area into the posterior eye and the accumulated ocular fluid is aspirated. The needle is withdrawn and a cotton-tipped applicator is used to apply pressure at the puncture site. The puncture site is checked for fluid leakage and antibiotic eye drops may be instilled.

Aspiration or release of vitreous, subretinal or choroidal fluid, pars plana approach

Sclera
Choroid
Retina
Lens
Cornea
Pars plana approach
Needle
Vitreous/subretinal/choroidal fluid may be aspirated

ICD-10-CM Diagnostic Codes

	Code	Description
⇄	C69.31	Malignant neoplasm of right choroid
	E08.311	Diabetes mellitus due to underlying condition with unspecified diabetic retinopathy with macular edema
	E08.319	Diabetes mellitus due to underlying condition with unspecified diabetic retinopathy without macular edema
❼⇄	E08.321	Diabetes mellitus due to underlying condition with mild nonproliferative diabetic retinopathy with macular edema
❼⇄	E08.329	Diabetes mellitus due to underlying condition with mild nonproliferative diabetic retinopathy without macular edema
❼⇄	E08.331	Diabetes mellitus due to underlying condition with moderate nonproliferative diabetic retinopathy with macular edema
❼⇄	E08.339	Diabetes mellitus due to underlying condition with moderate nonproliferative diabetic retinopathy without macular edema
❼⇄	E08.341	Diabetes mellitus due to underlying condition with severe nonproliferative diabetic retinopathy with macular edema
❼⇄	E08.349	Diabetes mellitus due to underlying condition with severe nonproliferative diabetic retinopathy without macular edema
❼⇄	E08.351	Diabetes mellitus due to underlying condition with proliferative diabetic retinopathy with macular edema
❼⇄	E08.352	Diabetes mellitus due to underlying condition with proliferative diabetic retinopathy with traction retinal detachment involving the macula
❼⇄	E08.353	Diabetes mellitus due to underlying condition with proliferative diabetic retinopathy with traction retinal detachment not involving the macula
❼⇄	E08.354	Diabetes mellitus due to underlying condition with proliferative diabetic retinopathy with combined traction retinal detachment and rhegmatogenous retinal detachment
❼⇄	E08.355	Diabetes mellitus due to underlying condition with stable proliferative diabetic retinopathy
❼⇄	E08.359	Diabetes mellitus due to underlying condition with proliferative diabetic retinopathy without macular edema
	E08.36	Diabetes mellitus due to underlying condition with diabetic cataract
	E08.39	Diabetes mellitus due to underlying condition with other diabetic ophthalmic complication
	E09.311	Drug or chemical induced diabetes mellitus with unspecified diabetic retinopathy with macular edema
❼⇄	E09.321	Drug or chemical induced diabetes mellitus with mild nonproliferative diabetic retinopathy with macular edema
❼⇄	E09.331	Drug or chemical induced diabetes mellitus with moderate nonproliferative diabetic retinopathy with macular edema
❼⇄	E09.341	Drug or chemical induced diabetes mellitus with severe nonproliferative diabetic retinopathy with macular edema
❼⇄	E09.351	Drug or chemical induced diabetes mellitus with proliferative diabetic retinopathy with macular edema
❼⇄	E09.359	Drug or chemical induced diabetes mellitus with proliferative diabetic retinopathy without macular edema
	E10.311	Type 1 diabetes mellitus with unspecified diabetic retinopathy with macular edema
	E10.319	Type 1 diabetes mellitus with unspecified diabetic retinopathy without macular edema
❼⇄	E10.321	Type 1 diabetes mellitus with mild nonproliferative diabetic retinopathy with macular edema
❼⇄	E10.329	Type 1 diabetes mellitus with mild nonproliferative diabetic retinopathy without macular edema
❼⇄	E10.331	Type 1 diabetes mellitus with moderate nonproliferative diabetic retinopathy with macular edema
❼⇄	E10.339	Type 1 diabetes mellitus with moderate nonproliferative diabetic retinopathy without macular edema
❼⇄	E10.341	Type 1 diabetes mellitus with severe nonproliferative diabetic retinopathy with macular edema
❼⇄	E10.349	Type 1 diabetes mellitus with severe nonproliferative diabetic retinopathy without macular edema
❼⇄	E10.351	Type 1 diabetes mellitus with proliferative diabetic retinopathy with macular edema
❼⇄	E10.359	Type 1 diabetes mellitus with proliferative diabetic retinopathy without macular edema
	E10.36	Type 1 diabetes mellitus with diabetic cataract
	E10.39	Type 1 diabetes mellitus with other diabetic ophthalmic complication
	E10.65	Type 1 diabetes mellitus with hyperglycemia
	E11.311	Type 2 diabetes mellitus with unspecified diabetic retinopathy with macular edema
	E11.319	Type 2 diabetes mellitus with unspecified diabetic retinopathy without macular edema
❼⇄	E11.321	Type 2 diabetes mellitus with mild nonproliferative diabetic retinopathy with macular edema
❼⇄	E11.329	Type 2 diabetes mellitus with mild nonproliferative diabetic retinopathy without macular edema
❼⇄	E11.331	Type 2 diabetes mellitus with moderate nonproliferative diabetic retinopathy with macular edema
❼⇄	E11.339	Type 2 diabetes mellitus with moderate nonproliferative diabetic retinopathy without macular edema
❼⇄	E11.341	Type 2 diabetes mellitus with severe nonproliferative diabetic retinopathy with macular edema
❼⇄	E11.349	Type 2 diabetes mellitus with severe nonproliferative diabetic retinopathy without macular edema
❼⇄	E11.351	Type 2 diabetes mellitus with proliferative diabetic retinopathy with macular edema

❼⇄	E11.359	Type 2 diabetes mellitus with proliferative diabetic retinopathy without macular edema
	E11.36	Type 2 diabetes mellitus with diabetic cataract
	E11.39	Type 2 diabetes mellitus with other diabetic ophthalmic complication
	E11.65	Type 2 diabetes mellitus with hyperglycemia
⇄	H11.031	Double pterygium of right eye
⇄	H27.01	Aphakia, right eye
⇄	H27.111	Subluxation of lens, right eye
⇄	H31.312	Expulsive choroidal hemorrhage, left eye
⇄	H31.322	Choroidal rupture, left eye
⇄	H31.402	Unspecified choroidal detachment, left eye
⇄	H31.411	Hemorrhagic choroidal detachment, right eye
⇄	H31.422	Serous choroidal detachment, left eye
⇄	H33.051	Total retinal detachment, right eye
⇄	H33.41	Traction detachment of retina, right eye
⇄	H35.21	Other non-diabetic proliferative retinopathy, right eye
❼⇄	H35.311	Nonexudative age-related macular degeneration, right eye
❼⇄	H35.312	Nonexudative age-related macular degeneration, left eye
❼⇄	H35.313	Nonexudative age-related macular degeneration, bilateral
❼⇄	H35.321	Exudative age-related macular degeneration, right eye
❼⇄	H35.322	Exudative age-related macular degeneration, left eye
❼⇄	H35.323	Exudative age-related macular degeneration, bilateral
⇄	H35.341	Macular cyst, hole, or pseudohole, right eye
⇄	H35.351	Cystoid macular degeneration, right eye
⇄	H35.371	Puckering of macula, right eye
⇄	H35.61	Retinal hemorrhage, right eye
	H35.81	Retinal edema
❼⇄	H40.111	Primary open-angle glaucoma, right eye
❼⇄	H40.112	Primary open-angle glaucoma, left eye
❼⇄	H40.113	Primary open-angle glaucoma, bilateral
	H43.9	Unspecified disorder of vitreous body
⇄	H44.001	Unspecified purulent endophthalmitis, right eye
⇄	H44.011	Panophthalmitis (acute), right eye
⇄	H44.021	Vitreous abscess (chronic), right eye
	H44.19	Other endophthalmitis
⇄	H44.2A1	Degenerative myopia with choroidal neovascularization, right eye
⇄	H44.2A2	Degenerative myopia with choroidal neovascularization, left eye
⇄	H44.2A3	Degenerative myopia with choroidal neovascularization, bilateral eye
⇄	H44.2B1	Degenerative myopia with macular hole, right eye
⇄	H44.2B2	Degenerative myopia with macular hole, left eye
⇄	H44.2B3	Degenerative myopia with macular hole, bilateral eye
⇄	H44.2E1	Degenerative myopia with other maculopathy, right eye
⇄	H44.2E2	Degenerative myopia with other maculopathy, left eye
⇄	H44.2E3	Degenerative myopia with other maculopathy, bilateral eye
⇄	H44.411	Flat anterior chamber hypotony of right eye
⇄	H44.421	Hypotony of right eye due to ocular fistula
	H59.41	Inflammation (infection) of postprocedural bleb, stage 1
	H59.42	Inflammation (infection) of postprocedural bleb, stage 2
	H59.43	Inflammation (infection) of postprocedural bleb, stage 3

ICD-10-CM Coding Notes

For codes requiring a 7th character extension, refer to your ICD-10-CM book. Review the character descriptions and coding guidelines for proper selection. For some procedures, only certain characters will apply.

CCI Edits

Refer to Appendix A for CCI edits.

Facility RVUs ▯

Code	Work	PE Facility	MP	Total Facility
67015	7.14	9.94	0.56	17.64

Non-facility RVUs ▯

Code	Work	PE Non-Facility	MP	Total Non-Facility
67015	7.14	9.94	0.56	17.64

Modifiers (PAR) ▯

Code	Mod 50	Mod 51	Mod 62	Mod 66	Mod 80
67015	1	2	1	0	1

Global Period

Code	Days
67015	090

67025

67025 Injection of vitreous substitute, pars plana or limbal approach (fluid-gas exchange), with or without aspiration (separate procedure)

AMA Coding Notes

Surgical Procedures on the Eye and Ocular Adnexa

(For diagnostic and treatment ophthalmological services, see Medicine, Ophthalmology, and 92002 et seq)

(Do not report code 69990 in addition to codes 65091-68850)

AMA *CPT® Assistant*

67025: Feb 18: 3, Aug 19: 11

Plain English Description

The vitreous humor is a clear substance of non-uniform density located in the posterior eye behind the lens. It is firmly attached to the anterior retina at the vitreous base. The consistency of vitreous humor is gel-like in early years and becomes more fluid like as a person ages. Vitreous humor may be lost due to eye injury or during vitrectomy, and replacement of the fluid with a vitreous substitute is necessary to relieve traction on the retina and allow a scar to form. Anesthetic drops are instilled and an antibacterial solution is used to wash the surface of the eye. An injection site is identified and marked in the area of the pars plana or limbus. A small-gauge needle attached to a syringe containing the vitreous substitute is inserted through the marked area into the posterior eye and the vitreous substitute is injected. Substances may include gas (sulfur hexafluoride, n-perfluoropropane), air, and/or oil (polydimethylsiloxane). The needle is withdrawn and a cotton-tipped applicator is used to apply pressure to the puncture site, which is then checked for fluid leakage. Antibiotic eye drops may be instilled.

Injection of vitreous substitute, pars plana/limbal approach, with/without aspiration

ICD-10-CM Diagnostic Codes

	Code	Description
	E08.311	Diabetes mellitus due to underlying condition with unspecified diabetic retinopathy with macular edema
	E08.319	Diabetes mellitus due to underlying condition with unspecified diabetic retinopathy without macular edema
➐⇄	E08.321	Diabetes mellitus due to underlying condition with mild nonproliferative diabetic retinopathy with macular edema
➐⇄	E08.329	Diabetes mellitus due to underlying condition with mild nonproliferative diabetic retinopathy without macular edema
➐⇄	E08.331	Diabetes mellitus due to underlying condition with moderate nonproliferative diabetic retinopathy with macular edema
➐⇄	E08.339	Diabetes mellitus due to underlying condition with moderate nonproliferative diabetic retinopathy without macular edema
➐⇄	E08.341	Diabetes mellitus due to underlying condition with severe nonproliferative diabetic retinopathy with macular edema
➐⇄	E08.349	Diabetes mellitus due to underlying condition with severe nonproliferative diabetic retinopathy without macular edema
➐⇄	E08.351	Diabetes mellitus due to underlying condition with proliferative diabetic retinopathy with macular edema
➐⇄	E08.352	Diabetes mellitus due to underlying condition with proliferative diabetic retinopathy with traction retinal detachment involving the macula
➐⇄	E08.353	Diabetes mellitus due to underlying condition with proliferative diabetic retinopathy with traction retinal detachment not involving the macula
➐⇄	E08.354	Diabetes mellitus due to underlying condition with proliferative diabetic retinopathy with combined traction retinal detachment and rhegmatogenous retinal detachment
➐⇄	E08.355	Diabetes mellitus due to underlying condition with stable proliferative diabetic retinopathy
➐⇄	E08.359	Diabetes mellitus due to underlying condition with proliferative diabetic retinopathy without macular edema
	E08.36	Diabetes mellitus due to underlying condition with diabetic cataract
➐⇄	E08.37	Diabetes mellitus due to underlying condition with diabetic macular edema, resolved following treatment
	E08.39	Diabetes mellitus due to underlying condition with other diabetic ophthalmic complication
	E08.65	Diabetes mellitus due to underlying condition with hyperglycemia
	E09.311	Drug or chemical induced diabetes mellitus with unspecified diabetic retinopathy with macular edema
	E09.319	Drug or chemical induced diabetes mellitus with unspecified diabetic retinopathy without macular edema
➐⇄	E09.321	Drug or chemical induced diabetes mellitus with mild nonproliferative diabetic retinopathy with macular edema
➐⇄	E09.329	Drug or chemical induced diabetes mellitus with mild nonproliferative diabetic retinopathy without macular edema
➐⇄	E09.331	Drug or chemical induced diabetes mellitus with moderate nonproliferative diabetic retinopathy with macular edema
➐⇄	E09.339	Drug or chemical induced diabetes mellitus with moderate nonproliferative diabetic retinopathy without macular edema
➐⇄	E09.341	Drug or chemical induced diabetes mellitus with severe nonproliferative diabetic retinopathy with macular edema
➐⇄	E09.349	Drug or chemical induced diabetes mellitus with severe nonproliferative diabetic retinopathy without macular edema
➐⇄	E09.351	Drug or chemical induced diabetes mellitus with proliferative diabetic retinopathy with macular edema
➐⇄	E09.352	Drug or chemical induced diabetes mellitus with proliferative diabetic retinopathy with traction retinal detachment involving the macula
➐⇄	E09.353	Drug or chemical induced diabetes mellitus with proliferative diabetic retinopathy with traction retinal detachment not involving the macula
➐⇄	E09.354	Drug or chemical induced diabetes mellitus with proliferative diabetic retinopathy with combined traction retinal detachment and rhegmatogenous retinal detachment
➐⇄	E09.355	Drug or chemical induced diabetes mellitus with stable proliferative diabetic retinopathy
➐⇄	E09.359	Drug or chemical induced diabetes mellitus with proliferative diabetic retinopathy without macular edema
	E09.36	Drug or chemical induced diabetes mellitus with diabetic cataract
➐⇄	E09.37	Drug or chemical induced diabetes mellitus with diabetic macular edema, resolved following treatment
	E09.39	Drug or chemical induced diabetes mellitus with other diabetic ophthalmic complication
	E10.311	Type 1 diabetes mellitus with unspecified diabetic retinopathy with macular edema
	E10.319	Type 1 diabetes mellitus with unspecified diabetic retinopathy without macular edema
➐⇄	E10.321	Type 1 diabetes mellitus with mild nonproliferative diabetic retinopathy with macular edema
➐⇄	E10.329	Type 1 diabetes mellitus with mild nonproliferative diabetic retinopathy without macular edema

➐⇄	E10.331	Type 1 diabetes mellitus with moderate nonproliferative diabetic retinopathy with macular edema
➐⇄	E10.339	Type 1 diabetes mellitus with moderate nonproliferative diabetic retinopathy without macular edema
➐⇄	E10.341	Type 1 diabetes mellitus with severe nonproliferative diabetic retinopathy with macular edema
➐⇄	E10.349	Type 1 diabetes mellitus with severe nonproliferative diabetic retinopathy without macular edema
➐⇄	E10.351	Type 1 diabetes mellitus with proliferative diabetic retinopathy with macular edema
➐⇄	E10.352	Type 1 diabetes mellitus with proliferative diabetic retinopathy with traction retinal detachment involving the macula
➐⇄	E10.353	Type 1 diabetes mellitus with proliferative diabetic retinopathy with traction retinal detachment not involving the macula
➐⇄	E10.354	Type 1 diabetes mellitus with proliferative diabetic retinopathy with combined traction retinal detachment and rhegmatogenous retinal detachment
➐⇄	E10.355	Type 1 diabetes mellitus with stable proliferative diabetic retinopathy
➐⇄	E10.359	Type 1 diabetes mellitus with proliferative diabetic retinopathy without macular edema
	E10.36	Type 1 diabetes mellitus with diabetic cataract
➐⇄	E10.37	Type 1 diabetes mellitus with diabetic macular edema, resolved following treatment
	E10.39	Type 1 diabetes mellitus with other diabetic ophthalmic complication
	E10.65	Type 1 diabetes mellitus with hyperglycemia
	E11.311	Type 2 diabetes mellitus with unspecified diabetic retinopathy with macular edema
	E11.319	Type 2 diabetes mellitus with unspecified diabetic retinopathy without macular edema
➐⇄	E11.321	Type 2 diabetes mellitus with mild nonproliferative diabetic retinopathy with macular edema
➐⇄	E11.329	Type 2 diabetes mellitus with mild nonproliferative diabetic retinopathy without macular edema
➐⇄	E11.331	Type 2 diabetes mellitus with moderate nonproliferative diabetic retinopathy with macular edema
➐⇄	E11.339	Type 2 diabetes mellitus with moderate nonproliferative diabetic retinopathy without macular edema
➐⇄	E11.341	Type 2 diabetes mellitus with severe nonproliferative diabetic retinopathy with macular edema
➐⇄	E11.349	Type 2 diabetes mellitus with severe nonproliferative diabetic retinopathy without macular edema
➐⇄	E11.351	Type 2 diabetes mellitus with proliferative diabetic retinopathy with macular edema
➐⇄	E11.352	Type 2 diabetes mellitus with proliferative diabetic retinopathy with traction retinal detachment involving the macula
➐⇄	E11.353	Type 2 diabetes mellitus with proliferative diabetic retinopathy with traction retinal detachment not involving the macula
➐⇄	E11.354	Type 2 diabetes mellitus with proliferative diabetic retinopathy with combined traction retinal detachment and rhegmatogenous retinal detachment
➐⇄	E11.355	Type 2 diabetes mellitus with stable proliferative diabetic retinopathy
➐⇄	E11.359	Type 2 diabetes mellitus with proliferative diabetic retinopathy without macular edema
	E11.36	Type 2 diabetes mellitus with diabetic cataract
➐⇄	E11.37	Type 2 diabetes mellitus with diabetic macular edema, resolved following treatment
	E11.39	Type 2 diabetes mellitus with other diabetic ophthalmic complication
	E11.65	Type 2 diabetes mellitus with hyperglycemia
⇄	H30.012	Focal chorioretinal inflammation, juxtapapillary, left eye
⇄	H30.022	Focal chorioretinal inflammation of posterior pole, left eye
⇄	H30.032	Focal chorioretinal inflammation, peripheral, left eye
⇄	H30.042	Focal chorioretinal inflammation, macular or paramacular, left eye
⇄	H30.102	Unspecified disseminated chorioretinal inflammation, left eye
⇄	H30.112	Disseminated chorioretinal inflammation of posterior pole, left eye
⇄	H30.122	Disseminated chorioretinal inflammation, peripheral, left eye
⇄	H30.132	Disseminated chorioretinal inflammation, generalized, left eye
⇄	H30.892	Other chorioretinal inflammations, left eye
⇄	H33.002	Unspecified retinal detachment with retinal break, left eye
⇄	H33.012	Retinal detachment with single break, left eye
⇄	H33.022	Retinal detachment with multiple breaks, left eye
⇄	H33.032	Retinal detachment with giant retinal tear, left eye
⇄	H33.052	Total retinal detachment, left eye
⇄	H33.312	Horseshoe tear of retina without detachment, left eye
⇄	H33.42	Traction detachment of retina, left eye
	H33.8	Other retinal detachments
⇄	H35.102	Retinopathy of prematurity, unspecified, left eye
⇄	H35.162	Retinopathy of prematurity, stage 5, left eye
➐⇄	H35.321	Exudative age-related macular degeneration, right eye
➐⇄	H35.322	Exudative age-related macular degeneration, left eye
➐⇄	H35.323	Exudative age-related macular degeneration, bilateral
⇄	H35.342	Macular cyst, hole, or pseudohole, left eye
⇄	H35.352	Cystoid macular degeneration, left eye
⇄	H35.372	Puckering of macula, left eye
⇄	H35.62	Retinal hemorrhage, left eye
	H35.81	Retinal edema
⇄	H43.12	Vitreous hemorrhage, left eye
⇄	H44.002	Unspecified purulent endophthalmitis, left eye
⇄	H44.012	Panophthalmitis (acute), left eye
⇄	H44.022	Vitreous abscess (chronic), left eye
⇄	H44.2A1	Degenerative myopia with choroidal neovascularization, right eye
⇄	H44.2A2	Degenerative myopia with choroidal neovascularization, left eye
⇄	H44.2A3	Degenerative myopia with choroidal neovascularization, bilateral eye
⇄	H44.2B1	Degenerative myopia with macular hole, right eye
⇄	H44.2B2	Degenerative myopia with macular hole, left eye
⇄	H44.2B3	Degenerative myopia with macular hole, bilateral eye
⇄	H44.2C1	Degenerative myopia with retinal detachment, right eye
⇄	H44.2C2	Degenerative myopia with retinal detachment, left eye
⇄	H44.2C3	Degenerative myopia with retinal detachment, bilateral eye
⇄	H44.2E1	Degenerative myopia with other maculopathy, right eye
⇄	H44.2E2	Degenerative myopia with other maculopathy, left eye
⇄	H44.2E3	Degenerative myopia with other maculopathy, bilateral eye

ICD-10-CM Coding Notes

For codes requiring a 7th character extension, refer to your ICD-10-CM book. Review the character descriptions and coding guidelines for proper selection. For some procedures, only certain characters will apply.

CCI Edits

Refer to Appendix A for CCI edits.

Facility RVUs

Code	Work	PE Facility	MP	Total Facility
67025	8.11	9.50	0.62	18.23

Non-facility RVUs

Code	Work	PE Non-Facility	MP	Total Non-Facility
67025	8.11	12.97	0.62	21.70

Modifiers (PAR)

Code	Mod 50	Mod 51	Mod 62	Mod 66	Mod 80
67025	1	2	1	0	1

Global Period

Code	Days
67025	090

67027

67027 Implantation of intravitreal drug delivery system (eg, ganciclovir implant), includes concomitant removal of vitreous

(For removal, use 67121)

AMA Coding Notes

Surgical Procedures on the Eye and Ocular Adnexa

(For diagnostic and treatment ophthalmological services, see Medicine, Ophthalmology, and 92002 et seq)

(Do not report code 69990 in addition to codes 65091-68850)

AMA *CPT® Assistant* ☐

67027: Nov 97: 23, Nov 98: 1, Feb 18: 3

Plain English Description

Implantable intravitreal drug delivery systems provide sustained release of a drug/medication to the posterior segment of the eye. This system may be used to treat conditions such as cytomegalovirus (CMV), macular degeneration, uveitis, diabetic retinopathy and retinal venous occlusions. Non-biodegradable implants include Vitrasert (contains the antiviral drug ganciclovir) and Retisert (contains the corticosteroid drug fluocinolone acetate). These devices can be implanted using local anesthesia in the ophthalmologist's office or same day surgery center. A 4-6 mm incision is made in the pars plana (area between the iris and sclera) near the cornea. A portion of the vitreous gel is removed and replaced with the implant. A suture is placed through a hub or tab on the implant and secured to the sclera. The pars plana incision is closed and saline is injected into the eye to return the intraocular pressure to normal. There are a number of implants that can be inserted into the posterior eye without an incision or removal of the vitreous gel. These include Iluvien, a non-biodegradable intravitreal implant containing the corticosteroid fluocinolone acetate, which is inserted using a 25-gauge needle through the area of the pars plana and the biodegradable intravitreal implant, Ozurdex (Posurdex) containing the corticosteroid dexamethasone, which is inserted using a customized 22-gauge applicator.

Implantation of intravitreal drug delivery system (eg, ganciclovir implant)

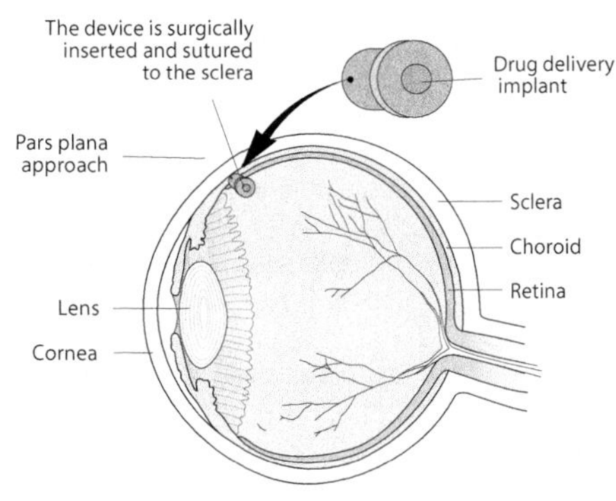

ICD-10-CM Diagnostic Codes

	Code	Description
	E08.311	Diabetes mellitus due to underlying condition with unspecified diabetic retinopathy with macular edema
	E08.319	Diabetes mellitus due to underlying condition with unspecified diabetic retinopathy without macular edema
❼⇄	E08.321	Diabetes mellitus due to underlying condition with mild nonproliferative diabetic retinopathy with macular edema
❼⇄	E08.329	Diabetes mellitus due to underlying condition with mild nonproliferative diabetic retinopathy without macular edema
❼⇄	E08.331	Diabetes mellitus due to underlying condition with moderate nonproliferative diabetic retinopathy with macular edema
❼⇄	E08.339	Diabetes mellitus due to underlying condition with moderate nonproliferative diabetic retinopathy without macular edema
❼⇄	E08.341	Diabetes mellitus due to underlying condition with severe nonproliferative diabetic retinopathy with macular edema
❼⇄	E08.349	Diabetes mellitus due to underlying condition with severe nonproliferative diabetic retinopathy without macular edema
❼⇄	E08.351	Diabetes mellitus due to underlying condition with proliferative diabetic retinopathy with macular edema
❼⇄	E08.352	Diabetes mellitus due to underlying condition with proliferative diabetic retinopathy with traction retinal detachment involving the macula
❼⇄	E08.353	Diabetes mellitus due to underlying condition with proliferative diabetic retinopathy with traction retinal detachment not involving the macula
❼⇄	E08.354	Diabetes mellitus due to underlying condition with proliferative diabetic retinopathy with combined traction retinal detachment and rhegmatogenous retinal detachment
❼⇄	E08.355	Diabetes mellitus due to underlying condition with stable proliferative diabetic retinopathy
❼⇄	E08.359	Diabetes mellitus due to underlying condition with proliferative diabetic retinopathy without macular edema
	E08.36	Diabetes mellitus due to underlying condition with diabetic cataract
❼⇄	E08.37	Diabetes mellitus due to underlying condition with diabetic macular edema, resolved following treatment
	E08.39	Diabetes mellitus due to underlying condition with other diabetic ophthalmic complication
	E08.65	Diabetes mellitus due to underlying condition with hyperglycemia
	E09.311	Drug or chemical induced diabetes mellitus with unspecified diabetic retinopathy with macular edema
	E09.319	Drug or chemical induced diabetes mellitus with unspecified diabetic retinopathy without macular edema
❼⇄	E09.321	Drug or chemical induced diabetes mellitus with mild nonproliferative diabetic retinopathy with macular edema
❼⇄	E09.329	Drug or chemical induced diabetes mellitus with mild nonproliferative diabetic retinopathy without macular edema
❼⇄	E09.331	Drug or chemical induced diabetes mellitus with moderate nonproliferative diabetic retinopathy with macular edema
❼⇄	E09.339	Drug or chemical induced diabetes mellitus with moderate nonproliferative diabetic retinopathy without macular edema
❼⇄	E09.341	Drug or chemical induced diabetes mellitus with severe nonproliferative diabetic retinopathy with macular edema
❼⇄	E09.349	Drug or chemical induced diabetes mellitus with severe nonproliferative diabetic retinopathy without macular edema
❼⇄	E09.351	Drug or chemical induced diabetes mellitus with proliferative diabetic retinopathy with macular edema
❼⇄	E09.352	Drug or chemical induced diabetes mellitus with proliferative diabetic retinopathy with traction retinal detachment involving the macula
❼⇄	E09.353	Drug or chemical induced diabetes mellitus with proliferative diabetic retinopathy with traction retinal detachment not involving the macula
❼⇄	E09.354	Drug or chemical induced diabetes mellitus with proliferative diabetic retinopathy with combined traction retinal detachment and rhegmatogenous retinal detachment
❼⇄	E09.355	Drug or chemical induced diabetes mellitus with stable proliferative diabetic retinopathy

❼⇄ E09.359 Drug or chemical induced diabetes mellitus with proliferative diabetic retinopathy without macular edema
❼⇄ E09.37 Drug or chemical induced diabetes mellitus with diabetic macular edema, resolved following treatment
E09.65 Drug or chemical induced diabetes mellitus with hyperglycemia
E10.311 Type 1 diabetes mellitus with unspecified diabetic retinopathy with macular edema
E10.319 Type 1 diabetes mellitus with unspecified diabetic retinopathy without macular edema
❼⇄ E10.321 Type 1 diabetes mellitus with mild nonproliferative diabetic retinopathy with macular edema
❼⇄ E10.329 Type 1 diabetes mellitus with mild nonproliferative diabetic retinopathy without macular edema
❼⇄ E10.331 Type 1 diabetes mellitus with moderate nonproliferative diabetic retinopathy with macular edema
❼⇄ E10.339 Type 1 diabetes mellitus with moderate nonproliferative diabetic retinopathy without macular edema
❼⇄ E10.341 Type 1 diabetes mellitus with severe nonproliferative diabetic retinopathy with macular edema
❼⇄ E10.349 Type 1 diabetes mellitus with severe nonproliferative diabetic retinopathy without macular edema
❼⇄ E10.351 Type 1 diabetes mellitus with proliferative diabetic retinopathy with macular edema
❼⇄ E10.352 Type 1 diabetes mellitus with proliferative diabetic retinopathy with traction retinal detachment involving the macula
❼⇄ E10.353 Type 1 diabetes mellitus with proliferative diabetic retinopathy with traction retinal detachment not involving the macula
❼⇄ E10.354 Type 1 diabetes mellitus with proliferative diabetic retinopathy with combined traction retinal detachment and rhegmatogenous retinal detachment
❼⇄ E10.355 Type 1 diabetes mellitus with stable proliferative diabetic retinopathy
❼⇄ E10.359 Type 1 diabetes mellitus with proliferative diabetic retinopathy without macular edema
E10.36 Type 1 diabetes mellitus with diabetic cataract
❼⇄ E10.37 Type 1 diabetes mellitus with diabetic macular edema, resolved following treatment
E10.39 Type 1 diabetes mellitus with other diabetic ophthalmic complication
E10.65 Type 1 diabetes mellitus with hyperglycemia
E11.311 Type 2 diabetes mellitus with unspecified diabetic retinopathy with macular edema
E11.319 Type 2 diabetes mellitus with unspecified diabetic retinopathy without macular edema
❼⇄ E11.321 Type 2 diabetes mellitus with mild nonproliferative diabetic retinopathy with macular edema
❼⇄ E11.329 Type 2 diabetes mellitus with mild nonproliferative diabetic retinopathy without macular edema
❼⇄ E11.331 Type 2 diabetes mellitus with moderate nonproliferative diabetic retinopathy with macular edema
❼⇄ E11.339 Type 2 diabetes mellitus with moderate nonproliferative diabetic retinopathy without macular edema
❼⇄ E11.341 Type 2 diabetes mellitus with severe nonproliferative diabetic retinopathy with macular edema
❼⇄ E11.349 Type 2 diabetes mellitus with severe nonproliferative diabetic retinopathy without macular edema
❼⇄ E11.351 Type 2 diabetes mellitus with proliferative diabetic retinopathy with macular edema
❼⇄ E11.352 Type 2 diabetes mellitus with proliferative diabetic retinopathy with traction retinal detachment involving the macula
❼⇄ E11.353 Type 2 diabetes mellitus with proliferative diabetic retinopathy with traction retinal detachment not involving the macula
❼⇄ E11.354 Type 2 diabetes mellitus with proliferative diabetic retinopathy with combined traction retinal detachment and rhegmatogenous retinal detachment
❼⇄ E11.355 Type 2 diabetes mellitus with stable proliferative diabetic retinopathy
❼⇄ E11.359 Type 2 diabetes mellitus with proliferative diabetic retinopathy without macular edema
E11.36 Type 2 diabetes mellitus with diabetic cataract
❼⇄ E11.37 Type 2 diabetes mellitus with diabetic macular edema, resolved following treatment
E11.39 Type 2 diabetes mellitus with other diabetic ophthalmic complication
E11.65 Type 2 diabetes mellitus with hyperglycemia
⇄ H20.11 Chronic iridocyclitis, right eye
⇄ H30.001 Unspecified focal chorioretinal inflammation, right eye
⇄ H30.011 Focal chorioretinal inflammation, juxtapapillary, right eye
⇄ H30.021 Focal chorioretinal inflammation of posterior pole, right eye
⇄ H30.031 Focal chorioretinal inflammation, peripheral, right eye
⇄ H30.041 Focal chorioretinal inflammation, macular or paramacular, right eye
⇄ H30.111 Disseminated chorioretinal inflammation of posterior pole, right eye
⇄ H30.121 Disseminated chorioretinal inflammation, peripheral right eye
⇄ H30.131 Disseminated chorioretinal inflammation, generalized, right eye
⇄ H30.891 Other chorioretinal inflammations, right eye
⇄ H33.011 Retinal detachment with single break, right eye
⇄ H33.021 Retinal detachment with multiple breaks, right eye
⇄ H33.031 Retinal detachment with giant retinal tear, right eye
⇄ H33.041 Retinal detachment with retinal dialysis, right eye
⇄ H33.051 Total retinal detachment, right eye
⇄ H33.301 Unspecified retinal break, right eye
H33.8 Other retinal detachments
⇄ H34.11 Central retinal artery occlusion, right eye
⇄ H34.211 Partial retinal artery occlusion, right eye
⇄ H34.231 Retinal artery branch occlusion, right eye
⇄ H34.8110 Central retinal vein occlusion, right eye, with macular edema
⇄ H34.8111 Central retinal vein occlusion, right eye, with retinal neovascularization
⇄ H34.8112 Central retinal vein occlusion, right eye, stable
⇄ H34.821 Venous engorgement, right eye
⇄ H34.8310 Tributary (branch) retinal vein occlusion, right eye, with macular edema
⇄ H34.8311 Tributary (branch) retinal vein occlusion, right eye, with retinal neovascularization
⇄ H34.8312 Tributary (branch) retinal vein occlusion, right eye, stable
H34.9 Unspecified retinal vascular occlusion
⇄ H35.021 Exudative retinopathy, right eye
⇄ H35.041 Retinal micro-aneurysms, unspecified, right eye
⇄ H35.051 Retinal neovascularization, unspecified, right eye
⇄ H35.061 Retinal vasculitis, right eye
⇄ H35.071 Retinal telangiectasis, right eye
H35.09 Other intraretinal microvascular abnormalities
⇄ H35.171 Retrolental fibroplasia, right eye
❼⇄ H35.321 Exudative age-related macular degeneration, right eye
❼⇄ H35.322 Exudative age-related macular degeneration, left eye
❼⇄ H35.323 Exudative age-related macular degeneration, bilateral
H35.81 Retinal edema
⇄ H44.001 Unspecified purulent endophthalmitis, right eye
⇄ H44.011 Panophthalmitis (acute), right eye
⇄ H44.021 Vitreous abscess (chronic), right eye
⇄ H44.2A1 Degenerative myopia with choroidal neovascularization, right eye
⇄ H44.2A2 Degenerative myopia with choroidal neovascularization, left eye

⇄	H44.2A3	Degenerative myopia with choroidal neovascularization, bilateral eye
⇄	H44.2B1	Degenerative myopia with macular hole, right eye
⇄	H44.2B2	Degenerative myopia with macular hole, left eye
⇄	H44.2B3	Degenerative myopia with macular hole, bilateral eye
⇄	H44.2C1	Degenerative myopia with retinal detachment, right eye
⇄	H44.2C2	Degenerative myopia with retinal detachment, left eye
⇄	H44.2C3	Degenerative myopia with retinal detachment, bilateral eye
⇄	H44.2E1	Degenerative myopia with other maculopathy, right eye
⇄	H44.2E2	Degenerative myopia with other maculopathy, left eye
⇄	H44.2E3	Degenerative myopia with other maculopathy, bilateral eye

ICD-10-CM Coding Notes

For codes requiring a 7th character extension, refer to your ICD-10-CM book. Review the character descriptions and coding guidelines for proper selection. For some procedures, only certain characters will apply.

CCI Edits

Refer to Appendix A for CCI edits.

Facility RVUs

Code	Work	PE Facility	MP	Total Facility
67027	11.62	12.00	0.90	24.52

Non-facility RVUs

Code	Work	PE Non-Facility	MP	Total Non-Facility
67027	11.62	12.00	0.90	24.52

Modifiers (PAR)

Code	Mod 50	Mod 51	Mod 62	Mod 66	Mod 80
67027	1	2	1	0	2

Global Period

Code	Days
67027	090

67028

67028 Intravitreal injection of a pharmacologic agent (separate procedure)

AMA Coding Notes

Surgical Procedures on the Eye and Ocular Adnexa

(For diagnostic and treatment ophthalmological services, see Medicine, Ophthalmology, and 92002 et seq)

(Do not report code 69990 in addition to codes 65091-68850)

AMA *CPT® Assistant* ▯

67028: Winter 90: 9, Oct 12: 15, Feb 18: 3

Plain English Description

Intravitreal injection of a pharmacologic agent (drug, medication) can be performed without an incision or removal of a portion of the vitreous gel. Intravitreal injected medications include Lucentis (Ranibizumab), a monoclonal antibody fragment that blocks vascular endothelial growth factor (VEGF) and is approved to treat neovascular (wet) age related macular degeneration (AMD) and macular edema following retinal vein occlusion. Macugen (pegaptanib sodium) and Eylea (Aflibercept) are VEGF antagonists also approved for the treatment of neovascular AMD. Avastin (Bevacizumab) a VEGF antagonist, is sometimes used "off label" to treat AMD by intravitreal injection. Intravitreal injections are performed outpatient in the physician's office. A topical ophthalmic anesthetic is placed in the eye and then the eye is cleansed with an antiseptic. An eyelid speculum is placed and the injections site(s) marked. A short 30-gauge needle is inserted into the mid-vitreous cavity, medication is injected and the needle is removed. Antibiotic eye drops may be instilled and the eye may be patched following the procedure.

Intravitreal injection of pharmacologic agent

Sclera
Choroid
Retina
Lens
Cornea
Pars plana approach
Pharmacologic agent is injected into the eye

ICD-10-CM Diagnostic Codes

	E08.311	Diabetes mellitus due to underlying condition with unspecified diabetic retinopathy with macular edema
	E08.319	Diabetes mellitus due to underlying condition with unspecified diabetic retinopathy without macular edema
❼⇄	E08.321	Diabetes mellitus due to underlying condition with mild nonproliferative diabetic retinopathy with macular edema
❼⇄	E08.329	Diabetes mellitus due to underlying condition with mild nonproliferative diabetic retinopathy without macular edema
❼⇄	E08.331	Diabetes mellitus due to underlying condition with moderate nonproliferative diabetic retinopathy with macular edema
❼⇄	E08.339	Diabetes mellitus due to underlying condition with moderate nonproliferative diabetic retinopathy without macular edema
❼⇄	E08.341	Diabetes mellitus due to underlying condition with severe nonproliferative diabetic retinopathy with macular edema
❼⇄	E08.349	Diabetes mellitus due to underlying condition with severe nonproliferative diabetic retinopathy without macular edema
❼⇄	E08.351	Diabetes mellitus due to underlying condition with proliferative diabetic retinopathy with macular edema
❼⇄	E08.352	Diabetes mellitus due to underlying condition with proliferative diabetic retinopathy with traction retinal detachment involving the macula
❼⇄	E08.353	Diabetes mellitus due to underlying condition with proliferative diabetic retinopathy with traction retinal detachment not involving the macula
❼⇄	E08.354	Diabetes mellitus due to underlying condition with proliferative diabetic retinopathy with combined traction retinal detachment and rhegmatogenous retinal detachment
❼⇄	E08.355	Diabetes mellitus due to underlying condition with stable proliferative diabetic retinopathy
❼⇄	E08.359	Diabetes mellitus due to underlying condition with proliferative diabetic retinopathy without macular edema
	E08.36	Diabetes mellitus due to underlying condition with diabetic cataract
❼⇄	E08.37	Diabetes mellitus due to underlying condition with diabetic macular edema, resolved following treatment
	E08.39	Diabetes mellitus due to underlying condition with other diabetic ophthalmic complication
	E08.65	Diabetes mellitus due to underlying condition with hyperglycemia
	E09.311	Drug or chemical induced diabetes mellitus with unspecified diabetic retinopathy with macular edema
	E09.319	Drug or chemical induced diabetes mellitus with unspecified diabetic retinopathy without macular edema
❼⇄	E09.321	Drug or chemical induced diabetes mellitus with mild nonproliferative diabetic retinopathy with macular edema
❼⇄	E09.329	Drug or chemical induced diabetes mellitus with mild nonproliferative diabetic retinopathy without macular edema
❼⇄	E09.331	Drug or chemical induced diabetes mellitus with moderate nonproliferative diabetic retinopathy with macular edema
❼⇄	E09.339	Drug or chemical induced diabetes mellitus with moderate nonproliferative diabetic retinopathy without macular edema
❼⇄	E09.341	Drug or chemical induced diabetes mellitus with severe nonproliferative diabetic retinopathy with macular edema
❼⇄	E09.349	Drug or chemical induced diabetes mellitus with severe nonproliferative diabetic retinopathy without macular edema
❼⇄	E09.351	Drug or chemical induced diabetes mellitus with proliferative diabetic retinopathy with macular edema
❼⇄	E09.352	Drug or chemical induced diabetes mellitus with proliferative diabetic retinopathy with traction retinal detachment involving the macula
❼⇄	E09.353	Drug or chemical induced diabetes mellitus with proliferative diabetic retinopathy with traction retinal detachment not involving the macula
❼⇄	E09.354	Drug or chemical induced diabetes mellitus with proliferative diabetic retinopathy with combined traction retinal detachment and rhegmatogenous retinal detachment
❼⇄	E09.355	Drug or chemical induced diabetes mellitus with stable proliferative diabetic retinopathy
❼⇄	E09.359	Drug or chemical induced diabetes mellitus with proliferative diabetic retinopathy without macular edema
	E09.36	Drug or chemical induced diabetes mellitus with diabetic cataract
❼⇄	E09.37	Drug or chemical induced diabetes mellitus with diabetic macular edema, resolved following treatment
	E09.39	Drug or chemical induced diabetes mellitus with other diabetic ophthalmic complication
	E09.65	Drug or chemical induced diabetes mellitus with hyperglycemia
	E10.311	Type 1 diabetes mellitus with unspecified diabetic retinopathy with macular edema
	E10.319	Type 1 diabetes mellitus with unspecified diabetic retinopathy without macular edema
❼⇄	E10.321	Type 1 diabetes mellitus with mild nonproliferative diabetic retinopathy with macular edema
❼⇄	E10.329	Type 1 diabetes mellitus with mild nonproliferative diabetic retinopathy without macular edema

- ❼⇄ E10.331 Type 1 diabetes mellitus with moderate nonproliferative diabetic retinopathy with macular edema
- ❼⇄ E10.339 Type 1 diabetes mellitus with moderate nonproliferative diabetic retinopathy without macular edema
- ❼⇄ E10.341 Type 1 diabetes mellitus with severe nonproliferative diabetic retinopathy with macular edema
- ❼⇄ E10.349 Type 1 diabetes mellitus with severe nonproliferative diabetic retinopathy without macular edema
- ❼⇄ E10.351 Type 1 diabetes mellitus with proliferative diabetic retinopathy with macular edema
- ❼⇄ E10.352 Type 1 diabetes mellitus with proliferative diabetic retinopathy with traction retinal detachment involving the macula
- ❼⇄ E10.353 Type 1 diabetes mellitus with proliferative diabetic retinopathy with traction retinal detachment not involving the macula
- ❼⇄ E10.354 Type 1 diabetes mellitus with proliferative diabetic retinopathy with combined traction retinal detachment and rhegmatogenous retinal detachment
- ❼⇄ E10.355 Type 1 diabetes mellitus with stable proliferative diabetic retinopathy
- ❼⇄ E10.359 Type 1 diabetes mellitus with proliferative diabetic retinopathy without macular edema
- E10.36 Type 1 diabetes mellitus with diabetic cataract
- ❼⇄ E10.37 Type 1 diabetes mellitus with diabetic macular edema, resolved following treatment
- E10.39 Type 1 diabetes mellitus with other diabetic ophthalmic complication
- E10.65 Type 1 diabetes mellitus with hyperglycemia
- E11.311 Type 2 diabetes mellitus with unspecified diabetic retinopathy with macular edema
- E11.319 Type 2 diabetes mellitus with unspecified diabetic retinopathy without macular edema
- ❼⇄ E11.321 Type 2 diabetes mellitus with mild nonproliferative diabetic retinopathy with macular edema
- ❼⇄ E11.329 Type 2 diabetes mellitus with mild nonproliferative diabetic retinopathy without macular edema
- ❼⇄ E11.331 Type 2 diabetes mellitus with moderate nonproliferative diabetic retinopathy with macular edema
- ❼⇄ E11.339 Type 2 diabetes mellitus with moderate nonproliferative diabetic retinopathy without macular edema
- ❼⇄ E11.341 Type 2 diabetes mellitus with severe nonproliferative diabetic retinopathy with macular edema
- ❼⇄ E11.349 Type 2 diabetes mellitus with severe nonproliferative diabetic retinopathy without macular edema
- ❼⇄ E11.351 Type 2 diabetes mellitus with proliferative diabetic retinopathy with macular edema
- ❼⇄ E11.352 Type 2 diabetes mellitus with proliferative diabetic retinopathy with traction retinal detachment involving the macula
- ❼⇄ E11.353 Type 2 diabetes mellitus with proliferative diabetic retinopathy with traction retinal detachment not involving the macula
- ❼⇄ E11.354 Type 2 diabetes mellitus with proliferative diabetic retinopathy with combined traction retinal detachment and rhegmatogenous retinal detachment
- ❼⇄ E11.355 Type 2 diabetes mellitus with stable proliferative diabetic retinopathy
- ❼⇄ E11.359 Type 2 diabetes mellitus with proliferative diabetic retinopathy without macular edema
- E11.36 Type 2 diabetes mellitus with diabetic cataract
- ❼⇄ E11.37 Type 2 diabetes mellitus with diabetic macular edema, resolved following treatment
- E11.39 Type 2 diabetes mellitus with other diabetic ophthalmic complication
- E11.65 Type 2 diabetes mellitus with hyperglycemia
- ⇄ H25.11 Age-related nuclear cataract, right eye
- ⇄ H30.002 Unspecified focal chorioretinal inflammation, left eye
- ⇄ H30.012 Focal chorioretinal inflammation, juxtapapillary, left eye
- ⇄ H30.022 Focal chorioretinal inflammation of posterior pole, left eye
- ⇄ H30.032 Focal chorioretinal inflammation, peripheral, left eye
- ⇄ H30.042 Focal chorioretinal inflammation, macular or paramacular, left eye
- ⇄ H30.102 Unspecified disseminated chorioretinal inflammation, left eye
- ⇄ H30.112 Disseminated chorioretinal inflammation of posterior pole, left eye
- ⇄ H30.122 Disseminated chorioretinal inflammation, peripheral, left eye
- ⇄ H30.132 Disseminated chorioretinal inflammation, generalized, left eye
- ⇄ H30.892 Other chorioretinal inflammations, left eye
- ⇄ H33.002 Unspecified retinal detachment with retinal break, left eye
- ⇄ H33.012 Retinal detachment with single break, left eye
- ⇄ H33.022 Retinal detachment with multiple breaks, left eye
- ⇄ H33.032 Retinal detachment with giant retinal tear, left eye
- ⇄ H33.042 Retinal detachment with retinal dialysis, left eye
- ⇄ H33.052 Total retinal detachment, left eye
- ⇄ H33.42 Traction detachment of retina, left eye
- H33.8 Other retinal detachments
- ⇄ H34.12 Central retinal artery occlusion, left eye
- ⇄ H34.212 Partial retinal artery occlusion, left eye
- ⇄ H34.232 Retinal artery branch occlusion, left eye
- ⇄ H34.8120 Central retinal vein occlusion, left eye, with macular edema
- ⇄ H34.8121 Central retinal vein occlusion, left eye, with retinal neovascularization
- ⇄ H34.8122 Central retinal vein occlusion, left eye, stable
- ⇄ H34.822 Venous engorgement, left eye
- ⇄ H34.8320 Tributary (branch) retinal vein occlusion, left eye, with macular edema
- ⇄ H34.8321 Tributary (branch) retinal vein occlusion, left eye, with retinal neovascularization
- ⇄ H34.8322 Tributary (branch) retinal vein occlusion, left eye, stable
- H34.9 Unspecified retinal vascular occlusion
- ⇄ H35.072 Retinal telangiectasis, left eye
- ❼⇄ H35.311 Nonexudative age-related macular degeneration, right eye
- ❼⇄ H35.312 Nonexudative age-related macular degeneration, left eye
- ❼⇄ H35.313 Nonexudative age-related macular degeneration, bilateral
- ❼⇄ H35.321 Exudative age-related macular degeneration, right eye
- ❼⇄ H35.322 Exudative age-related macular degeneration, left eye
- ❼⇄ H35.323 Exudative age-related macular degeneration, bilateral
- ⇄ H35.352 Cystoid macular degeneration, left eye
- ⇄ H35.372 Puckering of macula, left eye
- ⇄ H35.62 Retinal hemorrhage, left eye
- H35.81 Retinal edema
- ⇄ H43.812 Vitreous degeneration, left eye
- ⇄ H44.002 Unspecified purulent endophthalmitis, left eye
- ⇄ H44.012 Panophthalmitis (acute), left eye
- ⇄ H44.022 Vitreous abscess (chronic), left eye
- ⇄ H44.2A1 Degenerative myopia with choroidal neovascularization, right eye
- ⇄ H44.2A2 Degenerative myopia with choroidal neovascularization, left eye
- ⇄ H44.2A3 Degenerative myopia with choroidal neovascularization, bilateral eye
- ⇄ H44.2B1 Degenerative myopia with macular hole, right eye
- ⇄ H44.2B2 Degenerative myopia with macular hole, left eye
- ⇄ H44.2B3 Degenerative myopia with macular hole, bilateral eye
- ⇄ H44.2C1 Degenerative myopia with retinal detachment, right eye
- ⇄ H44.2C2 Degenerative myopia with retinal detachment, left eye
- ⇄ H44.2C3 Degenerative myopia with retinal detachment, bilateral eye
- ⇄ H44.2E1 Degenerative myopia with other maculopathy, right eye

⇄	H44.2E2	Degenerative myopia with other maculopathy, left eye
⇄	H44.2E3	Degenerative myopia with other maculopathy, bilateral eye

ICD-10-CM Coding Notes

For codes requiring a 7th character extension, refer to your ICD-10-CM book. Review the character descriptions and coding guidelines for proper selection. For some procedures, only certain characters will apply.

CCI Edits

Refer to Appendix A for CCI edits.

Facility RVUs ▯

Code	Work	PE Facility	MP	Total Facility
67028	1.44	1.10	0.11	2.65

Non-facility RVUs ▯

Code	Work	PE Non-Facility	MP	Total Non-Facility
67028	1.44	1.75	0.11	3.30

Modifiers (PAR) ▯

Code	Mod 50	Mod 51	Mod 62	Mod 66	Mod 80
67028	1	2	0	0	1

Global Period

Code	Days
67028	000

67030

67030 Discission of vitreous strands (without removal), pars plana approach

AMA Coding Notes

Surgical Procedures on the Eye and Ocular Adnexa

(For diagnostic and treatment ophthalmological services, see Medicine, Ophthalmology, and 92002 et seq)

(Do not report code 69990 in addition to codes 65091-68850)

Plain English Description

Vitreous strands may become incarcerated (trapped) in a corneoscleral wound or incision following surgery or trauma to the eye. This may lead to cystoid macular edema, loss of vision or the appearance of "floaters," dark shadowy areas in the visual field. With the patient supine and the eye prepared, an anterior limbal (pars plana) incision is made into the anterior chamber. The area is swept using a cyclodialysis spatula and the vitreous strands are pulled back into the posterior segment of the eye. The incision is then closed with 10-0 suture.

Discission/severing of vitreous strands/face adhesions/sheets/ membrane opacities

Vitreous strands are severed using an instrument (67030)
Pars plana approach
Sclera
Choroid
Retina
Lens
Cornea
Vitreous strands/face adhesions/sheets/ membrane opacities are severed using a laser (67031)
Vitreous fluid
Laser
Iris
Floaters

ICD-10-CM Diagnostic Codes

E08.311 Diabetes mellitus due to underlying condition with unspecified diabetic retinopathy with macular edema
E08.319 Diabetes mellitus due to underlying condition with unspecified diabetic retinopathy without macular edema
❼⇄ E08.321 Diabetes mellitus due to underlying condition with mild nonproliferative diabetic retinopathy with macular edema
❼⇄ E08.329 Diabetes mellitus due to underlying condition with mild nonproliferative diabetic retinopathy without macular edema
❼⇄ E08.331 Diabetes mellitus due to underlying condition with moderate nonproliferative diabetic retinopathy with macular edema
❼⇄ E08.339 Diabetes mellitus due to underlying condition with moderate nonproliferative diabetic retinopathy without macular edema
❼⇄ E08.341 Diabetes mellitus due to underlying condition with severe nonproliferative diabetic retinopathy with macular edema
❼⇄ E08.349 Diabetes mellitus due to underlying condition with severe nonproliferative diabetic retinopathy without macular edema
❼⇄ E08.351 Diabetes mellitus due to underlying condition with proliferative diabetic retinopathy with macular edema
❼⇄ E08.352 Diabetes mellitus due to underlying condition with proliferative diabetic retinopathy with traction retinal detachment involving the macula
❼⇄ E08.353 Diabetes mellitus due to underlying condition with proliferative diabetic retinopathy with traction retinal detachment not involving the macula
❼⇄ E08.354 Diabetes mellitus due to underlying condition with proliferative diabetic retinopathy with combined traction retinal detachment and rhegmatogenous retinal detachment
❼⇄ E08.355 Diabetes mellitus due to underlying condition with stable proliferative diabetic retinopathy
❼⇄ E08.359 Diabetes mellitus due to underlying condition with proliferative diabetic retinopathy without macular edema
E08.36 Diabetes mellitus due to underlying condition with diabetic cataract
❼⇄ E08.37 Diabetes mellitus due to underlying condition with diabetic macular edema, resolved following treatment
E08.39 Diabetes mellitus due to underlying condition with other diabetic ophthalmic complication
E08.65 Diabetes mellitus due to underlying condition with hyperglycemia
E09.311 Drug or chemical induced diabetes mellitus with unspecified diabetic retinopathy with macular edema
E09.319 Drug or chemical induced diabetes mellitus with unspecified diabetic retinopathy without macular edema
❼⇄ E09.321 Drug or chemical induced diabetes mellitus with mild nonproliferative diabetic retinopathy with macular edema
❼⇄ E09.329 Drug or chemical induced diabetes mellitus with mild nonproliferative diabetic retinopathy without macular edema
❼⇄ E09.331 Drug or chemical induced diabetes mellitus with moderate nonproliferative diabetic retinopathy with macular edema
❼⇄ E09.339 Drug or chemical induced diabetes mellitus with moderate nonproliferative diabetic retinopathy without macular edema
❼⇄ E09.341 Drug or chemical induced diabetes mellitus with severe nonproliferative diabetic retinopathy with macular edema
❼⇄ E09.349 Drug or chemical induced diabetes mellitus with severe nonproliferative diabetic retinopathy without macular edema
❼⇄ E09.351 Drug or chemical induced diabetes mellitus with proliferative diabetic retinopathy with macular edema
❼⇄ E09.352 Drug or chemical induced diabetes mellitus with proliferative diabetic retinopathy with traction retinal detachment involving the macula
❼⇄ E09.353 Drug or chemical induced diabetes mellitus with proliferative diabetic retinopathy with traction retinal detachment not involving the macula
❼⇄ E09.354 Drug or chemical induced diabetes mellitus with proliferative diabetic retinopathy with combined traction retinal detachment and rhegmatogenous retinal detachment
❼⇄ E09.355 Drug or chemical induced diabetes mellitus with stable proliferative diabetic retinopathy
❼⇄ E09.359 Drug or chemical induced diabetes mellitus with proliferative diabetic retinopathy without macular edema
E09.36 Drug or chemical induced diabetes mellitus with diabetic cataract
❼⇄ E09.37 Drug or chemical induced diabetes mellitus with diabetic macular edema, resolved following treatment
E09.39 Drug or chemical induced diabetes mellitus with other diabetic ophthalmic complication
E09.65 Drug or chemical induced diabetes mellitus with hyperglycemia
E10.311 Type 1 diabetes mellitus with unspecified diabetic retinopathy with macular edema
E10.319 Type 1 diabetes mellitus with unspecified diabetic retinopathy without macular edema
❼⇄ E10.321 Type 1 diabetes mellitus with mild nonproliferative diabetic retinopathy with macular edema
❼⇄ E10.329 Type 1 diabetes mellitus with mild nonproliferative diabetic retinopathy without macular edema
❼⇄ E10.331 Type 1 diabetes mellitus with moderate nonproliferative diabetic retinopathy with macular edema
❼⇄ E10.339 Type 1 diabetes mellitus with moderate nonproliferative diabetic retinopathy without macular edema

❼⇄ E10.341 Type 1 diabetes mellitus with severe nonproliferative diabetic retinopathy with macular edema

❼⇄ E10.349 Type 1 diabetes mellitus with severe nonproliferative diabetic retinopathy without macular edema

❼⇄ E10.351 Type 1 diabetes mellitus with proliferative diabetic retinopathy with macular edema

❼⇄ E10.352 Type 1 diabetes mellitus with proliferative diabetic retinopathy with traction retinal detachment involving the macula

❼⇄ E10.353 Type 1 diabetes mellitus with proliferative diabetic retinopathy with traction retinal detachment not involving the macula

❼⇄ E10.354 Type 1 diabetes mellitus with proliferative diabetic retinopathy with combined traction retinal detachment and rhegmatogenous retinal detachment

❼⇄ E10.355 Type 1 diabetes mellitus with stable proliferative diabetic retinopathy

❼⇄ E10.359 Type 1 diabetes mellitus with proliferative diabetic retinopathy without macular edema

E10.36 Type 1 diabetes mellitus with diabetic cataract

❼⇄ E10.37 Type 1 diabetes mellitus with diabetic macular edema, resolved following treatment

E10.39 Type 1 diabetes mellitus with other diabetic ophthalmic complication

E10.65 Type 1 diabetes mellitus with hyperglycemia

E11.311 Type 2 diabetes mellitus with unspecified diabetic retinopathy with macular edema

E11.319 Type 2 diabetes mellitus with unspecified diabetic retinopathy without macular edema

❼⇄ E11.321 Type 2 diabetes mellitus with mild nonproliferative diabetic retinopathy with macular edema

❼⇄ E11.329 Type 2 diabetes mellitus with mild nonproliferative diabetic retinopathy without macular edema

❼⇄ E11.331 Type 2 diabetes mellitus with moderate nonproliferative diabetic retinopathy with macular edema

❼⇄ E11.339 Type 2 diabetes mellitus with moderate nonproliferative diabetic retinopathy without macular edema

❼⇄ E11.341 Type 2 diabetes mellitus with severe nonproliferative diabetic retinopathy with macular edema

❼⇄ E11.349 Type 2 diabetes mellitus with severe nonproliferative diabetic retinopathy without macular edema

❼⇄ E11.351 Type 2 diabetes mellitus with proliferative diabetic retinopathy with macular edema

❼⇄ E11.352 Type 2 diabetes mellitus with proliferative diabetic retinopathy with traction retinal detachment involving the macula

❼⇄ E11.353 Type 2 diabetes mellitus with proliferative diabetic retinopathy with traction retinal detachment not involving the macula

❼⇄ E11.354 Type 2 diabetes mellitus with proliferative diabetic retinopathy with combined traction retinal detachment and rhegmatogenous retinal detachment

❼⇄ E11.355 Type 2 diabetes mellitus with stable proliferative diabetic retinopathy

❼⇄ E11.359 Type 2 diabetes mellitus with proliferative diabetic retinopathy without macular edema

E11.36 Type 2 diabetes mellitus with diabetic cataract

❼⇄ E11.37 Type 2 diabetes mellitus with diabetic macular edema, resolved following treatment

E11.39 Type 2 diabetes mellitus with other diabetic ophthalmic complication

E11.65 Type 2 diabetes mellitus with hyperglycemia

H18.20 Unspecified corneal edema

⇄ H20.11 Chronic iridocyclitis, right eye

⇄ H25.011 Cortical age-related cataract, right eye

⇄ H33.011 Retinal detachment with single break, right eye

⇄ H33.051 Total retinal detachment, right eye

⇄ H33.321 Round hole, right eye

⇄ H35.371 Puckering of macula, right eye

❼ H40.10 Unspecified open-angle glaucoma

⇄ H43.11 Vitreous hemorrhage, right eye

⇄ H43.312 Vitreous membranes and strands, left eye

⇄ H44.001 Unspecified purulent endophthalmitis, right eye

⇄ H54.0X33 Blindness right eye category 3, blindness left eye category 3

⇄ H54.0X34 Blindness right eye category 3, blindness left eye category 4

⇄ H54.0X35 Blindness right eye category 3, blindness left eye category 5

⇄ H54.0X43 Blindness right eye category 4, blindness left eye category 3

⇄ H54.0X44 Blindness right eye category 4, blindness left eye category 4

⇄ H54.0X45 Blindness right eye category 4, blindness left eye category 5

⇄ H54.0X53 Blindness right eye category 5, blindness left eye category 3

⇄ H54.0X54 Blindness right eye category 5, blindness left eye category 4

⇄ H54.0X55 Blindness right eye category 5, blindness left eye category 5

⇄ H54.1131 Blindness right eye category 3, low vision left eye category 1

⇄ H54.1132 Blindness right eye category 3, low vision left eye category 2

⇄ H54.1141 Blindness right eye category 4, low vision left eye category 1

⇄ H54.1142 Blindness right eye category 4, low vision left eye category 2

⇄ H54.1151 Blindness right eye category 5, low vision left eye category 1

⇄ H54.1152 Blindness right eye category 5, low vision left eye category 2

⇄ H54.1213 Low vision right eye category 1, blindness left eye category 3

⇄ H54.1214 Low vision right eye category 1, blindness left eye category 4

⇄ H54.1215 Low vision right eye category 1, blindness left eye category 5

⇄ H54.1223 Low vision right eye category 2, blindness left eye category 3

⇄ H54.1224 Low vision right eye category 2, blindness left eye category 4

⇄ H54.1225 Low vision right eye category 2, blindness left eye category 5

⇄ H54.2X11 Low vision right eye category 1, low vision left eye category 1

⇄ H54.2X12 Low vision right eye category 1, low vision left eye category 2

⇄ H54.2X21 Low vision right eye category 2, low vision left eye category 1

⇄ H54.2X22 Low vision right eye category 2, low vision left eye category 2

⇄ H54.413A Blindness right eye category 3, normal vision left eye

⇄ H54.414A Blindness right eye category 4, normal vision left eye

⇄ H54.415A Blindness right eye category 5, normal vision left eye

⇄ H54.42A3 Blindness left eye category 3, normal vision right eye

⇄ H54.42A4 Blindness left eye category 4, normal vision right eye

⇄ H54.42A5 Blindness left eye category 5, normal vision right eye

⇄ H54.511A Low vision right eye category 1, normal vision left eye

⇄ H54.512A Low vision right eye category 2, normal vision left eye

⇄ H54.52A1 Low vision left eye category 1, normal vision right eye

⇄ H54.52A2 Low vision left eye category 2, normal vision right eye

❼⇄ S01.112 Laceration without foreign body of left eyelid and periocular area

❼⇄ S01.131 Puncture wound without foreign body of right eyelid and periocular area

❼⇄ S01.141 Puncture wound with foreign body of right eyelid and periocular area

❼ T81.89 Other complications of procedures, not elsewhere classified

❼ T85.21 Breakdown (mechanical) of intraocular lens

❼ T85.22 Displacement of intraocular lens

❼ T85.29 Other mechanical complication of intraocular lens

ICD-10-CM Coding Notes

For codes requiring a 7th character extension, refer to your ICD-10-CM book. Review the character descriptions and coding guidelines for proper selection. For some procedures, only certain characters will apply.

CCI Edits

Refer to Appendix A for CCI edits.

Facility RVUs

Code	Work	PE Facility	MP	Total Facility
67030	6.11	9.68	0.45	16.24

Non-facility RVUs

Code	Work	PE Non-Facility	MP	Total Non-Facility
67030	6.11	9.68	0.45	16.24

Modifiers (PAR)

Code	Mod 50	Mod 51	Mod 62	Mod 66	Mod 80
67030	1	2	1	0	1

Global Period

Code	Days
67030	090

67031

67031 Severing of vitreous strands, vitreous face adhesions, sheets, membranes or opacities, laser surgery (1 or more stages)

AMA Coding Notes

Surgical Procedures on the Eye and Ocular Adnexa

(For diagnostic and treatment ophthalmological services, see Medicine, Ophthalmology, and 92002 et seq)

(Do not report code 69990 in addition to codes 65091-68850)

Plain English Description

The normal vitreous degenerates with age and the clear vitreous gel can dehydrate and clump together. These clumps (vitreous densities) cast shadows on the sensory retina causing "floaters" or dark shadowy areas in the visual field. Vitreous densities may also be caused by more complicated pathological conditions such as retinal tears and hemorrhage, inflammation and infection, diabetes and autoimmune disorders. Vitreolysis of the strands (vitreous densities) can be accomplished using a neodymium YAG laser. The procedure is performed in the physician's office with the patient seated before a slit lamp. A special contact lens is inserted to keep the eye immobile during the procedure. The laser beam is directed to the vitreous strand or area of density and concentrated energy vaporizes the material. The molecules are converted to a gas micro bubble, which is absorbed and disappears within a few hours of the procedure.

Discission/severing of vitreous strands/face adhesions/sheets/ membrane opacities

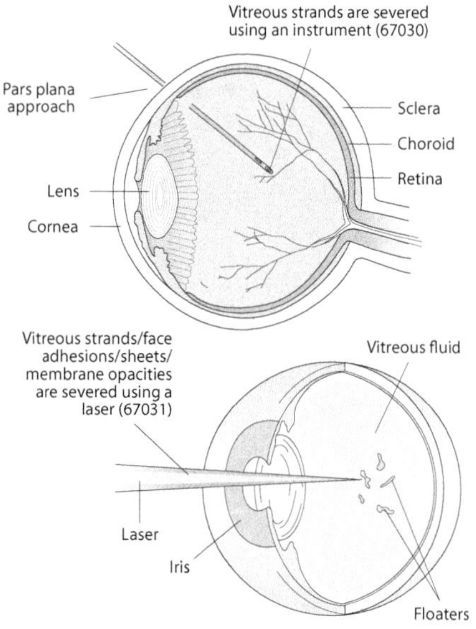

ICD-10-CM Diagnostic Codes

E08.311 Diabetes mellitus due to underlying condition with unspecified diabetic retinopathy with macular edema

E08.319 Diabetes mellitus due to underlying condition with unspecified diabetic retinopathy without macular edema

❼⇄ E08.321 Diabetes mellitus due to underlying condition with mild nonproliferative diabetic retinopathy with macular edema

❼⇄ E08.329 Diabetes mellitus due to underlying condition with mild nonproliferative diabetic retinopathy without macular edema

❼⇄ E08.331 Diabetes mellitus due to underlying condition with moderate nonproliferative diabetic retinopathy with macular edema

❼⇄ E08.339 Diabetes mellitus due to underlying condition with moderate nonproliferative diabetic retinopathy without macular edema

❼⇄ E08.341 Diabetes mellitus due to underlying condition with severe nonproliferative diabetic retinopathy with macular edema

❼⇄ E08.349 Diabetes mellitus due to underlying condition with severe nonproliferative diabetic retinopathy without macular edema

❼⇄ E08.351 Diabetes mellitus due to underlying condition with proliferative diabetic retinopathy with macular edema

❼⇄ E08.352 Diabetes mellitus due to underlying condition with proliferative diabetic retinopathy with traction retinal detachment involving the macula

❼⇄ E08.353 Diabetes mellitus due to underlying condition with proliferative diabetic retinopathy with traction retinal detachment not involving the macula

❼⇄ E08.354 Diabetes mellitus due to underlying condition with proliferative diabetic retinopathy with combined traction retinal detachment and rhegmatogenous retinal detachment

❼⇄ E08.355 Diabetes mellitus due to underlying condition with stable proliferative diabetic retinopathy

❼⇄ E08.359 Diabetes mellitus due to underlying condition with proliferative diabetic retinopathy without macular edema

E08.36 Diabetes mellitus due to underlying condition with diabetic cataract

❼⇄ E08.37 Diabetes mellitus due to underlying condition with diabetic macular edema, resolved following treatment

E08.39 Diabetes mellitus due to underlying condition with other diabetic ophthalmic complication

E08.65 Diabetes mellitus due to underlying condition with hyperglycemia

E09.311 Drug or chemical induced diabetes mellitus with unspecified diabetic retinopathy with macular edema

E09.319 Drug or chemical induced diabetes mellitus with unspecified diabetic retinopathy without macular edema

❼⇄ E09.321 Drug or chemical induced diabetes mellitus with mild nonproliferative diabetic retinopathy with macular edema

❼⇄ E09.329 Drug or chemical induced diabetes mellitus with mild nonproliferative diabetic retinopathy without macular edema

❼⇄ E09.331 Drug or chemical induced diabetes mellitus with moderate nonproliferative diabetic retinopathy with macular edema

❼⇄ E09.339 Drug or chemical induced diabetes mellitus with moderate nonproliferative diabetic retinopathy without macular edema

❼⇄ E09.341 Drug or chemical induced diabetes mellitus with severe nonproliferative diabetic retinopathy with macular edema

❼⇄ E09.349 Drug or chemical induced diabetes mellitus with severe nonproliferative diabetic retinopathy without macular edema

❼⇄ E09.351 Drug or chemical induced diabetes mellitus with proliferative diabetic retinopathy with macular edema

❼⇄ E09.352 Drug or chemical induced diabetes mellitus with proliferative diabetic retinopathy with traction retinal detachment involving the macula

❼⇄ E09.353 Drug or chemical induced diabetes mellitus with proliferative diabetic retinopathy with traction retinal detachment not involving the macula

❼⇄ E09.354 Drug or chemical induced diabetes mellitus with proliferative diabetic retinopathy with combined traction retinal detachment and rhegmatogenous retinal detachment

❼⇄ E09.355 Drug or chemical induced diabetes mellitus with stable proliferative diabetic retinopathy

❼⇄ E09.359 Drug or chemical induced diabetes mellitus with proliferative diabetic retinopathy without macular edema

E09.36 Drug or chemical induced diabetes mellitus with diabetic cataract

❼⇄ E09.37 Drug or chemical induced diabetes mellitus with diabetic macular edema, resolved following treatment

E09.39 Drug or chemical induced diabetes mellitus with other diabetic ophthalmic complication

E09.65 Drug or chemical induced diabetes mellitus with hyperglycemia

E10.311 Type 1 diabetes mellitus with unspecified diabetic retinopathy with macular edema

E10.319 Type 1 diabetes mellitus with unspecified diabetic retinopathy without macular edema

❼⇄ E10.321 Type 1 diabetes mellitus with mild nonproliferative diabetic retinopathy with macular edema

❼⇄ E10.329 Type 1 diabetes mellitus with mild nonproliferative diabetic retinopathy without macular edema

❼⇄ E10.331 Type 1 diabetes mellitus with moderate nonproliferative diabetic retinopathy with macular edema

❼⇄ E10.339 Type 1 diabetes mellitus with moderate nonproliferative diabetic retinopathy without macular edema

❼⇄ E10.341 Type 1 diabetes mellitus with severe nonproliferative diabetic retinopathy with macular edema

❼⇄ E10.349 Type 1 diabetes mellitus with severe nonproliferative diabetic retinopathy without macular edema

❼⇄ E10.351 Type 1 diabetes mellitus with proliferative diabetic retinopathy with macular edema

❼⇄ E10.352 Type 1 diabetes mellitus with proliferative diabetic retinopathy with traction retinal detachment involving the macula

❼⇄ E10.353 Type 1 diabetes mellitus with proliferative diabetic retinopathy with traction retinal detachment not involving the macula

❼⇄ E10.354 Type 1 diabetes mellitus with proliferative diabetic retinopathy with combined traction retinal detachment and rhegmatogenous retinal detachment

❼⇄ E10.355 Type 1 diabetes mellitus with stable proliferative diabetic retinopathy

❼⇄ E10.359 Type 1 diabetes mellitus with proliferative diabetic retinopathy without macular edema

E10.36 Type 1 diabetes mellitus with diabetic cataract

❼⇄ E10.37 Type 1 diabetes mellitus with diabetic macular edema, resolved following treatment

E10.39 Type 1 diabetes mellitus with other diabetic ophthalmic complication

E10.65 Type 1 diabetes mellitus with hyperglycemia

E11.311 Type 2 diabetes mellitus with unspecified diabetic retinopathy with macular edema

E11.319 Type 2 diabetes mellitus with unspecified diabetic retinopathy without macular edema

❼⇄ E11.321 Type 2 diabetes mellitus with mild nonproliferative diabetic retinopathy with macular edema

❼⇄ E11.329 Type 2 diabetes mellitus with mild nonproliferative diabetic retinopathy without macular edema

❼⇄ E11.331 Type 2 diabetes mellitus with moderate nonproliferative diabetic retinopathy with macular edema

❼⇄ E11.339 Type 2 diabetes mellitus with moderate nonproliferative diabetic retinopathy without macular edema

❼⇄ E11.341 Type 2 diabetes mellitus with severe nonproliferative diabetic retinopathy with macular edema

❼⇄ E11.349 Type 2 diabetes mellitus with severe nonproliferative diabetic retinopathy without macular edema

❼⇄ E11.351 Type 2 diabetes mellitus with proliferative diabetic retinopathy with macular edema

❼⇄ E11.352 Type 2 diabetes mellitus with proliferative diabetic retinopathy with traction retinal detachment involving the macula

❼⇄ E11.353 Type 2 diabetes mellitus with proliferative diabetic retinopathy with traction retinal detachment not involving the macula

❼⇄ E11.354 Type 2 diabetes mellitus with proliferative diabetic retinopathy with combined traction retinal detachment and rhegmatogenous retinal detachment

❼⇄ E11.355 Type 2 diabetes mellitus with stable proliferative diabetic retinopathy

❼⇄ E11.359 Type 2 diabetes mellitus with proliferative diabetic retinopathy without macular edema

E11.36 Type 2 diabetes mellitus with diabetic cataract

❼⇄ E11.37 Type 2 diabetes mellitus with diabetic macular edema, resolved following treatment

E11.39 Type 2 diabetes mellitus with other diabetic ophthalmic complication

E11.65 Type 2 diabetes mellitus with hyperglycemia

H20.00 Unspecified acute and subacute iridocyclitis

⇄ H21.42 Pupillary membranes, left eye

⇄ H21.512 Anterior synechiae (iris), left eye

⇄ H25.12 Age-related nuclear cataract, left eye

⇄ H26.492 Other secondary cataract, left eye

⇄ H35.351 Cystoid macular degeneration, right eye

❼⇄ H40.111 Primary open-angle glaucoma, right eye

❼⇄ H40.112 Primary open-angle glaucoma, left eye

❼⇄ H40.113 Primary open-angle glaucoma, bilateral

⇄ H43.02 Vitreous prolapse, left eye

⇄ H43.312 Vitreous membranes and strands, left eye

⇄ H44.2C1 Degenerative myopia with retinal detachment, right eye

⇄ H44.2C2 Degenerative myopia with retinal detachment, left eye

⇄ H44.2C3 Degenerative myopia with retinal detachment, bilateral eye

⇄ H52.222 Regular astigmatism, left eye

⇄ H54.0X33 Blindness right eye category 3, blindness left eye category 3

⇄ H54.0X34 Blindness right eye category 3, blindness left eye category 4

⇄ H54.0X35 Blindness right eye category 3, blindness left eye category 5

⇄ H54.0X43 Blindness right eye category 4, blindness left eye category 3

⇄ H54.0X44 Blindness right eye category 4, blindness left eye category 4

⇄ H54.0X45 Blindness right eye category 4, blindness left eye category 5

⇄ H54.0X53 Blindness right eye category 5, blindness left eye category 3

⇄ H54.0X54 Blindness right eye category 5, blindness left eye category 4

⇄ H54.0X55 Blindness right eye category 5, blindness left eye category 5

⇄ H54.1131 Blindness right eye category 3, low vision left eye category 1

⇄ H54.1132 Blindness right eye category 3, low vision left eye category 2

⇄ H54.1141 Blindness right eye category 4, low vision left eye category 1

⇄ H54.1142 Blindness right eye category 4, low vision left eye category 2

⇄ H54.1151 Blindness right eye category 5, low vision left eye category 1

⇄ H54.1152 Blindness right eye category 5, low vision left eye category 2

⇄ H54.1213 Low vision right eye category 1, blindness left eye category 3

⇄ H54.1214 Low vision right eye category 1, blindness left eye category 4

⇄ H54.1215 Low vision right eye category 1, blindness left eye category 5

⇄ H54.1223 Low vision right eye category 2, blindness left eye category 3

⇄ H54.1224 Low vision right eye category 2, blindness left eye category 4

⇄ H54.1225 Low vision right eye category 2, blindness left eye category 5

⇄ H54.2X11 Low vision right eye category 1, low vision left eye category 1

⇄ H54.2X12 Low vision right eye category 1, low vision left eye category 2

⇄ H54.2X21 Low vision right eye category 2, low vision left eye category 1

⇄ H54.2X22 Low vision right eye category 2, low vision left eye category 2

⇄ H54.413A Blindness right eye category 3, normal vision left eye

⇄ H54.414A Blindness right eye category 4, normal vision left eye

⇄ H54.415A Blindness right eye category 5, normal vision left eye

⇄ H54.42A3 Blindness left eye category 3, normal vision right eye

⇄ H54.42A4 Blindness left eye category 4, normal vision right eye

⇄ H54.42A5 Blindness left eye category 5, normal vision right eye

⇄ H54.511A Low vision right eye category 1, normal vision left eye

⇄ H54.512A Low vision right eye category 2, normal vision left eye

⇄ H54.52A1 Low vision left eye category 1, normal vision right eye

⇄ H54.52A2 Low vision left eye category 2, normal vision right eye

❼ T79.8 Other early complications of trauma

❼ T79.A9 Traumatic compartment syndrome of other sites

❼	T81.89	Other complications of procedures, not elsewhere classified
❼	T85.21	Breakdown (mechanical) of intraocular lens
❼	T85.22	Displacement of intraocular lens
❼	T85.29	Other mechanical complication of intraocular lens
	Z96.1	Presence of intraocular lens

ICD-10-CM Coding Notes

For codes requiring a 7th character extension, refer to your ICD-10-CM book. Review the character descriptions and coding guidelines for proper selection. For some procedures, only certain characters will apply.

CCI Edits

Refer to Appendix A for CCI edits.

Pub 100

67031: Pub 100-03, 1, 140.5

Facility RVUs ▯

Code	Work	PE Facility	MP	Total Facility
67031	4.47	5.45	0.34	10.26

Non-facility RVUs ▯

Code	Work	PE Non-Facility	MP	Total Non-Facility
67031	4.47	6.56	0.34	11.37

Modifiers (PAR) ▯

Code	Mod 50	Mod 51	Mod 62	Mod 66	Mod 80
67031	1	2	0	0	1

Global Period

Code	Days
67031	090

67036-67040

67036 Vitrectomy, mechanical, pars plana approach

67039 Vitrectomy, mechanical, pars plana approach; with focal endolaser photocoagulation

67040 Vitrectomy, mechanical, pars plana approach; with endolaser panretinal photocoagulation

AMA Coding Notes

Surgical Procedures on the Eye and Ocular Adnexa

(For diagnostic and treatment ophthalmological services, see Medicine, Ophthalmology, and 92002 et seq)

(Do not report code 69990 in addition to codes 65091-68850)

AMA *CPT® Assistant* ▯

67036: Fall 92: 6, Oct 08: 3

67039: Winter 90: 9, Sep 05: 12

67040: Winter 90: 9, Sep 05: 12, Jul 07: 12

Plain English Description

A mechanical vitrectomy using a pars plana approach is performed. The vitreous is a clear, gel-like substance that fills the center of the eye. Removal of the vitreous may be performed to treat hemorrhage, clear debris from the vitreous, remove scar tissue, or alleviate tension on the retina. Three tiny incisions are made in the eye in the pars plana, located in front of the ciliary body and behind the retina. A light pipe, an infusion port, and a vitrectomy device are then inserted. The inside of the eye is illuminated with the light pipe. The vitrectomy device, a microscopic oscillating cutting device, is activated and the vitreous gel is removed from the eye in a slow, controlled fashion. As the vitreous gel is removed, it is replaced with fluid through the infusion port to maintain proper pressure in the eye. When the vitreous has been extracted, the surgical instruments are removed. Use 67039 when repair of the retina using focal endolaser photocoagulation is also performed. A mechanical vitrectomy is performed as described above. An endoprobe is then inserted and small focal lesions of the retina are repaired using endolaser photocoagulation. Use 67040 when repair of the retina using panretinal endolaser photocoagulation is performed following the mechanical vitrectomy. An endoprobe is inserted and the entire retina is treated by photocoagulation.

Pars plana mechanical vitrectomy

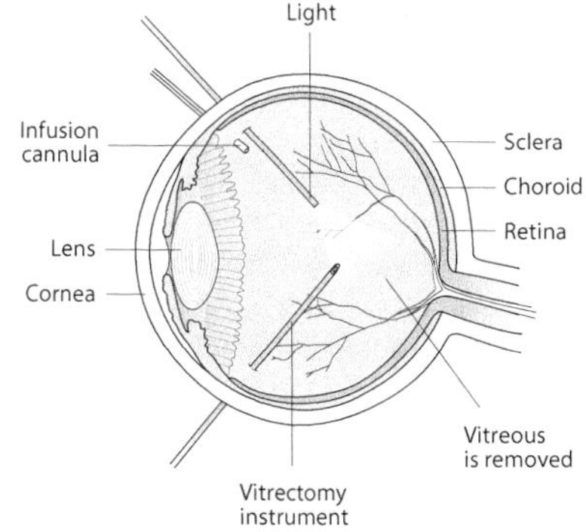

With focal endolaser (67039), or endolase panretinal (67040) photocoagulation

ICD-10-CM Diagnostic Codes

	E08.311	Diabetes mellitus due to underlying condition with unspecified diabetic retinopathy with macular edema
	E08.319	Diabetes mellitus due to underlying condition with unspecified diabetic retinopathy without macular edema
❼⇄	E08.321	Diabetes mellitus due to underlying condition with mild nonproliferative diabetic retinopathy with macular edema
❼⇄	E08.329	Diabetes mellitus due to underlying condition with mild nonproliferative diabetic retinopathy without macular edema
❼⇄	E08.331	Diabetes mellitus due to underlying condition with moderate nonproliferative diabetic retinopathy with macular edema
❼⇄	E08.339	Diabetes mellitus due to underlying condition with moderate nonproliferative diabetic retinopathy without macular edema
❼⇄	E08.341	Diabetes mellitus due to underlying condition with severe nonproliferative diabetic retinopathy with macular edema
❼⇄	E08.349	Diabetes mellitus due to underlying condition with severe nonproliferative diabetic retinopathy without macular edema
❼⇄	E08.351	Diabetes mellitus due to underlying condition with proliferative diabetic retinopathy with macular edema
❼⇄	E08.352	Diabetes mellitus due to underlying condition with proliferative diabetic retinopathy with traction retinal detachment involving the macula
❼⇄	E08.353	Diabetes mellitus due to underlying condition with proliferative diabetic retinopathy with traction retinal detachment not involving the macula
❼⇄	E08.354	Diabetes mellitus due to underlying condition with proliferative diabetic retinopathy with combined traction retinal detachment and rhegmatogenous retinal detachment
❼⇄	E08.355	Diabetes mellitus due to underlying condition with stable proliferative diabetic retinopathy
❼⇄	E08.359	Diabetes mellitus due to underlying condition with proliferative diabetic retinopathy without macular edema
	E08.36	Diabetes mellitus due to underlying condition with diabetic cataract
❼⇄	E08.37	Diabetes mellitus due to underlying condition with diabetic macular edema, resolved following treatment
	E08.39	Diabetes mellitus due to underlying condition with other diabetic ophthalmic complication
	E08.65	Diabetes mellitus due to underlying condition with hyperglycemia
	E09.311	Drug or chemical induced diabetes mellitus with unspecified diabetic retinopathy with macular edema
	E09.319	Drug or chemical induced diabetes mellitus with unspecified diabetic retinopathy without macular edema
❼⇄	E09.321	Drug or chemical induced diabetes mellitus with mild nonproliferative diabetic retinopathy with macular edema
❼⇄	E09.329	Drug or chemical induced diabetes mellitus with mild nonproliferative diabetic retinopathy without macular edema
❼⇄	E09.331	Drug or chemical induced diabetes mellitus with moderate nonproliferative diabetic retinopathy with macular edema
❼⇄	E09.339	Drug or chemical induced diabetes mellitus with moderate nonproliferative diabetic retinopathy without macular edema
❼⇄	E09.341	Drug or chemical induced diabetes mellitus with severe nonproliferative diabetic retinopathy with macular edema
❼⇄	E09.349	Drug or chemical induced diabetes mellitus with severe nonproliferative diabetic retinopathy without macular edema
❼⇄	E09.351	Drug or chemical induced diabetes mellitus with proliferative diabetic retinopathy with macular edema
❼⇄	E09.352	Drug or chemical induced diabetes mellitus with proliferative diabetic retinopathy with traction retinal detachment involving the macula
❼⇄	E09.353	Drug or chemical induced diabetes mellitus with proliferative diabetic retinopathy with traction retinal detachment not involving the macula
❼⇄	E09.354	Drug or chemical induced diabetes mellitus with proliferative diabetic retinopathy with combined traction retinal detachment and rhegmatogenous retinal detachment
❼⇄	E09.355	Drug or chemical induced diabetes mellitus with stable proliferative diabetic retinopathy

❼⇄	E09.359	Drug or chemical induced diabetes mellitus with proliferative diabetic retinopathy without macular edema
	E09.36	Drug or chemical induced diabetes mellitus with diabetic cataract
❼⇄	E09.37	Drug or chemical induced diabetes mellitus with diabetic macular edema, resolved following treatment
	E09.39	Drug or chemical induced diabetes mellitus with other diabetic ophthalmic complication
	E09.65	Drug or chemical induced diabetes mellitus with hyperglycemia
	E10.311	Type 1 diabetes mellitus with unspecified diabetic retinopathy with macular edema
	E10.319	Type 1 diabetes mellitus with unspecified diabetic retinopathy without macular edema
❼⇄	E10.321	Type 1 diabetes mellitus with mild nonproliferative diabetic retinopathy with macular edema
❼⇄	E10.329	Type 1 diabetes mellitus with mild nonproliferative diabetic retinopathy without macular edema
❼⇄	E10.331	Type 1 diabetes mellitus with moderate nonproliferative diabetic retinopathy with macular edema
❼⇄	E10.339	Type 1 diabetes mellitus with moderate nonproliferative diabetic retinopathy without macular edema
❼⇄	E10.341	Type 1 diabetes mellitus with severe nonproliferative diabetic retinopathy with macular edema
❼⇄	E10.349	Type 1 diabetes mellitus with severe nonproliferative diabetic retinopathy without macular edema
❼⇄	E10.351	Type 1 diabetes mellitus with proliferative diabetic retinopathy with macular edema
❼⇄	E10.352	Type 1 diabetes mellitus with proliferative diabetic retinopathy with traction retinal detachment involving the macula
❼⇄	E10.353	Type 1 diabetes mellitus with proliferative diabetic retinopathy with traction retinal detachment not involving the macula
❼⇄	E10.354	Type 1 diabetes mellitus with proliferative diabetic retinopathy with combined traction retinal detachment and rhegmatogenous retinal detachment
❼⇄	E10.355	Type 1 diabetes mellitus with stable proliferative diabetic retinopathy
❼⇄	E10.359	Type 1 diabetes mellitus with proliferative diabetic retinopathy without macular edema
	E10.36	Type 1 diabetes mellitus with diabetic cataract
❼⇄	E10.37	Type 1 diabetes mellitus with diabetic macular edema, resolved following treatment
	E10.39	Type 1 diabetes mellitus with other diabetic ophthalmic complication
	E10.65	Type 1 diabetes mellitus with hyperglycemia
	E11.311	Type 2 diabetes mellitus with unspecified diabetic retinopathy with macular edema
	E11.319	Type 2 diabetes mellitus with unspecified diabetic retinopathy without macular edema
❼⇄	E11.321	Type 2 diabetes mellitus with mild nonproliferative diabetic retinopathy with macular edema
❼⇄	E11.329	Type 2 diabetes mellitus with mild nonproliferative diabetic retinopathy without macular edema
❼⇄	E11.331	Type 2 diabetes mellitus with moderate nonproliferative diabetic retinopathy with macular edema
❼⇄	E11.339	Type 2 diabetes mellitus with moderate nonproliferative diabetic retinopathy without macular edema
❼⇄	E11.341	Type 2 diabetes mellitus with severe nonproliferative diabetic retinopathy with macular edema
❼⇄	E11.349	Type 2 diabetes mellitus with severe nonproliferative diabetic retinopathy without macular edema
❼⇄	E11.351	Type 2 diabetes mellitus with proliferative diabetic retinopathy with macular edema
❼⇄	E11.352	Type 2 diabetes mellitus with proliferative diabetic retinopathy with traction retinal detachment involving the macula
❼⇄	E11.353	Type 2 diabetes mellitus with proliferative diabetic retinopathy with traction retinal detachment not involving the macula
❼⇄	E11.354	Type 2 diabetes mellitus with proliferative diabetic retinopathy with combined traction retinal detachment and rhegmatogenous retinal detachment
❼⇄	E11.355	Type 2 diabetes mellitus with stable proliferative diabetic retinopathy
❼⇄	E11.359	Type 2 diabetes mellitus with proliferative diabetic retinopathy without macular edema
	E11.36	Type 2 diabetes mellitus with diabetic cataract
❼⇄	E11.37	Type 2 diabetes mellitus with diabetic macular edema, resolved following treatment
	E11.39	Type 2 diabetes mellitus with other diabetic ophthalmic complication
	E11.65	Type 2 diabetes mellitus with hyperglycemia
⇄	H21.331	Parasitic cyst of iris, ciliary body or anterior chamber, right eye
⇄	H27.01	Aphakia, right eye
⇄	H27.111	Subluxation of lens, right eye
⇄	H27.131	Posterior dislocation of lens, right eye
⇄	H31.011	Macula scars of posterior pole (postinflammatory) (post-traumatic), right eye
⇄	H33.121	Parasitic cyst of retina, right eye
⇄	H33.301	Unspecified retinal break, right eye
⇄	H33.331	Multiple defects of retina without detachment, right eye
❼⇄	H35.321	Exudative age-related macular degeneration, right eye
❼⇄	H35.322	Exudative age-related macular degeneration, left eye
❼⇄	H35.323	Exudative age-related macular degeneration, bilateral
⇄	H35.341	Macular cyst, hole, or pseudohole, right eye
⇄	H35.371	Puckering of macula, right eye
⇄	H35.61	Retinal hemorrhage, right eye
	H35.81	Retinal edema
⇄	H40.831	Aqueous misdirection, right eye
	H42	Glaucoma in diseases classified elsewhere
⇄	H43.01	Vitreous prolapse, right eye
⇄	H43.11	Vitreous hemorrhage, right eye
⇄	H43.21	Crystalline deposits in vitreous body, right eye
⇄	H43.311	Vitreous membranes and strands, right eye
⇄	H43.391	Other vitreous opacities, right eye
⇄	H44.001	Unspecified purulent endophthalmitis, right eye
⇄	H44.021	Vitreous abscess (chronic), right eye
⇄	H44.121	Parasitic endophthalmitis, unspecified, right eye
	H44.19	Other endophthalmitis
⇄	H59.021	Cataract (lens) fragments in eye following cataract surgery, right eye
	Q14.0	Congenital malformation of vitreous humor
❼	T85.21	Breakdown (mechanical) of intraocular lens
❼	T85.22	Displacement of intraocular lens
❼	T85.29	Other mechanical complication of intraocular lens

ICD-10-CM Coding Notes

For codes requiring a 7th character extension, refer to your ICD-10-CM book. Review the character descriptions and coding guidelines for proper selection. For some procedures, only certain characters will apply.

CCI Edits

Refer to Appendix A for CCI edits.

Pub 100

67036: Pub 100-03, 1, 80.11
67039: Pub 100-03, 1, 140.5, Pub 100-03, 1, 80.11
67040: Pub 100-03, 1, 140.5, Pub 100-03, 1, 80.11

Facility RVUs

Code	Work	PE Facility	MP	Total Facility
67036	12.13	12.85	0.95	25.93
67039	13.20	13.51	1.01	27.72
67040	14.50	14.32	1.11	29.93

Non-facility RVUs

Code	Work	PE Non-Facility	MP	Total Non-Facility
67036	12.13	12.85	0.95	25.93
67039	13.20	13.51	1.01	27.72
67040	14.50	14.32	1.11	29.93

Modifiers (PAR)

Code	Mod 50	Mod 51	Mod 62	Mod 66	Mod 80
67036	1	2	1	0	2
67039	1	2	1	0	2
67040	1	2	1	0	2

Global Period

Code	Days
67036	090
67039	090
67040	090

67041

67041 Vitrectomy, mechanical, pars plana approach; with removal of preretinal cellular membrane (eg, macular pucker)

AMA Coding Notes

Surgical Procedures on the Eye and Ocular Adnexa

(For diagnostic and treatment ophthalmological services, see Medicine, Ophthalmology, and 92002 et seq)

(Do not report code 69990 in addition to codes 65091-68850)

Plain English Description

A mechanical vitrectomy with removal of the preretinal cellular membrane (macular pucker) is performed via pars plana approach. The vitreous is a clear, gel-like substance that fills the center of the eye. It is removed prior to surgical treatment of macular pucker, also referred to as epiretinal membrane or preretinal membrane. A macular pucker occurs when the vitreous detaches from the retina, causing microscopic damage resulting in scar tissue at the site of the detachment. This can cause blurred or distorted vision. Three tiny incisions are made in the eye in the pars plana, located in front of the ciliary body and behind the retina. A light pipe, an infusion port, and a vitrectomy device are then inserted. The inside of the eye is illuminated with the light pipe. The vitrectomy device, a microscopic oscillating cutting device, is activated and vitreous gel is removed from the eye in a slow, controlled fashion. As the vitreous gel is removed, it is replaced with fluid through the infusion port to maintain proper pressure in the eye. The central vitreous is removed and the vitreous base is accessed. Using high magnification, the edge of the cellular membrane is elevated. Microforceps are introduced and the preretinal cellular membrane is elevated further and removed. The retina is examined for tearing before the surgical tools are removed.

Pars plana mechanical vitrectomy, with removal of preretinal cellular membrane

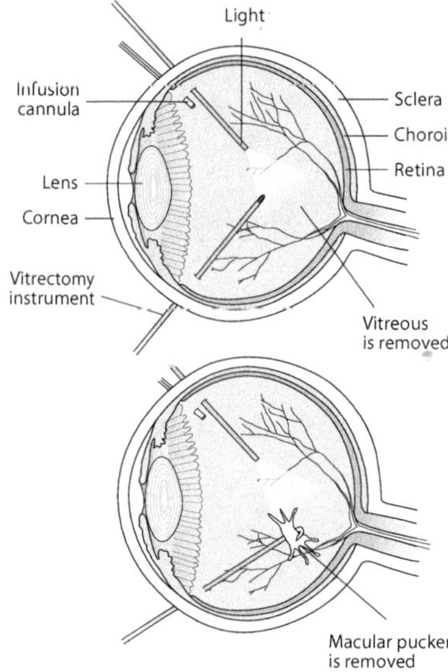

ICD-10-CM Diagnostic Codes

	Code	Description
	E08.311	Diabetes mellitus due to underlying condition with unspecified diabetic retinopathy with macular edema
	E08.319	Diabetes mellitus due to underlying condition with unspecified diabetic retinopathy without macular edema
➐⇄	E08.321	Diabetes mellitus due to underlying condition with mild nonproliferative diabetic retinopathy with macular edema
➐⇄	E08.329	Diabetes mellitus due to underlying condition with mild nonproliferative diabetic retinopathy without macular edema
➐⇄	E08.331	Diabetes mellitus due to underlying condition with moderate nonproliferative diabetic retinopathy with macular edema
➐⇄	E08.339	Diabetes mellitus due to underlying condition with moderate nonproliferative diabetic retinopathy without macular edema
➐⇄	E08.341	Diabetes mellitus due to underlying condition with severe nonproliferative diabetic retinopathy with macular edema
➐⇄	E08.349	Diabetes mellitus due to underlying condition with severe nonproliferative diabetic retinopathy without macular edema
➐⇄	E08.351	Diabetes mellitus due to underlying condition with proliferative diabetic retinopathy with macular edema
➐⇄	E08.352	Diabetes mellitus due to underlying condition with proliferative diabetic retinopathy with traction retinal detachment involving the macula
➐⇄	E08.353	Diabetes mellitus due to underlying condition with proliferative diabetic retinopathy with traction retinal detachment not involving the macula
➐⇄	E08.354	Diabetes mellitus due to underlying condition with proliferative diabetic retinopathy with combined traction retinal detachment and rhegmatogenous retinal detachment
➐⇄	E08.355	Diabetes mellitus due to underlying condition with stable proliferative diabetic retinopathy
➐⇄	E08.359	Diabetes mellitus due to underlying condition with proliferative diabetic retinopathy without macular edema
	E08.36	Diabetes mellitus due to underlying condition with diabetic cataract
➐⇄	E08.37	Diabetes mellitus due to underlying condition with diabetic macular edema, resolved following treatment
	E08.39	Diabetes mellitus due to underlying condition with other diabetic ophthalmic complication
	E08.65	Diabetes mellitus due to underlying condition with hyperglycemia
	E09.311	Drug or chemical induced diabetes mellitus with unspecified diabetic retinopathy with macular edema
	E09.319	Drug or chemical induced diabetes mellitus with unspecified diabetic retinopathy without macular edema
➐⇄	E09.321	Drug or chemical induced diabetes mellitus with mild nonproliferative diabetic retinopathy with macular edema
➐⇄	E09.329	Drug or chemical induced diabetes mellitus with mild nonproliferative diabetic retinopathy without macular edema
➐⇄	E09.331	Drug or chemical induced diabetes mellitus with moderate nonproliferative diabetic retinopathy with macular edema
➐⇄	E09.339	Drug or chemical induced diabetes mellitus with moderate nonproliferative diabetic retinopathy without macular edema
➐⇄	E09.341	Drug or chemical induced diabetes mellitus with severe nonproliferative diabetic retinopathy with macular edema
➐⇄	E09.349	Drug or chemical induced diabetes mellitus with severe nonproliferative diabetic retinopathy without macular edema
➐⇄	E09.351	Drug or chemical induced diabetes mellitus with proliferative diabetic retinopathy with macular edema
➐⇄	E09.352	Drug or chemical induced diabetes mellitus with proliferative diabetic retinopathy with traction retinal detachment involving the macula
➐⇄	E09.353	Drug or chemical induced diabetes mellitus with proliferative diabetic retinopathy with traction retinal detachment not involving the macula

	Code	Description
⑦⇄	E09.354	Drug or chemical induced diabetes mellitus with proliferative diabetic retinopathy with combined traction retinal detachment and rhegmatogenous retinal detachment
⑦⇄	E09.355	Drug or chemical induced diabetes mellitus with stable proliferative diabetic retinopathy
⑦⇄	E09.359	Drug or chemical induced diabetes mellitus with proliferative diabetic retinopathy without macular edema
	E09.36	Drug or chemical induced diabetes mellitus with diabetic cataract
⑦⇄	E09.37	Drug or chemical induced diabetes mellitus with diabetic macular edema, resolved following treatment
	E09.39	Drug or chemical induced diabetes mellitus with other diabetic ophthalmic complication
	E09.65	Drug or chemical induced diabetes mellitus with hyperglycemia
	E10.311	Type 1 diabetes mellitus with unspecified diabetic retinopathy with macular edema
	E10.319	Type 1 diabetes mellitus with unspecified diabetic retinopathy without macular edema
⑦⇄	E10.321	Type 1 diabetes mellitus with mild nonproliferative diabetic retinopathy with macular edema
⑦⇄	E10.329	Type 1 diabetes mellitus with mild nonproliferative diabetic retinopathy without macular edema
⑦⇄	E10.331	Type 1 diabetes mellitus with moderate nonproliferative diabetic retinopathy with macular edema
⑦⇄	E10.339	Type 1 diabetes mellitus with moderate nonproliferative diabetic retinopathy without macular edema
⑦⇄	E10.341	Type 1 diabetes mellitus with severe nonproliferative diabetic retinopathy with macular edema
⑦⇄	E10.349	Type 1 diabetes mellitus with severe nonproliferative diabetic retinopathy without macular edema
⑦⇄	E10.351	Type 1 diabetes mellitus with proliferative diabetic retinopathy with macular edema
⑦⇄	E10.352	Type 1 diabetes mellitus with proliferative diabetic retinopathy with traction retinal detachment involving the macula
⑦⇄	E10.353	Type 1 diabetes mellitus with proliferative diabetic retinopathy with traction retinal detachment not involving the macula
⑦⇄	E10.354	Type 1 diabetes mellitus with proliferative diabetic retinopathy with combined traction retinal detachment and rhegmatogenous retinal detachment
⑦⇄	E10.355	Type 1 diabetes mellitus with stable proliferative diabetic retinopathy
⑦⇄	E10.359	Type 1 diabetes mellitus with proliferative diabetic retinopathy without macular edema
	E10.36	Type 1 diabetes mellitus with diabetic cataract
⑦⇄	E10.37	Type 1 diabetes mellitus with diabetic macular edema, resolved following treatment
	E10.39	Type 1 diabetes mellitus with other diabetic ophthalmic complication
	E10.65	Type 1 diabetes mellitus with hyperglycemia
	E11.311	Type 2 diabetes mellitus with unspecified diabetic retinopathy with macular edema
	E11.319	Type 2 diabetes mellitus with unspecified diabetic retinopathy without macular edema
⑦⇄	E11.321	Type 2 diabetes mellitus with mild nonproliferative diabetic retinopathy with macular edema
⑦⇄	E11.329	Type 2 diabetes mellitus with mild nonproliferative diabetic retinopathy without macular edema
⑦⇄	E11.331	Type 2 diabetes mellitus with moderate nonproliferative diabetic retinopathy with macular edema
⑦⇄	E11.339	Type 2 diabetes mellitus with moderate nonproliferative diabetic retinopathy without macular edema
⑦⇄	E11.341	Type 2 diabetes mellitus with severe nonproliferative diabetic retinopathy with macular edema
⑦⇄	E11.349	Type 2 diabetes mellitus with severe nonproliferative diabetic retinopathy without macular edema
⑦⇄	E11.351	Type 2 diabetes mellitus with proliferative diabetic retinopathy with macular edema
⑦⇄	E11.352	Type 2 diabetes mellitus with proliferative diabetic retinopathy with traction retinal detachment involving the macula
⑦⇄	E11.353	Type 2 diabetes mellitus with proliferative diabetic retinopathy with traction retinal detachment not involving the macula
⑦⇄	E11.354	Type 2 diabetes mellitus with proliferative diabetic retinopathy with combined traction retinal detachment and rhegmatogenous retinal detachment
⑦⇄	E11.355	Type 2 diabetes mellitus with stable proliferative diabetic retinopathy
⑦⇄	E11.359	Type 2 diabetes mellitus with proliferative diabetic retinopathy without macular edema
	E11.36	Type 2 diabetes mellitus with diabetic cataract
⑦⇄	E11.37	Type 2 diabetes mellitus with diabetic macular edema, resolved following treatment
	E11.39	Type 2 diabetes mellitus with other diabetic ophthalmic complication
	E11.65	Type 2 diabetes mellitus with hyperglycemia
⇄	H33.002	Unspecified retinal detachment with retinal break, left eye
⇄	H33.012	Retinal detachment with single break, left eye
⇄	H33.022	Retinal detachment with multiple breaks, left eye
⇄	H33.032	Retinal detachment with giant retinal tear, left eye
⇄	H33.052	Total retinal detachment, left eye
⇄	H33.22	Serous retinal detachment, left eye
⇄	H33.42	Traction detachment of retina, left eye
	H33.8	Other retinal detachments
⇄	H35.22	Other non-diabetic proliferative retinopathy, left eye
⇄	H35.342	Macular cyst, hole, or pseudohole, left eye
⇄	H35.372	Puckering of macula, left eye
⇄	H35.722	Serous detachment of retinal pigment epithelium, left eye
⇄	H35.732	Hemorrhagic detachment of retinal pigment epithelium, left eye
⇄	H43.12	Vitreous hemorrhage, left eye
⇄	H43.312	Vitreous membranes and strands, left eye
⇄	H44.2C1	Degenerative myopia with retinal detachment, right eye
⇄	H44.2C2	Degenerative myopia with retinal detachment, left eye
⇄	H44.2C3	Degenerative myopia with retinal detachment, bilateral eye
⇄	H44.2E1	Degenerative myopia with other maculopathy, right eye
⇄	H44.2E2	Degenerative myopia with other maculopathy, left eye
⇄	H44.2E3	Degenerative myopia with other maculopathy, bilateral eye

ICD-10-CM Coding Notes

For codes requiring a 7th character extension, refer to your ICD-10-CM book. Review the character descriptions and coding guidelines for proper selection. For some procedures, only certain characters will apply.

CCI Edits

Refer to Appendix A for CCI edits.

Pub 100

67041: Pub 100-03, 1, 80.11

Facility RVUs

Code	Work	PE Facility	MP	Total Facility
67041	16.33	15.44	1.26	33.03

Non-facility RVUs

Code	Work	PE Non-Facility	MP	Total Non-Facility
67041	16.33	15.44	1.26	33.03

Modifiers (PAR)

Code	Mod 50	Mod 51	Mod 62	Mod 66	Mod 80
67041	1	2	1	0	2

Global Period

Code	Days
67041	090

67042

67042 Vitrectomy, mechanical, pars plana approach; with removal of internal limiting membrane of retina (eg, for repair of macular hole, diabetic macular edema), includes, if performed, intraocular tamponade (ie, air, gas or silicone oil)

AMA Coding Notes

Surgical Procedures on the Eye and Ocular Adnexa

(For diagnostic and treatment ophthalmological services, see Medicine, Ophthalmology, and 92002 et seq)

(Do not report code 69990 in addition to codes 65091-68850)

Plain English Description

A mechanical vitrectomy with peeling of the internal limiting membrane (ILM) for repair of a macular hole or diabetic macular edema is performed using a pars plana approach. The vitreous is a clear, gel-like substance that fills the center of the eye. It is removed prior to surgical treatment of a macular hole or diabetic macular edema. A macular hole occurs when the vitreous detaches from the retina, causing a tear that results in fluid leaking into the hole at the site of the detachment. Diabetic macular edema is caused by leaking vessels, resulting in retinal swelling (edema). In the case of macular holes, ILM peeling is performed to release macular traction and prevent recurrences with optimal visual recovery. Three tiny incisions are made in the eye in the pars plana, located in front of the ciliary body and behind the retina. A light pipe, an infusion port, and a vitrectomy device are then inserted. The inside of the eye is illuminated with the light pipe. The vitrectomy device, a microscopic oscillating cutting device, is activated and vitreous gel is removed from the eye in a slow, controlled fashion. As the vitreous gel is removed, it is replaced with fluid through the infusion port to maintain proper pressure in the eye. The posterior cortical vitreous is separated from the optic nerve head and posterior retina. Indocyanine green may be used to selectively stain the ILM, which is peeled by making a small opening and flap tear with vitreous forceps. A continuous, curvilinear tear is made completely around the macular hole. Air-fluid exchange is performed by injecting hexafluoride gas and the retina is examined for tearing. The patient must remain in the prone position for several days and anatomic closure occurs in about a month's time.

Pars plana mechanical vitrectomy, with removal of internal limiting membrane

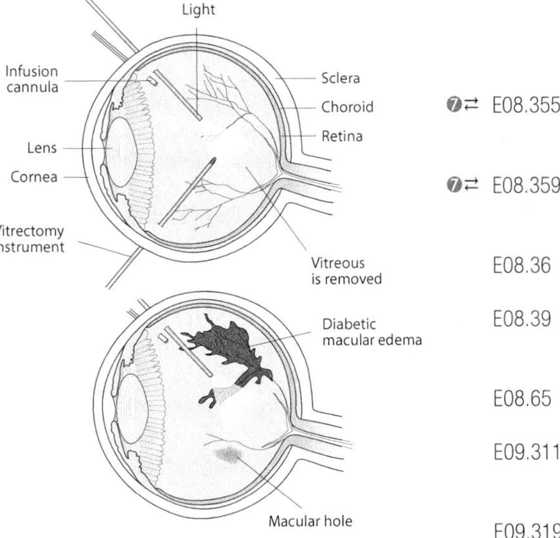

ICD-10-CM Diagnostic Codes

	E08.311	Diabetes mellitus due to underlying condition with unspecified diabetic retinopathy with macular edema
	E08.319	Diabetes mellitus due to underlying condition with unspecified diabetic retinopathy without macular edema
❼⇄	E08.321	Diabetes mellitus due to underlying condition with mild nonproliferative diabetic retinopathy with macular edema
❼⇄	E08.329	Diabetes mellitus due to underlying condition with mild nonproliferative diabetic retinopathy without macular edema
❼⇄	E08.331	Diabetes mellitus due to underlying condition with moderate nonproliferative diabetic retinopathy with macular edema
❼⇄	E08.339	Diabetes mellitus due to underlying condition with moderate nonproliferative diabetic retinopathy without macular edema
❼⇄	E08.341	Diabetes mellitus due to underlying condition with severe nonproliferative diabetic retinopathy with macular edema
❼⇄	E08.349	Diabetes mellitus due to underlying condition with severe nonproliferative diabetic retinopathy without macular edema
❼⇄	E08.351	Diabetes mellitus due to underlying condition with proliferative diabetic retinopathy with macular edema
❼⇄	E08.352	Diabetes mellitus due to underlying condition with proliferative diabetic retinopathy with traction retinal detachment involving the macula
❼⇄	E08.353	Diabetes mellitus due to underlying condition with proliferative diabetic retinopathy with traction retinal detachment not involving the macula
❼⇄	E08.354	Diabetes mellitus due to underlying condition with proliferative diabetic retinopathy with combined traction retinal detachment and rhegmatogenous retinal detachment
❼⇄	E08.355	Diabetes mellitus due to underlying condition with stable proliferative diabetic retinopathy
❼⇄	E08.359	Diabetes mellitus due to underlying condition with proliferative diabetic retinopathy without macular edema
	E08.36	Diabetes mellitus due to underlying condition with diabetic cataract
	E08.39	Diabetes mellitus due to underlying condition with other diabetic ophthalmic complication
	E08.65	Diabetes mellitus due to underlying condition with hyperglycemia
	E09.311	Drug or chemical induced diabetes mellitus with unspecified diabetic retinopathy with macular edema
	E09.319	Drug or chemical induced diabetes mellitus with unspecified diabetic retinopathy without macular edema
❼⇄	E09.321	Drug or chemical induced diabetes mellitus with mild nonproliferative diabetic retinopathy with macular edema
❼⇄	E09.329	Drug or chemical induced diabetes mellitus with mild nonproliferative diabetic retinopathy without macular edema
❼⇄	E09.331	Drug or chemical induced diabetes mellitus with moderate nonproliferative diabetic retinopathy with macular edema
❼⇄	E09.339	Drug or chemical induced diabetes mellitus with moderate nonproliferative diabetic retinopathy without macular edema
❼⇄	E09.341	Drug or chemical induced diabetes mellitus with severe nonproliferative diabetic retinopathy with macular edema
❼⇄	E09.349	Drug or chemical induced diabetes mellitus with severe nonproliferative diabetic retinopathy without macular edema
❼⇄	E09.351	Drug or chemical induced diabetes mellitus with proliferative diabetic retinopathy with macular edema
❼⇄	E09.359	Drug or chemical induced diabetes mellitus with proliferative diabetic retinopathy without macular edema
	E09.36	Drug or chemical induced diabetes mellitus with diabetic cataract
	E09.39	Drug or chemical induced diabetes mellitus with other diabetic ophthalmic complication
	E10.311	Type 1 diabetes mellitus with unspecified diabetic retinopathy with macular edema
	E10.319	Type 1 diabetes mellitus with unspecified diabetic retinopathy without macular edema
❼⇄	E10.321	Type 1 diabetes mellitus with mild nonproliferative diabetic retinopathy with macular edema

❼⇄	E10.329	Type 1 diabetes mellitus with mild nonproliferative diabetic retinopathy without macular edema
❼⇄	E10.331	Type 1 diabetes mellitus with moderate nonproliferative diabetic retinopathy with macular edema
❼⇄	E10.339	Type 1 diabetes mellitus with moderate nonproliferative diabetic retinopathy without macular edema
❼⇄	E10.341	Type 1 diabetes mellitus with severe nonproliferative diabetic retinopathy with macular edema
❼⇄	E10.349	Type 1 diabetes mellitus with severe nonproliferative diabetic retinopathy without macular edema
❼⇄	E10.351	Type 1 diabetes mellitus with proliferative diabetic retinopathy with macular edema
❼⇄	E10.359	Type 1 diabetes mellitus with proliferative diabetic retinopathy without macular edema
	E10.36	Type 1 diabetes mellitus with diabetic cataract
	E10.39	Type 1 diabetes mellitus with other diabetic ophthalmic complication
	E10.65	Type 1 diabetes mellitus with hyperglycemia
	E11.311	Type 2 diabetes mellitus with unspecified diabetic retinopathy with macular edema
	E11.319	Type 2 diabetes mellitus with unspecified diabetic retinopathy without macular edema
❼⇄	E11.321	Type 2 diabetes mellitus with mild nonproliferative diabetic retinopathy with macular edema
❼⇄	E11.329	Type 2 diabetes mellitus with mild nonproliferative diabetic retinopathy without macular edema
❼⇄	E11.331	Type 2 diabetes mellitus with moderate nonproliferative diabetic retinopathy with macular edema
❼⇄	E11.339	Type 2 diabetes mellitus with moderate nonproliferative diabetic retinopathy without macular edema
❼⇄	E11.341	Type 2 diabetes mellitus with severe nonproliferative diabetic retinopathy with macular edema
❼⇄	E11.349	Type 2 diabetes mellitus with severe nonproliferative diabetic retinopathy without macular edema
❼⇄	E11.351	Type 2 diabetes mellitus with proliferative diabetic retinopathy with macular edema
❼⇄	E11.359	Type 2 diabetes mellitus with proliferative diabetic retinopathy without macular edema
	E11.36	Type 2 diabetes mellitus with diabetic cataract
	E11.39	Type 2 diabetes mellitus with other diabetic ophthalmic complication
	E11.65	Type 2 diabetes mellitus with hyperglycemia
⇄	H35.341	Macular cyst, hole, or pseudohole, right eye
⇄	H35.351	Cystoid macular degeneration, right eye
	H35.82	Retinal ischemia
⇄	H44.2B1	Degenerative myopia with macular hole, right eye
⇄	H44.2B2	Degenerative myopia with macular hole, left eye
⇄	H44.2B3	Degenerative myopia with macular hole, bilateral eye
⇄	H44.2E1	Degenerative myopia with other maculopathy, right eye
⇄	H44.2E2	Degenerative myopia with other maculopathy, left eye
⇄	H44.2E3	Degenerative myopia with other maculopathy, bilateral eye

ICD-10-CM Coding Notes

For codes requiring a 7th character extension, refer to your ICD-10-CM book. Review the character descriptions and coding guidelines for proper selection. For some procedures, only certain characters will apply.

CCI Edits

Refer to Appendix A for CCI edits.

Pub 100

67042: Pub 100-03, 1, 80.11

Facility RVUs ▯

Code	Work	PE Facility	MP	Total Facility
67042	16.33	15.44	1.26	33.03

Non-facility RVUs ▯

Code	Work	PE Non-Facility	MP	Total Non-Facility
67042	16.33	15.44	1.26	33.03

Modifiers (PAR) ▯

Code	Mod 50	Mod 51	Mod 62	Mod 66	Mod 80
67042	1	2	1	0	2

Global Period

Code	Days
67042	090

67043

67043 Vitrectomy, mechanical, pars plana approach; with removal of subretinal membrane (eg, choroidal neovascularization), includes, if performed, intraocular tamponade (ie, air, gas or silicone oil) and laser photocoagulation

(For use of ophthalmic endoscope with 67036, 67039, 67040-67043, use 66990)

(For associated lensectomy, use 66850)

(For use of vitrectomy in retinal detachment surgery, see 67108, 67113)

(For associated removal of foreign body, see 65260, 65265)

(For unlisted procedures on vitreous, use 67299)

AMA Coding Notes

Surgical Procedures on the Eye and Ocular Adnexa

(For diagnostic and treatment ophthalmological services, see Medicine, Ophthalmology, and 92002 et seq)

(Do not report code 69990 in addition to codes 65091-68850)

Plain English Description

A mechanical vitrectomy with removal of the subretinal membrane for treatment of choroidal neovascularization (CNV) is performed using a pars plana approach. The vitreous is a clear, gel-like substance that fills the center of the eye. It is removed prior to surgical treatment of CNV—the growth of new blood vessels in the choroid resulting from a break in the structural layer beneath the retina (Bruch's membrane), which separates the choroidal or vascular layer from the retina. When a break occurs, the vascular in-growth of new blood vessels leak fluid or blood, causing distorted vision and scarring of the macula. CNV has a number of causes but occurs most often in patients with proliferative diabetic vitreoretinopathy, causing traction that results in retinal detachment, or giant retinal tears. CNV is a major cause of visual loss. Three tiny incisions are made in the eye in the pars plana, located in front of the ciliary body and behind the retina. A light pipe, an infusion port, and a vitrectomy device are then inserted. The inside of the eye is illuminated with the light pipe. The vitrectomy device, a microscopic oscillating cutting device, is activated and vitreous gel is removed from the eye in a slow, controlled fashion. As the vitreous gel is removed, it is replaced with fluid through the infusion port to maintain proper pressure in the eye. The retina is next incised (retinotomy) and the subretinal space is expanded. Using high magnification, micro forceps are introduced and the neovascular membrane is grasped and carefully removed from the subretinal space and then from the eye. The retina is examined for tearing. An intraocular tamponade may be performed using air, gas, or silicone oil if needed to prevent fluid from leaking into the retina.

Pars plana mechanical vitrectomy, with removal of subretinal membrane

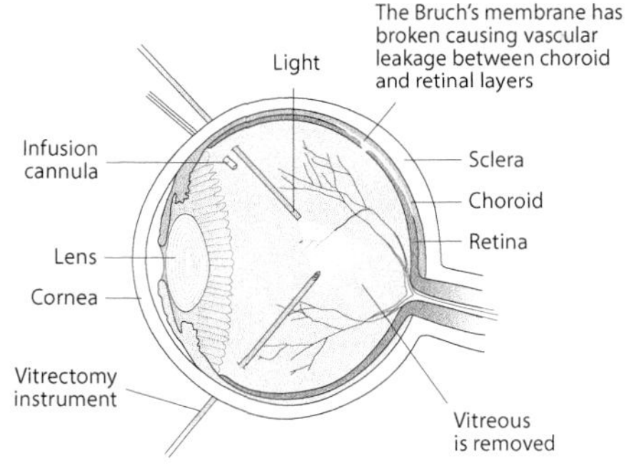

ICD-10-CM Diagnostic Codes

❼⇄	E08.341	Diabetes mellitus due to underlying condition with severe nonproliferative diabetic retinopathy with macular edema
❼⇄	E08.349	Diabetes mellitus due to underlying condition with severe nonproliferative diabetic retinopathy without macular edema
❼⇄	E08.351	Diabetes mellitus due to underlying condition with proliferative diabetic retinopathy with macular edema
❼⇄	E08.352	Diabetes mellitus due to underlying condition with proliferative diabetic retinopathy with traction retinal detachment involving the macula
❼⇄	E08.353	Diabetes mellitus due to underlying condition with proliferative diabetic retinopathy with traction retinal detachment not involving the macula
❼⇄	E08.354	Diabetes mellitus due to underlying condition with proliferative diabetic retinopathy with combined traction retinal detachment and rhegmatogenous retinal detachment
❼⇄	E08.355	Diabetes mellitus due to underlying condition with stable proliferative diabetic retinopathy
❼⇄	E08.359	Diabetes mellitus due to underlying condition with proliferative diabetic retinopathy without macular edema
❼⇄	E09.341	Drug or chemical induced diabetes mellitus with severe nonproliferative diabetic retinopathy with macular edema
❼⇄	E09.349	Drug or chemical induced diabetes mellitus with severe nonproliferative diabetic retinopathy without macular edema
❼⇄	E09.351	Drug or chemical induced diabetes mellitus with proliferative diabetic retinopathy with macular edema
❼⇄	E09.359	Drug or chemical induced diabetes mellitus with proliferative diabetic retinopathy without macular edema
❼⇄	E10.341	Type 1 diabetes mellitus with severe nonproliferative diabetic retinopathy with macular edema
❼⇄	E10.349	Type 1 diabetes mellitus with severe nonproliferative diabetic retinopathy without macular edema
❼⇄	E10.351	Type 1 diabetes mellitus with proliferative diabetic retinopathy with macular edema
❼⇄	E10.359	Type 1 diabetes mellitus with proliferative diabetic retinopathy without macular edema
❼⇄	E11.341	Type 2 diabetes mellitus with severe nonproliferative diabetic retinopathy with macular edema
❼⇄	E11.349	Type 2 diabetes mellitus with severe nonproliferative diabetic retinopathy without macular edema
❼⇄	E11.351	Type 2 diabetes mellitus with proliferative diabetic retinopathy with macular edema
❼⇄	E11.359	Type 2 diabetes mellitus with proliferative diabetic retinopathy without macular edema
⇄	H35.062	Retinal vasculitis, left eye
⇄	H35.072	Retinal telangiectasis, left eye
	H35.09	Other intraretinal microvascular abnormalities
⇄	H35.22	Other non-diabetic proliferative retinopathy, left eye
⇄	H35.3211	Exudative age-related macular degeneration, right eye, with active choroidal neovascularization
⇄	H35.3221	Exudative age-related macular degeneration, left eye, with active choroidal neovascularization
⇄	H35.3231	Exudative age-related macular degeneration, bilateral, with active choroidal neovascularization
⇄	H35.722	Serous detachment of retinal pigment epithelium, left eye
⇄	H35.732	Hemorrhagic detachment of retinal pigment epithelium, left eye
⇄	H43.12	Vitreous hemorrhage, left eye
⇄	H44.2A1	Degenerative myopia with choroidal neovascularization, right eye
⇄	H44.2A2	Degenerative myopia with choroidal neovascularization, left eye
⇄	H44.2A3	Degenerative myopia with choroidal neovascularization, bilateral eye

ICD-10-CM Coding Notes

For codes requiring a 7th character extension, refer to your ICD-10-CM book. Review the character descriptions and coding guidelines for proper selection. For some procedures, only certain characters will apply.

CCI Edits

Refer to Appendix A for CCI edits.

Pub 100

67043: Pub 100-03, 1, 80.11

Facility RVUs

Code	Work	PE Facility	MP	Total Facility
67043	17.40	16.10	1.33	34.83

Non-facility RVUs

Code	Work	PE Non-Facility	MP	Total Non-Facility
67043	17.40	16.10	1.33	34.83

Modifiers (PAR)

Code	Mod 50	Mod 51	Mod 62	Mod 66	Mod 80
67043	1	2	1	0	2

Global Period

Code	Days
67043	090

67101-67105

67101 Repair of retinal detachment, including drainage of subretinal fluid when performed; cryotherapy

67105 Repair of retinal detachment, including drainage of subretinal fluid when performed; photocoagulation

AMA Coding Notes

Repair Procedures on the Retina or Choroid

(If diathermy, cryotherapy and/or photocoagulation are combined, report under principal modality used)

Surgical Procedures on the Eye and Ocular Adnexa

(For diagnostic and treatment ophthalmological services, see Medicine, Ophthalmology, and 92002 et seq)

(Do not report code 69990 in addition to codes 65091-68850)

AMA *CPT® Assistant*

67101: Mar 98: 7, Jun 16: 6, Sep 16: 5, Feb 17: 14

67105: Mar 98: 7, Jun 16: 6, Sep 16: 5, Feb 17: 14

Plain English Description

Retinal detachment occurs when the retina separates from its normal position and the inner layers of the retina pull away from the choroid. Detachment results in blurred vision and if left untreated may cause blindness. A lid speculum is used to open the eyelids and expose the eye. In 67101, a freezing probe is used to treat the retinal detachment. Cryotherapy is performed to the outer surface of the eye through an intact sclera over the site of the retinal detachment. The cryotherapy probe is used to create a series of ice balls around the area of detachment. A lamellar scleral dissection is performed over the site of the detachment. As the frozen area over and around the detachment heals, scar tissue develops that helps secure the retina to the choroid. In 67105, a laser beam (photocoagulation) is directed through a contact lens or specially designed ophthalmoscope to the site of the retinal detachment. The laser beam is used to burn the tissue around the detachment resulting in scarring that secures the retina to the underlying choroid. Following the cryotherapy or photocoagulation, the physician may drain subretinal fluid. The sclera is incised over the area of retinal elevation and the choroid is punctured. Subretinal fluid is drained. When sufficient fluid has been expressed, the puncture site is dried and inspected to ensure that it has sealed. The scleral incision is closed with sutures.

Repair of retinal detachment, single/multiple sessions; cryotherapy/diathermy with/without drainage of subretinal fluid

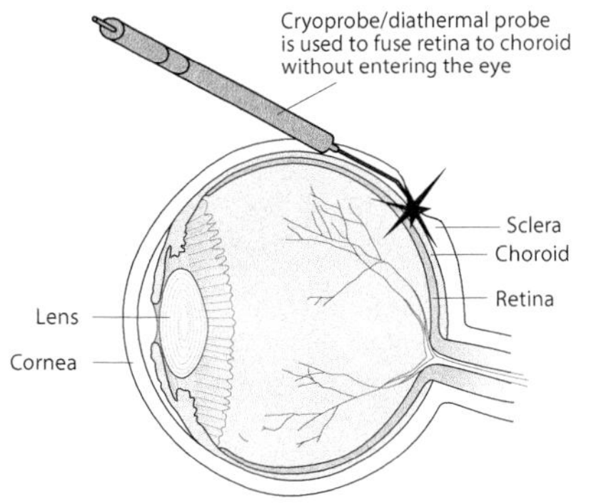

ICD-10-CM Diagnostic Codes

⇄	H33.011	Retinal detachment with single break, right eye
⇄	H33.021	Retinal detachment with multiple breaks, right eye
⇄	H33.031	Retinal detachment with giant retinal tear, right eye
⇄	H33.041	Retinal detachment with retinal dialysis, right eye
⇄	H33.051	Total retinal detachment, right eye
⇄	H33.21	Serous retinal detachment, right eye
⇄	H33.311	Horseshoe tear of retina without detachment, right eye
⇄	H33.41	Traction detachment of retina, right eye
	H33.8	Other retinal detachments
⇄	H35.101	Retinopathy of prematurity, unspecified, right eye
⇄	H35.341	Macular cyst, hole, or pseudohole, right eye
⇄	H35.351	Cystoid macular degeneration, right eye
⇄	H35.371	Puckering of macula, right eye
⇄	H35.721	Serous detachment of retinal pigment epithelium, right eye
⇄	H43.11	Vitreous hemorrhage, right eye
⇄	H43.811	Vitreous degeneration, right eye
⇄	H44.2C1	Degenerative myopia with retinal detachment, right eye
⇄	H44.2C2	Degenerative myopia with retinal detachment, left eye
⇄	H44.2C3	Degenerative myopia with retinal detachment, bilateral eye
⇄	H44.2E1	Degenerative myopia with other maculopathy, right eye
⇄	H44.2E2	Degenerative myopia with other maculopathy, left eye
⇄	H44.2E3	Degenerative myopia with other maculopathy, bilateral eye

CCI Edits

Refer to Appendix A for CCI edits.

Facility RVUs

Code	Work	PE Facility	MP	Total Facility
67101	3.50	4.45	0.25	8.20
67105	3.39	4.30	0.25	7.94

Non-facility RVUs

Code	Work	PE Non-Facility	MP	Total Non-Facility
67101	3.50	5.99	0.25	9.74
67105	3.39	4.97	0.25	8.61

Modifiers (PAR)

Code	Mod 50	Mod 51	Mod 62	Mod 66	Mod 80
67101	1	2	0	0	1
67105	1	2	0	0	1

Global Period

Code	Days
67101	010
67105	010

CPT® Procedural Coding

67107

67107 Repair of retinal detachment; scleral buckling (such as lamellar scleral dissection, imbrication or encircling procedure), including, when performed, implant, cryotherapy, photocoagulation, and drainage of subretinal fluid

AMA Coding Notes

Repair Procedures on the Retina or Choroid

(If diathermy, cryotherapy and/or photocoagulation are combined, report under principal modality used)

Surgical Procedures on the Eye and Ocular Adnexa

(For diagnostic and treatment ophthalmological services, see Medicine, Ophthalmology, and 92002 et seq)

(Do not report code 69990 in addition to codes 65091-68850)

AMA *CPT® Assistant* ▯

67107: Jun 16: 6, Sep 16: 5, Aug 19: 11

Plain English Description

Retinal detachment occurs when the retina separates from its normal position and the inner layers of the retina pull away from the choroid. Detachment results in blurred vision and if left untreated may cause blindness. A lid speculum is used to open the eyelids and expose the eye. Local anesthesia is administered. Scleral buckling is the most frequently performed procedure to treat retinal detachment. Scleral buckles are typically fabricated with silicone. Buckles come in a variety of types and shapes that are selected based on the size and location of the retinal defect. The retina is repaired as needed using a freezing probe (cryotherapy, cryopexy) or laser photocoagulation. Cryotherapy is performed to the outer surface of the eye through an intact sclera over the site of the retinal detachment. The cryotherapy probe is used to create a series of ice balls around the area of detachment. Alternatively, a laser beam (photocoagulation) is directed through a contact lens or specially designed ophthalmoscope to the site of the retinal detachment and used to burn the tissue around the detachment. As the frozen or burned area over and around the detachment heals, scar tissue develops that helps secure the retina to the choroid. Following the cryotherapy or laser photocoagulation, one of the rectus muscles is detached to access the sclera. The scleral buckle is then secured to the sclera. The buckle pushes the sclera toward the middle of the eye and relieves traction on the retina, which allows the retina to settle against the choroid and heal. The physician may also drain subretinal fluid. The sclera is incised over the area of retinal elevation and the choroid is punctured. Subretinal fluid is drained. When sufficient fluid has been expressed, the puncture site is dried and inspected to ensure that it has sealed. The scleral incision is closed with sutures.

Repair of retinal detachment; scleral buckling

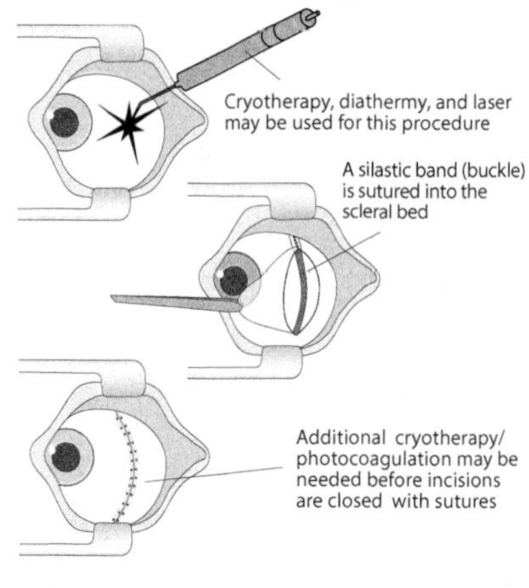
Cryotherapy, diathermy, and laser may be used for this procedure
A silastic band (buckle) is sutured into the scleral bed
Additional cryotherapy/ photocoagulation may be needed before incisions are closed with sutures

ICD-10-CM Diagnostic Codes

	Code	Description
	E08.311	Diabetes mellitus due to underlying condition with unspecified diabetic retinopathy with macular edema
	E08.319	Diabetes mellitus due to underlying condition with unspecified diabetic retinopathy without macular edema
➐⇄	E08.321	Diabetes mellitus due to underlying condition with mild nonproliferative diabetic retinopathy with macular edema
➐⇄	E08.329	Diabetes mellitus due to underlying condition with mild nonproliferative diabetic retinopathy without macular edema
➐⇄	E08.331	Diabetes mellitus due to underlying condition with moderate nonproliferative diabetic retinopathy with macular edema
➐⇄	E08.339	Diabetes mellitus due to underlying condition with moderate nonproliferative diabetic retinopathy without macular edema
➐⇄	E08.341	Diabetes mellitus due to underlying condition with severe nonproliferative diabetic retinopathy with macular edema
➐⇄	E08.349	Diabetes mellitus due to underlying condition with severe nonproliferative diabetic retinopathy without macular edema
➐⇄	E08.351	Diabetes mellitus due to underlying condition with proliferative diabetic retinopathy with macular edema
➐⇄	E08.352	Diabetes mellitus due to underlying condition with proliferative diabetic retinopathy with traction retinal detachment involving the macula
➐⇄	E08.353	Diabetes mellitus due to underlying condition with proliferative diabetic retinopathy with traction retinal detachment not involving the macula
➐⇄	E08.354	Diabetes mellitus due to underlying condition with proliferative diabetic retinopathy with combined traction retinal detachment and rhegmatogenous retinal detachment
➐⇄	E08.355	Diabetes mellitus due to underlying condition with stable proliferative diabetic retinopathy
➐⇄	E08.359	Diabetes mellitus due to underlying condition with proliferative diabetic retinopathy without macular edema
	E08.36	Diabetes mellitus due to underlying condition with diabetic cataract
➐⇄	E08.37	Diabetes mellitus due to underlying condition with diabetic macular edema, resolved following treatment
	E08.39	Diabetes mellitus due to underlying condition with other diabetic ophthalmic complication
	E08.65	Diabetes mellitus due to underlying condition with hyperglycemia
	E09.311	Drug or chemical induced diabetes mellitus with unspecified diabetic retinopathy with macular edema
	E09.319	Drug or chemical induced diabetes mellitus with unspecified diabetic retinopathy without macular edema
➐⇄	E09.321	Drug or chemical induced diabetes mellitus with mild nonproliferative diabetic retinopathy with macular edema
➐⇄	E09.329	Drug or chemical induced diabetes mellitus with mild nonproliferative diabetic retinopathy without macular edema
➐⇄	E09.331	Drug or chemical induced diabetes mellitus with moderate nonproliferative diabetic retinopathy with macular edema
➐⇄	E09.339	Drug or chemical induced diabetes mellitus with moderate nonproliferative diabetic retinopathy without macular edema
➐⇄	E09.341	Drug or chemical induced diabetes mellitus with severe nonproliferative diabetic retinopathy with macular edema
➐⇄	E09.349	Drug or chemical induced diabetes mellitus with severe nonproliferative diabetic retinopathy without macular edema
➐⇄	E09.351	Drug or chemical induced diabetes mellitus with proliferative diabetic retinopathy with macular edema
➐⇄	E09.352	Drug or chemical induced diabetes mellitus with proliferative diabetic retinopathy with traction retinal detachment involving the macula
➐⇄	E09.353	Drug or chemical induced diabetes mellitus with proliferative diabetic retinopathy with traction retinal detachment not involving the macula

❼⇄ E09.354 Drug or chemical induced diabetes mellitus with proliferative diabetic retinopathy with combined traction retinal detachment and rhegmatogenous retinal detachment

❼⇄ E09.355 Drug or chemical induced diabetes mellitus with stable proliferative diabetic retinopathy

❼⇄ E09.359 Drug or chemical induced diabetes mellitus with proliferative diabetic retinopathy without macular edema

E09.36 Drug or chemical induced diabetes mellitus with diabetic cataract

❼⇄ E09.37 Drug or chemical induced diabetes mellitus with diabetic macular edema, resolved following treatment

E09.39 Drug or chemical induced diabetes mellitus with other diabetic ophthalmic complication

E09.65 Drug or chemical induced diabetes mellitus with hyperglycemia

E10.311 Type 1 diabetes mellitus with unspecified diabetic retinopathy with macular edema

E10.319 Type 1 diabetes mellitus with unspecified diabetic retinopathy without macular edema

❼⇄ E10.321 Type 1 diabetes mellitus with mild nonproliferative diabetic retinopathy with macular edema

❼⇄ E10.329 Type 1 diabetes mellitus with mild nonproliferative diabetic retinopathy without macular edema

❼⇄ E10.331 Type 1 diabetes mellitus with moderate nonproliferative diabetic retinopathy with macular edema

❼⇄ E10.339 Type 1 diabetes mellitus with moderate nonproliferative diabetic retinopathy without macular edema

❼⇄ E10.341 Type 1 diabetes mellitus with severe nonproliferative diabetic retinopathy with macular edema

❼⇄ E10.349 Type 1 diabetes mellitus with severe nonproliferative diabetic retinopathy without macular edema

❼⇄ E10.351 Type 1 diabetes mellitus with proliferative diabetic retinopathy with macular edema

❼⇄ E10.352 Type 1 diabetes mellitus with proliferative diabetic retinopathy with traction retinal detachment involving the macula

❼⇄ E10.353 Type 1 diabetes mellitus with proliferative diabetic retinopathy with traction retinal detachment not involving the macula

❼⇄ E10.354 Type 1 diabetes mellitus with proliferative diabetic retinopathy with combined traction retinal detachment and rhegmatogenous retinal detachment

❼⇄ E10.355 Type 1 diabetes mellitus with stable proliferative diabetic retinopathy

❼⇄ E10.359 Type 1 diabetes mellitus with proliferative diabetic retinopathy without macular edema

E10.36 Type 1 diabetes mellitus with diabetic cataract

❼⇄ E10.37 Type 1 diabetes mellitus with diabetic macular edema, resolved following treatment

E10.39 Type 1 diabetes mellitus with other diabetic ophthalmic complication

E10.65 Type 1 diabetes mellitus with hyperglycemia

E11.311 Type 2 diabetes mellitus with unspecified diabetic retinopathy with macular edema

E11.319 Type 2 diabetes mellitus with unspecified diabetic retinopathy without macular edema

❼⇄ E11.321 Type 2 diabetes mellitus with mild nonproliferative diabetic retinopathy with macular edema

❼⇄ E11.329 Type 2 diabetes mellitus with mild nonproliferative diabetic retinopathy without macular edema

❼⇄ E11.331 Type 2 diabetes mellitus with moderate nonproliferative diabetic retinopathy with macular edema

❼⇄ E11.339 Type 2 diabetes mellitus with moderate nonproliferative diabetic retinopathy without macular edema

❼⇄ E11.341 Type 2 diabetes mellitus with severe nonproliferative diabetic retinopathy with macular edema

❼⇄ E11.349 Type 2 diabetes mellitus with severe nonproliferative diabetic retinopathy without macular edema

❼⇄ E11.351 Type 2 diabetes mellitus with proliferative diabetic retinopathy with macular edema

❼⇄ E11.352 Type 2 diabetes mellitus with proliferative diabetic retinopathy with traction retinal detachment involving the macula

❼⇄ E11.353 Type 2 diabetes mellitus with proliferative diabetic retinopathy with traction retinal detachment not involving the macula

❼⇄ E11.354 Type 2 diabetes mellitus with proliferative diabetic retinopathy with combined traction retinal detachment and rhegmatogenous retinal detachment

❼⇄ E11.355 Type 2 diabetes mellitus with stable proliferative diabetic retinopathy

❼⇄ E11.359 Type 2 diabetes mellitus with proliferative diabetic retinopathy without macular edema

E11.36 Type 2 diabetes mellitus with diabetic cataract

❼⇄ E11.37 Type 2 diabetes mellitus with diabetic macular edema, resolved following treatment

E11.39 Type 2 diabetes mellitus with other diabetic ophthalmic complication

E11.65 Type 2 diabetes mellitus with hyperglycemia

⇄ H33.012 Retinal detachment with single break, left eye

⇄ H33.022 Retinal detachment with multiple breaks, left eye

⇄ H33.032 Retinal detachment with giant retinal tear, left eye

⇄ H33.042 Retinal detachment with retinal dialysis, left eye

⇄ H33.052 Total retinal detachment, left eye

⇄ H33.102 Unspecified retinoschisis, left eye

⇄ H33.21 Serous retinal detachment, right eye

⇄ H33.302 Unspecified retinal break, left eye

⇄ H33.312 Horseshoe tear of retina without detachment, left eye

⇄ H33.42 Traction detachment of retina, left eye

H33.8 Other retinal detachments

⇄ H35.102 Retinopathy of prematurity, unspecified, left eye

⇄ H35.142 Retinopathy of prematurity, stage 3, left eye

⇄ H35.152 Retinopathy of prematurity, stage 4, left eye

⇄ H35.162 Retinopathy of prematurity, stage 5, left eye

⇄ H35.342 Macular cyst, hole, or pseudohole, left eye

⇄ H35.722 Serous detachment of retinal pigment epithelium, left eye

⇄ H35.732 Hemorrhagic detachment of retinal pigment epithelium, left eye

⇄ H44.2B1 Degenerative myopia with macular hole, right eye

⇄ H44.2B2 Degenerative myopia with macular hole, left eye

⇄ H44.2B3 Degenerative myopia with macular hole, bilateral eye

⇄ H44.2C1 Degenerative myopia with retinal detachment, right eye

⇄ H44.2C2 Degenerative myopia with retinal detachment, left eye

⇄ H44.2C3 Degenerative myopia with retinal detachment, bilateral eye

⇄ H44.2E1 Degenerative myopia with other maculopathy, right eye

⇄ H44.2E2 Degenerative myopia with other maculopathy, left eye

⇄ H44.2E3 Degenerative myopia with other maculopathy, bilateral eye

ICD-10-CM Coding Notes

For codes requiring a 7th character extension, refer to your ICD-10-CM book. Review the character descriptions and coding guidelines for proper selection. For some procedures, only certain characters will apply.

CCI Edits

Refer to Appendix A for CCI edits.

Facility RVUs

Code	Work	PE Facility	MP	Total Facility
67107	16.00	15.24	1.24	32.48

Non-facility RVUs

Code	Work	PE Non-Facility	MP	Total Non-Facility
67107	16.00	15.24	1.24	32.48

Modifiers (PAR)

Code	Mod 50	Mod 51	Mod 62	Mod 66	Mod 80
67107	1	2	1	0	2

Global Period

Code	Days
67107	090

67108

67108 Repair of retinal detachment; with vitrectomy, any method, including, when performed, air or gas tamponade, focal endolaser photocoagulation, cryotherapy, drainage of subretinal fluid, scleral buckling, and/or removal of lens by same technique

AMA Coding Notes

Repair Procedures on the Retina or Choroid

(If diathermy, cryotherapy and/or photocoagulation are combined, report under principal modality used)

Surgical Procedures on the Eye and Ocular Adnexa

(For diagnostic and treatment ophthalmological services, see Medicine, Ophthalmology, and 92002 et seq)

(Do not report code 69990 in addition to codes 65091-68850)

AMA *CPT® Assistant*

67108: Winter 90: 9, Mar 12: 9, Jun 16: 6, Sep 16: 5

Plain English Description

Retinal detachment occurs when the retina separates from its normal position and the inner layers of the retina pull away from the choroid. Detachment results in blurred vision and if left untreated may cause blindness. A lid speculum is used to open the eyelids and expose the eye. Local anesthesia is administered. Vitreous is a clear gel-like substance that fills the center of the eye. It is removed prior to the repair of the retinal detachment. To perform mechanical vitrectomy, three small incisions are made in the pars plana. A light pipe, an infusion port, and a vitrectomy device are inserted. The eye is illuminated with the light pipe. The vitrectomy device, a microscopic oscillating cutting device, is activated and vitreous is removed from the eye in a slow, controlled fashion. As the vitreous is removed, it is replaced with fluid to maintain proper eye pressure. Following removal of vitreous, the retina is repaired as needed using a freezing probe (cryotherapy, cryopexy) or laser photocoagulation. The lens may be removed to provide better access to the retina. Cryotherapy is performed to the outer surface of the eye through an intact sclera over the site of the retinal detachment. The cryotherapy probe is used to create a series of ice balls around the area of detachment. Alternatively, a laser beam (photocoagulation) is directed through a contact lens or specially designed ophthalmoscope to the site of the retinal detachment and used to burn the tissue around the detachment. As the frozen or burned area over and around the detachment heals, scar tissue develops that helps secure the retina to the choroid. If a scleral buckle is needed, one of the rectus muscles is detached to access the sclera. The buckle is then secured to the sclera. The buckle pushes the sclera toward the middle of the eye and relieves traction on the retina, which allows the retina to settle against the choroid and heal. An intraocular tamponade may be performed using air or gas to prevent fluid from leaking into the retina. The physician may also drain subretinal fluid. The sclera is incised over the area of retinal elevation and the choroid is punctured. Subretinal fluid is drained. When sufficient fluid has been expressed, the puncture site is dried and inspected to ensure that it has sealed. The scleral incision is closed with sutures.

Repair of detached retina; with vitrectomy

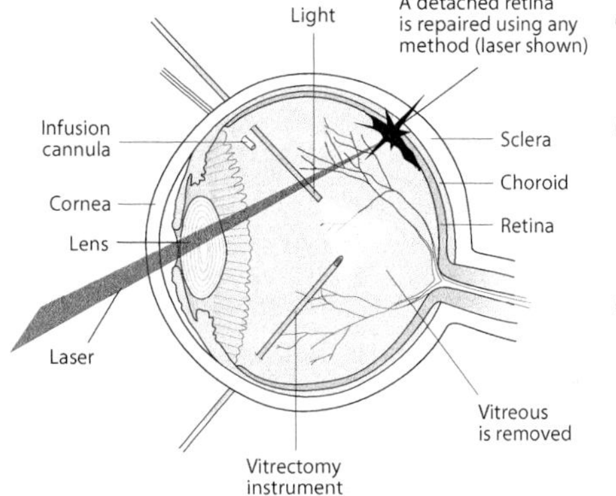

ICD-10-CM Diagnostic Codes

	Code	Description
	E08.311	Diabetes mellitus due to underlying condition with unspecified diabetic retinopathy with macular edema
	E08.319	Diabetes mellitus due to underlying condition with unspecified diabetic retinopathy without macular edema
❼⇄	E08.321	Diabetes mellitus due to underlying condition with mild nonproliferative diabetic retinopathy with macular edema
❼⇄	E08.329	Diabetes mellitus due to underlying condition with mild nonproliferative diabetic retinopathy without macular edema
❼⇄	E08.331	Diabetes mellitus due to underlying condition with moderate nonproliferative diabetic retinopathy with macular edema
❼⇄	E08.339	Diabetes mellitus due to underlying condition with moderate nonproliferative diabetic retinopathy without macular edema
❼⇄	E08.341	Diabetes mellitus due to underlying condition with severe nonproliferative diabetic retinopathy with macular edema
❼⇄	E08.349	Diabetes mellitus due to underlying condition with severe nonproliferative diabetic retinopathy without macular edema
	E08.35	Diabetes mellitus due to underlying condition with proliferative diabetic retinopathy
❼⇄	E08.351	Diabetes mellitus due to underlying condition with proliferative diabetic retinopathy with macular edema
❼⇄	E08.352	Diabetes mellitus due to underlying condition with proliferative diabetic retinopathy with traction retinal detachment involving the macula
❼⇄	E08.353	Diabetes mellitus due to underlying condition with proliferative diabetic retinopathy with traction retinal detachment not involving the macula
❼⇄	E08.354	Diabetes mellitus due to underlying condition with proliferative diabetic retinopathy with combined traction retinal detachment and rhegmatogenous retinal detachment
❼⇄	E08.355	Diabetes mellitus due to underlying condition with stable proliferative diabetic retinopathy
❼⇄	E08.359	Diabetes mellitus due to underlying condition with proliferative diabetic retinopathy without macular edema
	E08.36	Diabetes mellitus due to underlying condition with diabetic cataract
❼⇄	E08.37	Diabetes mellitus due to underlying condition with diabetic macular edema, resolved following treatment
	E08.39	Diabetes mellitus due to underlying condition with other diabetic ophthalmic complication
	E08.65	Diabetes mellitus due to underlying condition with hyperglycemia
	E09.311	Drug or chemical induced diabetes mellitus with unspecified diabetic retinopathy with macular edema
	E09.319	Drug or chemical induced diabetes mellitus with unspecified diabetic retinopathy without macular edema
❼⇄	E09.321	Drug or chemical induced diabetes mellitus with mild nonproliferative diabetic retinopathy with macular edema
❼⇄	E09.329	Drug or chemical induced diabetes mellitus with mild nonproliferative diabetic retinopathy without macular edema
❼⇄	E09.331	Drug or chemical induced diabetes mellitus with moderate nonproliferative diabetic retinopathy with macular edema
❼⇄	E09.339	Drug or chemical induced diabetes mellitus with moderate nonproliferative diabetic retinopathy without macular edema
❼⇄	E09.341	Drug or chemical induced diabetes mellitus with severe nonproliferative diabetic retinopathy with macular edema
❼⇄	E09.349	Drug or chemical induced diabetes mellitus with severe nonproliferative diabetic retinopathy without macular edema
❼⇄	E09.351	Drug or chemical induced diabetes mellitus with proliferative diabetic retinopathy with macular edema

	Code	Description
❼⇄	E09.359	Drug or chemical induced diabetes mellitus with proliferative diabetic retinopathy without macular edema
	E09.36	Drug or chemical induced diabetes mellitus with diabetic cataract
❼⇄	E09.37	Drug or chemical induced diabetes mellitus with diabetic macular edema, resolved following treatment
	E09.39	Drug or chemical induced diabetes mellitus with other diabetic ophthalmic complication
	E10.311	Type 1 diabetes mellitus with unspecified diabetic retinopathy with macular edema
	E10.319	Type 1 diabetes mellitus with unspecified diabetic retinopathy without macular edema
❼⇄	E10.321	Type 1 diabetes mellitus with mild nonproliferative diabetic retinopathy with macular edema
❼⇄	E10.329	Type 1 diabetes mellitus with mild nonproliferative diabetic retinopathy without macular edema
❼⇄	E10.331	Type 1 diabetes mellitus with moderate nonproliferative diabetic retinopathy with macular edema
❼⇄	E10.339	Type 1 diabetes mellitus with moderate nonproliferative diabetic retinopathy without macular edema
❼⇄	E10.341	Type 1 diabetes mellitus with severe nonproliferative diabetic retinopathy with macular edema
❼⇄	E10.349	Type 1 diabetes mellitus with severe nonproliferative diabetic retinopathy without macular edema
❼⇄	E10.351	Type 1 diabetes mellitus with proliferative diabetic retinopathy with macular edema
❼⇄	E10.359	Type 1 diabetes mellitus with proliferative diabetic retinopathy without macular edema
	E10.36	Type 1 diabetes mellitus with diabetic cataract
❼⇄	E10.37	Type 1 diabetes mellitus with diabetic macular edema, resolved following treatment
	E10.39	Type 1 diabetes mellitus with other diabetic ophthalmic complication
	E10.65	Type 1 diabetes mellitus with hyperglycemia
	E11.311	Type 2 diabetes mellitus with unspecified diabetic retinopathy with macular edema
	E11.319	Type 2 diabetes mellitus with unspecified diabetic retinopathy without macular edema
❼⇄	E11.321	Type 2 diabetes mellitus with mild nonproliferative diabetic retinopathy with macular edema
❼⇄	E11.329	Type 2 diabetes mellitus with mild nonproliferative diabetic retinopathy without macular edema
❼⇄	E11.331	Type 2 diabetes mellitus with moderate nonproliferative diabetic retinopathy with macular edema
❼⇄	E11.339	Type 2 diabetes mellitus with moderate nonproliferative diabetic retinopathy without macular edema
❼⇄	E11.341	Type 2 diabetes mellitus with severe nonproliferative diabetic retinopathy with macular edema
❼⇄	E11.349	Type 2 diabetes mellitus with severe nonproliferative diabetic retinopathy without macular edema
❼⇄	E11.351	Type 2 diabetes mellitus with proliferative diabetic retinopathy with macular edema
❼⇄	E11.359	Type 2 diabetes mellitus with proliferative diabetic retinopathy without macular edema
	E11.36	Type 2 diabetes mellitus with diabetic cataract
❼⇄	E11.37	Type 2 diabetes mellitus with diabetic macular edema, resolved following treatment
	E11.39	Type 2 diabetes mellitus with other diabetic ophthalmic complication
⇄	H33.011	Retinal detachment with single break, right eye
⇄	H33.021	Retinal detachment with multiple breaks, right eye
⇄	H33.031	Retinal detachment with giant retinal tear, right eye
⇄	H33.041	Retinal detachment with retinal dialysis, right eye
⇄	H33.051	Total retinal detachment, right eye
⇄	H33.21	Serous retinal detachment, right eye
⇄	H33.41	Traction detachment of retina, right eye
	H33.8	Other retinal detachments
⇄	H35.101	Retinopathy of prematurity, unspecified, right eye
⇄	H35.141	Retinopathy of prematurity, stage 3, right eye
⇄	H35.151	Retinopathy of prematurity, stage 4, right eye
⇄	H35.161	Retinopathy of prematurity, stage 5, right eye
⇄	H35.21	Other non-diabetic proliferative retinopathy, right eye
⇄	H35.341	Macular cyst, hole, or pseudohole, right eye
⇄	H35.371	Puckering of macula, right eye
⇄	H35.721	Serous detachment of retinal pigment epithelium, right eye
⇄	H35.731	Hemorrhagic detachment of retinal pigment epithelium, right eye
⇄	H43.11	Vitreous hemorrhage, right eye
⇄	H43.311	Vitreous membranes and strands, right eye
⇄	H44.2B1	Degenerative myopia with macular hole, right eye
⇄	H44.2B2	Degenerative myopia with macular hole, left eye
⇄	H44.2B3	Degenerative myopia with macular hole, bilateral eye
⇄	H44.2C1	Degenerative myopia with retinal detachment, right eye
⇄	H44.2C2	Degenerative myopia with retinal detachment, left eye
⇄	H44.2C3	Degenerative myopia with retinal detachment, bilateral eye
⇄	H44.2E1	Degenerative myopia with other maculopathy, right eye
⇄	H44.2E2	Degenerative myopia with other maculopathy, left eye
⇄	H44.2E3	Degenerative myopia with other maculopathy, bilateral eye

ICD-10-CM Coding Notes

For codes requiring a 7th character extension, refer to your ICD-10-CM book. Review the character descriptions and coding guidelines for proper selection. For some procedures, only certain characters will apply.

CCI Edits

Refer to Appendix A for CCI edits.

Pub 100

67108: Pub 100-03, 1, 80.11

Facility RVUs ▯

Code	Work	PE Facility	MP	Total Facility
67108	17.13	15.93	1.32	34.38

Non-facility RVUs ▯

Code	Work	PE Non-Facility	MP	Total Non-Facility
67108	17.13	15.93	1.32	34.38

Modifiers (PAR) ▯

Code	Mod 50	Mod 51	Mod 62	Mod 66	Mod 80
67108	1	2	1	0	2

Global Period

Code	Days
67108	090

67110

67110 Repair of retinal detachment; by injection of air or other gas (eg, pneumatic retinopexy)

(For aspiration or drainage of subretinal or subchoroidal fluid, use 67015)

AMA Coding Notes

Repair Procedures on the Retina or Choroid

(If diathermy, cryotherapy and/or photocoagulation are combined, report under principal modality used)

Surgical Procedures on the Eye and Ocular Adnexa

(For diagnostic and treatment ophthalmological services, see Medicine, Ophthalmology, and 92002 et seq)

(Do not report code 69990 in addition to codes 65091-68850)

AMA *CPT® Assistant* ▢

67110: Winter 90: 9, Sep 16: 5

Plain English Description

Retinal detachment occurs when the retina separates from its normal position and the inner layers of the retina pull away from the choroid. Detachment results in blurred vision and if left untreated may cause blindness. A lid speculum is used to open the eyelids and expose the eye. Local anesthetic is administered. Pneumatic retinopexy involves injecting air or another gas into the vitreal cavity at the site of the retinal detachment. The sclera is punctured and a needle advanced into the vitreous cavity. A gas bubble is injected. The head is positioned so that the gas bubble will move toward the area of detachment. The gas bubble then pushes the retina back against the choroid. Laser photocoagulation or cryotherapy may also be performed to seal the area of detachment. The patient may need to maintain the head in a certain position as much as possible for several weeks following the injection.

Repair of retinal detachment, by injection of air/gas (pneumatic retinopexy)

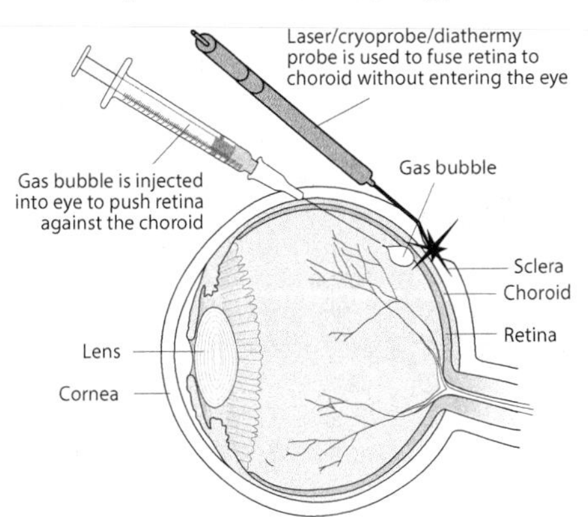

ICD-10-CM Diagnostic Codes

	Code	Description
❼⇄	E08.352	Diabetes mellitus due to underlying condition with proliferative diabetic retinopathy with traction retinal detachment involving the macula
❼⇄	E08.353	Diabetes mellitus due to underlying condition with proliferative diabetic retinopathy with traction retinal detachment not involving the macula
❼⇄	E08.354	Diabetes mellitus due to underlying condition with proliferative diabetic retinopathy with combined traction retinal detachment and rhegmatogenous retinal detachment
⇄	H33.012	Retinal detachment with single break, left eye
⇄	H33.02	Retinal detachment with multiple breaks
⇄	H33.022	Retinal detachment with multiple breaks, left eye
⇄	H33.032	Retinal detachment with giant retinal tear, left eye
⇄	H33.042	Retinal detachment with retinal dialysis, left eye
⇄	H33.052	Total retinal detachment, left eye
⇄	H33.102	Unspecified retinoschisis, left eye
⇄	H33.22	Serous retinal detachment, left eye
⇄	H33.312	Horseshoe tear of retina without detachment, left eye
⇄	H33.42	Traction detachment of retina, left eye
	H33.8	Other retinal detachments
⇄	H35.142	Retinopathy of prematurity, stage 3, left eye
⇄	H35.152	Retinopathy of prematurity, stage 4, left eye
⇄	H35.162	Retinopathy of prematurity, stage 5, left eye
⇄	H35.372	Puckering of macula, left eye
⇄	H35.722	Serous detachment of retinal pigment epithelium, left eye
⇄	H35.732	Hemorrhagic detachment of retinal pigment epithelium, left eye
⇄	H44.2C1	Degenerative myopia with retinal detachment, right eye
⇄	H44.2C2	Degenerative myopia with retinal detachment, left eye
⇄	H44.2C3	Degenerative myopia with retinal detachment, bilateral eye

ICD-10-CM Coding Notes

For codes requiring a 7th character extension, refer to your ICD-10-CM book. Review the character descriptions and coding guidelines for proper selection. For some procedures, only certain characters will apply.

CCI Edits

Refer to Appendix A for CCI edits.

Facility RVUs ▢

Code	Work	PE Facility	MP	Total Facility
67110	10.25	12.48	0.78	23.51

Non-facility RVUs ▢

Code	Work	PE Non-Facility	MP	Total Non-Facility
67110	10.25	14.93	0.78	25.96

Modifiers (PAR) ▢

Code	Mod 50	Mod 51	Mod 62	Mod 66	Mod 80
67110	1	2	0	0	1

Global Period

Code	Days
67110	090

67113

67113 Repair of complex retinal detachment (eg, proliferative vitreoretinopathy, stage C-1 or greater, diabetic traction retinal detachment, retinopathy of prematurity, retinal tear of greater than 90 degrees), with vitrectomy and membrane peeling, including, when performed, air, gas, or silicone oil tamponade, cryotherapy, endolaser photocoagulation, drainage of subretinal fluid, scleral buckling, and/or removal of lens

(To report vitrectomy, pars plana approach, other than in retinal detachment surgery, see 67036-67043)

(For use of ophthalmic endoscope with 67113, use 66990)

AMA Coding Notes

Repair Procedures on the Retina or Choroid

(If diathermy, cryotherapy and/or photocoagulation are combined, report under principal modality used)

Surgical Procedures on the Eye and Ocular Adnexa

(For diagnostic and treatment ophthalmological services, see Medicine, Ophthalmology, and 92002 et seq)

(Do not report code 69990 in addition to codes 65091-68850)

AMA *CPT® Assistant* ▯

67113: Jun 16: 6, Sep 16: 5

Plain English Description

A complex retinal detachment is repaired using multiple modalities including vitrectomy and membrane peeling. Complex retinal detachments are tears greater than 90 degrees or those resulting from conditions such as proliferative vitreoretinopathy with stage C-1 or greater, diabetic traction retinal detachment, or retinopathy of prematurity. Retinal detachment is the separation of the inner layers of the retina from the underlying choroid, also referred to as the retinal pigment epithelium (RPE), a vascular membrane that contains branched pigment cells lying between the retina and sclera. The conjunctiva is incised around the periphery of the cornea (peritomy). Tenon's capsule is peeled back and the rectus muscle is isolated. A vitrectomy device is inserted into the sclera. Two additional incisions are made in the sclera for a light pipe and infusion port. The inside of the eye is illuminated with the light pipe. The vitrectomy device, a microscopic oscillating cutting device, is activated and vitreous gel is removed from the center of the eye in a slow, controlled fashion. As the vitreous gel is removed, it is replaced with fluid through the infusion port to maintain proper pressure in the eye. The cellular membrane is then meticulously removed from the retinal surface and the retina is examined for tears. The posterior aspect of the retina may be opened (retinotomy), the subretinal fluid drained, and replaced with air, gas, or silicone oil to reattach the retina. Tears in the retina and the retinotomy are repaired using cryotherapy and/or endolaser photocoagulation. The lens may be removed to provide better access to the retina. Cryotherapy is performed to the outer surface of the eye through an intact sclera over the site of the retinal detachment. The cryotherapy probe is used to create a series of ice balls around the area of detachment. Alternatively, a laser beam (photocoagulation) is directed through a contact lens or specially designed ophthalmoscope to the site of the retinal detachment and used to burn the tissue around the detachment. As the frozen or burned area heals, scar tissue develops that helps secure the retina to the choroid. A scleral buckle comprised of silicone, rubber, sponge, or soft plastic, may also be secured to the sclera to relieve traction on the retinal detachment, allowing the retina to settle against the choroid and heal. Incisions in the sclera and conjunctiva are closed.

Repair of complex retinal detachment; with vitrectomy

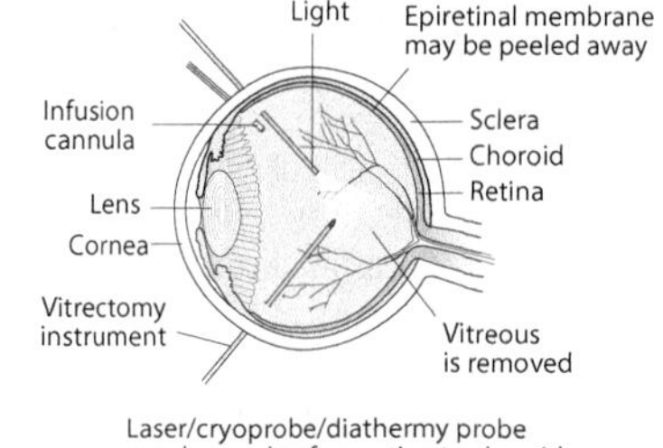

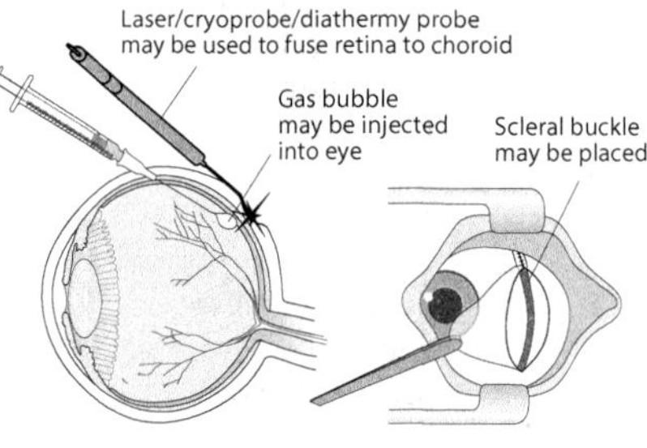

ICD-10-CM Diagnostic Codes

	Code	Description
	E08.311	Diabetes mellitus due to underlying condition with unspecified diabetic retinopathy with macular edema
	E08.319	Diabetes mellitus due to underlying condition with unspecified diabetic retinopathy without macular edema
❼⇄	E08.321	Diabetes mellitus due to underlying condition with mild nonproliferative diabetic retinopathy with macular edema
❼⇄	E08.329	Diabetes mellitus due to underlying condition with mild nonproliferative diabetic retinopathy without macular edema
❼⇄	E08.331	Diabetes mellitus due to underlying condition with moderate nonproliferative diabetic retinopathy with macular edema
❼⇄	E08.339	Diabetes mellitus due to underlying condition with moderate nonproliferative diabetic retinopathy without macular edema
❼⇄	E08.341	Diabetes mellitus due to underlying condition with severe nonproliferative diabetic retinopathy with macular edema
❼⇄	E08.349	Diabetes mellitus due to underlying condition with severe nonproliferative diabetic retinopathy without macular edema
❼⇄	E08.351	Diabetes mellitus due to underlying condition with proliferative diabetic retinopathy with macular edema
❼⇄	E08.352	Diabetes mellitus due to underlying condition with proliferative diabetic retinopathy with traction retinal detachment involving the macula
❼⇄	E08.353	Diabetes mellitus due to underlying condition with proliferative diabetic retinopathy with traction retinal detachment not involving the macula
❼⇄	E08.354	Diabetes mellitus due to underlying condition with proliferative diabetic retinopathy with combined traction retinal detachment and rhegmatogenous retinal detachment
❼⇄	E08.355	Diabetes mellitus due to underlying condition with stable proliferative diabetic retinopathy
❼⇄	E08.359	Diabetes mellitus due to underlying condition with proliferative diabetic retinopathy without macular edema
	E09.311	Drug or chemical induced diabetes mellitus with unspecified diabetic retinopathy with macular edema
	E09.319	Drug or chemical induced diabetes mellitus with unspecified diabetic retinopathy without macular edema
❼⇄	E09.321	Drug or chemical induced diabetes mellitus with mild nonproliferative diabetic retinopathy with macular edema
❼⇄	E09.329	Drug or chemical induced diabetes mellitus with mild nonproliferative diabetic retinopathy without macular edema
❼⇄	E09.331	Drug or chemical induced diabetes mellitus with moderate nonproliferative diabetic retinopathy with macular edema
❼⇄	E09.339	Drug or chemical induced diabetes mellitus with moderate nonproliferative diabetic retinopathy without macular edema
❼⇄	E09.341	Drug or chemical induced diabetes mellitus with severe nonproliferative diabetic retinopathy with macular edema

⑦⇄ E09.349 Drug or chemical induced diabetes mellitus with severe nonproliferative diabetic retinopathy without macular edema
⑦⇄ E09.351 Drug or chemical induced diabetes mellitus with proliferative diabetic retinopathy with macular edema
⑦⇄ E09.352 Drug or chemical induced diabetes mellitus with proliferative diabetic retinopathy with traction retinal detachment involving the macula
⑦⇄ E09.353 Drug or chemical induced diabetes mellitus with proliferative diabetic retinopathy with traction retinal detachment not involving the macula
⑦⇄ E09.354 Drug or chemical induced diabetes mellitus with proliferative diabetic retinopathy with combined traction retinal detachment and rhegmatogenous retinal detachment
⑦⇄ E09.359 Drug or chemical induced diabetes mellitus with proliferative diabetic retinopathy without macular edema
E10.311 Type 1 diabetes mellitus with unspecified diabetic retinopathy with macular edema
E10.319 Type 1 diabetes mellitus with unspecified diabetic retinopathy without macular edema
⑦⇄ E10.321 Type 1 diabetes mellitus with mild nonproliferative diabetic retinopathy with macular edema
⑦⇄ E10.329 Type 1 diabetes mellitus with mild nonproliferative diabetic retinopathy without macular edema
⑦⇄ E10.331 Type 1 diabetes mellitus with moderate nonproliferative diabetic retinopathy with macular edema
⑦⇄ E10.339 Type 1 diabetes mellitus with moderate nonproliferative diabetic retinopathy without macular edema
⑦⇄ E10.341 Type 1 diabetes mellitus with severe nonproliferative diabetic retinopathy with macular edema
⑦⇄ E10.349 Type 1 diabetes mellitus with severe nonproliferative diabetic retinopathy without macular edema
⑦⇄ E10.351 Type 1 diabetes mellitus with proliferative diabetic retinopathy with macular edema
⑦⇄ E10.352 Type 1 diabetes mellitus with proliferative diabetic retinopathy with traction retinal detachment involving the macula
⑦⇄ E10.353 Type 1 diabetes mellitus with proliferative diabetic retinopathy with traction retinal detachment not involving the macula
⑦⇄ E10.354 Type 1 diabetes mellitus with proliferative diabetic retinopathy with combined traction retinal detachment and rhegmatogenous retinal detachment
⑦⇄ E10.355 Type 1 diabetes mellitus with stable proliferative diabetic retinopathy
⑦⇄ E10.359 Type 1 diabetes mellitus with proliferative diabetic retinopathy without macular edema
E11.311 Type 2 diabetes mellitus with unspecified diabetic retinopathy with macular edema
E11.319 Type 2 diabetes mellitus with unspecified diabetic retinopathy without macular edema
⑦⇄ E11.321 Type 2 diabetes mellitus with mild nonproliferative diabetic retinopathy with macular edema
⑦⇄ E11.329 Type 2 diabetes mellitus with mild nonproliferative diabetic retinopathy without macular edema
⑦⇄ E11.331 Type 2 diabetes mellitus with moderate nonproliferative diabetic retinopathy with macular edema
⑦⇄ E11.339 Type 2 diabetes mellitus with moderate nonproliferative diabetic retinopathy without macular edema
⑦⇄ E11.341 Type 2 diabetes mellitus with severe nonproliferative diabetic retinopathy with macular edema
⑦⇄ E11.349 Type 2 diabetes mellitus with severe nonproliferative diabetic retinopathy without macular edema
⑦⇄ E11.351 Type 2 diabetes mellitus with proliferative diabetic retinopathy with macular edema
⑦⇄ E11.352 Type 2 diabetes mellitus with proliferative diabetic retinopathy with traction retinal detachment involving the macula
⑦⇄ E11.353 Type 2 diabetes mellitus with proliferative diabetic retinopathy with traction retinal detachment not involving the macula
⑦⇄ E11.354 Type 2 diabetes mellitus with proliferative diabetic retinopathy with combined traction retinal detachment and rhegmatogenous retinal detachment
⑦⇄ E11.355 Type 2 diabetes mellitus with stable proliferative diabetic retinopathy
⑦⇄ E11.359 Type 2 diabetes mellitus with proliferative diabetic retinopathy without macular edema
⇄ H35.022 Exudative retinopathy, left eye
⇄ H35.052 Retinal neovascularization, unspecified, left eye
H35.09 Other intraretinal microvascular abnormalities
⇄ H35.102 Retinopathy of prematurity, unspecified, left eye
⇄ H35.142 Retinopathy of prematurity, stage 3, left eye
⇄ H35.152 Retinopathy of prematurity, stage 4, left eye
⇄ H35.162 Retinopathy of prematurity, stage 5, left eye
⇄ H35.22 Other non-diabetic proliferative retinopathy, left eye
⇄ H44.2C1 Degenerative myopia with retinal detachment, right eye
⇄ H44.2C2 Degenerative myopia with retinal detachment, left eye
⇄ H44.2C3 Degenerative myopia with retinal detachment, bilateral eye

ICD-10-CM Coding Notes

For codes requiring a 7th character extension, refer to your ICD-10-CM book. Review the character descriptions and coding guidelines for proper selection. For some procedures, only certain characters will apply.

CCI Edits

Refer to Appendix A for CCI edits.

Pub 100

67113: Pub 100-03, 1, 80.11

Facility RVUs ▯

Code	Work	PE Facility	MP	Total Facility
67113	19.00	17.96	1.47	38.43

Non-facility RVUs ▯

Code	Work	PE Non-Facility	MP	Total Non-Facility
67113	19.00	17.96	1.47	38.43

Modifiers (PAR) ▯

Code	Mod 50	Mod 51	Mod 62	Mod 66	Mod 80
67113	1	2	1	0	2

Global Period

Code	Days
67113	090

67115

67115 Release of encircling material (posterior segment)

AMA Coding Notes

Repair Procedures on the Retina or Choroid

(If diathermy, cryotherapy and/or photocoagulation are combined, report under principal modality used)

Surgical Procedures on the Eye and Ocular Adnexa

(For diagnostic and treatment ophthalmological services, see Medicine, Ophthalmology, and 92002 et seq)

(Do not report code 69990 in addition to codes 65091-68850)

Plain English Description

Release of encircling material (scleral buckle) is typically performed for infection or intrusion of the buckle into the scleral tissue. A lid speculum is used to open the eyelids and expose the eye. Local anesthesia is administered. One of the rectus muscles is detached to access the sclera. The encircling material is then cut and removed. If the implant has intruded into the scleral tissue, it is removed using a device such as a fragmatome, which breaks up and aspirates the pieces of the device that have become embedded in the sclera. The rectus muscle is reattached.

Release of encircling material (posterior segment)

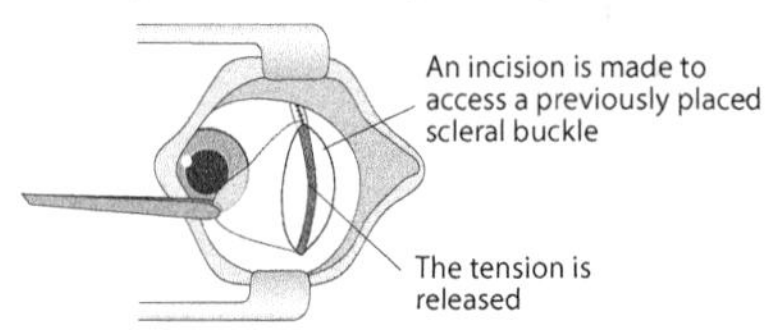
An incision is made to access a previously placed scleral buckle
The tension is released

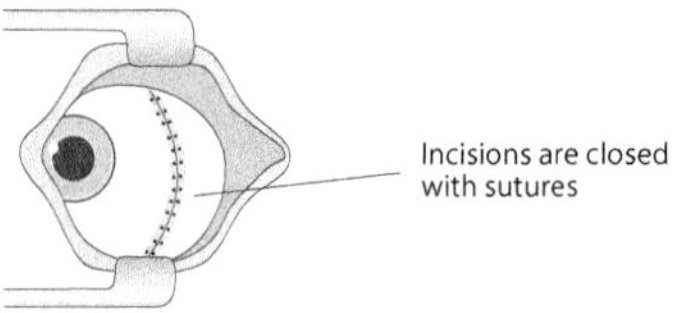
Incisions are closed with sutures

ICD-10-CM Diagnostic Codes

	Code	Description
❼⇄	T85.310	Breakdown (mechanical) of prosthetic orbit of right eye
❼⇄	T85.311	Breakdown (mechanical) of prosthetic orbit of left eye
❼⇄	T85.318	Breakdown (mechanical) of other ocular prosthetic devices, implants and grafts
❼⇄	T85.320	Displacement of prosthetic orbit of right eye
❼⇄	T85.321	Displacement of prosthetic orbit of left eye
❼⇄	T85.328	Displacement of other ocular prosthetic devices, implants and grafts
❼⇄	T85.390	Other mechanical complication of prosthetic orbit of right eye
❼⇄	T85.391	Other mechanical complication of prosthetic orbit of left eye
❼⇄	T85.398	Other mechanical complication of other ocular prosthetic devices, implants and grafts
⇄	T86.8421	Corneal transplant infection, right eye
⇄	T86.8422	Corneal transplant infection, left eye
⇄	T86.8423	Corneal transplant infection, bilateral
⇄	T86.8481	Other complications of corneal transplant, right eye
⇄	T86.8482	Other complications of corneal transplant, left eye
⇄	T86.8483	Other complications of corneal transplant, bilateral
	Z98.83	Filtering (vitreous) bleb after glaucoma surgery status

ICD-10-CM Coding Notes

For codes requiring a 7th character extension, refer to your ICD-10-CM book. Review the character descriptions and coding guidelines for proper selection. For some procedures, only certain characters will apply.

CCI Edits

Refer to Appendix A for CCI edits.

Facility RVUs ▯

Code	Work	PE Facility	MP	Total Facility
67115	6.11	7.84	0.45	14.40

Non-facility RVUs ▯

Code	Work	PE Non-Facility	MP	Total Non-Facility
67115	6.11	7.84	0.45	14.40

Modifiers (PAR) ▯

Code	Mod 50	Mod 51	Mod 62	Mod 66	Mod 80
67115	1	2	0	0	1

Global Period

Code	Days
67115	090

67120

67120 Removal of implanted material, posterior segment; extraocular

AMA Coding Notes

Repair Procedures on the Retina or Choroid

(If diathermy, cryotherapy and/or photocoagulation are combined, report under principal modality used)

Surgical Procedures on the Eye and Ocular Adnexa

(For diagnostic and treatment ophthalmological services, see Medicine, Ophthalmology, and 92002 et seq)

(Do not report code 69990 in addition to codes 65091-68850)

Plain English Description

A procedure is performed to remove extraocular or intraocular implanted material from the posterior segment of the eye. The posterior segment contains the anterior hyaloid membrane and the optical structures behind it including the vitreous humor, retina, choroid, and optic nerve. The most common materials removed are silicone oil and displaced intraocular lenses without performing a vitrectomy.

Removal of implanted material, posterior segment, extraocular

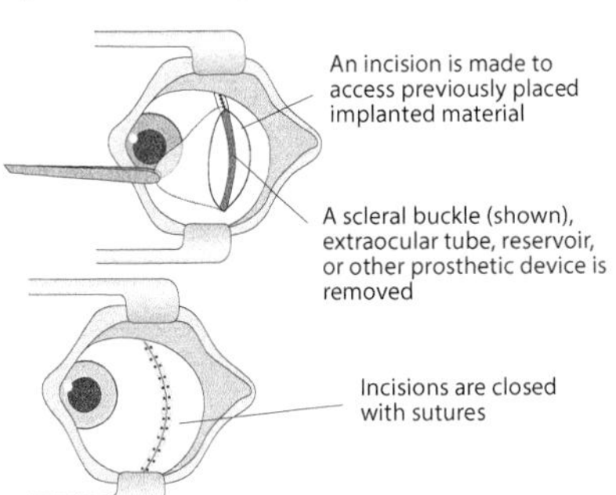
An incision is made to access previously placed implanted material
A scleral buckle (shown), extraocular tube, reservoir, or other prosthetic device is removed
Incisions are closed with sutures

ICD-10-CM Diagnostic Codes

⇄	H43.11	Vitreous hemorrhage, right eye
⇄	H43.12	Vitreous hemorrhage, left eye
⇄	H43.13	Vitreous hemorrhage, bilateral
⇄	H44.002	Unspecified purulent endophthalmitis, left eye
❼	T81.32	Disruption of internal operation (surgical) wound, not elsewhere classified
❼	T81.49	Infection following a procedure, other surgical site
❼⇄	T85.310	Breakdown (mechanical) of prosthetic orbit of right eye
❼⇄	T85.311	Breakdown (mechanical) of prosthetic orbit of left eye
❼⇄	T85.318	Breakdown (mechanical) of other ocular prosthetic devices, implants and grafts
❼⇄	T85.320	Displacement of prosthetic orbit of right eye
❼⇄	T85.321	Displacement of prosthetic orbit of left eye
❼⇄	T85.328	Displacement of other ocular prosthetic devices, implants and grafts
❼⇄	T85.390	Other mechanical complication of prosthetic orbit of right eye
❼⇄	T85.391	Other mechanical complication of prosthetic orbit of left eye
❼⇄	T85.398	Other mechanical complication of other ocular prosthetic devices, implants and grafts
⇄	T86.8421	Corneal transplant infection, right eye
⇄	T86.8422	Corneal transplant infection, left eye
⇄	T86.8423	Corneal transplant infection, bilateral
	Z96.1	Presence of intraocular lens
⇄	Z98.41	Cataract extraction status, right eye
⇄	Z98.42	Cataract extraction status, left eye
	Z98.83	Filtering (vitreous) bleb after glaucoma surgery status

ICD-10-CM Coding Notes

For codes requiring a 7th character extension, refer to your ICD-10-CM book. Review the character descriptions and coding guidelines for proper selection. For some procedures, only certain characters will apply.

CCI Edits

Refer to Appendix A for CCI edits.

Facility RVUs ▯

Code	Work	PE Facility	MP	Total Facility
67120	7.10	8.40	0.56	16.06

Non-facility RVUs ▯

Code	Work	PE Non-Facility	MP	Total Non-Facility
67120	7.10	12.01	0.56	19.67

Modifiers (PAR) ▯

Code	Mod 50	Mod 51	Mod 62	Mod 66	Mod 80
67120	1	2	1	0	1

Global Period

Code	Days
67120	090

67121

67121 Removal of implanted material, posterior segment; intraocular

(For removal from anterior segment, use 65920)

(For removal of foreign body, see 65260, 65265)

AMA Coding Notes

Repair Procedures on the Retina or Choroid

(If diathermy, cryotherapy and/or photocoagulation are combined, report under principal modality used)

Surgical Procedures on the Eye and Ocular Adnexa

(For diagnostic and treatment ophthalmological services, see Medicine, Ophthalmology, and 92002 et seq)

(Do not report code 69990 in addition to codes 65091-68850)

AMA *CPT® Assistant*

67121: Nov 97: 23, Nov 98: 19

Plain English Description

A procedure is performed to remove extraocular or intraocular implanted material from the posterior segment of the eye. The posterior segment contains the anterior hyaloid membrane and the optical structures behind it including the vitreous humor, retina, choroid, and optic nerve. The most common materials removed are silicone oil and displaced intraocular lenses without performing a vitrectomy.

Removal of implanted material; intraocular, posterior segment

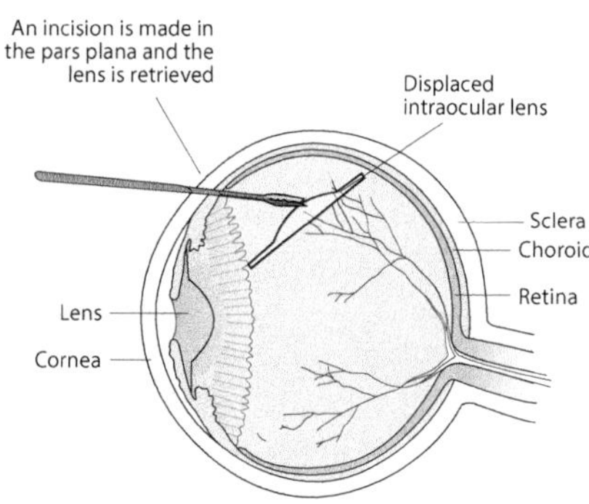
An incision is made in the pars plana and the lens is retrieved
Displaced intraocular lens
Sclera
Choroid
Retina
Lens
Cornea

ICD-10-CM Diagnostic Codes

	Code	Description
⇄	H27.01	Aphakia, right eye
⇄	H27.02	Aphakia, left eye
⇄	H27.03	Aphakia, bilateral
⇄	H27.111	Subluxation of lens, right eye
⇄	H27.112	Subluxation of lens, left eye
⇄	H27.113	Subluxation of lens, bilateral
⇄	H27.131	Posterior dislocation of lens, right eye
⇄	H27.132	Posterior dislocation of lens, left eye
⇄	H27.133	Posterior dislocation of lens, bilateral
❼	T81.32	Disruption of internal operation (surgical) wound, not elsewhere classified
❼	T81.49	Infection following a procedure, other surgical site
❼	T85.21	Breakdown (mechanical) of intraocular lens
❼	T85.22	Displacement of intraocular lens
❼	T85.29	Other mechanical complication of intraocular lens
❼⇄	T85.310	Breakdown (mechanical) of prosthetic orbit of right eye
❼⇄	T85.311	Breakdown (mechanical) of prosthetic orbit of left eye
❼⇄	T85.318	Breakdown (mechanical) of other ocular prosthetic devices, implants and grafts
❼⇄	T85.320	Displacement of prosthetic orbit of right eye
❼⇄	T85.321	Displacement of prosthetic orbit of left eye
❼⇄	T85.328	Displacement of other ocular prosthetic devices, implants and grafts
❼⇄	T85.390	Other mechanical complication of prosthetic orbit of right eye
❼⇄	T85.391	Other mechanical complication of prosthetic orbit of left eye
❼⇄	T85.398	Other mechanical complication of other ocular prosthetic devices, implants and grafts
⇄	T86.8421	Corneal transplant infection, right eye
⇄	T86.8422	Corneal transplant infection, left eye
⇄	T86.8423	Corneal transplant infection, bilateral
⇄	T86.8481	Other complications of corneal transplant, right eye
⇄	T86.8482	Other complications of corneal transplant, left eye
⇄	T86.8483	Other complications of corneal transplant, bilateral
	Z81.4	Family history of other substance abuse and dependence
	Z96.1	Presence of intraocular lens
⇄	Z98.41	Cataract extraction status, right eye
⇄	Z98.42	Cataract extraction status, left eye
	Z98.83	Filtering (vitreous) bleb after glaucoma surgery status

ICD-10-CM Coding Notes

For codes requiring a 7th character extension, refer to your ICD-10-CM book. Review the character descriptions and coding guidelines for proper selection. For some procedures, only certain characters will apply.

CCI Edits

Refer to Appendix A for CCI edits.

Facility RVUs

Code	Work	PE Facility	MP	Total Facility
67121	12.25	12.92	0.95	26.12

Non-facility RVUs

Code	Work	PE Non-Facility	MP	Total Non-Facility
67121	12.25	12.92	0.95	26.12

Modifiers (PAR)

Code	Mod 50	Mod 51	Mod 62	Mod 66	Mod 80
67121	1	2	1	0	2

Global Period

Code	Days
67121	090

67141-67145

▲ **67141 Prophylaxis of retinal detachment (eg, retinal break, lattice degeneration) without drainage; cryotherapy, diathermy**

▲ **67145 Prophylaxis of retinal detachment (eg, retinal break, lattice degeneration) without drainage; photocoagulation**

AMA Coding Notes

Surgical Procedures on the Eye and Ocular Adnexa

(For diagnostic and treatment ophthalmological services, see Medicine, Ophthalmology, and 92002 et seq)

(Do not report code 69990 in addition to codes 65091-68850)

AMA *CPT® Assistant* ▯

67141: Mar 98: 7, Oct 08: 3, Sep 16: 5

67145: Fall 92: 4, Mar 98: 7, Sep 16: 5

Plain English Description

Prophylactic management is performed on a break, hole, tear or lattice degeneration of the retina. Prophylactic treatment is required to prevent retinal detachment. A lid speculum is used to open the eyelids and expose the eye. Local anesthetic is administered. In 67141, a freezing probe (cryotherapy, cryopexy) or heat probe (diathermy) is used to treat the retinal defect. Cryotherapy is performed to the outer surface of the eye through an intact sclera over the site of the retinal defect. The cryotherapy probe is used to create a series of ice balls around the defect area. Diathermy uses radiofrequency current to generate heat and burn the region around the defect. Lamellar scleral dissection is performed over the site of the defect. Diathermy burns are placed in the scleral bed using a blunt-tipped electrode. As the frozen or burned area over and around the break, tear or degeneration heals, scar tissue develops that closes the defect and secures the retina to the choroid. In 67145, a laser beam (photocoagulation) is directed through a contact lens or specially designed ophthalmoscope to the site of the retinal defect. The laser beam is used to burn the tissue around the defect, resulting in scarring that secures the retina to the underlying choroid.

Prophylaxis of retinal detachment, without drainage, 1 or more sessions, cryotherapy/diathermy

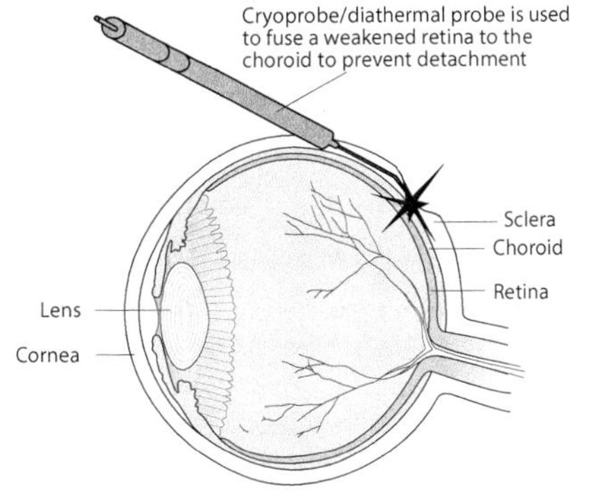
Cryoprobe/diathermal probe is used to fuse a weakened retina to the choroid to prevent detachment
Sclera
Choroid
Retina
Lens
Cornea

ICD-10-CM Diagnostic Codes

	Code	Description
⇄	H33.301	Unspecified retinal break, right eye
⇄	H33.302	Unspecified retinal break, left eye
⇄	H33.303	Unspecified retinal break, bilateral
⇄	H33.311	Horseshoe tear of retina without detachment, right eye
⇄	H33.312	Horseshoe tear of retina without detachment, left eye
⇄	H33.313	Horseshoe tear of retina without detachment, bilateral
⇄	H33.321	Round hole, right eye
⇄	H33.322	Round hole, left eye
⇄	H33.323	Round hole, bilateral
⇄	H33.331	Multiple defects of retina without detachment, right eye
⇄	H33.332	Multiple defects of retina without detachment, left eye
⇄	H33.333	Multiple defects of retina without detachment, bilateral
⇄	H35.341	Macular cyst, hole, or pseudohole, right eye
⇄	H35.342	Macular cyst, hole, or pseudohole, left eye
⇄	H35.343	Macular cyst, hole, or pseudohole, bilateral
⇄	H35.371	Puckering of macula, right eye
⇄	H35.372	Puckering of macula, left eye
⇄	H35.373	Puckering of macula, bilateral
⇄	H35.411	Lattice degeneration of retina, right eye
⇄	H35.412	Lattice degeneration of retina, left eye
⇄	H35.413	Lattice degeneration of retina, bilateral
⇄	H35.421	Microcystoid degeneration of retina, right eye
⇄	H35.422	Microcystoid degeneration of retina, left eye
⇄	H35.423	Microcystoid degeneration of retina, bilateral
⇄	H35.431	Paving stone degeneration of retina, right eye
⇄	H35.432	Paving stone degeneration of retina, left eye
⇄	H35.433	Paving stone degeneration of retina, bilateral
⇄	H35.441	Age-related reticular degeneration of retina, right eye
⇄	H35.442	Age-related reticular degeneration of retina, left eye
⇄	H35.443	Age-related reticular degeneration of retina, bilateral
⇄	H43.11	Vitreous hemorrhage, right eye
⇄	H43.12	Vitreous hemorrhage, left eye
⇄	H43.13	Vitreous hemorrhage, bilateral
⇄	H43.811	Vitreous degeneration, right eye
⇄	H43.812	Vitreous degeneration, left eye
⇄	H43.813	Vitreous degeneration, bilateral
⇄	H44.2B1	Degenerative myopia with macular hole, right eye
⇄	H44.2B2	Degenerative myopia with macular hole, left eye
⇄	H44.2B3	Degenerative myopia with macular hole, bilateral eye
⇄	H44.2E1	Degenerative myopia with other maculopathy, right eye
⇄	H44.2E2	Degenerative myopia with other maculopathy, left eye
⇄	H44.2E3	Degenerative myopia with other maculopathy, bilateral eye

CCI Edits

Refer to Appendix A for CCI edits.

Pub 100

67145: Pub 100-03, 1, 140.5

Facility RVUs ▯

Code	Work	PE Facility	MP	Total Facility
67141	2.53	3.54	0.20	6.27
67145	2.53	3.54	0.20	6.27

Non-facility RVUs ▯

Code	Work	PE Non-Facility	MP	Total Non-Facility
67141	2.53	5.15	0.20	7.88
67145	2.53	4.33	0.20	7.06

Modifiers (PAR) ▯

Code	Mod 50	Mod 51	Mod 62	Mod 66	Mod 80
67141	1	2	0	0	1
67145	1	2	0	0	1

Global Period

Code	Days
67141	010
67145	010

67208-67210

67208 Destruction of localized lesion of retina (eg, macular edema, tumors), 1 or more sessions; cryotherapy, diathermy

67210 Destruction of localized lesion of retina (eg, macular edema, tumors), 1 or more sessions; photocoagulation

AMA Coding Guideline

Destruction Procedures on the Retina or Choroid

Codes 67208, 67210, 67218, 67220, 67229 include treatment at one or more sessions that may occur at different encounters. These codes should be reported once during a defined treatment period.

AMA Coding Notes

Surgical Procedures on the Eye and Ocular Adnexa

(For diagnostic and treatment ophthalmological services, see Medicine, Ophthalmology, and 92002 et seq)

(Do not report code 69990 in addition to codes 65091-68850)

AMA *CPT® Assistant*

67208: Mar 98: 7, Nov 98: 19, Oct 08: 3

67210: Mar 98: 7, Nov 98: 19, Oct 08: 3, Jan 12: 3

Plain English Description

A lid speculum is used to open the eyelids and expose the eye. In 67208, a freezing probe (cryotherapy, cryopexy) or heat probe (diathermy) is used to destroy a localized lesion of the retina, such as a tumor or macular edema. Visual acuity is checked. The pupil is dilated and a local anesthetic administered to the surface of the retina. Cryotherapy is performed to the outer surface of the eye through an intact sclera over the site of the retinal lesion. The cryotherapy probe is positioned and the probe cooled to the desired temperature. Ice ball formation is monitored. Once the ice ball has encompassed the entire lesion, the tissue is warmed. This is repeated until the entire lesion has been destroyed. Diathermy uses a radiofrequency current to generate heat. A lamellar scleral dissection is performed over the site of the lesion. Diathermy burns are placed in the scleral bed at the site of the lesion using a blunt tipped electrode and the lesion is completely destroyed. In 67210, a laser beam (photocoagulation) is directed through a contact lens or specially designed ophthalmoscope to the site of the lesion. The laser beam is used to destroy the entire lesion.

Destruction of localized lesion of retina

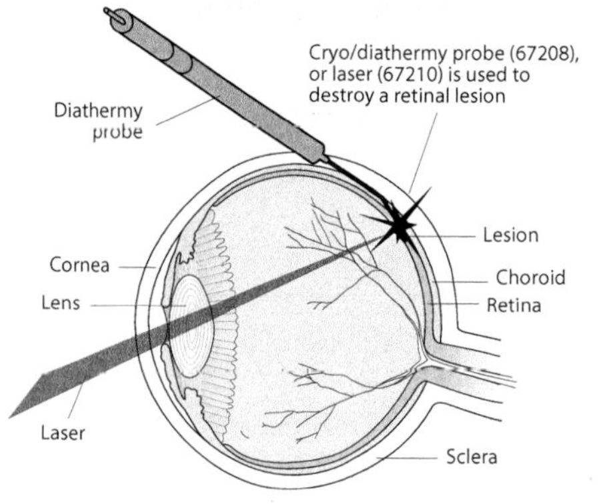

Cryo/diathermy probe (67208), or laser (67210) is used to destroy a retinal lesion
Diathermy probe
Lesion
Cornea
Choroid
Lens
Retina
Laser
Sclera

ICD-10-CM Diagnostic Codes

	Code	Description
⇄	C69.21	Malignant neoplasm of right retina
⇄	C69.31	Malignant neoplasm of right choroid
⇄	D09.21	Carcinoma in situ of right eye
	D18.09	Hemangioma of other sites
⇄	D31.21	Benign neoplasm of right retina
⇄	D31.31	Benign neoplasm of right choroid
	D48.7	Neoplasm of uncertain behavior of other specified sites
	D49.81	Neoplasm of unspecified behavior of retina and choroid
	E08.311	Diabetes mellitus due to underlying condition with unspecified diabetic retinopathy with macular edema
	E08.319	Diabetes mellitus due to underlying condition with unspecified diabetic retinopathy without macular edema
❼⇄	E08.321	Diabetes mellitus due to underlying condition with mild nonproliferative diabetic retinopathy with macular edema
❼⇄	E08.329	Diabetes mellitus due to underlying condition with mild nonproliferative diabetic retinopathy without macular edema
❼⇄	E08.331	Diabetes mellitus due to underlying condition with moderate nonproliferative diabetic retinopathy with macular edema
❼⇄	E08.339	Diabetes mellitus due to underlying condition with moderate nonproliferative diabetic retinopathy without macular edema
❼⇄	E08.341	Diabetes mellitus due to underlying condition with severe nonproliferative diabetic retinopathy with macular edema
❼⇄	E08.349	Diabetes mellitus due to underlying condition with severe nonproliferative diabetic retinopathy without macular edema
❼⇄	E08.351	Diabetes mellitus due to underlying condition with proliferative diabetic retinopathy with macular edema
❼⇄	E08.352	Diabetes mellitus due to underlying condition with proliferative diabetic retinopathy with traction retinal detachment involving the macula
❼⇄	E08.353	Diabetes mellitus due to underlying condition with proliferative diabetic retinopathy with traction retinal detachment not involving the macula
❼⇄	E08.354	Diabetes mellitus due to underlying condition with proliferative diabetic retinopathy with combined traction retinal detachment and rhegmatogenous retinal detachment
❼⇄	E08.355	Diabetes mellitus due to underlying condition with stable proliferative diabetic retinopathy
❼⇄	E08.359	Diabetes mellitus due to underlying condition with proliferative diabetic retinopathy without macular edema
	E08.36	Diabetes mellitus due to underlying condition with diabetic cataract
❼⇄	E08.37	Diabetes mellitus due to underlying condition with diabetic macular edema, resolved following treatment
	E08.39	Diabetes mellitus due to underlying condition with other diabetic ophthalmic complication
	E08.65	Diabetes mellitus due to underlying condition with hyperglycemia
	E09.311	Drug or chemical induced diabetes mellitus with unspecified diabetic retinopathy with macular edema
	E09.319	Drug or chemical induced diabetes mellitus with unspecified diabetic retinopathy without macular edema
❼⇄	E09.321	Drug or chemical induced diabetes mellitus with mild nonproliferative diabetic retinopathy with macular edema
❼⇄	E09.329	Drug or chemical induced diabetes mellitus with mild nonproliferative diabetic retinopathy without macular edema
❼⇄	E09.331	Drug or chemical induced diabetes mellitus with moderate nonproliferative diabetic retinopathy with macular edema
❼⇄	E09.339	Drug or chemical induced diabetes mellitus with moderate nonproliferative diabetic retinopathy without macular edema
❼⇄	E09.341	Drug or chemical induced diabetes mellitus with severe nonproliferative diabetic retinopathy with macular edema
❼⇄	E09.349	Drug or chemical induced diabetes mellitus with severe nonproliferative diabetic retinopathy without macular edema
❼⇄	E09.351	Drug or chemical induced diabetes mellitus with proliferative diabetic retinopathy with macular edema
❼⇄	E09.352	Drug or chemical induced diabetes mellitus with proliferative diabetic retinopathy with traction retinal detachment involving the macula

⑦⇄ E09.353 Drug or chemical induced diabetes mellitus with proliferative diabetic retinopathy with traction retinal detachment not involving the macula
⑦⇄ E09.354 Drug or chemical induced diabetes mellitus with proliferative diabetic retinopathy with combined traction retinal detachment and rhegmatogenous retinal detachment
⑦⇄ E09.355 Drug or chemical induced diabetes mellitus with stable proliferative diabetic retinopathy
⑦⇄ E09.359 Drug or chemical induced diabetes mellitus with proliferative diabetic retinopathy without macular edema
E09.36 Drug or chemical induced diabetes mellitus with diabetic cataract
⑦⇄ E09.37 Drug or chemical induced diabetes mellitus with diabetic macular edema, resolved following treatment
E09.39 Drug or chemical induced diabetes mellitus with other diabetic ophthalmic complication
E09.65 Drug or chemical induced diabetes mellitus with hyperglycemia
E10.311 Type 1 diabetes mellitus with unspecified diabetic retinopathy with macular edema
E10.319 Type 1 diabetes mellitus with unspecified diabetic retinopathy without macular edema
⑦⇄ E10.321 Type 1 diabetes mellitus with mild nonproliferative diabetic retinopathy with macular edema
⑦⇄ E10.329 Type 1 diabetes mellitus with mild nonproliferative diabetic retinopathy without macular edema
⑦⇄ E10.331 Type 1 diabetes mellitus with moderate nonproliferative diabetic retinopathy with macular edema
⑦⇄ E10.339 Type 1 diabetes mellitus with moderate nonproliferative diabetic retinopathy without macular edema
⑦⇄ E10.341 Type 1 diabetes mellitus with severe nonproliferative diabetic retinopathy with macular edema
⑦⇄ E10.349 Type 1 diabetes mellitus with severe nonproliferative diabetic retinopathy without macular edema
⑦⇄ E10.351 Type 1 diabetes mellitus with proliferative diabetic retinopathy with macular edema
⑦⇄ E10.352 Type 1 diabetes mellitus with proliferative diabetic retinopathy with traction retinal detachment involving the macula
⑦⇄ E10.353 Type 1 diabetes mellitus with proliferative diabetic retinopathy with traction retinal detachment not involving the macula
⑦⇄ E10.354 Type 1 diabetes mellitus with proliferative diabetic retinopathy with combined traction retinal detachment and rhegmatogenous retinal detachment
⑦⇄ E10.355 Type 1 diabetes mellitus with stable proliferative diabetic retinopathy
⑦⇄ E10.359 Type 1 diabetes mellitus with proliferative diabetic retinopathy without macular edema
E10.36 Type 1 diabetes mellitus with diabetic cataract
⑦⇄ E10.37 Type 1 diabetes mellitus with diabetic macular edema, resolved following treatment
E10.39 Type 1 diabetes mellitus with other diabetic ophthalmic complication
E10.65 Type 1 diabetes mellitus with hyperglycemia
E11.311 Type 2 diabetes mellitus with unspecified diabetic retinopathy with macular edema
E11.319 Type 2 diabetes mellitus with unspecified diabetic retinopathy without macular edema
⑦⇄ E11.321 Type 2 diabetes mellitus with mild nonproliferative diabetic retinopathy with macular edema
⑦⇄ E11.329 Type 2 diabetes mellitus with mild nonproliferative diabetic retinopathy without macular edema
⑦⇄ E11.331 Type 2 diabetes mellitus with moderate nonproliferative diabetic retinopathy with macular edema
⑦⇄ E11.339 Type 2 diabetes mellitus with moderate nonproliferative diabetic retinopathy without macular edema
⑦⇄ E11.341 Type 2 diabetes mellitus with severe nonproliferative diabetic retinopathy with macular edema
⑦⇄ E11.349 Type 2 diabetes mellitus with severe nonproliferative diabetic retinopathy without macular edema
⑦⇄ E11.351 Type 2 diabetes mellitus with proliferative diabetic retinopathy with macular edema
⑦⇄ E11.352 Type 2 diabetes mellitus with proliferative diabetic retinopathy with traction retinal detachment involving the macula
⑦⇄ E11.353 Type 2 diabetes mellitus with proliferative diabetic retinopathy with traction retinal detachment not involving the macula
⑦⇄ E11.354 Type 2 diabetes mellitus with proliferative diabetic retinopathy with combined traction retinal detachment and rhegmatogenous retinal detachment
⑦⇄ E11.355 Type 2 diabetes mellitus with stable proliferative diabetic retinopathy
⑦⇄ E11.359 Type 2 diabetes mellitus with proliferative diabetic retinopathy without macular edema
E11.36 Type 2 diabetes mellitus with diabetic cataract
⑦⇄ E11.37 Type 2 diabetes mellitus with diabetic macular edema, resolved following treatment
E11.39 Type 2 diabetes mellitus with other diabetic ophthalmic complication
E11.65 Type 2 diabetes mellitus with hyperglycemia
⇄ H34.11 Central retinal artery occlusion, right eye
⇄ H34.8110 Central retinal vein occlusion, right eye, with macular edema
⇄ H34.8111 Central retinal vein occlusion, right eye, with retinal neovascularization
⇄ H34.8112 Central retinal vein occlusion, right eye, stable
⇄ H35.051 Retinal neovascularization, unspecified, right eye
H35.09 Other intraretinal microvascular abnormalities
⇄ H35.341 Macular cyst, hole, or pseudohole, right eye
⇄ H35.351 Cystoid macular degeneration, right eye
⇄ H35.61 Retinal hemorrhage, right eye
⇄ H35.711 Central serous chorioretinopathy, right eye
⇄ H35.721 Serous detachment of retinal pigment epithelium, right eye
⇄ H35.731 Hemorrhagic detachment of retinal pigment epithelium, right eye
H35.81 Retinal edema
H35.89 Other specified retinal disorders
⇄ H44.2B1 Degenerative myopia with macular hole, right eye
⇄ H44.2B2 Degenerative myopia with macular hole, left eye
⇄ H44.2B3 Degenerative myopia with macular hole, bilateral eye
⇄ H44.2C1 Degenerative myopia with retinal detachment, right eye
⇄ H44.2C2 Degenerative myopia with retinal detachment, left eye
⇄ H44.2C3 Degenerative myopia with retinal detachment, bilateral eye
⇄ H44.2E1 Degenerative myopia with other maculopathy, right eye
⇄ H44.2E2 Degenerative myopia with other maculopathy, left eye
⇄ H44.2E3 Degenerative myopia with other maculopathy, bilateral eye
⇄ H54.0X33 Blindness right eye category 3, blindness left eye category 3
⇄ H54.0X34 Blindness right eye category 3, blindness left eye category 4
⇄ H54.0X35 Blindness right eye category 3, blindness left eye category 5
⇄ H54.0X43 Blindness right eye category 4, blindness left eye category 3
⇄ H54.0X44 Blindness right eye category 4, blindness left eye category 4
⇄ H54.0X45 Blindness right eye category 4, blindness left eye category 5
⇄ H54.0X53 Blindness right eye category 5, blindness left eye category 3
⇄ H54.0X54 Blindness right eye category 5, blindness left eye category 4
⇄ H54.0X55 Blindness right eye category 5, blindness left eye category 5
⇄ H54.1131 Blindness right eye category 3, low vision left eye category 1
⇄ H54.1132 Blindness right eye category 3, low vision left eye category 2
⇄ H54.1141 Blindness right eye category 4, low vision left eye category 1

⇄ H54.1142 Blindness right eye category 4, low vision left eye category 2
⇄ H54.1151 Blindness right eye category 5, low vision left eye category 1
⇄ H54.1152 Blindness right eye category 5, low vision left eye category 2
⇄ H54.1213 Low vision right eye category 1, blindness left eye category 3
⇄ H54.1214 Low vision right eye category 1, blindness left eye category 4
⇄ H54.1215 Low vision right eye category 1, blindness left eye category 5
⇄ H54.1223 Low vision right eye category 2, blindness left eye category 3
⇄ H54.1224 Low vision right eye category 2, blindness left eye category 4
⇄ H54.1225 Low vision right eye category 2, blindness left eye category 5
⇄ H54.2X11 Low vision right eye category 1, low vision left eye category 1
⇄ H54.2X12 Low vision right eye category 1, low vision left eye category 2
⇄ H54.2X21 Low vision right eye category 2, low vision left eye category 1
⇄ H54.2X22 Low vision right eye category 2, low vision left eye category 2
⇄ H54.413A Blindness right eye category 3, normal vision left eye
⇄ H54.414A Blindness right eye category 4, normal vision left eye
⇄ H54.415A Blindness right eye category 5, normal vision left eye
⇄ H54.42A3 Blindness left eye category 3, normal vision right eye
⇄ H54.42A4 Blindness left eye category 4, normal vision right eye
⇄ H54.42A5 Blindness left eye category 5, normal vision right eye
⇄ H54.511A Low vision right eye category 1, normal vision left eye
⇄ H54.512A Low vision right eye category 2, normal vision left eye
⇄ H54.52A1 Low vision left eye category 1, normal vision right eye
⇄ H54.52A2 Low vision left eye category 2, normal vision right eye

ICD-10-CM Coding Notes

For codes requiring a 7th character extension, refer to your ICD-10-CM book. Review the character descriptions and coding guidelines for proper selection. For some procedures, only certain characters will apply.

CCI Edits

Refer to Appendix A for CCI edits.

Facility RVUs ▯

Code	Work	PE Facility	MP	Total Facility
67208	7.65	8.45	0.60	16.70
67210	6.36	7.55	0.50	14.41

Non-facility RVUs ▯

Code	Work	PE Non-Facility	MP	Total Non-Facility
67208	7.65	9.25	0.60	17.50
67210	6.36	8.13	0.50	14.99

Modifiers (PAR) ▯

Code	Mod 50	Mod 51	Mod 62	Mod 66	Mod 80
67208	1	2	0	0	1
67210	1	2	0	0	1

Global Period

Code	Days
67208	090
67210	090

67218

67218 Destruction of localized lesion of retina (eg, macular edema, tumors), 1 or more sessions; radiation by implantation of source (includes removal of source)

AMA Coding Guideline
Destruction Procedures on the Retina or Choroid

Codes 67208, 67210, 67218, 67220, 67229 include treatment at one or more sessions that may occur at different encounters. These codes should be reported once during a defined treatment period.

AMA Coding Notes
Surgical Procedures on the Eye and Ocular Adnexa

(For diagnostic and treatment ophthalmological services, see Medicine, Ophthalmology, and 92002 et seq)

(Do not report code 69990 in addition to codes 65091-68850)

AMA *CPT® Assistant*

67218: Mar 98: 7, Oct 08: 3

Plain English Description

A procedure is performed to insert (or remove) a radioactive implant in the eye to treat macular edema and localized lesions of the choroid, retina, or iris such as tumors like melanoma. This treatment may be referred to as plaque radiotherapy, plaque brachytherapy, radiation implant, or radioactive source implantation. The device consists of a custom made, sealed metal plaque containing small radioactive seeds. The radioactive seeds deliver a precise dose of radiation to a prescribed area for a period of 4-7 days, after which the device is removed. An incision is made in the conjunctiva and the plaque is centered over the lesion and sutured to the sclera to keep it in place. The conjunctiva is then sutured closed and the eye is covered with a lead shield. At the conclusion of the treatment, the conjunctiva is incised, the plaque is removed, and the conjunctiva is closed again with sutures.

Destruction of localized lesion of retina, 1 or more sessions; radiation by implantation

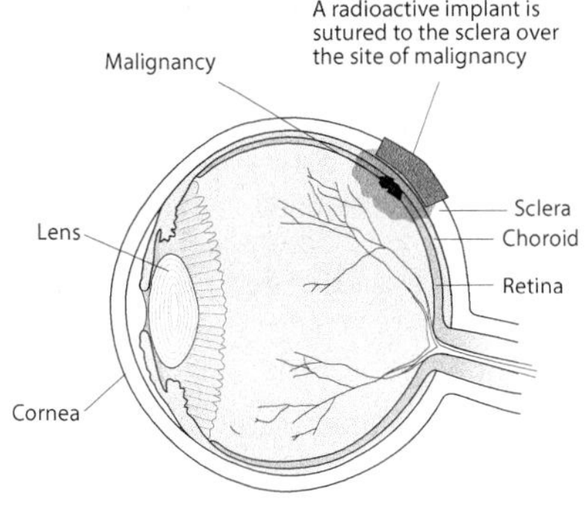
A radioactive implant is sutured to the sclera over the site of malignancy
Malignancy
Lens
Sclera
Choroid
Retina
Cornea

ICD-10-CM Diagnostic Codes

⇄ C69.22 Malignant neoplasm of left retina
⇄ D09.22 Carcinoma in situ of left eye
D18.09 Hemangioma of other sites
⇄ D31.22 Benign neoplasm of left retina
D48.7 Neoplasm of uncertain behavior of other specified sites
D49.81 Neoplasm of unspecified behavior of retina and choroid
E08.311 Diabetes mellitus due to underlying condition with unspecified diabetic retinopathy with macular edema
E08.319 Diabetes mellitus due to underlying condition with unspecified diabetic retinopathy without macular edema
➐⇄ E08.321 Diabetes mellitus due to underlying condition with mild nonproliferative diabetic retinopathy with macular edema
➐⇄ E08.329 Diabetes mellitus due to underlying condition with mild nonproliferative diabetic retinopathy without macular edema
➐⇄ E08.331 Diabetes mellitus due to underlying condition with moderate nonproliferative diabetic retinopathy with macular edema
➐⇄ E08.339 Diabetes mellitus due to underlying condition with moderate nonproliferative diabetic retinopathy without macular edema
➐⇄ E08.341 Diabetes mellitus due to underlying condition with severe nonproliferative diabetic retinopathy with macular edema
➐⇄ E08.349 Diabetes mellitus due to underlying condition with severe nonproliferative diabetic retinopathy without macular edema
➐⇄ E08.351 Diabetes mellitus due to underlying condition with proliferative diabetic retinopathy with macular edema
➐⇄ E08.352 Diabetes mellitus due to underlying condition with proliferative diabetic retinopathy with traction retinal detachment involving the macula
➐⇄ E08.353 Diabetes mellitus due to underlying condition with proliferative diabetic retinopathy with traction retinal detachment not involving the macula
➐⇄ E08.354 Diabetes mellitus due to underlying condition with proliferative diabetic retinopathy with combined traction retinal detachment and rhegmatogenous retinal detachment
➐⇄ E08.355 Diabetes mellitus due to underlying condition with stable proliferative diabetic retinopathy
➐⇄ E08.359 Diabetes mellitus due to underlying condition with proliferative diabetic retinopathy without macular edema
E08.36 Diabetes mellitus due to underlying condition with diabetic cataract
➐⇄ E08.37 Diabetes mellitus due to underlying condition with diabetic macular edema, resolved following treatment
E08.39 Diabetes mellitus due to underlying condition with other diabetic ophthalmic complication
E08.65 Diabetes mellitus due to underlying condition with hyperglycemia
E09.311 Drug or chemical induced diabetes mellitus with unspecified diabetic retinopathy with macular edema
E09.319 Drug or chemical induced diabetes mellitus with unspecified diabetic retinopathy without macular edema
➐⇄ E09.321 Drug or chemical induced diabetes mellitus with mild nonproliferative diabetic retinopathy with macular edema
➐⇄ E09.329 Drug or chemical induced diabetes mellitus with mild nonproliferative diabetic retinopathy without macular edema
➐⇄ E09.331 Drug or chemical induced diabetes mellitus with moderate nonproliferative diabetic retinopathy with macular edema
➐⇄ E09.339 Drug or chemical induced diabetes mellitus with moderate nonproliferative diabetic retinopathy without macular edema
➐⇄ E09.341 Drug or chemical induced diabetes mellitus with severe nonproliferative diabetic retinopathy with macular edema
➐⇄ E09.349 Drug or chemical induced diabetes mellitus with severe nonproliferative diabetic retinopathy without macular edema
➐⇄ E09.351 Drug or chemical induced diabetes mellitus with proliferative diabetic retinopathy with macular edema
➐⇄ E09.352 Drug or chemical induced diabetes mellitus with proliferative diabetic retinopathy with traction retinal detachment involving the macula
➐⇄ E09.353 Drug or chemical induced diabetes mellitus with proliferative diabetic retinopathy with traction retinal detachment not involving the macula

❼⇄ E09.354 Drug or chemical induced diabetes mellitus with proliferative diabetic retinopathy with combined traction retinal detachment and rhegmatogenous retinal detachment
❼⇄ E09.355 Drug or chemical induced diabetes mellitus with stable proliferative diabetic retinopathy
❼⇄ E09.359 Drug or chemical induced diabetes mellitus with proliferative diabetic retinopathy without macular edema
E09.36 Drug or chemical induced diabetes mellitus with diabetic cataract
❼⇄ E09.37 Drug or chemical induced diabetes mellitus with diabetic macular edema, resolved following treatment
E09.39 Drug or chemical induced diabetes mellitus with other diabetic ophthalmic complication
E09.65 Drug or chemical induced diabetes mellitus with hyperglycemia
E10.311 Type 1 diabetes mellitus with unspecified diabetic retinopathy with macular edema
E10.319 Type 1 diabetes mellitus with unspecified diabetic retinopathy without macular edema
❼⇄ E10.321 Type 1 diabetes mellitus with mild nonproliferative diabetic retinopathy with macular edema
❼⇄ E10.329 Type 1 diabetes mellitus with mild nonproliferative diabetic retinopathy without macular edema
❼⇄ E10.331 Type 1 diabetes mellitus with moderate nonproliferative diabetic retinopathy with macular edema
❼⇄ E10.339 Type 1 diabetes mellitus with moderate nonproliferative diabetic retinopathy without macular edema
❼⇄ E10.341 Type 1 diabetes mellitus with severe nonproliferative diabetic retinopathy with macular edema
❼⇄ E10.349 Type 1 diabetes mellitus with severe nonproliferative diabetic retinopathy without macular edema
❼⇄ E10.351 Type 1 diabetes mellitus with proliferative diabetic retinopathy with macular edema
❼⇄ E10.352 Type 1 diabetes mellitus with proliferative diabetic retinopathy with traction retinal detachment involving the macula
❼⇄ E10.353 Type 1 diabetes mellitus with proliferative diabetic retinopathy with traction retinal detachment not involving the macula
❼⇄ E10.354 Type 1 diabetes mellitus with proliferative diabetic retinopathy with combined traction retinal detachment and rhegmatogenous retinal detachment
❼⇄ E10.355 Type 1 diabetes mellitus with stable proliferative diabetic retinopathy
❼⇄ E10.359 Type 1 diabetes mellitus with proliferative diabetic retinopathy without macular edema
E10.36 Type 1 diabetes mellitus with diabetic cataract
❼⇄ E10.37 Type 1 diabetes mellitus with diabetic macular edema, resolved following treatment
E10.39 Type 1 diabetes mellitus with other diabetic ophthalmic complication
E10.65 Type 1 diabetes mellitus with hyperglycemia
E11.311 Type 2 diabetes mellitus with unspecified diabetic retinopathy with macular edema
E11.319 Type 2 diabetes mellitus with unspecified diabetic retinopathy without macular edema
❼⇄ E11.321 Type 2 diabetes mellitus with mild nonproliferative diabetic retinopathy with macular edema
❼⇄ E11.329 Type 2 diabetes mellitus with mild nonproliferative diabetic retinopathy without macular edema
❼⇄ E11.331 Type 2 diabetes mellitus with moderate nonproliferative diabetic retinopathy with macular edema
❼⇄ E11.339 Type 2 diabetes mellitus with moderate nonproliferative diabetic retinopathy without macular edema
❼⇄ E11.341 Type 2 diabetes mellitus with severe nonproliferative diabetic retinopathy with macular edema
❼⇄ E11.349 Type 2 diabetes mellitus with severe nonproliferative diabetic retinopathy without macular edema
❼⇄ E11.351 Type 2 diabetes mellitus with proliferative diabetic retinopathy with macular edema
❼⇄ E11.352 Type 2 diabetes mellitus with proliferative diabetic retinopathy with traction retinal detachment involving the macula
❼⇄ E11.353 Type 2 diabetes mellitus with proliferative diabetic retinopathy with traction retinal detachment not involving the macula
❼⇄ E11.354 Type 2 diabetes mellitus with proliferative diabetic retinopathy with combined traction retinal detachment and rhegmatogenous retinal detachment
❼⇄ E11.355 Type 2 diabetes mellitus with stable proliferative diabetic retinopathy
❼⇄ E11.359 Type 2 diabetes mellitus with proliferative diabetic retinopathy without macular edema
E11.36 Type 2 diabetes mellitus with diabetic cataract
❼⇄ E11.37 Type 2 diabetes mellitus with diabetic macular edema, resolved following treatment
E11.39 Type 2 diabetes mellitus with other diabetic ophthalmic complication
E11.65 Type 2 diabetes mellitus with hyperglycemia
⇄ H35.052 Retinal neovascularization, unspecified, left eye
H35.09 Other intraretinal microvascular abnormalities
H35.30 Unspecified macular degeneration
⇄ H35.352 Cystoid macular degeneration, left eye
⇄ H35.372 Puckering of macula, left eye
H35.81 Retinal edema
⇄ H44.2C1 Degenerative myopia with retinal detachment, right eye
⇄ H44.2C2 Degenerative myopia with retinal detachment, left eye
⇄ H44.2C3 Degenerative myopia with retinal detachment, bilateral eye

ICD-10-CM Coding Notes

For codes requiring a 7th character extension, refer to your ICD-10-CM book. Review the character descriptions and coding guidelines for proper selection. For some procedures, only certain characters will apply.

CCI Edits

Refer to Appendix A for CCI edits.

Facility RVUs

Code	Work	PE Facility	MP	Total Facility
67218	20.36	18.48	1.55	40.39

Non-facility RVUs

Code	Work	PE Non-Facility	MP	Total Non-Facility
67218	20.36	18.48	1.55	40.39

Modifiers (PAR)

Code	Mod 50	Mod 51	Mod 62	Mod 66	Mod 80
67218	1	2	0	0	1

Global Period

Code	Days
67218	090

67220

67220 Destruction of localized lesion of choroid (eg, choroidal neovascularization); photocoagulation (eg, laser), 1 or more sessions

AMA Coding Guideline

Destruction Procedures on the Retina or Choroid

Codes 67208, 67210, 67218, 67220, 67229 include treatment at one or more sessions that may occur at different encounters. These codes should be reported once during a defined treatment period.

AMA Coding Notes

Surgical Procedures on the Eye and Ocular Adnexa

(For diagnostic and treatment ophthalmological services, see Medicine, Ophthalmology, and 92002 et seq)

(Do not report code 69990 in addition to codes 65091-68850)

AMA *CPT® Assistant* ▢

67220: Nov 98: 19, Nov 99: 39, Feb 01: 8, Oct 08: 3, Jan 12: 3

Plain English Description

Destruction of a localized lesion of the choroid is performed in one or more sessions using photocoagulation. Laser photocoagulation uses a laser to physically ablate abnormal choroidal tissue, such as a choroidal neovascularization (CNV), a disorder in which new blood vessels originating in the choroid break through the Bruch membrane into the subretinal pigment epithelium or subretinal space. CNV is a major cause of vision loss. The lesion is delineated using fluorescein angiography and then destroyed using multiple laser burns. After each firing of the laser, the surgeon evaluates the burn area, the tissue's reaction to the burn, and the remaining extent of the lesion to be destroyed, including both thickness and diameter. The procedure is performed in one or more sessions during a defined treatment period that may occur at different encounters on different days.

Destruction of localized lesion of choroid 1 or more sessions; photocoagulation

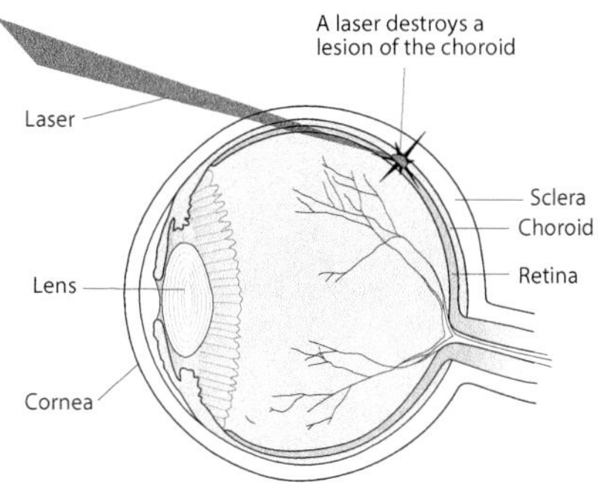

ICD-10-CM Diagnostic Codes

	Code	Description
	B39.3	Disseminated histoplasmosis capsulati
	B39.4	Histoplasmosis capsulati, unspecified
⇄	C69.31	Malignant neoplasm of right choroid
⇄	C69.32	Malignant neoplasm of left choroid
⇄	D09.21	Carcinoma in situ of right eye
⇄	D09.22	Carcinoma in situ of left eye
	D18.09	Hemangioma of other sites
⇄	D31.31	Benign neoplasm of right choroid
⇄	D31.32	Benign neoplasm of left choroid
	D48.7	Neoplasm of uncertain behavior of other specified sites
	D49.81	Neoplasm of unspecified behavior of retina and choroid
⇄	H31.091	Other chorioretinal scars, right eye
⇄	H31.092	Other chorioretinal scars, left eye
⇄	H31.093	Other chorioretinal scars, bilateral
⇄	H31.311	Expulsive choroidal hemorrhage, right eye
⇄	H31.312	Expulsive choroidal hemorrhage, left eye
⇄	H31.313	Expulsive choroidal hemorrhage, bilateral
⇄	H31.321	Choroidal rupture, right eye
⇄	H31.322	Choroidal rupture, left eye
⇄	H31.323	Choroidal rupture, bilateral
⇄	H31.411	Hemorrhagic choroidal detachment, right eye
⇄	H31.412	Hemorrhagic choroidal detachment, left eye
⇄	H31.413	Hemorrhagic choroidal detachment, bilateral
⇄	H31.421	Serous choroidal detachment, right eye
⇄	H31.422	Serous choroidal detachment, left eye
⇄	H31.423	Serous choroidal detachment, bilateral
	H31.8	Other specified disorders of choroid
	H32	Chorioretinal disorders in diseases classified elsewhere
⇄	H35.3211	Exudative age-related macular degeneration, right eye, with active choroidal neovascularization
⇄	H35.3212	Exudative age-related macular degeneration, right eye, with inactive choroidal neovascularization
⇄	H35.3221	Exudative age-related macular degeneration, left eye, with active choroidal neovascularization
⇄	H35.3222	Exudative age-related macular degeneration, left eye, with inactive choroidal neovascularization
⇄	H35.3231	Exudative age-related macular degeneration, bilateral, with active choroidal neovascularization
⇄	H35.3232	Exudative age-related macular degeneration, bilateral, with inactive choroidal neovascularization
⇄	H44.2A1	Degenerative myopia with choroidal neovascularization, right eye
⇄	H44.2A2	Degenerative myopia with choroidal neovascularization, left eye
⇄	H44.2A3	Degenerative myopia with choroidal neovascularization, bilateral eye
❼⇄	S05.11	Contusion of eyeball and orbital tissues, right eye
❼⇄	S05.12	Contusion of eyeball and orbital tissues, left eye
❼⇄	S05.31	Ocular laceration without prolapse or loss of intraocular tissue, right eye
❼⇄	S05.32	Ocular laceration without prolapse or loss of intraocular tissue, left eye
❼⇄	S05.61	Penetrating wound without foreign body of right eyeball
❼⇄	S05.62	Penetrating wound without foreign body of left eyeball
❼⇄	S05.8X1	Other injuries of right eye and orbit
❼⇄	S05.8X2	Other injuries of left eye and orbit

ICD-10-CM Coding Notes

For codes requiring a 7th character extension, refer to your ICD-10-CM book. Review the character descriptions and coding guidelines for proper selection. For some procedures, only certain characters will apply.

CCI Edits

Refer to Appendix A for CCI edits.

Pub 100

67220: Pub 100-03, 1, 140.5

Facility RVUs

Code	Work	PE Facility	MP	Total Facility
67220	6.36	7.55	0.50	14.41

Non-facility RVUs

Code	Work	PE Non-Facility	MP	Total Non-Facility
67220	6.36	8.58	0.50	15.44

Modifiers (PAR)

Code	Mod 50	Mod 51	Mod 62	Mod 66	Mod 80
67220	1	2	0	0	1

Global Period

Code	Days
67220	090

67221-67225

67221 Destruction of localized lesion of choroid (eg, choroidal neovascularization); photodynamic therapy (includes intravenous infusion)

✚ **67225 Destruction of localized lesion of choroid (eg, choroidal neovascularization); photodynamic therapy, second eye, at single session (List separately in addition to code for primary eye treatment)**

(Use 67225 in conjunction with 67221)

AMA Coding Guideline

Destruction Procedures on the Retina or Choroid

Codes 67208, 67210, 67218, 67220, 67229 include treatment at one or more sessions that may occur at different encounters. These codes should be reported once during a defined treatment period.

AMA Coding Notes

Surgical Procedures on the Eye and Ocular Adnexa

(For diagnostic and treatment ophthalmological services, see Medicine, Ophthalmology, and 92002 et seq)

(Do not report code 69990 in addition to codes 65091-68850)

AMA *CPT® Assistant* ▯

67221: Feb 01: 8, Sep 01: 10, Jun 02: 10, Feb 18: 10

67225: Jun 02: 10

Plain English Description

Destruction of a localized lesion of the choroid is performed using photodynamic therapy to ablate abnormal choroidal tissue, such as choroidal neovascularization (CNV), a disorder in which new blood vessels originating in the choroid break through the Bruch membrane into the subretinal pigment epithelium or subretinal space. CNV is a major cause of vision loss. Photodynamic therapy (PDT) uses a low-energy targeted laser light to activate a photoactive drug that is administered intravenously prior to PDT. The photoactive drug, Verteporfin, is administered by intravenous infusion over an approximate 10 min period 15 min prior to the initiation of PDT. The lesion is then destroyed using a contact lens and slit lamp to direct the low-energy laser at the targeted lesion. The procedure may be performed on one or both eyes during a single session. Use 67221 for PDT on the first eye and 67225 for PDT on the second eye performed during the same session.

Destruction of localized lesion of choroid; photodynamic therapy

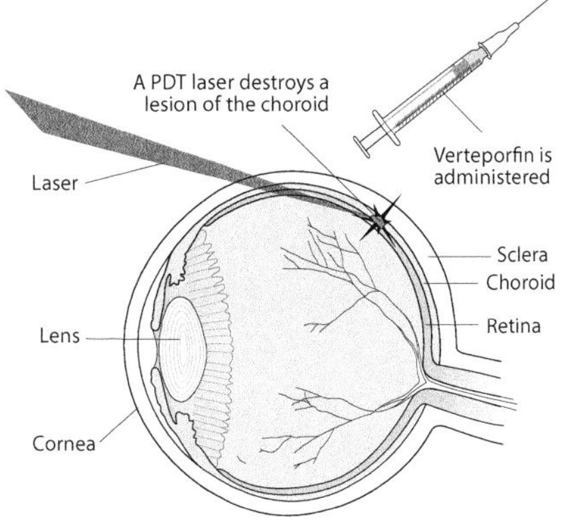

ICD-10-CM Diagnostic Codes

	B39.3	Disseminated histoplasmosis capsulati
	B39.4	Histoplasmosis capsulati, unspecified
⇄	C69.31	Malignant neoplasm of right choroid
⇄	C69.32	Malignant neoplasm of left choroid
⇄	D09.21	Carcinoma in situ of right eye
⇄	D09.22	Carcinoma in situ of left eye
	D18.09	Hemangioma of other sites
⇄	D31.31	Benign neoplasm of right choroid
⇄	D31.32	Benign neoplasm of left choroid
	D48.7	Neoplasm of uncertain behavior of other specified sites
	D49.81	Neoplasm of unspecified behavior of retina and choroid
	E08.39	Diabetes mellitus due to underlying condition with other diabetic ophthalmic complication
	E09.39	Drug or chemical induced diabetes mellitus with other diabetic ophthalmic complication
	E10.39	Type 1 diabetes mellitus with other diabetic ophthalmic complication
	E11.39	Type 2 diabetes mellitus with other diabetic ophthalmic complication
⇄	H31.091	Other chorioretinal scars, right eye
⇄	H31.092	Other chorioretinal scars, left eye
⇄	H31.093	Other chorioretinal scars, bilateral
⇄	H31.311	Expulsive choroidal hemorrhage, right eye
⇄	H31.312	Expulsive choroidal hemorrhage, left eye
⇄	H31.313	Expulsive choroidal hemorrhage, bilateral
⇄	H31.321	Choroidal rupture, right eye
⇄	H31.322	Choroidal rupture, left eye
⇄	H31.323	Choroidal rupture, bilateral
⇄	H31.411	Hemorrhagic choroidal detachment, right eye
⇄	H31.412	Hemorrhagic choroidal detachment, left eye
⇄	H31.413	Hemorrhagic choroidal detachment, bilateral
⇄	H31.421	Serous choroidal detachment, right eye
⇄	H31.422	Serous choroidal detachment, left eye
⇄	H31.423	Serous choroidal detachment, bilateral
	H31.8	Other specified disorders of choroid
	H32	Chorioretinal disorders in diseases classified elsewhere
⇄	H35.3211	Exudative age-related macular degeneration, right eye, with active choroidal neovascularization
⇄	H35.3212	Exudative age-related macular degeneration, right eye, with inactive choroidal neovascularization
⇄	H35.3221	Exudative age-related macular degeneration, left eye, with active choroidal neovascularization
⇄	H35.3222	Exudative age-related macular degeneration, left eye, with inactive choroidal neovascularization
⇄	H35.3231	Exudative age-related macular degeneration, bilateral, with active choroidal neovascularization
⇄	H35.3232	Exudative age-related macular degeneration, bilateral, with inactive choroidal neovascularization
⇄	H44.2A1	Degenerative myopia with choroidal neovascularization, right eye
⇄	H44.2A2	Degenerative myopia with choroidal neovascularization, left eye
⇄	H44.2A3	Degenerative myopia with choroidal neovascularization, bilateral eye
❼⇄	S05.11	Contusion of eyeball and orbital tissues, right eye
❼⇄	S05.12	Contusion of eyeball and orbital tissues, left eye
❼⇄	S05.31	Ocular laceration without prolapse or loss of intraocular tissue, right eye
❼⇄	S05.32	Ocular laceration without prolapse or loss of intraocular tissue, left eye
❼⇄	S05.61	Penetrating wound without foreign body of right eyeball
❼⇄	S05.62	Penetrating wound without foreign body of left eyeball
❼⇄	S05.8X1	Other injuries of right eye and orbit
❼⇄	S05.8X2	Other injuries of left eye and orbit

ICD-10-CM Coding Notes

For codes requiring a 7th character extension, refer to your ICD-10-CM book. Review the character descriptions and coding guidelines for proper selection. For some procedures, only certain characters will apply.

CCI Edits

Refer to Appendix A for CCI edits.

Pub 100

67221: , Pub 100-04, 32, 300.1, Pub 100-04, 32, 300.2

67225: , Pub 100-04, 32, 300.1, Pub 100-04, 32, 300.2

Facility RVUs 🗆

Code	Work	PE Facility	MP	Total Facility
67221	3.45	2.32	0.25	6.02
67225	0.47	0.29	0.04	0.80

Non-facility RVUs 🗆

Code	Work	PE Non-Facility	MP	Total Non-Facility
67221	3.45	4.24	0.25	7.94
67225	0.47	0.34	0.04	0.85

Modifiers (PAR) 🗆

Code	Mod 50	Mod 51	Mod 62	Mod 66	Mod 80
67221	0	2	0	0	1
67225	0	0	0	0	1

Global Period

Code	Days
67221	000
67225	ZZZ

67227

67227 Destruction of extensive or progressive retinopathy (eg, diabetic retinopathy), cryotherapy, diathermy

AMA Coding Guideline

Destruction Procedures on the Retina or Choroid

Codes 67208, 67210, 67218, 67220, 67229 include treatment at one or more sessions that may occur at different encounters. These codes should be reported once during a defined treatment period.

AMA Coding Notes

Surgical Procedures on the Eye and Ocular Adnexa

(For diagnostic and treatment ophthalmological services, see Medicine, Ophthalmology, and 92002 et seq)

(Do not report code 69990 in addition to codes 65091-68850)

AMA *CPT® Assistant*

67227: Mar 98: 7, Oct 08: 3

Plain English Description

Extensive or progressive retinopathy (diabetic retinopathy) is destroyed using extreme cold (cryotherapy) or extreme heat (diathermy) in 67227, or treated using photocoagulation in 67228. Extensive or progressive (diabetic) retinopathy is characterized by damage to the blood vessels, which swell and leak blood or cause new blood vessels to form on the surface of the retina. Visual acuity is checked. The pupil is dilated and a local anesthetic is administered. The cryoprobe or diathermy probe is briefly placed on the surface of the eye overlying the periphery of the retina and the damaged blood vessels are destroyed by freezing or heat. When laser photocoagulation is used for treatment, it is administered by a technique referred to as scatter laser treatment or pan retinal photocoagulation (PRP), in which as many as 2,000 burns are placed in the mid-periphery and periphery of the retina, taking care to avoid the area of central vision, the macula. The burns destroy oxygen-deprived retinal tissue, seal leaking blood vessels, and prevent the formation of new blood vessels. The procedure may be performed using a slit lamp delivery system, which requires placement of a fundus contact lens, or indirect delivery system.

Destruction of extensive or progressive retinopathy by cryotherapy or diathermy

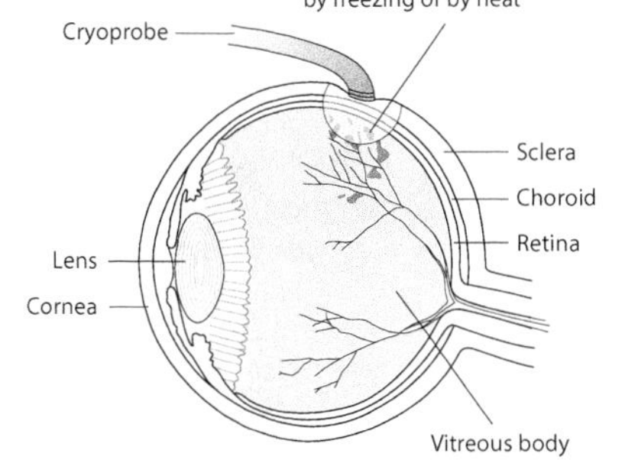
Small vessels that are leaking blood on the retina are destroyed by freezing or by heat
Cryoprobe
Sclera
Choroid
Retina
Lens
Cornea
Vitreous body

ICD-10-CM Diagnostic Codes

	Code	Description
⑦⇄	E08.331	Diabetes mellitus due to underlying condition with moderate nonproliferative diabetic retinopathy with macular edema
⑦⇄	E08.339	Diabetes mellitus due to underlying condition with moderate nonproliferative diabetic retinopathy without macular edema
⑦⇄	E08.341	Diabetes mellitus due to underlying condition with severe nonproliferative diabetic retinopathy with macular edema
⑦⇄	E08.349	Diabetes mellitus due to underlying condition with severe nonproliferative diabetic retinopathy without macular edema
⑦⇄	E08.351	Diabetes mellitus due to underlying condition with proliferative diabetic retinopathy with macular edema
⑦⇄	E08.352	Diabetes mellitus due to underlying condition with proliferative diabetic retinopathy with traction retinal detachment involving the macula
⑦⇄	E08.353	Diabetes mellitus due to underlying condition with proliferative diabetic retinopathy with traction retinal detachment not involving the macula
⑦⇄	E08.354	Diabetes mellitus due to underlying condition with proliferative diabetic retinopathy with combined traction retinal detachment and rhegmatogenous retinal detachment
⑦⇄	E08.355	Diabetes mellitus due to underlying condition with stable proliferative diabetic retinopathy
⑦⇄	E08.359	Diabetes mellitus due to underlying condition with proliferative diabetic retinopathy without macular edema
⑦⇄	E09.331	Drug or chemical induced diabetes mellitus with moderate nonproliferative diabetic retinopathy with macular edema
⑦⇄	E09.339	Drug or chemical induced diabetes mellitus with moderate nonproliferative diabetic retinopathy without macular edema
⑦⇄	E09.341	Drug or chemical induced diabetes mellitus with severe nonproliferative diabetic retinopathy with macular edema
⑦⇄	E09.349	Drug or chemical induced diabetes mellitus with severe nonproliferative diabetic retinopathy without macular edema
⑦⇄	E09.351	Drug or chemical induced diabetes mellitus with proliferative diabetic retinopathy with macular edema
⑦⇄	E09.352	Drug or chemical induced diabetes mellitus with proliferative diabetic retinopathy with traction retinal detachment involving the macula
⑦⇄	E09.353	Drug or chemical induced diabetes mellitus with proliferative diabetic retinopathy with traction retinal detachment not involving the macula
⑦⇄	E09.354	Drug or chemical induced diabetes mellitus with proliferative diabetic retinopathy with combined traction retinal detachment and rhegmatogenous retinal detachment
⑦⇄	E09.355	Drug or chemical induced diabetes mellitus with stable proliferative diabetic retinopathy
⑦⇄	E09.359	Drug or chemical induced diabetes mellitus with proliferative diabetic retinopathy without macular edema
⑦⇄	E10.331	Type 1 diabetes mellitus with moderate nonproliferative diabetic retinopathy with macular edema
⑦⇄	E10.339	Type 1 diabetes mellitus with moderate nonproliferative diabetic retinopathy without macular edema
⑦⇄	E10.341	Type 1 diabetes mellitus with severe nonproliferative diabetic retinopathy with macular edema
⑦⇄	E10.349	Type 1 diabetes mellitus with severe nonproliferative diabetic retinopathy without macular edema
⑦⇄	E10.351	Type 1 diabetes mellitus with proliferative diabetic retinopathy with macular edema
⑦⇄	E10.352	Type 1 diabetes mellitus with proliferative diabetic retinopathy with traction retinal detachment involving the macula
⑦⇄	E10.353	Type 1 diabetes mellitus with proliferative diabetic retinopathy with traction retinal detachment not involving the macula
⑦⇄	E10.354	Type 1 diabetes mellitus with proliferative diabetic retinopathy with combined traction retinal detachment and rhegmatogenous retinal detachment
⑦⇄	E10.355	Type 1 diabetes mellitus with stable proliferative diabetic retinopathy
⑦⇄	E10.359	Type 1 diabetes mellitus with proliferative diabetic retinopathy without macular edema
⑦⇄	E11.331	Type 2 diabetes mellitus with moderate nonproliferative diabetic retinopathy with macular edema

❼⇄	E11.339	Type 2 diabetes mellitus with moderate nonproliferative diabetic retinopathy without macular edema
❼⇄	E11.341	Type 2 diabetes mellitus with severe nonproliferative diabetic retinopathy with macular edema
❼⇄	E11.349	Type 2 diabetes mellitus with severe nonproliferative diabetic retinopathy without macular edema
❼⇄	E11.351	Type 2 diabetes mellitus with proliferative diabetic retinopathy with macular edema
❼⇄	E11.352	Type 2 diabetes mellitus with proliferative diabetic retinopathy with traction retinal detachment involving the macula
❼⇄	E11.353	Type 2 diabetes mellitus with proliferative diabetic retinopathy with traction retinal detachment not involving the macula
❼⇄	E11.354	Type 2 diabetes mellitus with proliferative diabetic retinopathy with combined traction retinal detachment and rhegmatogenous retinal detachment
❼⇄	E11.355	Type 2 diabetes mellitus with stable proliferative diabetic retinopathy
❼⇄	E11.359	Type 2 diabetes mellitus with proliferative diabetic retinopathy without macular edema
⇄	H34.8311	Tributary (branch) retinal vein occlusion, right eye, with retinal neovascularization
⇄	H35.021	Exudative retinopathy, right eye
⇄	H35.022	Exudative retinopathy, left eye
⇄	H35.032	Hypertensive retinopathy, left eye
⇄	H35.052	Retinal neovascularization, unspecified, left eye
⇄	H35.061	Retinal vasculitis, right eye
⇄	H35.062	Retinal vasculitis, left eye
⇄	H35.171	Retrolental fibroplasia, right eye
⇄	H35.21	Other non-diabetic proliferative retinopathy, right eye
⇄	H35.22	Other non-diabetic proliferative retinopathy, left eye
⇄	H43.11	Vitreous hemorrhage, right eye
⇄	H43.12	Vitreous hemorrhage, left eye
⇄	H54.1131	Blindness right eye category 3, low vision left eye category 1
⇄	H54.1132	Blindness right eye category 3, low vision left eye category 2
⇄	H54.1141	Blindness right eye category 4, low vision left eye category 1
⇄	H54.1142	Blindness right eye category 4, low vision left eye category 2
⇄	H54.1151	Blindness right eye category 5, low vision left eye category 1
⇄	H54.1152	Blindness right eye category 5, low vision left eye category 2
⇄	H54.1213	Low vision right eye category 1, blindness left eye category 3
⇄	H54.1214	Low vision right eye category 1, blindness left eye category 4
⇄	H54.1215	Low vision right eye category 1, blindness left eye category 5
⇄	H54.1223	Low vision right eye category 2, blindness left eye category 3
⇄	H54.1224	Low vision right eye category 2, blindness left eye category 4
⇄	H54.1225	Low vision right eye category 2, blindness left eye category 5
⇄	H54.2X11	Low vision right eye category 1, low vision left eye category 1
⇄	H54.2X12	Low vision right eye category 1, low vision left eye category 2
⇄	H54.2X21	Low vision right eye category 2, low vision left eye category 1
⇄	H54.2X22	Low vision right eye category 2, low vision left eye category 2
	H54.3	Unqualified visual loss, both eyes
⇄	H54.413A	Blindness right eye category 3, normal vision left eye
⇄	H54.414A	Blindness right eye category 4, normal vision left eye
⇄	H54.415A	Blindness right eye category 5, normal vision left eye
⇄	H54.42A3	Blindness left eye category 3, normal vision right eye
⇄	H54.42A4	Blindness left eye category 4, normal vision right eye
⇄	H54.42A5	Blindness left eye category 5, normal vision right eye
⇄	H54.511A	Low vision right eye category 1, normal vision left eye
⇄	H54.512A	Low vision right eye category 2, normal vision left eye
⇄	H54.52A1	Low vision left eye category 1, normal vision right eye
⇄	H54.52A2	Low vision left eye category 2, normal vision right eye
⇄	H54.61	Unqualified visual loss, right eye, normal vision left eye
	H54.8	Legal blindness, as defined in USA

ICD-10-CM Coding Notes

For codes requiring a 7th character extension, refer to your ICD-10-CM book. Review the character descriptions and coding guidelines for proper selection. For some procedures, only certain characters will apply.

CCI Edits

Refer to Appendix A for CCI edits.

Facility RVUs ▯

Code	Work	PE Facility	MP	Total Facility
67227	3.50	3.58	0.25	7.33

Non-facility RVUs ▯

Code	Work	PE Non-Facility	MP	Total Non-Facility
67227	3.50	4.83	0.25	8.58

Modifiers (PAR) ▯

Code	Mod 50	Mod 51	Mod 62	Mod 66	Mod 80
67227	1	2	0	0	1

Global Period

Code	Days
67227	010

67228

67228 Treatment of extensive or progressive retinopathy (eg, diabetic retinopathy), photocoagulation

AMA Coding Guideline

Destruction Procedures on the Retina or Choroid

Codes 67208, 67210, 67218, 67220, 67229 include treatment at one or more sessions that may occur at different encounters. These codes should be reported once during a defined treatment period.

AMA Coding Notes

Surgical Procedures on the Eye and Ocular Adnexa

(For diagnostic and treatment ophthalmological services, see Medicine, Ophthalmology, and 92002 et seq)

(Do not report code 69990 in addition to codes 65091-68850)

AMA *CPT® Assistant* ▢

67228: Mar 98: 7, Oct 08: 3

Plain English Description

Extensive or progressive retinopathy (diabetic retinopathy) is destroyed using extreme cold (cryotherapy) or extreme heat (diathermy) in 67227, or treated using photocoagulation in 67228. Extensive or progressive (diabetic) retinopathy is characterized by damage to the blood vessels, which swell and leak blood or cause new blood vessels to form on the surface of the retina. Visual acuity is checked. The pupil is dilated and a local anesthetic is administered. The cryoprobe or diathermy probe is briefly placed on the surface of the eye overlying the periphery of the retina and the damaged blood vessels are destroyed by freezing or heat. When laser photocoagulation is used for treatment, it is administered by a technique referred to as scatter laser treatment or pan retinal photocoagulation (PRP), in which as many as 2,000 burns are placed in the mid-periphery and periphery of the retina, taking care to avoid the area of central vision, the macula. The burns destroy oxygen-deprived retinal tissue, seal leaking blood vessels, and prevent the formation of new blood vessels. The procedure may be performed using a slit lamp delivery system, which requires placement of a fundus contact lens, or indirect delivery system.

Treatment of extensive/progressive retinopathy, photocoagulation

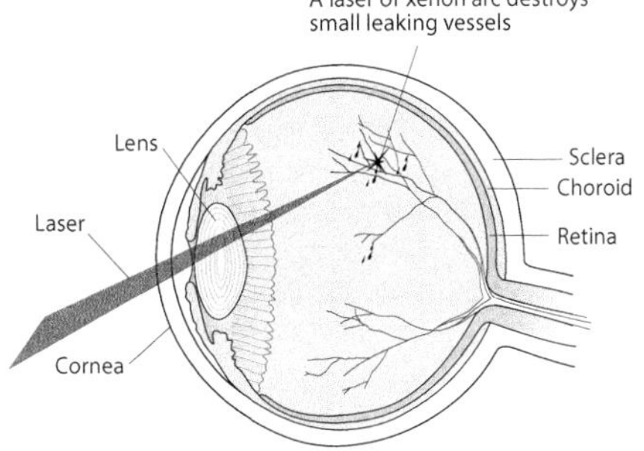

ICD-10-CM Diagnostic Codes

❼⇄ E08.331	Diabetes mellitus due to underlying condition with moderate nonproliferative diabetic retinopathy with macular edema
❼⇄ E08.339	Diabetes mellitus due to underlying condition with moderate nonproliferative diabetic retinopathy without macular edema
❼⇄ E08.341	Diabetes mellitus due to underlying condition with severe nonproliferative diabetic retinopathy with macular edema
❼⇄ E08.349	Diabetes mellitus due to underlying condition with severe nonproliferative diabetic retinopathy without macular edema
❼⇄ E08.351	Diabetes mellitus due to underlying condition with proliferative diabetic retinopathy with macular edema
❼⇄ E08.352	Diabetes mellitus due to underlying condition with proliferative diabetic retinopathy with traction retinal detachment involving the macula
❼⇄ E08.353	Diabetes mellitus due to underlying condition with proliferative diabetic retinopathy with traction retinal detachment not involving the macula
❼⇄ E08.354	Diabetes mellitus due to underlying condition with proliferative diabetic retinopathy with combined traction retinal detachment and rhegmatogenous retinal detachment
❼⇄ E08.355	Diabetes mellitus due to underlying condition with stable proliferative diabetic retinopathy
❼⇄ E08.359	Diabetes mellitus due to underlying condition with proliferative diabetic retinopathy without macular edema
❼⇄ E09.331	Drug or chemical induced diabetes mellitus with moderate nonproliferative diabetic retinopathy with macular edema
❼⇄ E09.339	Drug or chemical induced diabetes mellitus with moderate nonproliferative diabetic retinopathy without macular edema
❼⇄ E09.341	Drug or chemical induced diabetes mellitus with severe nonproliferative diabetic retinopathy with macular edema
❼⇄ E09.349	Drug or chemical induced diabetes mellitus with severe nonproliferative diabetic retinopathy without macular edema
❼⇄ E09.351	Drug or chemical induced diabetes mellitus with proliferative diabetic retinopathy with macular edema
❼⇄ E09.352	Drug or chemical induced diabetes mellitus with proliferative diabetic retinopathy with traction retinal detachment involving the macula
❼⇄ E09.353	Drug or chemical induced diabetes mellitus with proliferative diabetic retinopathy with traction retinal detachment not involving the macula
❼⇄ E09.354	Drug or chemical induced diabetes mellitus with proliferative diabetic retinopathy with combined traction retinal detachment and rhegmatogenous retinal detachment
❼⇄ E09.355	Drug or chemical induced diabetes mellitus with stable proliferative diabetic retinopathy
❼⇄ E09.359	Drug or chemical induced diabetes mellitus with proliferative diabetic retinopathy without macular edema
❼⇄ E10.331	Type 1 diabetes mellitus with moderate nonproliferative diabetic retinopathy with macular edema
❼⇄ E10.339	Type 1 diabetes mellitus with moderate nonproliferative diabetic retinopathy without macular edema
❼⇄ E10.341	Type 1 diabetes mellitus with severe nonproliferative diabetic retinopathy with macular edema
❼⇄ E10.349	Type 1 diabetes mellitus with severe nonproliferative diabetic retinopathy without macular edema
❼⇄ E10.351	Type 1 diabetes mellitus with proliferative diabetic retinopathy with macular edema
❼⇄ E10.352	Type 1 diabetes mellitus with proliferative diabetic retinopathy with traction retinal detachment involving the macula
❼⇄ E10.353	Type 1 diabetes mellitus with proliferative diabetic retinopathy with traction retinal detachment not involving the macula
❼⇄ E10.354	Type 1 diabetes mellitus with proliferative diabetic retinopathy with combined traction retinal detachment and rhegmatogenous retinal detachment
❼⇄ E10.355	Type 1 diabetes mellitus with stable proliferative diabetic retinopathy
❼⇄ E10.359	Type 1 diabetes mellitus with proliferative diabetic retinopathy without macular edema
❼⇄ E11.331	Type 2 diabetes mellitus with moderate nonproliferative diabetic retinopathy with macular edema
❼⇄ E11.339	Type 2 diabetes mellitus with moderate nonproliferative diabetic retinopathy without macular edema

❼⇄	E11.341	Type 2 diabetes mellitus with severe nonproliferative diabetic retinopathy with macular edema
❼⇄	E11.349	Type 2 diabetes mellitus with severe nonproliferative diabetic retinopathy without macular edema
❼⇄	E11.351	Type 2 diabetes mellitus with proliferative diabetic retinopathy with macular edema
❼⇄	E11.352	Type 2 diabetes mellitus with proliferative diabetic retinopathy with traction retinal detachment involving the macula
❼⇄	E11.353	Type 2 diabetes mellitus with proliferative diabetic retinopathy with traction retinal detachment not involving the macula
❼⇄	E11.354	Type 2 diabetes mellitus with proliferative diabetic retinopathy with combined traction retinal detachment and rhegmatogenous retinal detachment
❼⇄	E11.355	Type 2 diabetes mellitus with stable proliferative diabetic retinopathy
❼⇄	E11.359	Type 2 diabetes mellitus with proliferative diabetic retinopathy without macular edema
⇄	H35.022	Exudative retinopathy, left eye
⇄	H35.032	Hypertensive retinopathy, left eye
⇄	H35.052	Retinal neovascularization, unspecified, left eye
⇄	H35.062	Retinal vasculitis, left eye
⇄	H35.22	Other non-diabetic proliferative retinopathy, left eye
⇄	H43.12	Vitreous hemorrhage, left eye
⇄	H54.1131	Blindness right eye category 3, low vision left eye category 1
⇄	H54.1132	Blindness right eye category 3, low vision left eye category 2
⇄	H54.1141	Blindness right eye category 4, low vision left eye category 1
⇄	H54.1142	Blindness right eye category 4, low vision left eye category 2
⇄	H54.1151	Blindness right eye category 5, low vision left eye category 1
⇄	H54.1152	Blindness right eye category 5, low vision left eye category 2
⇄	H54.1213	Low vision right eye category 1, blindness left eye category 3
⇄	H54.1214	Low vision right eye category 1, blindness left eye category 4
⇄	H54.1215	Low vision right eye category 1, blindness left eye category 5
⇄	H54.1223	Low vision right eye category 2, blindness left eye category 3
⇄	H54.1224	Low vision right eye category 2, blindness left eye category 4
⇄	H54.1225	Low vision right eye category 2, blindness left eye category 5
⇄	H54.2X11	Low vision right eye category 1, low vision left eye category 1
⇄	H54.2X12	Low vision right eye category 1, low vision left eye category 2
⇄	H54.2X21	Low vision right eye category 2, low vision left eye category 1
⇄	H54.2X22	Low vision right eye category 2, low vision left eye category 2
	H54.3	Unqualified visual loss, both eyes
⇄	H54.413A	Blindness right eye category 3, normal vision left eye
⇄	H54.414A	Blindness right eye category 4, normal vision left eye
⇄	H54.415A	Blindness right eye category 5, normal vision left eye
⇄	H54.42A3	Blindness left eye category 3, normal vision right eye
⇄	H54.42A4	Blindness left eye category 4, normal vision right eye
⇄	H54.42A5	Blindness left eye category 5, normal vision right eye
⇄	H54.511A	Low vision right eye category 1, normal vision left eye
⇄	H54.512A	Low vision right eye category 2, normal vision left eye
⇄	H54.52A1	Low vision left eye category 1, normal vision right eye
⇄	H54.52A2	Low vision left eye category 2, normal vision right eye
	H54.8	Legal blindness, as defined in USA

ICD-10-CM Coding Notes

For codes requiring a 7th character extension, refer to your ICD-10-CM book. Review the character descriptions and coding guidelines for proper selection. For some procedures, only certain characters will apply.

CCI Edits

Refer to Appendix A for CCI edits.

Facility RVUs ☐

Code	Work	PE Facility	MP	Total Facility
67228	4.39	4.04	0.34	8.77

Non-facility RVUs ☐

Code	Work	PE Non-Facility	MP	Total Non-Facility
67228	4.39	5.14	0.34	9.87

Modifiers (PAR) ☐

Code	Mod 50	Mod 51	Mod 62	Mod 66	Mod 80
67228	1	2	0	0	1

Global Period

Code	Days
67228	010

67229

67229 Treatment of extensive or progressive retinopathy, 1 or more sessions, preterm infant (less than 37 weeks gestation at birth), performed from birth up to 1 year of age (eg, retinopathy of prematurity), photocoagulation or cryotherapy

(For bilateral procedure, use modifier 50 with 67208, 67210, 67218, 67220, 67227, 67228, 67229)

(For unlisted procedures on retina, use 67299)

AMA Coding Guideline

Destruction Procedures on the Retina or Choroid

Codes 67208, 67210, 67218, 67220, 67229 include treatment at one or more sessions that may occur at different encounters. These codes should be reported once during a defined treatment period.

AMA Coding Notes

Surgical Procedures on the Eye and Ocular Adnexa

(For diagnostic and treatment ophthalmological services, see Medicine, Ophthalmology, and 92002 et seq)

(Do not report code 69990 in addition to codes 65091-68850)

Plain English Description

Extensive progressive retinopathy of a preterm infant (retinopathy of prematurity) is treated by photocoagulation or cryotherapy in one or more sessions. A preterm infant is defined as being less than 37 weeks gestation at birth. The procedure may be performed from birth up to one year of age. Retinopathy of prematurity (ROP), also referred to as retrolental fibroplasia, primarily affects premature infants that are less than 31 weeks gestation and weigh less than 1250 grams (2.75 pounds) at birth. ROP is characterized by the failure of blood vessels in the retina to reach the periphery and an abnormal proliferation of blood vessels where they terminate. These fragile blood vessels may leak, causing scarring and traction on the retina that may cause it to detach, resulting in vision impairment or blindness. A topical anesthetic is administered. Mydriatic drops are applied to dilate the pupil as needed. Scleral depression is applied to position the eye. Regions of normal, abnormal, and absent vascularization are identified. If cryotherapy (freezing) is used to destroy the abnormal vasculature or avascular regions in the retina, a cryoprobe is briefly placed on the surface of the eye overlying the regions of abnormal or absent vasculature in the retina. If laser photocoagulation is used, as many as 1,500 burns may be applied to the abnormal vasculature or avascular regions in the retina using an indirect ophthalmoscopic laser delivery system. Care is taken to avoid damage to the iris and crystalline lens. Both laser treatment and cryotherapy destroy the peripheral areas of the retina that have no normal vasculature. Care is taken to preserve the area of central vision (macula).

Treatment of extensive/progressive retinopathy, photocoagulation

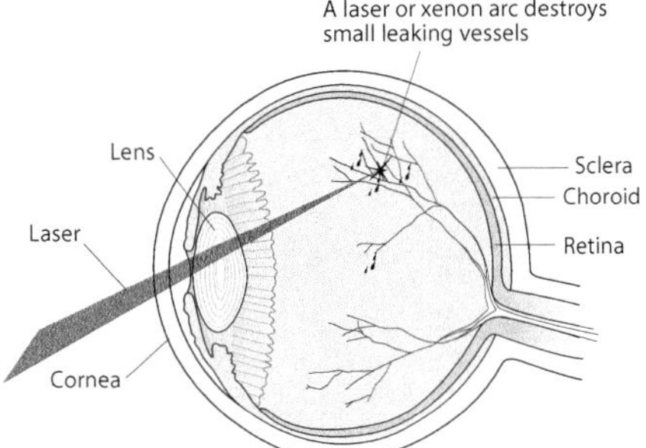

Photocoagulation/cryotherapy preterm infant (67229)

ICD-10-CM Diagnostic Codes

	Code	Description
⇄	H35.101	Retinopathy of prematurity, unspecified, right eye
⇄	H35.111	Retinopathy of prematurity, stage 0, right eye
⇄	H35.121	Retinopathy of prematurity, stage 1, right eye
⇄	H35.131	Retinopathy of prematurity, stage 2, right eye
⇄	H35.141	Retinopathy of prematurity, stage 3, right eye
⇄	H35.151	Retinopathy of prematurity, stage 4, right eye
⇄	H35.161	Retinopathy of prematurity, stage 5, right eye
⇄	H35.171	Retrolental fibroplasia, right eye
⇄	H35.21	Other non-diabetic proliferative retinopathy, right eye
	P07.00	Extremely low birth weight newborn, unspecified weight
	P07.01	Extremely low birth weight newborn, less than 500 grams
	P07.02	Extremely low birth weight newborn, 500-749 grams
	P07.03	Extremely low birth weight newborn, 750-999 grams
	P07.10	Other low birth weight newborn, unspecified weight
	P07.14	Other low birth weight newborn, 1000-1249 grams
	P07.15	Other low birth weight newborn, 1250-1499 grams
	P07.16	Other low birth weight newborn, 1500-1749 grams
	P07.17	Other low birth weight newborn, 1750-1999 grams
	P07.18	Other low birth weight newborn, 2000-2499 grams
	P07.20	Extreme immaturity of newborn, unspecified weeks of gestation
	P07.21	Extreme immaturity of newborn, gestational age less than 23 completed weeks
	P07.22	Extreme immaturity of newborn, gestational age 23 completed weeks
	P07.23	Extreme immaturity of newborn, gestational age 24 completed weeks
	P07.24	Extreme immaturity of newborn, gestational age 25 completed weeks
	P07.25	Extreme immaturity of newborn, gestational age 26 completed weeks
	P07.26	Extreme immaturity of newborn, gestational age 27 completed weeks
	P07.30	Preterm newborn, unspecified weeks of gestation
	P07.31	Preterm newborn, gestational age 28 completed weeks
	P07.32	Preterm newborn, gestational age 29 completed weeks
	P07.33	Preterm newborn, gestational age 30 completed weeks
	P07.34	Preterm newborn, gestational age 31 completed weeks
	P07.35	Preterm newborn, gestational age 32 completed weeks
	P07.36	Preterm newborn, gestational age 33 completed weeks
	P07.37	Preterm newborn, gestational age 34 completed weeks
	P07.38	Preterm newborn, gestational age 35 completed weeks
	P07.39	Preterm newborn, gestational age 36 completed weeks

CCI Edits

Refer to Appendix A for CCI edits.

Facility RVUs ▢

Code	Work	PE Facility	MP	Total Facility
67229	16.30	15.93	1.26	33.49

Non-facility RVUs ▢

Code	Work	PE Non-Facility	MP	Total Non-Facility
67229	16.30	15.93	1.26	33.49

Modifiers (PAR) ▢

Code	Mod 50	Mod 51	Mod 62	Mod 66	Mod 80
67229	1	2	0	0	1

Global Period

Code	Days
67229	090

CPT® Procedural Coding

67250-67255

67250 Scleral reinforcement (separate procedure); without graft

67255 Scleral reinforcement (separate procedure); with graft

(Do not report 67255 in conjunction with 66180, 66185)

(For repair scleral staphyloma, use 66225)

AMA Coding Notes

Repair Procedures on the Posterior Sclera of the Eye

(For excision lesion sclera, use 66130)

Surgical Procedures on the Eye and Ocular Adnexa

(For diagnostic and treatment ophthalmological services, see Medicine, Ophthalmology, and 92002 et seq)

(Do not report code 69990 in addition to codes 65091-68850)

AMA *CPT® Assistant* ▢

67255: Jun 12: 15, Jan 15: 10

Plain English Description

Scleral reinforcement is performed in a separate procedure to treat high myopia and help prevent damage to the macula associated with this condition. A lid speculum is used to open the eyelids and expose the eye. Local anesthesia is administered. The conjunctiva and Tenon's capsule are incised about 6 mm from the corneal limbus. The lateral, superior and inferior recti muscles are separated using a strabismus hook. Connective tissue is dissected away from the posterior pole and inferior oblique muscle. In 67250, the sclera is reinforced without the use of a graft. This involves creating an indentation in the posterior aspect of the sclera. In this procedure, the thinned weakened region of the posterior sclera is oversewn with a thick piece of rubber or sponge material, which causes the posterior region to indent or buckle. A strip of synthetic material may be used to create a sling, which provides additional support of the posterior sclera. The sling is passed under the separated muscles along the posterior pole of the eye. The sling is sutured to the anteromedial and anterolateral sclera. In 67255, a graft is used to reinforce the sclera. Once the posterior aspect of the sclera has been exposed, an allograft, usually donor sclera, is used to reinforce the weak sclera at the back of the eye. The graft is sutured to the healthy, stronger anterior sclera. The muscles are repaired and the Tenon's capsule and conjunctive closed.

Scleral reinforcement with/without graft

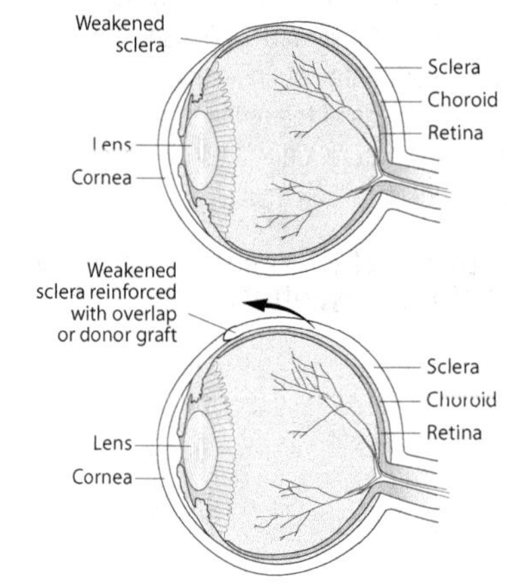

Sclera is incised and overlapped for reinforcement (67250); use code 67255 when a donor graft is used.

ICD-10-CM Diagnostic Codes

	Code	Description
	H35.40	Unspecified peripheral retinal degeneration
	H35.50	Unspecified hereditary retinal dystrophy
⇄	H43.812	Vitreous degeneration, left eye
⇄	H44.21	Degenerative myopia, right eye
⇄	H44.22	Degenerative myopia, left eye
⇄	H44.23	Degenerative myopia, bilateral
⇄	H44.2A1	Degenerative myopia with choroidal neovascularization, right eye
⇄	H44.2A2	Degenerative myopia with choroidal neovascularization, left eye
⇄	H44.2A3	Degenerative myopia with choroidal neovascularization, bilateral eye
⇄	H44.2B1	Degenerative myopia with macular hole, right eye
⇄	H44.2B2	Degenerative myopia with macular hole, left eye
⇄	H44.2B3	Degenerative myopia with macular hole, bilateral eye
⇄	H44.2C1	Degenerative myopia with retinal detachment, right eye
⇄	H44.2C2	Degenerative myopia with retinal detachment, left eye
⇄	H44.2C3	Degenerative myopia with retinal detachment, bilateral eye
⇄	H44.2D1	Degenerative myopia with foveoschisis, right eye
⇄	H44.2D2	Degenerative myopia with foveoschisis, left eye
⇄	H44.2D3	Degenerative myopia with foveoschisis, bilateral eye
⇄	H44.2E1	Degenerative myopia with other maculopathy, right eye
⇄	H44.2E2	Degenerative myopia with other maculopathy, left eye
⇄	H44.2E3	Degenerative myopia with other maculopathy, bilateral eye

CCI Edits

Refer to Appendix A for CCI edits.

Facility RVUs ▢

Code	Work	PE Facility	MP	Total Facility
67250	9.61	16.47	0.73	26.81
67255	8.38	10.92	0.65	19.95

Non-facility RVUs ▢

Code	Work	PE Non-Facility	MP	Total Non-Facility
67250	9.61	16.47	0.73	26.81
67255	8.38	10.92	0.65	19.95

Modifiers (PAR) ▢

Code	Mod 50	Mod 51	Mod 62	Mod 66	Mod 80
67250	1	2	1	0	1
67255	1	2	1	0	2

Global Period

Code	Days
67250	090
67255	090

67311-67316

67311 Strabismus surgery, recession or resection procedure; 1 horizontal muscle

67312 Strabismus surgery, recession or resection procedure; 2 horizontal muscles

67314 Strabismus surgery, recession or resection procedure; 1 vertical muscle (excluding superior oblique)

67316 Strabismus surgery, recession or resection procedure; 2 or more vertical muscles (excluding superior oblique)

(For adjustable sutures, use 67335 in addition to codes 67311-67334 for primary procedure reflecting number of muscles operated on)

AMA Coding Notes

Surgical Procedures on the Eye and Ocular Adnexa

(For diagnostic and treatment ophthalmological services, see Medicine, Ophthalmology, and 92002 et seq)

(Do not report code 69990 in addition to codes 65091-68850)

AMA *CPT® Assistant*

67311: Summer 93: 20, Mar 97: 5, Nov 98: 19, Sep 02: 10, Jan 17: 7

67312: Summer 93: 20, Mar 97: 5

67314: Summer 93: 20, Mar 97: 5

67316: Summer 93: 20, Mar 97: 5

Plain English Description

The eye has six extraocular muscles that control eye movement. If a muscle is too strong, it can cause the eye to turn in, turn out, or rotate too high or too low. If a muscle is too weak, the eyes may be misaligned. For an extraocular muscle that is too strong, a recession procedure of the affected eye is performed. For an extraocular muscle that is too weak, a recession procedure of the opposing eye is performed. In a recession procedure, the extraocular muscle is detached from the eye and reattached farther back on the eye to weaken the strength of the stronger muscle relative to the opposing weaker muscle. Alternatively a resection procedure may be used to strengthen an eye muscle and correct misalignment of the eye. Resection involves detaching the eye muscle from the eye and reattaching it in a new location. A small incision is made in the conjunctiva over the extraocular muscle. The muscle is detached from the globe. The eye muscle is then reattached with sutures farther back on the globe or in a new location to correct the misalignment of the eyes. The incision in the conjunctiva is closed. Use 67311 if recession or resection is performed on either the lateral or medial rectus muscle. Use 67312 if the procedure is performed on both the lateral and medial rectus muscle of the same eye. Use 67314 if the procedure is performed on either the superior or inferior rectus muscle. Use 67316 if the procedure is performed on both the superior and inferior rectus muscles of the same eye.

Strabismus surgery, recession/ resection, horizontal muscle

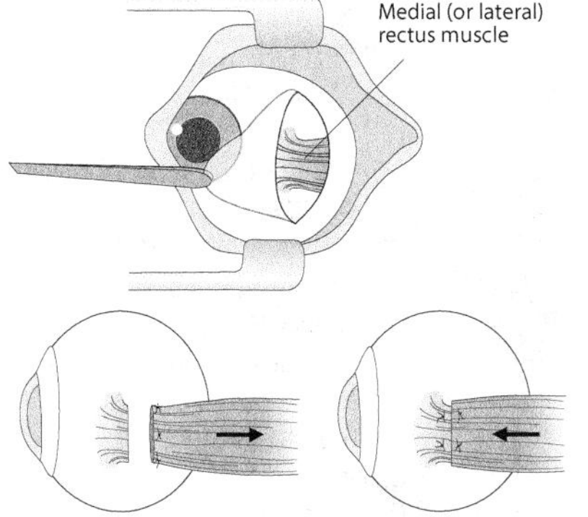

One (67311), or two (67312) horizontal muscles; either superior/inferior rectus muscle (67314); both superior/inferior rectus muscles (67316)

ICD-10-CM Diagnostic Codes

⇄	H49.01	Third [oculomotor] nerve palsy, right eye
⇄	H49.02	Third [oculomotor] nerve palsy, left eye
⇄	H49.03	Third [oculomotor] nerve palsy, bilateral
⇄	H49.21	Sixth [abducent] nerve palsy, right eye
⇄	H49.22	Sixth [abducent] nerve palsy, left eye
⇄	H49.23	Sixth [abducent] nerve palsy, bilateral
⇄	H50.011	Monocular esotropia, right eye
⇄	H50.021	Monocular esotropia with A pattern, right eye
⇄	H50.031	Monocular esotropia with V pattern, right eye
	H50.05	Alternating esotropia
⇄	H50.111	Monocular exotropia, right eye
⇄	H50.121	Monocular exotropia with A pattern, right eye
⇄	H50.131	Monocular exotropia with V pattern, right eye
⇄	H50.141	Monocular exotropia with other noncomitancies, right eye
	H50.15	Alternating exotropia
	H50.16	Alternating exotropia with A pattern
	H50.17	Alternating exotropia with V pattern
	H50.18	Alternating exotropia with other noncomitancies
⇄	H50.21	Vertical strabismus, right eye
⇄	H50.311	Intermittent monocular esotropia, right eye
	H50.32	Intermittent alternating esotropia
⇄	H50.331	Intermittent monocular exotropia, right eye
	H50.34	Intermittent alternating exotropia
	H50.43	Accommodative component in esotropia
	H50.89	Other specified strabismus
	H53.19	Other subjective visual disturbances
	H53.2	Diplopia
	R29.891	Ocular torticollis

CCI Edits

Refer to Appendix A for CCI edits.

Facility RVUs

Code	Work	PE Facility	MP	Total Facility
67311	5.93	7.61	0.44	13.98
67312	9.50	9.01	0.73	19.24
67314	5.93	9.63	0.44	16.00
67316	10.31	9.48	0.79	20.58

Non-facility RVUs

Code	Work	PE Non-Facility	MP	Total Non-Facility
67311	5.93	7.61	0.44	13.98
67312	9.50	9.01	0.73	19.24
67314	5.93	9.63	0.44	16.00
67316	10.31	9.48	0.79	20.58

Modifiers (PAR)

Code	Mod 50	Mod 51	Mod 62	Mod 66	Mod 80
67311	1	2	0	0	1
67312	1	2	1	0	1
67314	1	2	0	0	1
67316	1	2	0	0	0

Global Period

Code	Days
67311	090
67312	090
67314	090
67316	090

67318

67318 Strabismus surgery, any procedure, superior oblique muscle

AMA Coding Notes

Surgical Procedures on the Eye and Ocular Adnexa

(For diagnostic and treatment ophthalmological services, see Medicine, Ophthalmology, and 92002 et seq)

(Do not report code 69990 in addition to codes 65091-68850)

AMA *CPT® Assistant* ▢

67318: Summer 93: 20, Mar 97: 5, Nov 98: 19

Plain English Description

The superior oblique muscle of the eye attaches to the superolateral aspect of the globe, passes through a tendon called the trochlea at the medial (nasal) aspect of the orbit and then attaches to the posterior aspect of the orbit. Because this code is for any procedure on the superior oblique muscle the exact procedure performed will depend on the condition being treated. One procedure, called the Harada-Ito procedure, is used to treat misalignment of the eye due to cranial nerve IV palsy. An incision is made in the conjunctiva over the superior oblique muscle. The superior oblique tendon is split and the anterior fibers are moved in an anterior and lateral direction and reattached to the globe. The conjunctival incision is closed with sutures.

Strabismus surgery, any procedure; superior oblique muscle

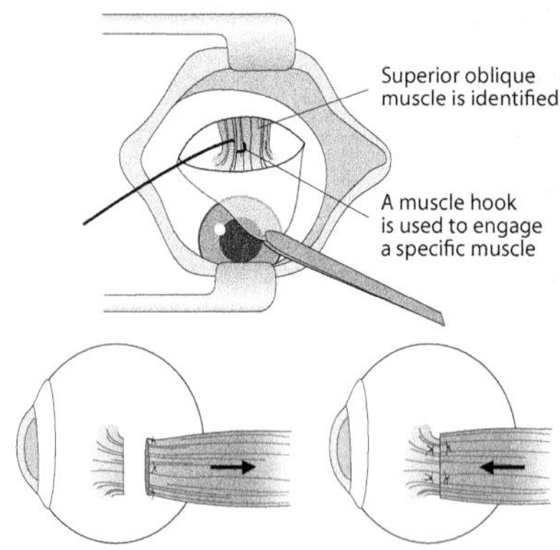
Superior oblique muscle is identified
A muscle hook is used to engage a specific muscle
Recession procedure
Resection procedure

The superior oblique muscle is adjusted.

ICD-10-CM Diagnostic Codes

⇄	H49.11	Fourth [trochlear] nerve palsy, right eye
⇄	H49.12	Fourth [trochlear] nerve palsy, left eye
⇄	H49.13	Fourth [trochlear] nerve palsy, bilateral
⇄	H49.41	Progressive external ophthalmoplegia, right eye
⇄	H49.42	Progressive external ophthalmoplegia, left eye
⇄	H49.43	Progressive external ophthalmoplegia, bilateral
⇄	H49.881	Other paralytic strabismus, right eye
⇄	H49.882	Other paralytic strabismus, left eye
⇄	H49.883	Other paralytic strabismus, bilateral
⇄	H50.021	Monocular esotropia with A pattern, right eye
⇄	H50.022	Monocular esotropia with A pattern, left eye
⇄	H50.121	Monocular exotropia with A pattern, right eye
⇄	H50.122	Monocular exotropia with A pattern, left eye
	H50.16	Alternating exotropia with A pattern
⇄	H50.21	Vertical strabismus, right eye
⇄	H50.22	Vertical strabismus, left eye
⇄	H50.411	Cyclotropia, right eye
⇄	H50.412	Cyclotropia, left eye
⇄	H50.611	Brown's sheath syndrome, right eye
⇄	H50.612	Brown's sheath syndrome, left eye
	H53.2	Diplopia
	R29.891	Ocular torticollis

CCI Edits

Refer to Appendix A for CCI edits.

Facility RVUs ▢

Code	Work	PE Facility	MP	Total Facility
67318	9.80	9.36	0.75	19.91

Non-facility RVUs ▢

Code	Work	PE Non-Facility	MP	Total Non-Facility
67318	9.80	9.36	0.75	19.91

Modifiers (PAR) ▢

Code	Mod 50	Mod 51	Mod 62	Mod 66	Mod 80
67318	1	2	1	0	1

Global Period

Code	Days
67318	090

67320

✚ **67320 Transposition procedure (eg, for paretic extraocular muscle), any extraocular muscle (specify) (List separately in addition to code for primary procedure)**

(Use 67320 in conjunction with 67311-67318)

AMA Coding Notes

Surgical Procedures on the Eye and Ocular Adnexa

(For diagnostic and treatment ophthalmological services, see Medicine, Ophthalmology, and 92002 et seq)

(Do not report code 69990 in addition to codes 65091-68850)

AMA *CPT® Assistant*

67320: Summer 93: 20, Mar 97: 5

Plain English Description

Transposition of the extraocular muscles involves detaching and moving an extraocular muscle to a new location on the globe. This type of procedure is performed at the time of another separately reportable strabismus procedure. It may be performed to treat paralysis or paresis of an extraocular muscle caused by damage to one of the cranial nerves (CN III, CN IV, or CN VI). A conjunctival incision is made over the extraocular muscle or muscles that are to be detached. The muscle(s) is detached from the globe, moved to a new position, and secured to the globe with sutures. The conjunctival incision is closed.

Transposition procedure, any extraocular muscle

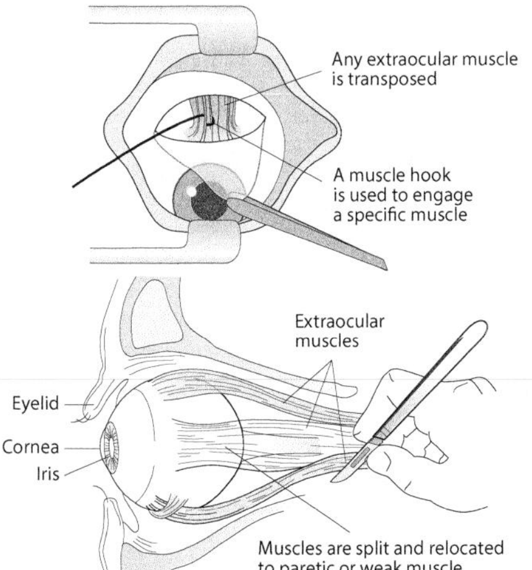
Any extraocular muscle is transposed
A muscle hook is used to engage a specific muscle
Extraocular muscles
Eyelid
Cornea
Iris
Muscles are split and relocated to paretic or weak muscle

ICD-10-CM Diagnostic Codes

See Primary Procedure code for crosswalks.

CCI Edits

Refer to Appendix A for CCI edits.

Facility RVUs

Code	Work	PE Facility	MP	Total Facility
67320	3.00	4.16	0.23	7.39

Non-facility RVUs

Code	Work	PE Non-Facility	MP	Total Non-Facility
67320	3.00	4.16	0.23	7.39

Modifiers (PAR)

Code	Mod 50	Mod 51	Mod 62	Mod 66	Mod 80
67320	0	0	0	0	1

Global Period

Code	Days
67320	ZZZ

67331-67332

✚ **67331 Strabismus surgery on patient with previous eye surgery or injury that did not involve the extraocular muscles (List separately in addition to code for primary procedure)**

(Use 67331 in conjunction with 67311-67318)

✚ **67332 Strabismus surgery on patient with scarring of extraocular muscles (eg, prior ocular injury, strabismus or retinal detachment surgery) or restrictive myopathy (eg, dysthyroid ophthalmopathy) (List separately in addition to code for primary procedure)**

(Use 67332 in conjunction with 67311-67318)

AMA Coding Notes

Surgical Procedures on the Eye and Ocular Adnexa

(For diagnostic and treatment ophthalmological services, see Medicine, Ophthalmology, and 92002 et seq)

(Do not report code 69990 in addition to codes 65091-68850)

AMA *CPT® Assistant* ▯

67331: Summer 93: 20, Mar 97: 5

67332: Summer 93: 20, Mar 97: 5

Plain English Description

Strabismus surgery on a patient who has had a previous procedure on the eye is technically more difficult. An incision is made in the conjunctiva over the affected extraocular muscle and the muscle insertion site is exposed. Scar tissue and adhesions are released and old suture material removed as needed. The separately reportable recession, resection or other strabismus procedure on the eye is then performed. Use 67331 for strabismus surgery on a patient with previous eye surgery or an eye injury that did not involve the extraocular muscles Use 67332 for strabismus surgery on a patient with scarring of the extraocular muscles due to previous ocular injury or strabismus or retinal detachment surgery on patients with restrictive myopathy.

Strabismus surgery, on patient with previous eye surgery/injury

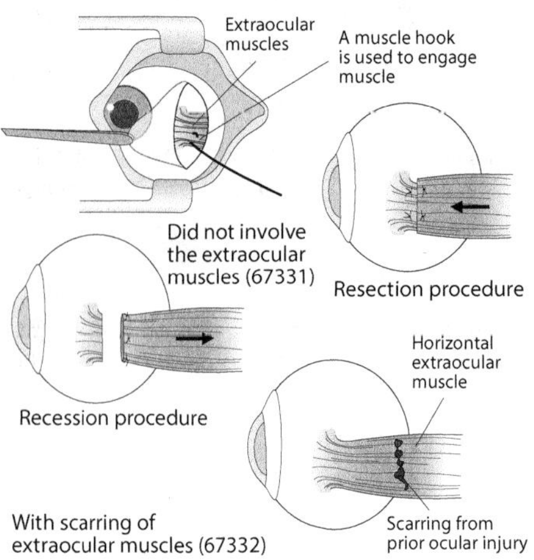

ICD-10-CM Diagnostic Codes

See Primary Procedure code for crosswalks.

CCI Edits

Refer to Appendix A for CCI edits.

Facility RVUs ▯

Code	Work	PE Facility	MP	Total Facility
67331	2.00	4.85	0.17	7.02
67332	3.50	3.86	0.25	7.61

Non-facility RVUs ▯

Code	Work	PE Non-Facility	MP	Total Non-Facility
67331	2.00	4.85	0.17	7.02
67332	3.50	3.86	0.25	7.61

Modifiers (PAR) ▯

Code	Mod 50	Mod 51	Mod 62	Mod 66	Mod 80
67331	1	0	1	0	1
67332	1	0	1	0	1

Global Period

Code	Days
67331	ZZZ
67332	ZZZ

67334-67335

✚ **67334 Strabismus surgery by posterior fixation suture technique, with or without muscle recession (List separately in addition to code for primary procedure)**

(Use 67334 in conjunction with 67311-67318)

✚ **67335 Placement of adjustable suture(s) during strabismus surgery, including postoperative adjustment(s) of suture(s) (List separately in addition to code for specific strabismus surgery)**

(Use 67335 in conjunction with 67311-67334)

AMA Coding Notes

Surgical Procedures on the Eye and Ocular Adnexa

(For diagnostic and treatment ophthalmological services, see Medicine, Ophthalmology, and 92002 et seq)

(Do not report code 69990 in addition to codes 65091-68850)

AMA *CPT® Assistant* ▯

67334: Summer 93: 20, Mar 97: 5
67335: Summer 93: 20, Mar 97: 5

Plain English Description

Two suture techniques that are sometimes used for strabismus surgery and increase the technical difficulty of the procedure include posterior fixation suture technique and adjustable sutures. In 67334, posterior fixation suture is performed. This suture technique is used to limit the action of the extraocular muscle or make the muscle work harder in its field of action without changing the primary position of the muscle. Posterior fixation suturing is usually used in the fixing eye. The extra work required of the muscle in the fixing eye causes extra innervation and has a straightening effect on the fellow eye. The eye muscle is exposed in a separately reportable primary procedure. Once the necessary components of the primary procedure have been completed the physician places posterior fixation sutures through the borders of the extraocular muscle. If posterior fixation is required on the lateral rectus muscle, the inferior oblique insertion is dissected from the lateral rectus muscle and the sutures are then placed. If posterior fixation is performed on the superior rectus, the fixation suture is placed behind the superior oblique muscle. If posterior fixation is performed on the inferior rectus, the inferior oblique and Lockwood's ligament are retracted and the fixation sutures placed. The primary procedure is completed and the operative incisions are closed. In 67335, adjustable sutures are placed. The eye muscle is exposed and a separately reportable recession or resection procedure is performed. Instead of placing permanent knots in the sutures, the physician places temporary suture knots. The physician then evaluates the eyes several hours after the surgery. Anesthetic eye drops are applied. If the eye alignment is good, permanent knots are tied. If the eye needs some additional realignment, the adjustable suture is used to modify the muscle tension. Once the eyes are aligned, permanent knots are tied.

Strabismus surgery by posterior fixation suture technique; placement of adjustable suture(s) during strabismus surgery

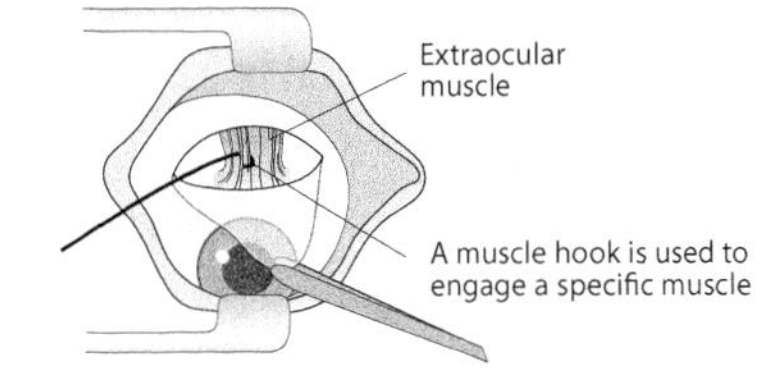
Extraocular muscle
A muscle hook is used to engage a specific muscle

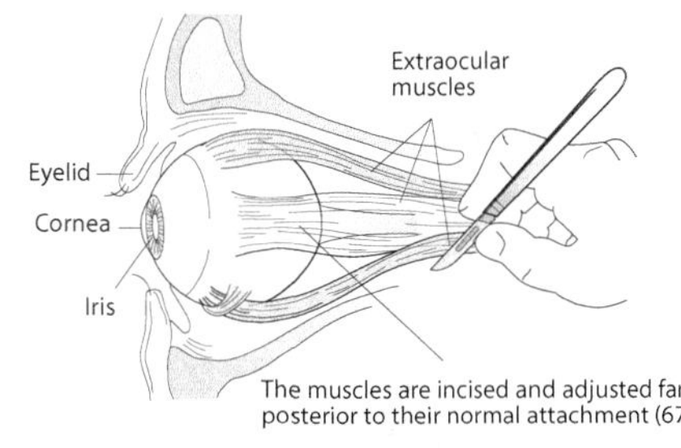
Extraocular muscles
Eyelid
Cornea
Iris
The muscles are incised and adjusted far posterior to their normal attachment (67334).

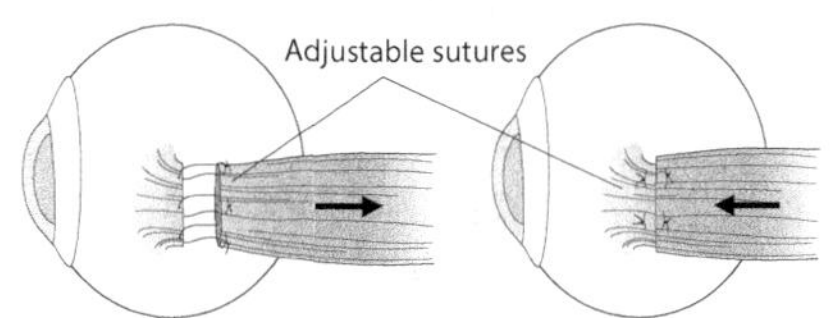
Adjustable sutures

Adjustable sutures are placed during strabismus surgery that are re-adjusted after anesthesia has worn off (67335).

ICD-10-CM Diagnostic Codes

See Primary Procedure code for crosswalks.

CCI Edits

Refer to Appendix A for CCI edits.

Facility RVUs ▯

Code	Work	PE Facility	MP	Total Facility
67334	2.06	4.69	0.17	6.92
67335	3.23	1.96	0.25	5.44

Non-facility RVUs ▯

Code	Work	PE Non-Facility	MP	Total Non-Facility
67334	2.06	4.69	0.17	6.92
67335	3.23	1.96	0.25	5.44

Modifiers (PAR) ▯

Code	Mod 50	Mod 51	Mod 62	Mod 66	Mod 80
67334	1	0	1	0	1
67335	1	0	1	0	1

Global Period

Code	Days
67334	ZZZ
67335	ZZZ

67340

+ 67340 Strabismus surgery involving exploration and/or repair of detached extraocular muscle(s) (List separately in addition to code for primary procedure)

(Use 67340 in conjunction with 67311-67334)

AMA Coding Notes

Surgical Procedures on the Eye and Ocular Adnexa

(For diagnostic and treatment ophthalmological services, see Medicine, Ophthalmology, and 92002 et seq)

(Do not report code 69990 in addition to codes 65091-68850)

AMA *CPT® Assistant* ☐

67340: Summer 93: 20, Mar 97: 5

Plain English Description

During a separately reportable primary strabismus surgery, the physician explores the eye to find a detached extraocular muscle and/or repair it. Extraocular muscles may become detached following a previous recession or resection procedure, due to facial or ocular trauma, or during a surgical misadventure. The conjunctiva is incised over the affected extraocular muscle. Often there is extensive scar tissue from previous surgeries or from the eye injury that must be dissected. The orbit is explored and an attempt made to locate the eye muscle. If the eye muscle cannot be retrieved a separately reportable transposition procedure may be required. If the eye muscle is located it is carefully inspected to determine if it can be reattached. If it cannot be reattached due to traumatic injury or damage from previous surgeries, a separately reportable transposition procedure is performed. If it can be reattached the muscle is debrided and sutured to any remaining muscle at the insertion site or sutured to the globe in a new location. The primary strabismus procedure is then completed.

Strabismus surgery; exploration/repair detached extraocular muscle(s)

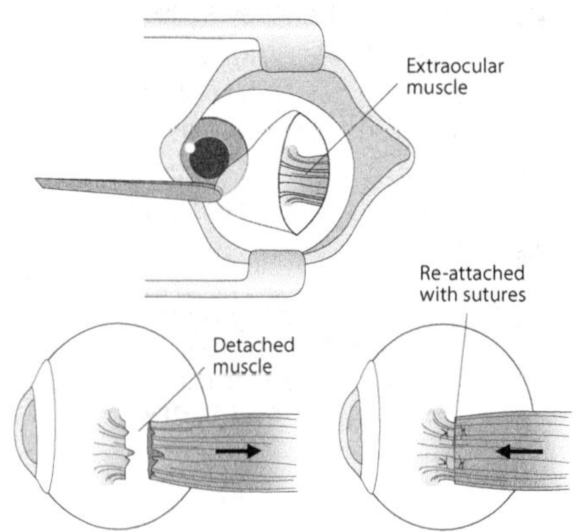

Extensive dissection may be necessary to locate and retrieve the detached muscle.

ICD-10-CM Diagnostic Codes

See Primary Procedure code for crosswalks.

CCI Edits

Refer to Appendix A for CCI edits.

Facility RVUs ☐

Code	Work	PE Facility	MP	Total Facility
67340	5.00	3.08	0.39	8.47

Non-facility RVUs ☐

Code	Work	PE Non-Facility	MP	Total Non-Facility
67340	5.00	3.08	0.39	8.47

Modifiers (PAR) ☐

Code	Mod 50	Mod 51	Mod 62	Mod 66	Mod 80
67340	0	0	0	0	2

Global Period

Code	Days
67340	ZZZ

67343

67343 Release of extensive scar tissue without detaching extraocular muscle (separate procedure)

(Use 67343 in conjunction with 67311-67340, when such procedures are performed other than on the affected muscle)

AMA Coding Notes

Surgical Procedures on the Eye and Ocular Adnexa

(For diagnostic and treatment ophthalmological services, see Medicine, Ophthalmology, and 92002 et seq)

(Do not report code 69990 in addition to codes 65091-68850)

AMA *CPT® Assistant*

67343: Summer 93: 20, Mar 97: 5

Plain English Description

Eye movement may be affected by extensive scar tissue from a previous injury or previous eye surgery. An incision is made over the affected extraocular muscle. The muscle is exposed and inspected. Leaving the eye muscle attached to the globe, the surgeon addresses the scar tissue that is causing the impaired eye movement. Adhesions between the eye muscle and surrounding structures are lysed. The conjunctiva is closed.

Release of extensive scar tissue without detaching extraocular muscle

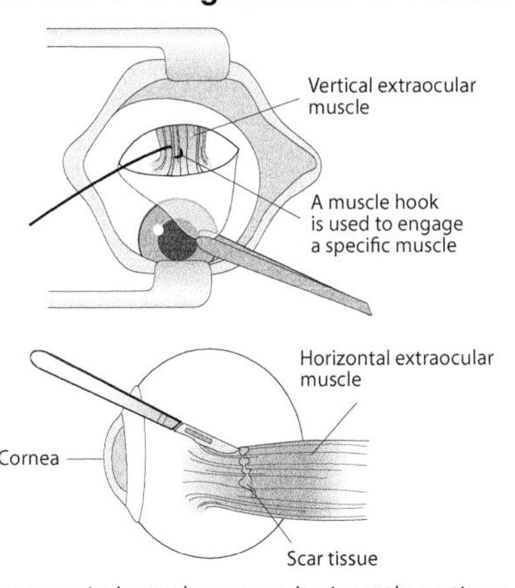

During a vertical muscle surgery, horizontal scar tissue is excised, or during horizontal surgery, vertical scar tissue is excised.

ICD-10-CM Diagnostic Codes

	H01.8	Other specified inflammations of eyelid
	H02.89	Other specified disorders of eyelid
⇄	H50.012	Monocular esotropia, left eye
	H50.05	Alternating esotropia
	H50.10	Unspecified exotropia
⇄	H50.112	Monocular exotropia, left eye
⇄	H50.22	Vertical strabismus, left eye
⇄	H50.312	Intermittent monocular esotropia, left eye
	H50.60	Mechanical strabismus, unspecified
	H50.69	Other mechanical strabismus
	H53.2	Diplopia
⇄	H57.12	Ocular pain, left eye
	H57.89	Other specified disorders of eye and adnexa
	M35.4	Diffuse (eosinophilic) fasciitis
	M62.28	Nontraumatic ischemic infarction of muscle, other site
❼⇄	S01.112	Laceration without foreign body of left eyelid and periocular area
❼⇄	S01.122	Laceration with foreign body of left eyelid and periocular area
❼⇄	S01.132	Puncture wound without foreign body of left eyelid and periocular area
❼⇄	S01.142	Puncture wound with foreign body of left eyelid and periocular area
❼⇄	S01.152	Open bite of left eyelid and periocular area
❼	T81.89	Other complications of procedures, not elsewhere classified

ICD-10-CM Coding Notes

For codes requiring a 7th character extension, refer to your ICD-10-CM book. Review the character descriptions and coding guidelines for proper selection. For some procedures, only certain characters will apply.

CCI Edits

Refer to Appendix A for CCI edits.

Facility RVUs

Code	Work	PE Facility	MP	Total Facility
67343	8.47	10.28	0.67	19.42

Non-facility RVUs

Code	Work	PE Non-Facility	MP	Total Non-Facility
67343	8.47	10.28	0.67	19.42

Modifiers (PAR)

Code	Mod 50	Mod 51	Mod 62	Mod 66	Mod 80
67343	1	2	1	0	1

Global Period

Code	Days
67343	090

67345

67345 Chemodenervation of extraocular muscle

(For chemodenervation for blepharospasm and other neurological disorders, see 64612 and 64616)

AMA Coding Notes

Surgical Procedures on the Eye and Ocular Adnexa

(For diagnostic and treatment ophthalmological services, see Medicine, Ophthalmology, and 92002 et seq)

(Do not report code 69990 in addition to codes 65091-68850)

AMA *CPT® Assistant* ▢

67345: Summer 93: 20, Mar 97: 5, Apr 00: 2, Feb 10: 13, Dec 13: 10, May 14: 5

Plain English Description

Chemodenervation of extraocular muscles involves the injection of botulinum toxin type A (BTA) into one or more eye muscles, which temporarily paralyzes the muscles. Chemodenervation is used to treat paralytic strabismus. The botulinum toxin is injected into the unopposed antagonist of the paralyzed muscle, which causes paralysis of that muscle as well and corrects the strabismus. Injection is performed under electromyographic (EMG) control. An electrode is placed on the forehead. Anesthetic eye drops are administered and an eye speculum placed to keep the eyelids open. Additional local anesthetic is applied with a cotton swab at the planned conjunctival injection site. A needle electrode is attached to a syringe and to the EMG device. The needle is inserted through the conjunctiva and into the eye muscle close to the insertion site. The patient is instructed to move the eye and movement is monitored by the EMG device. The needle is adjusted as needed. Once the needle is properly placed the botulinum toxin is injected. Alternatively, the procedure may be performed under direct vision. The conjunctiva is incised over the extraocular muscle. The muscle is engaged on a muscle hook and the botulinum toxin injected. The conjunctival incision is closed.

Chemodenervation of extraocular muscle

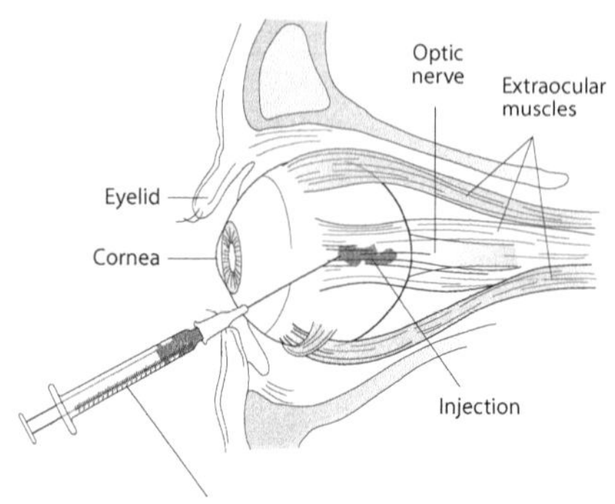

Botulinum toxin is injected into the muscle to achieve temporary paralysis.

ICD-10-CM Diagnostic Codes

	G24.1	Genetic torsion dystonia
	G24.4	Idiopathic orofacial dystonia
	G24.5	Blepharospasm
	G51.2	Melkersson's syndrome
⇄	G51.31	Clonic hemifacial spasm, right
⇄	G51.32	Clonic hemifacial spasm, left
⇄	G51.33	Clonic hemifacial spasm, bilateral
⇄	G51.39	Clonic hemifacial spasm, unspecified
	G51.4	Facial myokymia
	G51.8	Other disorders of facial nerve
⇄	H49.01	Third [oculomotor] nerve palsy, right eye
⇄	H49.11	Fourth [trochlear] nerve palsy, right eye
⇄	H49.21	Sixth [abducent] nerve palsy, right eye
⇄	H49.41	Progressive external ophthalmoplegia, right eye
⇄	H49.881	Other paralytic strabismus, right eye
⇄	H50.012	Monocular esotropia, left eye
⇄	H50.021	Monocular esotropia with A pattern, right eye
⇄	H50.031	Monocular esotropia with V pattern, right eye
⇄	H50.041	Monocular esotropia with other noncomitancies, right eye
	H50.05	Alternating esotropia
	H50.06	Alternating esotropia with A pattern
	H50.07	Alternating esotropia with V pattern
⇄	H50.111	Monocular exotropia, right eye
⇄	H50.121	Monocular exotropia with A pattern, right eye
⇄	H50.131	Monocular exotropia with V pattern, right eye
⇄	H50.141	Monocular exotropia with other noncomitancies, right eye
	H50.15	Alternating exotropia
	H50.16	Alternating exotropia with A pattern
	H50.17	Alternating exotropia with V pattern
	H50.18	Alternating exotropia with other noncomitancies

CCI Edits

Refer to Appendix A for CCI edits.

Facility RVUs ▢

Code	Work	PE Facility	MP	Total Facility
67345	3.01	2.87	0.40	6.28

Non-facility RVUs ▢

Code	Work	PE Non-Facility	MP	Total Non-Facility
67345	3.01	3.69	0.40	7.10

Modifiers (PAR) ▢

Code	Mod 50	Mod 51	Mod 62	Mod 66	Mod 80
67345	1	2	0	0	1

Global Period

Code	Days
67345	010

67346

67346 Biopsy of extraocular muscle

(For repair of wound, extraocular muscle, tendon or Tenon's capsule, use 65290)

AMA Coding Notes

Surgical Procedures on the Eye and Ocular Adnexa

(For diagnostic and treatment ophthalmological services, see Medicine, Ophthalmology, and 92002 et seq)

(Do not report code 69990 in addition to codes 65091-68850)

Plain English Description

An extraocular muscle is biopsied. An ocular speculum is placed to hold the patient's eye open and incisions are made through the conjunctiva and sclera to expose the muscle. The target biopsy muscle is isolated and a small sampling of the muscle tissue is carefully removed so that the excision will not harm the overall function of the eye muscle. The wound is closed.

Biopsy of extraocular muscle

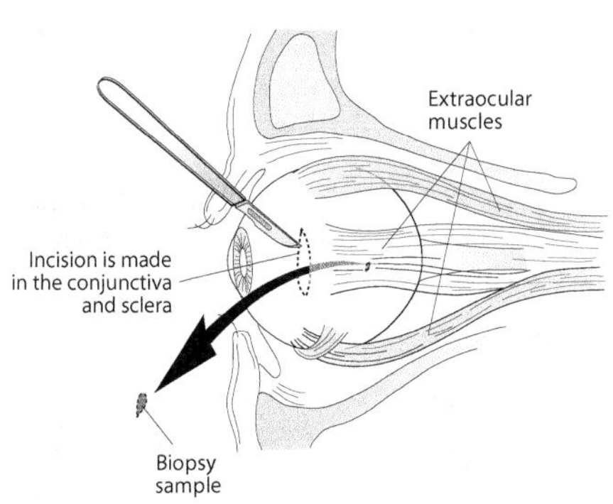

A scalpel is used to excise a small portion of the muscle for biopsy.

ICD-10-CM Diagnostic Codes

⇄	H49.32	Total (external) ophthalmoplegia, left eye
	H50.89	Other specified strabismus
	H51.0	Palsy (spasm) of conjugate gaze
	H51.11	Convergence insufficiency
	H51.12	Convergence excess
⇄	H51.22	Internuclear ophthalmoplegia, left eye
	H51.9	Unspecified disorder of binocular movement

CCI Edits

Refer to Appendix A for CCI edits.

Facility RVUs ▯

Code	Work	PE Facility	MP	Total Facility
67346	2.87	2.41	0.22	5.50

Non-facility RVUs ▯

Code	Work	PE Non-Facility	MP	Total Non-Facility
67346	2.87	2.41	0.22	5.50

Modifiers (PAR) ▯

Code	Mod 50	Mod 51	Mod 62	Mod 66	Mod 80
67346	1	2	0	0	0

Global Period

Code	Days
67346	000

67400-67405

67400 Orbitotomy without bone flap (frontal or transconjunctival approach); for exploration, with or without biopsy

67405 Orbitotomy without bone flap (frontal or transconjunctival approach); with drainage only

AMA Coding Notes

Surgical Procedures on the Eye and Ocular Adnexa

(For diagnostic and treatment ophthalmological services, see Medicine, Ophthalmology, and 92002 et seq)

(Do not report code 69990 in addition to codes 65091-68850)

Plain English Description

The orbit is explored and other procedures, such as biopsy or drainage, performed via a frontal or transconjunctival approach without creating a bone flap. The exact procedure depends on the site of the lesion or other abnormality. A transconjunctival approach may be performed via an incision in the upper or lower conjunctival fornix. Soft tissues are dissected and the area of interest exposed. In 67400, the upper or lower aspect of the orbit is explored and any abnormalities noted. Tissue samples are obtained as needed and sent for separately reportable pathology evaluation. In 67405, a fluid collection is located, tissues incised, and the fluid is drained. Fluid samples may be sent for separately reportable laboratory evaluation. Soft tissues and the conjunctiva are closed in layers.

Orbitotomy without bone flap (frontal/transconjunctival approach) exploration/biopsy/drainage

Incisions
Orbit
Orbital bone
Orbit is explored biopsy/drainage is performed

Exploration with/without biopsy use code 67400; for drainage only use code 67405

ICD-10-CM Diagnostic Codes

⇄	C69.61	Malignant neoplasm of right orbit
⇄	C69.62	Malignant neoplasm of left orbit
⇄	C69.81	Malignant neoplasm of overlapping sites of right eye and adnexa
⇄	C69.82	Malignant neoplasm of overlapping sites of left eye and adnexa
	C79.49	Secondary malignant neoplasm of other parts of nervous system
⇄	D09.21	Carcinoma in situ of right eye
⇄	D09.22	Carcinoma in situ of left eye
⇄	D31.61	Benign neoplasm of unspecified site of right orbit
⇄	D31.62	Benign neoplasm of unspecified site of left orbit
	D48.7	Neoplasm of uncertain behavior of other specified sites
	D49.89	Neoplasm of unspecified behavior of other specified sites
⇄	H05.011	Cellulitis of right orbit
⇄	H05.012	Cellulitis of left orbit
⇄	H05.013	Cellulitis of bilateral orbits
⇄	H05.021	Osteomyelitis of right orbit
⇄	H05.022	Osteomyelitis of left orbit
⇄	H05.023	Osteomyelitis of bilateral orbits
⇄	H05.031	Periostitis of right orbit
⇄	H05.032	Periostitis of left orbit
⇄	H05.033	Periostitis of bilateral orbits
	H05.10	Unspecified chronic inflammatory disorders of orbit
⇄	H05.121	Orbital myositis, right orbit
⇄	H05.122	Orbital myositis, left orbit
⇄	H05.123	Orbital myositis, bilateral
⇄	H05.231	Hemorrhage of right orbit
⇄	H05.232	Hemorrhage of left orbit
⇄	H05.233	Hemorrhage of bilateral orbit
⇄	H05.811	Cyst of right orbit
⇄	H05.812	Cyst of left orbit
⇄	H05.813	Cyst of bilateral orbits
	H05.89	Other disorders of orbit
⇄	H53.131	Sudden visual loss, right eye
	H53.71	Glare sensitivity
	H53.72	Impaired contrast sensitivity
	H53.8	Other visual disturbances
⇄	H57.11	Ocular pain, right eye
	H57.89	Other specified disorders of eye and adnexa
⇄	H59.111	Intraoperative hemorrhage and hematoma of right eye and adnexa complicating an ophthalmic procedure
⇄	H59.112	Intraoperative hemorrhage and hematoma of left eye and adnexa complicating an ophthalmic procedure
⇄	H59.113	Intraoperative hemorrhage and hematoma of eye and adnexa complicating an ophthalmic procedure, bilateral
⇄	H59.121	Intraoperative hemorrhage and hematoma of right eye and adnexa complicating other procedure
⇄	H59.122	Intraoperative hemorrhage and hematoma of left eye and adnexa complicating other procedure
⇄	H59.123	Intraoperative hemorrhage and hematoma of eye and adnexa complicating other procedure, bilateral
⇄	H59.311	Postprocedural hemorrhage of right eye and adnexa following an ophthalmic procedure
⇄	H59.312	Postprocedural hemorrhage of left eye and adnexa following an ophthalmic procedure
⇄	H59.313	Postprocedural hemorrhage of eye and adnexa following an ophthalmic procedure, bilateral
⇄	H59.321	Postprocedural hemorrhage of right eye and adnexa following other procedure
⇄	H59.322	Postprocedural hemorrhage of left eye and adnexa following other procedure
⇄	H59.323	Postprocedural hemorrhage of eye and adnexa following other procedure, bilateral
❼	T81.49	Infection following a procedure, other surgical site

ICD-10-CM Coding Notes

For codes requiring a 7th character extension, refer to your ICD-10-CM book. Review the character descriptions and coding guidelines for proper selection. For some procedures, only certain characters will apply.

CCI Edits

Refer to Appendix A for CCI edits.

Facility RVUs ▯

Code	Work	PE Facility	MP	Total Facility
67400	11.20	18.58	0.89	30.67
67405	9.20	16.74	0.86	26.80

Non-facility RVUs ▯

Code	Work	PE Non-Facility	MP	Total Non-Facility
67400	11.20	18.58	0.89	30.67
67405	9.20	16.74	0.86	26.80

Modifiers (PAR) ▯

Code	Mod 50	Mod 51	Mod 62	Mod 66	Mod 80
67400	1	2	1	0	1
67405	1	2	0	0	1

Global Period

Code	Days
67400	090
67405	090

67412-67413

67412 Orbitotomy without bone flap (frontal or transconjunctival approach); with removal of lesion

67413 Orbitotomy without bone flap (frontal or transconjunctival approach); with removal of foreign body

AMA Coding Notes

Surgical Procedures on the Eye and Ocular Adnexa

(For diagnostic and treatment ophthalmological services, see Medicine, Ophthalmology, and 92002 et seq)

(Do not report code 69990 in addition to codes 65091-68850)

Plain English Description

The orbit is explored and other procedures, such as removal of a lesion or foreign body, performed via a frontal or transconjunctival approach without creating a bone flap. The exact procedure depends on the site of the lesion or foreign body. A transconjunctival approach may be performed via an incision in the upper or lower conjunctival fornix. Soft tissues are dissected and the area of interest exposed. In 67412, the upper or lower aspect of the orbit is explored and the lesion is located. The cystic or solid tumor is carefully dissected free of surrounding tissue taking care to remove all abnormal tissue along with a margin of normal tissue. The cystic or solid tumor is sent for separately reportable pathology evaluation. In 67413, a foreign body is located, grasped with forceps and removed. Alternatively, the foreign body may be carefully dissected from surrounding tissue and removed. The wound is flushed with sterile saline or antibiotic solution as needed. Soft tissues and the conjunctiva are closed in layers.

Orbitotomy without bone flap (frontal/transconjunctival approach) removal of lesion/foreign body

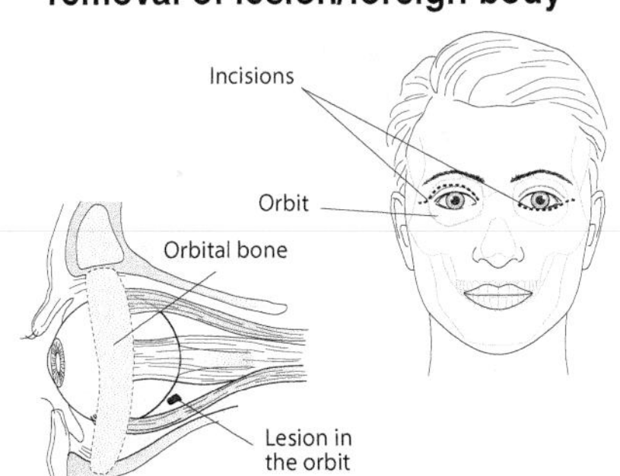

A lesion (67412), or foreign body (67413) is removed from the orbit.

ICD-10-CM Diagnostic Codes

⇄ C69.61 Malignant neoplasm of right orbit
⇄ C69.62 Malignant neoplasm of left orbit
⇄ D09.21 Carcinoma in situ of right eye
⇄ D09.22 Carcinoma in situ of left eye
D18.09 Hemangioma of other sites
⇄ D31.61 Benign neoplasm of unspecified site of right orbit
⇄ D31.62 Benign neoplasm of unspecified site of left orbit
D48.7 Neoplasm of uncertain behavior of other specified sites
D49.2 Neoplasm of unspecified behavior of bone, soft tissue, and skin
D49.89 Neoplasm of unspecified behavior of other specified sites
⇄ H05.51 Retained (old) foreign body following penetrating wound of right orbit
⇄ H05.52 Retained (old) foreign body following penetrating wound of left orbit
⇄ H05.811 Cyst of right orbit
⇄ H05.812 Cyst of left orbit
⇄ H05.813 Cyst of bilateral orbits
H57.89 Other specified disorders of eye and adnexa
Q85.00 Neurofibromatosis, unspecified
Q85.01 Neurofibromatosis, type 1
❼⇄ S05.41 Penetrating wound of orbit with or without foreign body, right eye
❼⇄ S05.42 Penetrating wound of orbit with or without foreign body, left eye
Z18.01 Retained depleted uranium fragments
Z18.09 Other retained radioactive fragments
Z18.10 Retained metal fragments, unspecified
Z18.11 Retained magnetic metal fragments
Z18.12 Retained nonmagnetic metal fragments
Z18.2 Retained plastic fragments
Z18.31 Retained animal quills or spines
Z18.32 Retained tooth
Z18.33 Retained wood fragments
Z18.39 Other retained organic fragments
Z18.81 Retained glass fragments
Z18.83 Retained stone or crystalline fragments
Z18.89 Other specified retained foreign body fragments

ICD-10-CM Coding Notes

For codes requiring a 7th character extension, refer to your ICD-10-CM book. Review the character descriptions and coding guidelines for proper selection. For some procedures, only certain characters will apply.

CCI Edits

Refer to Appendix A for CCI edits.

Facility RVUs

Code	Work	PE Facility	MP	Total Facility
67412	10.30	18.35	0.87	29.52
67413	10.24	17.49	0.89	28.62

Non-facility RVUs

Code	Work	PE Non-Facility	MP	Total Non-Facility
67412	10.30	18.35	0.87	29.52
67413	10.24	17.49	0.89	28.62

Modifiers (PAR)

Code	Mod 50	Mod 51	Mod 62	Mod 66	Mod 80
67412	1	2	1	0	1
67413	1	2	0	0	2

Global Period

Code	Days
67412	090
67413	090

67414

67414 Orbitotomy without bone flap (frontal or transconjunctival approach); with removal of bone for decompression

AMA Coding Notes

Surgical Procedures on the Eye and Ocular Adnexa

(For diagnostic and treatment ophthalmological services, see Medicine, Ophthalmology, and 92002 et seq)

(Do not report code 69990 in addition to codes 65091-68850)

AMA *CPT® Assistant* ▯

67414: Jul 99: 10

Plain English Description

The orbit is explored and orbital decompression with removal of bone performed via a frontal or transconjunctival approach without creating a bone flap. The exact procedure depends on the compartment of the eye requiring decompression. A transconjunctival approach may be performed via an incision in the upper or lower conjunctival fornix. Soft tissues are dissected and the area of interest exposed. The upper or lower aspect of the orbit is explored and the region requiring decompression identified. The orbital bone is exposed and the periosteum incised. Holes are drilled in the orbital bone and the holes are connected using an oscillating saw or osteotome. The area of bone causing the compression of the orbit is excised. Soft tissues and the conjunctiva are closed in layers.

Orbitotomy without bone flap (frontal/transconjunctival approach) with removal of bone for decompression

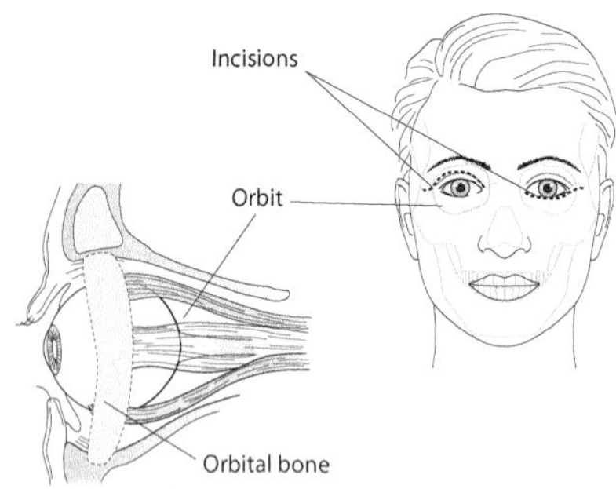

A piece of the orbital bone is excised for decompression.

ICD-10-CM Diagnostic Codes

	Code	Description
	E05.00	Thyrotoxicosis with diffuse goiter without thyrotoxic crisis or storm
	E05.01	Thyrotoxicosis with diffuse goiter with thyrotoxic crisis or storm
	E05.10	Thyrotoxicosis with toxic single thyroid nodule without thyrotoxic crisis or storm
	E05.11	Thyrotoxicosis with toxic single thyroid nodule with thyrotoxic crisis or storm
	E05.20	Thyrotoxicosis with toxic multinodular goiter without thyrotoxic crisis or storm
	E05.21	Thyrotoxicosis with toxic multinodular goiter with thyrotoxic crisis or storm
	E05.30	Thyrotoxicosis from ectopic thyroid tissue without thyrotoxic crisis or storm
	E05.31	Thyrotoxicosis from ectopic thyroid tissue with thyrotoxic crisis or storm
	E05.40	Thyrotoxicosis factitia without thyrotoxic crisis or storm
	E05.41	Thyrotoxicosis factitia with thyrotoxic crisis or storm
	E05.80	Other thyrotoxicosis without thyrotoxic crisis or storm
	E05.81	Other thyrotoxicosis with thyrotoxic crisis or storm
	E05.90	Thyrotoxicosis, unspecified without thyrotoxic crisis or storm
	E05.91	Thyrotoxicosis, unspecified with thyrotoxic crisis or storm
⇄	H05.221	Edema of right orbit
⇄	H05.222	Edema of left orbit
⇄	H05.223	Edema of bilateral orbit
⇄	H05.241	Constant exophthalmos, right eye
⇄	H05.242	Constant exophthalmos, left eye
⇄	H05.243	Constant exophthalmos, bilateral
⇄	H05.321	Deformity of right orbit due to bone disease
⇄	H05.322	Deformity of left orbit due to bone disease
⇄	H05.323	Deformity of bilateral orbits due to bone disease
⇄	H05.331	Deformity of right orbit due to trauma or surgery
⇄	H05.332	Deformity of left orbit due to trauma or surgery
⇄	H05.333	Deformity of bilateral orbits due to trauma or surgery
⇄	H05.341	Enlargement of right orbit
⇄	H05.342	Enlargement of left orbit
⇄	H05.343	Enlargement of bilateral orbits
⇄	H05.351	Exostosis of right orbit
⇄	H05.352	Exostosis of left orbit
⇄	H05.353	Exostosis of bilateral orbits
⇄	H05.821	Myopathy of extraocular muscles, right orbit
⇄	H05.822	Myopathy of extraocular muscles, left orbit
⇄	H05.823	Myopathy of extraocular muscles, bilateral
	H05.89	Other disorders of orbit
⇄	H53.131	Sudden visual loss, right eye
⇄	H53.132	Sudden visual loss, left eye
⇄	H53.133	Sudden visual loss, bilateral
⇄	H53.141	Visual discomfort, right eye
⇄	H53.142	Visual discomfort, left eye
⇄	H53.143	Visual discomfort, bilateral
⇄	H57.11	Ocular pain, right eye
⇄	H57.12	Ocular pain, left eye
⇄	H57.13	Ocular pain, bilateral
	P72.1	Transitory neonatal hyperthyroidism

CCI Edits

Refer to Appendix A for CCI edits.

Facility RVUs ▯

Code	Work	PE Facility	MP	Total Facility
67414	17.94	23.54	1.81	43.29

Non-facility RVUs ▯

Code	Work	PE Non-Facility	MP	Total Non-Facility
67414	17.94	23.54	1.81	43.29

Modifiers (PAR) ▯

Code	Mod 50	Mod 51	Mod 62	Mod 66	Mod 80
67414	1	2	1	0	2

Global Period

Code	Days
67414	090

67415

67415 Fine needle aspiration of orbital contents

(For exenteration, enucleation, and repair, see 65101 et seq; for optic nerve decompression, use 67570)

AMA Coding Notes

Surgical Procedures on the Eye and Ocular Adnexa

(For diagnostic and treatment ophthalmological services, see Medicine, Ophthalmology, and 92002 et seq)

(Do not report code 69990 in addition to codes 65091-68850)

Plain English Description

A mass or lesion is evaluated using fine needle aspiration of orbital contents. The eyelid overlying the area of interest is cleansed. Local anesthetic eye drops or gel may be used for patient comfort. The eye is held in place using firm pressure and the needle is inserted through the eyelid and into the mass or lesion. Once the needle is located in the desired region, the syringe plunger is retracted. The needle is moved back and forth within the desired region while maintaining negative pressure in the syringe. Once sufficient aspirate is obtained, the needle is removed and slides are prepared and a separately reportable evaluation of the fine needle aspirate is performed.

Fine needle aspiration of orbital contents

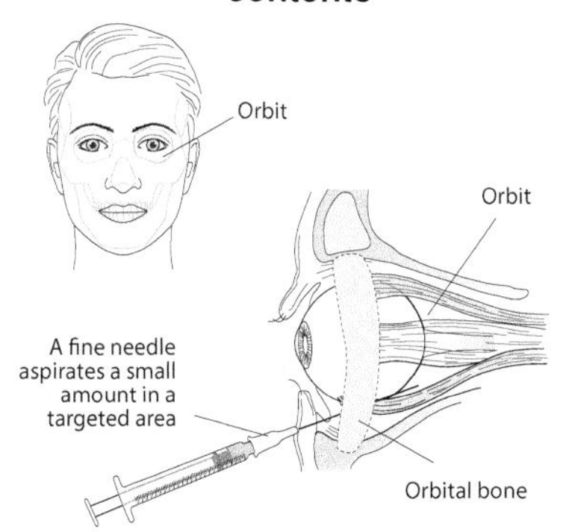

No incision or repair is required.

ICD-10-CM Diagnostic Codes

	Code	Description
	A49.01	Methicillin susceptible Staphylococcus aureus infection, unspecified site
	A49.02	Methicillin resistant Staphylococcus aureus infection, unspecified site
	B95.0	Streptococcus, group A, as the cause of diseases classified elsewhere
	B95.61	Methicillin susceptible Staphylococcus aureus infection as the cause of diseases classified elsewhere
	B95.62	Methicillin resistant Staphylococcus aureus infection as the cause of diseases classified elsewhere
⇄	C69.61	Malignant neoplasm of right orbit
⇄	C69.62	Malignant neoplasm of left orbit
⇄	C69.81	Malignant neoplasm of overlapping sites of right eye and adnexa
⇄	C69.82	Malignant neoplasm of overlapping sites of left eye and adnexa
	C79.49	Secondary malignant neoplasm of other parts of nervous system
⇄	D31.61	Benign neoplasm of unspecified site of right orbit
⇄	D31.62	Benign neoplasm of unspecified site of left orbit
	D48.7	Neoplasm of uncertain behavior of other specified sites
	D49.81	Neoplasm of unspecified behavior of retina and choroid
	D49.89	Neoplasm of unspecified behavior of other specified sites
⇄	H05.011	Cellulitis of right orbit
⇄	H05.012	Cellulitis of left orbit
⇄	H05.013	Cellulitis of bilateral orbits
	H05.20	Unspecified exophthalmos
⇄	H05.221	Edema of right orbit
⇄	H05.222	Edema of left orbit
⇄	H05.223	Edema of bilateral orbit

CCI Edits

Refer to Appendix A for CCI edits.

Facility RVUs ▢

Code	Work	PE Facility	MP	Total Facility
67415	1.76	1.08	0.12	2.96

Non-facility RVUs ▢

Code	Work	PE Non-Facility	MP	Total Non-Facility
67415	1.76	1.08	0.12	2.96

Modifiers (PAR) ▢

Code	Mod 50	Mod 51	Mod 62	Mod 66	Mod 80
67415	1	2	0	0	0

Global Period

Code	Days
67415	000

67420-67430

67420 Orbitotomy with bone flap or window, lateral approach (eg, Kroenlein); with removal of lesion

67430 Orbitotomy with bone flap or window, lateral approach (eg, Kroenlein); with removal of foreign body

AMA Coding Notes

Surgical Procedures on the Eye and Ocular Adnexa

(For diagnostic and treatment ophthalmological services, see Medicine, Ophthalmology, and 92002 et seq)

(Do not report code 69990 in addition to codes 65091-68850)

Plain English Description

The orbit is explored and definitive procedures such as removal of a lesion or foreign body performed via a lateral approach with creation of a bone flap or window. A lazy-S incision is made in the upper eyelid crease. The lateral rectus muscle is exposed and retracted. Soft tissues are dissected and the underlying zygomatic bone is exposed. The periosteum is incised and the edges undermined to expose the hard cortical bone of the zygoma. Holes are drilled and the holes connected using an oscillating saw to create a bone window or flap. The periorbita is incised. Underlying fat and soft tissue attachments are dissected and the orbit is exposed. In 67420, a lesion is removed. The lesion may be cystic or solid and may involve soft tissue and/or bony structures. The lesion is carefully dissected free of surrounding tissue taking care to remove all abnormal tissue along with a margin of normal tissue. The lesion is sent for separately reportable pathology evaluation. In 67430, a foreign body is located, grasped with forceps and removed. Alternatively, the foreign body may be carefully dissected from surrounding tissue and removed. The wound is flushed with sterile saline or antibiotic solution as needed. Orbital tissues are reapproximated and the periorbita is closed. The bone window or flap is replaced and secured with miniplates and screws. The periosteum is closed. Soft tissues and the skin of the eyelid are closed in layers.

Orbitotomy with bone flap/window, lateral approach (eg, Kroenlein); with removal of lesion/foreign body

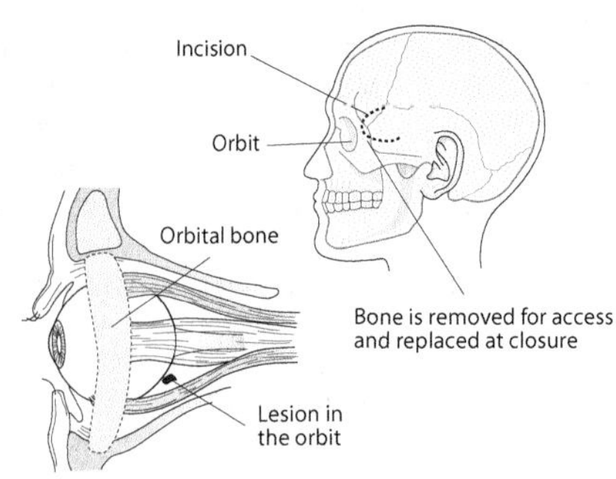

A lesion (67420), or foreign body (67430) is removed from the orbit.

ICD-10-CM Diagnostic Codes

⇄	C69.61	Malignant neoplasm of right orbit
⇄	C69.62	Malignant neoplasm of left orbit
⇄	D09.21	Carcinoma in situ of right eye
⇄	D09.22	Carcinoma in situ of left eye
	D16.4	Benign neoplasm of bones of skull and face
	D18.09	Hemangioma of other sites
⇄	D31.61	Benign neoplasm of unspecified site of right orbit
⇄	D31.62	Benign neoplasm of unspecified site of left orbit
	D48.7	Neoplasm of uncertain behavior of other specified sites
	D49.2	Neoplasm of unspecified behavior of bone, soft tissue, and skin
	D49.89	Neoplasm of unspecified behavior of other specified sites
⇄	H05.51	Retained (old) foreign body following penetrating wound of right orbit
⇄	H05.52	Retained (old) foreign body following penetrating wound of left orbit
⇄	H05.811	Cyst of right orbit
⇄	H05.812	Cyst of left orbit
⇄	H05.813	Cyst of bilateral orbits
	H57.89	Other specified disorders of eye and adnexa
	Q85.00	Neurofibromatosis, unspecified
	Q85.01	Neurofibromatosis, type 1
❼⇄	S05.41	Penetrating wound of orbit with or without foreign body, right eye
❼⇄	S05.42	Penetrating wound of orbit with or without foreign body, left eye
	Z18.01	Retained depleted uranium fragments
	Z18.09	Other retained radioactive fragments
	Z18.10	Retained metal fragments, unspecified
	Z18.11	Retained magnetic metal fragments
	Z18.12	Retained nonmagnetic metal fragments
	Z18.2	Retained plastic fragments
	Z18.31	Retained animal quills or spines
	Z18.32	Retained tooth
	Z18.33	Retained wood fragments
	Z18.39	Other retained organic fragments
	Z18.81	Retained glass fragments
	Z18.83	Retained stone or crystalline fragments
	Z18.89	Other specified retained foreign body fragments

ICD-10-CM Coding Notes

For codes requiring a 7th character extension, refer to your ICD-10-CM book. Review the character descriptions and coding guidelines for proper selection. For some procedures, only certain characters will apply.

CCI Edits

Refer to Appendix A for CCI edits.

Facility RVUs ▯

Code	Work	PE Facility	MP	Total Facility
67420	21.87	27.49	2.01	51.37
67430	15.29	24.51	1.18	40.98

Non-facility RVUs ▯

Code	Work	PE Non-Facility	MP	Total Non-Facility
67420	21.87	27.49	2.01	51.37
67430	15.29	24.51	1.18	40.98

Modifiers (PAR) ▯

Code	Mod 50	Mod 51	Mod 62	Mod 66	Mod 80
67420	1	2	1	0	2
67430	1	2	0	0	2

Global Period

Code	Days
67420	090
67430	090

● New ▲ Revised ✚ Add On ⊘Modifier 51 Exempt ★Telemedicine ▯ CPT QuickRef ⁄FDA Pending ⇄ Laterality ❼ Seventh Character ♂Male ♀Female

67440

67440 Orbitotomy with bone flap or window, lateral approach (eg, Kroenlein); with drainage

AMA Coding Notes

Surgical Procedures on the Eye and Ocular Adnexa

(For diagnostic and treatment ophthalmological services, see Medicine, Ophthalmology, and 92002 et seq)

(Do not report code 69990 in addition to codes 65091-68850)

Plain English Description

The orbit is explored and drainage of a fluid collection performed via a lateral approach with creation of a bone flap or window. A lazy-S incision is made in the upper eyelid crease. The lateral rectus muscle is exposed and retracted. Soft tissues are dissected and the underlying zygomatic bone is exposed. The periosteum is incised and the edges undermined to expose the hard cortical bone of the zygoma. Holes are drilled and the holes connected using an oscillating saw to create a bone window or flap. The periorbita is incised. Underlying fat and soft tissue attachments are dissected and the orbit is exposed. The fluid collection is located, tissues incised, and the fluid drained. The operative site is flushed with sterile saline or antibiotic solution as needed. Orbital tissues are reapproximated and the periorbita is closed. The bone window or flap is replaced and secured with miniplates and screws. The periosteum is closed. Soft tissues and the skin of the eyelid are closed in layers.

Orbitotomy with bone flap/window, lateral approach (eg, Kroenlein); with drainage

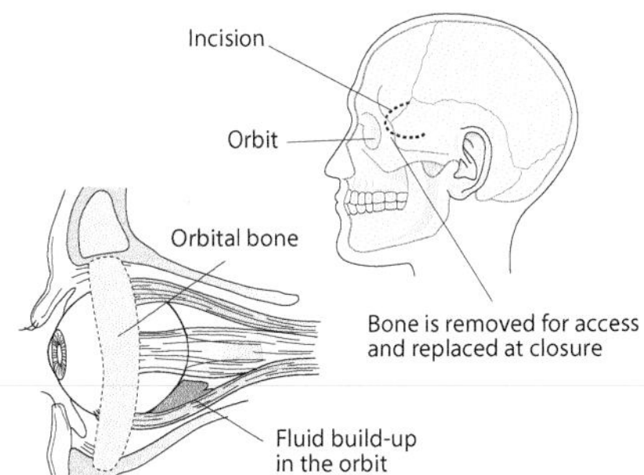

A fluid build-up is accessed and removed from the orbit.

ICD-10-CM Diagnostic Codes

⇄	H05.011	Cellulitis of right orbit
⇄	H05.012	Cellulitis of left orbit
⇄	H05.013	Cellulitis of bilateral orbits
⇄	H05.021	Osteomyelitis of right orbit
⇄	H05.022	Osteomyelitis of left orbit
⇄	H05.023	Osteomyelitis of bilateral orbits
⇄	H05.031	Periostitis of right orbit
⇄	H05.032	Periostitis of left orbit
⇄	H05.033	Periostitis of bilateral orbits
	H05.10	Unspecified chronic inflammatory disorders of orbit
⇄	H05.121	Orbital myositis, right orbit
⇄	H05.122	Orbital myositis, left orbit
⇄	H05.123	Orbital myositis, bilateral
⇄	H05.231	Hemorrhage of right orbit
⇄	H05.232	Hemorrhage of left orbit
⇄	H05.233	Hemorrhage of bilateral orbit
⇄	H05.811	Cyst of right orbit
⇄	H05.812	Cyst of left orbit
⇄	H05.813	Cyst of bilateral orbits
	H05.89	Other disorders of orbit
⇄	H59.111	Intraoperative hemorrhage and hematoma of right eye and adnexa complicating an ophthalmic procedure
⇄	H59.112	Intraoperative hemorrhage and hematoma of left eye and adnexa complicating an ophthalmic procedure
⇄	H59.113	Intraoperative hemorrhage and hematoma of eye and adnexa complicating an ophthalmic procedure, bilateral
⇄	H59.121	Intraoperative hemorrhage and hematoma of right eye and adnexa complicating other procedure
⇄	H59.122	Intraoperative hemorrhage and hematoma of left eye and adnexa complicating other procedure
⇄	H59.123	Intraoperative hemorrhage and hematoma of eye and adnexa complicating other procedure, bilateral
⇄	H59.311	Postprocedural hemorrhage of right eye and adnexa following an ophthalmic procedure
⇄	H59.312	Postprocedural hemorrhage of left eye and adnexa following an ophthalmic procedure
⇄	H59.313	Postprocedural hemorrhage of eye and adnexa following an ophthalmic procedure, bilateral
⇄	H59.321	Postprocedural hemorrhage of right eye and adnexa following other procedure
⇄	H59.322	Postprocedural hemorrhage of left eye and adnexa following other procedure
⇄	H59.323	Postprocedural hemorrhage of eye and adnexa following other procedure, bilateral
❼	T81.49	Infection following a procedure, other surgical site

ICD-10-CM Coding Notes

For codes requiring a 7th character extension, refer to your ICD-10-CM book. Review the character descriptions and coding guidelines for proper selection. For some procedures, only certain characters will apply.

CCI Edits

Refer to Appendix A for CCI edits.

Facility RVUs ▯

Code	Work	PE Facility	MP	Total Facility
67440	14.84	23.79	1.16	39.79

Non-facility RVUs ▯

Code	Work	PE Non-Facility	MP	Total Non-Facility
67440	14.84	23.79	1.16	39.79

Modifiers (PAR) ▯

Code	Mod 50	Mod 51	Mod 62	Mod 66	Mod 80
67440	1	2	1	0	2

Global Period

Code	Days
67440	090

67445

67445 Orbitotomy with bone flap or window, lateral approach (eg, Kroenlein); with removal of bone for decompression

(For optic nerve sheath decompression, use 67570)

AMA Coding Notes

Surgical Procedures on the Eye and Ocular Adnexa

(For diagnostic and treatment ophthalmological services, see Medicine, Ophthalmology, and 92002 et seq)

(Do not report code 69990 in addition to codes 65091-68850)

AMA *CPT® Assistant* ▢

67445: Dec 19: 14

Plain English Description

The orbit is explored and orbital decompression with removal of bone performed via a lateral approach with creation of a bone flap or window. A lazy-S incision is made in the upper eyelid crease. The lateral rectus muscle is exposed and retracted. Soft tissues are dissected and the underlying zygomatic bone is exposed. The periosteum is incised and the edges undermined to expose the hard cortical bone of the zygoma. Holes are drilled and the holes connected using an oscillating saw to create a bone window or flap. The periorbita is incised. Underlying fat and soft tissue attachments are dissected and the orbit is exposed. Soft tissues are dissected and the area of interest exposed. The orbit is explored and the region requiring decompression identified. The orbital bone is exposed and the periosteum incised. Holes are drilled in the orbital bone and the holes are connected using an oscillating saw or osteotome. The area of bone causing the compression of the orbit is excised. Orbital tissues are reapproximated and the periorbita is closed. The zygomatic bone window or flap is replaced and secured with miniplates and screws. The periosteum is closed. Soft tissues and the skin of the eyelid are closed in layers.

Orbitotomy with bone flap/window, lateral approach (eg, Kroenlein); with removal of bone for decompression

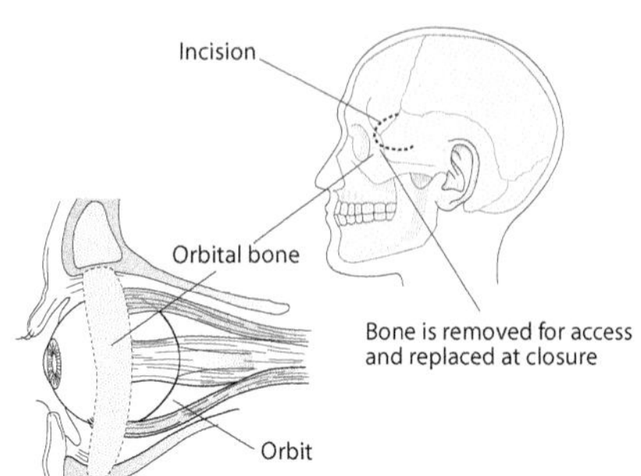

A piece of the orbital bone is excised for decompression.

ICD-10-CM Diagnostic Codes

	Code	Description
	E05.00	Thyrotoxicosis with diffuse goiter without thyrotoxic crisis or storm
	E05.01	Thyrotoxicosis with diffuse goiter with thyrotoxic crisis or storm
	E05.10	Thyrotoxicosis with toxic single thyroid nodule without thyrotoxic crisis or storm
	E05.11	Thyrotoxicosis with toxic single thyroid nodule with thyrotoxic crisis or storm
	E05.20	Thyrotoxicosis with toxic multinodular goiter without thyrotoxic crisis or storm
	E05.21	Thyrotoxicosis with toxic multinodular goiter with thyrotoxic crisis or storm
	E05.80	Other thyrotoxicosis without thyrotoxic crisis or storm
	E05.81	Other thyrotoxicosis with thyrotoxic crisis or storm
	E05.90	Thyrotoxicosis, unspecified without thyrotoxic crisis or storm
	E05.91	Thyrotoxicosis, unspecified with thyrotoxic crisis or storm
⇄	H05.221	Edema of right orbit
⇄	H05.222	Edema of left orbit
⇄	H05.223	Edema of bilateral orbit
⇄	H05.241	Constant exophthalmos, right eye
⇄	H05.242	Constant exophthalmos, left eye
⇄	H05.243	Constant exophthalmos, bilateral
⇄	H05.321	Deformity of right orbit due to bone disease
⇄	H05.322	Deformity of left orbit due to bone disease
⇄	H05.323	Deformity of bilateral orbits due to bone disease
⇄	H05.331	Deformity of right orbit due to trauma or surgery
⇄	H05.332	Deformity of left orbit due to trauma or surgery
⇄	H05.333	Deformity of bilateral orbits due to trauma or surgery
⇄	H05.341	Enlargement of right orbit
⇄	H05.342	Enlargement of left orbit
⇄	H05.343	Enlargement of bilateral orbits
⇄	H05.351	Exostosis of right orbit
⇄	H05.352	Exostosis of left orbit
⇄	H05.353	Exostosis of bilateral orbits
⇄	H05.821	Myopathy of extraocular muscles, right orbit
⇄	H05.822	Myopathy of extraocular muscles, left orbit
⇄	H05.823	Myopathy of extraocular muscles, bilateral
	H05.89	Other disorders of orbit
⇄	H53.131	Sudden visual loss, right eye
⇄	H53.132	Sudden visual loss, left eye
⇄	H53.133	Sudden visual loss, bilateral
⇄	H53.141	Visual discomfort, right eye
⇄	H53.142	Visual discomfort, left eye
⇄	H53.143	Visual discomfort, bilateral
⇄	H57.11	Ocular pain, right eye
⇄	H57.12	Ocular pain, left eye
⇄	H57.13	Ocular pain, bilateral
	P72.1	Transitory neonatal hyperthyroidism

CCI Edits

Refer to Appendix A for CCI edits.

Facility RVUs ▢

Code	Work	PE Facility	MP	Total Facility
67445	19.12	24.36	1.57	45.05

Non-facility RVUs ▢

Code	Work	PE Non-Facility	MP	Total Non-Facility
67445	19.12	24.36	1.57	45.05

Modifiers (PAR) ▢

Code	Mod 50	Mod 51	Mod 62	Mod 66	Mod 80
67445	1	2	1	0	2

Global Period

Code	Days
67445	090

67450

67450 Orbitotomy with bone flap or window, lateral approach (eg, Kroenlein); for exploration, with or without biopsy

(For orbitotomy, transcranial approach, see 61330, 61333)

(For orbital implant, see 67550, 67560)

(For removal of eyeball or for repair after removal, see 65091-65175)

AMA Coding Notes

Surgical Procedures on the Eye and Ocular Adnexa

(For diagnostic and treatment ophthalmological services, see Medicine, Ophthalmology, and 92002 et seq)

(Do not report code 69990 in addition to codes 65091-68850)

Plain English Description

The orbit is explored and tissue samples obtained as needed via a lateral approach with creation of a bone flap or window. A lazy-S incision is made in the upper eyelid crease. The lateral rectus muscle is exposed and retracted. Soft tissues are dissected and the underlying zygomatic bone is exposed. The periosteum is incised and the edges undermined to expose the hard cortical bone of the zygoma. Holes are drilled and the holes connected using an oscillating saw to create a bone window or flap. The periorbita is incised. Underlying fat and soft tissue attachments are dissected and the orbit is exposed. Soft tissues are dissected and the area of interest exposed. The orbit is explored and any abnormalities noted. Tissue samples are obtained as needed and sent for separately reportable pathology evaluation. Orbital tissues are reapproximated and the periorbita is closed. The zygomatic bone window or flap is replaced and secured with miniplates and screws. The periosteum is closed. Soft tissues and the skin of the eyelid are closed in layers.

Orbitotomy with bone flap/window, lateral approach (eg, Kroenlein); for exploration with/without biopsy

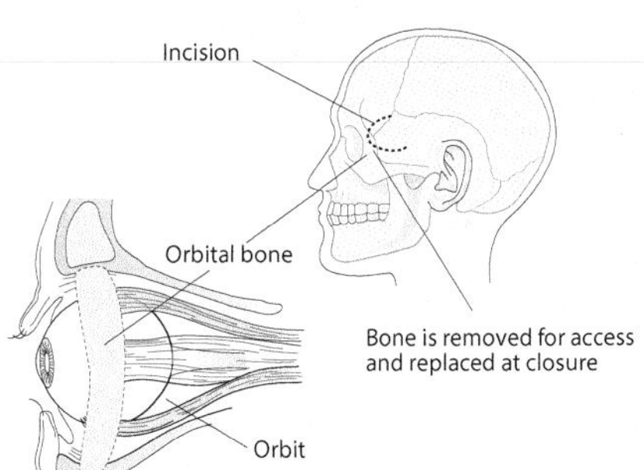

The orbital area is accessed and explored; bone/tissue may be taken for biopsy.

ICD-10-CM Diagnostic Codes

	C41.0	Malignant neoplasm of bones of skull and face
⇄	C69.61	Malignant neoplasm of right orbit
⇄	C69.62	Malignant neoplasm of left orbit
	C79.49	Secondary malignant neoplasm of other parts of nervous system
⇄	D09.21	Carcinoma in situ of right eye
⇄	D09.22	Carcinoma in situ of left eye
	D16.4	Benign neoplasm of bones of skull and face
⇄	D31.61	Benign neoplasm of unspecified site of right orbit
⇄	D31.62	Benign neoplasm of unspecified site of left orbit
⇄	H53.131	Sudden visual loss, right eye
⇄	H53.132	Sudden visual loss, left eye
⇄	H53.141	Visual discomfort, right eye
⇄	H53.142	Visual discomfort, left eye
⇄	H53.143	Visual discomfort, bilateral
	H53.71	Glare sensitivity
	H53.72	Impaired contrast sensitivity
	H53.8	Other visual disturbances
⇄	H57.11	Ocular pain, right eye
⇄	H57.12	Ocular pain, left eye
⇄	H57.13	Ocular pain, bilateral
	H57.89	Other specified disorders of eye and adnexa

CCI Edits

Refer to Appendix A for CCI edits.

Facility RVUs

Code	Work	PE Facility	MP	Total Facility
67450	15.41	24.58	1.18	41.17

Non-facility RVUs

Code	Work	PE Non-Facility	MP	Total Non-Facility
67450	15.41	24.58	1.18	41.17

Modifiers (PAR)

Code	Mod 50	Mod 51	Mod 62	Mod 66	Mod 80
67450	1	2	1	0	2

Global Period

Code	Days
67450	090

67500-67505

67500 Retrobulbar injection; medication (separate procedure, does not include supply of medication)

67505 Retrobulbar injection; alcohol

AMA Coding Notes

Surgical Procedures on the Eye and Ocular Adnexa

(For diagnostic and treatment ophthalmological services, see Medicine, Ophthalmology, and 92002 et seq)

(Do not report code 69990 in addition to codes 65091-68850)

AMA *CPT® Assistant*

67500: Nov 12: 10

Plain English Description

An injection into the retrobulbar region of the eye is performed. The skin over the lateral aspect of the lower lid is cleansed and a local anesthetic administered as needed. The needle is inserted through the skin of the eyelid slightly lateral of the midline of the eye. The needle is inserted straight down through the septum and then the needle is redirected upward until the needle is in the free space of the retrobulbar region. The plunger is withdrawn to ensure the needle is not in a blood vessel or other vital structure of the eye. The medication or alcohol mixture is then injected into the retrobulbar space. The needle is withdrawn. Gentle pressure is applied over the injection site. Use 67500 for injection of medication. Use 67505 for injection of alcohol.

Retrobulbar injection; medicine/alcohol

Medicine (67500), or alcohol (67505) is injected into the orbit through the lower eyelid

Eyelid

Cornea

Injection

Extraocular muscles

ICD-10-CM Diagnostic Codes

	A18.54	Tuberculous iridocyclitis
	B39.9	Histoplasmosis, unspecified
	D86.89	Sarcoidosis of other sites
	E08.311	Diabetes mellitus due to underlying condition with unspecified diabetic retinopathy with macular edema
	E08.319	Diabetes mellitus due to underlying condition with unspecified diabetic retinopathy without macular edema
⑦⇄	E08.321	Diabetes mellitus due to underlying condition with mild nonproliferative diabetic retinopathy with macular edema
⑦⇄	E08.329	Diabetes mellitus due to underlying condition with mild nonproliferative diabetic retinopathy without macular edema
⑦⇄	E08.331	Diabetes mellitus due to underlying condition with moderate nonproliferative diabetic retinopathy with macular edema
⑦⇄	E08.339	Diabetes mellitus due to underlying condition with moderate nonproliferative diabetic retinopathy without macular edema
⑦⇄	E08.341	Diabetes mellitus due to underlying condition with severe nonproliferative diabetic retinopathy with macular edema
⑦⇄	E08.349	Diabetes mellitus due to underlying condition with severe nonproliferative diabetic retinopathy without macular edema
⑦⇄	E08.351	Diabetes mellitus due to underlying condition with proliferative diabetic retinopathy with macular edema
⑦⇄	E08.352	Diabetes mellitus due to underlying condition with proliferative diabetic retinopathy with traction retinal detachment involving the macula
⑦⇄	E08.353	Diabetes mellitus due to underlying condition with proliferative diabetic retinopathy with traction retinal detachment not involving the macula
⑦⇄	E08.354	Diabetes mellitus due to underlying condition with proliferative diabetic retinopathy with combined traction retinal detachment and rhegmatogenous retinal detachment
⑦⇄	E08.355	Diabetes mellitus due to underlying condition with stable proliferative diabetic retinopathy
⑦⇄	E08.359	Diabetes mellitus due to underlying condition with proliferative diabetic retinopathy without macular edema
	E08.36	Diabetes mellitus due to underlying condition with diabetic cataract
	E08.39	Diabetes mellitus due to underlying condition with other diabetic ophthalmic complication
	E09.311	Drug or chemical induced diabetes mellitus with unspecified diabetic retinopathy with macular edema
	E09.319	Drug or chemical induced diabetes mellitus with unspecified diabetic retinopathy without macular edema
⑦⇄	E09.321	Drug or chemical induced diabetes mellitus with mild nonproliferative diabetic retinopathy with macular edema
⑦⇄	E09.329	Drug or chemical induced diabetes mellitus with mild nonproliferative diabetic retinopathy without macular edema
⑦⇄	E09.331	Drug or chemical induced diabetes mellitus with moderate nonproliferative diabetic retinopathy with macular edema
⑦⇄	E09.339	Drug or chemical induced diabetes mellitus with moderate nonproliferative diabetic retinopathy without macular edema
⑦⇄	E09.341	Drug or chemical induced diabetes mellitus with severe nonproliferative diabetic retinopathy with macular edema
⑦⇄	E09.349	Drug or chemical induced diabetes mellitus with severe nonproliferative diabetic retinopathy without macular edema
⑦⇄	E09.351	Drug or chemical induced diabetes mellitus with proliferative diabetic retinopathy with macular edema
⑦⇄	E09.352	Drug or chemical induced diabetes mellitus with proliferative diabetic retinopathy with traction retinal detachment involving the macula
⑦⇄	E09.353	Drug or chemical induced diabetes mellitus with proliferative diabetic retinopathy with traction retinal detachment not involving the macula
⑦⇄	E09.354	Drug or chemical induced diabetes mellitus with proliferative diabetic retinopathy with combined traction retinal detachment and rhegmatogenous retinal detachment
⑦⇄	E09.355	Drug or chemical induced diabetes mellitus with stable proliferative diabetic retinopathy
⑦⇄	E09.359	Drug or chemical induced diabetes mellitus with proliferative diabetic retinopathy without macular edema
	E09.36	Drug or chemical induced diabetes mellitus with diabetic cataract
	E09.39	Drug or chemical induced diabetes mellitus with other diabetic ophthalmic complication
	E10.311	Type 1 diabetes mellitus with unspecified diabetic retinopathy with macular edema
	E10.319	Type 1 diabetes mellitus with unspecified diabetic retinopathy without macular edema
⑦⇄	E10.321	Type 1 diabetes mellitus with mild nonproliferative diabetic retinopathy with macular edema
⑦⇄	E10.329	Type 1 diabetes mellitus with mild nonproliferative diabetic retinopathy without macular edema
⑦⇄	E10.331	Type 1 diabetes mellitus with moderate nonproliferative diabetic retinopathy with macular edema
⑦⇄	E10.339	Type 1 diabetes mellitus with moderate nonproliferative diabetic retinopathy without macular edema
⑦⇄	E10.341	Type 1 diabetes mellitus with severe nonproliferative diabetic retinopathy with macular edema
⑦⇄	E10.349	Type 1 diabetes mellitus with severe nonproliferative diabetic retinopathy without macular edema

● New ▲ Revised ✚ Add On ⊘Modifier 51 Exempt ★Telemedicine ▯CPT QuickRef ⁄FDA Pending ⇄ Laterality ⑦Seventh Character ♂Male ♀Female

❼⇄ E10.351 Type 1 diabetes mellitus with proliferative diabetic retinopathy with macular edema
❼⇄ E10.352 Type 1 diabetes mellitus with proliferative diabetic retinopathy with traction retinal detachment involving the macula
❼⇄ E10.353 Type 1 diabetes mellitus with proliferative diabetic retinopathy with traction retinal detachment not involving the macula
❼⇄ E10.354 Type 1 diabetes mellitus with proliferative diabetic retinopathy with combined traction retinal detachment and rhegmatogenous retinal detachment
❼⇄ E10.355 Type 1 diabetes mellitus with stable proliferative diabetic retinopathy
❼⇄ E10.359 Type 1 diabetes mellitus with proliferative diabetic retinopathy without macular edema
E10.36 Type 1 diabetes mellitus with diabetic cataract
E10.39 Type 1 diabetes mellitus with other diabetic ophthalmic complication
E10.65 Type 1 diabetes mellitus with hyperglycemia
E11.311 Type 2 diabetes mellitus with unspecified diabetic retinopathy with macular edema
E11.319 Type 2 diabetes mellitus with unspecified diabetic retinopathy without macular edema
❼⇄ E11.321 Type 2 diabetes mellitus with mild nonproliferative diabetic retinopathy with macular edema
❼⇄ E11.329 Type 2 diabetes mellitus with mild nonproliferative diabetic retinopathy without macular edema
❼⇄ E11.331 Type 2 diabetes mellitus with moderate nonproliferative diabetic retinopathy with macular edema
❼⇄ E11.339 Type 2 diabetes mellitus with moderate nonproliferative diabetic retinopathy without macular edema
❼⇄ E11.341 Type 2 diabetes mellitus with severe nonproliferative diabetic retinopathy with macular edema
❼⇄ E11.349 Type 2 diabetes mellitus with severe nonproliferative diabetic retinopathy without macular edema
❼⇄ E11.351 Type 2 diabetes mellitus with proliferative diabetic retinopathy with macular edema
❼⇄ E11.352 Type 2 diabetes mellitus with proliferative diabetic retinopathy with traction retinal detachment involving the macula
❼⇄ E11.353 Type 2 diabetes mellitus with proliferative diabetic retinopathy with traction retinal detachment not involving the macula
❼⇄ E11.354 Type 2 diabetes mellitus with proliferative diabetic retinopathy with combined traction retinal detachment and rhegmatogenous retinal detachment
❼⇄ E11.355 Type 2 diabetes mellitus with stable proliferative diabetic retinopathy
❼⇄ E11.359 Type 2 diabetes mellitus with proliferative diabetic retinopathy without macular edema
E11.36 Type 2 diabetes mellitus with diabetic cataract
E11.39 Type 2 diabetes mellitus with other diabetic ophthalmic complication
E11.65 Type 2 diabetes mellitus with hyperglycemia
⇄ H18.11 Bullous keratopathy, right eye
H20.9 Unspecified iridocyclitis
⇄ H21.1X1 Other vascular disorders of iris and ciliary body, right eye
⇄ H25.011 Cortical age-related cataract, right eye
⇄ H25.11 Age-related nuclear cataract, right eye
⇄ H25.811 Combined forms of age-related cataract, right eye
H25.89 Other age-related cataract
⇄ H30.21 Posterior cyclitis, right eye
H32 Chorioretinal disorders in diseases classified elsewhere
⇄ H33.21 Serous retinal detachment, right eye
⇄ H35.051 Retinal neovascularization, unspecified, right eye
❼⇄ H35.321 Exudative age-related macular degeneration, right eye
❼⇄ H35.322 Exudative age-related macular degeneration, left eye
❼⇄ H35.323 Exudative age-related macular degeneration, bilateral
⇄ H35.351 Cystoid macular degeneration, right eye
⇄ H35.361 Drusen (degenerative) of macula, right eye
⇄ H35.371 Puckering of macula, right eye
H35.81 Retinal edema
❼⇄ H40.111 Primary open-angle glaucoma, right eye
❼⇄ H40.112 Primary open-angle glaucoma, left eye
❼⇄ H40.113 Primary open-angle glaucoma, bilateral
⇄ H40.831 Aqueous misdirection, right eye
⇄ H43.11 Vitreous hemorrhage, right eye
⇄ H44.2C1 Degenerative myopia with retinal detachment, right eye
⇄ H44.2C2 Degenerative myopia with retinal detachment, left eye
⇄ H44.2C3 Degenerative myopia with retinal detachment, bilateral eye
⇄ H44.2E1 Degenerative myopia with other maculopathy, right eye
⇄ H44.2E2 Degenerative myopia with other maculopathy, left eye
⇄ H44.2E3 Degenerative myopia with other maculopathy, bilateral eye
T86.890 Other transplanted tissue rejection
T86.891 Other transplanted tissue failure
T86.892 Other transplanted tissue infection
T86.898 Other complications of other transplanted tissue

ICD-10-CM Coding Notes

For codes requiring a 7th character extension, refer to your ICD-10-CM book. Review the character descriptions and coding guidelines for proper selection. For some procedures, only certain characters will apply.

CCI Edits

Refer to Appendix A for CCI edits.

Facility RVUs ▯

Code	Work	PE Facility	MP	Total Facility
67500	1.18	0.55	0.09	1.82
67505	1.18	0.82	0.09	2.09

Non-facility RVUs ▯

Code	Work	PE Non-Facility	MP	Total Non-Facility
67500	1.18	0.95	0.09	2.22
67505	1.18	1.26	0.09	2.53

Modifiers (PAR) ▯

Code	Mod 50	Mod 51	Mod 62	Mod 66	Mod 80
67500	1	2	0	0	1
67505	1	2	0	0	1

Global Period

Code	Days
67500	000
67505	000

67515

67515 Injection of medication or other substance into Tenon's capsule

(For subconjunctival injection, use 68200)

AMA Coding Notes

Surgical Procedures on the Eye and Ocular Adnexa

(For diagnostic and treatment ophthalmological services, see Medicine, Ophthalmology, and 92002 et seq)

(Do not report code 69990 in addition to codes 65091-68850)

AMA *CPT® Assistant* ▯

67515: Nov 12: 10

Plain English Description

The Tenon's capsule is a thin fascial sheath that envelopes the eyeball and separates it from the orbital fat. The inner surface is smooth and shiny and is separated from the outer surface of the sclera by a potential space called the episcleral or sub-Tenon's space. The fascial sheath and the sclera are actually attached to each other by fine bands of connective tissue. The anterior aspect of the fascial sheath is attached to the sclera about 1.5 cm posterior to the corneoscleral junction. In the posterior aspect the sheath fuses with the meninges around the optic nerve and with the sclera where the optic nerve exits the eyeball. The tendons of all six extrinsic eye muscles pierce the sheath and the fascial sheath forms a tubular sleeve around the tendons. To perform Tenon's capsule injection, local anesthetic eye drops are administered. An eyelid speculum is placed to keep the lids open. As the patient looks upwards and outwards, the Tenon's capsule and sclera are grasped with a forceps. A small incision may be made. A blunt, curved sub-Tenon's capsule cannula is mounted on a syringe and inserted along the curvature of the sclera. The cannula is passed into the posterior sub-Tenon's space. The medication or other substance is injected. The cannula is removed and pressure applied over the globe so that the substance injected will spread throughout the capsule.

Injection of medication or other substance into Tenon's capsule

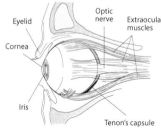

The physician injects medication or another substance into the thin sac that surrounds the eye and allows it to move in the eye socket.

ICD-10-CM Diagnostic Codes

	B39.4	Histoplasmosis capsulati, unspecified
	B39.9	Histoplasmosis, unspecified
	E08.311	Diabetes mellitus due to underlying condition with unspecified diabetic retinopathy with macular edema
	E08.319	Diabetes mellitus due to underlying condition with unspecified diabetic retinopathy without macular edema
❼⇄	E08.321	Diabetes mellitus due to underlying condition with mild nonproliferative diabetic retinopathy with macular edema
❼⇄	E08.329	Diabetes mellitus due to underlying condition with mild nonproliferative diabetic retinopathy without macular edema
❼⇄	E08.331	Diabetes mellitus due to underlying condition with moderate nonproliferative diabetic retinopathy with macular edema
❼⇄	E08.339	Diabetes mellitus due to underlying condition with moderate nonproliferative diabetic retinopathy without macular edema
❼⇄	E08.341	Diabetes mellitus due to underlying condition with severe nonproliferative diabetic retinopathy with macular edema
❼⇄	E08.349	Diabetes mellitus due to underlying condition with severe nonproliferative diabetic retinopathy without macular edema
❼⇄	E08.351	Diabetes mellitus due to underlying condition with proliferative diabetic retinopathy with macular edema
❼⇄	E08.352	Diabetes mellitus due to underlying condition with proliferative diabetic retinopathy with traction retinal detachment involving the macula
❼⇄	E08.353	Diabetes mellitus due to underlying condition with proliferative diabetic retinopathy with traction retinal detachment not involving the macula
❼⇄	E08.354	Diabetes mellitus due to underlying condition with proliferative diabetic retinopathy with combined traction retinal detachment and rhegmatogenous retinal detachment
❼⇄	E08.355	Diabetes mellitus due to underlying condition with stable proliferative diabetic retinopathy
❼⇄	E08.359	Diabetes mellitus due to underlying condition with proliferative diabetic retinopathy without macular edema
	E08.36	Diabetes mellitus due to underlying condition with diabetic cataract
	E08.39	Diabetes mellitus due to underlying condition with other diabetic ophthalmic complication
	E09.311	Drug or chemical induced diabetes mellitus with unspecified diabetic retinopathy with macular edema
	E09.319	Drug or chemical induced diabetes mellitus with unspecified diabetic retinopathy without macular edema
❼⇄	E09.321	Drug or chemical induced diabetes mellitus with mild nonproliferative diabetic retinopathy with macular edema
❼⇄	E09.329	Drug or chemical induced diabetes mellitus with mild nonproliferative diabetic retinopathy without macular edema
❼⇄	E09.331	Drug or chemical induced diabetes mellitus with moderate nonproliferative diabetic retinopathy with macular edema
❼⇄	E09.339	Drug or chemical induced diabetes mellitus with moderate nonproliferative diabetic retinopathy without macular edema
❼⇄	E09.341	Drug or chemical induced diabetes mellitus with severe nonproliferative diabetic retinopathy with macular edema
❼⇄	E09.349	Drug or chemical induced diabetes mellitus with severe nonproliferative diabetic retinopathy without macular edema
❼⇄	E09.351	Drug or chemical induced diabetes mellitus with proliferative diabetic retinopathy with macular edema
❼⇄	E09.352	Drug or chemical induced diabetes mellitus with proliferative diabetic retinopathy with traction retinal detachment involving the macula
❼⇄	E09.353	Drug or chemical induced diabetes mellitus with proliferative diabetic retinopathy with traction retinal detachment not involving the macula
❼⇄	E09.354	Drug or chemical induced diabetes mellitus with proliferative diabetic retinopathy with combined traction retinal detachment and rhegmatogenous retinal detachment
❼⇄	E09.355	Drug or chemical induced diabetes mellitus with stable proliferative diabetic retinopathy
❼⇄	E09.359	Drug or chemical induced diabetes mellitus with proliferative diabetic retinopathy without macular edema
	E09.36	Drug or chemical induced diabetes mellitus with diabetic cataract
	E09.39	Drug or chemical induced diabetes mellitus with other diabetic ophthalmic complication
	E10.311	Type 1 diabetes mellitus with unspecified diabetic retinopathy with macular edema
	E10.319	Type 1 diabetes mellitus with unspecified diabetic retinopathy without macular edema
❼⇄	E10.321	Type 1 diabetes mellitus with mild nonproliferative diabetic retinopathy with macular edema
❼⇄	E10.329	Type 1 diabetes mellitus with mild nonproliferative diabetic retinopathy without macular edema
❼⇄	E10.331	Type 1 diabetes mellitus with moderate nonproliferative diabetic retinopathy with macular edema

⑦⇄ E10.339 Type 1 diabetes mellitus with moderate nonproliferative diabetic retinopathy without macular edema
⑦⇄ E10.341 Type 1 diabetes mellitus with severe nonproliferative diabetic retinopathy with macular edema
⑦⇄ E10.349 Type 1 diabetes mellitus with severe nonproliferative diabetic retinopathy without macular edema
⑦⇄ E10.351 Type 1 diabetes mellitus with proliferative diabetic retinopathy with macular edema
⑦⇄ E10.352 Type 1 diabetes mellitus with proliferative diabetic retinopathy with traction retinal detachment involving the macula
⑦⇄ E10.353 Type 1 diabetes mellitus with proliferative diabetic retinopathy with traction retinal detachment not involving the macula
⑦⇄ E10.354 Type 1 diabetes mellitus with proliferative diabetic retinopathy with combined traction retinal detachment and rhegmatogenous retinal detachment
⑦⇄ E10.355 Type 1 diabetes mellitus with stable proliferative diabetic retinopathy
⑦⇄ E10.359 Type 1 diabetes mellitus with proliferative diabetic retinopathy without macular edema
E10.36 Type 1 diabetes mellitus with diabetic cataract
E10.39 Type 1 diabetes mellitus with other diabetic ophthalmic complication
E10.65 Type 1 diabetes mellitus with hyperglycemia
E11.311 Type 2 diabetes mellitus with unspecified diabetic retinopathy with macular edema
E11.319 Type 2 diabetes mellitus with unspecified diabetic retinopathy without macular edema
⑦⇄ E11.321 Type 2 diabetes mellitus with mild nonproliferative diabetic retinopathy with macular edema
⑦⇄ E11.329 Type 2 diabetes mellitus with mild nonproliferative diabetic retinopathy without macular edema
⑦⇄ E11.331 Type 2 diabetes mellitus with moderate nonproliferative diabetic retinopathy with macular edema
⑦⇄ E11.339 Type 2 diabetes mellitus with moderate nonproliferative diabetic retinopathy without macular edema
⑦⇄ E11.341 Type 2 diabetes mellitus with severe nonproliferative diabetic retinopathy with macular edema
⑦⇄ E11.349 Type 2 diabetes mellitus with severe nonproliferative diabetic retinopathy without macular edema
⑦⇄ E11.351 Type 2 diabetes mellitus with proliferative diabetic retinopathy with macular edema
⑦⇄ E11.352 Type 2 diabetes mellitus with proliferative diabetic retinopathy with traction retinal detachment involving the macula
⑦⇄ E11.353 Type 2 diabetes mellitus with proliferative diabetic retinopathy with traction retinal detachment not involving the macula
⑦⇄ E11.354 Type 2 diabetes mellitus with proliferative diabetic retinopathy with combined traction retinal detachment and rhegmatogenous retinal detachment
⑦⇄ E11.355 Type 2 diabetes mellitus with stable proliferative diabetic retinopathy
⑦⇄ E11.359 Type 2 diabetes mellitus with proliferative diabetic retinopathy without macular edema
E11.36 Type 2 diabetes mellitus with diabetic cataract
E11.39 Type 2 diabetes mellitus with other diabetic ophthalmic complication
E11.65 Type 2 diabetes mellitus with hyperglycemia
⇄ H00.024 Hordeolum internum left upper eyelid
⇄ H00.025 Hordeolum internum left lower eyelid
⇄ H20.012 Primary iridocyclitis, left eye
⇄ H20.022 Recurrent acute iridocyclitis, left eye
⇄ H20.12 Chronic iridocyclitis, left eye
⇄ H25.12 Age-related nuclear cataract, left eye
⇄ H30.22 Posterior cyclitis, left eye
H32 Chorioretinal disorders in diseases classified elsewhere
H33.8 Other retinal detachments
⑦⇄ H34.832 Tributary (branch) retinal vein occlusion, left eye
⑦⇄ H35.311 Nonexudative age-related macular degeneration, right eye
⑦⇄ H35.312 Nonexudative age-related macular degeneration, left eye
⑦⇄ H35.313 Nonexudative age-related macular degeneration, bilateral
⑦⇄ H35.321 Exudative age-related macular degeneration, right eye
⑦⇄ H35.322 Exudative age-related macular degeneration, left eye
⑦⇄ H35.323 Exudative age-related macular degeneration, bilateral
⇄ H35.352 Cystoid macular degeneration, left eye
⇄ H35.372 Puckering of macula, left eye
H35.81 Retinal edema
⑦⇄ H40.111 Primary open-angle glaucoma, right eye
⑦⇄ H40.112 Primary open-angle glaucoma, left eye
⑦⇄ H40.113 Primary open-angle glaucoma, bilateral
⇄ H44.2A1 Degenerative myopia with choroidal neovascularization, right eye
⇄ H44.2A2 Degenerative myopia with choroidal neovascularization, left eye
⇄ H44.2A3 Degenerative myopia with choroidal neovascularization, bilateral eye
⇄ H44.2B1 Degenerative myopia with macular hole, right eye
⇄ H44.2B2 Degenerative myopia with macular hole, left eye
⇄ H44.2B3 Degenerative myopia with macular hole, bilateral eye
⇄ H44.2C1 Degenerative myopia with retinal detachment, right eye
⇄ H44.2C2 Degenerative myopia with retinal detachment, left eye
⇄ H44.2C3 Degenerative myopia with retinal detachment, bilateral eye
⇄ H44.2E1 Degenerative myopia with other maculopathy, right eye
⇄ H44.2E2 Degenerative myopia with other maculopathy, left eye
⇄ H44.2E3 Degenerative myopia with other maculopathy, bilateral eye
⇄ H57.12 Ocular pain, left eye

ICD-10-CM Coding Notes

For codes requiring a 7th character extension, refer to your ICD-10-CM book. Review the character descriptions and coding guidelines for proper selection. For some procedures, only certain characters will apply.

CCI Edits

Refer to Appendix A for CCI edits.

Facility RVUs ▯

Code	Work	PE Facility	MP	Total Facility
67515	0.75	0.55	0.07	1.37

Non-facility RVUs ▯

Code	Work	PE Non-Facility	MP	Total Non-Facility
67515	0.75	0.70	0.07	1.52

Modifiers (PAR) ▯

Code	Mod 50	Mod 51	Mod 62	Mod 66	Mod 80
67515	1	2	0	0	1

Global Period

Code	Days
67515	000

67550-67560

67550 Orbital implant (implant outside muscle cone); insertion

67560 Orbital implant (implant outside muscle cone); removal or revision

(For ocular implant (implant inside muscle cone), see 65093-65105, 65130-65175)

(For treatment of fractures of malar area, orbit, see 21355 et seq)

AMA Coding Notes

Surgical Procedures on the Eye and Ocular Adnexa

(For diagnostic and treatment ophthalmological services, see Medicine, Ophthalmology, and 92002 et seq)

(Do not report code 69990 in addition to codes 65091-68850)

Plain English Description

An orbital implant located outside the muscle cone is inserted, removed or revised. Implants placed outside the muscle cone are typically used for patients with extensive loss of tissue in the orbit due to trauma, surgery or radiation treatment. The physician works with an anaplastologist to determine the type and position of the implant. This procedure may be performed in one or two stages. The first part of the procedure consists of placing one or more titanium implants into the bone to which the prosthesis will be attached. A skin incision is made at the planned implant site. Soft tissues are dissected and the orbital periosteum is exposed. One or more implant sites in the bone are prepared, which involves incising the periosteum and then creating burr holes. The periosteum is incised in a cruciate fashion and the edges are raised. A drill is used to create a burr hole in the orbital bone. Soft tissues are then prepared. All hair follicles around the implant site are removed. The subcutaneous tissue is reduced to minimize skin mobility at the implant site. The periosteum is trimmed down to the innermost layer. The implant is then seated in the bone using a specially designed drill. This is repeated until all the implant components are in place. The soft tissue and skin around the implants is then closed. In a one-stage procedure, healing abutments are placed until the implants have osseointegrated. The wound is dressed. In a two-stage procedure, a cover screw is inserted into the implant and the soft tissue and skin is closed over the bone and the implants. Approximately 4-6 months later once the implants have osseointegrated. The skin is incised and the cover screws removed. The skin and soft tissues are repaired and abutments placed. Healing caps are attached to the abutments and a dressing applied. Once healing is complete the orbital implant, which has been fabricated in a separately reportable procedure, is attached to the abutments. Use 67550 for insertion of orbital implant. Use 67560 if complications arise and the orbital implant must be removed or revised. Removal is typically performed for infection. The abutments are removed. The bone implants are exposed and the removed. All infected tissue is debrided. A drain is placed as needed. Soft tissue and skin are closed around the drain. Revision may be required if there is excessive skin mobility at the implant site causing irritation. The abutments are removed and the implants are exposed and inspected. The subcutaneous tissue may be thinned to prevent mobility and irritation of the overlying skin or other revision measures performed. The skin is closed over the implants and the abutments replaced.

Orbital implant (implant outside muscle cone) insertion/removal/revision

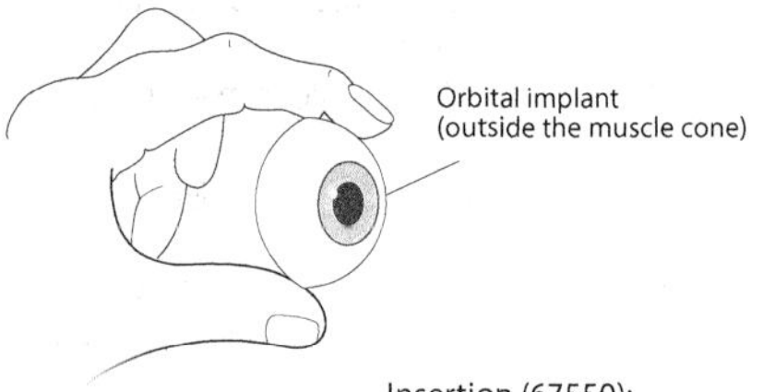

ICD-10-CM Diagnostic Codes

⇄	H05.331	Deformity of right orbit due to trauma or surgery
⇄	H05.332	Deformity of left orbit due to trauma or surgery
⇄	H05.333	Deformity of bilateral orbits due to trauma or surgery
➐	S07.1	Crushing injury of skull
➐	T20.39	Burn of third degree of multiple sites of head, face, and neck
➐	T20.79	Corrosion of third degree of multiple sites of head, face, and neck
➐⇄	T85.310	Breakdown (mechanical) of prosthetic orbit of right eye
➐⇄	T85.320	Displacement of prosthetic orbit of right eye
➐⇄	T85.390	Other mechanical complication of prosthetic orbit of right eye
➐	T85.79	Infection and inflammatory reaction due to other internal prosthetic devices, implants and grafts
⇄	Z44.21	Encounter for fitting and adjustment of artificial right eye
	Z85.840	Personal history of malignant neoplasm of eye
	Z97.0	Presence of artificial eye

ICD-10-CM Coding Notes

For codes requiring a 7th character extension, refer to your ICD-10-CM book. Review the character descriptions and coding guidelines for proper selection. For some procedures, only certain characters will apply.

CCI Edits

Refer to Appendix A for CCI edits.

Facility RVUs ▢

Code	Work	PE Facility	MP	Total Facility
67550	11.77	19.33	1.00	32.10
67560	12.18	19.60	1.00	32.78

Non-facility RVUs ▢

Code	Work	PE Non-Facility	MP	Total Non-Facility
67550	11.77	19.33	1.00	32.10
67560	12.18	19.60	1.00	32.78

Modifiers (PAR) ▢

Code	Mod 50	Mod 51	Mod 62	Mod 66	Mod 80
67550	1	2	1	0	1
67560	1	2	0	0	0

Global Period

Code	Days
67550	090
67560	090

67570

67570 Optic nerve decompression (eg, incision or fenestration of optic nerve sheath)

AMA Coding Notes

Surgical Procedures on the Eye and Ocular Adnexa

(For diagnostic and treatment ophthalmological services, see Medicine, Ophthalmology, and 92002 et seq)

(Do not report code 69990 in addition to codes 65091-68850)

Plain English Description

Optic nerve decompression may be needed following a traumatic closed head injury causing traumatic optic neuropathy, papilledema accompanying pseudotumor cerebri, also referred to as idiopathic intracranial hypertension, or other condition causing compression of the optic nerve with associated loss of vision. The optic nerve may be approached via a transfrontal craniotomy, extranasal or intranasal transethmoidal approach, or lateral facial approach. If a transfrontal craniotomy is performed, the skin is incised over the affected eye and dissection carried down to the frontal bone. Burr holes are drilled and the holes connected using an oscillating saw or craniotome. A bone flap is elevated. The orbit is exposed and the optic nerve identified. The bone of the optic canal around the optic nerve is thinned as needed to widen the canal. The Zinn rings and the optic nerve sheath are incised to allow decompression of the nerve. Once the decompression is complete, the bone flap is replaced and secured with miniplates and screws. Soft tissue and skin are closed in layers. If an extranasal or intranasal ethmoidal approach is used, a total ethmoidectomy is performed and the orbital apex exposed. The optic nerve is located and exposed. The medial optic canal is enlarged with a burr followed by bone curettage. The nerve is then decompressed as described above.

Optic nerve decompression (eg, incision/fenestration of optic nerve sheath)

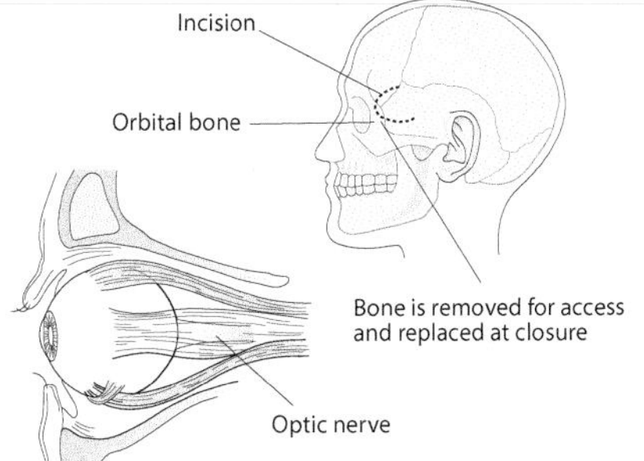

The optic nerve is accessed and perforated for decompression.

ICD-10-CM Diagnostic Codes

	Code	Description
	G93.2	Benign intracranial hypertension
⇄	H46.01	Optic papillitis, right eye
⇄	H46.02	Optic papillitis, left eye
⇄	H46.03	Optic papillitis, bilateral
	H46.8	Other optic neuritis
	H46.9	Unspecified optic neuritis
⇄	H47.021	Hemorrhage in optic nerve sheath, right eye
⇄	H47.022	Hemorrhage in optic nerve sheath, left eye
⇄	H47.023	Hemorrhage in optic nerve sheath, bilateral
⇄	H47.091	Other disorders of optic nerve, not elsewhere classified, right eye
⇄	H47.092	Other disorders of optic nerve, not elsewhere classified, left eye
⇄	H47.093	Other disorders of optic nerve, not elsewhere classified, bilateral
	H47.10	Unspecified papilledema
	H47.11	Papilledema associated with increased intracranial pressure
	I67.4	Hypertensive encephalopathy
❼	S06.1X0	Traumatic cerebral edema without loss of consciousness
❼⇄	S06.340	Traumatic hemorrhage of right cerebrum without loss of consciousness
❼⇄	S06.350	Traumatic hemorrhage of left cerebrum without loss of consciousness
❼	S06.360	Traumatic hemorrhage of cerebrum, unspecified, without loss of consciousness
❼	S06.5X0	Traumatic subdural hemorrhage without loss of consciousness
❼	S06.6X0	Traumatic subarachnoid hemorrhage without loss of consciousness
❼	S06.9X0	Unspecified intracranial injury without loss of consciousness

ICD-10-CM Coding Notes

For codes requiring a 7th character extension, refer to your ICD-10-CM book. Review the character descriptions and coding guidelines for proper selection. For some procedures, only certain characters will apply.

CCI Edits

Refer to Appendix A for CCI edits.

Facility RVUs ▯

Code	Work	PE Facility	MP	Total Facility
67570	14.40	23.55	2.93	40.88

Non-facility RVUs ▯

Code	Work	PE Non-Facility	MP	Total Non-Facility
67570	14.40	23.55	2.93	40.88

Modifiers (PAR) ▯

Code	Mod 50	Mod 51	Mod 62	Mod 66	Mod 80
67570	1	2	1	0	2

Global Period

Code	Days
67570	090

67700

67700 Blepharotomy, drainage of abscess, eyelid

AMA Coding Notes

Surgical Procedures on the Eye and Ocular Adnexa

(For diagnostic and treatment ophthalmological services, see Medicine, Ophthalmology, and 92002 et seq)

(Do not report code 69990 in addition to codes 65091-68850)

AMA *CPT® Assistant*

67700: Mar 13: 6

Plain English Description

A blepharotomy is performed to drain an eyelid abscess. The skin overlying the abscess is cleansed and a local anesthetic injected. An incision is made over the area of greatest fluctuance and the abscess is drained.

Blepharotomy, drainage of abscess, eyelid

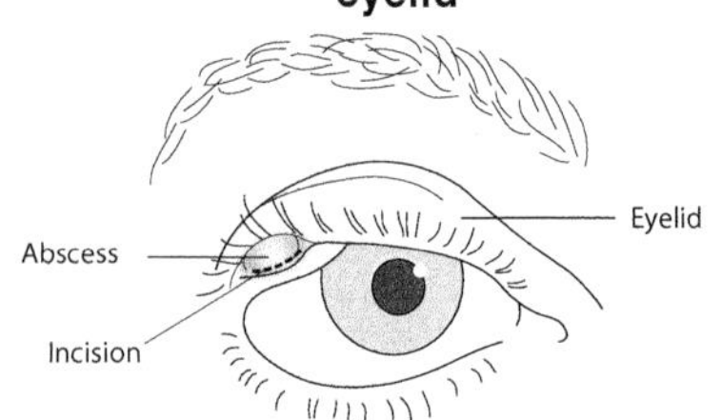

The physician makes an incision to drain an abscess on the eyelid.

ICD-10-CM Diagnostic Codes

⇄	H00.011	Hordeolum externum right upper eyelid
⇄	H00.012	Hordeolum externum right lower eyelid
⇄	H00.021	Hordeolum internum right upper eyelid
⇄	H00.022	Hordeolum internum right lower eyelid
⇄	H00.031	Abscess of right upper eyelid
⇄	H00.032	Abscess of right lower eyelid
⇄	H00.034	Abscess of left upper eyelid
⇄	H00.035	Abscess of left lower eyelid
⇄	H00.11	Chalazion right upper eyelid
⇄	H00.12	Chalazion right lower eyelid
⇄	H00.14	Chalazion left upper eyelid
⇄	H00.15	Chalazion left lower eyelid
⇄	H01.001	Unspecified blepharitis right upper eyelid
⇄	H01.002	Unspecified blepharitis right lower eyelid
⇄	H01.004	Unspecified blepharitis left upper eyelid
⇄	H01.005	Unspecified blepharitis left lower eyelid
⇄	H01.00A	Unspecified blepharitis right eye, upper and lower eyelids
⇄	H01.00B	Unspecified blepharitis left eye, upper and lower eyelids
⇄	H01.011	Ulcerative blepharitis right upper eyelid
⇄	H01.012	Ulcerative blepharitis right lower eyelid
⇄	H01.014	Ulcerative blepharitis left upper eyelid
⇄	H01.015	Ulcerative blepharitis left lower eyelid
⇄	H01.01A	Ulcerative blepharitis right eye, upper and lower eyelids
⇄	H01.01B	Ulcerative blepharitis left eye, upper and lower eyelids
	H01.8	Other specified inflammations of eyelid
	H01.9	Unspecified inflammation of eyelid

CCI Edits

Refer to Appendix A for CCI edits.

Facility RVUs

Code	Work	PE Facility	MP	Total Facility
67700	1.40	1.85	0.11	3.36

Non-facility RVUs

Code	Work	PE Non-Facility	MP	Total Non-Facility
67700	1.40	7.06	0.11	8.57

Modifiers (PAR)

Code	Mod 50	Mod 51	Mod 62	Mod 66	Mod 80
67700	1	2	0	0	1

Global Period

Code	Days
67700	010

67710

67710 Severing of tarsorrhaphy

AMA Coding Notes

Surgical Procedures on the Eye and Ocular Adnexa

(For diagnostic and treatment ophthalmological services, see Medicine, Ophthalmology, and 92002 et seq)

(Do not report code 69990 in addition to codes 65091-68850)

AMA *CPT® Assistant* ▯

67710: Mar 13: 6

Plain English Description

The physician removes sutures that were previously placed in the eyelids to close them. Suturing of the eyelids, also referred to as tarsorrhaphy, is a rare procedure used to protect the eye following an eye injury, due to a corneal disease that has caused inflammation of the cornea, due to dendritic ulcers caused by a virus, or for other conditions that require closure of the eyelid. The sutures are cut and removed.

Severing of tarsorrhaphy

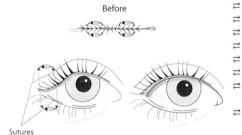

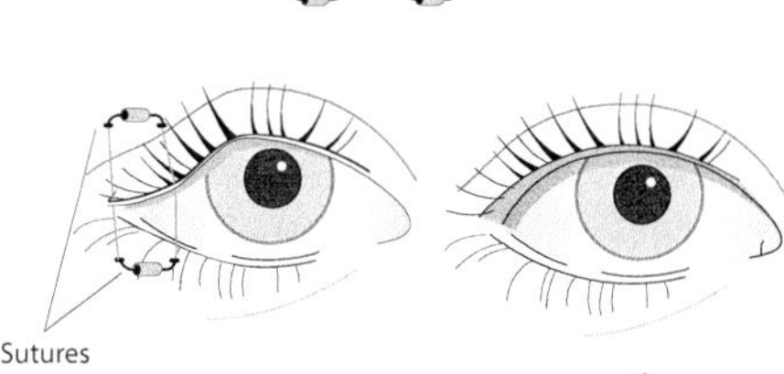

The physician reverses a procedure in which the eyelids are partially sewn shut to protect the eye.

ICD-10-CM Diagnostic Codes

	Code	Description
	B00.52	Herpesviral keratitis
	B02.33	Zoster keratitis
	E05.00	Thyrotoxicosis with diffuse goiter without thyrotoxic crisis or storm
	E05.01	Thyrotoxicosis with diffuse goiter with thyrotoxic crisis or storm
	G50.8	Other disorders of trigeminal nerve
	G51.0	Bell's palsy
	G51.8	Other disorders of facial nerve
	G51.9	Disorder of facial nerve, unspecified
⇄	H02.151	Paralytic ectropion of right upper eyelid
⇄	H02.152	Paralytic ectropion of right lower eyelid
⇄	H02.154	Paralytic ectropion of left upper eyelid
⇄	H02.155	Paralytic ectropion of left lower eyelid
⇄	H02.221	Mechanical lagophthalmos right upper eyelid
⇄	H02.222	Mechanical lagophthalmos right lower eyelid
⇄	H02.224	Mechanical lagophthalmos left upper eyelid
⇄	H02.225	Mechanical lagophthalmos left lower eyelid
⇄	H02.22A	Mechanical lagophthalmos right eye, upper and lower eyelids
⇄	H02.22B	Mechanical lagophthalmos left eye, upper and lower eyelids
⇄	H02.231	Paralytic lagophthalmos right upper eyelid
⇄	H02.232	Paralytic lagophthalmos right lower eyelid
⇄	H02.234	Paralytic lagophthalmos left upper eyelid
⇄	H02.235	Paralytic lagophthalmos left lower eyelid
⇄	H02.23A	Paralytic lagophthalmos right eye, upper and lower eyelids
⇄	H02.23B	Paralytic lagophthalmos left eye, upper and lower eyelids
⇄	H02.524	Blepharophimosis left upper eyelid
⇄	H02.525	Blepharophimosis left lower eyelid
⇄	H04.121	Dry eye syndrome of right lacrimal gland
⇄	H04.122	Dry eye syndrome of left lacrimal gland
⇄	H04.123	Dry eye syndrome of bilateral lacrimal glands
⇄	H16.011	Central corneal ulcer, right eye
⇄	H16.012	Central corneal ulcer, left eye
⇄	H16.041	Marginal corneal ulcer, right eye
⇄	H16.042	Marginal corneal ulcer, left eye
⇄	H16.111	Macular keratitis, right eye
⇄	H16.112	Macular keratitis, left eye
⇄	H16.141	Punctate keratitis, right eye
⇄	H16.142	Punctate keratitis, left eye
⇄	H16.211	Exposure keratoconjunctivitis, right eye
⇄	H16.212	Exposure keratoconjunctivitis, left eye
⇄	H16.231	Neurotrophic keratoconjunctivitis, right eye
⇄	H16.232	Neurotrophic keratoconjunctivitis, left eye
⇄	H18.792	Other corneal deformities, left eye
	M35.01	Sjögren syndrome with keratoconjunctivitis
➐⇄	S04.51	Injury of facial nerve, right side
➐⇄	S04.52	Injury of facial nerve, left side
➐	T81.89	Other complications of procedures, not elsewhere classified
⇄	T86.848	Other complications of corneal transplant
	Z48.02	Encounter for removal of sutures
	Z48.89	Encounter for other specified surgical aftercare

ICD-10-CM Coding Notes

For codes requiring a 7th character extension, refer to your ICD-10-CM book. Review the character descriptions and coding guidelines for proper selection. For some procedures, only certain characters will apply.

CCI Edits

Refer to Appendix A for CCI edits.

Facility RVUs ▯

Code	Work	PE Facility	MP	Total Facility
67710	1.07	1.67	0.09	2.83

Non-facility RVUs ▯

Code	Work	PE Non-Facility	MP	Total Non-Facility
67710	1.07	6.16	0.09	7.32

Modifiers (PAR) ▯

Code	Mod 50	Mod 51	Mod 62	Mod 66	Mod 80
67710	1	2	0	0	1

Global Period

Code	Days
67710	010

67715

67715 Canthotomy (separate procedure)

(For canthoplasty, use 67950)

(For division of symblepharon, use 68340)

AMA Coding Notes

Surgical Procedures on the Eye and Ocular Adnexa

(For diagnostic and treatment ophthalmological services, see Medicine, Ophthalmology, and 92002 et seq)

(Do not report code 69990 in addition to codes 65091-68850)

AMA *CPT® Assistant* ▯

67715: Mar 13: 6

Plain English Description

Canthotomy is typically performed on the lateral canthus to relieve pressure and swelling in the eye following trauma. The skin on the lateral aspect of the eye is crimped with a hemostat for 1-2 minutes to help achieve hemostasis and to mark the line of the incision. The hemostat is released and a forceps is used to elevate the skin around the lateral aspect of the eye. Scissors are used to make the incision beginning at the lateral canthus and extending laterally outward from the eye. If this does not relieve the pressure and swelling the lateral canthus tendon is exposed and divided. The incision is left open until the pressure and swelling subsides.

Canthotomy
(separate procedure)

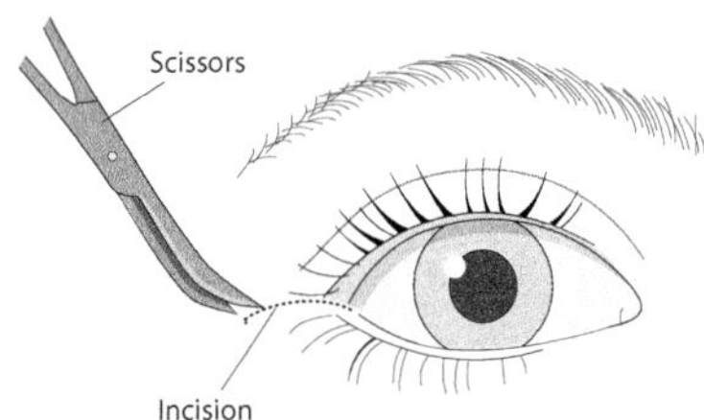

Scissors cut the lateral canthus to further divide the upper and lower lid.

ICD-10-CM Diagnostic Codes

⇄	H02.521	Blepharophimosis right upper eyelid
⇄	H02.522	Blepharophimosis right lower eyelid
⇄	H02.524	Blepharophimosis left upper eyelid
⇄	H02.525	Blepharophimosis left lower eyelid
⇄	H05.011	Cellulitis of right orbit
⇄	H05.012	Cellulitis of left orbit
⇄	H05.231	Hemorrhage of right orbit
⇄	H05.232	Hemorrhage of left orbit
	H05.89	Other disorders of orbit
❼⇄	S00.11	Contusion of right eyelid and periocular area
❼⇄	S00.12	Contusion of left eyelid and periocular area
❼⇄	S05.11	Contusion of eyeball and orbital tissues, right eye
❼⇄	S05.12	Contusion of eyeball and orbital tissues, left eye
❼	S07.0	Crushing injury of face

ICD-10-CM Coding Notes

For codes requiring a 7th character extension, refer to your ICD-10-CM book. Review the character descriptions and coding guidelines for proper selection. For some procedures, only certain characters will apply.

CCI Edits

Refer to Appendix A for CCI edits.

Facility RVUs ▯

Code	Work	PE Facility	MP	Total Facility
67715	1.27	1.70	0.17	3.14

Non-facility RVUs ▯

Code	Work	PE Non-Facility	MP	Total Non-Facility
67715	1.27	6.51	0.17	7.95

Modifiers (PAR) ▯

Code	Mod 50	Mod 51	Mod 62	Mod 66	Mod 80
67715	1	2	0	0	1

Global Period

Code	Days
67715	010

67800-67808

67800 **Excision of chalazion; single**

67801 **Excision of chalazion; multiple, same lid**

67805 **Excision of chalazion; multiple, different lids**

67808 **Excision of chalazion; under general anesthesia and/or requiring hospitalization, single or multiple**

AMA Coding Guideline

Excision and Destruction Procedures on the Eyelids

Codes for removal of lesion include more than skin (ie, involving lid margin, tarsus, and/or palpebral conjunctiva).

AMA Coding Notes

Excision and Destruction Procedures on the Eyelids

(For removal of lesion, involving mainly skin of eyelid, see 11310-11313; 11440-11446, 11640-11646; 17000-17004)

(For repair of wounds, blepharoplasty, grafts, reconstructive surgery, see 67930-67975)

Surgical Procedures on the Eye and Ocular Adnexa

(For diagnostic and treatment ophthalmological services, see Medicine, Ophthalmology, and 92002 et seq)

(Do not report code 69990 in addition to codes 65091-68850)

AMA *CPT® Assistant* ☐

67800: Sep 99: 10

67805: Sep 99: 10

Plain English Description

The physician excises one or more chalazia. A chalazion is an inflammatory lesion of the eyelid caused by obstruction of a sebaceous gland that may be superficial or deep depending on which gland is blocked. Superficial chalazia may be removed under local anesthesia while deep chalazia may require a hospitalization and a general anesthetic. A vertical incision is made in the palpebral conjunctival surface. The chalazion is removed by curettage or by dissecting the lesion from surrounding tissue. If a deep chalazion involving a meibomian gland is excised, the physician may cauterize or remove the meibomian gland. If the chalazion extends to the skin, it may be removed via an incision in the skin of the eyelid rather than the conjunctiva. For chalazia removed using a local anesthetic without hospitalization, use 67800 for excision of a single chalazion; 67801 for multiple chalazia of the same eyelid; and 67805 for multiple chalazia involving both eyelids. When removal of one or more chalazia requires general anesthesia and/or hospitalization, use 67808.

Excision of chalazion

Removal of small mass in eyelid

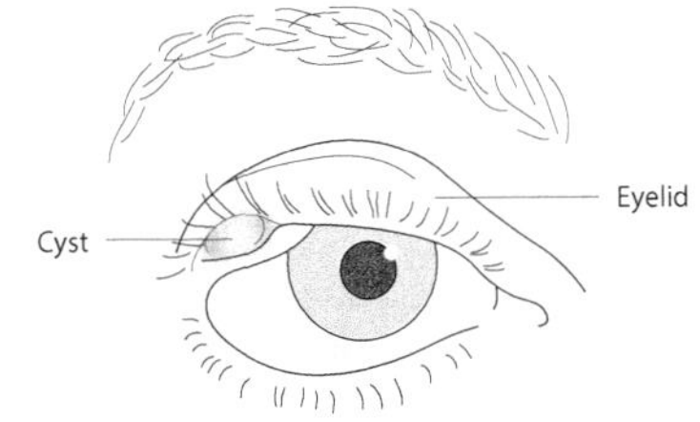

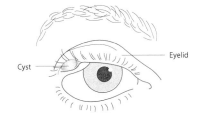

Single (67800); multiple same lid (67801); multiple different lids (67805); single or multiple under general anesthesia and/or requiring hospital visit (67808)

ICD-10-CM Diagnostic Codes

⇄	H00.11	Chalazion right upper eyelid
⇄	H00.12	Chalazion right lower eyelid
⇄	H00.14	Chalazion left upper eyelid
⇄	H00.15	Chalazion left lower eyelid

CCI Edits

Refer to Appendix A for CCI edits.

Facility RVUs ☐

Code	Work	PE Facility	MP	Total Facility
67800	1.41	1.44	0.11	2.96
67801	1.91	1.75	0.14	3.80
67805	2.27	2.28	0.19	4.74
67808	4.60	5.67	0.37	10.64

Non-facility RVUs ☐

Code	Work	PE Non-Facility	MP	Total Non-Facility
67800	1.41	2.24	0.11	3.76
67801	1.91	2.70	0.14	4.75
67805	2.27	3.48	0.19	5.94
67808	4.60	5.67	0.37	10.64

Modifiers (PAR) ☐

Code	Mod 50	Mod 51	Mod 62	Mod 66	Mod 80
67800	0	2	0	0	1
67801	0	2	0	0	1
67805	0	2	0	0	1
67808	0	2	0	0	1

Global Period

Code	Days
67800	010
67801	010
67805	010
67808	090

67810

67810 Incisional biopsy of eyelid skin including lid margin

(For biopsy of skin of the eyelid, see 11102, 11103, 11104, 11105, 11106, 11107)

AMA Coding Notes

Surgical Procedures on the Eye and Ocular Adnexa

(For diagnostic and treatment ophthalmological services, see Medicine, Ophthalmology, and 92002 et seq)

(Do not report code 69990 in addition to codes 65091-68850)

AMA *CPT® Assistant* ▯

67810: Dec 04: 19, Feb 13: 16, Mar 13: 6

Plain English Description

An incisional biopsy of the eyelid is performed. The mass or lesion in the eyelid is identified. The skin is disinfected over the planned biopsy site and a local anesthetic is injected. An incision is made through the skin and a tissue sample is obtained from the mass or lesion. The incision is closed with sutures. The tissue sample is sent to the laboratory for separately reportable histological evaluation.

Biopsy of eyelid

Lesion or mass

Eyelid

The physician takes a tissue sample from the eyelid for examination and diagnosis.

ICD-10-CM Diagnostic Codes

	Code	Description
⇄	C43.111	Malignant melanoma of right upper eyelid, including canthus
⇄	C43.112	Malignant melanoma of right lower eyelid, including canthus
⇄	C43.121	Malignant melanoma of left upper eyelid, including canthus
⇄	C43.122	Malignant melanoma of left lower eyelid, including canthus
⇄	C44.1021	Unspecified malignant neoplasm of skin of right upper eyelid, including canthus
⇄	C44.1022	Unspecified malignant neoplasm of skin of right lower eyelid, including canthus
⇄	C44.1091	Unspecified malignant neoplasm of skin of left upper eyelid, including canthus
⇄	C44.1092	Unspecified malignant neoplasm of skin of left lower eyelid, including canthus
⇄	C44.1121	Basal cell carcinoma of skin of right upper eyelid, including canthus
⇄	C44.1122	Basal cell carcinoma of skin of right lower eyelid, including canthus
⇄	C44.1191	Basal cell carcinoma of skin of left upper eyelid, including canthus
⇄	C44.1192	Basal cell carcinoma of skin of left lower eyelid, including canthus
⇄	C44.1221	Squamous cell carcinoma of skin of right upper eyelid, including canthus
⇄	C44.1222	Squamous cell carcinoma of skin of right lower eyelid, including canthus
⇄	C44.1291	Squamous cell carcinoma of skin of left upper eyelid, including canthus
⇄	C44.1292	Squamous cell carcinoma of skin of left lower eyelid, including canthus
⇄	C44.1321	Sebaceous cell carcinoma of skin of right upper eyelid, including canthus
⇄	C44.1322	Sebaceous cell carcinoma of skin of right lower eyelid, including canthus
⇄	C44.1391	Sebaceous cell carcinoma of skin of left upper eyelid, including canthus
⇄	C44.1392	Sebaceous cell carcinoma of skin of left lower eyelid, including canthus
⇄	C44.1921	Other specified malignant neoplasm of skin of right upper eyelid, including canthus
⇄	C44.1922	Other specified malignant neoplasm of skin of right lower eyelid, including canthus
⇄	C44.1991	Other specified malignant neoplasm of skin of left upper eyelid, including canthus
⇄	C44.1992	Other specified malignant neoplasm of skin of left lower eyelid, including canthus
⇄	C4A.111	Merkel cell carcinoma of right upper eyelid, including canthus
⇄	C4A.112	Merkel cell carcinoma of right lower eyelid, including canthus
⇄	C4A.121	Merkel cell carcinoma of left upper eyelid, including canthus
⇄	C4A.122	Merkel cell carcinoma of left lower eyelid, including canthus
⇄	D03.111	Melanoma in situ of right upper eyelid, including canthus
⇄	D03.112	Melanoma in situ of right lower eyelid, including canthus
⇄	D03.121	Melanoma in situ of left upper eyelid, including canthus
⇄	D03.122	Melanoma in situ of left lower eyelid, including canthus
⇄	D04.111	Carcinoma in situ of skin of right upper eyelid, including canthus
⇄	D04.112	Carcinoma in situ of skin of right lower eyelid, including canthus
⇄	D04.121	Carcinoma in situ of skin of left upper eyelid, including canthus
⇄	D04.122	Carcinoma in situ of skin of left lower eyelid, including canthus
⇄	D22.111	Melanocytic nevi of right upper eyelid, including canthus
⇄	D22.112	Melanocytic nevi of right lower eyelid, including canthus
⇄	D22.121	Melanocytic nevi of left upper eyelid, including canthus
⇄	D22.122	Melanocytic nevi of left lower eyelid, including canthus
⇄	D23.111	Other benign neoplasm of skin of right upper eyelid, including canthus
⇄	D23.112	Other benign neoplasm of skin of right lower eyelid, including canthus
⇄	D23.121	Other benign neoplasm of skin of left upper eyelid, including canthus
⇄	D23.122	Other benign neoplasm of skin of left lower eyelid, including canthus

CCI Edits

Refer to Appendix A for CCI edits.

Facility RVUs ▯

Code	Work	PE Facility	MP	Total Facility
67810	1.18	0.69	0.11	1.98

Non-facility RVUs ▯

Code	Work	PE Non-Facility	MP	Total Non-Facility
67810	1.18	4.26	0.11	5.55

Modifiers (PAR) ▯

Code	Mod 50	Mod 51	Mod 62	Mod 66	Mod 80
67810	1	2	0	0	1

Global Period

Code	Days
67810	000

67820-67835

67820 Correction of trichiasis; epilation, by forceps only

67825 Correction of trichiasis; epilation by other than forceps (eg, by electrosurgery, cryotherapy, laser surgery)

67830 Correction of trichiasis; incision of lid margin

67835 Correction of trichiasis; incision of lid margin, with free mucous membrane graft

AMA Coding Guideline

Excision and Destruction Procedures on the Eyelids

Codes for removal of lesion include more than skin (ie, involving lid margin, tarsus, and/or palpebral conjunctiva).

AMA Coding Notes

Excision and Destruction Procedures on the Eyelids

(For removal of lesion, involving mainly skin of eyelid, see 11310-11313; 11440-11446, 11640-11646; 17000-17004)

(For repair of wounds, blepharoplasty, grafts, reconstructive surgery, see 67930-67975)

Surgical Procedures on the Eye and Ocular Adnexa

(For diagnostic and treatment ophthalmological services, see Medicine, Ophthalmology, and 92002 et seq)

(Do not report code 69990 in addition to codes 65091-68850)

AMA *CPT® Assistant*

67820: Jul 98: 10

67825: Jul 98: 10

Plain English Description

Trichiasis is a common eyelid abnormality characterized by an inward orientation of the lashes toward the globe. This causes irritation of the eye. Treatment depends on whether only a segment of the eyelid is involved or whether the lashes on the entire eyelid are misdirected. Removal of the eyelashes, also called epilation, is typically performed when only a segment of the eyelid is involved, while incision with or without grafting is performed when a larger portion of the eyelid is affected. In 67820, the eyelashes are removed using forceps. The eyelid is everted. Each misdirected eyelash is grasped and removed under microscopic visualization. In 67825, the eyelashes are removed using another technique. Typically, the lashes along with the lash follicle are destroyed. If cryosurgery is performed the lash and follicle are destroyed by freezing with liquid nitrogen or a cryoprobe. If electrosurgery is used a thermal electrocautery device is used. Radiofrequency ablation uses a small-gauge wire introduced alongside the lash down to the follicle. The radiofrequency device is activated and the tissue coagulated thereby destroying the lash and hair follicle. Alternatively, an Argon laser may be used to destroy the lash and follicle. In 67830, the lid margin is strategically incised to release scar tissue that may have formed and to redirect the lashes away from the globe. The incision is left open to heal by secondary intention. In 67835, the lid margin is incised as described above and a free mucosal graft used to repair the defect. A split thickness mucous membrane graft is harvested from the lower lip or other site using a mucotome. The graft is configured to the desired size and shape to fit the defect in the lid margin. The graft is sutured to the lid margin at the site of the surgically created defect.

Correction of trichiasis, epilation, by forceps; incision of lid margin

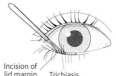

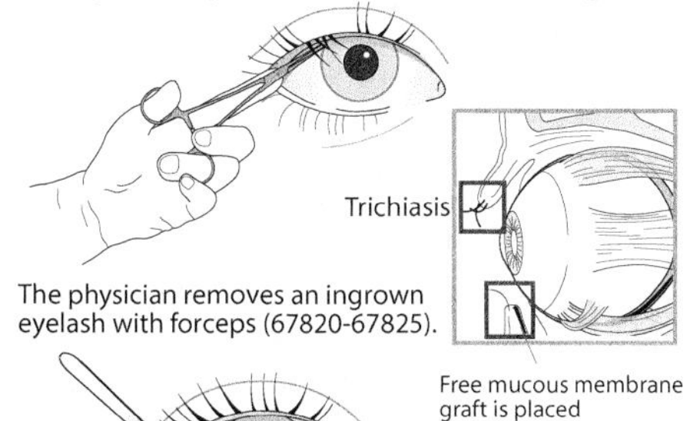

ICD-10-CM Diagnostic Codes

⇄	H02.051	Trichiasis without entropion right upper eyelid
⇄	H02.052	Trichiasis without entropion right lower eyelid
⇄	H02.054	Trichiasis without entropion left upper eyelid
⇄	H02.055	Trichiasis without entropion left lower eyelid
⇄	H02.861	Hypertrichosis of right upper eyelid
⇄	H02.862	Hypertrichosis of right lower eyelid
⇄	H02.864	Hypertrichosis of left upper eyelid
⇄	H02.865	Hypertrichosis of left lower eyelid
	H02.89	Other specified disorders of eyelid
	Q10.3	Other congenital malformations of eyelid

CCI Edits

Refer to Appendix A for CCI edits.

Pub 100

67825: Pub 100-03, 1, 140.5

Facility RVUs

Code	Work	PE Facility	MP	Total Facility
67820	0.32	0.30	0.02	0.64
67825	1.43	1.98	0.11	3.52
67830	1.75	2.08	0.12	3.95
67835	5.70	6.64	0.42	12.76

Non-facility RVUs

Code	Work	PE Non-Facility	MP	Total Non-Facility
67820	0.32	0.22	0.02	0.56
67825	1.43	2.43	0.11	3.97
67830	1.75	6.19	0.12	8.06
67835	5.70	6.64	0.42	12.76

Modifiers (PAR)

Code	Mod 50	Mod 51	Mod 62	Mod 66	Mod 80
67820	1	2	0	0	1
67825	1	2	0	0	1
67830	1	2	0	0	1
67835	1	2	0	0	0

Global Period

Code	Days
67820	000
67825	010
67830	010
67835	090

67840

67840 Excision of lesion of eyelid (except chalazion) without closure or with simple direct closure

(For excision and repair of eyelid by reconstructive surgery, see 67961, 67966)

AMA Coding Guideline

Excision and Destruction Procedures on the Eyelids

Codes for removal of lesion include more than skin (ie, involving lid margin, tarsus, and/or palpebral conjunctiva).

AMA Coding Notes

Excision and Destruction Procedures on the Eyelids

(For removal of lesion, involving mainly skin of eyelid, see 11310-11313; 11440-11446, 11640-11646; 17000-17004)

(For repair of wounds, blepharoplasty, grafts, reconstructive surgery, see 67930-67975)

Surgical Procedures on the Eye and Ocular Adnexa

(For diagnostic and treatment ophthalmological services, see Medicine, Ophthalmology, and 92002 et seq)

(Do not report code 69990 in addition to codes 65091-68850)

Plain English Description

A lesion of the eyelid other than a chalazion is excised without closure or with simple direct closure. The skin over the lesion is disinfected and a local anesthetic injected. An incision is made through the skin and the lesion is excised along with a margin of healthy tissue. The excised tissue is sent to the laboratory for separately reportable histological evaluation. The incision may be left open to heal by secondary intention or sutured using simple, single layer, direct closure.

Excision of lesion of eyelid

Lesion

ICD-10-CM Diagnostic Codes

	Code	Description
	B08.1	Molluscum contagiosum
⇄	C43.111	Malignant melanoma of right upper eyelid, including canthus
⇄	C43.112	Malignant melanoma of right lower eyelid, including canthus
⇄	C43.121	Malignant melanoma of left upper eyelid, including canthus
⇄	C43.122	Malignant melanoma of left lower eyelid, including canthus
⇄	C44.1021	Unspecified malignant neoplasm of skin of right upper eyelid, including canthus
⇄	C44.1022	Unspecified malignant neoplasm of skin of right lower eyelid, including canthus
⇄	C44.1091	Unspecified malignant neoplasm of skin of left upper eyelid, including canthus
⇄	C44.1092	Unspecified malignant neoplasm of skin of left lower eyelid, including canthus
⇄	C44.1121	Basal cell carcinoma of skin of right upper eyelid, including canthus
⇄	C44.1122	Basal cell carcinoma of skin of right lower eyelid, including canthus
⇄	C44.1191	Basal cell carcinoma of skin of left upper eyelid, including canthus
⇄	C44.1192	Basal cell carcinoma of skin of left lower eyelid, including canthus
⇄	C44.1221	Squamous cell carcinoma of skin of right upper eyelid, including canthus
⇄	C44.1222	Squamous cell carcinoma of skin of right lower eyelid, including canthus
⇄	C44.1291	Squamous cell carcinoma of skin of left upper eyelid, including canthus
⇄	C44.1292	Squamous cell carcinoma of skin of left lower eyelid, including canthus
⇄	C44.1321	Sebaceous cell carcinoma of skin of right upper eyelid, including canthus
⇄	C44.1322	Sebaceous cell carcinoma of skin of right lower eyelid, including canthus
⇄	C44.1391	Sebaceous cell carcinoma of skin of left upper eyelid, including canthus
⇄	C44.1392	Sebaceous cell carcinoma of skin of left lower eyelid, including canthus
⇄	C44.1921	Other specified malignant neoplasm of skin of right upper eyelid, including canthus
⇄	C44.1922	Other specified malignant neoplasm of skin of right lower eyelid, including canthus
⇄	C44.1991	Other specified malignant neoplasm of skin of left upper eyelid, including canthus
⇄	C44.1992	Other specified malignant neoplasm of skin of left lower eyelid, including canthus
⇄	C4A.111	Merkel cell carcinoma of right upper eyelid, including canthus
⇄	C4A.112	Merkel cell carcinoma of right lower eyelid, including canthus
⇄	C4A.121	Merkel cell carcinoma of left upper eyelid, including canthus
⇄	C4A.122	Merkel cell carcinoma of left lower eyelid, including canthus
⇄	D03.111	Melanoma in situ of right upper eyelid, including canthus
⇄	D03.112	Melanoma in situ of right lower eyelid, including canthus
⇄	D03.121	Melanoma in situ of left upper eyelid, including canthus
⇄	D03.122	Melanoma in situ of left lower eyelid, including canthus
⇄	D04.111	Carcinoma in situ of skin of right upper eyelid, including canthus
⇄	D04.112	Carcinoma in situ of skin of right lower eyelid, including canthus
⇄	D04.121	Carcinoma in situ of skin of left upper eyelid, including canthus
⇄	D04.122	Carcinoma in situ of skin of left lower eyelid, including canthus
	D17.0	Benign lipomatous neoplasm of skin and subcutaneous tissue of head, face and neck
	D18.01	Hemangioma of skin and subcutaneous tissue
⇄	D22.111	Melanocytic nevi of right upper eyelid, including canthus
⇄	D22.112	Melanocytic nevi of right lower eyelid, including canthus
⇄	D22.121	Melanocytic nevi of left upper eyelid, including canthus
⇄	D22.122	Melanocytic nevi of left lower eyelid, including canthus
⇄	D23.111	Other benign neoplasm of skin of right upper eyelid, including canthus
⇄	D23.112	Other benign neoplasm of skin of right lower eyelid, including canthus
⇄	D23.121	Other benign neoplasm of skin of left upper eyelid, including canthus
⇄	D23.122	Other benign neoplasm of skin of left lower eyelid, including canthus
⇄	H00.011	Hordeolum externum right upper eyelid
⇄	H00.012	Hordeolum externum right lower eyelid
⇄	H00.014	Hordeolum externum left upper eyelid
⇄	H00.015	Hordeolum externum left lower eyelid
⇄	H00.021	Hordeolum internum right upper eyelid
⇄	H00.022	Hordeolum internum right lower eyelid
⇄	H00.024	Hordeolum internum left upper eyelid
⇄	H00.025	Hordeolum internum left lower eyelid
⇄	H02.61	Xanthelasma of right upper eyelid
⇄	H02.62	Xanthelasma of right lower eyelid
⇄	H02.64	Xanthelasma of left upper eyelid
⇄	H02.65	Xanthelasma of left lower eyelid
	L57.0	Actinic keratosis
	L72.0	Epidermal cyst
	L82.1	Other seborrheic keratosis
	Q82.5	Congenital non-neoplastic nevus

CCI Edits

Refer to Appendix A for CCI edits.

Facility RVUs □

Code	Work	PE Facility	MP	Total Facility
67840	2.09	2.29	0.18	4.56

Non-facility RVUs □

Code	Work	PE Non-Facility	MP	Total Non-Facility
67840	2.09	6.12	0.18	8.39

Modifiers (PAR) □

Code	Mod 50	Mod 51	Mod 62	Mod 66	Mod 80
67840	1	2	0	0	1

Global Period

Code	Days
67840	010

67850

67850 Destruction of lesion of lid margin (up to 1 cm)

(For Mohs micrographic surgery, see 17311-17315)

(For initiation or follow-up care of topical chemotherapy (eg, 5-FU or similar agents), see appropriate office visits)

AMA Coding Guideline

Excision and Destruction Procedures on the Eyelids

Codes for removal of lesion include more than skin (ie, involving lid margin, tarsus, and/or palpebral conjunctiva).

AMA Coding Notes

Excision and Destruction Procedures on the Eyelids

(For removal of lesion, involving mainly skin of eyelid, see 11310-11313; 11440-11446, 11640-11646; 17000-17004)

(For repair of wounds, blepharoplasty, grafts, reconstructive surgery, see 67930-67975)

Surgical Procedures on the Eye and Ocular Adnexa

(For diagnostic and treatment ophthalmological services, see Medicine, Ophthalmology, and 92002 et seq)

(Do not report code 69990 in addition to codes 65091-68850)

Plain English Description

The physician destroys a lesion of the lid margin of 1 cm or less. The lesion is examined and the most appropriate form of destruction is determined. Local anesthesia is administered as needed. The lesion may be destroyed using a chemical compound, cryosurgery, electrosurgery, or other technique. Cryosurgery is performed using liquid nitrogen to freeze the lesion. A series of freeze-thaw cycles may be required to completely destroy the lesion. Electrosurgery uses heat applied to the lesion(s) with a high frequency current that passes through a metal probe or needle.

Destruction of lesion of lid margin

(Up to one centimeter)

Lesion

Methods include: chemical compound; cryosurgery; electrosurgery

ICD-10-CM Diagnostic Codes

	B08.1	Molluscum contagiosum
⇄	C43.111	Malignant melanoma of right upper eyelid, including canthus
⇄	C43.112	Malignant melanoma of right lower eyelid, including canthus
⇄	C43.121	Malignant melanoma of left upper eyelid, including canthus
⇄	C43.122	Malignant melanoma of left lower eyelid, including canthus
⇄	C44.1021	Unspecified malignant neoplasm of skin of right upper eyelid, including canthus
⇄	C44.1022	Unspecified malignant neoplasm of skin of right lower eyelid, including canthus
⇄	C44.1091	Unspecified malignant neoplasm of skin of left upper eyelid, including canthus
⇄	C44.1092	Unspecified malignant neoplasm of skin of left lower eyelid, including canthus
⇄	C44.1121	Basal cell carcinoma of skin of right upper eyelid, including canthus
⇄	C44.1122	Basal cell carcinoma of skin of right lower eyelid, including canthus
⇄	C44.1191	Basal cell carcinoma of skin of left upper eyelid, including canthus
⇄	C44.1192	Basal cell carcinoma of skin of left lower eyelid, including canthus
⇄	C44.1221	Squamous cell carcinoma of skin of right upper eyelid, including canthus
⇄	C44.1222	Squamous cell carcinoma of skin of right lower eyelid, including canthus
⇄	C44.1291	Squamous cell carcinoma of skin of left upper eyelid, including canthus
⇄	C44.1292	Squamous cell carcinoma of skin of left lower eyelid, including canthus
⇄	C44.1321	Sebaceous cell carcinoma of skin of right upper eyelid, including canthus
⇄	C44.1322	Sebaceous cell carcinoma of skin of right lower eyelid, including canthus
⇄	C44.1391	Sebaceous cell carcinoma of skin of left upper eyelid, including canthus
⇄	C44.1392	Sebaceous cell carcinoma of skin of left lower eyelid, including canthus
⇄	C44.1921	Other specified malignant neoplasm of skin of right upper eyelid, including canthus
⇄	C44.1922	Other specified malignant neoplasm of skin of right lower eyelid, including canthus
⇄	C44.1991	Other specified malignant neoplasm of skin of left upper eyelid, including canthus
⇄	C44.1992	Other specified malignant neoplasm of skin of left lower eyelid, including canthus
⇄	C4A.111	Merkel cell carcinoma of right upper eyelid, including canthus
⇄	C4A.112	Merkel cell carcinoma of right lower eyelid, including canthus
⇄	C4A.121	Merkel cell carcinoma of left upper eyelid, including canthus
⇄	C4A.122	Merkel cell carcinoma of left lower eyelid, including canthus
⇄	D03.111	Melanoma in situ of right upper eyelid, including canthus
⇄	D03.112	Melanoma in situ of right lower eyelid, including canthus
⇄	D03.121	Melanoma in situ of left upper eyelid, including canthus
⇄	D03.122	Melanoma in situ of left lower eyelid, including canthus
⇄	D04.111	Carcinoma in situ of skin of right upper eyelid, including canthus
⇄	D04.112	Carcinoma in situ of skin of right lower eyelid, including canthus
⇄	D04.121	Carcinoma in situ of skin of left upper eyelid, including canthus
⇄	D04.122	Carcinoma in situ of skin of left lower eyelid, including canthus
	D17.0	Benign lipomatous neoplasm of skin and subcutaneous tissue of head, face and neck
	D18.01	Hemangioma of skin and subcutaneous tissue
⇄	D22.111	Melanocytic nevi of right upper eyelid, including canthus
⇄	D22.112	Melanocytic nevi of right lower eyelid, including canthus
⇄	D22.121	Melanocytic nevi of left upper eyelid, including canthus
⇄	D22.122	Melanocytic nevi of left lower eyelid, including canthus
⇄	D23.111	Other benign neoplasm of skin of right upper eyelid, including canthus
⇄	D23.112	Other benign neoplasm of skin of right lower eyelid, including canthus
⇄	D23.121	Other benign neoplasm of skin of left upper eyelid, including canthus
⇄	D23.122	Other benign neoplasm of skin of left lower eyelid, including canthus
⇄	H00.011	Hordeolum externum right upper eyelid
⇄	H00.012	Hordeolum externum right lower eyelid
⇄	H00.014	Hordeolum externum left upper eyelid
⇄	H00.015	Hordeolum externum left lower eyelid
⇄	H00.021	Hordeolum internum right upper eyelid
⇄	H00.022	Hordeolum internum right lower eyelid
⇄	H00.024	Hordeolum internum left upper eyelid
⇄	H00.025	Hordeolum internum left lower eyelid
⇄	H02.61	Xanthelasma of right upper eyelid
⇄	H02.62	Xanthelasma of right lower eyelid
⇄	H02.64	Xanthelasma of left upper eyelid
⇄	H02.65	Xanthelasma of left lower eyelid
	L57.0	Actinic keratosis
	L72.0	Epidermal cyst
	L82.1	Other seborrheic keratosis
	Q82.5	Congenital non-neoplastic nevus

CCI Edits

Refer to Appendix A for CCI edits.

Facility RVUs

Code	Work	PE Facility	MP	Total Facility
67850	1.74	1.90	0.12	3.76

Non-facility RVUs

Code	Work	PE Non-Facility	MP	Total Non-Facility
67850	1.74	4.55	0.12	6.41

Modifiers (PAR)

Code	Mod 50	Mod 51	Mod 62	Mod 66	Mod 80
67850	1	2	0	0	1

Global Period

Code	Days
67850	010

CPT® Procedural Coding

67875

67875 Temporary closure of eyelids by suture (eg, Frost suture)

AMA Coding Notes

Surgical Procedures on the Eye and Ocular Adnexa

(For diagnostic and treatment ophthalmological services, see Medicine, Ophthalmology, and 92002 et seq)

(Do not report code 69990 in addition to codes 65091-68850)

AMA *CPT® Assistant* ▢

67875: Winter 90: 9

Plain English Description

The upper and lower eyelids are temporarily sutured together usually following an injury. Suturing the eyelids together or passing sutures through the lower lid and then taping the suture ends to the forehead (Frost suture) protects the eye while the injury heals. To suture the upper and lower lids together, sutures are placed through the upper and lower lid margins and the sutures are tied so that the eyelids will remain closed. Frost suture involves passing sutures through the lower eyelid only. Tension is then applied to the suture ends to close the lower lid and the ends of the suture material are secured with tape to the forehead.

Temporary closure of eyelids by suture (eg, Frost suture)

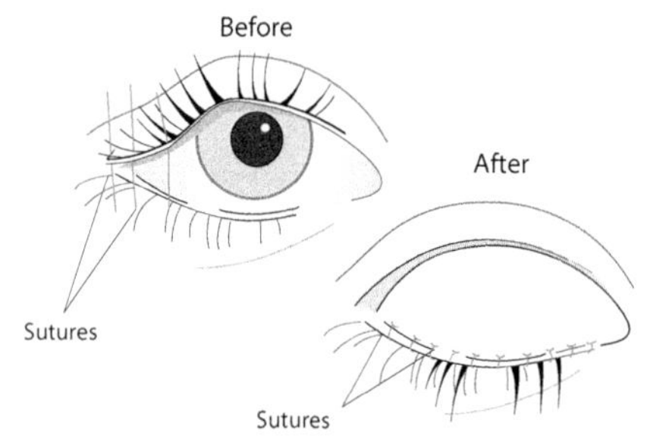

The eyelids are temporarily sutured closed, usually over a bolster to prevent erosion of the suture through the lid.

ICD-10-CM Diagnostic Codes

	Code	Description
	G51.0	Bell's palsy
⇄	H02.051	Trichiasis without entropion right upper eyelid
⇄	H02.052	Trichiasis without entropion right lower eyelid
⇄	H02.054	Trichiasis without entropion left upper eyelid
⇄	H02.055	Trichiasis without entropion left lower eyelid
⇄	H02.111	Cicatricial ectropion of right upper eyelid
⇄	H02.112	Cicatricial ectropion of right lower eyelid
⇄	H02.114	Cicatricial ectropion of left upper eyelid
⇄	H02.115	Cicatricial ectropion of left lower eyelid
⇄	H02.131	Senile ectropion of right upper eyelid
⇄	H02.132	Senile ectropion of right lower eyelid
⇄	H02.134	Senile ectropion of left upper eyelid
⇄	H02.135	Senile ectropion of left lower eyelid
⇄	H02.211	Cicatricial lagophthalmos right upper eyelid
⇄	H02.213	Cicatricial lagophthalmos right eye, unspecified eyelid
⇄	H02.214	Cicatricial lagophthalmos left upper eyelid
⇄	H02.215	Cicatricial lagophthalmos left lower eyelid
⇄	H02.531	Eyelid retraction right upper eyelid
⇄	H02.532	Eyelid retraction right lower eyelid
⇄	H02.534	Eyelid retraction left upper eyelid
⇄	H02.535	Eyelid retraction left lower eyelid
⇄	H04.121	Dry eye syndrome of right lacrimal gland
⇄	H04.122	Dry eye syndrome of left lacrimal gland
⇄	H04.123	Dry eye syndrome of bilateral lacrimal glands
⇄	H11.421	Conjunctival edema, right eye
⇄	H11.422	Conjunctival edema, left eye
⇄	H11.423	Conjunctival edema, bilateral
⇄	H16.011	Central corneal ulcer, right eye
⇄	H16.012	Central corneal ulcer, left eye
⇄	H16.013	Central corneal ulcer, bilateral
⇄	H16.031	Corneal ulcer with hypopyon, right eye
⇄	H16.032	Corneal ulcer with hypopyon, left eye
⇄	H16.033	Corneal ulcer with hypopyon, bilateral
⇄	H16.071	Perforated corneal ulcer, right eye
⇄	H16.072	Perforated corneal ulcer, left eye
⇄	H16.073	Perforated corneal ulcer, bilateral
⇄	H16.211	Exposure keratoconjunctivitis, right eye
⇄	H16.212	Exposure keratoconjunctivitis, left eye
⇄	H16.213	Exposure keratoconjunctivitis, bilateral
⇄	H16.231	Neurotrophic keratoconjunctivitis, right eye
⇄	H16.232	Neurotrophic keratoconjunctivitis, left eye
⇄	H16.233	Neurotrophic keratoconjunctivitis, bilateral
⇄	H49.41	Progressive external ophthalmoplegia, right eye
⇄	H49.42	Progressive external ophthalmoplegia, left eye
⇄	H49.43	Progressive external ophthalmoplegia, bilateral
	M35.01	Sjögren syndrome with keratoconjunctivitis
❼⇄	S05.21	Ocular laceration and rupture with prolapse or loss of intraocular tissue, right eye
❼⇄	S05.22	Ocular laceration and rupture with prolapse or loss of intraocular tissue, left eye
❼⇄	S05.31	Ocular laceration without prolapse or loss of intraocular tissue, right eye
❼⇄	S05.32	Ocular laceration without prolapse or loss of intraocular tissue, left eye
❼⇄	S05.51	Penetrating wound with foreign body of right eyeball
❼⇄	S05.52	Penetrating wound with foreign body of left eyeball
❼⇄	S05.61	Penetrating wound without foreign body of right eyeball
❼⇄	S05.62	Penetrating wound without foreign body of left eyeball
❼⇄	S05.71	Avulsion of right eye
❼⇄	S05.72	Avulsion of left eye
❼⇄	T15.01	Foreign body in cornea, right eye
❼⇄	T15.02	Foreign body in cornea, left eye
❼⇄	T15.11	Foreign body in conjunctival sac, right eye
❼⇄	T15.12	Foreign body in conjunctival sac, left eye

ICD-10-CM Coding Notes

For codes requiring a 7th character extension, refer to your ICD-10-CM book. Review the character descriptions and coding guidelines for proper selection. For some procedures, only certain characters will apply.

CCI Edits

Refer to Appendix A for CCI edits.

Facility RVUs ▢

Code	Work	PE Facility	MP	Total Facility
67875	1.35	1.29	0.11	2.75

Non-facility RVUs ▢

Code	Work	PE Non-Facility	MP	Total Non-Facility
67875	1.35	3.97	0.11	5.43

Modifiers (PAR) ▢

Code	Mod 50	Mod 51	Mod 62	Mod 66	Mod 80
67875	1	2	0	0	1

Global Period

Code	Days
67875	000

67880-67882

67880 Construction of intermarginal adhesions, median tarsorrhaphy, or canthorrhaphy

67882 Construction of intermarginal adhesions, median tarsorrhaphy, or canthorrhaphy; with transposition of tarsal plate

(For severing of tarsorrhaphy, use 67710)

(For canthoplasty, reconstruction canthus, use 67950)

(For canthotomy, use 67715)

AMA Coding Notes

Surgical Procedures on the Eye and Ocular Adnexa

(For diagnostic and treatment ophthalmological services, see Medicine, Ophthalmology, and 92002 et seq)

(Do not report code 69990 in addition to codes 65091-68850)

Plain English Description

The eyelids consist of multiple tissue layers with the most superficial layer being the skin followed by the orbicularis muscle, tarsus, and conjunctiva. The tarsi, also referred to as the tarsal plates, are composed of dense fibrous tissue that gives the upper and lower eyelids their shape. The upper eyelid has a crescent shape and the lower eyelid has a rectangular shape. In 67880, a median tarsorrhaphy or canthorrhaphy is performed. Median tarsorrhaphy involves creating adhesions between the upper and lower lid margins at the midline. It is performed to protect the cornea. Canthorrhaphy is the creation of adhesions at the corners, also called the medial and lateral canthus, of the eye. To perform median tarsorrhaphy, a narrow strip of skin is excised from the upper and lower lids at the midline. The skin is incised just posterior to the eyelashes. The surgically created wounds in the upper and lower lid are then approximated and secured using interrupted sutures. Canthorrhaphy is performed in the same manner except a strip of skin is removed from the upper and lower lid at the medial or lateral canthus and the surgical wounds are then approximated and secured with sutures. In 67882, median tarsorrhaphy or canthorrhaphy is performed in conjunction with transposition of the tarsal plate. The tarsal plate is exposed and repositioned usually to allow better closure of the eyelid.

Construction of intermarginal adhesions, median tarsorrhaphy/ canthorrhaphy; with transposition of tarsal plate

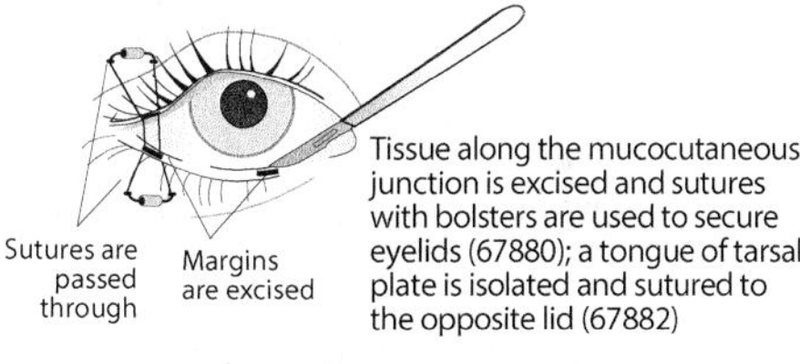

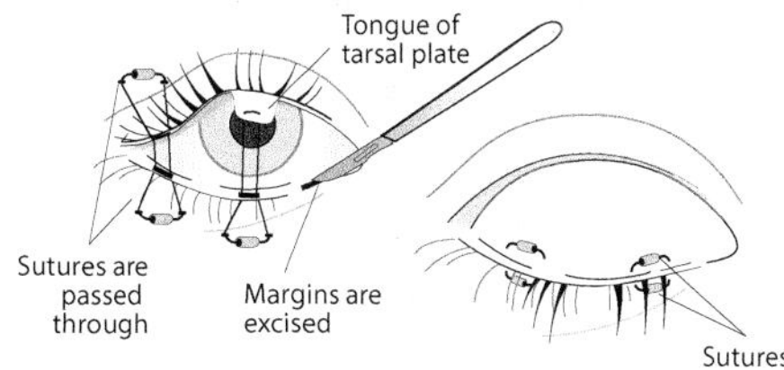

ICD-10-CM Diagnostic Codes

	G51.0	Bell's palsy
	G51.9	Disorder of facial nerve, unspecified
⇄	H02.111	Cicatricial ectropion of right upper eyelid
⇄	H02.112	Cicatricial ectropion of right lower eyelid
⇄	H02.131	Senile ectropion of right upper eyelid
⇄	H02.132	Senile ectropion of right lower eyelid
⇄	H02.221	Mechanical lagophthalmos right upper eyelid
⇄	H02.222	Mechanical lagophthalmos right lower eyelid
⇄	H02.231	Paralytic lagophthalmos right upper eyelid
⇄	H02.232	Paralytic lagophthalmos right lower eyelid
⇄	H02.31	Blepharochalasis right upper eyelid
⇄	H02.32	Blepharochalasis right lower eyelid
❼	T20.29	Burn of second degree of multiple sites of head, face, and neck
❼	T20.39	Burn of third degree of multiple sites of head, face, and neck
❼⇄	T26.91	Corrosion of right eye and adnexa, part unspecified

ICD-10-CM Coding Notes

For codes requiring a 7th character extension, refer to your ICD-10-CM book. Review the character descriptions and coding guidelines for proper selection. For some procedures, only certain characters will apply.

CCI Edits

Refer to Appendix A for CCI edits.

Facility RVUs ▯

Code	Work	PE Facility	MP	Total Facility
67880	4.60	5.67	0.37	10.64
67882	6.02	7.11	0.47	13.60

Non-facility RVUs ▯

Code	Work	PE Non-Facility	MP	Total Non-Facility
67880	4.60	8.79	0.37	13.76
67882	6.02	10.29	0.47	16.78

Modifiers (PAR) ▯

Code	Mod 50	Mod 51	Mod 62	Mod 66	Mod 80
67880	1	2	0	0	1
67882	1	2	0	0	1

Global Period

Code	Days
67880	090
67882	090

67900

67900 Repair of brow ptosis (supraciliary, mid-forehead or coronal approach)

(For forehead rhytidectomy, use 15824)

AMA Coding Notes

Surgical Procedures on the Eye and Ocular Adnexa

(For diagnostic and treatment ophthalmological services, see Medicine, Ophthalmology, and 92002 et seq)

(Do not report code 69990 in addition to codes 65091-68850)

Plain English Description

The physician repairs a sagging eyelid by making an incision in the forehead and pulling the skin upwards. Brow ptosis repair may be performed to correct laxity of forehead muscles and the descent of periorbital soft tissue causing functional visual impairment in the peripheral and superior visual fields. The procedure can be approached through a supraciliary incision along the superior border of the eyebrow, through preexisting horizontal mid-forehead furrows, or through a coronal scalp incision along the hairline. For all approaches, the skin is carefully marked with the patient upright before local anesthetic is injected. The supraciliary approach is appropriate for unilateral or bilateral brow ptosis. The skin is incised along the marked line(s) above the eyebrow and extended to find the frontalis muscle. Excess skin and subcutaneous tissue are excised en bloc. For the mid-forehead approach, a skin incision is made along the marked line(s) and carried down through the subcutaneous tissue to expose the corrugator supercilii and procerus muscles. This muscle complex is removed by incising the subgalea at the level of the glabella. The skin is trimmed before approximating the superior and inferior edges of the incision and closing in layers. The coronal approach near the hairline starts at the midline and extends laterally on each side to the anterior or superior reflection of the ear, incising the skin and galea. The temporalis fascia is identified and spared along with the superficial temporalis vessels. The galea is retracted to expose the underlying pericranium and a coronal flap is developed while preserving the seventh nerve near the orbital rims. The flap is turned down to allow further dissection in the subgaleal avascular plane with preservation of the frontal branch of the facial nerve. A dissector is used to expose the supraorbital neovascular bundles and the flap is turned down completely to expose the supraorbital rim, periosteum over the zygomatic process of the frontal bone laterally, and the superior aspect of the nasal bone in the glabellar region medially. The procerus, corrugator supercilii, and orbital orbicularis muscles are then elevated with the forehead skin and frontalis muscle, and the muscle complex is completely excised. The skin is pulled superiorly and trimmed. Vertical incisions are made anteriorly in the coronal flaps and additional skin is trimmed. The apex of each incision is approximated to the posterior skin with sutures and excess skin and galea are trimmed as necessary. The galea is closed with sutures followed by closure of the skin with sutures or staples.

Repair of brow ptosis (supraciliary, mid-forehead/coronal approach)

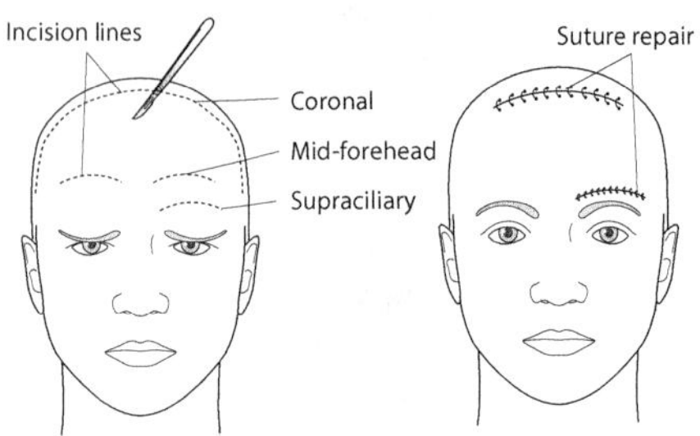

A droopy brow is repaired by excising excessive tissue and reapproximating its position.

ICD-10-CM Diagnostic Codes

⇄	H57.811	Brow ptosis, right
⇄	H57.812	Brow ptosis, left
⇄	H57.813	Brow ptosis, bilateral
	Q10.0	Congenital ptosis

CCI Edits

Refer to Appendix A for CCI edits.

Facility RVUs ☐

Code	Work	PE Facility	MP	Total Facility
67900	6.82	7.21	0.61	14.64

Non-facility RVUs ☐

Code	Work	PE Non-Facility	MP	Total Non-Facility
67900	6.82	11.69	0.61	19.12

Modifiers (PAR) ☐

Code	Mod 50	Mod 51	Mod 62	Mod 66	Mod 80
67900	1	2	0	0	1

Global Period

Code	Days
67900	090

67901-67902

67901 Repair of blepharoptosis; frontalis muscle technique with suture or other material (eg, banked fascia)

67902 Repair of blepharoptosis; frontalis muscle technique with autologous fascial sling (includes obtaining fascia)

AMA Coding Notes

Surgical Procedures on the Eye and Ocular Adnexa

(For diagnostic and treatment ophthalmological services, see Medicine, Ophthalmology, and 92002 et seq)

(Do not report code 69990 in addition to codes 65091-68850)

AMA *CPT® Assistant*

67901: Sep 00: 7, Oct 06: 11, Jul 17: 10

67902: Sep 00: 7, Oct 06: 11

Plain English Description

The physician repairs a blepharoptosis, which is a sagging of the upper eyelid caused by weakness of the levator palpebrae muscle, by frontalis muscle technique using suture or other material such as a Silastic rod or banked fascia. A shield is placed over the cornea. A skin incision is made just above the central portion of the eyebrow. Three small subcutaneous incisions are made in the upper eyelid in the pretarsal region just below the lid crease, one located medially, one centrally and one in the lateral aspect. A needle is then passed through the incision above the eyebrow between the orbicularis and levator muscles and through the medial eyelid incision. A length of Silastic rod or banked fascia may be threaded through the needle and retrieved through the incision above the eyebrow. The suture material, rod, or banked fascia is then threaded horizontally across the tarsus, exiting at the previously made below crease incision in the central aspect of the eyelid. The suture material, rod, or banked fascia is then passed through the previously made below crease lateral eyelid incision. The suture, rod, or banked fascia is secured by taking an intratarsal bite along each of three below crease incisions. A needle is then passed through the incision above the eyebrow and the suture, rod, or banked fascia retrieved at the lateral aspect of the tarsus. If a Silastic rod has been used, a Silastic sleeve is placed over the incision above the eyebrow and the rod passed through the sleeve. The tension of the suture, rod, or banked fascia is adjusted to the proper tension and suture, banked fascia or rod and sleeve secured to the deep frontalis muscle. The skin incisions are closed. In 67902, the physician repairs a blepharoptosis using a frontalis muscle technique with an autologous fascial sling. A fascia lata graft is harvested from the lateral thigh using a fascia stripper. The repair is performed as described except that a Silastic sleeve is not used. The lid level is adjusted and the fascia lata strip tied at each end. The fascial knot is reinforced at each end and anchored to the frontalis muscle on the upper edge of the incision above the eyebrow.

Repair of blepharoptosis; frontalis muscle technique

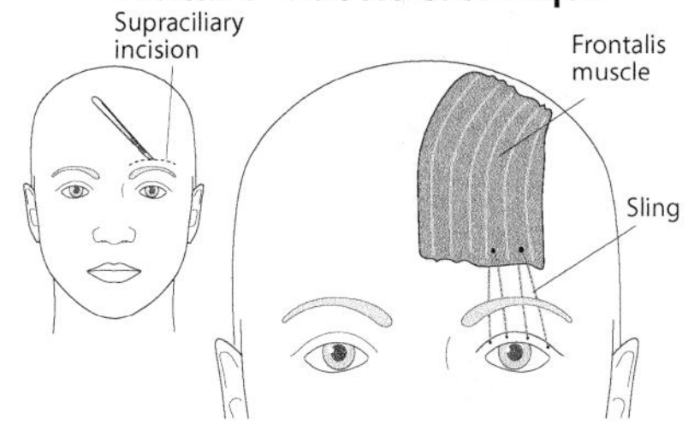

A sling is created using banked fascia from a cadaver/Mersilene (67901), or fascia obtained from the patient's thigh (67902).

ICD-10-CM Diagnostic Codes

⇄	H02.31	Blepharochalasis right upper eyelid
⇄	H02.32	Blepharochalasis right lower eyelid
⇄	H02.34	Blepharochalasis left upper eyelid
⇄	H02.35	Blepharochalasis left lower eyelid
⇄	H02.401	Unspecified ptosis of right eyelid
⇄	H02.402	Unspecified ptosis of left eyelid
⇄	H02.403	Unspecified ptosis of bilateral eyelids
⇄	H02.411	Mechanical ptosis of right eyelid
⇄	H02.412	Mechanical ptosis of left eyelid
⇄	H02.413	Mechanical ptosis of bilateral eyelids
⇄	H02.421	Myogenic ptosis of right eyelid
⇄	H02.422	Myogenic ptosis of left eyelid
⇄	H02.423	Myogenic ptosis of bilateral eyelids
⇄	H02.431	Paralytic ptosis of right eyelid
⇄	H02.432	Paralytic ptosis of left eyelid
⇄	H02.433	Paralytic ptosis of bilateral eyelids
⇄	H02.521	Blepharophimosis right upper eyelid
⇄	H02.522	Blepharophimosis right lower eyelid
⇄	H02.524	Blepharophimosis left upper eyelid
⇄	H02.525	Blepharophimosis left lower eyelid
	H02.70	Unspecified degenerative disorders of eyelid and periocular area
⇄	H02.831	Dermatochalasis of right upper eyelid
⇄	H02.832	Dermatochalasis of right lower eyelid
⇄	H02.834	Dermatochalasis of left upper eyelid
⇄	H02.835	Dermatochalasis of left lower eyelid
	Q10.0	Congenital ptosis
	Q10.3	Other congenital malformations of eyelid

CCI Edits

Refer to Appendix A for CCI edits.

Facility RVUs

Code	Work	PE Facility	MP	Total Facility
67901	7.59	8.90	0.62	17.11
67902	9.82	10.45	0.77	21.04

Non-facility RVUs

Code	Work	PE Non-Facility	MP	Total Non-Facility
67901	7.59	15.30	0.62	23.51
67902	9.82	10.45	0.77	21.04

Modifiers (PAR)

Code	Mod 50	Mod 51	Mod 62	Mod 66	Mod 80
67901	1	2	0	0	1
67902	1	2	1	0	1

Global Period

Code	Days
67901	090
67902	090

67903-67904

67903 Repair of blepharoptosis; (tarso) levator resection or advancement, internal approach

67904 Repair of blepharoptosis; (tarso) levator resection or advancement, external approach

AMA Coding Notes

Surgical Procedures on the Eye and Ocular Adnexa

(For diagnostic and treatment ophthalmological services, see Medicine, Ophthalmology, and 92002 et seq)

(Do not report code 69990 in addition to codes 65091-68850)

AMA *CPT® Assistant* ▯

67903: Sep 00: 7, Oct 06: 11

67904: Sep 00: 7, Oct 06: 11, Aug 11: 8

Plain English Description

The physician repairs a blepharoptosis, which is a sagging of the upper eyelid caused by weakness of the levator palpebrae muscle, by tarso levator resection or advancement using an internal (67903) or external (67904) approach. A local anesthetic is injected into the upper eyelid. Measurements are taken to determine the amount of resection or advancement required. In 67903, the eyelid is everted and traction sutures placed in the upper eyelid. The planned incision lines are marked using previously obtained measurements and the conjunctiva incised for an internal approach. In 67904, a shield is placed over the cornea. An incision is made in the skin of the upper eyelid fold for an external approach. The anterior tarsal surface and levator aponeurosis are exposed by incising the orbicularis along the superior tarsal border and traversing the eyelid horizontally. Using the previously made measurements, the tarsal plate is incised and a spindle-shaped section of tarsus and aponeurosis excised. A suture is placed anteriorly through the tarsus along the central portion of the superior edge and then passed through the superior edge of the levator aponeurosis. Two additional sutures are placed medially and laterally using the same technique. The sutures are temporarily tied and the lid contour assessed. The sutures are adjusted until an ideal lid shape is attained and the sutures are then permanently tied. The lid crease skin incision or conjunctival incision is closed.

Repair of blepharoptosis; (tarso) levator advancement/resection

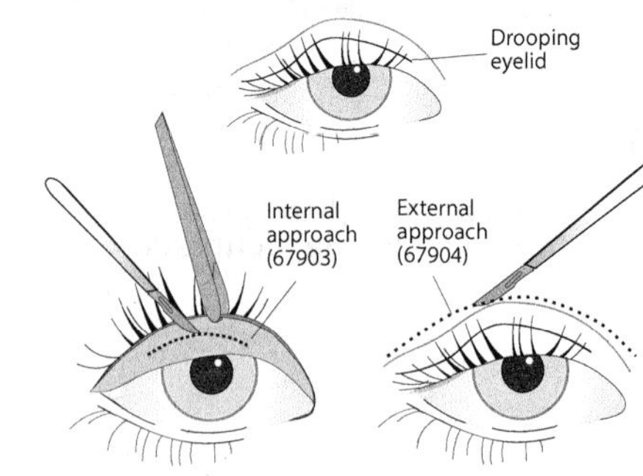

ICD-10-CM Diagnostic Codes

⇄	H02.31	Blepharochalasis right upper eyelid
⇄	H02.32	Blepharochalasis right lower eyelid
⇄	H02.34	Blepharochalasis left upper eyelid
⇄	H02.35	Blepharochalasis left lower eyelid
⇄	H02.401	Unspecified ptosis of right eyelid
⇄	H02.402	Unspecified ptosis of left eyelid
⇄	H02.403	Unspecified ptosis of bilateral eyelids
⇄	H02.411	Mechanical ptosis of right eyelid
⇄	H02.412	Mechanical ptosis of left eyelid
⇄	H02.413	Mechanical ptosis of bilateral eyelids
⇄	H02.421	Myogenic ptosis of right eyelid
⇄	H02.422	Myogenic ptosis of left eyelid
⇄	H02.423	Myogenic ptosis of bilateral eyelids
⇄	H02.431	Paralytic ptosis of right eyelid
⇄	H02.432	Paralytic ptosis of left eyelid
⇄	H02.433	Paralytic ptosis of bilateral eyelids
⇄	H02.521	Blepharophimosis right upper eyelid
⇄	H02.522	Blepharophimosis right lower eyelid
⇄	H02.524	Blepharophimosis left upper eyelid
⇄	H02.525	Blepharophimosis left lower eyelid
	H02.70	Unspecified degenerative disorders of eyelid and periocular area
⇄	H02.831	Dermatochalasis of right upper eyelid
⇄	H02.832	Dermatochalasis of right lower eyelid
⇄	H02.834	Dermatochalasis of left upper eyelid
⇄	H02.835	Dermatochalasis of left lower eyelid
	Q10.0	Congenital ptosis
	Q10.3	Other congenital malformations of eyelid

CCI Edits

Refer to Appendix A for CCI edits.

Facility RVUs ▯

Code	Work	PE Facility	MP	Total Facility
67903	6.51	6.86	0.54	13.91
67904	7.97	8.59	0.66	17.22

Non-facility RVUs ▯

Code	Work	PE Non-Facility	MP	Total Non-Facility
67903	6.51	10.72	0.54	17.77
67904	7.97	13.15	0.66	21.78

Modifiers (PAR) ▯

Code	Mod 50	Mod 51	Mod 62	Mod 66	Mod 80
67903	1	2	1	0	1
67904	1	2	1	0	1

Global Period

Code	Days
67903	090
67904	090

67906

67906 Repair of blepharoptosis; superior rectus technique with fascial sling (includes obtaining fascia)

AMA Coding Notes

Surgical Procedures on the Eye and Ocular Adnexa

(For diagnostic and treatment ophthalmological services, see Medicine, Ophthalmology, and 92002 et seq)

(Do not report code 69990 in addition to codes 65091-68850)

AMA *CPT® Assistant*

67906: Sep 00: 7, Oct 06: 11

Plain English Description

The physician repairs a blepharoptosis, which is a sagging of the upper eyelid caused by weakness of the levator palpebrae muscle, by a superior rectus technique with a fascial sling. A fascia lata graft is harvested from the lateral thigh using a fascia stripper. Alternatively, a length of banked fascia may be used. A skin incision is made over the superior rectus muscle of the eye. One or more small subcutaneous incisions are made in the upper eyelid in the pretarsal region just below the lid crease. A needle is then passed through the incision above the superior rectus. The fascial graft is threaded through the needle and retrieved through the incision over the superior rectus. The fascia is then threaded through the eyelid between the orbicularis and levator muscles and then horizontally across the tarsus, exiting in the upper eyelid. The fascia is then passed through the previously made incision(s) below the eyelid crease. The fascia is secured by taking an intratarsal bite along the crease incision(s). A needle is then passed through the incision over the superior rectus and the fascia is retrieved at the lateral aspect of the tarsus. The fascia is adjusted to the proper tension and secured in the superior rectus muscle. The skin incisions are closed. This code should be chosen carefully, as the superior rectus technique is considered outmoded and has been replaced by levator resection and advancement procedures.

Repair of blepharoptosis; superior rectus technique with fascial sling

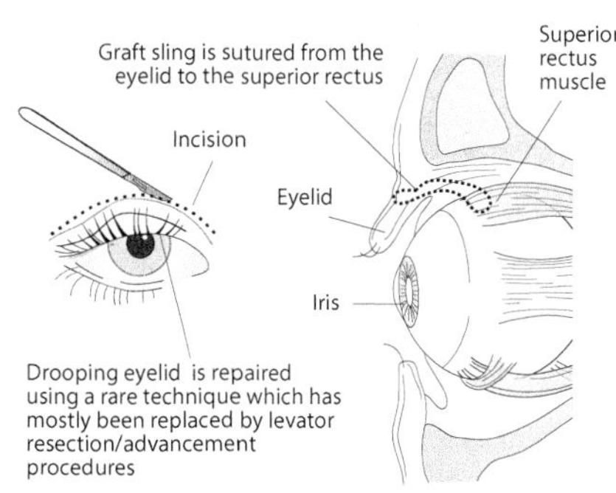

ICD-10-CM Diagnostic Codes

⇄	H02.401	Unspecified ptosis of right eyelid
⇄	H02.402	Unspecified ptosis of left eyelid
⇄	H02.411	Mechanical ptosis of right eyelid
⇄	H02.412	Mechanical ptosis of left eyelid
⇄	H02.413	Mechanical ptosis of bilateral eyelids
⇄	H02.421	Myogenic ptosis of right eyelid
⇄	H02.422	Myogenic ptosis of left eyelid
⇄	H02.423	Myogenic ptosis of bilateral eyelids
⇄	H02.431	Paralytic ptosis of right eyelid
⇄	H02.432	Paralytic ptosis of left eyelid
⇄	H02.433	Paralytic ptosis of bilateral eyelids
	Q10.0	Congenital ptosis

CCI Edits

Refer to Appendix A for CCI edits.

Facility RVUs

Code	Work	PE Facility	MP	Total Facility
67906	6.93	7.13	0.55	14.61

Non-facility RVUs

Code	Work	PE Non-Facility	MP	Total Non-Facility
67906	6.93	7.13	0.55	14.61

Modifiers (PAR)

Code	Mod 50	Mod 51	Mod 62	Mod 66	Mod 80
67906	1	2	0	0	1

Global Period

Code	Days
67906	090

67908

67908 Repair of blepharoptosis; conjunctivo-tarso-Muller's muscle-levator resection (eg, Fasanella-Servat type)

AMA Coding Notes

Surgical Procedures on the Eye and Ocular Adnexa

(For diagnostic and treatment ophthalmological services, see Medicine, Ophthalmology, and 92002 et seq)

(Do not report code 69990 in addition to codes 65091-68850)

AMA *CPT® Assistant* ▢

67908: Sep 00: 7, Oct 06: 11, Mar 21: 11

Plain English Description

The physician repairs a blepharoptosis, which is a sagging of the upper eyelid caused by weakness of the levator palpebrae muscle, by conjunctivo-tarso-Muller's muscle levator resection, also referred to as a Muller muscle conjunctiva repair (MMCR) or Fasanella-Servat repair. The upper eyelid is everted and the tarsal plate is exposed. Three temporary traction sutures are placed close to the folded superior margin of the tarsal plate, one medially, one laterally, and one in the central aspect. These sutures lift and hold up the portion of the tarsal plate to be excised. The ends of the sutures are clamped with artery forceps. Three additional temporary traction sutures are placed close to the margin of the everted lid, emerging near the superior fornix aligned with the first three sutures. These three sutures lift and support the conjunctival and tarsal wedge for suturing. The planned incision lines are marked using previously obtained measurements. A blade breaker knife is used to make an incision in the form of a groove. Scissor tips are placed in the groove and the tarsal plate is excised. The wound is then repaired with a continuous buried suture temporarily tied at both ends. The lid shape is assessed and adjustments are made as needed until an ideal lid shape has been attained. The sutures are permanently tied with small knots that are buried at each end. The temporary traction sutures are removed and the lid crease skin incision is closed. If a modified or sutureless Fasanella-Servat repair is performed, hemostat forceps are used to grasp the tarsoconjunctival Muller complex along the marked lines and the hemostat forceps are left in place for 60 seconds. When the hemostat is removed, it leaves behind a broad ischemic groove of tissue that is then excised. Suture repair is not required as the compressed groove located at the site of the forceps acts as a mechanical suture.

Repair of blepharoptosis; conjunctivo-tarso-Muller's muscle-levator resection

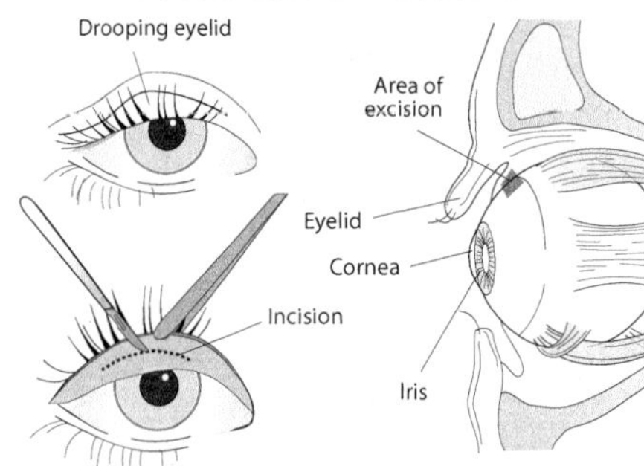

The eyelid is repaired by an incision in the everted eyelid. Tissue excised includes conjunctiva, tarsus, and Muller's muscle.

ICD-10-CM Diagnostic Codes

⇄	H02.401	Unspecified ptosis of right eyelid
⇄	H02.402	Unspecified ptosis of left eyelid
⇄	H02.403	Unspecified ptosis of bilateral eyelids
⇄	H02.411	Mechanical ptosis of right eyelid
⇄	H02.412	Mechanical ptosis of left eyelid
⇄	H02.413	Mechanical ptosis of bilateral eyelids
⇄	H02.421	Myogenic ptosis of right eyelid
⇄	H02.422	Myogenic ptosis of left eyelid
⇄	H02.423	Myogenic ptosis of bilateral eyelids
⇄	H02.431	Paralytic ptosis of right eyelid
⇄	H02.432	Paralytic ptosis of left eyelid
⇄	H02.433	Paralytic ptosis of bilateral eyelids
	Q10.1	Congenital ectropion
	Q10.3	Other congenital malformations of eyelid

CCI Edits

Refer to Appendix A for CCI edits.

Facility RVUs ▢

Code	Work	PE Facility	MP	Total Facility
67908	5.30	6.81	0.40	12.51

Non-facility RVUs ▢

Code	Work	PE Non-Facility	MP	Total Non-Facility
67908	5.30	10.27	0.40	15.97

Modifiers (PAR) ▢

Code	Mod 50	Mod 51	Mod 62	Mod 66	Mod 80
67908	1	2	0	0	1

Global Period

Code	Days
67908	090

67909

67909 Reduction of overcorrection of ptosis

AMA Coding Notes

Surgical Procedures on the Eye and Ocular Adnexa

(For diagnostic and treatment ophthalmological services, see Medicine, Ophthalmology, and 92002 et seq)

(Do not report code 69990 in addition to codes 65091-68850)

Plain English Description

Ptosis refers to sagging or drooping of the upper eyelid. Ptosis can be corrected surgically, but some patients experience an overcorrection of the ptosis. Overcorrection can make it impossible to completely close the eye, which can cause dry eye and damage to the cornea. The old incision is reopened. The levator aponeurosis is exposed and released. The tension of the levator is adjusted until the eyelid is in a more normal position and the eyelid can be closed completely. The levator is then reattached more superiorly on the tarsus or to the Muller muscle or conjunctiva. The surgical wound is closed in layers.

Reduction of overcorrection of ptosis

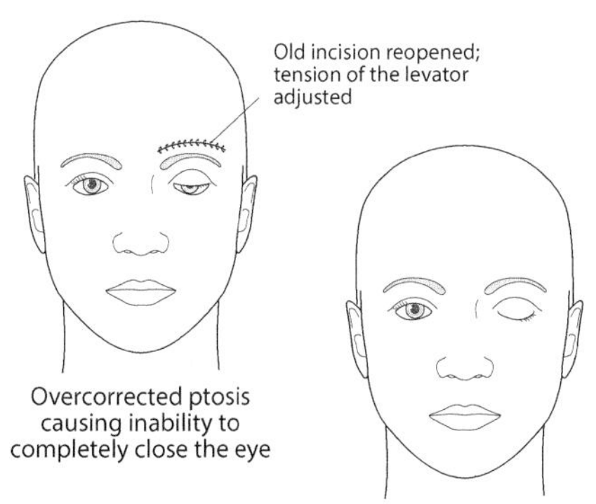
Old incision reopened; tension of the levator adjusted
Overcorrected ptosis causing inability to completely close the eye
Eyelid able to close completely

ICD-10-CM Diagnostic Codes

	Code	Description
⇄	H02.31	Blepharochalasis right upper eyelid
⇄	H02.34	Blepharochalasis left upper eyelid
⇄	H02.401	Unspecified ptosis of right eyelid
⇄	H02.402	Unspecified ptosis of left eyelid
⇄	H02.403	Unspecified ptosis of bilateral eyelids
⇄	H02.411	Mechanical ptosis of right eyelid
⇄	H02.412	Mechanical ptosis of left eyelid
⇄	H02.413	Mechanical ptosis of bilateral eyelids
⇄	H02.421	Myogenic ptosis of right eyelid
⇄	H02.422	Myogenic ptosis of left eyelid
⇄	H02.423	Myogenic ptosis of bilateral eyelids
⇄	H02.431	Paralytic ptosis of right eyelid
⇄	H02.432	Paralytic ptosis of left eyelid
⇄	H02.433	Paralytic ptosis of bilateral eyelids
⇄	H02.831	Dermatochalasis of right upper eyelid
⇄	H02.834	Dermatochalasis of left upper eyelid
	H59.89	Other postprocedural complications and disorders of eye and adnexa, not elsewhere classified
	Q10.0	Congenital ptosis
	Q10.3	Other congenital malformations of eyelid
➐	T88.8	Other specified complications of surgical and medical care, not elsewhere classified

ICD-10-CM Coding Notes

For codes requiring a 7th character extension, refer to your ICD-10-CM book. Review the character descriptions and coding guidelines for proper selection. For some procedures, only certain characters will apply.

CCI Edits

Refer to Appendix A for CCI edits.

Facility RVUs ▯

Code	Work	PE Facility	MP	Total Facility
67909	5.57	6.63	0.50	12.70

Non-facility RVUs ▯

Code	Work	PE Non-Facility	MP	Total Non-Facility
67909	5.57	10.13	0.50	16.20

Modifiers (PAR) ▯

Code	Mod 50	Mod 51	Mod 62	Mod 66	Mod 80
67909	1	2	0	0	1

Global Period

Code	Days
67909	090

67911

67911 Correction of lid retraction

(For obtaining autologous graft materials, see 15769, 20920, 20922)

(For correction of lid defects using fat harvested via liposuction technique, see 15773, 15774)

(For correction of trichiasis by mucous membrane graft, use 67835)

AMA Coding Notes

Surgical Procedures on the Eye and Ocular Adnexa

(For diagnostic and treatment ophthalmological services, see Medicine, Ophthalmology, and 92002 et seq)

(Do not report code 69990 in addition to codes 65091-68850)

Plain English Description

The upper and lower eyelid can be affected by lid retraction. Lower eyelid retraction is caused by relaxation of the support system of the eye and also by shrinkage of the tissue layers that include skin, muscle, and retractor muscles. Lower lid retraction causes an inability to completely close the eye with exposure of the sclera below the cornea. Lower lid retraction may be due to aging, thyroid disease, or a complication of lower eyelid blepharoplasty. Upper lid retraction causes exposure of the sclera above the cornea and is most often caused by thyroid disease. The exact procedure performed for correction of lid retraction depends on whether the upper or lower eyelid is affected, as well as the cause, extent, and any unique individual characteristics of the lid retraction. Correction of upper lid retraction is performed through a transconjunctival or transcutaneous approach. Muller's muscle is exposed and excised. The levator aponeurosis may also be resected. Adjustable sutures are then used to adjust the eyelid position. Alternatively, an autogenous graft may be harvested usually from the hard palate or synthetic graft material may be used to support the eyelid and adjust the height. Lower lid retraction is corrected via a transconjunctival approach. Lower lid support structures may be reconstructed or reinforced. Repair may require skin grafting, placement of an another type of autogenous graft, or reinforcement with synthetic material. The lower lid height is adjusted as needed and the surgical wound is closed in layers.

Correction of lid retraction

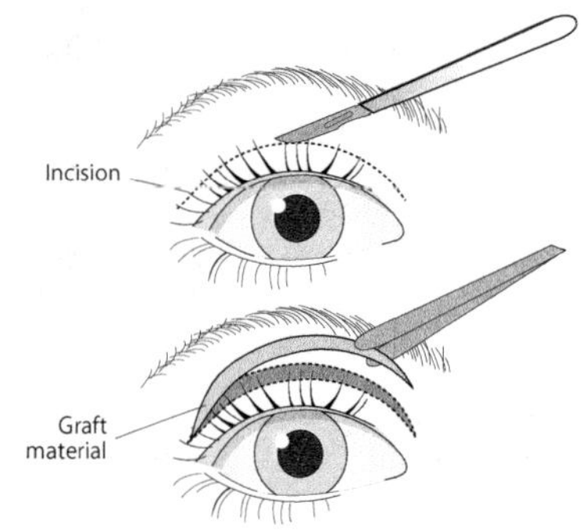

A graft is inserted into the tarsal plate.

ICD-10-CM Diagnostic Codes

	Code	Description
	E05.00	Thyrotoxicosis with diffuse goiter without thyrotoxic crisis or storm
	E05.01	Thyrotoxicosis with diffuse goiter with thyrotoxic crisis or storm
	G51.0	Bell's palsy
⇄	H02.531	Eyelid retraction right upper eyelid
⇄	H02.532	Eyelid retraction right lower eyelid
⇄	H02.534	Eyelid retraction left upper eyelid
⇄	H02.535	Eyelid retraction left lower eyelid
	H02.89	Other specified disorders of eyelid
	H05.89	Other disorders of orbit
	Q10.3	Other congenital malformations of eyelid
⇄	S01.101S	Unspecified open wound of right eyelid and periocular area, sequela
⇄	S01.102S	Unspecified open wound of left eyelid and periocular area, sequela

CCI Edits

Refer to Appendix A for CCI edits.

Facility RVUs ▯

Code	Work	PE Facility	MP	Total Facility
67911	7.50	8.07	0.60	16.17

Non-facility RVUs ▯

Code	Work	PE Non-Facility	MP	Total Non-Facility
67911	7.50	8.07	0.60	16.17

Modifiers (PAR) ▯

Code	Mod 50	Mod 51	Mod 62	Mod 66	Mod 80
67911	1	2	0	0	1

Global Period

Code	Days
67911	090

67912

67912 Correction of lagophthalmos, with implantation of upper eyelid lid load (eg, gold weight)

AMA Coding Notes

Surgical Procedures on the Eye and Ocular Adnexa

(For diagnostic and treatment ophthalmological services, see Medicine, Ophthalmology, and 92002 et seq)

(Do not report code 69990 in addition to codes 65091-68850)

AMA *CPT® Assistant* ▢

67912: May 04: 12, Aug 04: 10, Oct 06: 11

Plain English Description

Lagophthalmos affects the orbicularis muscle of the eyelid and is a form of facial paralysis that is characterized by the inability to completely close the upper eyelid. Surgical correction is performed when the paralysis is persistent or permanent and involves placement of a small, pure gold weight in the upper eyelid. The upper eyelid is prepared and a local anesthetic injected. A small incision is made in the upper eyelid crease or just above the eyelashes. A small pocket is created inside the lid and an implant of appropriate weight is placed in the pocket. The weight is secured with sutures. The lid incision is closed. A protective eye pad is placed over the eyelid.

Correction of lagophthalmos, implant of upper eyelid load

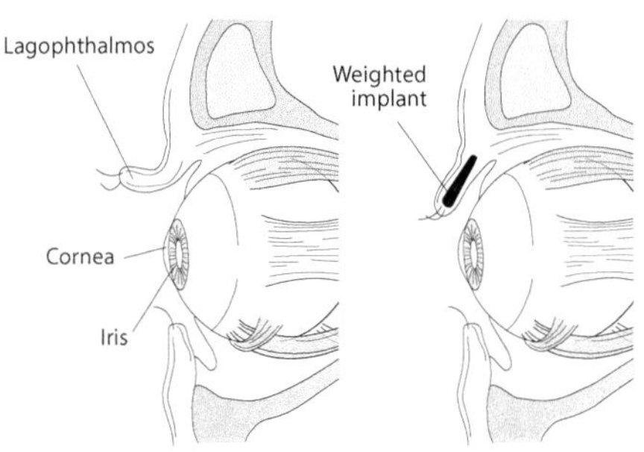

A weight or load device is inserted for gravity-assisted closure.

ICD-10-CM Diagnostic Codes

	G50.8	Other disorders of trigeminal nerve
	G51.0	Bell's palsy
⇄	G51.31	Clonic hemifacial spasm, right
⇄	G51.32	Clonic hemifacial spasm, left
	G51.8	Other disorders of facial nerve
	G71.02	Facioscapulohumeral muscular dystrophy
⇄	H02.201	Unspecified lagophthalmos right upper eyelid
⇄	H02.204	Unspecified lagophthalmos left upper eyelid
⇄	H02.231	Paralytic lagophthalmos right upper eyelid
⇄	H02.234	Paralytic lagophthalmos left upper eyelid
➐⇄	S04.31	Injury of trigeminal nerve, right side
➐⇄	S04.32	Injury of trigeminal nerve, left side
➐⇄	S04.51	Injury of facial nerve, right side
➐⇄	S04.52	Injury of facial nerve, left side

ICD-10-CM Coding Notes

For codes requiring a 7th character extension, refer to your ICD-10-CM book. Review the character descriptions and coding guidelines for proper selection. For some procedures, only certain characters will apply.

CCI Edits

Refer to Appendix A for CCI edits.

Facility RVUs ▢

Code	Work	PE Facility	MP	Total Facility
67912	6.36	7.09	0.66	14.11

Non-facility RVUs ▢

Code	Work	PE Non-Facility	MP	Total Non-Facility
67912	6.36	20.14	0.66	27.16

Modifiers (PAR) ▢

Code	Mod 50	Mod 51	Mod 62	Mod 66	Mod 80
67912	1	2	0	0	1

Global Period

Code	Days
67912	090

67914-67915

67914 Repair of ectropion; suture
67915 Repair of ectropion; thermocauterization

AMA Coding Notes
Surgical Procedures on the Eye and Ocular Adnexa

(For diagnostic and treatment ophthalmological services, see Medicine, Ophthalmology, and 92002 et seq)

(Do not report code 69990 in addition to codes 65091-68850)

Plain English Description

An ectropion is a condition in which the lid margin is everted, which means that it is turned outward and away from the globe. When the lid margin is everted, the cornea is exposed, excessive tearing occurs, changes occur in the palpebral conjunctiva, and vision loss may occur. Ectropion is more common in the lower eyelid. A local anesthetic or nerve block is employed for pain control. In 67914, the ectropion is treated by suturing the eyelid at the site of the ectropion. Sutures are placed through the inferior border of the tarsus and exit at the skin surface near the orbital rim. The edges of the conjunctiva are approximated and secured with sutures. In 67915, thermocauterization is performed. A corneal protector is placed over the globe. The eyelid is everted and electrocautery applied at the junction of the conjunctiva and lower margin of the lower margin of the tarsus.

Repair of ectropion

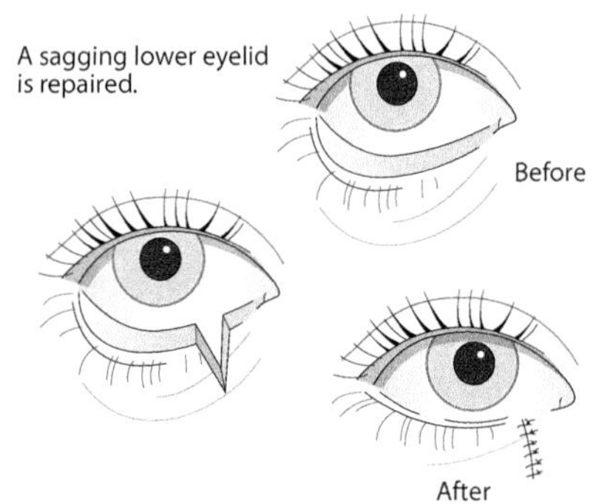
A sagging lower eyelid is repaired.
Before
After

Use code 67914 if sutures are used and code 67915 if a heat probe is used to repair the eyelid.

ICD-10-CM Diagnostic Codes

⇄ H02.101 Unspecified ectropion of right upper eyelid
⇄ H02.102 Unspecified ectropion of right lower eyelid
⇄ H02.104 Unspecified ectropion of left upper eyelid
⇄ H02.105 Unspecified ectropion of left lower eyelid
⇄ H02.111 Cicatricial ectropion of right upper eyelid
⇄ H02.112 Cicatricial ectropion of right lower eyelid
⇄ H02.114 Cicatricial ectropion of left upper eyelid
⇄ H02.115 Cicatricial ectropion of left lower eyelid
⇄ H02.121 Mechanical ectropion of right upper eyelid
⇄ H02.122 Mechanical ectropion of right lower eyelid
⇄ H02.124 Mechanical ectropion of left upper eyelid
⇄ H02.125 Mechanical ectropion of left lower eyelid
⇄ H02.131 Senile ectropion of right upper eyelid
⇄ H02.132 Senile ectropion of right lower eyelid
⇄ H02.134 Senile ectropion of left upper eyelid
⇄ H02.135 Senile ectropion of left lower eyelid
⇄ H02.141 Spastic ectropion of right upper eyelid
⇄ H02.142 Spastic ectropion of right lower eyelid
⇄ H02.144 Spastic ectropion of left upper eyelid
⇄ H02.145 Spastic ectropion of left lower eyelid
⇄ H02.151 Paralytic ectropion of right upper eyelid
⇄ H02.152 Paralytic ectropion of right lower eyelid
⇄ H02.154 Paralytic ectropion of left upper eyelid
⇄ H02.155 Paralytic ectropion of left lower eyelid
⇄ H04.521 Eversion of right lacrimal punctum
⇄ H04.522 Eversion of left lacrimal punctum
⇄ H04.523 Eversion of bilateral lacrimal punctum
⇄ H16.201 Unspecified keratoconjunctivitis, right eye
⇄ H16.202 Unspecified keratoconjunctivitis, left eye
⇄ H16.203 Unspecified keratoconjunctivitis, bilateral
⇄ H16.211 Exposure keratoconjunctivitis, right eye
⇄ H16.212 Exposure keratoconjunctivitis, left eye
⇄ H16.213 Exposure keratoconjunctivitis, bilateral

CCI Edits

Refer to Appendix A for CCI edits.

Facility RVUs ▯

Code	Work	PE Facility	MP	Total Facility
67914	3.75	5.42	0.32	9.49
67915	2.03	3.55	0.17	5.75

Non-facility RVUs ▯

Code	Work	PE Non-Facility	MP	Total Non-Facility
67914	3.75	10.45	0.32	14.52
67915	2.03	7.24	0.17	9.44

Modifiers (PAR) ▯

Code	Mod 50	Mod 51	Mod 62	Mod 66	Mod 80
67914	1	2	0	0	1
67915	1	2	0	0	1

Global Period

Code	Days
67914	090
67915	090

67916-67917

67916 Repair of ectropion; excision tarsal wedge

67917 Repair of ectropion; extensive (eg, tarsal strip operations)

(For correction of everted punctum, use 68705)

AMA Coding Notes

Surgical Procedures on the Eye and Ocular Adnexa

(For diagnostic and treatment ophthalmological services, see Medicine, Ophthalmology, and 92002 et seq)

(Do not report code 69990 in addition to codes 65091-68850)

AMA *CPT® Assistant* ▯

67916: Feb 04: 11, May 04: 12, Feb 05: 16, Oct 06: 11

67917: Feb 04: 11, May 04: 12, Oct 06: 11, Feb 20: 13, Mar 20: 14

Plain English Description

An ectropion is a condition in which the lid margin is everted, which means that it is turned outward and away from the globe. When the lid margin is everted, the cornea is exposed, excessive tearing occurs, changes occur in the palpebral conjunctiva, and vision loss may occur. Ectropion is more common in the lower eyelid. Local anesthesia is administered and supplemented with a nerve block as needed. A corneal shield is placed.

In 67916, a tarsal wedge is excised. A V-shaped incision is made over the ectropion and a wedge of the tarsal plate is excised. The open wedge in the tarsal plate is then closed with sutures. The skin is closed. In 67917, an extensive repair is performed such as a tarsal strip procedure. The exact procedure performed depends on the site and severity of the ectropion. To perform a lateral tarsal strip procedure, the lateral canthus is incised and the lower lid mobilized. If excess skin is present it is excised. The lid margin is split and the meibomian orifices of the lateral strip are trimmed off. The lateral conjunctiva is inspected and scraped to prevent formation of epithelial inclusion cysts. The lateral strip of tarsus is sutured to periosteum of the lateral orbital rim near the Whitnall's tubercle. The surgical wound is closed in layers.

Repair of ectropion

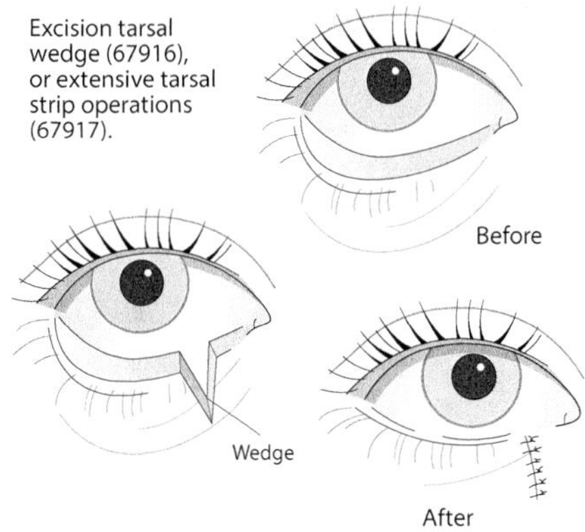

ICD-10-CM Diagnostic Codes

⇄	H02.101	Unspecified ectropion of right upper eyelid
⇄	H02.102	Unspecified ectropion of right lower eyelid
⇄	H02.104	Unspecified ectropion of left upper eyelid
⇄	H02.105	Unspecified ectropion of left lower eyelid
⇄	H02.111	Cicatricial ectropion of right upper eyelid
⇄	H02.112	Cicatricial ectropion of right lower eyelid
⇄	H02.114	Cicatricial ectropion of left upper eyelid
⇄	H02.115	Cicatricial ectropion of left lower eyelid
⇄	H02.121	Mechanical ectropion of right upper eyelid
⇄	H02.122	Mechanical ectropion of right lower eyelid
⇄	H02.124	Mechanical ectropion of left upper eyelid
⇄	H02.125	Mechanical ectropion of left lower eyelid
⇄	H02.131	Senile ectropion of right upper eyelid
⇄	H02.132	Senile ectropion of right lower eyelid
⇄	H02.134	Senile ectropion of left upper eyelid
⇄	H02.135	Senile ectropion of left lower eyelid
⇄	H02.141	Spastic ectropion of right upper eyelid
⇄	H02.142	Spastic ectropion of right lower eyelid
⇄	H02.144	Spastic ectropion of left upper eyelid
⇄	H02.145	Spastic ectropion of left lower eyelid
⇄	H02.151	Paralytic ectropion of right upper eyelid
⇄	H02.152	Paralytic ectropion of right lower eyelid
⇄	H02.154	Paralytic ectropion of left upper eyelid
⇄	H02.155	Paralytic ectropion of left lower eyelid
⇄	H04.521	Eversion of right lacrimal punctum
⇄	H04.522	Eversion of left lacrimal punctum
⇄	H04.523	Eversion of bilateral lacrimal punctum
⇄	H16.201	Unspecified keratoconjunctivitis, right eye
⇄	H16.202	Unspecified keratoconjunctivitis, left eye
⇄	H16.203	Unspecified keratoconjunctivitis, bilateral
⇄	H16.211	Exposure keratoconjunctivitis, right eye
⇄	H16.212	Exposure keratoconjunctivitis, left eye
⇄	H16.213	Exposure keratoconjunctivitis, bilateral

CCI Edits

Refer to Appendix A for CCI edits.

Facility RVUs ▯

Code	Work	PE Facility	MP	Total Facility
67916	5.48	6.50	0.44	12.42
67917	5.93	6.77	0.50	13.20

Non-facility RVUs ▯

Code	Work	PE Non-Facility	MP	Total Non-Facility
67916	5.48	12.18	0.44	18.10
67917	5.93	12.06	0.50	18.49

Modifiers (PAR) ▯

Code	Mod 50	Mod 51	Mod 62	Mod 66	Mod 80
67916	1	2	0	0	1
67917	1	2	0	0	1

Global Period

Code	Days
67916	090
67917	090

67921-67922

67921 Repair of entropion; suture
67922 Repair of entropion; thermocauterization

AMA Coding Notes

Surgical Procedures on the Eye and Ocular Adnexa

(For diagnostic and treatment ophthalmological services, see Medicine, Ophthalmology, and 92002 et seq)

(Do not report code 69990 in addition to codes 65091-68850)

Plain English Description

Entropion is a condition in which the eyelid margin rotates inward toward the surface of the eye causing the eyelashes and eyelid to rub against the conjunctiva and cornea. The resulting irritation may progress to corneal abrasion and ulceration. Entropions are most commonly seen in the lower eyelid of elderly individuals. A local anesthetic is injected into the eyelid. In 67921, a suture repair of the entropion is performed. Paired full-thickness sutures are placed from the conjunctival side of the eyelid just below the tarsal border, exiting out through the skin of the eyelid. The sutures are angled so that the exit site on the eyelid is closer to the lid margin, in order to cause eversion of the inverted eyelid. The externalized ends of the paired sutures are tied and remain in place for up to 2 weeks. Suture repair of an entropion is typically performed as a temporary measure until definitive, permanent repair of the entropion can be accomplished. In 67922, thermocauterization is performed. A corneal protector is placed over the globe. The eyelid is everted and electrocautery strategically applied so that when the burned tissue heals, scar tissue will form and the eyelid tissue will retract causing the inverted eyelid to assume a normal position against the globe.

Repair of entropion, suture; thermocauterization

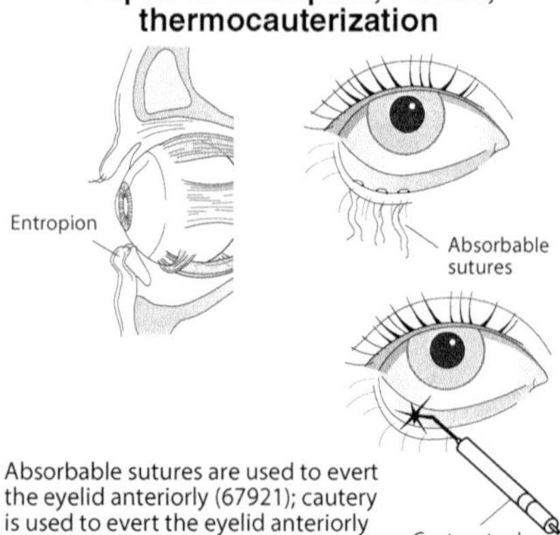

Absorbable sutures are used to evert the eyelid anteriorly (67921); cautery is used to evert the eyelid anteriorly by shrinking the tissue (67922).

ICD-10-CM Diagnostic Codes

⇄	H02.011	Cicatricial entropion of right upper eyelid
⇄	H02.012	Cicatricial entropion of right lower eyelid
⇄	H02.014	Cicatricial entropion of left upper eyelid
⇄	H02.015	Cicatricial entropion of left lower eyelid
⇄	H02.021	Mechanical entropion of right upper eyelid
⇄	H02.022	Mechanical entropion of right lower eyelid
⇄	H02.024	Mechanical entropion of left upper eyelid
⇄	H02.025	Mechanical entropion of left lower eyelid
⇄	H02.031	Senile entropion of right upper eyelid
⇄	H02.032	Senile entropion of right lower eyelid
⇄	H02.034	Senile entropion of left upper eyelid
⇄	H02.035	Senile entropion of left lower eyelid
⇄	H02.041	Spastic entropion of right upper eyelid
⇄	H02.042	Spastic entropion of right lower eyelid
⇄	H02.044	Spastic entropion of left upper eyelid
⇄	H02.045	Spastic entropion of left lower eyelid

CCI Edits

Refer to Appendix A for CCI edits.

Facility RVUs ▯

Code	Work	PE Facility	MP	Total Facility
67921	3.47	5.27	0.25	8.99
67922	2.03	3.56	0.17	5.76

Non-facility RVUs ▯

Code	Work	PE Non-Facility	MP	Total Non-Facility
67921	3.47	10.49	0.25	14.21
67922	2.03	6.94	0.17	9.14

Modifiers (PAR) ▯

Code	Mod 50	Mod 51	Mod 62	Mod 66	Mod 80
67921	1	2	0	0	1
67922	1	2	0	0	1

Global Period

Code	Days
67921	090
67922	090

67923-67924

67923 Repair of entropion; excision tarsal wedge

67924 Repair of entropion; extensive (eg, tarsal strip or capsulopalpebral fascia repairs operation)

(For repair of cicatricial ectropion or entropion requiring scar excision or skin graft, see also 67961 et seq)

AMA Coding Notes

Surgical Procedures on the Eye and Ocular Adnexa

(For diagnostic and treatment ophthalmological services, see Medicine, Ophthalmology, and 92002 et seq)

(Do not report code 69990 in addition to codes 65091-68850)

AMA *CPT® Assistant* ▢

67923: May 04: 12, Oct 06: 11

67924: May 04: 12, Oct 06: 11

Plain English Description

Entropion is a condition in which the eyelid margin rotates inward toward the surface of the eye causing the eyelashes and eyelid to rub against the conjunctiva and cornea. The resulting irritation may progress to corneal abrasion and ulceration. Entropions are most commonly seen in the lower eyelid of elderly individuals. A local anesthetic is injected into the eyelid. Local anesthesia is administered and supplemented with a nerve block as needed. A corneal shield is placed. In 67923, a tarsal wedge is excised. A V-shaped incision is made over the entropion and a wedge of the tarsal plate is excised. The open wedge in the tarsal plate is then closed with sutures. The skin is closed. In 67924, an extensive repair is performed such as a tarsal strip procedure or capsulopalpebral fascia repair. The exact procedure performed depends on the site and severity of the entropion. To perform a lateral tarsal strip procedure, the lateral canthus is incised and the lower lid mobilized. If excess skin is present, it is excised. The lid margin is split and the meibomian orifices of the lateral strip are trimmed off. The lateral conjunctiva is inspected and scraped to prevent formation of epithelial inclusion cysts. The lateral strip of tarsus is sutured to the periosteum of the lateral orbital rim near the Whitnall's tubercle. The surgical wound is closed in layers. If the entropion is due to horizontal and vertical laxity of the eyelid, medial and/or lateral canthal tightening may be performed using a tarsal strip procedure followed by vertical shortening and reattachment of the lower eyelid retractors to the inferior border of the tarsus.

Repair of entropion

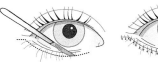

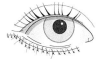

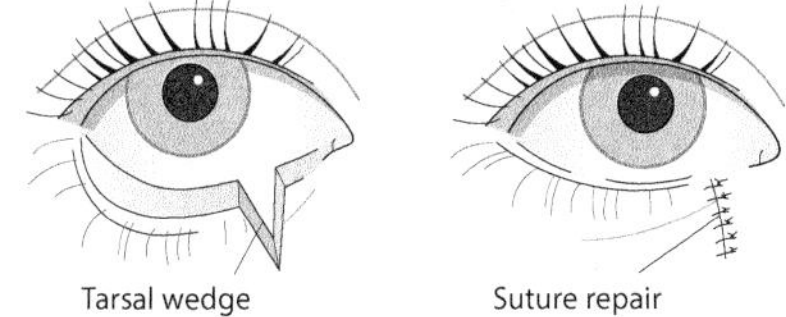

Excision tarsal wedge (67923)

Incision (up to 80% width of eyelid)

Suture repair

Extensive repairs (67924)

ICD-10-CM Diagnostic Codes

⇄	H02.011	Cicatricial entropion of right upper eyelid
⇄	H02.012	Cicatricial entropion of right lower eyelid
⇄	H02.014	Cicatricial entropion of left upper eyelid
⇄	H02.015	Cicatricial entropion of left lower eyelid
⇄	H02.021	Mechanical entropion of right upper eyelid
⇄	H02.022	Mechanical entropion of right lower eyelid
⇄	H02.024	Mechanical entropion of left upper eyelid
⇄	H02.025	Mechanical entropion of left lower eyelid
⇄	H02.031	Senile entropion of right upper eyelid
⇄	H02.032	Senile entropion of right lower eyelid
⇄	H02.034	Senile entropion of left upper eyelid
⇄	H02.035	Senile entropion of left lower eyelid
⇄	H02.041	Spastic entropion of right upper eyelid
⇄	H02.042	Spastic entropion of right lower eyelid
⇄	H02.044	Spastic entropion of left upper eyelid
⇄	H02.045	Spastic entropion of left lower eyelid

CCI Edits

Refer to Appendix A for CCI edits.

Facility RVUs ▢

Code	Work	PE Facility	MP	Total Facility
67923	5.48	6.51	0.42	12.41
67924	5.93	6.78	0.47	13.18

Non-facility RVUs ▢

Code	Work	PE Non-Facility	MP	Total Non-Facility
67923	5.48	12.19	0.42	18.09
67924	5.93	12.85	0.47	19.25

Modifiers (PAR) ▢

Code	Mod 50	Mod 51	Mod 62	Mod 66	Mod 80
67923	1	2	0	0	1
67924	1	2	0	0	1

Global Period

Code	Days
67923	090
67924	090

CPT® Procedural Coding

67930-67935

67930 Suture of recent wound, eyelid, involving lid margin, tarsus, and/or palpebral conjunctiva direct closure; partial thickness

67935 Suture of recent wound, eyelid, involving lid margin, tarsus, and/or palpebral conjunctiva direct closure; full thickness

AMA Coding Guideline

Reconstruction Procedures on the Eyelids

Codes for blepharoplasty involve more than skin (ie, involving lid margin, tarsus, and/or palpebral conjunctiva).

AMA Coding Notes

Surgical Procedures on the Eye and Ocular Adnexa

(For diagnostic and treatment ophthalmological services, see Medicine, Ophthalmology, and 92002 et seq)

(Do not report code 69990 in addition to codes 65091-68850)

Plain English Description

The eyelids consist of multiple tissue layers with the most superficial layer being the skin followed by the orbicularis muscle, tarsus, and conjunctiva. Repair of wounds involving more than the skin require layered closure. Anesthetic eye drops or other topical anesthetic is administered. The corneal protector is placed over the globe. The wound is cleansed and any debris is removed. Damaged tissue is debrided. The lid margin is realigned by placing three marginal sutures. The first suture passes through the plane of the meibomian orifices. The other two sutures are placed anterior and posterior to the first. If the lid margin is involved, it is repaired with mattress sutures. Another technique is to use a single vertical-mattress suture to realign the lid margin. If the tarsus is involved, sutures are placed through the tarsus with the knotted ends directed away from the cornea. If the palpebral conjunctiva is involved, it is repaired with sutures. The skin is then closed. Use 67930, if the wound involves only a partial-thickness injury extending only part of the way through the eyelid. Use 67935 if the wound extends through the entire eyelid.

Suture of recent wound, eyelid partial/full thickness

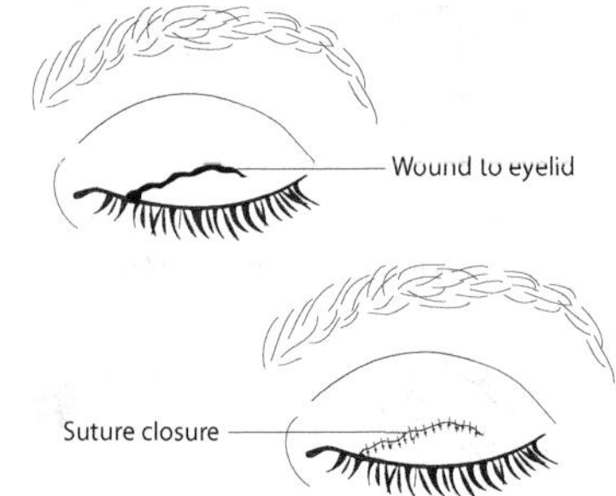

A wound involving lid margin/palpebral conjunctiva/tarsus is repaired with sutures; partial (67930), or full (67935) thickness.

ICD-10-CM Diagnostic Codes

❼⇄	S01.101	Unspecified open wound of right eyelid and periocular area
❼⇄	S01.102	Unspecified open wound of left eyelid and periocular area
❼⇄	S01.111	Laceration without foreign body of right eyelid and periocular area
❼⇄	S01.112	Laceration without foreign body of left eyelid and periocular area
❼⇄	S01.121	Laceration with foreign body of right eyelid and periocular area
❼⇄	S01.122	Laceration with foreign body of left eyelid and periocular area
❼⇄	S01.131	Puncture wound without foreign body of right eyelid and periocular area
❼⇄	S01.132	Puncture wound without foreign body of left eyelid and periocular area
❼⇄	S01.141	Puncture wound with foreign body of right eyelid and periocular area
❼⇄	S01.142	Puncture wound with foreign body of left eyelid and periocular area
❼⇄	S01.151	Open bite of right eyelid and periocular area
❼⇄	S01.152	Open bite of left eyelid and periocular area

ICD-10-CM Coding Notes

For codes requiring a 7th character extension, refer to your ICD-10-CM book. Review the character descriptions and coding guidelines for proper selection. For some procedures, only certain characters will apply.

CCI Edits

Refer to Appendix A for CCI edits.

Facility RVUs ▯

Code	Work	PE Facility	MP	Total Facility
67930	3.65	2.89	0.29	6.83
67935	6.36	5.82	0.57	12.75

Non-facility RVUs ▯

Code	Work	PE Non-Facility	MP	Total Non-Facility
67930	3.65	7.01	0.29	10.95
67935	6.36	10.72	0.57	17.65

Modifiers (PAR) ▯

Code	Mod 50	Mod 51	Mod 62	Mod 66	Mod 80
67930	1	2	0	0	1
67935	1	2	0	0	1

Global Period

Code	Days
67930	010
67935	090

67938

67938 Removal of embedded foreign body, eyelid

(For repair of skin of eyelid, see 12011-12018, 12051-12057, 13151-13153)

(For tarsorrhaphy, canthorrhaphy, see 67880, 67882)

(For repair of blepharoptosis and lid retraction, see 67901-67911)

(For blepharoplasty for entropion, ectropion, see 67916, 67917, 67923, 67924)

(For correction of blepharochalasis (blepharorhytidectomy), see 15820-15823)

(For repair of skin of eyelid, adjacent tissue transfer, see 14060, 14061; preparation for graft, use 15004; free graft, see 15120, 15121, 15260, 15261)

(For excision of lesion of eyelid, use 67800 et seq)

(For repair of lacrimal canaliculi, use 68700)

AMA Coding Guideline

Reconstruction Procedures on the Eyelids

Codes for blepharoplasty involve more than skin (ie, involving lid margin, tarsus, and/or palpebral conjunctiva).

AMA Coding Notes

Surgical Procedures on the Eye and Ocular Adnexa

(For diagnostic and treatment ophthalmological services, see Medicine, Ophthalmology, and 92002 et seq)

(Do not report code 69990 in addition to codes 65091-68850)

AMA *CPT® Assistant* ▢

67938: May 14: 5

Plain English Description

An embedded foreign body is removed from the eyelid. A topical anesthetic is administered. A corneal protector is placed over the globe. The wound is cleansed and any debris removed. The eyelid is inspected to try to identify the entry site of the foreign body. If the entry site cannot be identified a chalazion curette may be used to palpate the eyelid and help locate the foreign body. Once the foreign body is identified, the entry wound is enlarged or an incision is made in the eyelid and the foreign body is removed. The entry wound or incision is repaired with tissue glue or sutures.

Removal of embedded foreign body, eyelid

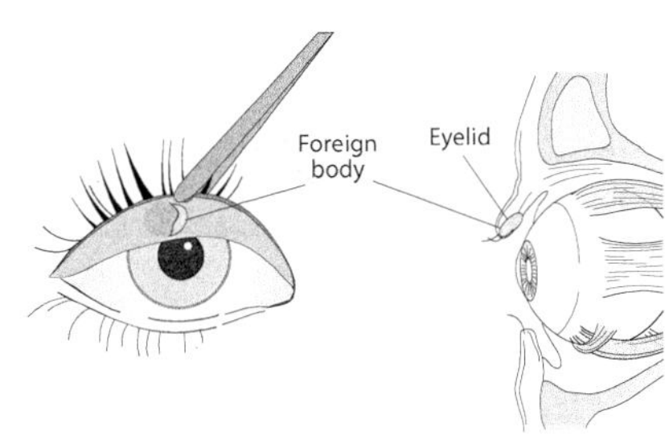

ICD-10-CM Diagnostic Codes

⇄	H02.811	Retained foreign body in right upper eyelid
⇄	H02.812	Retained foreign body in right lower eyelid
⇄	H02.814	Retained foreign body in left upper eyelid
⇄	H02.815	Retained foreign body in left lower eyelid
❼⇄	S01.121	Laceration with foreign body of right eyelid and periocular area
❼⇄	S01.122	Laceration with foreign body of left eyelid and periocular area
❼⇄	S01.141	Puncture wound with foreign body of right eyelid and periocular area
❼⇄	S01.142	Puncture wound with foreign body of left eyelid and periocular area
❼⇄	T15.81	Foreign body in other and multiple parts of external eye, right eye
❼⇄	T15.82	Foreign body in other and multiple parts of external eye, left eye
	Z18.10	Retained metal fragments, unspecified
	Z18.11	Retained magnetic metal fragments
	Z18.12	Retained nonmagnetic metal fragments
	Z18.2	Retained plastic fragments
	Z18.31	Retained animal quills or spines
	Z18.32	Retained tooth
	Z18.33	Retained wood fragments
	Z18.39	Other retained organic fragments
	Z18.81	Retained glass fragments
	Z18.83	Retained stone or crystalline fragments
	Z18.89	Other specified retained foreign body fragments
	Z18.9	Retained foreign body fragments, unspecified material

ICD-10-CM Coding Notes

For codes requiring a 7th character extension, refer to your ICD-10-CM book. Review the character descriptions and coding guidelines for proper selection. For some procedures, only certain characters will apply.

CCI Edits

Refer to Appendix A for CCI edits.

Facility RVUs ▢

Code	Work	PE Facility	MP	Total Facility
67938	1.38	1.93	0.09	3.40

Non-facility RVUs ▢

Code	Work	PE Non-Facility	MP	Total Non-Facility
67938	1.38	6.73	0.09	8.20

Modifiers (PAR) ▢

Code	Mod 50	Mod 51	Mod 62	Mod 66	Mod 80
67938	1	2	0	0	1

Global Period

Code	Days
67938	010

67950

67950 Canthoplasty (reconstruction of canthus)

AMA Coding Guideline

Reconstruction Procedures on the Eyelids

Codes for blepharoplasty involve more than skin (ie, involving lid margin, tarsus, and/or palpebral conjunctiva).

AMA Coding Notes

Surgical Procedures on the Eye and Ocular Adnexa

(For diagnostic and treatment ophthalmological services, see Medicine, Ophthalmology, and 92002 et seq)

(Do not report code 69990 in addition to codes 65091-68850)

Plain English Description

Canthoplasty is performed to reconstruct the medial or lateral canthus, which is the point where the upper and lower eyelids meet. The medial canthus contains the medial canthal ligament that attaches to the orbit forming the bony attachment of the eyelids and the lacrimal drainage and collecting system. The lateral canthus consists of four structures, the lateral canthal tendon, Lockwood's ligament, cheek ligaments of the lateral rectus muscle, and the lateral horn of the levator aponeurosis. The exact procedure depends on which canthus is involved and the nature of the injury. If the medial canthus has been injured, it may be reconstructed using a full-thickness skin graft, upper eyelid transposition flap, or a rotation or transposition flap from the glabella. If a skin graft is used it is harvested, prepared for grafting, and sutured over the defect. If a flap from the upper eyelid or glabella is used, the flap configuration is determined, the skin is incised, and the incision is carried down to subcutaneous tissues. The flap is developed. Glabellar flaps require thinning to maintain the proper contour and skin thickness around the eye. If the medial canthal supports (ligaments and tendons) have been damaged they are reconstructed so that the eyelid will properly oppose the globe. The flap is then rotated or transferred and sutured to surrounding tissue. The flap must be configured in a way that allows reconstruction of the canthus and coverage of the defect. If the lateral canthus has been injured it is typically repaired with a cheek rotation flap. The location, shape, and size of the flap depend on the characteristics of the defect and the available donor site. Extensive defects involving the ligaments may require development of a periosteal strip from the zygomatic arch to provide support to the lateral canthus. Once the supporting structures have been repaired, the flap is positioned and sutured over the defect and the donor site is repaired.

Canthoplasty

ICD-10-CM Diagnostic Codes

⇄	C43.112	Malignant melanoma of right lower eyelid, including canthus
⇄	C43.122	Malignant melanoma of left lower eyelid, including canthus
⇄	C44.1122	Basal cell carcinoma of skin of right lower eyelid, including canthus
⇄	C44.1192	Basal cell carcinoma of skin of left lower eyelid, including canthus
⇄	C44.1222	Squamous cell carcinoma of skin of right lower eyelid, including canthus
⇄	C44.1292	Squamous cell carcinoma of skin of left lower eyelid, including canthus
⇄	C44.1322	Sebaceous cell carcinoma of skin of right lower eyelid, including canthus
⇄	C44.1392	Sebaceous cell carcinoma of skin of left lower eyelid, including canthus
⇄	C44.1922	Other specified malignant neoplasm of skin of right lower eyelid, including canthus
⇄	C44.1992	Other specified malignant neoplasm of skin of left lower eyelid, including canthus
⇄	C4A.112	Merkel cell carcinoma of right lower eyelid, including canthus
⇄	C4A.122	Merkel cell carcinoma of left lower eyelid, including canthus
⇄	D03.112	Melanoma in situ of right lower eyelid, including canthus
⇄	D03.122	Melanoma in situ of left lower eyelid, including canthus
⇄	D04.112	Carcinoma in situ of skin of right lower eyelid, including canthus
⇄	D04.122	Carcinoma in situ of skin of left lower eyelid, including canthus
⇄	D22.112	Melanocytic nevi of right lower eyelid, including canthus
⇄	D22.122	Melanocytic nevi of left lower eyelid, including canthus
⇄	H02.012	Cicatricial entropion of right lower eyelid
⇄	H02.015	Cicatricial entropion of left lower eyelid
⇄	H02.022	Mechanical entropion of right lower eyelid
⇄	H02.025	Mechanical entropion of left lower eyelid
⇄	H02.032	Senile entropion of right lower eyelid
⇄	H02.035	Senile entropion of left lower eyelid
⇄	H02.042	Spastic entropion of right lower eyelid
⇄	H02.045	Spastic entropion of left lower eyelid
⇄	H02.112	Cicatricial ectropion of right lower eyelid
⇄	H02.115	Cicatricial ectropion of left lower eyelid
⇄	H02.122	Mechanical ectropion of right lower eyelid
⇄	H02.125	Mechanical ectropion of left lower eyelid
⇄	H02.132	Senile ectropion of right lower eyelid
⇄	H02.135	Senile ectropion of left lower eyelid
⇄	H02.142	Spastic ectropion of right lower eyelid
⇄	H02.145	Spastic ectropion of left lower eyelid
⇄	H02.152	Paralytic ectropion of right lower eyelid
⇄	H02.155	Paralytic ectropion of left lower eyelid
⇄	H02.222	Mechanical lagophthalmos right lower eyelid
⇄	H02.225	Mechanical lagophthalmos left lower eyelid
⇄	H02.232	Paralytic lagophthalmos right lower eyelid
⇄	H02.235	Paralytic lagophthalmos left lower eyelid
⇄	H02.32	Blepharochalasis right lower eyelid
⇄	H02.35	Blepharochalasis left lower eyelid
⇄	H02.401	Unspecified ptosis of right eyelid
⇄	H02.402	Unspecified ptosis of left eyelid
⇄	H02.421	Myogenic ptosis of right eyelid
⇄	H02.422	Myogenic ptosis of left eyelid
⇄	H02.522	Blepharophimosis right lower eyelid
⇄	H02.525	Blepharophimosis left lower eyelid
⇄	H02.532	Eyelid retraction right lower eyelid
⇄	H02.535	Eyelid retraction left lower eyelid
	H02.89	Other specified disorders of eyelid
⇄	H04.151	Secondary lacrimal gland atrophy, right lacrimal gland
⇄	H04.152	Secondary lacrimal gland atrophy, left lacrimal gland
⇄	H05.211	Displacement (lateral) of globe, right eye
⇄	H05.212	Displacement (lateral) of globe, left eye
⇄	H05.411	Enophthalmos due to atrophy of orbital tissue, right eye
⇄	H05.421	Enophthalmos due to trauma or surgery, right eye
	Q10.0	Congenital ptosis
	Q10.2	Congenital entropion
	Q10.3	Other congenital malformations of eyelid
❼⇄	S01.111	Laceration without foreign body of right eyelid and periocular area
❼⇄	S01.112	Laceration without foreign body of left eyelid and periocular area
❼⇄	S01.121	Laceration with foreign body of right eyelid and periocular area
❼⇄	S01.122	Laceration with foreign body of left eyelid and periocular area

➐⇄	S01.131	Puncture wound without foreign body of right eyelid and periocular area
➐⇄	S01.132	Puncture wound without foreign body of left eyelid and periocular area
➐⇄	S01.141	Puncture wound with foreign body of right eyelid and periocular area
➐⇄	S01.142	Puncture wound with foreign body of left eyelid and periocular area
➐⇄	S01.151	Open bite of right eyelid and periocular area
➐⇄	S01.152	Open bite of left eyelid and periocular area
➐	T20.39	Burn of third degree of multiple sites of head, face, and neck
➐	T20.79	Corrosion of third degree of multiple sites of head, face, and neck
➐⇄	T26.01	Burn of right eyelid and periocular area
➐⇄	T26.02	Burn of left eyelid and periocular area
➐⇄	T26.51	Corrosion of right eyelid and periocular area
➐⇄	T26.52	Corrosion of left eyelid and periocular area
	Z85.820	Personal history of malignant melanoma of skin
	Z85.828	Personal history of other malignant neoplasm of skin
	Z85.840	Personal history of malignant neoplasm of eye

ICD-10-CM Coding Notes

For codes requiring a 7th character extension, refer to your ICD-10-CM book. Review the character descriptions and coding guidelines for proper selection. For some procedures, only certain characters will apply.

CCI Edits

Refer to Appendix A for CCI edits.

Facility RVUs

Code	Work	PE Facility	MP	Total Facility
67950	5.99	6.86	0.54	13.39

Non-facility RVUs

Code	Work	PE Non-Facility	MP	Total Non-Facility
67950	5.99	10.72	0.54	17.25

Modifiers (PAR)

Code	Mod 50	Mod 51	Mod 62	Mod 66	Mod 80
67950	1	2	1	0	1

Global Period

Code	Days
67950	090

67961-67966

67961 Excision and repair of eyelid, involving lid margin, tarsus, conjunctiva, canthus, or full thickness, may include preparation for skin graft or pedicle flap with adjacent tissue transfer or rearrangement; up to one-fourth of lid margin

67966 Excision and repair of eyelid, involving lid margin, tarsus, conjunctiva, canthus, or full thickness, may include preparation for skin graft or pedicle flap with adjacent tissue transfer or rearrangement; over one-fourth of lid margin

(For canthoplasty, use 67950)

(For free skin grafts, see 15120, 15121, 15260, 15261)

(For tubed pedicle flap preparation, use 15576; for delay, use 15630; for attachment, use 15650)

AMA Coding Guideline

Reconstruction Procedures on the Eyelids

Codes for blepharoplasty involve more than skin (ie, involving lid margin, tarsus, and/or palpebral conjunctiva).

AMA Coding Notes

Surgical Procedures on the Eye and Ocular Adnexa

(For diagnostic and treatment ophthalmological services, see Medicine, Ophthalmology, and 92002 et seq)

(Do not report code 69990 in addition to codes 65091-68850)

AMA *CPT® Assistant* ☐

67966: Nov 12: 13

Plain English Description

A lesion of the eyelid involving the lid margin, tarsus, conjunctiva, canthus, or the full thickness of the eyelid is excised and the surgical defect repaired using a skin graft or pedicle flap or some type of tissue transfer or rearrangement. Most lesions requiring excision of deeper eyelid tissues are malignant in nature and include basal cell carcinoma, squamous cell carcinoma, sebaceous carcinoma, and melanoma. The lesion is excised along with a margin of healthy tissue. Separately reportable pathological examination is performed to ensure that the margins are clean. If the margins are not clean, the excision is extended until clean margins are obtained. The eyelid is then reconstructed. The technique varies based on whether the upper or lower eyelid is reconstructed and the site of the defect on the lid itself (medial, central or lateral aspect). If a skin graft is used, an appropriate donor site is selected and the skin graft is harvested. The skin graft is prepared, placed over the defect, and sutured in place. If a pedicle flap is used, the configuration of the flap is determined. The skin and deeper tissues are incised and the flap is elevated and rotated over the defect. The flap is secured with sutures. The defect created by the creation of the flap is closed in layers. Use 67961 for excision of a lesion and repair of the surgical defect involving up to one-fourth (1/4) of the lid margin. Use 67966 when the surgical procedure involves over one-fourth of the lid margin.

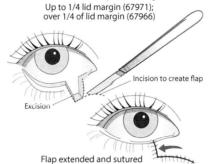

Excision and repair of eyelid

Up to 1/4 lid margin (67971); over 1/4 of lid margin (67966)

Incision to create flap

Excision

Flap extended and sutured

Excision and repair is made to eyelid involving lid margin/tarsus/conjuctiva/canthus or full thickness.

ICD-10-CM Diagnostic Codes

	Code	Description
➐⇄	S01.101	Unspecified open wound of right eyelid and periocular area
➐⇄	S01.102	Unspecified open wound of left eyelid and periocular area
➐⇄	S01.111	Laceration without foreign body of right eyelid and periocular area
➐⇄	S01.112	Laceration without foreign body of left eyelid and periocular area
➐⇄	S01.121	Laceration with foreign body of right eyelid and periocular area
➐⇄	S01.122	Laceration with foreign body of left eyelid and periocular area
➐⇄	S01.131	Puncture wound without foreign body of right eyelid and periocular area
➐⇄	S01.132	Puncture wound without foreign body of left eyelid and periocular area
➐⇄	S01.141	Puncture wound with foreign body of right eyelid and periocular area
➐⇄	S01.142	Puncture wound with foreign body of left eyelid and periocular area
➐⇄	S01.151	Open bite of right eyelid and periocular area
➐⇄	S01.152	Open bite of left eyelid and periocular area
➐	T20.39	Burn of third degree of multiple sites of head, face, and neck
➐	T20.79	Corrosion of third degree of multiple sites of head, face, and neck
➐⇄	T26.01	Burn of right eyelid and periocular area
➐⇄	T26.02	Burn of left eyelid and periocular area
➐⇄	T26.51	Corrosion of right eyelid and periocular area
➐⇄	T26.52	Corrosion of left eyelid and periocular area

ICD-10-CM Coding Notes

For codes requiring a 7th character extension, refer to your ICD-10-CM book. Review the character descriptions and coding guidelines for proper selection. For some procedures, only certain characters will apply.

CCI Edits

Refer to Appendix A for CCI edits.

Facility RVUs ☐

Code	Work	PE Facility	MP	Total Facility
67961	5.86	6.79	0.47	13.12
67966	8.97	9.21	0.73	18.91

Non-facility RVUs ☐

Code	Work	PE Non-Facility	MP	Total Non-Facility
67961	5.86	10.97	0.47	17.30
67966	8.97	13.12	0.73	22.82

Modifiers (PAR) ☐

Code	Mod 50	Mod 51	Mod 62	Mod 66	Mod 80
67961	1	2	0	0	0
67966	1	2	0	0	1

Global Period

Code	Days
67961	090
67966	090

67971-67975

67971 Reconstruction of eyelid, full thickness by transfer of tarsoconjunctival flap from opposing eyelid; up to two-thirds of eyelid, 1 stage or first stage

67973 Reconstruction of eyelid, full thickness by transfer of tarsoconjunctival flap from opposing eyelid; total eyelid, lower, 1 stage or first stage

67974 Reconstruction of eyelid, full thickness by transfer of tarsoconjunctival flap from opposing eyelid; total eyelid, upper, 1 stage or first stage

67975 Reconstruction of eyelid, full thickness by transfer of tarsoconjunctival flap from opposing eyelid; second stage

AMA Coding Guideline

Reconstruction Procedures on the Eyelids

Codes for blepharoplasty involve more than skin (ie, involving lid margin, tarsus, and/or palpebral conjunctiva).

AMA Coding Notes

Surgical Procedures on the Eye and Ocular Adnexa

(For diagnostic and treatment ophthalmological services, see Medicine, Ophthalmology, and 92002 et seq)

(Do not report code 69990 in addition to codes 65091-68850)

Plain English Description

A tarsoconjunctival flap from the opposing eyelid is used to reconstruct the eyelid defect following trauma or extensive surgical excision of a lesion. This is known as a lid-sharing reconstruction technique. The exact technique depends on whether the upper or lower eyelid is being reconstructed. A common technique for reconstruction of the lower eyelid is the tarsoconjunctival bridge flap, also called a modified Hughes procedure. A traction suture is placed in the upper eyelid margin. The upper eyelid is everted and the tarsus and conjunctiva of the upper eyelid are incised horizontally 4 mm proximal to the lid margin. The tarsus and conjunctiva are dissected away from the levator aponeurosis and the Muller muscle to create the flap. The flap is advanced to the defect in the lower eyelid. The edges of the flap are sutured to the medial and lateral remnants of the lower lid tarsus and the lower lid conjunctiva. The flap is then covered by a skin graft harvested from the upper eyelid or retroauricular region. Alternatively, the locally based skin flap may be advanced over the tarsoconjunctival flap. The flap is left in place for 4-6 weeks to develop lower lid blood supply to the flap. In the second stage of the procedure a grooved director is inserted under the flap and anterior to the globe. The flap is divided. Conjunctiva is sutured to the reconstructed lower lid margin. The Muller muscle and levator aponeurosis are dissected away from the overlying skin and allowed to retract. The remainder of the pedicled upper lid flap is reattached to the upper lid. A common technique for reconstructing the upper eyelid is the Cutler-Beard procedure. A skin-muscle-conjunctival flap is developed using the lower lid leaving the lower lid margin intact. The flap is advanced into the defect of the upper lid and sutured to the defect margins using a technique similar to that used for lower lid defects. The flap is left in place for 6-8 weeks. During the second stage of the procedure, the flap is divided at the planned reconstructed upper lid margin and the remainder of the pedicled flap reattached to the lower eyelid. Use 67971 for reconstruction of up to two-thirds of the upper or lower eyelid, 1 stage or first stage. Use 67973 for total lower eyelid reconstruction, 1 stage or first stage. Use 67974 for total upper eyelid, 1 stage or first stage. Use 67975 for the second stage of a two-stage procedure.

Reconstruction of eyelid, full thickness

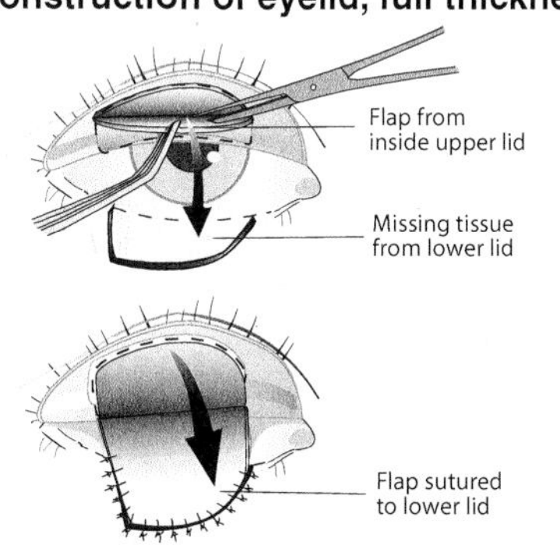

Up to two-thirds eyelid, first stage (67971); total eyelid, lower, first stage (67973); total eyelid, upper, first stage (67974); second stage (67975)

ICD-10-CM Diagnostic Codes

	Q10.3	Other congenital malformations of eyelid
➐⇄	S01.101	Unspecified open wound of right eyelid and periocular area
➐⇄	S01.102	Unspecified open wound of left eyelid and periocular area
➐⇄	S01.111	Laceration without foreign body of right eyelid and periocular area
➐⇄	S01.112	Laceration without foreign body of left eyelid and periocular area
➐⇄	S01.121	Laceration with foreign body of right eyelid and periocular area
➐⇄	S01.122	Laceration with foreign body of left eyelid and periocular area
➐⇄	S01.131	Puncture wound without foreign body of right eyelid and periocular area
➐⇄	S01.132	Puncture wound without foreign body of left eyelid and periocular area
➐⇄	S01.141	Puncture wound with foreign body of right eyelid and periocular area
➐⇄	S01.142	Puncture wound with foreign body of left eyelid and periocular area
➐⇄	S01.151	Open bite of right eyelid and periocular area
➐⇄	S01.152	Open bite of left eyelid and periocular area
➐	T20.39	Burn of third degree of multiple sites of head, face, and neck
➐	T20.79	Corrosion of third degree of multiple sites of head, face, and neck
➐⇄	T26.01	Burn of right eyelid and periocular area
➐⇄	T26.02	Burn of left eyelid and periocular area
➐⇄	T26.51	Corrosion of right eyelid and periocular area
➐⇄	T26.52	Corrosion of left eyelid and periocular area

ICD-10-CM Coding Notes

For codes requiring a 7th character extension, refer to your ICD-10-CM book. Review the character descriptions and coding guidelines for proper selection. For some procedures, only certain characters will apply.

CCI Edits

Refer to Appendix A for CCI edits.

Facility RVUs

Code	Work	PE Facility	MP	Total Facility
67971	10.01	9.97	0.84	20.82
67973	13.13	12.55	1.05	26.73
67974	13.10	12.53	1.04	26.67
67975	9.35	9.58	0.78	19.71

Non-facility RVUs

Code	Work	PE Non-Facility	MP	Total Non-Facility
67971	10.01	9.97	0.84	20.82
67973	13.13	12.55	1.05	26.73
67974	13.10	12.53	1.04	26.67
67975	9.35	9.58	0.78	19.71

Modifiers (PAR)

Code	Mod 50	Mod 51	Mod 62	Mod 66	Mod 80
67971	1	2	1	0	1
67973	1	2	1	0	2
67974	1	2	1	0	2
67975	1	2	0	0	1

Global Period

Code	Days
67971	090
67973	090
67974	090
67975	090

68020

68020 Incision of conjunctiva, drainage of cyst

AMA Coding Notes

Surgical Procedures on the Conjunctiva

(For removal of foreign body, see 65205 et seq)

Surgical Procedures on the Eye and Ocular Adnexa

(For diagnostic and treatment ophthalmological services, see Medicine, Ophthalmology, and 92002 et seq)

(Do not report code 69990 in addition to codes 65091-68850)

Plain English Description

A conjunctival cyst is a thin walled, fluid-filled sac located on the surface of the clear vascular tissue that covers the eye. The cyst may be congenital or acquired and usually results from friction to the tissue. To drain the cyst, ocular anesthetic eye drops are first instilled and the sac is grasped with forceps. The sac is then incised using a needle, scissors, knife blade, or curette and the fluid is drained. Hemostasis is achieved using electrocautery and the incision is closed with fibrin glue.

Incision/drainage conjunctival cyst

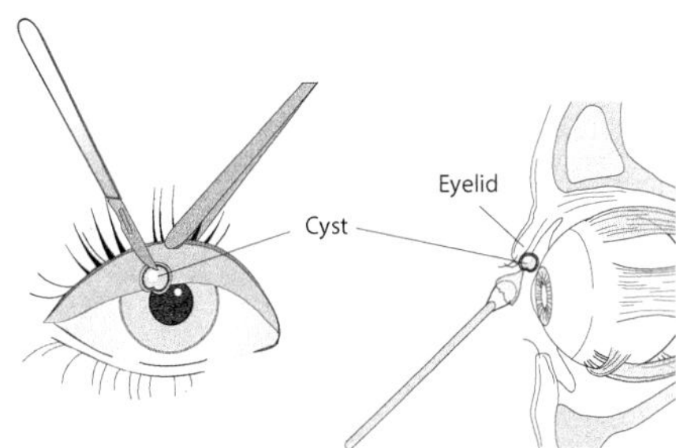

The cyst is incised and the contents are drained using a cotton-tipped probe or curette.

ICD-10-CM Diagnostic Codes

⇄	H11.122	Conjunctival concretions, left eye
⇄	H11.442	Conjunctival cysts, left eye

CCI Edits

Refer to Appendix A for CCI edits.

Facility RVUs

Code	Work	PE Facility	MP	Total Facility
68020	1.42	1.68	0.10	3.20

Non-facility RVUs

Code	Work	PE Non-Facility	MP	Total Non-Facility
68020	1.42	2.02	0.10	3.54

Modifiers (PAR)

Code	Mod 50	Mod 51	Mod 62	Mod 66	Mod 80
68020	1	2	0	0	1

Global Period

Code	Days
68020	010

68040

68040 Expression of conjunctival follicles (eg, for trachoma)

(To report automated evacuation of meibomian glands, use 0207T)

(For manual evacuation of meibomian glands, use 0563T)

AMA Coding Notes

Surgical Procedures on the Conjunctiva

(For removal of foreign body, see 65205 et seq)

Surgical Procedures on the Eye and Ocular Adnexa

(For diagnostic and treatment ophthalmological services, see Medicine, Ophthalmology, and 92002 et seq)

(Do not report code 69990 in addition to codes 65091-68850)

AMA *CPT® Assistant* ▢

68040: May 14: 5

Plain English Description

Expression of conjunctival follicles is performed to treat follicular conjunctivitis. Follicular conjunctivitis is usually caused by a viral or bacterial infection with the most common type requiring expression or drainage of the follicles being caused by Chlamydia trachomatis. Anesthetic drops are administered or another type of local anesthetic applied as needed. The eyelid is everted and the follicles inspected. Manual pressure is applied to express purulent matter from the follicles.

Expression of conjunctival follicles (eg, for trachoma)

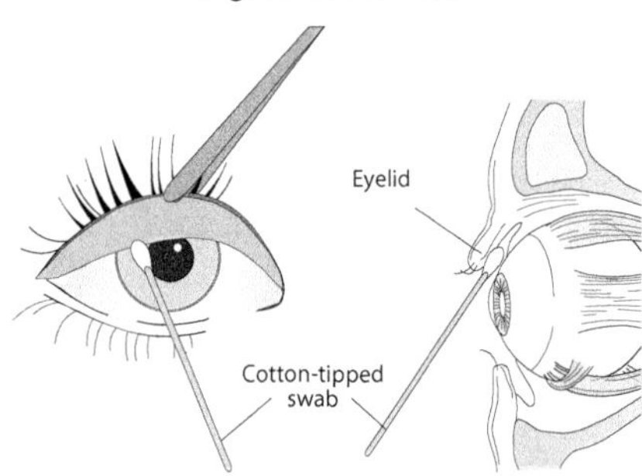

Granulations are removed using a cotton-tipped swab or a curette.

ICD-10-CM Diagnostic Codes

	A71.0	Initial stage of trachoma
	A71.1	Active stage of trachoma
	A71.9	Trachoma, unspecified
	A74.0	Chlamydial conjunctivitis
	B94.0	Sequelae of trachoma
⇄	H10.011	Acute follicular conjunctivitis, right eye
⇄	H10.012	Acute follicular conjunctivitis, left eye
⇄	H10.013	Acute follicular conjunctivitis, bilateral
⇄	H10.021	Other mucopurulent conjunctivitis, right eye
⇄	H10.022	Other mucopurulent conjunctivitis, left eye
⇄	H10.023	Other mucopurulent conjunctivitis, bilateral
	P39.1	Neonatal conjunctivitis and dacryocystitis

CCI Edits

Refer to Appendix A for CCI edits.

Facility RVUs ▢

Code	Work	PE Facility	MP	Total Facility
68040	0.85	0.49	0.04	1.38

Non-facility RVUs ▢

Code	Work	PE Non-Facility	MP	Total Non-Facility
68040	0.85	0.92	0.04	1.81

Modifiers (PAR) ▢

Code	Mod 50	Mod 51	Mod 62	Mod 66	Mod 80
68040	1	2	0	0	1

Global Period

Code	Days
68040	000

68100

68100 Biopsy of conjunctiva

AMA Coding Notes

Surgical Procedures on the Conjunctiva

(For removal of foreign body, see 65205 et seq)

Surgical Procedures on the Eye and Ocular Adnexa

(For diagnostic and treatment ophthalmological services, see Medicine, Ophthalmology, and 92002 et seq)

(Do not report code 69990 in addition to codes 65091-68850)

Plain English Description

The physician biopsies the conjunctiva. The conjunctiva is the mucous membrane covering the anterior surface of the eyeball (bulbar conjunctiva) and the posterior surface of the eyelid (palpebral conjunctiva). A biopsy may be performed when there is a lesion present or to help diagnose the cause of persistent conjunctivitis. A conjunctival biopsy may also be performed to aid in the diagnosis of some systemic diseases such as sarcoidosis, ocular pemphigoid, Stevens-Johnson syndrome, or amyloidosis. Anesthetic eye drops are instilled to numb the eye. A forceps is used to grasp the conjunctiva and a small piece of tissue is removed with scissors. The tissue sample is sent to the laboratory for separately reportable histological evaluation. Antibiotic ointment is applied to the biopsy site. An eye patch is applied as needed.

Biopsy of conjunctiva

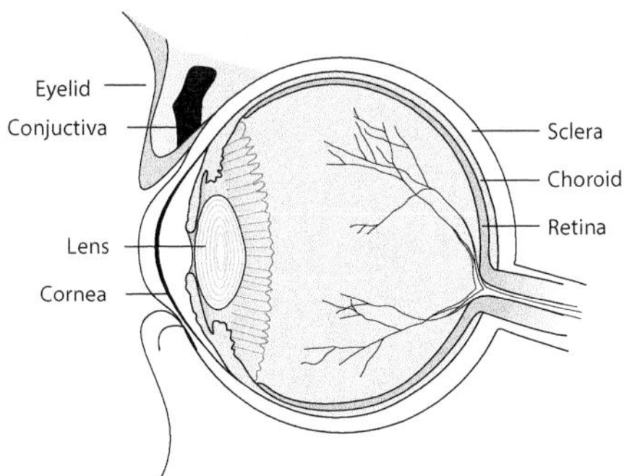

The physician takes a tissue sample from the inner eyelid.

ICD-10-CM Diagnostic Codes

⇄	C69.02	Malignant neoplasm of left conjunctiva
	C79.32	Secondary malignant neoplasm of cerebral meninges
⇄	D09.22	Carcinoma in situ of left eye
⇄	D31.02	Benign neoplasm of left conjunctiva
	D48.7	Neoplasm of uncertain behavior of other specified sites
	D49.89	Neoplasm of unspecified behavior of other specified sites
⇄	H11.152	Pinguecula, left eye
⇄	H11.242	Scarring of conjunctiva, left eye
⇄	H11.442	Conjunctival cysts, left eye
	H11.89	Other specified disorders of conjunctiva
⇄	H16.22	Keratoconjunctivitis sicca, not specified as Sjögren's

CCI Edits

Refer to Appendix A for CCI edits.

Facility RVUs

Code	Work	PE Facility	MP	Total Facility
68100	1.35	1.29	0.11	2.75

Non-facility RVUs

Code	Work	PE Non-Facility	MP	Total Non-Facility
68100	1.35	3.92	0.11	5.38

Modifiers (PAR)

Code	Mod 50	Mod 51	Mod 62	Mod 66	Mod 80
68100	1	2	0	0	1

Global Period

Code	Days
68100	000

68110-68130

68110 Excision of lesion, conjunctiva; up to 1 cm

68115 Excision of lesion, conjunctiva; over 1 cm

68130 Excision of lesion, conjunctiva; with adjacent sclera

AMA Coding Notes

Surgical Procedures on the Conjunctiva

(For removal of foreign body, see 65205 et seq)

Surgical Procedures on the Eye and Ocular Adnexa

(For diagnostic and treatment ophthalmological services, see Medicine, Ophthalmology, and 92002 et seq)

(Do not report code 69990 in addition to codes 65091-68850)

AMA *CPT® Assistant* ▯

68110: Jan 17: 7, Feb 18: 11

68115: Feb 18: 11

Plain English Description

Some of the more common types of conjunctival lesions requiring excision include benign squamous cell and limbal papillomas, and malignant primary acquired melanosis, conjunctival melanoma, and squamous cell carcinoma. Anesthetic drops or another type of local anesthesia is administered. The conjunctiva is inspected and the extent of the excision determined. The lesion is then excised along with a margin of healthy tissue. The tissue is sent for separately reportable pathological evaluation and to ensure that the margins are clear. Additional tissue is excised as needed including scleral tissue until clear margins have been obtained. Use 68110 for a conjunctival lesion up to 1 cm; use 68115 for a conjunctival lesion over 1 cm; and use 68130 for a lesion that requires excision of adjacent scleral tissue.

Excision of lesion, conjunctiva

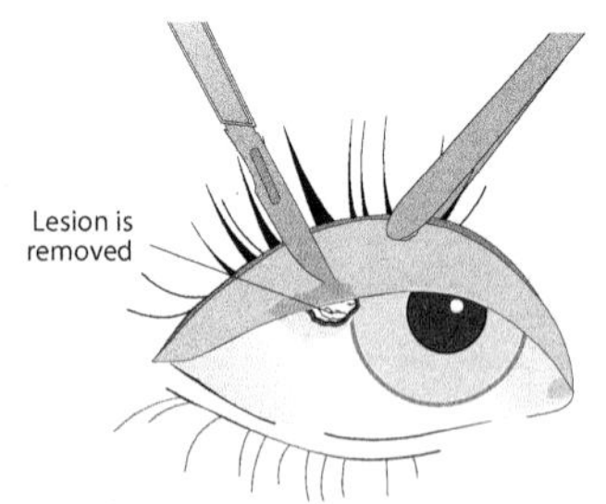

Lesion up to 1cm is removed (68110); lesion greater than 1cm is removed (68115); lesion is removed along with adjacent sclera (68130)

ICD-10-CM Diagnostic Codes

⇄	C69.01	Malignant neoplasm of right conjunctiva
⇄	C69.41	Malignant neoplasm of right ciliary body
⇄	D09.21	Carcinoma in situ of right eye
⇄	D31.01	Benign neoplasm of right conjunctiva
⇄	D31.41	Benign neoplasm of right ciliary body
	D48.7	Neoplasm of uncertain behavior of other specified sites
	D49.89	Neoplasm of unspecified behavior of other specified sites
⇄	H11.121	Conjunctival concretions, right eye
⇄	H11.221	Conjunctival granuloma, right eye
⇄	H11.431	Conjunctival hyperemia, right eye
⇄	H11.441	Conjunctival cysts, right eye
⇄	H11.821	Conjunctivochalasis, right eye
	H11.89	Other specified disorders of conjunctiva

CCI Edits

Refer to Appendix A for CCI edits.

Facility RVUs ▯

Code	Work	PE Facility	MP	Total Facility
68110	1.82	2.32	0.12	4.26
68115	2.41	2.68	0.20	5.29
68130	5.10	6.44	0.39	11.93

Non-facility RVUs ▯

Code	Work	PE Non-Facility	MP	Total Non-Facility
68110	1.82	5.06	0.12	7.00
68115	2.41	7.32	0.20	9.93
68130	5.10	10.82	0.39	16.31

Modifiers (PAR) ▯

Code	Mod 50	Mod 51	Mod 62	Mod 66	Mod 80
68110	1	2	0	0	1
68115	1	2	0	0	1
68130	1	2	0	0	1

Global Period

Code	Days
68110	010
68115	010
68130	090

68135

68135 Destruction of lesion, conjunctiva

AMA Coding Notes

Surgical Procedures on the Conjunctiva

(For removal of foreign body, see 65205 et seq)

Surgical Procedures on the Eye and Ocular Adnexa

(For diagnostic and treatment ophthalmological services, see Medicine, Ophthalmology, and 92002 et seq)

(Do not report code 69990 in addition to codes 65091-68850)

Plain English Description

A lesion of the conjunctiva is destroyed. Destruction may be performed using a laser, electrocautery, cryotherapy, chemical agent, or other method. Anesthetic drops or another type of local anesthesia is administered. The conjunctival lesion is inspected and the most effective method of destruction determined. Laser destruction uses a laser beam focused on the lesion. Electrocautery destroys the lesion using a heat probe. Cryotherapy uses liquid nitrogen to freeze the lesion. Chemical destruction involves the use of a chemical or pharmacologic agent.

Destruction of lesion, conjunctiva

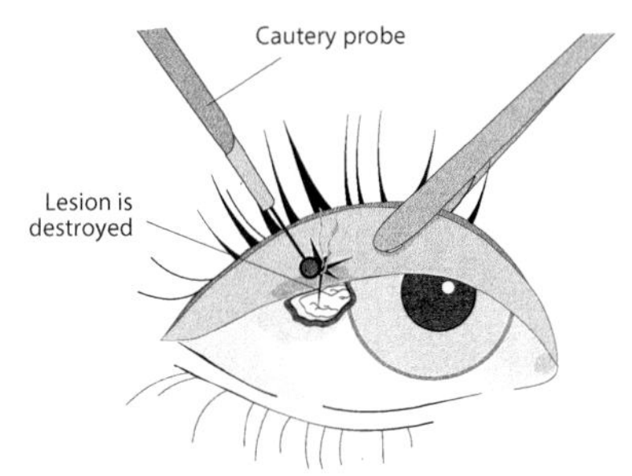

ICD-10-CM Diagnostic Codes

	Code	Description
⇄	C69.02	Malignant neoplasm of left conjunctiva
⇄	D09.22	Carcinoma in situ of left eye
⇄	D31.02	Benign neoplasm of left conjunctiva
	D48.7	Neoplasm of uncertain behavior of other specified sites
	D49.89	Neoplasm of unspecified behavior of other specified sites
⇄	H11.122	Conjunctival concretions, left eye
⇄	H11.212	Conjunctival adhesions and strands (localized), left eye
⇄	H11.222	Conjunctival granuloma, left eye
⇄	H11.242	Scarring of conjunctiva, left eye
⇄	H11.412	Vascular abnormalities of conjunctiva, left eye
⇄	H11.432	Conjunctival hyperemia, left eye
⇄	H11.442	Conjunctival cysts, left eye

CCI Edits

Refer to Appendix A for CCI edits.

Facility RVUs ▯

Code	Work	PE Facility	MP	Total Facility
68135	1.89	2.29	0.12	4.30

Non-facility RVUs ▯

Code	Work	PE Non-Facility	MP	Total Non-Facility
68135	1.89	2.55	0.12	4.56

Modifiers (PAR) ▯

Code	Mod 50	Mod 51	Mod 62	Mod 66	Mod 80
68135	1	2	0	0	1

Global Period

Code	Days
68135	010

68200

68200 Subconjunctival injection

AMA Coding Notes

Injection Procedures on the Conjunctiva

(For injection into Tenon's capsule or retrobulbar injection, see 67500-67515)

Surgical Procedures on the Conjunctiva

(For removal of foreign body, see 65205 et seq)

Surgical Procedures on the Eye and Ocular Adnexa

(For diagnostic and treatment ophthalmological services, see Medicine, Ophthalmology, and 92002 et seq)

(Do not report code 69990 in addition to codes 65091-68850)

AMA *CPT® Assistant* ▯

68200: Aug 03: 15, Nov 12: 10

Plain English Description

A subconjunctival injection is administered usually to treat severe inflammation or infection. Local anesthetic drops are administered. The site of the injection, usually the upper or lower fornix is identified. The needle is advanced through the conjunctiva and into the space between the conjunctiva and the sclera. The substance is then injected slowly, which will cause a ballooning effect between the conjunctiva and sclera. The needle is removed, the eye closed, and an eye pad applied until the fluid disperses and the ballooning subsides. The eye pad may be secured and left in place for several hours.

Subconjunctival injection

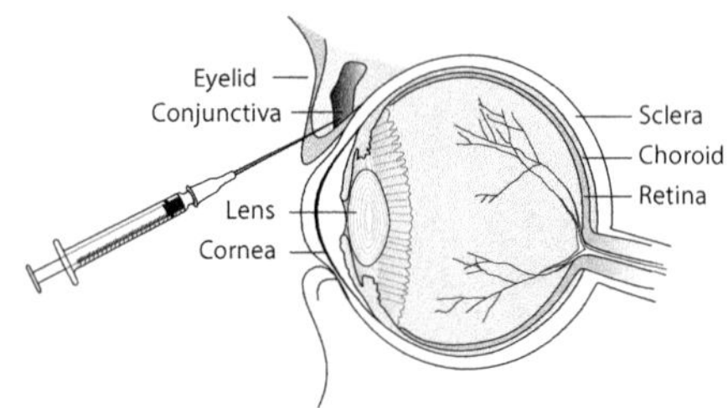

The physician injects a substance under the top layer of tissue on the inside of the eyelid.

ICD-10-CM Diagnostic Codes

	Code	Description
	A51.43	Secondary syphilitic oculopathy
⇄	C69.01	Malignant neoplasm of right conjunctiva
⇄	D09.21	Carcinoma in situ of right eye
⇄	D31.01	Benign neoplasm of right conjunctiva
	D48.7	Neoplasm of uncertain behavior of other specified sites
	D49.9	Neoplasm of unspecified behavior of unspecified site
⇄	H11.221	Conjunctival granuloma, right eye
⇄	H11.241	Scarring of conjunctiva, right eye
⇄	H11.31	Conjunctival hemorrhage, right eye
⇄	H11.411	Vascular abnormalities of conjunctiva, right eye
⇄	H11.421	Conjunctival edema, right eye
⇄	H11.431	Conjunctival hyperemia, right eye
⇄	H11.441	Conjunctival cysts, right eye
⇄	H11.821	Conjunctivochalasis, right eye
	H11.89	Other specified disorders of conjunctiva
⇄	H16.211	Exposure keratoconjunctivitis, right eye
⇄	H16.311	Corneal abscess, right eye
⇄	H44.111	Panuveitis, right eye
⇄	H44.131	Sympathetic uveitis, right eye
	H59.40	Inflammation (infection) of postprocedural bleb, unspecified
	H59.41	Inflammation (infection) of postprocedural bleb, stage 1
	H59.42	Inflammation (infection) of postprocedural bleb, stage 2
	H59.43	Inflammation (infection) of postprocedural bleb, stage 3
	L12.1	Cicatricial pemphigoid

CCI Edits

Refer to Appendix A for CCI edits.

Facility RVUs ▯

Code	Work	PE Facility	MP	Total Facility
68200	0.49	0.46	0.04	0.99

Non-facility RVUs ▯

Code	Work	PE Non-Facility	MP	Total Non-Facility
68200	0.49	0.69	0.04	1.22

Modifiers (PAR) ▯

Code	Mod 50	Mod 51	Mod 62	Mod 66	Mod 80
68200	1	2	0	0	1

Global Period

Code	Days
68200	000

68320-68325

68320 Conjunctivoplasty; with conjunctival graft or extensive rearrangement

68325 Conjunctivoplasty; with buccal mucous membrane graft (includes obtaining graft)

AMA Coding Notes

Conjunctivoplasty Procedures

(For wound repair, see 65270-65273)

Surgical Procedures on the Conjunctiva

(For removal of foreign body, see 65205 et seq)

Surgical Procedures on the Eye and Ocular Adnexa

(For diagnostic and treatment ophthalmological services, see Medicine, Ophthalmology, and 92002 et seq)

(Do not report code 69990 in addition to codes 65091-68850)

AMA *CPT® Assistant* ▯

68320: Feb 04: 11

Plain English Description

Conjunctivoplasty is performed to treat a number of conditions including redundant conjunctiva, lesions of the conjunctiva, and hyperemia of conjunctival blood vessels. A subconjunctival injection may be used to elevate the conjunctiva off of the sclera. The redundant or abnormal conjunctival tissue is excised. In 68320, the remaining conjunctiva is then rearranged or a conjunctival graft is harvested from the contralateral eye and used to repair the defect. If the conjunctiva is rearranged, one or more conjunctival flaps are configured, raised, and repositioned over the sclera. The flap is secured with sutures or tissue glue. If a conjunctival graft from the contralateral eye is used, the conjunctival harvest site is marked with a pen or keratotomy marker. The conjunctiva at the donor site is elevated using a subconjunctival injection of balanced salt solution and a local anesthetic. The lateral borders of the graft are incised in a radial fashion. The tissue between the incisions at the lateral borders is undermined using blunt dissection. Dissection is carried in an anterior direction to the conjunctival insertion at the limbus and then beyond the limbus into the peripheral cornea. The conjunctival graft including the superficial epithelial corneal tissue is then excised. The donor site may be left to heal by secondary intention or the conjunctiva may be advanced to cover a portion of the donor site to minimize pain and inflammation. The graft is then placed over the surgically created defect in the opposite eye. In 68325, a buccal mucous membrane graft is used to repair the defect and is usually taken from the lower lip. A split thickness mucous membrane graft is harvested using a mucotome. The graft is configured to the desired size and shape to fit the defect in the conjunctiva. The graft is sutured to the conjunctiva and/or sclera.

Conjunctivoplasty

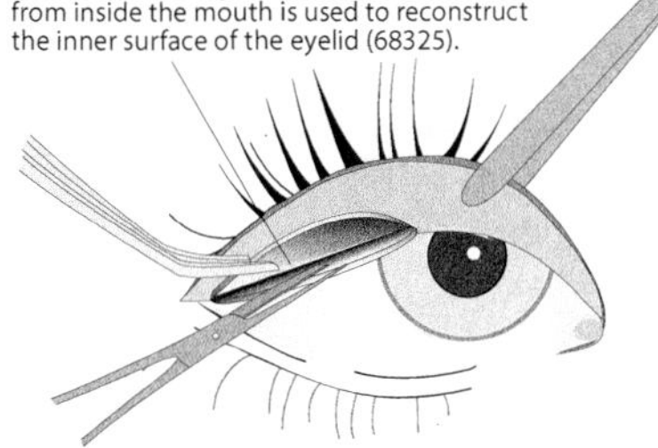

The inner surface of the eyelid is extensively reconstructed, or grafted (68320); graft obtained from inside the mouth is used to reconstruct the inner surface of the eyelid (68325).

ICD-10-CM Diagnostic Codes

	B94.0	Sequelae of trachoma
⇄	C69.01	Malignant neoplasm of right conjunctiva
⇄	C69.02	Malignant neoplasm of left conjunctiva
⇄	D09.21	Carcinoma in situ of right eye
⇄	D09.22	Carcinoma in situ of left eye
⇄	D31.01	Benign neoplasm of right conjunctiva
⇄	D31.02	Benign neoplasm of left conjunctiva
	D48.7	Neoplasm of uncertain behavior of other specified sites
⇄	H02.011	Cicatricial entropion of right upper eyelid
⇄	H02.012	Cicatricial entropion of right lower eyelid
⇄	H02.014	Cicatricial entropion of left upper eyelid
⇄	H02.015	Cicatricial entropion of left lower eyelid
⇄	H02.051	Trichiasis without entropion right upper eyelid
⇄	H02.052	Trichiasis without entropion right lower eyelid
⇄	H02.054	Trichiasis without entropion left upper eyelid
⇄	H02.055	Trichiasis without entropion left lower eyelid
⇄	H02.101	Unspecified ectropion of right upper eyelid
⇄	H02.102	Unspecified ectropion of right lower eyelid
⇄	H02.104	Unspecified ectropion of left upper eyelid
⇄	H02.105	Unspecified ectropion of left lower eyelid
⇄	H02.111	Cicatricial ectropion of right upper eyelid
⇄	H02.112	Cicatricial ectropion of right lower eyelid
⇄	H02.114	Cicatricial ectropion of left upper eyelid
⇄	H02.115	Cicatricial ectropion of left lower eyelid
⇄	H02.131	Senile ectropion of right upper eyelid
⇄	H02.132	Senile ectropion of right lower eyelid
⇄	H02.134	Senile ectropion of left upper eyelid
⇄	H02.135	Senile ectropion of left lower eyelid
⇄	H02.531	Eyelid retraction right upper eyelid
⇄	H02.532	Eyelid retraction right lower eyelid
⇄	H02.534	Eyelid retraction left upper eyelid
⇄	H02.535	Eyelid retraction left lower eyelid
⇄	H04.151	Secondary lacrimal gland atrophy, right lacrimal gland
⇄	H04.152	Secondary lacrimal gland atrophy, left lacrimal gland
⇄	H04.153	Secondary lacrimal gland atrophy, bilateral lacrimal glands
⇄	H04.221	Epiphora due to insufficient drainage, right side
⇄	H04.222	Epiphora due to insufficient drainage, left side
⇄	H04.223	Epiphora due to insufficient drainage, bilateral
⇄	H04.521	Eversion of right lacrimal punctum
⇄	H04.522	Eversion of left lacrimal punctum
⇄	H04.523	Eversion of bilateral lacrimal punctum
⇄	H04.561	Stenosis of right lacrimal punctum
⇄	H04.562	Stenosis of left lacrimal punctum
⇄	H04.563	Stenosis of bilateral lacrimal punctum
⇄	H10.211	Acute toxic conjunctivitis, right eye
⇄	H10.212	Acute toxic conjunctivitis, left eye
⇄	H10.213	Acute toxic conjunctivitis, bilateral
⇄	H10.221	Pseudomembranous conjunctivitis, right eye
⇄	H10.222	Pseudomembranous conjunctivitis, left eye
⇄	H10.223	Pseudomembranous conjunctivitis, bilateral
⇄	H11.211	Conjunctival adhesions and strands (localized), right eye
⇄	H11.212	Conjunctival adhesions and strands (localized), left eye
⇄	H11.213	Conjunctival adhesions and strands (localized), bilateral
⇄	H11.221	Conjunctival granuloma, right eye
⇄	H11.222	Conjunctival granuloma, left eye
⇄	H11.223	Conjunctival granuloma, bilateral
⇄	H11.231	Symblepharon, right eye
⇄	H11.232	Symblepharon, left eye
⇄	H11.233	Symblepharon, bilateral
⇄	H11.241	Scarring of conjunctiva, right eye
⇄	H11.242	Scarring of conjunctiva, left eye
⇄	H11.243	Scarring of conjunctiva, bilateral
⇄	H11.431	Conjunctival hyperemia, right eye
⇄	H11.432	Conjunctival hyperemia, left eye
⇄	H11.433	Conjunctival hyperemia, bilateral
⇄	H11.441	Conjunctival cysts, right eye
⇄	H11.442	Conjunctival cysts, left eye
⇄	H11.443	Conjunctival cysts, bilateral
⇄	H15.841	Scleral ectasia, right eye
⇄	H15.842	Scleral ectasia, left eye
⇄	H15.843	Scleral ectasia, bilateral
⇄	H44.421	Hypotony of right eye due to ocular fistula
⇄	H44.422	Hypotony of left eye due to ocular fistula
⇄	H44.423	Hypotony of eye due to ocular fistula, bilateral
	H44.89	Other disorders of globe
	Q10.1	Congenital ectropion
	Q10.2	Congenital entropion
	Q10.3	Other congenital malformations of eyelid

	Code	Description
	Q10.6	Other congenital malformations of lacrimal apparatus
	Q10.7	Congenital malformation of orbit
❼⇄	S01.111	Laceration without foreign body of right eyelid and periocular area
❼⇄	S01.112	Laceration without foreign body of left eyelid and periocular area
❼⇄	S01.121	Laceration with foreign body of right eyelid and periocular area
❼⇄	S01.122	Laceration with foreign body of left eyelid and periocular area
❼⇄	S01.131	Puncture wound without foreign body of right eyelid and periocular area
❼⇄	S01.132	Puncture wound without foreign body of left eyelid and periocular area
❼⇄	S01.141	Puncture wound with foreign body of right eyelid and periocular area
❼⇄	S01.142	Puncture wound with foreign body of left eyelid and periocular area
❼⇄	S01.151	Open bite of right eyelid and periocular area
❼⇄	S01.152	Open bite of left eyelid and periocular area
❼⇄	S05.31	Ocular laceration without prolapse or loss of intraocular tissue, right eye
❼⇄	S05.32	Ocular laceration without prolapse or loss of intraocular tissue, left eye
❼⇄	T26.11	Burn of cornea and conjunctival sac, right eye
❼⇄	T26.12	Burn of cornea and conjunctival sac, left eye
❼⇄	T26.61	Corrosion of cornea and conjunctival sac, right eye
❼⇄	T26.62	Corrosion of cornea and conjunctival sac, left eye
	Z85.831	Personal history of malignant neoplasm of soft tissue
	Z85.89	Personal history of malignant neoplasm of other organs and systems

ICD-10-CM Coding Notes

For codes requiring a 7th character extension, refer to your ICD-10-CM book. Review the character descriptions and coding guidelines for proper selection. For some procedures, only certain characters will apply.

CCI Edits

Refer to Appendix A for CCI edits.

Facility RVUs

Code	Work	PE Facility	MP	Total Facility
68320	6.64	8.43	0.54	15.61
68325	8.63	9.65	0.66	18.94

Non-facility RVUs

Code	Work	PE Non-Facility	MP	Total Non-Facility
68320	6.64	14.76	0.54	21.94
68325	8.63	9.65	0.66	18.94

Modifiers (PAR)

Code	Mod 50	Mod 51	Mod 62	Mod 66	Mod 80
68320	1	2	1	0	1
68325	1	2	1	0	1

Global Period

Code	Days
68320	090
68325	090

68326-68328

68326 Conjunctivoplasty, reconstruction cul-de-sac; with conjunctival graft or extensive rearrangement

68328 Conjunctivoplasty, reconstruction cul-de-sac; with buccal mucous membrane graft (includes obtaining graft)

AMA Coding Notes

Conjunctivoplasty Procedures

(For wound repair, see 65270-65273)

Surgical Procedures on the Conjunctiva

(For removal of foreign body, see 65205 et seq)

Surgical Procedures on the Eye and Ocular Adnexa

(For diagnostic and treatment ophthalmological services, see Medicine, Ophthalmology, and 92002 et seq)

(Do not report code 69990 in addition to codes 65091-68850)

Plain English Description

Conjunctivoplasty with reconstruction of the cul-de-sac is performed to treat a number of conditions including redundant conjunctiva, lesions of the conjunctiva, and hyperemia of conjunctival blood vessels. The cul-de-sac, also referred to as the conjunctival fornix is the site where the conjunctiva of the globe meets the conjunctiva of the eyelid.
A subconjunctival injection may be used to elevate the conjunctiva off of the sclera. The redundant or abnormal conjunctival tissue is excised.
In 68326, the remaining conjunctiva is then rearranged or a conjunctival graft is harvested from the contralateral eye and used to repair the defect including the defect in the cul-de-sac.
If the conjunctiva is rearranged, one or more conjunctival flaps are configured, raised and repositioned over the sclera and cul-de-sac.
The flap is secured with sutures or tissue glue.
If a conjunctival graft from the contralateral eye is used, the conjunctival harvest site is marked with a pen or keratotomy marker. The conjunctiva at the donor site is elevated using a subconjunctival injection of balanced salt solution and a local anesthetic. The lateral borders of the graft are incised in a radial fashion. The tissue between the incisions at the lateral borders is undermined using blunt dissection. Dissection is carried in an anterior direction to the conjunctival insertion at the limbus and then beyond the limbus into the peripheral cornea. The conjunctival graft including the superficial epithelial corneal tissue is then excised. The donor site may be left to heal by secondary intention or the conjunctiva may be advanced to cover a portion of the donor site to minimize pain and inflammation. The graft is then placed over the surgically created conjunctival defect in the opposite eye. In 68328, a buccal mucous membrane graft is used to repair a conjunctival defect that includes the cul-de-sac. The graft is usually taken from the lower lip. A split thickness mucous membrane graft is harvested using a mucotome. The graft is configured to the desired size and shape to fit the defect in the conjunctiva including the defect in the cul-de-sac. The graft is sutured to the conjunctiva and/or sclera including the defect in the cul-de-sac.

Conjunctivoplasty, reconstruction cul-de-sac

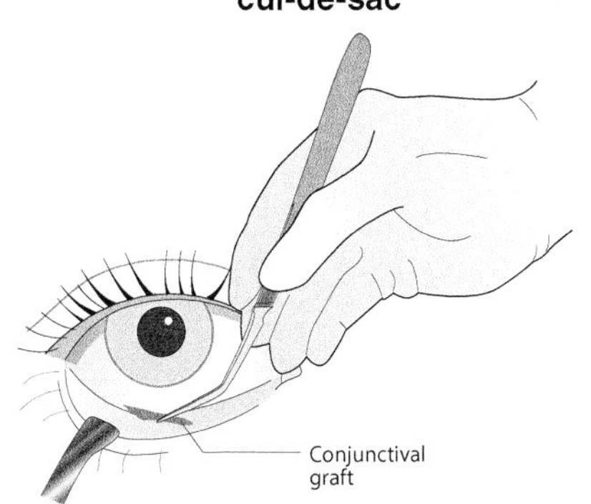

The conjunctival cul-de-sac is repaired with a graft obtained from another eyelid (68326); graft obtained from inside the mouth (68328).

ICD-10-CM Diagnostic Codes

⇄	C69.01	Malignant neoplasm of right conjunctiva
⇄	D09.21	Carcinoma in situ of right eye
⇄	D31.01	Benign neoplasm of right conjunctiva
	D48.7	Neoplasm of uncertain behavior of other specified sites
	D49.89	Neoplasm of unspecified behavior of other specified sites
⇄	H02.011	Cicatricial entropion of right upper eyelid
⇄	H02.012	Cicatricial entropion of right lower eyelid
⇄	H02.031	Senile entropion of right upper eyelid
⇄	H02.032	Senile entropion of right lower eyelid
⇄	H02.051	Trichiasis without entropion right upper eyelid
⇄	H02.052	Trichiasis without entropion right lower eyelid
⇄	H02.131	Senile ectropion of right upper eyelid
⇄	H02.132	Senile ectropion of right lower eyelid
⇄	H02.141	Spastic ectropion of right upper eyelid
⇄	H02.142	Spastic ectropion of right lower eyelid
⇄	H02.531	Eyelid retraction right upper eyelid
⇄	H02.532	Eyelid retraction right lower eyelid
⇄	H10.211	Acute toxic conjunctivitis, right eye
⇄	H11.221	Conjunctival granuloma, right eye
⇄	H11.231	Symblepharon, right eye
⇄	H11.241	Scarring of conjunctiva, right eye
⇄	H11.431	Conjunctival hyperemia, right eye
⇄	H11.441	Conjunctival cysts, right eye
⇄	H11.821	Conjunctivochalasis, right eye
⇄	H16.211	Exposure keratoconjunctivitis, right eye
⇄	H44.421	Hypotony of right eye due to ocular fistula
	H44.89	Other disorders of globe
	Q10.1	Congenital ectropion
	Q10.2	Congenital entropion
	Q10.3	Other congenital malformations of eyelid
	Q10.6	Other congenital malformations of lacrimal apparatus
	Q10.7	Congenital malformation of orbit
➐⇄	S01.111	Laceration without foreign body of right eyelid and periocular area
➐⇄	S01.121	Laceration with foreign body of right eyelid and periocular area
➐⇄	S01.131	Puncture wound without foreign body of right eyelid and periocular area
➐⇄	S01.141	Puncture wound with foreign body of right eyelid and periocular area
➐⇄	S01.151	Open bite of right eyelid and periocular area
➐⇄	S05.21	Ocular laceration and rupture with prolapse or loss of intraocular tissue, right eye
➐⇄	S05.31	Ocular laceration without prolapse or loss of intraocular tissue, right eye
➐⇄	T26.11	Burn of cornea and conjunctival sac, right eye
➐⇄	T26.61	Corrosion of cornea and conjunctival sac, right eye
➐⇄	T85.310	Breakdown (mechanical) of prosthetic orbit of right eye
➐⇄	T85.320	Displacement of prosthetic orbit of right eye
➐⇄	T85.390	Other mechanical complication of prosthetic orbit of right eye
	Z85.831	Personal history of malignant neoplasm of soft tissue
	Z85.89	Personal history of malignant neoplasm of other organs and systems

ICD-10-CM Coding Notes

For codes requiring a 7th character extension, refer to your ICD-10-CM book. Review the character descriptions and coding guidelines for proper selection. For some procedures, only certain characters will apply.

CCI Edits

Refer to Appendix A for CCI edits.

Facility RVUs

Code	Work	PE Facility	MP	Total Facility
68326	8.42	9.52	0.66	18.60
68328	9.45	10.13	0.84	20.42

Non-facility RVUs

Code	Work	PE Non-Facility	MP	Total Non-Facility
68326	8.42	9.52	0.66	18.60
68328	9.45	10.13	0.84	20.42

Modifiers (PAR)

Code	Mod 50	Mod 51	Mod 62	Mod 66	Mod 80
68326	1	2	0	0	1
68328	1	2	0	0	0

Global Period

Code	Days
68326	090
68328	090

68330-68340

68330 Repair of symblepharon; conjunctivoplasty, without graft

68335 Repair of symblepharon; with free graft conjunctiva or buccal mucous membrane (includes obtaining graft)

68340 Repair of symblepharon; division of symblepharon, with or without insertion of conformer or contact lens

AMA Coding Notes

Conjunctivoplasty Procedures

(For wound repair, see 65270-65273)

Surgical Procedures on the Conjunctiva

(For removal of foreign body, see 65205 et seq)

Surgical Procedures on the Eye and Ocular Adnexa

(For diagnostic and treatment ophthalmological services, see Medicine, Ophthalmology, and 92002 et seq)

(Do not report code 69990 in addition to codes 65091-68850)

Plain English Description

A symblepharon is the formation of adhesions or scar tissue between the palpebral conjunctiva of the eyelid and the bulbar conjunctiva of the globe and is typically secondary to trauma or infection. Symblepharon formation can affect eye movement, prevent the eyelids from closing or opening completely, and can cause double vision. In 68330, a symblepharon is repaired without a graft. The adhesions between the palpebral and bulbar conjunctiva are released and the fibrous tissue is carefully dissected from normal conjunctiva and excised. Adjacent healthy conjunctiva is advanced over the site where the adhesions were excised and secured with sutures. In 68335, the symblepharon is excised as described above and a free conjunctival graft or buccal mucous membrane graft is used to repair the defect. If a conjunctival graft from the contralateral eye is used, the conjunctival harvest site is marked with a pen or keratotomy marker. The conjunctiva at the donor site is elevated using a subconjunctival injection of balanced salt solution and a local anesthetic. The lateral borders of the graft are incised in a radial fashion. The tissue between the incisions at the lateral borders is undermined using blunt dissection. Dissection is carried in an anterior direction to the conjunctival insertion at the limbus and then beyond the limbus into the peripheral cornea. The conjunctival graft including the superficial epithelial corneal tissue is then excised. The donor site may be left to heal by secondary intention or the conjunctiva may be advanced to cover a portion of the donor site to minimize pain and inflammation. The graft is then placed over the surgically created conjunctival defect in the opposite eye. If a buccal mucous membrane graft is used to repair a conjunctival defect, the graft is usually taken from the lower lip. A split thickness mucous membrane graft is harvested using a mucotome. The graft is configured to the desired size and shape to fit the defect in the conjunctiva. The graft is sutured to the conjunctiva and/or sclera including the defect in the cul-de-sac. In 68340, the symblepharon is divided. The adhesions between the palpebral and bulbar conjunctiva are released and the fibrous tissue is carefully dissected from normal conjunctiva and excised. The site may be left open to heal by secondary intention or a conformer or contact lens inserted. If a conformer or contact lens is inserted, the eye is measured and a properly sized conformer or lens is selected and inserted into the eye to maintain separation between the conjunctiva of the lid and the globe while the conjunctiva heals. The conformer or lens is permanently removed 4-12 weeks later.

Repair of symblepharon

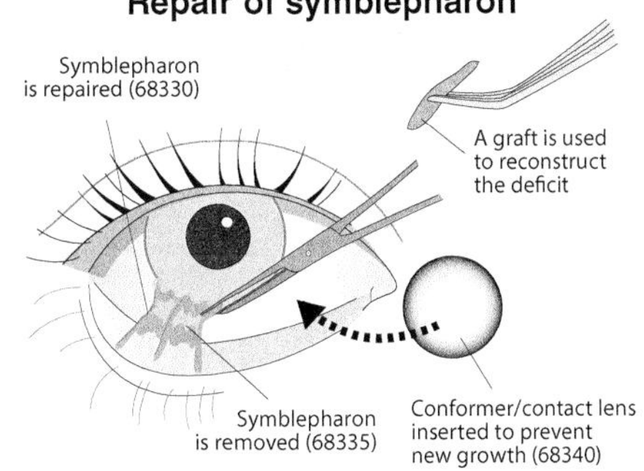

The fibrous adhesion is repaired without a graft (68330); a graft is used to reconstruct the deficit (68335); conformer or contact lens may be inserted to prevent new growth (68340).

ICD-10-CM Diagnostic Codes

	Code	Description
	B94.0	Sequelae of trachoma
⇄	H11.231	Symblepharon, right eye
⇄	H11.232	Symblepharon, left eye
⇄	H11.233	Symblepharon, bilateral

CCI Edits

Refer to Appendix A for CCI edits.

Facility RVUs ☐

Code	Work	PE Facility	MP	Total Facility
68330	5.78	7.06	0.43	13.27
68335	8.46	9.54	0.65	18.65
68340	4.97	6.14	0.40	11.51

Non-facility RVUs ☐

Code	Work	PE Non-Facility	MP	Total Non-Facility
68330	5.78	12.16	0.43	18.37
68335	8.46	9.54	0.65	18.65
68340	4.97	12.55	0.40	17.92

Modifiers (PAR) ☐

Code	Mod 50	Mod 51	Mod 62	Mod 66	Mod 80
68330	1	2	0	0	0
68335	1	2	1	0	1
68340	1	2	0	0	0

Global Period

Code	Days
68330	090
68335	090
68340	090

68360-68362

68360 Conjunctival flap; bridge or partial (separate procedure)

68362 Conjunctival flap; total (such as Gunderson thin flap or purse string flap)

(For conjunctival flap for perforating injury, see 65280, 65285)

(For repair of operative wound, use 66250)

(For removal of conjunctival foreign body, see 65205, 65210)

AMA Coding Notes

Surgical Procedures on the Conjunctiva

(For removal of foreign body, see 65205 et seq)

Surgical Procedures on the Eye and Ocular Adnexa

(For diagnostic and treatment ophthalmological services, see Medicine, Ophthalmology, and 92002 et seq)

(Do not report code 69990 in addition to codes 65091-68850)

Plain English Description

A conjunctival flap either partial or total may be used for treatment of corneal ulcers. Anesthetic eye drops are administered. An eye speculum is inserted and any diseased tissue is excised. The size and location of the defect is evaluated and the optimal site and configuration of the flap is determined. In 68360, a bridge or partial conjunctival flap is used. A subconjunctival injection containing lidocaine and epinephrine is injected to elevate the conjunctiva that will be used to configure the flap. Incisions are strategically placed and the flap is raised and mobilized. The flap is rotated over the defect taking care to maintain blood supply to the flap. The flap is secured with sutures. In 68362, a total conjunctival flap, also referred to as a Gunderson thin flap is prepared. A 360-degree peritomy is performed. Tissue from the upper bulbar conjunctiva is mobilized. Damaged corneal epithelium is excised. The flap is secured to the lower limbal conjunctiva. This type of flap covers the entire cornea.

Conjunctival flap

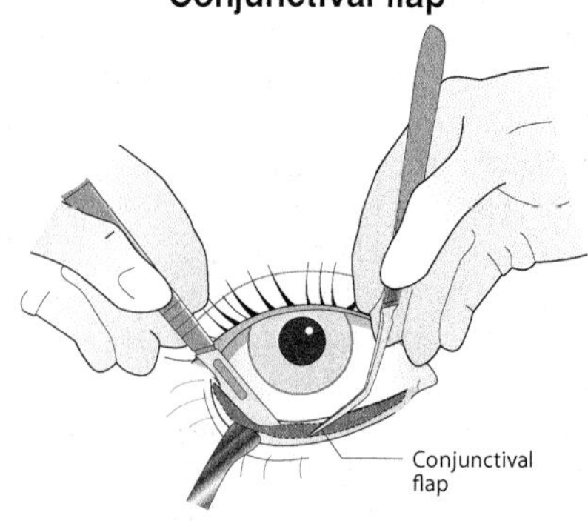

A small piece of the inner eyelid is removed to be used as a graft (68360); the entire inner eyelid is removed to be used as a graft (68362).

ICD-10-CM Diagnostic Codes

	B94.0	Sequelae of trachoma
⇄	C69.81	Malignant neoplasm of overlapping sites of right eye and adnexa
⇄	C69.82	Malignant neoplasm of overlapping sites of left eye and adnexa
⇄	D31.01	Benign neoplasm of right conjunctiva
⇄	D31.02	Benign neoplasm of left conjunctiva
	D48.7	Neoplasm of uncertain behavior of other specified sites
	D49.89	Neoplasm of unspecified behavior of other specified sites
	E50.3	Vitamin A deficiency with corneal ulceration and xerosis
⇄	H11.021	Central pterygium of right eye
⇄	H11.022	Central pterygium of left eye
⇄	H11.023	Central pterygium of eye, bilateral
⇄	H11.031	Double pterygium of right eye
⇄	H11.032	Double pterygium of left eye
⇄	H11.033	Double pterygium of eye, bilateral
⇄	H11.041	Peripheral pterygium, stationary, right eye
⇄	H11.042	Peripheral pterygium, stationary, left eye
⇄	H11.043	Peripheral pterygium, stationary, bilateral
⇄	H11.051	Peripheral pterygium, progressive, right eye
⇄	H11.052	Peripheral pterygium, progressive, left eye
⇄	H11.053	Peripheral pterygium, progressive, bilateral
⇄	H11.061	Recurrent pterygium of right eye
⇄	H11.062	Recurrent pterygium of left eye
⇄	H11.063	Recurrent pterygium of eye, bilateral
⇄	H11.221	Conjunctival granuloma, right eye
⇄	H11.222	Conjunctival granuloma, left eye
⇄	H11.223	Conjunctival granuloma, bilateral
⇄	H11.241	Scarring of conjunctiva, right eye
⇄	H11.242	Scarring of conjunctiva, left eye
⇄	H11.243	Scarring of conjunctiva, bilateral
⇄	H11.441	Conjunctival cysts, right eye
⇄	H11.442	Conjunctival cysts, left eye
⇄	H11.443	Conjunctival cysts, bilateral
⇄	H11.811	Pseudopterygium of conjunctiva, right eye
⇄	H11.812	Pseudopterygium of conjunctiva, left eye
⇄	H11.813	Pseudopterygium of conjunctiva, bilateral
⇄	H16.011	Central corneal ulcer, right eye
⇄	H16.012	Central corneal ulcer, left eye
⇄	H16.013	Central corneal ulcer, bilateral
⇄	H16.021	Ring corneal ulcer, right eye
⇄	H16.022	Ring corneal ulcer, left eye
⇄	H16.023	Ring corneal ulcer, bilateral
⇄	H16.041	Marginal corneal ulcer, right eye
⇄	H16.042	Marginal corneal ulcer, left eye
⇄	H16.043	Marginal corneal ulcer, bilateral
⇄	H16.061	Mycotic corneal ulcer, right eye
⇄	H16.062	Mycotic corneal ulcer, left eye
⇄	H16.063	Mycotic corneal ulcer, bilateral
⇄	H16.071	Perforated corneal ulcer, right eye
⇄	H16.072	Perforated corneal ulcer, left eye
⇄	H16.073	Perforated corneal ulcer, bilateral
⇄	H16.121	Filamentary keratitis, right eye
⇄	H16.122	Filamentary keratitis, left eye
⇄	H16.123	Filamentary keratitis, bilateral
⇄	H44.421	Hypotony of right eye due to ocular fistula
⇄	H44.422	Hypotony of left eye due to ocular fistula
⇄	H44.423	Hypotony of eye due to ocular fistula, bilateral
❼⇄	S05.31	Ocular laceration without prolapse or loss of intraocular tissue, right eye
❼⇄	S05.32	Ocular laceration without prolapse or loss of intraocular tissue, left eye
	Z85.840	Personal history of malignant neoplasm of eye

ICD-10-CM Coding Notes

For codes requiring a 7th character extension, refer to your ICD-10-CM book. Review the character descriptions and coding guidelines for proper selection. For some procedures, only certain characters will apply.

CCI Edits

Refer to Appendix A for CCI edits.

Facility RVUs

Code	Work	PE Facility	MP	Total Facility
68360	5.17	6.28	0.40	11.85
68362	8.61	9.63	0.66	18.90

Non-facility RVUs

Code	Work	PE Non-Facility	MP	Total Non-Facility
68360	5.17	10.44	0.40	16.01
68362	8.61	9.63	0.66	18.90

Modifiers (PAR)

Code	Mod 50	Mod 51	Mod 62	Mod 66	Mod 80
68360	1	2	0	0	1
68362	1	2	1	0	1

Global Period

Code	Days
68360	090
68362	090

68371

68371 Harvesting conjunctival allograft, living donor

AMA Coding Notes

Surgical Procedures on the Conjunctiva

(For removal of foreign body, see 65205 et seq)

Surgical Procedures on the Eye and Ocular Adnexa

(For diagnostic and treatment ophthalmological services, see Medicine, Ophthalmology, and 92002 et seq)

(Do not report code 69990 in addition to codes 65091-68850)

AMA *CPT® Assistant* ▯

68371: May 04: 10

Plain English Description

The eye from which the conjunctival allograft is to be obtained is prepared and draped and the conjunctival harvest sites marked with a pen or keratotomy marker. The conjunctiva at the donor site is elevated using a subconjunctival injection of balanced salt solution and a local anesthetic. The lateral borders of the graft are incised in a radial fashion. The tissue between the incisions at the lateral borders is undermined using blunt dissection. Dissection is carried in an anterior direction to the conjunctival insertion at the limbus and then beyond the limbus into the peripheral cornea. The conjunctival graft including the superficial epithelial corneal tissue is then excised. The donor site may be left to heal by secondary intention or the conjunctiva may be advanced to cover a portion of the donor site to minimize pain and inflammation at the donor site. The graft is placed in preservation solution with the epithelial side up and transported to the recipient surgical suite.

Harvesting conjunctival allograft

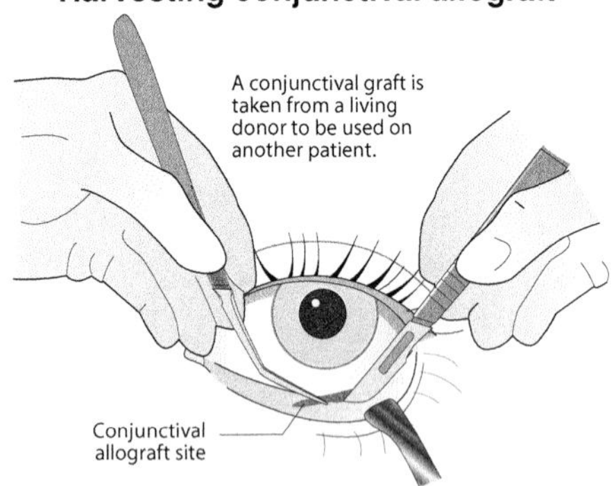
A conjunctival graft is taken from a living donor to be used on another patient.
Conjunctival allograft site

ICD-10-CM Diagnostic Codes

Z52.89 Donor of other specified organs or tissues

CCI Edits

Refer to Appendix A for CCI edits.

Facility RVUs ▯

Code	Work	PE Facility	MP	Total Facility
68371	5.09	6.46	0.39	11.94

Non-facility RVUs ▯

Code	Work	PE Non-Facility	MP	Total Non-Facility
68371	5.09	6.46	0.39	11.94

Modifiers (PAR) ▯

Code	Mod 50	Mod 51	Mod 62	Mod 66	Mod 80
68371	1	2	0	0	1

Global Period

Code	Days
68371	010

68400-68420

68400 Incision, drainage of lacrimal gland

68420 Incision, drainage of lacrimal sac (dacryocystotomy or dacryocystostomy)

AMA Coding Notes

Surgical Procedures on the Conjunctiva

(For removal of foreign body, see 65205 et seq)

Surgical Procedures on the Eye and Ocular Adnexa

(For diagnostic and treatment ophthalmological services, see Medicine, Ophthalmology, and 92002 et seq)

(Do not report code 69990 in addition to codes 65091-68850)

Plain English Description

An abscess or other accumulation of fluid in the lacrimal gland or lacrimal sac is treated with incision and drainage. In 68400, the upper eyelid is cleansed and a local anesthetic is administered as needed. The area of fluctuance in the lacrimal gland is incised and drained. Any loculations are disrupted using blunt and sharp dissection. The area is flushed with antibiotic solution as needed. The incision may be left open or a drain may be placed and the skin closed around the drain. In 68420, the inner aspect of the lower eyelid is cleansed and a local anesthetic administered as needed. A stab incision is made over the area of fluctuance and fluid is drained.

Incision, drainage of lacrimal sac

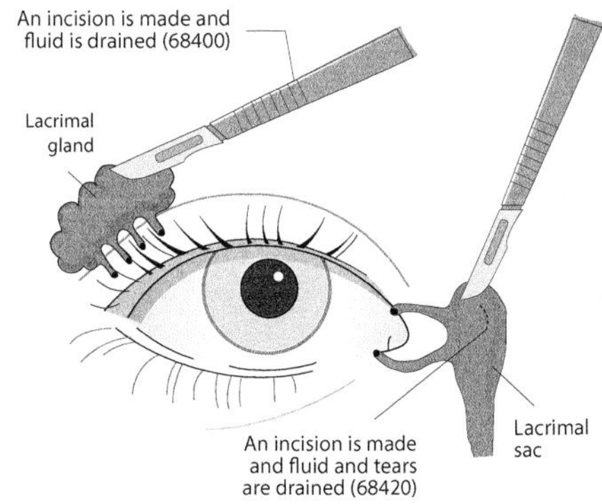

ICD-10-CM Diagnostic Codes

⇄	H04.011	Acute dacryoadenitis, right lacrimal gland
⇄	H04.012	Acute dacryoadenitis, left lacrimal gland
⇄	H04.013	Acute dacryoadenitis, bilateral lacrimal glands
⇄	H04.021	Chronic dacryoadenitis, right lacrimal gland
⇄	H04.022	Chronic dacryoadenitis, left lacrimal gland
⇄	H04.023	Chronic dacryoadenitis, bilateral lacrimal gland
⇄	H04.111	Dacryops of right lacrimal gland
⇄	H04.112	Dacryops of left lacrimal gland
⇄	H04.113	Dacryops of bilateral lacrimal glands
⇄	H04.131	Lacrimal cyst, right lacrimal gland
⇄	H04.132	Lacrimal cyst, left lacrimal gland
⇄	H04.133	Lacrimal cyst, bilateral lacrimal glands
⇄	H04.221	Epiphora due to insufficient drainage, right side
⇄	H04.222	Epiphora due to insufficient drainage, left side
⇄	H04.223	Epiphora due to insufficient drainage, bilateral
⇄	H04.311	Phlegmonous dacryocystitis of right lacrimal passage
⇄	H04.321	Acute dacryocystitis of right lacrimal passage
⇄	H04.331	Acute lacrimal canaliculitis of right lacrimal passage
⇄	H04.411	Chronic dacryocystitis of right lacrimal passage
⇄	H04.531	Neonatal obstruction of right nasolacrimal duct
⇄	H04.561	Stenosis of right lacrimal punctum
	Q10.5	Congenital stenosis and stricture of lacrimal duct
	Q10.6	Other congenital malformations of lacrimal apparatus

CCI Edits

Refer to Appendix A for CCI edits.

Facility RVUs ☐

Code	Work	PE Facility	MP	Total Facility
68400	1.74	1.90	0.12	3.76
68420	2.35	2.27	0.20	4.82

Non-facility RVUs ☐

Code	Work	PE Non-Facility	MP	Total Non-Facility
68400	1.74	7.01	0.12	8.87
68420	2.35	7.39	0.20	9.94

Modifiers (PAR) ☐

Code	Mod 50	Mod 51	Mod 62	Mod 66	Mod 80
68400	1	2	0	0	1
68420	1	2	0	0	1

Global Period

Code	Days
68400	010
68420	010

68440

68440 Snip incision of lacrimal punctum

AMA Coding Notes

Surgical Procedures on the Conjunctiva

(For removal of foreign body, see 65205 et seq)

Surgical Procedures on the Eye and Ocular Adnexa

(For diagnostic and treatment ophthalmological services, see Medicine, Ophthalmology, and 92002 et seq)

(Do not report code 69990 in addition to codes 65091-68850)

Plain English Description

Stenosis of the lacrimal punctum is treated by using a snipping procedure to widen the opening. This procedure may also be referred to as a one-snip, two-snip, or three-snip procedure, or a snip punctoplasty. Stenosis may result from an infection, a rare systemic condition such as porphyria cutanea tarda or acrodermatitis enteropathica, trauma, thermal or chemical burn, topical or systemic chemotherapy, or radiation therapy. The skin around the eye is cleansed and a local anesthetic injected subcutaneously below the lower punctum. The punctum is located and dilated. Toothed microforceps are inserted through the punctum and the posterior wall of the ampulla grasped. Vannas scissors are passed into the ampulla. A one-snip procedure involves a single vertical snip down the posterior aspect of the ampulla. A two-snip procedure uses a second snip down the canalicula. A three-snip procedure uses two downward snips along the posterior aspect of the ampulla and a third across the bottom joining the two downward snips.

Snip incision of lacrimal punctum

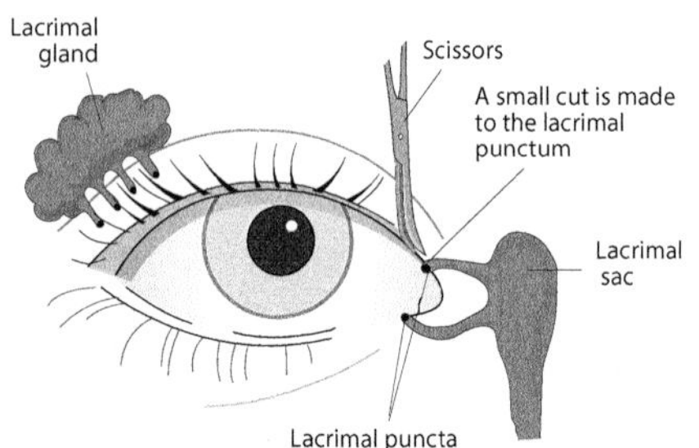

ICD-10-CM Diagnostic Codes

- ⇄ H04.121 Dry eye syndrome of right lacrimal gland
- ⇄ H04.122 Dry eye syndrome of left lacrimal gland
- ⇄ H04.123 Dry eye syndrome of bilateral lacrimal glands
- ⇄ H04.151 Secondary lacrimal gland atrophy, right lacrimal gland
- ⇄ H04.152 Secondary lacrimal gland atrophy, left lacrimal gland
- ⇄ H04.153 Secondary lacrimal gland atrophy, bilateral lacrimal glands
- ⇄ H04.211 Epiphora due to excess lacrimation, right lacrimal gland
- ⇄ H04.212 Epiphora due to excess lacrimation, left lacrimal gland
- ⇄ H04.213 Epiphora due to excess lacrimation, bilateral lacrimal glands
- ⇄ H04.221 Epiphora due to insufficient drainage, right side
- ⇄ H04.222 Epiphora due to insufficient drainage, left side
- ⇄ H04.223 Epiphora due to insufficient drainage, bilateral
- ⇄ H04.331 Acute lacrimal canaliculitis of right lacrimal passage
- ⇄ H04.332 Acute lacrimal canaliculitis of left lacrimal passage
- ⇄ H04.333 Acute lacrimal canaliculitis of bilateral lacrimal passages
- ⇄ H04.411 Chronic dacryocystitis of right lacrimal passage
- ⇄ H04.412 Chronic dacryocystitis of left lacrimal passage
- ⇄ H04.413 Chronic dacryocystitis of bilateral lacrimal passages
- ⇄ H04.421 Chronic lacrimal canaliculitis of right lacrimal passage
- ⇄ H04.422 Chronic lacrimal canaliculitis of left lacrimal passage
- ⇄ H04.423 Chronic lacrimal canaliculitis of bilateral lacrimal passages
- ⇄ H04.521 Eversion of right lacrimal punctum
- ⇄ H04.522 Eversion of left lacrimal punctum
- ⇄ H04.523 Eversion of bilateral lacrimal punctum
- ⇄ H04.541 Stenosis of right lacrimal canaliculi
- ⇄ H04.542 Stenosis of left lacrimal canaliculi
- ⇄ H04.543 Stenosis of bilateral lacrimal canaliculi
- ⇄ H04.551 Acquired stenosis of right nasolacrimal duct
- ⇄ H04.552 Acquired stenosis of left nasolacrimal duct
- ⇄ H04.553 Acquired stenosis of bilateral nasolacrimal duct

CCI Edits

Refer to Appendix A for CCI edits.

Facility RVUs ▯

Code	Work	PE Facility	MP	Total Facility
68440	0.99	1.81	0.09	2.89

Non-facility RVUs ▯

Code	Work	PE Non-Facility	MP	Total Non-Facility
68440	0.99	1.96	0.09	3.04

Modifiers (PAR) ▯

Code	Mod 50	Mod 51	Mod 62	Mod 66	Mod 80
68440	1	2	0	0	1

Global Period

Code	Days
68440	010

68500-68505

68500 Excision of lacrimal gland (dacryoadenectomy), except for tumor; total

68505 Excision of lacrimal gland (dacryoadenectomy), except for tumor; partial

AMA Coding Notes

Surgical Procedures on the Conjunctiva

(For removal of foreign body, see 65205 et seq)

Surgical Procedures on the Eye and Ocular Adnexa

(For diagnostic and treatment ophthalmological services, see Medicine, Ophthalmology, and 92002 et seq)

(Do not report code 69990 in addition to codes 65091-68850)

Plain English Description

Part or all of the lacrimal (tear) gland is excised for a condition other than a tumor. The skin is cleansed over the eye. A local anesthetic is injected. An incision is made over the temporal aspect of the eye. The temporal muscle is exposed and retracted laterally to the expose the lacrimal gland. In 68500, the entire lacrimal gland is dissected free of surrounding tissue and excised. In 68505, part of the lacrimal gland, usually the palpebral lobe is dissected and excised. The operative wound is closed in layers.

Excision of lacrimal gland

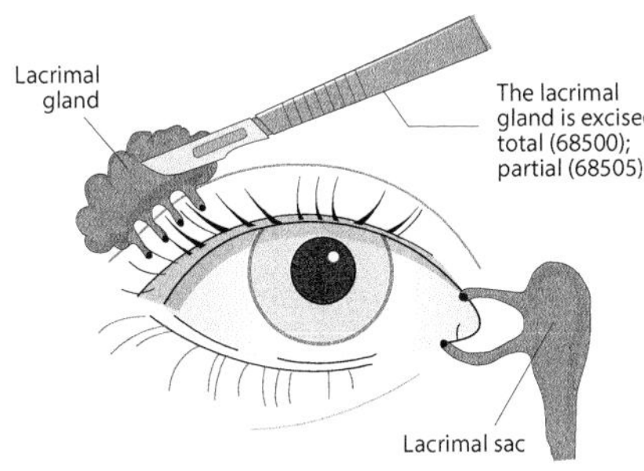
Lacrimal gland
The lacrimal gland is excised total (68500); partial (68505)
Lacrimal sac

ICD-10-CM Diagnostic Codes

	Code	Description
⇄	H04.021	Chronic dacryoadenitis, right lacrimal gland
⇄	H04.022	Chronic dacryoadenitis, left lacrimal gland
⇄	H04.023	Chronic dacryoadenitis, bilateral lacrimal gland
⇄	H04.031	Chronic enlargement of right lacrimal gland
⇄	H04.032	Chronic enlargement of left lacrimal gland
⇄	H04.033	Chronic enlargement of bilateral lacrimal glands
⇄	H04.111	Dacryops of right lacrimal gland
⇄	H04.112	Dacryops of left lacrimal gland
⇄	H04.113	Dacryops of bilateral lacrimal glands
⇄	H04.131	Lacrimal cyst, right lacrimal gland
⇄	H04.132	Lacrimal cyst, left lacrimal gland
⇄	H04.133	Lacrimal cyst, bilateral lacrimal glands
⇄	H04.141	Primary lacrimal gland atrophy, right lacrimal gland
⇄	H04.142	Primary lacrimal gland atrophy, left lacrimal gland
⇄	H04.143	Primary lacrimal gland atrophy, bilateral lacrimal glands
⇄	H04.151	Secondary lacrimal gland atrophy, right lacrimal gland
⇄	H04.152	Secondary lacrimal gland atrophy, left lacrimal gland
⇄	H04.153	Secondary lacrimal gland atrophy, bilateral lacrimal glands
⇄	H04.211	Epiphora due to excess lacrimation, right lacrimal gland
⇄	H04.212	Epiphora due to excess lacrimation, left lacrimal gland
⇄	H04.213	Epiphora due to excess lacrimation, bilateral lacrimal glands

CCI Edits

Refer to Appendix A for CCI edits.

Facility RVUs ▯

Code	Work	PE Facility	MP	Total Facility
68500	12.77	17.37	0.99	31.13
68505	12.69	17.32	0.98	30.99

Non-facility RVUs ▯

Code	Work	PE Non-Facility	MP	Total Non-Facility
68500	12.77	17.37	0.99	31.13
68505	12.69	17.32	0.98	30.99

Modifiers (PAR) ▯

Code	Mod 50	Mod 51	Mod 62	Mod 66	Mod 80
68500	1	2	0	0	1
68505	1	2	0	0	1

Global Period

Code	Days
68500	090
68505	090

68510

68510 Biopsy of lacrimal gland

AMA Coding Notes

Surgical Procedures on the Conjunctiva

(For removal of foreign body, see 65205 et seq)

Surgical Procedures on the Eye and Ocular Adnexa

(For diagnostic and treatment ophthalmological services, see Medicine, Ophthalmology, and 92002 et seq)

(Do not report code 69990 in addition to codes 65091-68850)

Plain English Description

The skin is cleansed over the eye. A local anesthetic is injected. An incision is made over the temporal aspect of the eye. The temporal muscle is exposed and retracted laterally to the expose the lacrimal gland. The lacrimal gland is inspected. One or more tissue samples are obtained from the lacrimal gland and sent to the laboratory for separately reportable pathology examination. The operative wound is closed in layers.

Biopsy of lacrimal gland

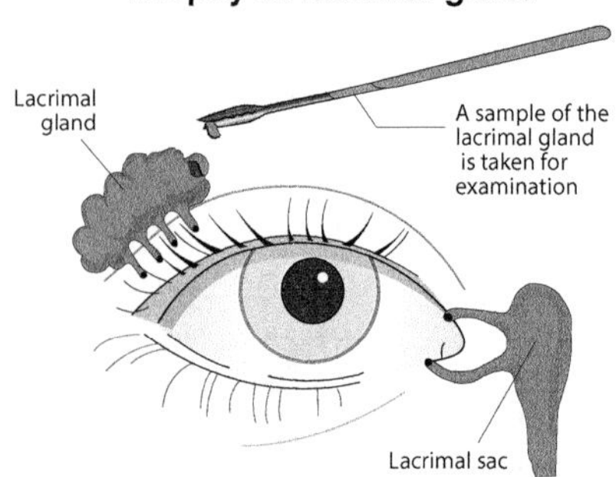
Lacrimal gland
A sample of the lacrimal gland is taken for examination
Lacrimal sac

ICD-10-CM Diagnostic Codes

⇄	C69.52	Malignant neoplasm of left lacrimal gland and duct
⇄	D09.22	Carcinoma in situ of left eye
⇄	D31.52	Benign neoplasm of left lacrimal gland and duct
	D48.7	Neoplasm of uncertain behavior of other specified sites
	D49.89	Neoplasm of unspecified behavior of other specified sites
⇄	H04.132	Lacrimal cyst, left lacrimal gland
⇄	H04.412	Chronic dacryocystitis of left lacrimal passage

CCI Edits

Refer to Appendix A for CCI edits.

Facility RVUs ▯

Code	Work	PE Facility	MP	Total Facility
68510	4.60	3.30	0.37	8.27

Non-facility RVUs ▯

Code	Work	PE Non-Facility	MP	Total Non-Facility
68510	4.60	8.42	0.37	13.39

Modifiers (PAR) ▯

Code	Mod 50	Mod 51	Mod 62	Mod 66	Mod 80
68510	1	2	0	0	0

Global Period

Code	Days
68510	000

68520

68520 Excision of lacrimal sac (dacryocystectomy)

AMA Coding Notes

Surgical Procedures on the Conjunctiva

(For removal of foreign body, see 65205 et seq)

Surgical Procedures on the Eye and Ocular Adnexa

(For diagnostic and treatment ophthalmological services, see Medicine, Ophthalmology, and 92002 et seq)

(Do not report code 69990 in addition to codes 65091-68850)

Plain English Description

The skin around the eye is cleansed. A local anesthetic is injected subcutaneously around the lacrimal sac. An incision is made over the inner aspect of the lower eyelid, and the lacrimal sac, nasolacrimal duct, and canaliculi are exposed. The lacrimal sac is excised. The proximal end of the nasolacrimal duct is cauterized. The canaliculi are probed and if the superior or inferior canaliculus is patent they are cauterized. If a fistula is present it is also excised. The surgical wound is closed and a dressing applied.

Excision of lacrimal sac

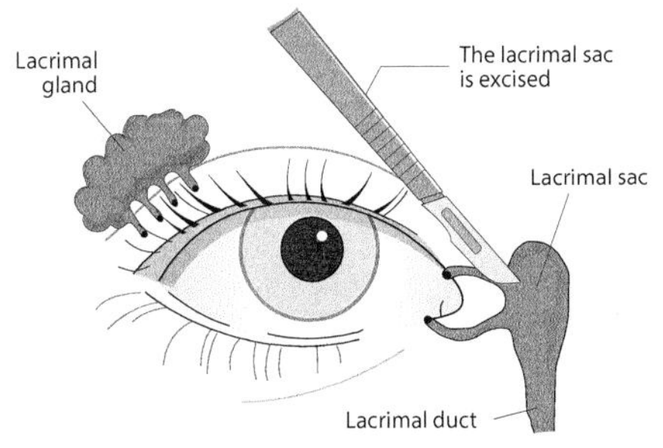

ICD-10-CM Diagnostic Codes

⇄	C69.51	Malignant neoplasm of right lacrimal gland and duct
⇄	C69.52	Malignant neoplasm of left lacrimal gland and duct
⇄	D09.21	Carcinoma in situ of right eye
⇄	D09.22	Carcinoma in situ of left eye
⇄	D31.51	Benign neoplasm of right lacrimal gland and duct
⇄	D31.52	Benign neoplasm of left lacrimal gland and duct
⇄	H04.221	Epiphora due to insufficient drainage, right side
⇄	H04.222	Epiphora due to insufficient drainage, left side
⇄	H04.223	Epiphora due to insufficient drainage, bilateral
⇄	H04.411	Chronic dacryocystitis of right lacrimal passage
⇄	H04.412	Chronic dacryocystitis of left lacrimal passage
⇄	H04.413	Chronic dacryocystitis of bilateral lacrimal passages
⇄	H04.551	Acquired stenosis of right nasolacrimal duct
⇄	H04.552	Acquired stenosis of left nasolacrimal duct
⇄	H04.553	Acquired stenosis of bilateral nasolacrimal duct
⇄	H04.571	Stenosis of right lacrimal sac
⇄	H04.572	Stenosis of left lacrimal sac
⇄	H04.573	Stenosis of bilateral lacrimal sac
	Q10.6	Other congenital malformations of lacrimal apparatus

CCI Edits

Refer to Appendix A for CCI edits.

Facility RVUs ☐

Code	Work	PE Facility	MP	Total Facility
68520	8.78	12.13	0.72	21.63

Non-facility RVUs ☐

Code	Work	PE Non-Facility	MP	Total Non-Facility
68520	8.78	12.13	0.72	21.63

Modifiers (PAR) ☐

Code	Mod 50	Mod 51	Mod 62	Mod 66	Mod 80
68520	1	2	0	0	0

Global Period

Code	Days
68520	090

68525

68525 Biopsy of lacrimal sac

AMA Coding Notes

Surgical Procedures on the Conjunctiva

(For removal of foreign body, see 65205 et seq)

Surgical Procedures on the Eye and Ocular Adnexa

(For diagnostic and treatment ophthalmological services, see Medicine, Ophthalmology, and 92002 et seq)

(Do not report code 69990 in addition to codes 65091-68850)

Plain English Description

The skin around the eye is cleansed. A local anesthetic is injected subcutaneously around the lacrimal sac. An incision is made over the inner aspect of the lower eyelid, and the lacrimal sac, nasolacrimal duct, and canaliculi exposed. The lacrimal sac and surrounding structures are inspected. One or two tissue samples are obtained from the lacrimal sac and sent to the laboratory for separately reportable pathology examination. The operative wound is closed in layers.

Biopsy of lacrimal sac

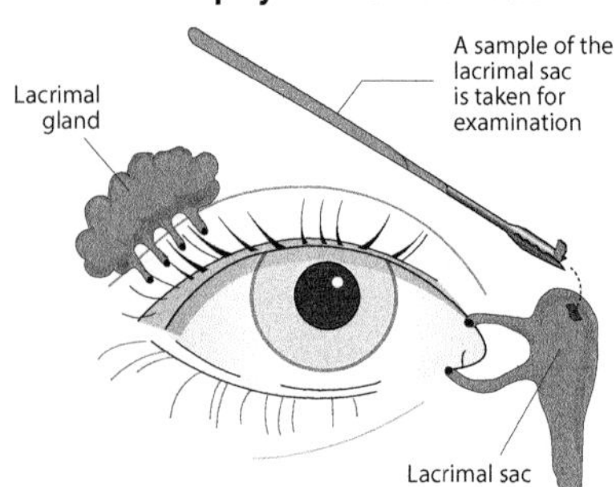
Lacrimal gland
A sample of the lacrimal sac is taken for examination
Lacrimal sac

ICD-10-CM Diagnostic Codes

⇄ C69.52 Malignant neoplasm of left lacrimal gland and duct
⇄ D09.22 Carcinoma in situ of left eye
⇄ D31.52 Benign neoplasm of left lacrimal gland and duct
D48.7 Neoplasm of uncertain behavior of other specified sites
D49.89 Neoplasm of unspecified behavior of other specified sites
⇄ H04.002 Unspecified dacryoadenitis, left lacrimal gland
⇄ H04.012 Acute dacryoadenitis, left lacrimal gland
⇄ H04.022 Chronic dacryoadenitis, left lacrimal gland
⇄ H04.032 Chronic enlargement of left lacrimal gland
⇄ H04.112 Dacryops of left lacrimal gland
⇄ H04.122 Dry eye syndrome of left lacrimal gland
⇄ H04.132 Lacrimal cyst, left lacrimal gland
⇄ H04.142 Primary lacrimal gland atrophy, left lacrimal gland
⇄ H04.152 Secondary lacrimal gland atrophy, left lacrimal gland
⇄ H04.162 Lacrimal gland dislocation, left lacrimal gland
⇄ H04.222 Epiphora due to insufficient drainage, left side
⇄ H04.312 Phlegmonous dacryocystitis of left lacrimal passage
⇄ H04.322 Acute dacryocystitis of left lacrimal passage
⇄ H04.332 Acute lacrimal canaliculitis of left lacrimal passage
⇄ H04.412 Chronic dacryocystitis of left lacrimal passage
⇄ H04.512 Dacryolith of left lacrimal passage
⇄ H04.532 Neonatal obstruction of left nasolacrimal duct
⇄ H04.542 Stenosis of left lacrimal canaliculi
⇄ H04.552 Acquired stenosis of left nasolacrimal duct
⇄ H04.572 Stenosis of left lacrimal sac
⇄ H04.612 Lacrimal fistula left lacrimal passage
H04.69 Other changes of lacrimal passages
⇄ H04.812 Granuloma of left lacrimal passage
⇄ H04.819 Granuloma of unspecified lacrimal passage
H04.89 Other disorders of lacrimal system

CCI Edits

Refer to Appendix A for CCI edits.

Facility RVUs ▢

Code	Work	PE Facility	MP	Total Facility
68525	4.42	2.68	0.39	7.49

Non-facility RVUs ▢

Code	Work	PE Non-Facility	MP	Total Non-Facility
68525	4.42	2.68	0.39	7.49

Modifiers (PAR) ▢

Code	Mod 50	Mod 51	Mod 62	Mod 66	Mod 80
68525	1	2	1	0	1

Global Period

Code	Days
68525	000

68530

68530 Removal of foreign body or dacryolith, lacrimal passages

AMA Coding Notes

Surgical Procedures on the Conjunctiva

(For removal of foreign body, see 65205 et seq)

Surgical Procedures on the Eye and Ocular Adnexa

(For diagnostic and treatment ophthalmological services, see Medicine, Ophthalmology, and 92002 et seq)

(Do not report code 69990 in addition to codes 65091-68850)

Plain English Description

A foreign body or dacryolith is removed from the lacrimal passages. A dacryolith is a concretion or stone that has formed in the lacrimal system. An incision is made over the affected lacrimal passage and the foreign body or dacryolith is located. An incision is made into the affected lacrimal structure and the foreign body or dacryolith is removed. The lacrimal structure is repaired with sutures.

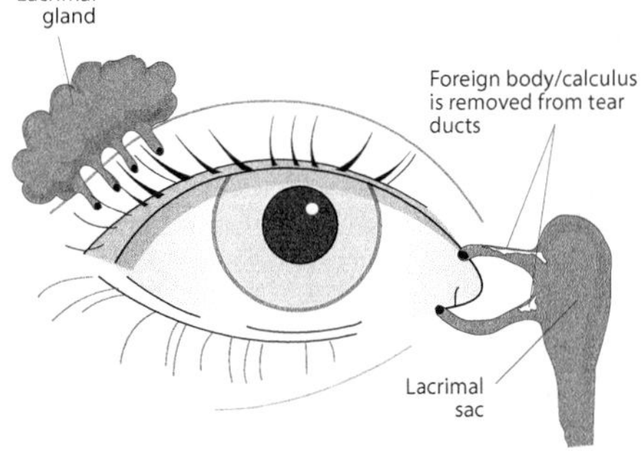

ICD-10-CM Diagnostic Codes

⇄	H04.201	Unspecified epiphora, right side
⇄	H04.202	Unspecified epiphora, left side
⇄	H04.203	Unspecified epiphora, bilateral
⇄	H04.221	Epiphora due to insufficient drainage, right side
⇄	H04.222	Epiphora due to insufficient drainage, left side
⇄	H04.223	Epiphora due to insufficient drainage, bilateral
⇄	H04.511	Dacryolith of right lacrimal passage
⇄	H04.512	Dacryolith of left lacrimal passage
⇄	H04.513	Dacryolith of bilateral lacrimal passages
❼⇄	T15.81	Foreign body in other and multiple parts of external eye, right eye
❼⇄	T15.82	Foreign body in other and multiple parts of external eye, left eye

ICD-10-CM Coding Notes

For codes requiring a 7th character extension, refer to your ICD-10-CM book. Review the character descriptions and coding guidelines for proper selection. For some procedures, only certain characters will apply.

CCI Edits

Refer to Appendix A for CCI edits.

Facility RVUs ☐

Code	Work	PE Facility	MP	Total Facility
68530	3.70	3.33	0.28	7.31

Non-facility RVUs ☐

Code	Work	PE Non-Facility	MP	Total Non-Facility
68530	3.70	8.91	0.28	12.89

Modifiers (PAR) ☐

Code	Mod 50	Mod 51	Mod 62	Mod 66	Mod 80
68530	1	2	0	0	1

Global Period

Code	Days
68530	010

CPT® Procedural Coding

68540-68550

68540 Excision of lacrimal gland tumor; frontal approach

68550 Excision of lacrimal gland tumor; involving osteotomy

AMA Coding Notes

Surgical Procedures on the Conjunctiva

(For removal of foreign body, see 65205 et seq)

Surgical Procedures on the Eye and Ocular Adnexa

(For diagnostic and treatment ophthalmological services, see Medicine, Ophthalmology, and 92002 et seq)

(Do not report code 69990 in addition to codes 65091-68850)

Plain English Description

The lacrimal gland is a bilobed gland located in the superotemporal aspect of the orbit. The two lobes consisting of the larger orbital lobe and smaller palpebral lobe are separated by the lateral horn of the levator aponeurosis. The palpebral lobe can be identified in the lateral fornix with the lid everted on an external eye exam. The orbital lobe lies behind the orbital bone and is not visible on external eye exam. Lesions of the lacrimal gland may be inflammatory or neoplastic. Inflammatory lesions include dacryoadenitis, sarcoidosis, and orbital inflammatory pseudotumor. Benign neoplastic lesions include pleomorphic adenoma, benign reactive lymphoid hyperplasia, and oncocytomas. Malignant neoplastic lesions include adenoid cystic carcinoma, squamous cell carcinoma, adenocarcinoma, mucoepidermoid carcinoma, and malignant lymphomas. In 68540, using an anterior or frontal approach, the eyelid is sutured closed and a skin incision is made over crease of the upper eyelid. Soft tissues are dissected and the lacrimal gland is exposed. The lacrimal gland is dissected free of surrounding tissues and excised. Separately reportable frozen sections are evaluated by a pathologist to determine if the margins are clean. If the margins are not clean surrounding tissue is excised until the margins are clean. The surgical wound is closed in layers. In 68550, the tumor excision is performed as described above except that any involved bone is also excised using a bone saw or osteotome.

Excision of lacrimal gland tumor, frontal approach or involving osteotomy

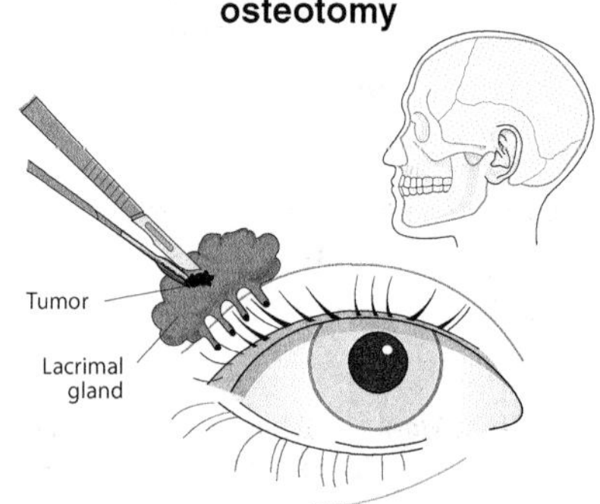

Accessed through the face, a tumor is removed from the lacrimal gland (68540); a tumor is removed from the lacrimal gland requiring access through the bone of the eye socket (68550).

ICD-10-CM Diagnostic Codes

⇄	C69.51	Malignant neoplasm of right lacrimal gland and duct
⇄	C69.52	Malignant neoplasm of left lacrimal gland and duct
⇄	D09.21	Carcinoma in situ of right eye
⇄	D09.22	Carcinoma in situ of left eye
⇄	D31.51	Benign neoplasm of right lacrimal gland and duct
⇄	D31.52	Benign neoplasm of left lacrimal gland and duct
	D48.7	Neoplasm of uncertain behavior of other specified sites
	D49.89	Neoplasm of unspecified behavior of other specified sites

CCI Edits

Refer to Appendix A for CCI edits.

Facility RVUs ▢

Code	Work	PE Facility	MP	Total Facility
68540	12.18	15.64	0.95	28.77
68550	15.16	19.52	1.17	35.85

Non-facility RVUs ▢

Code	Work	PE Non-Facility	MP	Total Non-Facility
68540	12.18	15.64	0.95	28.77
68550	15.16	19.52	1.17	35.85

Modifiers (PAR) ▢

Code	Mod 50	Mod 51	Mod 62	Mod 66	Mod 80
68540	1	2	1	0	1
68550	1	2	0	0	1

Global Period

Code	Days
68540	090
68550	090

68700

68700 Plastic repair of canaliculi

AMA Coding Notes

Surgical Procedures on the Conjunctiva

(For removal of foreign body, see 65205 et seq)

Surgical Procedures on the Eye and Ocular Adnexa

(For diagnostic and treatment ophthalmological services, see Medicine, Ophthalmology, and 92002 et seq)

(Do not report code 69990 in addition to codes 65091-68850)

Plain English Description

An injury to the canaliculus is repaired. The canaliculi are the mucosal ducts at the medial aspect of the eye that drain tears from the eye. The punctum is dilated and a probe passed through the punctum into the canaliculus. The severed ends of the canaliculus are identified. A surgical microscope or loupes may be used to provide better visualization. The ends are reapproximated and repaired with sutures.

Plastic repair of canaliculi

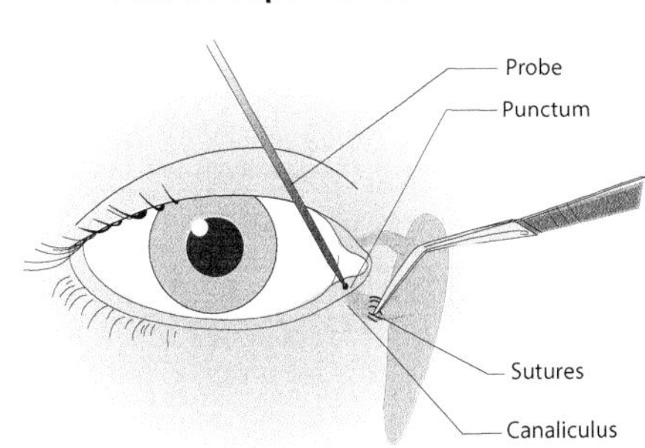

ICD-10-CM Diagnostic Codes

- ⇄ C69.51 Malignant neoplasm of right lacrimal gland and duct
- ⇄ D09.21 Carcinoma in situ of right eye
- ⇄ D31.51 Benign neoplasm of right lacrimal gland and duct
- D48.9 Neoplasm of uncertain behavior, unspecified
- D49.89 Neoplasm of unspecified behavior of other specified sites
- ⇄ H04.211 Epiphora due to excess lacrimation, right lacrimal gland
- ⇄ H04.221 Epiphora due to insufficient drainage, right side
- ⇄ H04.311 Phlegmonous dacryocystitis of right lacrimal passage
- ⇄ H04.321 Acute dacryocystitis of right lacrimal passage
- ⇄ H04.331 Acute lacrimal canaliculitis of right lacrimal passage
- ⇄ H04.411 Chronic dacryocystitis of right lacrimal passage
- ⇄ H04.421 Chronic lacrimal canaliculitis of right lacrimal passage
- ⇄ H04.531 Neonatal obstruction of right nasolacrimal duct
- ⇄ H04.541 Stenosis of right lacrimal canaliculi
- ⇄ H04.551 Acquired stenosis of right nasolacrimal duct
- ⇄ H04.561 Stenosis of right lacrimal punctum
- ⇄ H04.571 Stenosis of right lacrimal sac
- ⇄ H04.611 Lacrimal fistula right lacrimal passage
- Q10.4 Absence and agenesis of lacrimal apparatus
- Q10.5 Congenital stenosis and stricture of lacrimal duct
- Q10.6 Other congenital malformations of lacrimal apparatus
- ❼⇄ S01.111 Laceration without foreign body of right eyelid and periocular area
- ❼⇄ S01.121 Laceration with foreign body of right eyelid and periocular area
- ❼⇄ S01.131 Puncture wound without foreign body of right eyelid and periocular area
- ❼⇄ S01.141 Puncture wound with foreign body of right eyelid and periocular area
- ❼⇄ S01.151 Open bite of right eyelid and periocular area

ICD-10-CM Coding Notes

For codes requiring a 7th character extension, refer to your ICD-10-CM book. Review the character descriptions and coding guidelines for proper selection. For some procedures, only certain characters will apply.

CCI Edits

Refer to Appendix A for CCI edits.

Facility RVUs ▯

Code	Work	PE Facility	MP	Total Facility
68700	7.87	8.94	0.61	17.42

Non-facility RVUs ▯

Code	Work	PE Non-Facility	MP	Total Non-Facility
68700	7.87	8.94	0.61	17.42

Modifiers (PAR) ▯

Code	Mod 50	Mod 51	Mod 62	Mod 66	Mod 80
68700	1	2	0	0	1

Global Period

Code	Days
68700	090

68705

68705 Correction of everted punctum, cautery

AMA Coding Notes

Surgical Procedures on the Conjunctiva

(For removal of foreign body, see 65205 et seq)

Surgical Procedures on the Eye and Ocular Adnexa

(For diagnostic and treatment ophthalmological services, see Medicine, Ophthalmology, and 92002 et seq)

(Do not report code 69990 in addition to codes 65091-68850)

AMA *CPT® Assistant* ▯

68705: Feb 20: 13

Plain English Description

The inferior punctum is normally oriented posteriorly and is in contact with the globe. An everted punctum turns outward and away from the globe. A probe is passed through the punctum and into the canaliculus. The lower lid is everted and strategically cauterized so that when the cautery site heals and scar tissue forms, the tissue will contract and pull the punctum back into a more normal posterior position that is in contact with the globe.

Correction of everted punctum, cautery

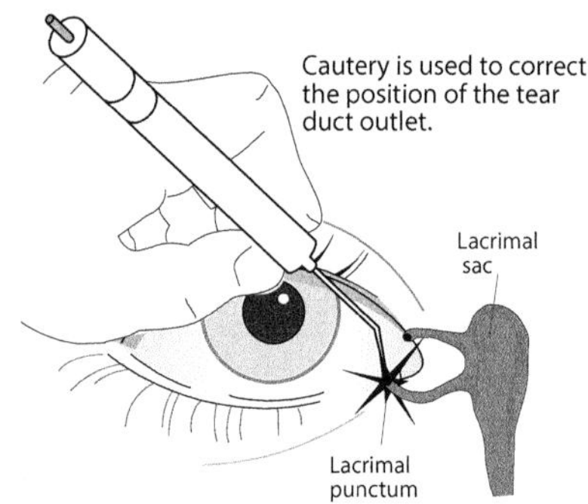
Cautery is used to correct the position of the tear duct outlet.
Lacrimal sac
Lacrimal punctum

ICD-10-CM Diagnostic Codes

⇄	H04.522	Eversion of left lacrimal punctum
⇄	H04.552	Acquired stenosis of left nasolacrimal duct
⇄	H04.562	Stenosis of left lacrimal punctum

CCI Edits

Refer to Appendix A for CCI edits.

Facility RVUs ▯

Code	Work	PE Facility	MP	Total Facility
68705	2.11	2.50	0.18	4.79

Non-facility RVUs ▯

Code	Work	PE Non-Facility	MP	Total Non-Facility
68705	2.11	5.53	0.18	7.82

Modifiers (PAR) ▯

Code	Mod 50	Mod 51	Mod 62	Mod 66	Mod 80
68705	1	2	0	0	1

Global Period

Code	Days
68705	010

68720

68720 Dacryocystorhinostomy (fistulization of lacrimal sac to nasal cavity)

AMA Coding Notes

Surgical Procedures on the Conjunctiva

(For removal of foreign body, see 65205 et seq)

Surgical Procedures on the Eye and Ocular Adnexa

(For diagnostic and treatment ophthalmological services, see Medicine, Ophthalmology, and 92002 et seq)

(Do not report code 69990 in addition to codes 65091-68850)

AMA *CPT® Assistant*

68720: Sep 01: 10, Jul 03: 15, Aug 03: 14, Aug 09: 11

Plain English Description

Dacryocystorhinostomy is performed to treat epiphora (excessive tearing) caused by blockage of the lacrimal passages. The nose is packed for 10 minutes with a solution containing epinephrine and Xylocaine. A fiberoptic light probe is passed through the punctum, into the upper or lower canaliculus, and then into the lacrimal sac. The light can be seen through the nose mucosa at the posterior end of the lacrimal sac. A circle of nasal mucosa of 1-cm diameter is excised and the underlying bone exposed. The bone is removed with a drill. The lacrimal sac is opened. Metal stents attached to Silastic tubing are passed through the upper and lower canaliculi and the distal ends guided into the nasal passage. The metal stents are severed and the tubing is secured with sutures. The tubing keeps the lacrimal sac open so that tears drain into the nose.

Dacryocystorhinostomy
(fistula of lacrimal sac to nasal cavity)

ICD-10-CM Diagnostic Codes

⇄ H04.211 Epiphora due to excess lacrimation, right lacrimal gland
⇄ H04.212 Epiphora due to excess lacrimation, left lacrimal gland
⇄ H04.213 Epiphora due to excess lacrimation, bilateral lacrimal glands
⇄ H04.221 Epiphora due to insufficient drainage, right side
⇄ H04.222 Epiphora due to insufficient drainage, left side
⇄ H04.223 Epiphora due to insufficient drainage, bilateral
⇄ H04.311 Phlegmonous dacryocystitis of right lacrimal passage
⇄ H04.312 Phlegmonous dacryocystitis of left lacrimal passage
⇄ H04.313 Phlegmonous dacryocystitis of bilateral lacrimal passages
⇄ H04.321 Acute dacryocystitis of right lacrimal passage
⇄ H04.322 Acute dacryocystitis of left lacrimal passage
⇄ H04.323 Acute dacryocystitis of bilateral lacrimal passages
⇄ H04.331 Acute lacrimal canaliculitis of right lacrimal passage
⇄ H04.332 Acute lacrimal canaliculitis of left lacrimal passage
⇄ H04.333 Acute lacrimal canaliculitis of bilateral lacrimal passages
⇄ H04.411 Chronic dacryocystitis of right lacrimal passage
⇄ H04.412 Chronic dacryocystitis of left lacrimal passage
⇄ H04.413 Chronic dacryocystitis of bilateral lacrimal passages
⇄ H04.431 Chronic lacrimal mucocele of right lacrimal passage
⇄ H04.432 Chronic lacrimal mucocele of left lacrimal passage
⇄ H04.433 Chronic lacrimal mucocele of bilateral lacrimal passages
⇄ H04.531 Neonatal obstruction of right nasolacrimal duct
⇄ H04.532 Neonatal obstruction of left nasolacrimal duct
⇄ H04.533 Neonatal obstruction of bilateral nasolacrimal duct
⇄ H04.541 Stenosis of right lacrimal canaliculi
⇄ H04.542 Stenosis of left lacrimal canaliculi
⇄ H04.543 Stenosis of bilateral lacrimal canaliculi
⇄ H04.551 Acquired stenosis of right nasolacrimal duct
⇄ H04.552 Acquired stenosis of left nasolacrimal duct
⇄ H04.553 Acquired stenosis of bilateral nasolacrimal duct
⇄ H04.561 Stenosis of right lacrimal punctum
⇄ H04.562 Stenosis of left lacrimal punctum
⇄ H04.563 Stenosis of bilateral lacrimal punctum
⇄ H04.571 Stenosis of right lacrimal sac
⇄ H04.572 Stenosis of left lacrimal sac
⇄ H04.573 Stenosis of bilateral lacrimal sac
Q10.4 Absence and agenesis of lacrimal apparatus
Q10.5 Congenital stenosis and stricture of lacrimal duct
Q10.6 Other congenital malformations of lacrimal apparatus

CCI Edits

Refer to Appendix A for CCI edits.

Facility RVUs

Code	Work	PE Facility	MP	Total Facility
68720	9.96	12.98	0.79	23.73

Non-facility RVUs

Code	Work	PE Non-Facility	MP	Total Non-Facility
68720	9.96	12.98	0.79	23.73

Modifiers (PAR)

Code	Mod 50	Mod 51	Mod 62	Mod 66	Mod 80
68720	1	2	1	0	2

Global Period

Code	Days
68720	090

68745-68750

68745 Conjunctivorhinostomy (fistulization of conjunctiva to nasal cavity); without tube

68750 Conjunctivorhinostomy (fistulization of conjunctiva to nasal cavity); with insertion of tube or stent

AMA Coding Notes

Surgical Procedures on the Conjunctiva

(For removal of foreign body, see 65205 et seq)

Surgical Procedures on the Eye and Ocular Adnexa

(For diagnostic and treatment ophthalmological services, see Medicine, Ophthalmology, and 92002 et seq)

(Do not report code 69990 in addition to codes 65091-68850)

Plain English Description

Conjunctivorhinostomy is performed to treat epiphora (excessive tearing) caused by blockage of the upper lacrimal structures including the punctum and canaliculi. An incision is made in the lower lid conjunctival sac and mucosal flaps are raised. In 68745, the frontal process of the maxillary bone is perforated and a passageway opened between the conjunctival sac and nasal fossa. In 68750, a tube is passed through the surgically created mucosal opening under the soft tissues of the face over the maxillary bone and into the nasal atrium. This creates a passageway from the lacrimal lake to the nasal atrium. The tube is secured with sutures.

Conjunctivorhinostomy
(fistulization of conjuctiva to nasal cavity)

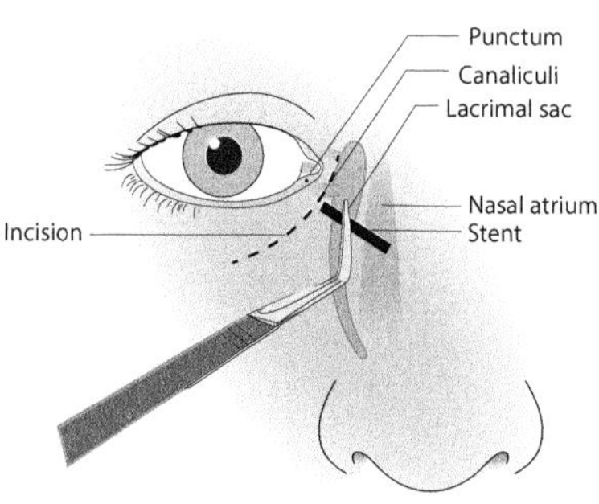

Without tube (68745); with insertion of tube or stent (68750)

ICD-10-CM Diagnostic Codes

⇄	H04.222	Epiphora due to insufficient drainage, left side
⇄	H04.312	Phlegmonous dacryocystitis of left lacrimal passage
⇄	H04.322	Acute dacryocystitis of left lacrimal passage
⇄	H04.332	Acute lacrimal canaliculitis of left lacrimal passage
⇄	H04.412	Chronic dacryocystitis of left lacrimal passage
⇄	H04.432	Chronic lacrimal mucocele of left lacrimal passage
⇄	H04.532	Neonatal obstruction of left nasolacrimal duct
⇄	H04.542	Stenosis of left lacrimal canaliculi
⇄	H04.552	Acquired stenosis of left nasolacrimal duct
⇄	H04.572	Stenosis of left lacrimal sac
	Q10.4	Absence and agenesis of lacrimal apparatus
	Q10.5	Congenital stenosis and stricture of lacrimal duct
	Q10.6	Other congenital malformations of lacrimal apparatus

CCI Edits

Refer to Appendix A for CCI edits.

Facility RVUs ▯

Code	Work	PE Facility	MP	Total Facility
68745	9.90	13.18	0.76	23.84
68750	10.10	14.29	0.85	25.24

Non-facility RVUs ▯

Code	Work	PE Non-Facility	MP	Total Non-Facility
68745	9.90	13.18	0.76	23.84
68750	10.10	14.29	0.85	25.24

Modifiers (PAR) ▯

Code	Mod 50	Mod 51	Mod 62	Mod 66	Mod 80
68745	1	2	1	0	2
68750	1	2	1	0	2

Global Period

Code	Days
68745	090
68750	090

68760-68761

68760 Closure of the lacrimal punctum; by thermocauterization, ligation, or laser surgery

68761 Closure of the lacrimal punctum; by plug, each

(For insertion and removal of drug-eluting implant into lacrimal canaliculus for intraocular pressure, use 68841)

(For placement of drug-eluting insert under the eyelid[s], see 0444T, 0445T)

AMA Coding Notes

Surgical Procedures on the Conjunctiva

(For removal of foreign body, see 65205 et seq)

Surgical Procedures on the Eye and Ocular Adnexa

(For diagnostic and treatment ophthalmological services, see Medicine, Ophthalmology, and 92002 et seq)

(Do not report code 69990 in addition to codes 65091-68850)

AMA *CPT® Assistant* ☐

68761: Jun 96: 10, Jan 07: 28

Plain English Description

The lacrimal punctum is closed to treat dry eye syndrome. Anesthetic eye drops or other local anesthesia is applied to the conjunctiva near the punctum. In 68760, the punctum is closed by thermocauterization, ligation, or laser surgery. If thermocauterization is used, the electrocautery device is activated and the punctum burned to cause scarring and closure of the punctum. Ligation involves suturing the punctum closed. Laser surgery involves activating the laser and destroying the punctual opening. In 68761, a plug is placed in the punctum. The punctum is inspected and dilated as needed. The lid is pulled away from the globe. The implant is grasped with fine forceps and inserted into the punctum and the lid is manipulated until the plug is in the proper position.

Closure of lacrimal punctum

Cautery instrument

Cautery/laser/ligation is used to close the tear duct outlet (68760).

Lacrimal sac

Lacrimal punctum

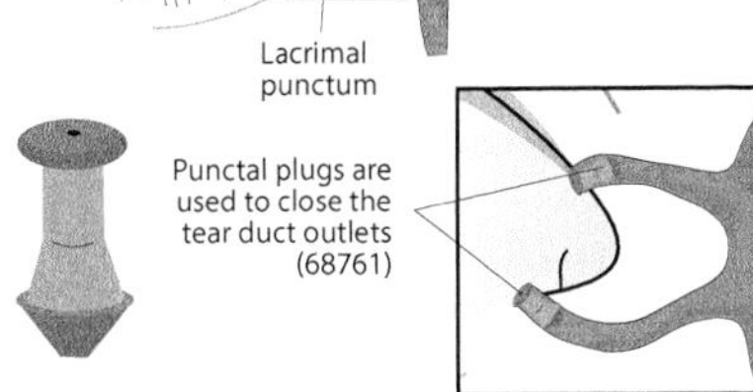
Punctal plugs are used to close the tear duct outlets (68761)

ICD-10-CM Diagnostic Codes

	Code	Description
⇄	H04.121	Dry eye syndrome of right lacrimal gland
⇄	H04.122	Dry eye syndrome of left lacrimal gland
⇄	H04.123	Dry eye syndrome of bilateral lacrimal glands
⇄	H16.121	Filamentary keratitis, right eye
⇄	H16.122	Filamentary keratitis, left eye
⇄	H16.123	Filamentary keratitis, bilateral
⇄	H16.141	Punctate keratitis, right eye
⇄	H16.142	Punctate keratitis, left eye
⇄	H16.143	Punctate keratitis, bilateral
⇄	H16.211	Exposure keratoconjunctivitis, right eye
⇄	H16.212	Exposure keratoconjunctivitis, left eye
⇄	H16.213	Exposure keratoconjunctivitis, bilateral
⇄	H16.221	Keratoconjunctivitis sicca, not specified as Sjögren's, right eye
⇄	H16.222	Keratoconjunctivitis sicca, not specified as Sjögren's, left eye
⇄	H16.223	Keratoconjunctivitis sicca, not specified as Sjögren's, bilateral
	H16.8	Other keratitis
⇄	H18.831	Recurrent erosion of cornea, right eye
⇄	H18.832	Recurrent erosion of cornea, left eye
⇄	H18.833	Recurrent erosion of cornea, bilateral
	M35.01	Sjögren syndrome with keratoconjunctivitis

CCI Edits

Refer to Appendix A for CCI edits.

Pub 100

68760: Pub 100-03, 1, 140.5

Facility RVUs ☐

Code	Work	PE Facility	MP	Total Facility
68760	1.78	2.29	0.12	4.19
68761	1.41	1.91	0.09	3.41

Non-facility RVUs ☐

Code	Work	PE Non-Facility	MP	Total Non-Facility
68760	1.78	4.64	0.12	6.54
68761	1.41	2.84	0.09	4.34

Modifiers (PAR) ☐

Code	Mod 50	Mod 51	Mod 62	Mod 66	Mod 80
68760	1	2	0	0	1
68761	1	2	0	0	0

Global Period

Code	Days
68760	010
68761	010

68770

68770 Closure of lacrimal fistula (separate procedure)

AMA Coding Notes

Surgical Procedures on the Conjunctiva

(For removal of foreign body, see 65205 et seq)

Surgical Procedures on the Eye and Ocular Adnexa

(For diagnostic and treatment ophthalmological services, see Medicine, Ophthalmology, and 92002 et seq)

(Do not report code 69990 in addition to codes 65091-68850)

Plain English Description

Lacrimal fistulas may be congenital or acquired. Congenital fistulas may be open or closed. Open fistulous tracts appear as a small hole inferior to the medial canthus, and tears or other fluid drains from the fistula onto the skin. Closed fistulous tracts end in a blind sac and do not drain. Acquired fistulas may result from trauma or disease such as an infection. A local anesthetic is administered and the fistulous tract inspected. The fistula is then obliterated using electrocautery, laser surgery, or other technique.

Closure of lacrimal fistula

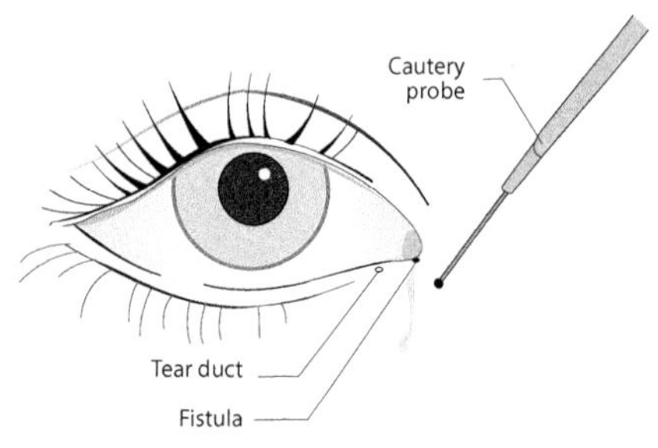

A lacrimal fistula is closed using cautery, laser, or another technique.

ICD-10-CM Diagnostic Codes

⇄	H04.611	Lacrimal fistula right lacrimal passage
⇄	H04.612	Lacrimal fistula left lacrimal passage
⇄	H04.613	Lacrimal fistula bilateral lacrimal passages
	Q10.4	Absence and agenesis of lacrimal apparatus
	Q10.5	Congenital stenosis and stricture of lacrimal duct
	Q10.6	Other congenital malformations of lacrimal apparatus

CCI Edits

Refer to Appendix A for CCI edits.

Facility RVUs ☐

Code	Work	PE Facility	MP	Total Facility
68770	8.29	9.20	0.64	18.13

Non-facility RVUs ☐

Code	Work	PE Non-Facility	MP	Total Non-Facility
68770	8.29	9.20	0.64	18.13

Modifiers (PAR) ☐

Code	Mod 50	Mod 51	Mod 62	Mod 66	Mod 80
68770	1	2	0	0	0

Global Period

Code	Days
68770	090

68801

68801 Dilation of lacrimal punctum, with or without irrigation

(To report a bilateral procedure, use 68801 with modifier 50)

AMA Coding Notes

Surgical Procedures on the Conjunctiva

(For removal of foreign body, see 65205 et seq)

Surgical Procedures on the Eye and Ocular Adnexa

(For diagnostic and treatment ophthalmological services, see Medicine, Ophthalmology, and 92002 et seq)

(Do not report code 69990 in addition to codes 65091-68850)

Plain English Description

Dilation of the lacrimal punctum is performed to treat stenosis or obstruction. A local anesthetic is administered. The punctum is inspected. A dilator is passed into the punctum and the narrowed region is dilated. The dilator is removed and the punctum is cannulated and flushed as needed with an irrigation solution.

Dilation of lacrimal punctum

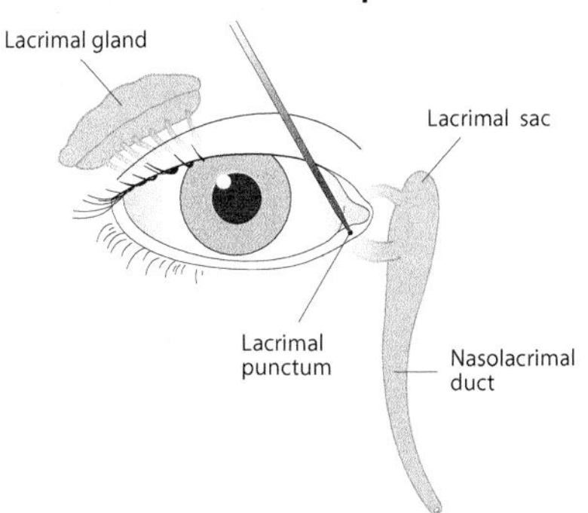

A plastic probe, catheter, or large suture is inserted into the lacrimal punctum to increase the size of the opening.

ICD-10-CM Diagnostic Codes

⇄ H04.221 Epiphora due to insufficient drainage, right side
⇄ H04.222 Epiphora due to insufficient drainage, left side
⇄ H04.223 Epiphora due to insufficient drainage, bilateral
⇄ H04.301 Unspecified dacryocystitis of right lacrimal passage
⇄ H04.302 Unspecified dacryocystitis of left lacrimal passage
⇄ H04.303 Unspecified dacryocystitis of bilateral lacrimal passages
⇄ H04.311 Phlegmonous dacryocystitis of right lacrimal passage
⇄ H04.312 Phlegmonous dacryocystitis of left lacrimal passage
⇄ H04.313 Phlegmonous dacryocystitis of bilateral lacrimal passages
⇄ H04.321 Acute dacryocystitis of right lacrimal passage
⇄ H04.322 Acute dacryocystitis of left lacrimal passage
⇄ H04.323 Acute dacryocystitis of bilateral lacrimal passages
⇄ H04.331 Acute lacrimal canaliculitis of right lacrimal passage
⇄ H04.332 Acute lacrimal canaliculitis of left lacrimal passage
⇄ H04.333 Acute lacrimal canaliculitis of bilateral lacrimal passages
⇄ H04.411 Chronic dacryocystitis of right lacrimal passage
⇄ H04.412 Chronic dacryocystitis of left lacrimal passage
⇄ H04.413 Chronic dacryocystitis of bilateral lacrimal passages
⇄ H04.421 Chronic lacrimal canaliculitis of right lacrimal passage
⇄ H04.422 Chronic lacrimal canaliculitis of left lacrimal passage
⇄ H04.423 Chronic lacrimal canaliculitis of bilateral lacrimal passages
⇄ H04.431 Chronic lacrimal mucocele of right lacrimal passage
⇄ H04.432 Chronic lacrimal mucocele of left lacrimal passage
⇄ H04.433 Chronic lacrimal mucocele of bilateral lacrimal passages
⇄ H04.511 Dacryolith of right lacrimal passage
⇄ H04.512 Dacryolith of left lacrimal passage
⇄ H04.513 Dacryolith of bilateral lacrimal passages
⇄ H04.531 Neonatal obstruction of right nasolacrimal duct
⇄ H04.532 Neonatal obstruction of left nasolacrimal duct
⇄ H04.533 Neonatal obstruction of bilateral nasolacrimal duct
⇄ H04.541 Stenosis of right lacrimal canaliculi
⇄ H04.542 Stenosis of left lacrimal canaliculi
⇄ H04.543 Stenosis of bilateral lacrimal canaliculi
⇄ H04.551 Acquired stenosis of right nasolacrimal duct
⇄ H04.552 Acquired stenosis of left nasolacrimal duct
⇄ H04.553 Acquired stenosis of bilateral nasolacrimal duct
⇄ H04.561 Stenosis of right lacrimal punctum
⇄ H04.571 Stenosis of right lacrimal sac
⇄ H04.572 Stenosis of left lacrimal sac
⇄ H04.573 Stenosis of bilateral lacrimal sac
H04.69 Other changes of lacrimal passages
H04.89 Other disorders of lacrimal system
P39.1 Neonatal conjunctivitis and dacryocystitis
Q10.5 Congenital stenosis and stricture of lacrimal duct
Q10.6 Other congenital malformations of lacrimal apparatus

CCI Edits

Refer to Appendix A for CCI edits.

Facility RVUs ▯

Code	Work	PE Facility	MP	Total Facility
68801	0.82	1.40	0.05	2.27

Non-facility RVUs ▯

Code	Work	PE Non-Facility	MP	Total Non-Facility
68801	0.82	1.96	0.05	2.83

Modifiers (PAR) ▯

Code	Mod 50	Mod 51	Mod 62	Mod 66	Mod 80
68801	1	2	0	0	1

Global Period

Code	Days
68801	010

68810-68816

68810 Probing of nasolacrimal duct, with or without irrigation

(For bilateral procedure, report 68810 with modifier 50)

68811 Probing of nasolacrimal duct, with or without irrigation; requiring general anesthesia

(For bilateral procedure, report 68811 with modifier 50)

68815 Probing of nasolacrimal duct, with or without irrigation; with insertion of tube or stent

(See also 92018)

(For bilateral procedure, report 68815 with modifier 50)

(For insertion and removal of drug-eluting implant into lacrimal canaliculus for intraocular pressure, use 68841)

(For placement of drug-eluting insert under the eyelid[s], see 0444T, 0445T)

68816 Probing of nasolacrimal duct, with or without irrigation; with transluminal balloon catheter dilation

(Do not report 68816 in conjunction with 68810, 68811, 68815)

(For bilateral procedure, report 68816 with modifier 50)

AMA Coding Notes

Surgical Procedures on the Conjunctiva

(For removal of foreign body, see 65205 et seq)

Surgical Procedures on the Eye and Ocular Adnexa

(For diagnostic and treatment ophthalmological services, see Medicine, Ophthalmology, and 92002 et seq)

(Do not report code 69990 in addition to codes 65091-68850)

AMA *CPT® Assistant* ▯

68810: Nov 02: 11, Oct 08: 3

68811: Nov 02: 11, Oct 08: 3

68815: Nov 02: 11, Oct 08: 3, Aug 09: 11, Nov 10: 9

Plain English Description

The nasolacrimal duct is probed with or without irrigation in 68810. Probing of the nasolacrimal duct (NLD), also called the tear duct, is typically performed to treat a congenital obstruction in children or, less commonly, to treat an acquired obstruction in adults. Congenital NLD obstruction is characterized by failure of the NLD to open into the nose. Most congenital obstructions resolve spontaneously by 12 months of age. If the NLD is still obstructed at 12 months, it may be treated by inserting a probe into the duct to identify and open the area of obstruction or stenosis. The puncta are dilated. A probe is inserted and passed through the duct until it can be visualized in the nose or can be touched by a second probe passed through the nasal punctum. The probe(s) is removed. The duct may be irrigated with saline solution containing fluorescein dye to flush debris or an obstructing stone or concretion from the duct. Use 68811 if the procedure is performed under general anesthesia. Use 68815 if probing and irrigation are followed by insertion of a tube or stent, also referred to as silicone tube intubation, placed in the tear duct to stretch it. The tube is left in place for approximately 6 months and removed in a separately reportable procedure. Use 68816 if the probing and irrigation are followed by transluminal balloon dilation. A deflated balloon catheter is inserted into the nasolacrimal duct through the opening in the corner of the eye. The presence of the catheter in the duct is confirmed and the balloon is inflated to expand the tear duct for 90 seconds. The balloon is then deflated and reinflated for 60 seconds. The balloon is retracted to a point slightly higher in the duct and two inflation/deflation cycles are again performed before the deflated balloon catheter is removed.

Probing of nasolacrimal duct, with or without irrigation

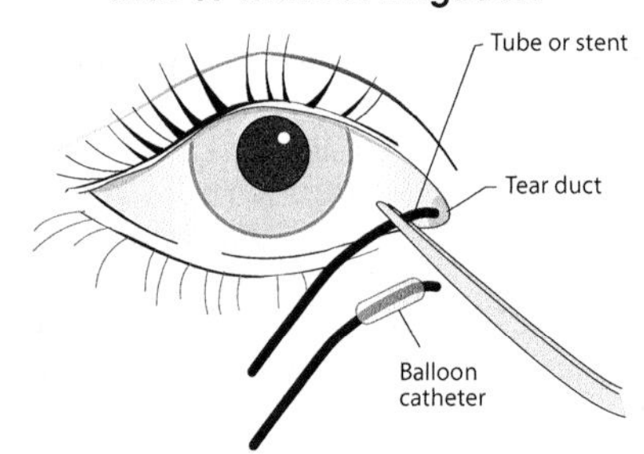

With or without irrigation (68810); requiring general anesthesia (68811); with insertion of tube or stent (68815); with transluminal balloon catheter dilation (68816)

ICD-10-CM Diagnostic Codes

⇄	H04.221	Epiphora due to insufficient drainage, right side
⇄	H04.222	Epiphora due to insufficient drainage, left side
⇄	H04.223	Epiphora due to insufficient drainage, bilateral
⇄	H04.301	Unspecified dacryocystitis of right lacrimal passage
⇄	H04.302	Unspecified dacryocystitis of left lacrimal passage
⇄	H04.303	Unspecified dacryocystitis of bilateral lacrimal passages
⇄	H04.311	Phlegmonous dacryocystitis of right lacrimal passage
⇄	H04.312	Phlegmonous dacryocystitis of left lacrimal passage
⇄	H04.313	Phlegmonous dacryocystitis of bilateral lacrimal passages
⇄	H04.321	Acute dacryocystitis of right lacrimal passage
⇄	H04.322	Acute dacryocystitis of left lacrimal passage
⇄	H04.323	Acute dacryocystitis of bilateral lacrimal passages
⇄	H04.331	Acute lacrimal canaliculitis of right lacrimal passage
⇄	H04.332	Acute lacrimal canaliculitis of left lacrimal passage
⇄	H04.333	Acute lacrimal canaliculitis of bilateral lacrimal passages
⇄	H04.411	Chronic dacryocystitis of right lacrimal passage
⇄	H04.412	Chronic dacryocystitis of left lacrimal passage
⇄	H04.413	Chronic dacryocystitis of bilateral lacrimal passages
⇄	H04.421	Chronic lacrimal canaliculitis of right lacrimal passage
⇄	H04.422	Chronic lacrimal canaliculitis of left lacrimal passage
⇄	H04.423	Chronic lacrimal canaliculitis of bilateral lacrimal passages
⇄	H04.431	Chronic lacrimal mucocele of right lacrimal passage
⇄	H04.432	Chronic lacrimal mucocele of left lacrimal passage
⇄	H04.433	Chronic lacrimal mucocele of bilateral lacrimal passages
⇄	H04.511	Dacrylolith of right lacrimal passage
⇄	H04.512	Dacrylolith of left lacrimal passage
⇄	H04.513	Dacrylolith of bilateral lacrimal passages
⇄	H04.531	Neonatal obstruction of right nasolacrimal duct
⇄	H04.532	Neonatal obstruction of left nasolacrimal duct
⇄	H04.533	Neonatal obstruction of bilateral nasolacrimal duct
⇄	H04.541	Stenosis of right lacrimal canaliculi
⇄	H04.542	Stenosis of left lacrimal canaliculi
⇄	H04.543	Stenosis of bilateral lacrimal canaliculi
⇄	H04.551	Acquired stenosis of right nasolacrimal duct
⇄	H04.552	Acquired stenosis of left nasolacrimal duct
⇄	H04.553	Acquired stenosis of bilateral nasolacrimal duct
⇄	H04.571	Stenosis of right lacrimal sac
⇄	H04.572	Stenosis of left lacrimal sac
⇄	H04.573	Stenosis of bilateral lacrimal sac
⇄	H04.611	Lacrimal fistula right lacrimal passage
⇄	H04.612	Lacrimal fistula left lacrimal passage
⇄	H04.613	Lacrimal fistula bilateral lacrimal passages
	H04.69	Other changes of lacrimal passages
⇄	H04.811	Granuloma of right lacrimal passage
⇄	H04.812	Granuloma of left lacrimal passage
⇄	H04.813	Granuloma of bilateral lacrimal passages
	H04.89	Other disorders of lacrimal system
	P39.1	Neonatal conjunctivitis and dacryocystitis
	Q10.5	Congenital stenosis and stricture of lacrimal duct
	Q10.6	Other congenital malformations of lacrimal apparatus

CCI Edits

Refer to Appendix A for CCI edits.

Facility RVUs

Code	Work	PE Facility	MP	Total Facility
68810	1.54	2.03	0.11	3.68
68811	1.74	2.02	0.12	3.88
68815	2.70	3.50	0.22	6.42
68816	2.10	2.27	0.18	4.55

Non-facility RVUs

Code	Work	PE Non-Facility	MP	Total Non-Facility
68810	1.54	3.09	0.11	4.74
68811	1.74	2.02	0.12	3.88
68815	2.70	8.30	0.22	11.22
68816	2.10	23.97	0.18	26.25

Modifiers (PAR)

Code	Mod 50	Mod 51	Mod 62	Mod 66	Mod 80
68810	1	2	0	0	1
68811	1	2	0	0	1
68815	1	2	0	0	1
68816	1	2	0	0	1

Global Period

Code	Days
68810	010
68811	010
68815	010
68816	010

CPT® Procedural Coding

68840

68840 Probing of lacrimal canaliculi, with or without irrigation

AMA Coding Notes

Surgical Procedures on the Conjunctiva

(For removal of foreign body, see 65205 et seq)

Surgical Procedures on the Eye and Ocular Adnexa

(For diagnostic and treatment ophthalmological services, see Medicine, Ophthalmology, and 92002 et seq)

(Do not report code 69990 in addition to codes 65091-68850)

Plain English Description

The canaliculi are the mucosal ducts at the medial aspect of the eye that drain tears from the eye. There are two canaliculi in each eye, one in the upper and lower lid referred to as the superior and inferior canaliculi, respectively. A local anesthetic is administered. The punctum is dilated and a probe passed through the punctum into the superior and/or inferior canaliculus. The superior and/or inferior canaliculus are cannulated and flushed as needed with an irrigation solution.

Probing of lacrimal canaliculi, with or without irrigation

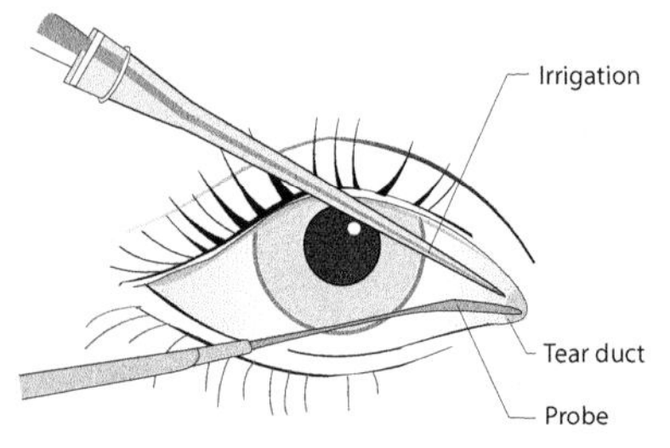

ICD-10-CM Diagnostic Codes

⇄	H04.221	Epiphora due to insufficient drainage, right side
⇄	H04.222	Epiphora due to insufficient drainage, left side
⇄	H04.223	Epiphora due to insufficient drainage, bilateral
⇄	H04.301	Unspecified dacryocystitis of right lacrimal passage
⇄	H04.302	Unspecified dacryocystitis of left lacrimal passage
⇄	H04.303	Unspecified dacryocystitis of bilateral lacrimal passages
⇄	H04.311	Phlegmonous dacryocystitis of right lacrimal passage
⇄	H04.312	Phlegmonous dacryocystitis of left lacrimal passage
⇄	H04.313	Phlegmonous dacryocystitis of bilateral lacrimal passages
⇄	H04.321	Acute dacryocystitis of right lacrimal passage
⇄	H04.322	Acute dacryocystitis of left lacrimal passage
⇄	H04.323	Acute dacryocystitis of bilateral lacrimal passages
⇄	H04.331	Acute lacrimal canaliculitis of right lacrimal passage
⇄	H04.332	Acute lacrimal canaliculitis of left lacrimal passage
⇄	H04.333	Acute lacrimal canaliculitis of bilateral lacrimal passages
⇄	H04.411	Chronic dacryocystitis of right lacrimal passage
⇄	H04.412	Chronic dacryocystitis of left lacrimal passage
⇄	H04.413	Chronic dacryocystitis of bilateral lacrimal passages
⇄	H04.421	Chronic lacrimal canaliculitis of right lacrimal passage
⇄	H04.422	Chronic lacrimal canaliculitis of left lacrimal passage
⇄	H04.423	Chronic lacrimal canaliculitis of bilateral lacrimal passages
⇄	H04.431	Chronic lacrimal mucocele of right lacrimal passage
⇄	H04.432	Chronic lacrimal mucocele of left lacrimal passage
⇄	H04.433	Chronic lacrimal mucocele of bilateral lacrimal passages
⇄	H04.511	Dacryolith of right lacrimal passage
⇄	H04.512	Dacryolith of left lacrimal passage
⇄	H04.513	Dacryolith of bilateral lacrimal passages
⇄	H04.521	Eversion of right lacrimal punctum
⇄	H04.522	Eversion of left lacrimal punctum
⇄	H04.523	Eversion of bilateral lacrimal punctum
⇄	H04.531	Neonatal obstruction of right nasolacrimal duct
⇄	H04.532	Neonatal obstruction of left nasolacrimal duct
⇄	H04.533	Neonatal obstruction of bilateral nasolacrimal duct
⇄	H04.541	Stenosis of right lacrimal canaliculi
⇄	H04.542	Stenosis of left lacrimal canaliculi
⇄	H04.543	Stenosis of bilateral lacrimal canaliculi
⇄	H04.551	Acquired stenosis of right nasolacrimal duct
⇄	H04.552	Acquired stenosis of left nasolacrimal duct
⇄	H04.553	Acquired stenosis of bilateral nasolacrimal duct
⇄	H04.561	Stenosis of right lacrimal punctum
⇄	H04.562	Stenosis of left lacrimal punctum
⇄	H04.563	Stenosis of bilateral lacrimal punctum
⇄	H04.611	Lacrimal fistula right lacrimal passage
⇄	H04.612	Lacrimal fistula left lacrimal passage
⇄	H04.613	Lacrimal fistula bilateral lacrimal passages
	H04.69	Other changes of lacrimal passages
⇄	H04.811	Granuloma of right lacrimal passage
⇄	H04.812	Granuloma of left lacrimal passage
⇄	H04.813	Granuloma of bilateral lacrimal passages
	P39.1	Neonatal conjunctivitis and dacryocystitis

CCI Edits

Refer to Appendix A for CCI edits.

Facility RVUs ▯

Code	Work	PE Facility	MP	Total Facility
68840	1.30	1.98	0.10	3.38

Non-facility RVUs ▯

Code	Work	PE Non-Facility	MP	Total Non-Facility
68840	1.30	2.50	0.10	3.90

Modifiers (PAR) ▯

Code	Mod 50	Mod 51	Mod 62	Mod 66	Mod 80
68840	1	2	0	0	1

Global Period

Code	Days
68840	010

68841

● **68841 Insertion of drug-eluting implant, including punctal dilation when performed, into lacrimal canaliculus, each**

(For placement of drug-eluting ocular insert under the eyelid[s], see 0444T, 0445T)

(Report drug-eluting implant separately with 99070 or appropriate supply code)

AMA Coding Notes

Surgical Procedures on the Conjunctiva

(For removal of foreign body, see 65205 et seq)

Surgical Procedures on the Eye and Ocular Adnexa

(For diagnostic and treatment ophthalmological services, see Medicine, Ophthalmology, and 92002 et seq)

(Do not report code 69990 in addition to codes 65091-68850)

Plain English Description

A procedure is performed to insert drug-eluting intracanalicular plug(s). The superior and inferior lacrimal canals connect to the lacrimal puncta, located at the inner aspect of each eye. Tears drain from the lacrimal lake and collect in the lacrimal puncta. The implant, or plug, is comprised of an absorbable polyethylene glycol hydrogel impregnated with a drug such as dexamethasone or travoprost. It is inserted into the lacrimal canaliculus to treat postoperative inflammation and pain (dexamethasone) or glaucoma and ocular hypertension (travoprost). The implant provides sustained release of medication, which is absorbed by the eye and exits via the nasolacrimal system. After the prescribed course of treatment, the implant is usually absorbed completely. A visualization agent is present in the implant to monitor its retention or aid in removal prior to completing the course of treatment. Report code 68841 for insertion of each implant.

ICD-10-CM Diagnostic Codes

	G89.18	Other acute postprocedural pain
⇄	H40.051	Ocular hypertension, right eye
⇄	H40.052	Ocular hypertension, left eye
⇄	H40.053	Ocular hypertension, bilateral
	H40.10X1	Unspecified open-angle glaucoma, mild stage
	H40.10X2	Unspecified open-angle glaucoma, moderate stage
	H40.10X3	Unspecified open-angle glaucoma, severe stage
	H40.10X4	Unspecified open-angle glaucoma, indeterminate stage
⇄	H40.1111	Primary open-angle glaucoma, right eye, mild stage
⇄	H40.1112	Primary open-angle glaucoma, right eye, moderate stage
⇄	H40.1113	Primary open-angle glaucoma, right eye, severe stage
⇄	H40.1114	Primary open-angle glaucoma, right eye, indeterminate stage
⇄	H40.1121	Primary open-angle glaucoma, left eye, mild stage
⇄	H40.1122	Primary open-angle glaucoma, left eye, moderate stage
⇄	H40.1123	Primary open-angle glaucoma, left eye, severe stage
⇄	H40.1124	Primary open-angle glaucoma, left eye, indeterminate stage
⇄	H40.1131	Primary open-angle glaucoma, bilateral, mild stage
⇄	H40.1132	Primary open-angle glaucoma, bilateral, moderate stage
⇄	H40.1133	Primary open-angle glaucoma, bilateral, severe stage
⇄	H40.1134	Primary open-angle glaucoma, bilateral, indeterminate stage
⇄	H59.031	Cystoid macular edema following cataract surgery, right eye
⇄	H59.032	Cystoid macular edema following cataract surgery, left eye
⇄	H59.033	Cystoid macular edema following cataract surgery, bilateral
⇄	H59.091	Other disorders of the right eye following cataract surgery
⇄	H59.092	Other disorders of the left eye following cataract surgery
⇄	H59.093	Other disorders of the eye following cataract surgery, bilateral
	H59.89	Other postprocedural complications and disorders of eye and adnexa, not elsewhere classified
	Z96.1	Presence of intraocular lens

CCI Edits

Refer to Appendix A for CCI edits.

Facility RVUs ▢

Code	Work	PE Facility	MP	Total Facility
68841	0.49	0.41	0.04	0.94

Non-facility RVUs ▢

Code	Work	PE Non-Facility	MP	Total Non-Facility
68841	0.49	0.58	0.04	1.11

Modifiers (PAR) ▢

Code	Mod 50	Mod 51	Mod 62	Mod 66	Mod 80
68841					

Global Period

Code	Days
68841	000

68850

68850 Injection of contrast medium for dacryocystography

(For radiological supervision and interpretation, see 70170, 78660)

AMA Coding Notes

Surgical Procedures on the Conjunctiva

(For removal of foreign body, see 65205 et seq)

Surgical Procedures on the Eye and Ocular Adnexa

(For diagnostic and treatment ophthalmological services, see Medicine, Ophthalmology, and 92002 et seq)

(Do not report code 69990 in addition to codes 65091-68850)

AMA *CPT® Assistant* ▢

68850: Feb 01: 9

Plain English Description

Dacryocystography is a radiologic examination performed on the nasolacrimal ducts, (tear ducts) after the injection of a contrast medium, to evaluate excessive tearing and assess patency or other pathology of the lacrimal drainage system. Dacryocystography is also used for pre- and post-operative evaluation. The patient may initially have separately reportable panoramic radiography of the face. Anesthetic drops are instilled into the eyes, the lacrimal canaliculi are cannulated, and water-soluble or oil-based contrast medium is injected. Radiographic images are obtained at different degrees or oblique angles to show the lacrimal pathways. This code reports the contrast medium injection and necessary cannulation portion of the procedure only.

Injection of contrast medium for dacryocystography

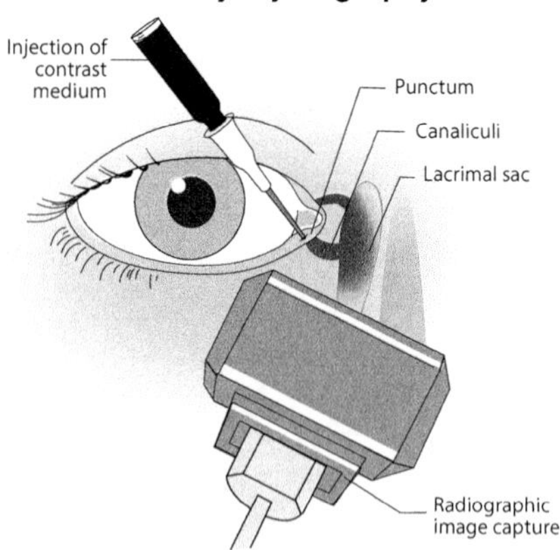

ICD-10-CM Diagnostic Codes

	Code	Description
⇄	C69.51	Malignant neoplasm of right lacrimal gland and duct
⇄	C69.52	Malignant neoplasm of left lacrimal gland and duct
⇄	D31.51	Benign neoplasm of right lacrimal gland and duct
⇄	D31.52	Benign neoplasm of left lacrimal gland and duct
⇄	H04.221	Epiphora due to insufficient drainage, right side
⇄	H04.222	Epiphora due to insufficient drainage, left side
⇄	H04.223	Epiphora due to insufficient drainage, bilateral
⇄	H04.511	Dacryolith of right lacrimal passage
⇄	H04.512	Dacryolith of left lacrimal passage
⇄	H04.513	Dacryolith of bilateral lacrimal passages
⇄	H04.531	Neonatal obstruction of right nasolacrimal duct
⇄	H04.532	Neonatal obstruction of left nasolacrimal duct
⇄	H04.533	Neonatal obstruction of bilateral nasolacrimal duct
⇄	H04.551	Acquired stenosis of right nasolacrimal duct
⇄	H04.552	Acquired stenosis of left nasolacrimal duct
⇄	H04.553	Acquired stenosis of bilateral nasolacrimal duct
⇄	H04.571	Stenosis of right lacrimal sac
⇄	H04.572	Stenosis of left lacrimal sac
⇄	H04.573	Stenosis of bilateral lacrimal sac
⇄	H04.611	Lacrimal fistula right lacrimal passage
⇄	H04.612	Lacrimal fistula left lacrimal passage
⇄	H04.613	Lacrimal fistula bilateral lacrimal passages
⇄	H04.811	Granuloma of right lacrimal passage
⇄	H04.812	Granuloma of left lacrimal passage
⇄	H04.813	Granuloma of bilateral lacrimal passages
	H04.9	Disorder of lacrimal system, unspecified
	Q10.4	Absence and agenesis of lacrimal apparatus
	Q10.5	Congenital stenosis and stricture of lacrimal duct
	Q10.6	Other congenital malformations of lacrimal apparatus

CCI Edits

Refer to Appendix A for CCI edits.

Facility RVUs ▢

Code	Work	PE Facility	MP	Total Facility
68850	0.80	0.64	0.08	1.52

Non-facility RVUs ▢

Code	Work	PE Non-Facility	MP	Total Non-Facility
68850	0.80	0.87	0.08	1.75

Modifiers (PAR) ▢

Code	Mod 50	Mod 51	Mod 62	Mod 66	Mod 80
68850	1	2	0	0	1

Global Period

Code	Days
68850	000

76510-76512

76510 Ophthalmic ultrasound, diagnostic; B-scan and quantitative A-scan performed during the same patient encounter

76511 Ophthalmic ultrasound, diagnostic; quantitative A-scan only

76512 Ophthalmic ultrasound, diagnostic; B-scan (with or without superimposed non-quantitative A-scan)

Plain English Description

Ophthalmic ultrasound (US) uses high frequency sound waves to produce images and may be used to evaluate acute vision-threatening conditions or abnormal pathology found during a routine eye examination. The fluid-filled structure of the eye provides excellent acoustics, making detailed imaging possible with US. Ultrasound may be used as the principle diagnostic tool for anomalies within the eye or as a supplement to MRI and CT. An A-scan (time amplitude) US creates vertical lines along a baseline by using thin, parallel, sound beams directed toward a small area of tissue. The A-scan image represents tissue interfacing and is very useful for distinguishing intraocular tumors, extraocular muscles, and the optic nerve, as well as measuring lacrimal gland thickness, evaluating the paranasal sinus and nasolacrimal systems, and post-sclera and sub Tenon's space. A B-scan (brightness amplitude) US uses an oscillating beam of sound with the echoes appearing as pixel images on a computer screen. A B-scan can be used to analyze intraocular structures for shape and anatomical relationships, identify foreign bodies, unusual deposits of calcium, anterior orbital tumors, myositis-induced tendon thickening, and enlargement of the superior ophthalmic vein. B-scan complements A-scan and the two can be superimposed on each other to aid in the diagnosis of ocular tumors, tissue detachment, cataracts, and traumatic injury. Code 76510 is used when B-scan and quantitative A-scan diagnostic ophthalmic ultrasound is performed during the same procedure. Code 76511 is used for quantitative A-scan only. Code 76512 is used for B-scan with or without superimposed non-quantitative A-Scan.

RVUs

Code	Work	PE	PE Non-Facility	MP	Total Non-Facility	Total Facility	Global
76510	0.70	1.33	1.33	0.02	2.05	2.05	XXX
76511	0.64	1.01	1.01	0.02	1.67	1.67	XXX
76512	0.56	0.83	0.83	0.02	1.41	1.41	XXX

76513

76513 Ophthalmic ultrasound, diagnostic; anterior segment ultrasound, immersion (water bath) B-scan or high resolution biomicroscopy, unilateral or bilateral

(For scanning computerized ophthalmic diagnostic imaging of the anterior and posterior segments using technology other than ultrasound, see 92132, 92133, 92134)

Plain English Description

Diagnostic ophthalmic ultrasound of the anterior segment may be accomplished using water bath immersion B-scan technique or high resolution biomicroscopy. For water bath immersion, a plastic eye cup containing a coupling medium such as methylcellulose or normal saline is inserted between the lids. The eye is then examined using B-scan ultrasound. High resolution biomicroscopy uses a higher frequency ultrasound transducer fitted into a B-mode clinical scanner to produce fine resolution images of the eye. Both techniques are useful when detailed images of the cornea, iris, sclera, ciliary bodies, or zonules are required. Clinical application includes measurement of the anterior chamber depth prior to cataract surgery and intraocular lens (IOL) implantation, assessment of the iridocorneal angle in patients with glaucoma, characterizing cystic and solid lesions in suspected tumors, identifying ocular foreign bodies, and mapping anterior and posterior corneal elevations for refractive surgery. Immersion B-scan also has the capability of scanning through opaque matter such as scars and cataracts.

RVUs

Code	Work	PE	PE Non-Facility	MP	Total Non-Facility	Total Facility	Global
76513	0.60	1.62	1.62	0.02	2.24	2.24	XXX

76514

76514 Ophthalmic ultrasound, diagnostic; corneal pachymetry, unilateral or bilateral (determination of corneal thickness)

(Do not report 76514 in conjunction with 0402T)

Plain English Description

Diagnostic ophthalmic ultrasound (US) for corneal pachymetry may be performed unilaterally or bilaterally and is used to measure corneal thickness. This non-invasive US technique is accomplished by placing the US probe directly onto the anesthetized central cornea of the eye to capture an ultra-high definition echogram (corneal A-scan) that measures the thickness of the cornea in micrometers. The corneal waveform of one echogram can be superimposed on others to monitor changes over time. Ultrasonic corneal pachymetry may be used to diagnose bullous keratopathy, corneal edema, or suspected glaucoma; to monitor patients with Fuchs' endothelial dystrophy or posterior polymorphous dystrophy; and to evaluate pre/post corneal refractive surgery or rejection status post penetrating keratoplasty.

RVUs

Code	Work	PE	PE Non-Facility	MP	Total Non-Facility	Total Facility	Global
76514	0.14	0.18	0.18	0.02	0.34	0.34	XXX

76516-76519

76516 Ophthalmic biometry by ultrasound echography, A-scan

76519 Ophthalmic biometry by ultrasound echography, A-scan; with intraocular lens power calculation

(For partial coherence interferometry, use 92136)

Plain English Description

Ophthalmic biometry by ultrasound (US) echography uses a single dimension, amplitude (A-scan) modulated sound beam from the tip of an US probe to measure the length of the eye and then calculate refractive power. Biometry may be used to diagnose common sight disorders but is most often employed to calculate the power of an intraocular lens (IOL) implant. The cornea and crystalline lens provide the refractive power of the eye. When a cataract is removed, the lens must be replaced with an IOL. The measurements obtained from A-scan and keratometry are applied to a simple formula that calculates the power of IOL necessary for the patient to ensure optimal sight in the treated eye. Code 76516 is used for ophthalmic biometry (A-scan) only. Code 76519 is used for ophthalmic biometry (A-scan) with intraocular lens power calculation.

RVUs

Code	Work	PE	PE Non-Facility	MP	Total Non-Facility	Total Facility	Global
76516	0.40	0.95	0.95	0.02	1.37	1.37	XXX
76519	0.54	1.42	1.42	0.02	1.98	1.98	XXX

76529

76529 Ophthalmic ultrasonic foreign body localization

Plain English Description

Ophthalmic ultrasound to localize a foreign body is a non-invasive procedure that uses a transducer probe placed firmly against the closed eye to deliver high frequency sound waves and create a gray scale image of the eye structure. Ultrasound can often identify radiolucent objects not seen on X-ray or CT scans. In addition to identifying the anatomic location and size and shape of the foreign body, the procedure can assess the extent and severity of intraocular trauma and help determine management of the injury. With the eye closed, ultrasonic conduction gel is applied over the eyelid and the globe is scanned in both the sagittal and transverse planes. The naturally fluid-filled eye structure provides a good acoustic window and image detail. Both the injured and non-injured eye may be scanned for comparison.

RVUs

Code	Work	PE	PE Non-Facility	MP	Total Non-Facility	Total Facility	Global
76529	0.57	1.95	1.95	0.02	2.54	2.54	XXX

80158

80158 Cyclosporine

Plain English Description

A blood test performed to measure cyclosporine levels. Cyclosporine, also known as Sandimmune, Gengraf, or Neoral, can be administered in oral and injectable form and RESTASIS in ophthalmic solution, is an immunosuppressant drug that affects the ability of certain WBCs in the body to recognize and respond to transplanted bone marrow and organs such as kidney, liver, heart, and lung. The drug may also be used to treat rheumatoid arthritis, psoriasis, aplastic anemia, and Crohn's disease. The ophthalmic solution is used to increase tear production in keratoconjunctivitis sicca (severe dry eyes). For transplant patients, the therapeutic levels may be assessed daily at the start of therapy, taper to 1 to 2 times per week and finally to once every 1 to 2 months. For routine monitoring the specimen is collected 12 hours after a dose. In new transplant, patient's peak levels may be drawn 2 hours after a dose and trough levels immediately prior to a dose. A blood sample is obtained by a separately reportable venipuncture. Whole blood is then tested using liquid chromatography-tandem mass spectrometry. Sandimmune may be tested with chromatographic or immunoassay technique and the results will be somewhat different. Make note of the technique used when comparing results with previous levels.

RVUs

Code	Work	PE	PE Non-Facility	MP	Total Non-Facility	Total Facility	Global
80158	0.00	0.00	0.00	0.00	0.00	0.00	XXX

81290

81290 *MCOLN1 (mucolipin 1)* (eg, Mucolipidosis, type IV) gene analysis, common variants (eg, IVS3-2A>G, del6.4kb)

Plain English Description

Molecular genetic testing is performed to identify a specific mutation of the MCOLN1 gene, which provides instruction to make the mucolipin 1 protein responsible for the transport of fat and protein across the membrane of lysosomes and endosomes, structures that digest and recycle cellular material. A lysosomal storage disorder, mucolipidosis, type IV, results when the mutated gene fails to produce an adequate amount of functional mucolipin-1 causing a buildup of fat and protein inside the lysosomes/ endosomes. The mucolipin-1 protein is necessary for the development and maintenance of brain/nerve cells, light sensitive retinal tissue in the eye, and cells that produce digestive acids. The disease is autosomal recessive. Individuals with mutation of the MCOLN1 gene from both parents develop Mucolipidosis, type IV. Individuals who receive the MCOLN1 mutation from only one parent are carriers of the disease. The disorder is found most commonly in people of Ashkenazi Jewish descent (Central and Eastern European). The gene is located on chromosome 19 and there are 2 common variants in the Ashkenazi Jewish population, c.406-2A>G, which changes a nucleotide by splice mutation at intron 3 and prematurely stops production of mucolipin 1, and g.511_6943del, which deletes a large piece of DNA on the MCOLN1 gene. Both of these mutations cause the mucolipin 1 protein to be abnormally short and nonfunctional. Symptoms of typical mucolipidosis, type IV begin in the first year of life and include psychomotor delay, progressive vision loss, achlorhydria (decreased stomach acid), hypotonia leading to spasticity and muscle stiffness, elevated serum gastrin levels, and anemia. Individuals with the disorder have a shortened lifespan. Atypical mucolipidosis, type IV will display milder (Typical) symptoms beginning in the first decade of life. Molecular genetic testing is indicated in individuals with symptoms associated with lysosomal storage disorders or when there is a family history of the disease.

RVUs

Code	Work	PE	PE Non-Facility	MP	Total Non-Facility	Total Facility	Global
81290	0.00	0.00	0.00	0.00	0.00	0.00	XXX

81434

81434 Hereditary retinal disorders (eg, retinitis pigmentosa, Leber congenital amaurosis, cone-rod dystrophy), genomic sequence analysis panel, must include sequencing of at least 15 genes, including *ABCA4, CNGA1, CRB1, EYS, PDE6A, PDE6B, PRPF31, PRPH2, RDH12, RHO, RP1, RP2, RPE65, RPGR,* and *USH2A*

Plain English Description

Molecular genetic testing is performed to identify hereditary retinal disorders including retinitis pigmentosa, Leber congenital amaurosis, and cone-rod dystrophy using a genomic sequence analysis panel. Hereditary retinal disorders may be present at birth or develop later in life and are characterized by vision loss, including night blindness and vision distortion. Targeted gene segments (exons) extracted from the DNA in a whole blood specimen are enriched using hybridization. The captured regions undergo next generation sequencing to detect gene mutations. Genetic testing may be used to confirm a clinical diagnosis for a syndromic or non-syndromic eye disorder or to identify adults who may carry familial germ line mutations in their DNA.

RVUs

Code	Work	PE	PE Non-Facility	MP	Total Non-Facility	Total Facility	Global
81434	0.00	0.00	0.00	0.00	0.00	0.00	XXX

81460

81460 Whole mitochondrial genome (eg, Leigh syndrome, mitochondrial encephalomyopathy, lactic acidosis, and stroke-like episodes [MELAS], myoclonic epilepsy with ragged-red fibers [MERFF], neuropathy, ataxia, and retinitis pigmentosa [NARP], Leber hereditary optic neuropathy [LHON]), genomic sequence, must include sequence analysis of entire mitochondrial genome with heteroplasmy detection

Plain English Description

Molecular genetic testing is performed on the whole mitochondrial genome to identify mutations in mitochondrial DNA (mtDNA). The mitochondrial genome contains 37 genes in a double stranded circle of DNA. These genes are all critical to mitochondrial function and may contain point mutations, deletions, duplications, or complex rearrangements. Disorders of mtDNA are heterogeneous with a maternal line of inheritance. Mitochondrial disorders primarily affect high energy-demanding tissues such as muscles and nerves and can involve multi-systems especially in children. The symptoms and severity of a mitochondrial disorder can vary between family members with the same mutation/disease. In contrast with nuclear gene (nDNA) where mutations are present in 0, 1, or 2 copies of the organelle, mutations of mtDNA can be present in any fraction of the total organelle. This property is known as heteroplasmy. The severity of mitochondrial disease is largely a function of the degree of heteroplasmy—the greater the degree of heteroplasmy, the more severe the symptoms of mitochondrial disease. Disorders associated with mtDNA point mutations include Leigh syndrome, mitochondrial encephalomyopathy, lactic acidosis, and stroke-like episodes (MELAS); myoclonic epilepsy with ragged-red fibers (MERFF); neuropathy, ataxia, and retinitis pigmentosa (NARP); Leber hereditary optic neuropathy (LHON); and aminoglycoside-induced and nonsyndromic hearing loss. A blood sample, skin, or tissue sample is used for analysis of the entire mitochondrial genome, identifying mutations in any fraction. Amplification of the entire mitochondrial genome is accomplished using long range polymerase chain reaction (LRPCR) followed by next generation sequencing (NGS)/massively parallel sequencing to identify mutations within the mitochondrial genome known to be associated with mitochondrial disease. This is usually performed on patients with negative results from targeted gene mutation analysis for specific mitochondrial diseases and/or for predictive testing of at risk family members.

RVUs

Code	Work	PE	PE Non-Facility	MP	Total Non-Facility	Total Facility	Global
81460	0.00	0.00	0.00	0.00	0.00	0.00	XXX

81465

81465 Whole mitochondrial genome large deletion analysis panel (eg, Kearns-Sayre syndrome, chronic progressive external ophthalmoplegia), including heteroplasmy detection, if performed

Plain English Description

Molecular genetic testing is performed on the whole mitochondrial genome to identify large deletion mutations in mitochondrial DNA (mtDNA). The mitochondrial genome contains 37 genes in a double stranded circle of DNA. These genes are all critical to mitochondrial function and may contain point mutations, deletions, duplications, or complex rearrangements. Disorders of mtDNA are heterogeneous with a maternal line of inheritance. Mitochondrial disorders primarily affect high energy-demanding tissues such as muscles and nerves and can involve multi-systems especially in children. The symptoms and severity of a mitochondrial disorder can vary between family members with the same mutation/disease. In contrast with nuclear DNA (nDNA) where mutations are present in 0, 1, or 2 copies of the organelle, mutations of mtDNA can be present in any fraction of the total organelle. This property is known as heteroplasmy. The severity of mitochondrial disease is largely a function of the degree of heteroplasmy, the greater the degree of heteroplasmy, the more severe the symptoms of mitochondrial disease. Disorders associated with mtDNA large deletion mutations include Kearns-Sayre syndrome (KSS) and chronic progressive external ophthalmoplegia (CPEO). A blood, skin, or tissue sample is analyzed on the whole mitochondrial genome for large deletion mutations, which are detected using gel electrophoresis followed by localization of the detected deletions on the mtDNA by next generation sequencing (NGS).

RVUs

Code	Work	PE	PE Non-Facility	MP	Total Non-Facility	Total Facility	Global
81465	0.00	0.00	0.00	0.00	0.00	0.00	XXX

81552

81552 Oncology (uveal melanoma), mRNA, gene expression profiling by real-time RT-PCR of 15 genes (12 content and 3 housekeeping), utilizing fine needle aspirate or formalin-fixed paraffin-embedded tissue, algorithm reported as risk of metastasis

Plain English Description

Molecular genetic testing is performed on formalin-fixed paraffin-embedded (FFPE) tissue or fine needle aspirate from uveal or choroidal melanomas to identify messenger RNA (mRNA) in 15 genes (12 content genes and 3 housekeeping genes) and predict the likelihood of metastasis. Uveal melanoma is a very rare malignancy; however, the disease has a metastatic rate of 50% within 3 years. Using reverse transcriptase-polymerase chain reaction (RT-PCR) the test measures mRNA at a given point in time to identify current disease status and assist in making a prediction of response to treatment. An algorithm is created from the genetic information in mRNA and a risk score for metastasis is assigned.

RVUs

Code	Work	PE	PE Non-Facility	MP	Total Non-Facility	Total Facility	Global
81552	0.00	0.00	0.00	0.00	0.00	0.00	XXX

83861

83861 Microfluidic analysis utilizing an integrated collection and analysis device, tear osmolarity

(Microglobulin, beta-2, use 82232)

(For microfluidic tear osmolarity of both eyes, report 83861 twice)

Plain English Description

Microfluidic analysis of tear osmolarity is performed to evaluate dry eye disease. Hyperosmolarity is a condition in which the quantity or quality of secreted tears is compromised and this condition is a primary indicator of dry eye disease. Tears perform essential functions such as maintaining eye surface integrity, protecting against infection, and preserving visual acuity. When the quantity or quality of the tears secreted is disrupted, deficient, or absent, damage to the ocular surface can occur including eye infections, desiccation of the corneal epithelium, and ulceration or perforation of the cornea. A sample of tear film is collected from each eye using an integrated collection and analysis device. The tear film sample from one eye is placed in the analysis device, which evaluates a predetermined set of criteria related to the tear film and displays the osmolarity measurement on a display panel. This is repeated with the sample from the second eye. The osmolarity measurement of the eye with the highest level of hyperosmolarity is used to determine whether the patient has normal osmolarity or whether dry eye disease is present. The measurement determines the degree of dry eye disease, which is classified as mild, moderate, or severe.

RVUs

Code	Work	PE	PE Non-Facility	MP	Total Non-Facility	Total Facility	Global
83861	0.00	0.00	0.00	0.00	0.00	0.00	XXX

84590

84590 Vitamin A

(Vitamin B-1, use 84425)
(Vitamin B-2, use 84252)
(Vitamin B-6, use 84207)
(Vitamin B-12, use 82607)
(Vitamin C, use 82180)
(Vitamin D, see 82306, 82652)
(Vitamin E, use 84446)

Plain English Description

A blood test is performed to measure vitamin A (retinol) levels. Retinol is the storage form of vitamin A found in the body. It produces the pigment found in the eye (retina) and is necessary for the maintenance of healthy eyes, skin, teeth, mucous membranes, and soft tissue. Decreased levels may contribute to infections and vision problems, even blindness. Levels may be elevated with renal compromise (kidney disease) and certain drug interactions. A blood sample is obtained by separately reportable venipuncture. Serum/plasma is tested using quantitative high performance liquid chromatography.

RVUs

Code	Work	PE	PE Non-Facility	MP	Total Non-Facility	Total Facility	Global
84590	0.00	0.00	0.00	0.00	0.00	0.00	XXX

86609

86609 Antibody; bacterium, not elsewhere specified

Plain English Description

A blood sample is tested for antibodies to bacteria not specified in any other code. Some of the commonly tested antibodies reported with this code include listeria, mycobacterium tuberculosis, and toxic shock syndrome antibody. A humoral immunity panel, which tests for multiple organisms in patients with chronic and recurrent infections also includes tests for bacteria not listed in other codes. Methodology depends on the antibody being tested. Listeria uses complement fixation. Mycobacterium tuberculosis uses enzyme-linked immunosorbent assay (ELISA). Toxic shock syndrome uses multi-analyte immunodetection (MAID). IgG antibody is the most common antibody class tested. This code may be reported multiple times depending on how many organisms are tested, the number of antibody classes (IgG, IgM), and the different methodologies used for each organism.

RVUs

Code	Work	PE	PE Non-Facility	MP	Total Non-Facility	Total Facility	Global
86609	0.00	0.00	0.00	0.00	0.00	0.00	XXX

86628

86628 Antibody; Candida

(For skin test, candida, use 86485)

Plain English Description

A blood sample is tested for antibodies to Candida, a fungus normally present on the skin and in mucous membranes such as the vagina, mouth, or rectum. Candida becomes an infectious agent only when a change in body chemistry allows the fungus to grow out of control and is referred to as Candidiasis moniliasis. Individuals on antibiotics and those who are immunocompromised are susceptible to Candida infection as are infants. Typically, the infection is localized in the mouth, skin, nails, or vagina; less commonly, the esophagus and gastrointestinal tract are affected. However, Candida can also infect the blood and cause damage to the kidneys, heart, lungs, eyes, or brain. There are several methods available to test for Candida infection including immunodiffusion and enzyme-linked immunosorbent assay (ELISA). Tests for Candida by ELISA generally measure IgA, IgG, and IgM antibodies and each immunoglobulin class (IgA, IgG, and/or IgM) tested is reported separately.

RVUs

Code	Work	PE	PE Non-Facility	MP	Total Non-Facility	Total Facility	Global
86628	0.00	0.00	0.00	0.00	0.00	0.00	XXX

86682

86682 Antibody; helminth, not elsewhere specified

Plain English Description

A laboratory test is performed to measure helminth antibodies, not elsewhere specified. Helminth or parasitic worms are numerous and code 86682 may be applied when testing for IgG antibodies in serum to the following: Cysticercosis, Toxocara, Schistosoma, Strongyloides, Filaria, and Echinococcus. Cysticercosis is a parasitic infection of the brain, muscle, or other tissue caused by the tapeworm Taenia solium, that infects humans who ingest the larvae. Toxocara are round worms found primarily in dogs and cats that invades the intestine of the host animal and is shed in their feces. Human infection is often asymptomatic but may present with vision loss, eye inflammation, and retinal damage, or liver and central nervous system symptoms causing fever, fatigue, cough, wheezing, or abdominal pain. The schistosoma parasite is not found in the United States but is endemic in other areas of the world. The larvae breed in freshwater snails where water has been contaminated. The parasite enters the body through skin penetration causing a rash and/or itching at the site followed later by fever, chills, cough, and muscle aches. The worm migrates to the liver and bladder causing inflammation and scarring. Filaria is a thread-like worm that can infect humans through the bite of tropical mosquitoes. The parasite migrates to lymphatic tissue causing lymphedema. Echinococcus is a tiny parasitic tapeworm carried by dogs, sheep, cattle, goats, and pigs that can cause cystic disease in humans in the lungs, liver, and other organs.

RVUs

Code	Work	PE	PE Non-Facility	MP	Total Non-Facility	Total Facility	Global
86682	0.00	0.00	0.00	0.00	0.00	0.00	XXX

86738

86738 Antibody; mycoplasma

Plain English Description

A laboratory test is performed to measure mycoplasma antibodies. Mycoplasma is the smallest free living organism and lacks a cell wall around the cell membrane, making it unaffected by many antibiotics, such as penicillin and other beta lactams that target cell wall synthesis. This genus of bacteria is responsible for a wide range of infections. M. pneumoniae is commonly found in the mucosa of the throat, respiratory tract, and genitourinary system. It is often identified as the infective agent in "atypical" pneumonia, a mild, self-limiting illness characterized by bronchitis, runny nose, and cough. It can also cause ophthalmic manifestations such as conjunctivitis, swelling of the optic disk, iritis, retinal hemorrhage, and optic neuropathy. M. hominis and Ureaplasma urealyticum are genital mycoplasmas associated with sexually transmitted diseases that cause urethritis and vaginitis, and can be passed to newborns during delivery. Infants and immunocompromised individuals are at risk for chronic or more severe infection. The mycoplasma organism is difficult to culture and antibody testing may be used to identify it as the probable cause of an illness. A positive IgM antibody titer suggests current or recent infection. A positive IgG antibody titer is present in over 50 percent of all serum samples and suggests past exposure. IgA antibody titers may be tested for in conjunction with IgM and IgG. A blood sample is obtained by separately reportable venipuncture. Serum is tested for IgM/IgG/IgA antibodies using semi-quantitative enzyme-linked immunosorbent assay.

RVUs

Code	Work	PE	PE Non-Facility	MP	Total Non-Facility	Total Facility	Global
86738	0.00	0.00	0.00	0.00	0.00	0.00	XXX

87101-87103

87101 Culture, fungi (mold or yeast) isolation, with presumptive identification of isolates; skin, hair, or nail

87102 Culture, fungi (mold or yeast) isolation, with presumptive identification of isolates; other source (except blood)

87103 Culture, fungi (mold or yeast) isolation, with presumptive identification of isolates; blood

Plain English Description

A laboratory test is performed to isolate and presumptively identify fungi (mold or yeast) in skin, hair, nails (87101), blood (87103), or other body source (87102). This test may be used to diagnose the presence of a fungal infection or manage an acute, chronic, or recurring condition or disease. Hair samples are obtained by plucking diseased follicle(s), skin samples by scraping cells from the outer edge of the lesion(s), and nail samples by scraping friable material from beneath the nail edge or scraping/clipping the diseased portion of the nail. Blood is obtained by venipuncture or central line draw, and other body fluids such as bone marrow or vaginal fluid are acquired for testing as appropriate. Hair, skin, nails, and other body fluids are cultured on agar plates for the growth/presence of fungi in the sample. Blood is collected in a blood culture monitoring system with microscopic, biochemical DNA probes and chromatography identification techniques to isolate mold or yeast colonies in the sample. The mold or yeast present in the sample is presumptively identified; however, additional laboratory tests may be required for positive identification of the yeast or mold isolate in the culture.

RVUs

Code	Work	PE	PE Non-Facility	MP	Total Non-Facility	Total Facility	Global
87101	0.00	0.00	0.00	0.00	0.00	0.00	XXX
87102	0.00	0.00	0.00	0.00	0.00	0.00	XXX
87103	0.00	0.00	0.00	0.00	0.00	0.00	XXX

87106-87107

87106 Culture, fungi, definitive identification, each organism; yeast

87107 Culture, fungi, definitive identification, each organism; mold

Plain English Description

A laboratory test is performed to definitively identify the pure isolate(s) of yeast and/or filamentous fungi (mold) grown in culture. This test may be used to diagnose fungal or yeast infection and/or manage an acute, chronic, or recurring condition or disease. Yeast and mold are identified using macroscopic and microscopic morphology, and pathogen identification is confirmed using nucleic acid hybridization probes, D2rDNA gene sequencing, real-time polymerase chain reaction (RT-PCR), or MALDI-TOF mass spectrometry. A separate code is reported for each organism identified. When multiple colonies are present in the culture, the code(s) may be reported more than once. Code 87106 is used when identifying yeast genus and species. Code 87107 is used when identifying mold genus and species.

RVUs

Code	Work	PE	PE Non-Facility	MP	Total Non-Facility	Total Facility	Global
87106	0.00	0.00	0.00	0.00	0.00	0.00	XXX
87107	0.00	0.00	0.00	0.00	0.00	0.00	XXX

87109

87109 Culture, mycoplasma, any source

Plain English Description

A laboratory test is performed to culture mycoplasma from any source. Mycoplasma is the smallest of free-living organisms, lacking a cell wall and able to replicate without a host. The two most common species are *M. pneumoniae* and *M. hominis. M. pneumoniae* causes atypical pneumonia, mild upper respiratory infections such as tracheobronchitis, and ocular infection such as conjunctivitis, iritis, swelling of the optic disc, and less commonly optic nerve atrophy and retinal exudate or hemorrhaging. *M. hominis* causes adult urogenital tract infection and neonatal respiratory infection. The appropriate fluid or tissue sample is first acquired. Fluid samples may include ocular fluid, respiratory secretions such as throat or nasopharyngeal swab/aspirate and bronchial lavage washings, pleural fluid, pericardial fluid, synovial fluid, amniotic fluid, cerebrospinal fluid, urine, vaginal/cervical/urethral swab, semen, or prostatic fluid. Tissue samples may include lung, placenta, endometrium, fallopian tube, bone, and urinary calculi. The fluid or tissue sample is placed in a culture medium and allowed to grow for a number of days. The cells are then examined under a microscope to identify the mycoplasma organism.

RVUs

Code	Work	PE	PE Non-Facility	MP	Total Non-Facility	Total Facility	Global
87109	0.00	0.00	0.00	0.00	0.00	0.00	XXX

87118

87118 Culture, mycobacterial, definitive identification, each isolate

Plain English Description

A laboratory test is performed to culture and definitively identify mycobacteria in each isolate. Mycobacteria are aerobic, non-motile, characteristically acid fast bacilli that have a thick, waxy, hydrophobic cell wall making it difficult to culture and treat infections caused by the organism. Body fluid sources such as cerebrospinal fluid, gastric aspirate, respiratory secretions, bronchial washings or brushings, sputum, urine, or corneal wash is collected by separately reported procedure. The fluid sample is placed in a culture medium and allowed to grow for a number of days. The cells are then examined using Matrix Assisted Laser Desorption/Ionization-Time of Flight to identify the definitive mycobacteria species such as *M. tuberculosis* complex, *M. avium* complex, *M. kansasii*, and *M. gordonae*.

RVUs

Code	Work	PE	PE Non-Facility	MP	Total Non-Facility	Total Facility	Global
87118	0.00	0.00	0.00	0.00	0.00	0.00	XXX

87205

87205 Smear, primary source with interpretation; Gram or Giemsa stain for bacteria, fungi, or cell types

Plain English Description

A laboratory test is performed to identify bacteria, fungi, or cell types in pus, normally sterile body fluid(s), or aspirated material using Gram or Giemsa stain technique. Gram staining is a differential technique used to classify bacteria into gram-positive (Gram+) or gram-negative (Gram-) groups. Gram+ bacteria have a thick layer of peptidoglycan in the cell wall, which stains purple. Giemsa technique is used in cytogenetics for chromosome staining; in histopathology to detect trichomonas, some spirochetes, protozoans, malaria, and other parasites; and as a stain for peripheral blood and bone marrow to differentiate cell types, such as erythrocytes, platelets, lymphocyte cytoplasm, monocyte cytoplasm, and leukocyte nuclear chromatin. A drop of suspended culture or cell material is applied in a thin layer to a slide using an inoculation hook and fixed with heat. The material is stained and the slide is examined under a microscope. The bacteria, fungi, or cells are identified, counted, and a written report of the findings is made.

RVUs

Code	Work	PE	PE Non-Facility	MP	Total Non-Facility	Total Facility	Global
87205	0.00	0.00	0.00	0.00	0.00	0.00	XXX

87206

87206 Smear, primary source with interpretation; fluorescent and/or acid fast stain for bacteria, fungi, parasites, viruses or cell types

Plain English Description

A laboratory test is performed to identify bacteria, fungi, parasites, viruses, or cell types in body fluid such as gastric aspirate, urine, vitreous, cerebrospinal fluid, respiratory secretions, and body tissue using fluorescent and/or acid fast stain technique. Acid fast stain technique uses auramine O to color the cells of sputum or respiratory secretions to identify mycoplasma and actinomycetes. KOH stain and Calcofluor White stain can be used to identify free living amoebae in cerebrospinal fluid (CSF), corneal scrapings, vitreous fluid, and tissue. A drop of suspended culture or cell material is applied in a thin layer to a slide using an inoculation hook and fixed with heat. The material is stained and the slide is examined under a microscope. The bacteria, fungi, parasites, viruses or cell types are identified, counted, and a written report of the findings is made.

RVUs

Code	Work	PE	PE Non-Facility	MP	Total Non-Facility	Total Facility	Global
87206	0.00	0.00	0.00	0.00	0.00	0.00	XXX

87207-87209

87207 Smear, primary source with interpretation; special stain for inclusion bodies or parasites (eg, malaria, coccidia, microsporidia, trypanosomes, herpes viruses)

(For direct smears with concentration and identification, use 87177)

(For thick smear preparation, use 87015)

(For fat, meat, fibers, nasal eosinophils, and starch, see miscellaneous section)

87209 Smear, primary source with interpretation; complex special stain (eg, trichrome, iron hemotoxylin) for ova and parasites

Plain English Description

A laboratory test is performed to identify inclusion bodies or parasites/eggs in blood, stool, urine, sputum, duodenal aspirate, liver or pancreatic aspirate, cerebrospinal fluid (CSF), nasal secretions, corneal/conjunctival scrapings or biopsy tissue material using special stain (Giemsa, Giemsa-Wright, Tzanck) (87207), or complex special stain (trichrome, iron hematoxylin, 87209). Blood may be examined for malarial parasites, trypanosomes, and microfilaria. Stool, sputum, corneal/conjunctival scrapings, biliary, and pancreatic aspirate may be examined for microsporidia. Urine may be examined for schistosoma. Sputum may be tested for Ascaris lumbricoides larvae, Strongyloides filariform larvae, hookworm larvae, Paragonimus westermani ova, Echinococcus granulosus hooklets, Entamoeba histolytica, and cryptosporidium. Liver and lung abscess aspirates may be tested for E. histolytica. Blood is drawn via fingerstick and droplets are placed on slides in both thin and thick layers; other cell material is applied in a thin layer to a slide using an inoculation hook and fixed with heat. The material is stained and the slide is examined under a microscope. The inclusion bodies, ova, or parasites are identified, counted, and a written report of the findings is made.

RVUs

Code	Work	PE	PE Non-Facility	MP	Total Non-Facility	Total Facility	Global
87207	0.00	0.00	0.00	0.00	0.00	0.00	XXX
87209	0.00	0.00	0.00	0.00	0.00	0.00	XXX

87590-87592

87590 Infectious agent detection by nucleic acid (DNA or RNA); Neisseria gonorrhoeae, direct probe technique

87591 Infectious agent detection by nucleic acid (DNA or RNA); Neisseria gonorrhoeae, amplified probe technique

87592 Infectious agent detection by nucleic acid (DNA or RNA); Neisseria gonorrhoeae, quantification

Plain English Description

Neisseria gonorrhoeae (N. gonorrhoeae) causes gonorrhea, a sexually transmitted disease (STD) that is spread through direct contact and can infect the reproductive tract, mouth, throat, eyes, and anus. N. gonorrhoeae often causes no symptoms in women, but can cause irreversible damage to the reproductive tract of women, which can result in infertility. In men, symptoms include burning, itching, and discharge of the urethra, but men rarely suffer reproductive damage from the infection. Some types of nucleic acid tests are rapid tests that may be performed in the physician office using a test kit. A swab is used to obtain a specimen from the cervix, male urethra, mouth, throat, or eye. In 87590, the exact methodology is dependent on the test kit used as there are several manufacturers. One test kit uses a nucleic acid hybridization method. A single stranded chemiluminescent DNA probe is used that is complementary to the ribosomal RNA of the N. gonorrhoeae organism. Lysate is used to rupture cells and release nucleic acids. The ribosomal RNA from the organism then combines with the labeled DNA probe to form a stable DNA:RNA hybrid. The presence of DNA:RNA hybrids is then detected using a luminometer. In 87591, an amplification technique, such as polymerase chain reaction (PCR) or transcription mediated amplification (TMA), is used to create copies of the N. gonorrhoeae nucleic acids. Amplification is used when there may be low levels of the suspected microorganism in the specimen that would not be detected using a direct probe. The N. gonorrhoeae nucleic acid is then detected using a variety of techniques. In 87592, the amplified product is quantified to provide an assessment of how many N. gonorrhoeae organisms are present. Quantification may be used to evaluate severity of infection and response to treatment.

RVUs

Code	Work	PE	PE Non-Facility	MP	Total Non-Facility	Total Facility	Global
87590	0.00	0.00	0.00	0.00	0.00	0.00	XXX
87591	0.00	0.00	0.00	0.00	0.00	0.00	XXX
87592	0.00	0.00	0.00	0.00	0.00	0.00	XXX

87809

▲ 87809 Infectious agent antigen detection by immunoassay with direct optical (ie, visual) observation; adenovirus

Plain English Description

Infectious agent antigen detection of adenovirus is performed by immunoassay with direct optical observation. Adenoviral infections are caused by a group of viruses that can infect the membranes of the respiratory tract, eyes, intestines, and urinary tract. This code reports a rapid detection technique for adenovirus infections of the eye. The lower eyelid is pulled back to expose the inner fornix. A sample collection pad provided with the rapid test kit is dabbed on the inside of the lower eyelid until it is saturated. The pad is then processed per the rapid test kit instructions by placing it in a buffer solution for the specified amount of time, waiting for the results to develop, and then reading the results visually to determine the presence of adenovirus eye infection.

RVUs

Code	Work	PE	PE Non-Facility	MP	Total Non-Facility	Total Facility	Global
87809	0.00	0.00	0.00	0.00	0.00	0.00	XXX

87850

▲ 87850 Infectious agent antigen detection by immunoassay with direct optical (ie, visual) observation; Neisseria gonorrhoeae

Plain English Description

Neisseria gonorrhoeae causes gonorrhea, a sexually transmitted disease spread through direct contact that can infect the reproductive tract, mouth, throat, eyes, and anus. Neisseria gonorrhoeae often causes no symptoms in women, but can cause irreversible damage to the female reproductive tract, which can result in infertility. In men, symptoms include urethral burning, itching, and discharge, but men rarely suffer reproductive damage from the infection. A swab is used to obtain a specimen from the cervix, male urethra, mouth, throat, or eye. Alternatively, a urine sample may be obtained. This test is a rapid, qualitative sandwich immunoassay that detects gonorrhea antigen in the specimen. The specimen is placed in a tube containing a reagent that extracts the gonorrhea antigen. Monoclonal and polyclonal antibodies are then used to identify Neisseria gonorrhoeae. If the sample contains the antigen, the test strip, line, or dot will change color as will a second control strip, line, or dot, indicating a positive result.

RVUs

Code	Work	PE	PE Non-Facility	MP	Total Non-Facility	Total Facility	Global
87850	0.00	0.00	0.00	0.00	0.00	0.00	XXX

92002

92002 Ophthalmological services: medical examination and evaluation with initiation of diagnostic and treatment program; intermediate, new patient

(Do not report 92002 in conjunction with 99173, 99174, 99177, 0469T)

Plain English Description

An intermediate level of general ophthalmological services is provided to a new patient. A new patient is one who has not received any services from that physician or other physicians of the same specialty belonging to the same group practice for three years. For an intermediate level service, the ophthalmologist focuses on evaluating a new condition or an existing condition now complicated by a new diagnosis or management problem, which need not necessarily be related to the primary diagnosis. The intermediate evaluation includes a history and general medical observations; external ocular and adnexal exam; the use of slit lamp; routine ophthalmoscopy; biomicroscopy and tonometry for conditions that do not require comprehensive care; keratometry; retinoscopy; and the use of mydriasis to facilitate routine ophthalmoscopy by dilating the pupils to help visualize the ocular media and fundus. Following diagnostic evaluation, the physician initiates a diagnostic treatment program that includes any necessary medication prescriptions and arranging for additional special services, consultations, laboratory tests, or radiology services.

RVUs

Code	Work	PE	PE Non-Facility	MP	Total Non-Facility	Total Facility	Global
92002	0.88	0.44	1.61	0.04	2.53	1.36	XXX

92004

92004 Ophthalmological services: medical examination and evaluation with initiation of diagnostic and treatment program; comprehensive, new patient, 1 or more visits

(Do not report 92004 in conjunction with 99173, 99174, 99177, 0469T)

Plain English Description

A comprehensive level of general ophthalmological services is provided to a new patient within the course of 1 or more visits. The entire service reported with 92004 need not be performed in a single session.
A comprehensive evaluation describes a general diagnostic evaluation of the complete visual system. It includes a history and general medical observations; external ocular and adnexal exam that includes lids, lashes, brows, eye alignment and motility, conjunctiva, cornea, and iris; the use of slit lamp;

examination of the gross visual field or visual acuity of each eye; sensorimotor examination, routine ophthalmoscopy to examine the ocular media, retina, and optic nerve; tonometry; keratometry; retinoscopy; biomicroscopy for acute, complicated conditions; and the use of mydriasis or cycloplegia to facilitate the exam. A mydriatic agent may be used to dilate the pupils to help visualize the ocular media and fundus. A cycloplegic agent is used to temporarily paralyze the ciliary muscle and dilate the pupil for accommodation. Following diagnostic evaluation, the physician initiates a diagnostic treatment program that includes any necessary medication prescription and arranging for additional special services, consultations, laboratory tests, or radiology services.

RVUs

Code	Work	PE	PE Non-Facility	MP	Total Non-Facility	Total Facility	Global
92004	1.82	0.90	2.52	0.05	4.39	2.77	XXX

92012

92012 Ophthalmological services: medical examination and evaluation, with initiation or continuation of diagnostic and treatment program; intermediate, established patient

(Do not report 92012 in conjunction with 99173, 99174, 99177, 0469T)

Plain English Description

An intermediate level of general ophthalmological services is provided to an established patient. For an intermediate level service, the ophthalmologist focuses on evaluating a new condition or an existing condition now complicated by a new diagnosis or management problem, which need not necessarily be related to the primary diagnosis. The intermediate evaluation includes a history or interval history and general medical observations; external ocular and adnexal exam; the use of slit lamp; routine ophthalmoscopy; biomicroscopy and tonometry for conditions that do not require comprehensive care; keratometry; retinoscopy; and the use of mydriasis to facilitate routine ophthalmoscopy by dilating the pupils to help visualize the ocular media and fundus. Following diagnostic evaluation, the physician either initiates a new diagnostic treatment program or makes arrangements for continuation of an established program. This may include medication prescription and arranging for additional special services, consultations, laboratory tests, or radiology services.

RVUs

Code	Work	PE	PE Non-Facility	MP	Total Non-Facility	Total Facility	Global
92012	0.92	0.52	1.66	0.04	2.62	1.48	XXX

92014

92014 Ophthalmological services: medical examination and evaluation, with initiation or continuation of diagnostic and treatment program; comprehensive, established patient, 1 or more visits

(Do not report 92014 in conjunction with 99173, 99174, 99177, 0469T)

(For surgical procedures, see Surgery, Eye and Ocular Adnexa, 65091 et seq)

Plain English Description

A comprehensive level of general ophthalmological services is provided to an established patient within the course of 1 or more visits. The entire service reported with 92014 need not be performed in a single session. A comprehensive evaluation describes a general diagnostic evaluation of the complete visual system. It includes a history or interval history and general medical observations; external ocular and adnexal exam that includes lids, lashes, brows, eye alignment and motility, conjunctiva, cornea, and iris; the use of slit lamp; examination of the gross visual field or visual acuity of each eye; sensorimotor examination, routine ophthalmoscopy to examine the ocular media, retina, and optic nerve; tonometry in the established patient, such as for known cataract; keratometry; retinoscopy; biomicroscopy for acute, complicated conditions; and the use of mydriasis or cycloplegia to facilitate the exam. A mydriatic agent may be used to dilate the pupils to help visualize the ocular media and fundus. A cycloplegic agent is used to temporarily paralyze the ciliary muscle and dilate the pupil for accommodation. Following diagnostic evaluation, the physician either initiates a new diagnostic treatment program or makes arrangements for continuation of an established program. This may include medication prescription, and arranging for additional special services, consultations, laboratory tests, or radiology services.

RVUs

Code	Work	PE	PE Non-Facility	MP	Total Non-Facility	Total Facility	Global
92014	1.42	0.76	2.24	0.05	3.71	2.23	XXX

92015

92015 Determination of refractive state

(Do not report 92015 in conjunction with 99173, 99174, 99177)

(For instrument-based ocular screening, use 99174, 99177)

Plain English Description

The provider examines the patient's eyes for refractive errors in conditions such as hyperopia, myopia, and astigmatism. Refraction is the ability of the eye to refract or deflect light that enters it from a straight path to focus an image on the retina. This refractive ability is what determines the patient's need for glasses or contact lenses and the appropriate prescription. Lens prescription includes the specification of lens type (monofocal, bifocal, other), lens power, axis, prism, absorptive power, impact resistance, and other factors. The patient sits in a chair behind a special device called a phoropter, or refractor, and looks through it while focusing on an eye chart. The provider moves lenses with different strengths into place and the patient determines when the chart appears more or less clear. For those with normal uncorrected vision, the refractive error is zero. Those with a refractive error achieve the best corrected visual acuity through the refractive test using different combinations of lenses. The examiner may also use a keratometer to measure the curvature of the surface of the cornea, or a retinoscope to shine light into the patient's eye and observe the reflex off the retina. The streak or spot of light is moved across the pupil as the examiner observes this reflex, then uses the phoropter to move different lenses over the eye to neutralize the reflex.

RVUs

Code	Work	PE	PE Non-Facility	MP	Total Non-Facility	Total Facility	Global
92015	0.38	0.15	0.16	0.04	0.58	0.57	XXX

92018-92019

92018 Ophthalmological examination and evaluation, under general anesthesia, with or without manipulation of globe for passive range of motion or other manipulation to facilitate diagnostic examination; complete

92019 Ophthalmological examination and evaluation, under general anesthesia, with or without manipulation of globe for passive range of motion or other manipulation to facilitate diagnostic examination; limited

Plain English Description

Prior to administration of general anesthesia for an ophthalmological examination and evaluation, mydriatic eye drops are instilled to dilate the pupil and an intravenous line is placed. Once the pupils are adequately dilated, a general anesthetic is administered. Using an ocular microscope, the anterior portion of the eye is examined, including the cornea, iris, and lens. Eye pressure is measured and eye measurements are taken, including eye length and width and corneal thickness. Refraction is performed as needed to determine the correct eyeglass prescription. The posterior portion of the eye is examined including the retina, optic disc, and optic nerve. Photos are taken as needed. Any abnormalities are noted. Use 92018 for a complete examination under anesthesia and 92019 for a limited examination. Both 92018 and 92019 report bilateral procedures.

RVUs

Code	Work	PE	PE Non-Facility	MP	Total Non-Facility	Total Facility	Global
92018	2.50	1.42	1.42	0.10	4.02	4.02	XXX
92019	1.31	0.72	0.72	0.05	2.08	2.08	XXX

92020

92020 Gonioscopy (separate procedure)

(Do not report 92020 in conjunction with 0621T, 0622T)

(For gonioscopy under general anesthesia, use 92018)

Plain English Description

Gonioscopy is an eye exam that is performed to look at the anterior chamber of the eye between the cornea and the iris to check for glaucoma or birth defects that may cause glaucoma; view the iridocorneal angle to see if drainage is open, closed, or nearly closed; and identify any scarring or damage. Gonioscopy can help the doctor determine which kind of glaucoma is present and can also help treat glaucoma by aiming a laser light at the drainage angle through a special lens during gonioscopy to decrease pressure within the eye. The patient may lie down or sit in a chair with the chin and forehead supported while looking straight ahead. The eyes are numbed with drops. A lens is placed lightly onto the front of the eye and a slit lamp is used to look in the eye. A narrow beam of light is then directed into the eye and the doctor looks through the slit lamp to view the width of the iridocorneal drainage angle.

RVUs

Code	Work	PE	PE Non-Facility	MP	Total Non-Facility	Total Facility	Global
92020	0.37	0.21	0.44	0.01	0.82	0.59	XXX

92025

92025 Computerized corneal topography, unilateral or bilateral, with interpretation and report

(Do not report 92025 in conjunction with 65710-65771)

(92025 is not used for manual keratoscopy, which is part of a single system Evaluation and Management or ophthalmological service)

Plain English Description

Computerized corneal topography is also known as computer assisted keratography or videokeratography. This is a method of measuring the curvature of the cornea. A special instrument projects rings of light onto the eye, which are reflected back to the device, which then creates a color-coded map of the cornea's surface with a cross-sectional profile. Defects such as scarring, astigmatism, and other abnormal curvatures of the eye can be detected using this method, which is commonly performed prior to corrective eye surgery, such as LASIK.

RVUs

Code	Work	PE	PE Non-Facility	MP	Total Non-Facility	Total Facility	Global
92025	0.35	0.69	0.69	0.02	1.06	1.06	XXX

92060

92060 Sensorimotor examination with multiple measurements of ocular deviation (eg, restrictive or paretic muscle with diplopia) with interpretation and report (separate procedure)

Plain English Description

An extended sensorimotor examination is performed to evaluate eye movement. The test is performed bilaterally. Motor function is tested by taking ocular alignment measurements as the eyes focus on different locations. More than one field of gaze is tested at distance and/or near. In adults and children who are old enough and able to respond, at least one sensory test, such as Titmus fly, Worth 4 dot, Maddox rod, or Bagolini lens test, is also performed. Any deviations in normal eye movements are documented. Test results are interpreted and a report of findings provided.

RVUs

Code	Work	PE	PE Non-Facility	MP	Total Non-Facility	Total Facility	Global
92060	0.69	1.13	1.13	0.02	1.84	1.84	XXX

92065

▲ **92065 Orthoptic training**

Plain English Description

Individual orthoptic training sessions are given to improve eye muscle function. The physician prescribes specific eye movement and focusing exercises aimed at improving visual tracking and correcting ocular problems, such as uncoordinated eye movement (amblyopia, strabismus) and defects in binocular vision (convergence insufficiency, convergence excess). Convergence insufficiency is a disorder in which the eyes' ability to turn inward toward each other when looking at near objects is impaired. The physician determines the appropriate eye exercises and trains the patient to do the therapy. A wide variety of techniques and equipment is employed and may include the use of prisms, pencil push-ups, special tinted lenses, color cards, penlights and mirrors, video games, and tracing pictures. Some visual therapy may be performed mainly in the office, while other exercises may be assigned to continue at home.

RVUs

Code	Work	PE	PE Non-Facility	MP	Total Non-Facility	Total Facility	Global
92065	0.37	1.16	1.16	0.02	1.55	1.55	XXX

92071-92072

92071 Fitting of contact lens for treatment of ocular surface disease

(Do not report 92071 in conjunction with 92072)

(Report supply of lens separately with 99070 or appropriate supply code)

92072 Fitting of contact lens for management of keratoconus, initial fitting

(For subsequent fittings, report using evaluation and management services or general ophthalmological services)

(Do not report 92072 in conjunction with 92071)

(Report supply of lens separately with 99070 or appropriate supply code)

Plain English Description

Contact lenses are fitted for the purpose of treating a disease. Fitting includes instruction for the wearer and training on use. Supply of the lenses and any incidental revision during the fitting and training are included. Lens fitting reported with these codes is not for vision correction. In 92071, the lens is fitted to help treat diseases of the ocular surface such as corneal abrasions, keratitis, corneal ulcers, bullous keratopathy, and recurrent corneal erosion. These conditions are treated with bandage soft contact lenses (BSCL) to help heal the cornea. These lenses can relieve pain, encourage epithelial growth and migration, deliver antibiotics, and allow for oxygen transmissibility. The type and extent of corneal wound is assessed along with pain level. The hydrogel or silicone hydrogel lens is then fitted for complete corneal coverage and centered with minimal movement. Additional topical antibiotics and oral analgesics may be utilized. In 92072, an initial fitting is performed for management of keratoconus, which is a progressive eye condition affecting the cornea. The normally spherical shaped cornea thins and becomes cone-shaped and irregular. This causes blurred and distorted vision. There are several different types of lenses available for correction of keratoconus. The exact fitting technique depends on the type of lens selected. The stage of the disease is evaluated. The lens is then selected based on corneal topography studies and the practitioner's evaluation. A trial lens is selected and the fit is checked. This is repeated until the best fitting lens is identified. The patient may need to return to fine-tune the lens selection and fit.

RVUs

Code	Work	PE	PE Non-Facility	MP	Total Non-Facility	Total Facility	Global
92071	0.61	0.31	0.44	0.02	1.07	0.94	XXX
92072	1.97	0.77	1.72	0.04	3.73	2.78	XXX

92081

92081 Visual field examination, unilateral or bilateral, with interpretation and report; limited examination (eg, tangent screen, Autoplot, arc perimeter, or single stimulus level automated test, such as Octopus 3 or 7 equivalent)

Plain English Description

A visual-field examination tests the total area in which the patient can see objects within the peripheral vision while focusing on a central point. This is performed for one or both eyes and tests for blind spots or loss of peripheral vision. One eye is tested with the other completely covered. A limited examination is reported for using a wide-field screening protocol that evaluates the static field of vision and is essentially a screening test at a single stimulus level. This includes a tangent screen test in which the patient sits 3 feet away from a target painted on a screen, stares at the centered target, and tells the examiner when he/she sees objects that move into the side vision. Automated perimetry may be performed in which the patient sits in front of a concave dome staring at an object in the center and presses a button whenever a small flash of light is seen in the peripheral vision. Interpretation of the results and a written report is included.

RVUs

Code	Work	PE	PE Non-Facility	MP	Total Non-Facility	Total Facility	Global
92081	0.30	0.65	0.65	0.02	0.97	0.97	XXX

92082

92082 Visual field examination, unilateral or bilateral, with interpretation and report; intermediate examination (eg, at least 2 isopters on Goldmann perimeter, or semiquantitative, automated suprathreshold screening program, Humphrey suprathreshold automatic diagnostic test, Octopus program 33)

Plain English Description

A visual-field examination tests the total area in which the patient can see objects within the peripheral vision while focusing on a central point. This is performed for one or both eyes to test for loss of peripheral vision and detect causative conditions, such as glaucomatous optic nerve damage and retinal disease. One eye is completely covered while the other is tested. An intermediate examination evaluates the full visual field using manual perimetry tests, such as 2 isopters on Goldman perimeter or an equivalent test, automated suprathreshold Humphrey testing or semiquantitative screening program, and automated testing at 2 or 3 threshold-related luminance levels such as Octopus program 33. The Octopus and the Humphrey-Zeiss field analyzer are popular devices that test static perimetry. These automated devices run a choice of programs by an onboard computer and employ stationary pinpoint light sources or dots projected within a large, white bowl. The patient focuses on a central point and pushes a button when he/she sees the light or movement in different locations. The computer stores the data and generates a vision field report. The traditional Goldman perimeter is a kinetic perimetry test process that utilizes moving light sources. A trained technician moves the light source and monitors that the patient maintains central focus fixation throughout the test and then produces a map of peripheral vision perception. Interpretation and report is included.

RVUs

Code	Work	PE	PE Non-Facility	MP	Total Non-Facility	Total Facility	Global
92082	0.40	0.94	0.94	0.02	1.36	1.36	XXX

92083

92083 Visual field examination, unilateral or bilateral, with interpretation and report; extended examination (eg, Goldmann visual fields with at least 3 isopters plotted and static determination within the central 30°, or quantitative, automated threshold perimetry, Octopus program G-1, 32 or 42, Humphrey visual field analyzer full threshold programs 30-2, 24-2, or 30/60-2)

(Gross visual field testing (eg, confrontation testing) is a part of general ophthalmological services and is not reported separately)

(For visual field assessment by patient activated data transmission to a remote surveillance center, see 0378T, 0379T)

Plain English Description

A visual field examination tests the total area in which the patient can see objects within the peripheral vision while focusing on a central point. One or both eyes are tested for loss of peripheral vision and causative conditions, such as glaucomatous optic nerve damage and retinal disease. One eye is completely covered while the other is tested. An extended examination includes more comprehensive quantitative automated perimetry tests with multilevel threshold testing or manual perimetry tests with 3 isopters on Goldman visual field and static determination within central 30 degrees. The Octopus and the Humphrey-Zeiss field analyzer are popular automated devices that test static perimetry running a choice of programs (such as Octopus program G-1, 32, or 42 or Humphrey full threshold programs 30-2, 24-2, or 30/60-2) by an onboard computer. They employ stationary pinpoint light sources or dots projected within a large, white bowl. The patient focuses on a central point and pushes a button when he/she sees the light or movement in different locations or at different intensities. The computer stores the data and generates a vision field report. The traditional Goldman perimeter is a kinetic perimetry test process that utilizes moving light sources. A trained technician moves the light source and monitors that the patient maintains central focus fixation throughout the test. A map of peripheral vision perception intensity within specified degrees is then produced. Interpretation and report is included.

RVUs

Code	Work	PE	PE Non-Facility	MP	Total Non-Facility	Total Facility	Global
92083	0.50	1.32	1.32	0.02	1.84	1.84	XXX

92100

92100 Serial tonometry (separate procedure) with multiple measurements of intraocular pressure over an extended time period with interpretation and report, same day (eg, diurnal curve or medical treatment of acute elevation of intraocular pressure)

(For monitoring of intraocular pressure for 24 hours or longer, use 0329T)

(Ocular blood flow measurements are reported with 0198T. Single-episode tonometry is a component of general ophthalmological service or E/M service)

Plain English Description

Serial tonometry is used to determine the pressure of intraocular fluid in the diagnosis of certain conditions, such as glaucoma). Serial tonometry includes a series of pressure checks over the course of a day to measure peaks and acute elevations in intraocular pressure (diurnal curve). There are a variety of methods used, such as Goldmann's, applanation, and Perkins. Goldmann's is the most widely accepted type of tonometry and uses a technique where an area is flattened and force is applied to measure intraocular pressure. In applanation, a topical anesthetic is introduced into the eye. A disinfected prism is then mounted on the tonometer and placed against the cornea. A cobalt blue filter is used to view the green semi-circles. The tonometer head is adjusted until the inner edges of the green semi-circles meet. A Perkins tonometer is a portable tonometer, used for children, patients unable to undergo a slit lamp examination and those in a supine position.

RVUs

Code	Work	PE	PE Non-Facility	MP	Total Non-Facility	Total Facility	Global
92100	0.61	0.31	1.87	0.02	2.50	0.94	XXX

92132

92132 Scanning computerized ophthalmic diagnostic imaging, anterior segment, with interpretation and report, unilateral or bilateral

(For specular microscopy and endothelial cell analysis, use 92286)

(For tear film imaging, use 0330T)

Plain English Description

This procedure may also be referred to as optical coherence tomography, which is a noninvasive, noncontact imaging technique that allows visualization of anterior segment structures using backscattering of light. The procedure is used to diagnose glaucoma and selected macular abnormalities. The procedure may be performed on one or both eyes. The patient is seated in front of the scanning device and is instructed to fixate on a target contained in the scanning system. The scanner is aligned and centered and the scan is obtained. The scanned images are reviewed and accepted. The physician then reviews the images, using the computerized scanning software to help analyze the images and assist in diagnosis and treatment planning. The physician identifies key landmarks and takes measurements required to formulate a diagnosis and assist with treatment planning. The physician interprets the results of the scan and provides a written report of findings.

RVUs

Code	Work	PE	PE Non-Facility	MP	Total Non-Facility	Total Facility	Global
92132	0.30	0.60	0.60	0.02	0.92	0.92	XXX

92133-92134

92133 Scanning computerized ophthalmic diagnostic imaging, posterior segment, with interpretation and report, unilateral or bilateral; optic nerve

92134 Scanning computerized ophthalmic diagnostic imaging, posterior segment, with interpretation and report, unilateral or bilateral; retina

(Do not report 92133 and 92134 at the same patient encounter)

(For scanning computerized ophthalmic diagnostic imaging of the optic nerve and retina, see 92133, 92134)

Plain English Description

These tests may be performed on one or both eyes to evaluate diseases affecting the optic nerve or retina. Two different types of laser scanning devices are available, confocal laser scanning ophthalmoscopy (topography) and scanning laser polarimetry. Confocal laser scanning topography uses stereoscopic videographic digitized images to calculate measurements of anterior or posterior eye structures. Scanning laser polarimetry measures the change in linear polarization of light. This device employs a polarimeter, an optical device, and a scanning laser ophthalmoscope. The patient is told to fixate on an internal target generated by the computer. Multiple radial scans of the posterior segment of the eye are obtained. Scans may be obtained of the optic nerve head (92133) or the retina (92134). Digitized images are displayed on a monitor. The computer calculates optic nerve head measurements, retinal thickness, or other measurements. The digitized images and measurements are evaluated by the physician and then interpreted, with a written report provided.

RVUs

Code	Work	PE	PE Non-Facility	MP	Total Non-Facility	Total Facility	Global
92133	0.40	0.66	0.66	0.02	1.08	1.08	XXX
92134	0.45	0.72	0.72	0.02	1.19	1.19	XXX

92136

92136 Ophthalmic biometry by partial coherence interferometry with intraocular lens power calculation

(For tear film imaging, use 0330T)

Plain English Description

Ophthalmic biometry by partial coherence interferometry is performed preoperatively to calculate the intraocular lens power needed to attain optimal refraction following cataract surgery. This procedure may also be referred to as optical or ocular coherence biometry (OCB) or laser Doppler interferometry. In order to calculate the correct intraocular lens power, three measurements are needed -- axial eye length, the corneal radius, and the anterior chamber length. Partial coherence interferometry measures the axial length of the eye. The axial eye length is calculated by illuminating the eye using a laser Doppler. Light from the laser Doppler is passed through a beam splitting prism and is then reflected at both the cornea and the retinal pigment epithelium. Interference of the reflected light from the cornea and retinal pigment epithelium is detected by a photodetector and processed by the device computer, which measures the path difference between the cornea and the retinal pigment epithelium. These measurements are then used to calculate the axial length, which is displayed graphically. The same device is used to measure the corneal radius using keratometry and the anterior chamber length using a slit lamp illumination.

RVUs

Code	Work	PE	PE Non-Facility	MP	Total Non-Facility	Total Facility	Global
92136	0.54	0.90	0.90	0.02	1.46	1.46	XXX

92145

92145 Corneal hysteresis determination, by air impulse stimulation, unilateral or bilateral, with interpretation and report

Plain English Description

Corneal hysteresis (CH) is a viscoelastic property that can be measured by sending an external shear force in the form of a puff of air toward the cornea causing it to flatten, called applanate, and then using an infrared beam to track the change in shape. The CH is calculated as the difference in air pressure between force in and force out applanation and is used to determine the stiffness or rigidity of the cornea and its resistance to intraocular pressure (IOP). CH can provide independent information that will aide in the diagnosis and management of glaucoma and may also help identify eyes at risk for keratoconus. CH may be used with topographic measurements to determine the geometric attributes of the eye, or to monitor the accuracy of tonometers and provide corneal compensated intraocular pressure (IOPcc) measurement.

RVUs

Code	Work	PE	PE Non-Facility	MP	Total Non-Facility	Total Facility	Global
92145	0.10	0.25	0.25	0.02	0.37	0.37	XXX

92201-92202

92201 Ophthalmoscopy, extended; with retinal drawing and scleral depression of peripheral retinal disease (eg, for retinal tear, retinal detachment, retinal tumor) with interpretation and report, unilateral or bilateral

92202 Ophthalmoscopy, extended; with drawing of optic nerve or macula (eg, for glaucoma, macular pathology, tumor) with interpretation and report, unilateral or bilateral

(Do not report 92201, 92202 in conjunction with 92250)

Plain English Description

Extended ophthalmoscopy is a detailed examination of the inside of the back of the eye (fundus) and other structures, including the retina, optic disc, choroid, and blood vessels, that goes beyond an intermediate or comprehensive general ophthalmological exam. This is done for severe posterior segment pathology. Eyedrops are given to dilate the pupil and numb the eye surface. An ophthalmoscope about the size of a flashlight is used that shines a beam of light through the pupil and has several different tiny lenses through which the doctor examines the eye. The microscope of a slit lamp and a tiny lens may also be used. The physician exams the back of the eye and makes a retinal drawing in 92201, or a drawing of the optic nerve or macula in 92202, using standard colors and labeling that details the extent of retinal detachment, location of holes or tears, areas of traction, vitreous opacities, hemorrhaging, lesions or tumors, and any other appropriate documentation for specific conditions, such as glaucoma in which cupping, disc rim, pallor, slope, and any pathology around the optic nerve should be identified.
In 92201, scleral depression is done for a better examination of the peripheral fundus to help diagnose retinal lesions, holes, tears, or adhesions that may go undetected. The tip of the scleral depressor is inserted between the globe and the orbit to displace the retina with an inward elevation. An interpretation is written that provides pertinent conclusions, impressions, and findings.

RVUs

Code	Work	PE	PE Non-Facility	MP	Total Non-Facility	Total Facility	Global
92201	0.40	0.24	0.30	0.02	0.72	0.66	XXX
92202	0.26	0.15	0.19	0.01	0.46	0.42	XXX

92227-92229

★ **92227 Imaging of retina for detection or monitoring of disease; with remote clinical staff review and report, unilateral or bilateral**

(Do not report 92227 in conjunction with 92133, 92134, 92228, 92229, 92250)

★ **92228 Imaging of retina for detection or monitoring of disease; with remote physician or other qualified health care professional interpretation and report, unilateral or bilateral**

(Do not report 92228 in conjunction with 92133, 92134, 92227, 92229, 92250)

92229 Imaging of retina for detection or monitoring of disease; point-of-care automated analysis and report, unilateral or bilateral

(Do not report 92229 in conjunction with 92133, 92134, 92227, 92228, 92250)

Plain English Description

Remote retinal imaging is performed on one or both eyes to screen for retinopathy in at risk patients, such as those with diabetes, or to evaluate and monitor active retinal disease. The retinal images are obtained by a provider at one facility, and then either transmitted electronically to be reviewed and interpreted at another site, or the images are analyzed by the computer program at the point of care. One or both pupils are dilated. Images are obtained using a computerized retinal imaging system. Most systems automatically center on the pupil, illuminate the retina, focus, estimate visual acuity, and then obtain digital images of the retina. The digital images are electronically transmitted to the eye center. For 92227, the images are reviewed by clinical staff and a report is provided. For 92228, the images are reviewed by an ophthalmologist or other qualified health care professional under the direction of a retinal specialist and an interpretation of findings is provided in a written report. In 92229, the report is automatically generated at the point of care after the images are analyzed by the computerized system.

RVUs

Code	Work	PE	PE Non-Facility	MP	Total Non-Facility	Total Facility	Global
92227	0.00	0.46	0.46	0.01	0.47	0.47	XXX
92228	0.32	0.56	0.56	0.02	0.90	0.90	XXX
92229	0.00	1.35	1.35	0.01	1.36	1.36	XXX

92230

92230 Fluorescein angioscopy with interpretation and report

Plain English Description

Fluorescein angioscopy is performed using a modified microscope to study capillary vessels and assess or evaluate lesions in the eye and around the retinal periphery. A fluorescein dye is injected into a peripheral vein or fluorescence sodium salt can also be applied externally. An indirect ophthalmoscope is used to shine light into the eye. The fluorescent dye or sodium allows the vascular area that is being examined to light up and appear in relation to the color and be demarcated against surrounded areas and landmarks. One technique uses a cobalt blue filter that is carefully adjusted so only blue light illuminates the retina and partial fluorescence appears through the microscope, causing a blue image that identifies the location of retinal lesions. Other types of interference bandpass filters, such as a barrier filter, may be used to block out all light from the fluorescence, except at a specific wavelength. Acidic, yellowish green fluorescent sodium is used to identify corneal trauma and injury. Digital imaging is produced that can be stored, printed, and transferred. The physician provides a written interpretation and report of the findings.

RVUs

Code	Work	PE	PE Non-Facility	MP	Total Non-Facility	Total Facility	Global
92230	0.60	0.31	2.24	0.04	2.88	0.95	XXX

92235-92242

92235 Fluorescein angiography (includes multiframe imaging) with interpretation and report, unilateral or bilateral

(When fluorescein and indocyanine-green angiography are performed at the same patient encounter, use 92242)

92240 Indocyanine-green angiography (includes multiframe imaging) with interpretation and report, unilateral or bilateral

(When indocyanine-green and fluorescein angiography are performed at the same patient encounter, use 92242)

92242 Fluorescein angiography and indocyanine-green angiography (includes multiframe imaging) performed at the same patient encounter with interpretation and report, unilateral or bilateral

(To report fluorescein angiography and indocyanine-green angiography not performed at the same patient encounter, see 92235, 92240)

Plain English Description

In 92235, fluorescein angiography is used in the diagnosis and treatment of retinal disorders. Fluorescein is a fluorescent dye that is injected into the bloodstream and used to highlight the blood vessels of the retina. In 92240, indocyanine-green angiography is used in the evaluation of the retina and the choroid for diseases such as macular degeneration, abnormal vessel growth, macular edema, and retinal detachment. The test is performed using indocyanine green dye that fluoresces in the infrared spectrum and allows imaging through pigmentation, fluid, and collections of blood in the retina and choroid. To perform either test, the pupil is dilated using Mydriatic drops and fundal photographs are obtained prior to the infusion of fluorescein or indocyanine-green (ICG). A bolus of fluorescein or ICG is then injected into a peripheral vein, usually in the arm, and fundus photographs are obtained using a rapid sequence or video camera as the fluorescein flows through the blood vessels in the retina, or the ICG flows through the blood vessels in the retina and the choroid. The photographs or video images are then reviewed by the physician and any retinal abnormalities or retinal and choroid abnormalities are identified. A written interpretation of findings is provided, which may be for one eye or both eyes. Report 92242 when both the fluorescein angiography and the indocyanine-green angiography test are performed during the same patient encounter.

RVUs

Code	Work	PE	PE Non-Facility	MP	Total Non-Facility	Total Facility	Global
92235	0.75	2.92	2.92	0.02	3.69	3.69	XXX
92240	0.80	4.82	4.82	0.10	5.72	5.72	XXX
92242	0.95	6.38	6.38	0.05	7.38	7.38	XXX

92250

92250 Fundus photography with interpretation and report

Plain English Description

Fundus photography is the use of a retinal camera to take pictures of the inside of the back of the eye. Fundus photography may look at the optic nerve, macula, vitreous, the retina, and its vasculature. The highly specialized retinal camera is mounted on a microscope that contains high-powered, intricate lenses and mirrors. The lenses capture images of the back of the eye when light is focused through the cornea, the pupil, and the lens. The pupils are dilated with drops to prevent them from constricting at the bright light. The patient is instructed to stare at one fixation point to keep the eyes still. Pictures are then taken as a series of flashes of bright light are focused through the eye and camera lens. Fundus photography is performed to evaluate abnormalities, follow the progress of a disease, assess therapeutic effects and surgical treatments, and plan for future treatment. Diseases that indicate a need for fundus photography include retinal neoplasms, macular degeneration, diabetic retinopathy, glaucoma, multiple sclerosis, and other central nervous system problems.

RVUs

Code	Work	PE	PE Non-Facility	MP	Total Non-Facility	Total Facility	Global
92250	0.40	0.67	0.67	0.02	1.09	1.09	XXX

92260

92260 Ophthalmodynamometry

(For ophthalmoscopy under general anesthesia, use 92018)

Plain English Description

Ophthalmodynamometry (ODM) is a method for measuring blood pressure within the central retinal artery or vein. This noninvasive method involves an ophthalmoscopic examination of the central retinal artery/vein while intraocular pressure is induced and gradually increased. The eyes are dilated and numbing drops are instilled. An ophthalmodynamometer is then used to exert pressure on the globe towards the center of the eyeball. The patient holds the gaze fixed straight ahead with the other eye. The calibrated plunger transmits the extent of eye compression to a unit scale on the ophthalmodynamometer. The reading is noted when the central retinal artery ceases pulsation and becomes completely collapsed and blanched by the pressure applied to give the systolic measurement. The pressure applied is slowly lessened and the reading is noted again when the artery first begins to pulsate after collapse and complete interruption of blood flow. This number is the diastolic pressure measurement. The average diastolic value of retinal pressure is 47 mm/Hg and the systolic value is 78 mm/Hg. Measurements are used to detect retinal hypertension and to test for the presence of disease in the internal carotid artery as the two measurements are correlated. Blood pressure measured in the central retinal vein is used as a non-invasive method for screening cases of suspected elevated intracranial pressure (ICP). The pressure in the central retinal vein depends on ICP because the optic nerve is surrounded by cerebrospinal fluid and when the vein collapses or pulsates, the ICP is at least equal to or greater than the pressure within the optic nerve.

RVUs

Code	Work	PE	PE Non-Facility	MP	Total Non-Facility	Total Facility	Global
92260	0.20	0.10	0.37	0.01	0.58	0.31	XXX

92265

92265 Needle oculoelectromyography, 1 or more extraocular muscles, 1 or both eyes, with interpretation and report

Plain English Description

Needle oculoelectromyography is performed to evaluate nerve and muscle function of the eye muscles. This test is commonly performed in the diagnosis and evaluation of myasthenia gravis as well as other neuromuscular conditions effecting eye movement. This test is typically performed using single fiber electromyography (EMG), which uses a very fine needle to evaluate function in a single muscle fiber. The recording needle electrode is inserted into the targeted nerve-muscle communication point in the selected extraocular muscle. The electrode cable is attached to a recording device with a visual display. Electrical activity of the muscle is recorded. Action potential is tested by stimulating the muscle fiber. Action potential evaluates the ability of muscle fibers to respond to nerve stimulation. The EMG recording is displayed graphically as a wave form. The physician reviews the needle EMG recording and provides a written report of findings.

RVUs

Code	Work	PE	PE Non-Facility	MP	Total Non-Facility	Total Facility	Global
92265	0.81	1.70	1.70	0.02	2.53	2.53	XXX

92270

92270 Electro-oculography with interpretation and report

(For vestibular function tests with recording, see 92537, 92538, 92540, 92541, 92542, 92544, 92545, 92546, 92547, 92548)

(Do not report 92270 in conjunction with 92537, 92538, 92540, 92541, 92542, 92544, 92545, 92546, 92547, 92548, 92549)

(To report saccadic eye movement testing with recording, use 92700)

Plain English Description

Electro-oculography (EOG) is used to evaluate function of the retinal pigment epithelium (RPE) of the eye. The test records changes in electrical potential across the RPE as the eye adapts to periods of dark and light. The RPE is a pigmented cell layer lying just outside the retina that is located between the vascular layer of the choroid and the light sensitive outer segments of the photoreceptors. The RPE along with the photoreceptors play a critical role in the maintenance of visual function. To perform EOG, the pupils are dilated. Pairs of electrodes are placed on the skin usually medial and lateral to the eye. The patient is positioned in a head and chin rest within a full-field dome with two red fixation lights located to the left and right of center. Dark phase adaptation is tested first. The dome is programmed for complete darkness with maximal dimming of the fixation lights. The fixation lights are then alternately activated, prompting the patient to move the eyes from side to side to focus on the activated light. The dark phase lasts for 15 minutes, with the fixation lights alternating from side to side for 10 seconds a minute during which recordings are taken alternating with 50 seconds of complete darkness. The light phase is tested next and also lasts 15 minutes. The dome background lights are turned on and light phase testing is performed in the same manner with 10 seconds of alternating fixation lights followed by 50 seconds of light. Upon completion of the procedure, the EOG recording is evaluated for dark/light adaptation. Dark adaptation is identified as a decrease in resting potential, which typically reaches a minimum called the dark trough after several minutes. Light adaptation is identified as an increase in resting potential called the light peak that drops off as the retina adapts to light. Specific parameters are calculated either manually or using computer algorithms, which include the Arden (light/dark) ratio), the dark trough amplitude, the time from light phase initiation to light peak, the pupil size, and the type of adapting light source. A written report of findings is provided.

RVUs

Code	Work	PE	PE Non-Facility	MP	Total Non-Facility	Total Facility	Global
92270	0.81	2.36	2.36	0.03	3.20	3.20	XXX

92273-92274

92273 Electroretinography (ERG), with interpretation and report; full field (ie, ffERG, flash ERG, Ganzfeld ERG)

92274 Electroretinography (ERG), with interpretation and report; multifocal (mfERG)

(For pattern ERG, use 0509T)

(For electronystagmography for vestibular function studies, see 92541 et seq)

(For ophthalmic echography (diagnostic ultrasound), see 76511-76529)

Plain English Description

Electroretinography (ERG) is performed to diagnose and evaluate conditions affecting the retina and optic nerve by measuring the electrical activity generated by retinal cells in response to light stimulus. Mydriatic drops are instilled to dilate the pupil. The patient is dark or light adapted for several minutes first, depending on the protocol. ERG electrodes are then placed on the surface of the eye using dim red illumination. There are several types of electrodes that can be used including contact lens electrodes placed over the cornea, or gold Mylar tape containing electrodes placed between the lower lid and the sclera or cornea. The electrodes are connected to a recording device. The head is kept stationary using head and chin supports. The eye is then stimulated by flashes of light from a bright light source such as LEDs, a strobe lamp, or a full-field dome with its own light source. The response to light flashes are first recorded in the dark and then with background lighting. The flash of light causes an electrical response in the retina that is captured by the electrodes, recorded, and represented digitally as a waveform. For conventional, full field, or flash ERG (92273), the summation of electrical response from the entire retina is evoked by a flash light (Ganzfeld stimulus bow) scattered throughout the eye. This ERG can record the response from the entire retina but will not detect local responses. In multifocal ERG (mfERG), many areas of the retina are stimulated by multiple sequences at the same time and the electrical responses from different regions of the retina are recorded simultaneously. Following completion of the test, two components are typically evaluated, the a-wave and b-wave correlating to the health of the photoreceptors in the outer retina and the health of the inner layers of the retina. A written interpretation of findings is provided.

RVUs

Code	Work	PE	PE Non-Facility	MP	Total Non-Facility	Total Facility	Global
92273	0.69	3.01	3.01	0.03	3.73	3.73	XXX
92274	0.61	1.92	1.92	0.02	2.55	2.55	XXX

92283

92283 Color vision examination, extended, eg, anomaloscope or equivalent

(Color vision testing with pseudoisochromatic plates [such as HRR or Ishihara] is not reported separately. It is included in the appropriate general or ophthalmological service, or 99172)

Plain English Description

A test is performed to determine whether color vision is within the normal range. Individuals who do not see all colors in the spectrum in the usual way suffer from a vision deficit called color blindness. Color vision deficits are caused by color sensing pigment deficiencies in the cone cells of the eye. The most common type of color vision deficit is called protanomaly, which is the reduced ability to process red light. Two less common types are deuteranomaly, which is the reduced ability to process green light and tritanomaly, which is the reduced ability to process blue light. The severity of each of these types of color vision deficits can vary significantly. In very rare cases, an individual may see no color at all, only shades of gray. An anomaloscope uses two light sources that display light of different colors and different brightness side-by-side. The light on one side must be blended to match the color and brightness of the opposite side. The patient is familiarized with the controls on the anomaloscope. Lights in the red and green spectrums are displayed and the patient turns the dials until a color and brightness match is perceived. The patient may also indicate that no match can be made. An initial review of results is made and if a color vision deficit is noted, the anomaloscope is recalibrated to test for the severity of the specific color deficit detected. The test results are displayed graphically to show deviations from normal color and brightness perception and the severity of the color vision deficit. The test may be repeated with colors in the blue and yellow spectrums. The physician reviews the test results and provides a written test of findings.

RVUs

Code	Work	PE	PE Non-Facility	MP	Total Non-Facility	Total Facility	Global
92283	0.17	1.40	1.40	0.02	1.59	1.59	XXX

92284

92284 Dark adaptation examination with interpretation and report

Plain English Description

Dark adaptation tests the ability of the eyes to recover sensitivity in the dark following exposure to bright light. Light and dark vision is mediated by cone and rod cells in the retina. Cone cells mediate vision in well-lit conditions, while rod cells mediate vision in low-light conditions. During dark adaption, following exposure to bright light, the eye adapts by shifting from cone cells to rod cells to mediate vision. However, this does not happen instantaneously. Depending on the intensity of the light and the duration of exposure it can take the eye up to 50 minutes to make a complete shift from cone cells to rod cells. During this time, dark vision gradually improves as the eye adapts to the dark. To test for dark adaptation, the patient is first exposed to bright light for about 5 minutes. The light source is turned off and the time it takes for the eye to adapt to the dark and reach peak dark or low-light vision is determined. This is accomplished by exposing the eye to flashes of light of varying intensities in the newly darkened environment. The patient is cued when a flash of light occurs and must indicate whether or not the flash was seen. If the patient is not able to see the flash, a higher intensity flash is used until the patient indicates that the flash can be seen. The flashes of light continue but are reduced in intensity to determine the lowest level of intensity that can be seen during dark adaptation. The time it takes to reach the lowest level of light intensity that is able to be seen is the dark adaptation time. The results are displayed graphically and a written interpretation of findings is provided.

RVUs

Code	Work	PE	PE Non-Facility	MP	Total Non-Facility	Total Facility	Global
92284	0.24	1.43	1.43	0.03	1.70	1.70	XXX

92285

92285 External ocular photography with interpretation and report for documentation of medical progress (eg, close-up photography, slit lamp photography, goniophotography, stereo-photography)

(For tear film imaging, use 0330T)

(For meibomian gland imaging, use 0507T)

Plain English Description

External ocular photography is performed to document and track conditions or injuries affecting the external structures of the eye, including the eyelids, lashes, sclerae, conjunctiva, and cornea. It may also be used for some structures of the anterior chamber, including the iris and filtration angle. Photography may be performed using a slit lamp, goniophotography, stereo photography, or close-up photography. Pictures may be stored as prints, slides, videotape, or digital media. The physician reviews the external ocular photographs and describes the findings, compares them to previously obtained photographs, and notes any resolution, progression, or late effects of the condition or injury.

RVUs

Code	Work	PE	PE Non-Facility	MP	Total Non-Facility	Total Facility	Global
92285	0.05	0.61	0.61	0.02	0.68	0.68	XXX

92286-92287

92286 Anterior segment imaging with interpretation and report; with specular microscopy and endothelial cell analysis

92287 Anterior segment imaging with interpretation and report; with fluorescein angiography

Plain English Description

Anterior segment imaging is performed to evaluate the integrity of the cornea, iris and other anterior segment structures. In 92286, anterior segment imaging is performed with specular microscopy and endothelial cell analysis of the cornea. The cornea has several layers including epithelium, stroma, and a single-celled endothelial layer with the endothelium being the most posterior layer. The health of the endothelial layer is critical for maintaining visual acuity. The endothelial cells prevent aqueous humor from entering the cornea and pump fluid from the corneal stroma into the anterior chamber. Maintaining the cornea in a relatively dehydrated state is necessary for corneal clarity. However, because the corneal endothelial cells do not replicate, if they are destroyed by disease or surgery, the remaining cells must spread out to cover an increased surface area. As the total number of endothelial cells decrease, the endothelial layer can no longer maintain the dehydrated state and the cornea becomes cloudy resulting in loss of visual acuity. Specular microscopy provides a magnified view of a small area of corneal endothelial cells. Images obtained using specular microscopy are recorded on videotape or photographic film. Endothelial cell density and configuration are evaluated and cell counts are provided. The images are compared with any previous images and changes documented. In 92287, anterior segment imaging is performed with fluorescein angiography to evaluate the iris and other anterior segment structures. An intravenous injection of sodium fluorescein is administered. Serial images of the anterior segment are obtained beginning 8 to 10 seconds following fluorescein injection and continuing until 1 minute after injection. Additional images may be obtained 5 to 10 minutes after injection. The images are viewed and a written interpretation of findings is provided.

RVUs

Code	Work	PE	PE Non-Facility	MP	Total Non-Facility	Total Facility	Global
92286	0.40	0.73	0.73	0.02	1.15	1.15	XXX
92287	0.81	4.48	4.48	0.03	5.32	5.32	XXX

92310-92313

92310 Prescription of optical and physical characteristics of and fitting of contact lens, with medical supervision of adaptation; corneal lens, both eyes, except for aphakia

(For prescription and fitting of 1 eye, add modifier 52)

92311 Prescription of optical and physical characteristics of and fitting of contact lens, with medical supervision of adaptation; corneal lens for aphakia, 1 eye

92312 Prescription of optical and physical characteristics of and fitting of contact lens, with medical supervision of adaptation; corneal lens for aphakia, both eyes

92313 Prescription of optical and physical characteristics of and fitting of contact lens, with medical supervision of adaptation; corneoscleral lens

Plain English Description

Based on the patient's vision needs, the medical provider selects the best contact lens options for the patient. The provider discusses the pros and cons of the different types of contact lenses available and assists the patient in selecting the type of lens that will best meet his/her needs. The provider specifies the optical and physical characteristics of the selected lenses, such as power, size, curvature, flexibility (hard/soft), and gas-permeability. The lenses are inserted by the provider and the fit of the selected lenses is checked. Adjustments are made as needed to achieve the best visual acuity and the most comfortable fit. The patient is then instructed on how to insert and remove the lenses and practices inserting and removing the lenses under the guidance of the provider. The patient may be given sample contact lenses by different manufacturers to try for a period of time so that the lenses that best meet the patient's needs can be determined. During the trial period, incidental revisions to the optical and physical characteristics of the lenses may be made to improve visual acuity or comfort. All services are performed by the medical provider. Use code 92310 for corneal lenses for both eyes to correct a condition other than aphakia. Use code 92311 for a lens prescribed to treat aphakia in one eye, or code 92312 when lenses are prescribed to treat bilateral aphakia. Use code 92313 for a corneoscleral lens.

RVUs

Code	Work	PE	PE Non-Facility	MP	Total Non-Facility	Total Facility	Global
92310	1.17	0.45	1.74	0.10	3.01	1.72	XXX
92311	1.08	0.43	2.03	0.02	3.13	1.53	XXX
92312	1.26	0.49	2.35	0.02	3.63	1.77	XXX
92313	0.92	0.33	2.03	0.01	2.96	1.26	XXX

92314-92317

92314 Prescription of optical and physical characteristics of contact lens, with medical supervision of adaptation and direction of fitting by independent technician; corneal lens, both eyes except for aphakia

(For prescription and fitting of 1 eye, add modifier 52)

92315 Prescription of optical and physical characteristics of contact lens, with medical supervision of adaptation and direction of fitting by independent technician; corneal lens for aphakia, 1 eye

92316 Prescription of optical and physical characteristics of contact lens, with medical supervision of adaptation and direction of fitting by independent technician; corneal lens for aphakia, both eyes

92317 Prescription of optical and physical characteristics of contact lens, with medical supervision of adaptation and direction of fitting by independent technician; corneoscleral lens

Plain English Description

Based on the patient's vision needs, the medical provider selects the best contact lens options for the patient. The provider discusses the pros and cons of the different types of contact lenses available and assists the patient in selecting the type of lens that will best meet his/her needs. The provider specifies the optical and physical characteristics of the selected lenses, such as power, size, curvature, flexibility (hard/soft), and gas-permeability. The lenses are inserted by the provider and the fit of the selected lenses is checked. Adjustments are made as needed to achieve the best visual acuity and the most comfortable fit. An independent technician then works with the patient, providing instruction on how to insert and remove the lenses. The technician observes and assists the patient as needed while the patient practices inserting and removing the lenses. The patient may be given sample contact lenses by different manufacturers to try for a period of time so that the lenses that best meet the patient's needs can be determined. During the trial period, incidental revisions to the optical and physical characteristics of the lenses may be made to improve visual acuity or comfort. Use code 92314 for corneal lenses for both eyes to correct a condition other than aphakia. Use code 92315 for a lens prescribed to treat aphakia in one eye, or code 92316 when lenses are prescribed to treat bilateral aphakia. Use code 92317 for a corneoscleral lens.

RVUs

Code	Work	PE	PE Non-Facility	MP	Total Non-Facility	Total Facility	Global
92314	0.69	0.27	1.87	0.07	2.63	1.03	XXX
92315	0.45	0.15	1.98	0.01	2.44	0.61	XXX
92316	0.68	0.23	2.32	0.01	3.01	0.92	XXX
92317	0.45	0.15	2.10	0.01	2.56	0.61	XXX

92325

92325 Modification of contact lens (separate procedure), with medical supervision of adaptation

Plain English Description

Modification of the contact lens is performed during a separate procedure to improve the function, fit, and/or comfort of the lens. The medical provider evaluates the current fit of the contact lens and queries the patient regarding visual acuity and the comfort of the lens. The provider determines what modifications should be made. Possible modifications include reducing the overall lens diameter; reducing the optical zone diameter; flattening the peripheral curves; blending the peripheral curves; polishing the edges, anterior, and posterior surfaces; or modifying the lens power. The provider makes the necessary lens modifications, checks the fit and comfort, and then checks visual acuity.

RVUs

Code	Work	PE	PE Non-Facility	MP	Total Non-Facility	Total Facility	Global
92325	0.00	1.35	1.35	0.01	1.36	1.36	XXX

92326

92326 Replacement of contact lens

Plain English Description

A contact lens is replaced due to damage or loss, or because of problems related to fit, comfort, or vision. If the contact lens has been damaged or lost, the provider verifies the optical and physical characteristics and provides a replacement prescription. If the contact lens needs to be replaced because of poor fit, discomfort, or vision problems, the provider determines what changes should be made, which may include a different brand or type of contact lens, and a new prescription is provided. The patient may be given a trial supply of the new brand or type of lens to see if the new lens eliminates the problems that the patient was experiencing with the previous lens.

RVUs

Code	Work	PE	PE Non-Facility	MP	Total Non-Facility	Total Facility	Global
92326	0.00	1.15	1.15	0.01	1.16	1.16	XXX

92340-92342

92340 Fitting of spectacles, except for aphakia; monofocal

92341 Fitting of spectacles, except for aphakia; bifocal

92342 Fitting of spectacles, except for aphakia; multifocal, other than bifocal

Plain English Description

Following a separately reportable eye examination of a patient needing corrective lenses for a condition other than aphakia, the patient meets with an eyeglass (spectacle) technician who evaluates anatomical facial characteristics and determines the correct frame size. The technician measures the anatomical facial characteristics, including the distance between the pupils, and submits the measurements to a laboratory for manufacture of the lenses and insertion into the selected frame. The lab returns the completed eyeglasses to the technician, and the patient then returns for fitting of the eyeglasses. The fit of the bridge and the nose pads are evaluated and modified as necessary. The fit of the temples and the temple arms that curve around the ear are inspected and adjusted as needed. The technician makes sure that the frame is level on the face and makes adjustments to the nose pads and/or temple arms as needed. Use code 92340 for fitting of monofocal lenses, code 92341 for bifocal lenses, and code 93242 for other multifocal lenses.

RVUs

Code	Work	PE	PE Non-Facility	MP	Total Non-Facility	Total Facility	Global
92340	0.37	0.14	0.61	0.04	1.02	0.55	XXX
92341	0.47	0.18	0.65	0.04	1.16	0.69	XXX
92342	0.53	0.20	0.67	0.04	1.24	0.77	XXX

92352-92353

92352 Fitting of spectacle prosthesis for aphakia; monofocal
92353 Fitting of spectacle prosthesis for aphakia; multifocal

Plain English Description

Following a separately reportable eye examination of a patient with aphakia (absence of the lens), the patient meets with a technician who evaluates anatomical facial characteristics and fits the spectacle prosthesis. The technician first determines the correct frame size by measuring the anatomical facial characteristics, including the distance between the pupils. The specifications are then submitted to a laboratory for manufacture of the prosthetic lenses and insertion into the selected frame. The lab returns the completed prosthetic spectacles to the technician, and the patient then returns for fitting. The fit of the bridge and the nose pads are evaluated and modified as necessary. The fit of the temples and the temple arms that curve around the ear are inspected and adjusted as needed. The technician makes sure that the frame is level on the face and makes adjustments to the nose pads and/or temple arms as needed. Use code 92352 for fitting of monofocal spectacle prosthetic lenses and code 93253 for multifocal spectacle prosthetic lenses.

RVUs

Code	Work	PE	PE Non-Facility	MP	Total Non-Facility	Total Facility	Global
92352	0.37	0.14	0.95	0.04	1.36	0.55	XXX
92353	0.50	0.19	1.00	0.04	1.54	0.73	XXX

92354-92355

92354 Fitting of spectacle mounted low vision aid; single element system
92355 Fitting of spectacle mounted low vision aid; telescopic or other compound lens system

Plain English Description

A technician fits a spectacle mounted low vision aid to the patient's eyeglasses (spectacles). Spectacle mounted low vision aids protrude from the frame. They may be designed for use with one or both eyes. Low vision aids may magnify objects. They may be telescopes, which aid distance vision, or microscopes that aid close-up vision. The existing frame is evaluated for proper fit and comfort. The low vision aid is then attached to the spectacles and the patient is instructed on proper use. The patient tests the low vision aid by using a reading card, holding it against the tip of the nose, and then pushing the card away until the words come in to focus. The distance needed to achieve the best focus is dependent on the size of the print or object the patient is reading or looking at. Use code 92354 for a single element low vision aid system, such as a magnifier. Use 92355 for a telescopic, microscopic, or other compound lens system.

RVUs

Code	Work	PE	PE Non-Facility	MP	Total Non-Facility	Total Facility	Global
92354	0.00	0.38	0.38	0.01	0.39	0.39	XXX
92355	0.00	0.59	0.59	0.02	0.61	0.61	XXX

92358

92358 Prosthesis service for aphakia, temporary (disposable or loan, including materials)

Plain English Description

A patient, whose natural lens has been removed, is fitted for a temporary lens that attaches to the patient's spectacles. The fit of the patient's current spectacles is checked and adjustments are made as needed to ensure that the best fit is achieved. The temporary prosthetic lens is positioned over the lens in the patient's current spectacles and secured. The temporary lens is only capable of providing the patient with somewhat improved vision. It does not completely correct vision. The patient is instructed on the characteristics of the temporary lens and assured that the permanent prosthetic lens will provide better visual acuity.

RVUs

Code	Work	PE	PE Non-Facility	MP	Total Non-Facility	Total Facility	Global
92358	0.00	0.31	0.31	0.01	0.32	0.32	XXX

92370-92371

92370 Repair and refitting spectacles; except for aphakia
92371 Repair and refitting spectacles; spectacle prosthesis for aphakia

Plain English Description

The patient's existing spectacles that have been damaged or that do not fit properly are repaired and refitted. This may involve replacement of nose pads or hinges or repair of broken rims, bridges, temples, or temple arms. Once the repairs are made, the technician makes sure that the frame is level on the face and makes adjustments to the nose pads and/or temple arms as needed. Report 92370 when this is performed for spectacles except for aphakia, and use code 92371 when this is performed for spectacle prosthetic lenses for aphakia.

RVUs

Code	Work	PE	PE Non-Facility	MP	Total Non-Facility	Total Facility	Global
92370	0.32	0.12	0.56	0.04	0.92	0.48	XXX
92371	0.00	0.32	0.32	0.01	0.33	0.33	XXX

92534

92534 Optokinetic nystagmus test

Plain English Description

An optokinetic nystagmus (OKN) test is performed. The patient is placed in front of a rotating drum of alternating black and white vertical strips and told not to focus on any one stripe. The physician observes the eyes and notes the response. The rotation is reversed and the process is repeated. The OKN test generates eye movements that resemble nystagmus. The physician observes the eye movement and evaluates the symmetry of the response. If the response is not symmetrical, it may be indicative of central nervous system pathology. The physician analyzes and interprets the results of the test.

RVUs

Code	Work	PE	PE Non-Facility	MP	Total Non-Facility	Total Facility	Global
92534	0.00	0.00	0.00	0.00	0.00	0.00	XXX

92540

92540 Basic vestibular evaluation, includes spontaneous nystagmus test with eccentric gaze fixation nystagmus, with recording, positional nystagmus test, minimum of 4 positions, with recording, optokinetic nystagmus test, bidirectional foveal and peripheral stimulation, with recording, and oscillating tracking test, with recording

(Do not report 92540 in conjunction with 92270, 92541, 92542, 92544, 92545)

Plain English Description

A vestibular evaluation is performed for nystagmus, which is a rapid, involuntary movement of the eye. Nystagmus tests are performed to identify the presence of a vestibular disorder characterized by vertigo (dizziness) and balance disturbance including the inability to maintain balance, to stand upright, or to walk with a normal gait. The physician first observes eye movement with the naked eye. The tests are performed with recording using electronystagmography (ENG). Horizontal electrodes are placed on the skin at the inner and outer aspect of each eye. A spontaneous nystagmus test with eccentric gaze and fixation is performed. For gaze testing, the patient first looks straight ahead for 30 seconds and then fixates on a target 30 degrees to the right for 10 seconds. The gaze is then returned to center. This is repeated with gaze directed to the left, up, and down. A positional nystagmus test is performed in a minimum of four positions to identify vertigo and nystagmus associated with certain movements of the head or body. Positional nystagmus is associated with disorders of function of the semicircular canals of the middle ear. Standard testing positions include head hanging forward, supine, supine with head turned to right, supine with head turned to left, lateral left, lateral right, or any other position that causes dizziness. Eye movement is recorded. A minimum of four positions are tested and any abnormal eye movement noted. An optokinetic nystagmus (OKN) test with bidirectional, foveal, or peripheral stimulation is performed. Eye movements are recorded and measured as the patient watches a series of targets moving simultaneously to the right and then to the left. The types of targets used include stripes on a rotating drum, a stream of lighted dots across a light bar, or a full-field array of moving stars or trees. The targets are moved at a rate of 300, 400, or 600 feet per second. This test generates eye movements that resemble nystagmus. The physician evaluates the symmetry of the response. If the response is not symmetrical it may be indicative of central nervous system pathology. An oscillating tracking test is performed. The test evaluates the patient's ability to keep a moving visual target registered on the fovea. The patient tracks a pendulum, metronome, light, or computer generated stimulus as it moves back and forth along a smooth arc or path. Eye movement is recorded. A computer is used to calculate the gain, expressed as target velocity divided by eye velocity. This calculation is compared to age-matched norms. Upon completion of the vestibular evaluation, the recordings are reviewed and interpreted, and the physician provides a written report of findings.

RVUs

Code	Work	PE	PE Non-Facility	MP	Total Non-Facility	Total Facility	Global
92540	1.50	1.72	1.72	0.05	3.27	3.27	XXX

92544

92544 Optokinetic nystagmus test, bidirectional, foveal or peripheral stimulation, with recording

(Do not report 92544 in conjunction with 92270, 92540 or the set of 92541, 92542, and 92545)

Plain English Description

An optokinetic nystagmus (OKN) test with bidirectional, foveal, or peripheral stimulation is performed with recording using electronystagmography (ENG). Horizontal electrodes are placed on the skin at the inner and outer aspect of each eye. Eye movements are recorded and measured as the patient watches a series of targets moving simultaneously to the right. The types of targets used include stripes on a rotating drum, a stream of lighted dots across a light bar, or a full-field array of moving stars or trees. The targets are moved at a rate of 300, 400, or 600 feet per second. The movement is then reversed and the procedure is repeated as the targets move simultaneously to the left. Eye movements are generated that resemble nystagmus. The physician reviews the recording and evaluates the symmetry of the response. If the response is not symmetrical, it may be indicative of central nervous system pathology.

RVUs

Code	Work	PE	PE Non-Facility	MP	Total Non-Facility	Total Facility	Global
92544	0.27	0.24	0.24	0.02	0.53	0.53	XXX

92545

92545 Oscillating tracking test, with recording

(Do not report 92545 in conjunction with 92270, 92540 or the set of 92541, 92542, and 92544)

Plain English Description

An oscillating tracking test is performed with recording using electronystagmography (ENG). Horizontal electrodes are placed on the skin at the inner and outer aspect of each eye. The test evaluates the patient's ability to keep a moving visual target registered on the fovea. The patient tracks a pendulum, metronome, light, or computer generated stimulus as it moves back and forth along a smooth pendular path. Eye movement is recorded. A computer is used to calculate the gain, expressed as target velocity, divided by eye velocity. This calculation is compared to age-matched norms. The physician reviews and interprets the results.

RVUs

Code	Work	PE	PE Non-Facility	MP	Total Non-Facility	Total Facility	Global
92545	0.25	0.23	0.23	0.02	0.50	0.50	XXX

92546

92546 Sinusoidal vertical axis rotational testing

(Do not report 92546 in conjunction with 92270)

Plain English Description

A sinusoidal vertical axis rotational test is performed with recording using electronystagmography (ENG). The test evaluates the integrity of the vestibular-ocular system. The test reflects the relationship between natural head and eye movements involved in the balance mechanism. Horizontal electrodes are placed on the skin at the inner and outer aspect of each eye. The patient sits in a rotational chair. A slow, harmonic acceleration rotation lasting 30-40 minutes is typically performed under computer control and eye movement is recorded. The physician reviews the recording and analyzes and interprets the results.

RVUs

Code	Work	PE	PE Non-Facility	MP	Total Non-Facility	Total Facility	Global
92546	0.29	3.38	3.38	0.03	3.70	3.70	XXX

99024

99024 Postoperative follow-up visit, normally included in the surgical package, to indicate that an evaluation and management service was performed during a postoperative period for a reason(s) related to the original procedure

(As a component of a surgical "package," see Surgery Guidelines)

Plain English Description

Postoperative follow-up visit, normally included as a part of the surgical codes, reporting an evaluation and management service given for a reason(s) related to the surgical procedure provided as an adjunct to the basic services.

RVUs

Code	Work	PE	PE Non-Facility	MP	Total Non-Facility	Total Facility	Global
99024	0.00	0.00	0.00	0.00	0.00	0.00	XXX

99071

99071 Educational supplies, such as books, tapes, and pamphlets, for the patient's education at cost to physician or other qualified health care professional

Plain English Description

Educational supplies are provided at the expense of the physician or other qualified health care professional and the patient is then billed for those educational supplies. This code may be used to bill for books, tapes, pamphlets, or other educational material.

RVUs

Code	Work	PE	PE Non-Facility	MP	Total Non-Facility	Total Facility	Global
99071	0.00	0.00	0.00	0.00	0.00	0.00	XXX

99151-99153

⊘ **99151 Moderate sedation services provided by the same physician or other qualified health care professional performing the diagnostic or therapeutic service that the sedation supports, requiring the presence of an independent trained observer to assist in the monitoring of the patient's level of consciousness and physiological status; initial 15 minutes of intraservice time, patient younger than 5 years of age**

⊘ **99152 Moderate sedation services provided by the same physician or other qualified health care professional performing the diagnostic or therapeutic service that the sedation supports, requiring the presence of an independent trained observer to assist in the monitoring of the patient's level of consciousness and physiological status; initial 15 minutes of intraservice time, patient age 5 years or older**

✚ **99153 Moderate sedation services provided by the same physician or other qualified health care professional performing the diagnostic or therapeutic service that the sedation supports, requiring the presence of an independent trained observer to assist in the monitoring of the patient's level of consciousness and physiological status; each additional 15 minutes intraservice time (List separately in addition to code for primary service)**

(Use 99153 in conjunction with 99151, 99152)

(Do not report 99153 in conjunction with 99155, 99156)

Plain English Description

Moderate sedation services are provided by the same physician or other qualified health care professional who is performing the diagnostic or therapeutic service requiring the sedation with an independent trained observer to assist in monitoring the patient. A patient assessment is performed. An intravenous line is inserted and fluids are administered as needed. A sedative agent is then administered. The patient is maintained under moderate sedation, with monitoring of the patient's consciousness level and physiological status that includes oxygen saturation, heart rate, and blood pressure. Following completion of the procedure, the physician or other qualified health care professional continues to monitor the patient until the patient has recovered from the sedation and can be turned over to nursing staff for continued care. Use 99151 for the first 15 minutes of intraservice time for a patient younger than 5 years old; 99152 for the first 15 minutes of intraservice time for a patient age 5 years or older; and 99153 for each additional 15 minutes.

RVUs

Code	Work	PE	PE Non-Facility	MP	Total Non-Facility	Total Facility	Global
99151	0.50	0.19	1.52	0.04	2.06	0.73	XXX
99152	0.25	0.08	1.22	0.04	1.51	0.37	XXX
99153	0.00	0.30	0.30	0.02	0.32	0.32	ZZZ

99155-99157

99155 Moderate sedation services provided by a physician or other qualified health care professional other than the physician or other qualified health care professional performing the diagnostic or therapeutic service that the sedation supports; initial 15 minutes of intraservice time, patient younger than 5 years of age

99156 Moderate sedation services provided by a physician or other qualified health care professional other than the physician or other qualified health care professional performing the diagnostic or therapeutic service that the sedation supports; initial 15 minutes of intraservice time, patient age 5 years or older

+ 99157 Moderate sedation services provided by a physician or other qualified health care professional other than the physician or other qualified health care professional performing the diagnostic or therapeutic service that the sedation supports; each additional 15 minutes intraservice time (List separately in addition to code for primary service)

(Use 99157 in conjunction with 99155, 99156)

(Do not report 99157 in conjunction with 99151, 99152)

Plain English Description

Moderate sedation services are provided by a physician or other qualified health care professional other than the one performing the diagnostic or therapeutic service requiring the sedation. A patient assessment is performed. An intravenous line is inserted and fluids are administered as needed. A sedative agent is then administered. The patient is maintained under moderate sedation, with monitoring of the patient's consciousness level and physiological status that includes oxygen saturation, heart rate, and blood pressure. Following completion of the procedure, the physician or other qualified health care professional continues to monitor the patient until the patient has recovered from the sedation and can be turned over to nursing staff for continued care. Use 99155 for the first 15 minutes of intraservice time for a patient younger than 5 years old; 99156 for the first 15 minutes of intraservice time for a patient age 5 years or older; and 99157 for each additional 15 minutes.

RVUs

Code	Work	PE	PE Non-Facility	MP	Total Non-Facility	Total Facility	Global
99155	1.90	0.32	0.32	0.21	2.43	2.43	XXX
99156	1.65	0.40	0.40	0.18	2.23	2.23	XXX
99157	1.25	0.46	0.46	0.11	1.82	1.82	ZZZ

99172

99172 Visual function screening, automated or semi-automated bilateral quantitative determination of visual acuity, ocular alignment, color vision by pseudoisochromatic plates, and field of vision (may include all or some screening of the determination[s] for contrast sensitivity, vision under glare)

(This service must employ graduated visual acuity stimuli that allow a quantitative determination of visual acuity [eg, Snellen chart]. This service may not be used in addition to a general ophthalmological service or an E/M service)

(Do not report 99172 in conjunction with 99173, 99174, 99177, 0469T)

Plain English Description

A vision function screening test is performed including automated or semi-automated bilateral quantitative determination of visual acuity, ocular alignment, color vision by pseudoisochromatic plates, and field of vision. The test may also include screening for determination of contrast sensitivity and vision under glare. This type of vision test is performed primarily on individuals whose occupations require that specific vision parameters be met for safety purposes. Typically, the specific vision requirements for the job are stated in the screening request so that the most appropriate evaluation of vision function is performed. Visual acuity is checked using a method that allows a quantitative determination, such as a Snellen chart. Both near and far vision may be evaluated, i.e., from 14 in to 20 ft. Ocular alignment tests extraocular muscle balance for both vertical and lateral phorias. Testing for phorias evaluates the relative directions assumed by the eyes during binocular fixation in the absence of a fusion stimulus. Color vision is evaluated using pseudoisochromatic plates to determine any color deficiencies. One type commonly used is the Ishihara color test. Pseudoisochromatic plates are composed of differently shaded dots that contain a number within the dot pattern. In a color vision deficient person, the number will not be visible on one or more of the plates. Field of vision testing is performed to determine if peripheral vision is normal. This may be accomplished using an apparatus onto which lights are projected. The patient fixates on a central spot and then indicates when he/she sees a small spot of light off to the side. Another method is to use a screen on which a white spot is moved horizontally and the patient indicates when the spot disappears. If needed, contrast sensitivity is tested to determine how well the patient sees low contrast images under conditions of low visibility. There are a number of tests available for contrast sensitivity including Pelli-Robson test, Bailey-Lovie chart, and Vision Contrast Test System (VCTS). Individuals with poor contrast sensitivity may fail to see edges, borders, or variations in brightness. Testing vision under glare may be performed using a Brightness Acuity Tester, which simulates three bright light conditions, including bright overhead sunlight, partly cloudy day, and bright overhead artificial light. If vision is diminished under these conditions, a glare disability may be present. The physician or technician performing the visual function screening interprets the results and provides a written report of findings.

RVUs

Code	Work	PE	PE Non-Facility	MP	Total Non-Facility	Total Facility	Global
99172	0.00	0.00	0.00	0.00	0.00	0.00	XXX

99173

99173 Screening test of visual acuity, quantitative, bilateral

(The screening test used must employ graduated visual acuity stimuli that allow a quantitative estimate of visual acuity [eg, Snellen chart]. Other identifiable services unrelated to this screening test provided at the same time may be reported separately [eg, preventive medicine services]. When acuity is measured as part of a general ophthalmological service or of an E/M service of the eye, it is a diagnostic examination and not a screening test.)

(Do not report 99173 in conjunction with 99172, 99174, 99177)

Plain English Description

A bilateral quantitative visual acuity screening test is performed, primarily on children, and used to test visual acuity only. Visual acuity is checked using a method that allows quantitative determination, such as a Snellen chart, which determines the smallest letters that the patient can read 14 to 20 feet away. Each eye is checked individually. Near vision may also be checked using a card held 14 inches away. In younger children, symbols, numbers, or gratings may be used instead of letters. Gratings are used to test vision in infants and consist of one gray and one black and white striped stimulus. The gray stimulus is placed over the striped stimulus. As the gray stimulus is slowly moved to expose the striped stimulus, an infant with normal vision will follow the striped stimulus. The physician or technician performing the visual acuity screening interprets the results and provides a written report of findings.

RVUs

Code	Work	PE	PE Non-Facility	MP	Total Non-Facility	Total Facility	Global
99173	0.00	0.08	0.08	0.01	0.09	0.09	XXX

99174

99174 Instrument-based ocular screening (eg, photoscreening, automated-refraction), bilateral; with remote analysis and report

(Do not report 99174 in conjunction with 92002-92014, 99172, 99173, 99177)

Plain English Description

Instrument based ocular screening such as photoscreening or automated refraction is performed on both eyes. Ocular photoscreening with interpretation and report is performed on an infant or child to screen for amblyogenic factors that reduce, dim, or blur vision, such as esotropia, exotropia, anisometropia, cataracts, ptosis, hyperopia, and myopia. Ocular photoscreening uses a specialized camera to detect and record eye reflexes in response to stimuli. The ocular photoscreening system is set up and the patient is positioned so that images can be obtained. Depending on the specific ocular photoscreening system used, the images may be reviewed by the physician, transmitted to a screening laboratory to be read analyzed remotely, and a report of findings submitted back to the physician (99174), or an automated analysis may be performed on site (99177) and the data provided to the physician. Automated refraction is performed with an automated refraction system that is used to obtain an auto-refractor reading, which is then analyzed by the software. A reading is also taken from the patient's glasses. Patient information is entered into the software. An automated phoropter is then used to obtain subjective refractions of both eyes. The results are compared with the automated refraction and the patient is again tested using the automated and subjective test results to ensure that the subjective testing results are those that the patient feels provide the best correction.

RVUs

Code	Work	PE	PE Non-Facility	MP	Total Non-Facility	Total Facility	Global
99174	0.00	0.16	0.16	0.01	0.17	0.17	XXX

99177

99177 Instrument-based ocular screening (eg, photoscreening, automated-refraction), bilateral; with on-site analysis

(Do not report 99177 in conjunction with 92002-92014, 99172, 99173, 99174)

(For retinal polarization scan, use 0469T)

Plain English Description

Instrument based ocular screening such as photoscreening or automated refraction is performed on both eyes. Ocular photoscreening with interpretation and report is performed on an infant or child to screen for amblyogenic factors that reduce, dim, or blur vision, such as esotropia, exotropia, anisometropia, cataracts, ptosis, hyperopia, and myopia. Ocular photoscreening uses a specialized camera to detect and record eye reflexes in response to stimuli. The ocular photoscreening system is set up and the patient is positioned so that images can be obtained. Depending on the specific ocular photoscreening system used, the images may be reviewed by the physician, transmitted to a screening laboratory to be read analyzed remotely, and a report of findings submitted back to the physician (99174), or an automated analysis may be performed on site (99177) and the data provided to the physician. Automated refraction is performed with an automated refraction system that is used to obtain an auto-refractor reading, which is then analyzed by the software. A reading is also taken from the patient's glasses. Patient information is entered into the software. An automated phoropter is then used to obtain subjective refractions of both eyes. The results are compared with the automated refraction and the patient is again tested using the automated and subjective test results to ensure that the subjective testing results are those that the patient feels provide the best correction.

RVUs

Code	Work	PE	PE Non-Facility	MP	Total Non-Facility	Total Facility	Global
99177	0.00	0.13	0.13	0.01	0.14	0.14	XXX

0100T

0100T Placement of a subconjunctival retinal prosthesis receiver and pulse generator, and implantation of intraocular retinal electrode array, with vitrectomy

(For initial programming of implantable intraocular retinal electrode array device, use 0472T)

Plain English Description

The placement of a subconjunctival retinal prosthesis receiver and pulse generator, and implantation of an intra-ocular retinal electrode array (artificial retina) may be used to restore sight to patients with blindness caused by retinal disease such as retinitis pigmentosa, hereditary retinal degeneration, and some forms of macular degeneration. The full device consists of an external video camera mounted on eyeglass frames that captures and feeds images to an external microcomputer worn on the body for processing. Signals are transmitted to the wireless receiver located in the subconjunctival space and the electrode array centered on the central macula and tacked to the retina. The system stimulates retinal ganglion cells and photoreceptor function. The conjunctiva and tenon layers are incised to expose the sclera. Vitrectomy is performed by making three small incisions (sclerotomies) in the pars plana just behind the iris and in front of the retina. A light pipe is inserted into one incision, a fluid infusion port is established in a second incision, and the vitrector is inserted through the third incision. The vitreous humor, a clear jelly-like substance is carefully cut and removed using suction. A saline solution is infused to maintain pressure and protect the retina, the light sensing tissue lining the back of the eye. The vitrector is removed and the receiver and electrode array are inserted and tacked into place on the retina. The fluid infusion line is removed after insuring that adequate fluid pressure has been established in the eye. The light pipe is removed and the sclerotomies are closed followed by closure of the tenon layers and the conjunctiva.

RVUs

Code	Work	PE	PE Non-Facility	MP	Total Non-Facility	Total Facility	Global
0100T	0.00	0.00	0.00	0.00	0.00	0.00	XXX

0198T

0198T Measurement of ocular blood flow by repetitive intraocular pressure sampling, with interpretation and report

(For tremor measurement with accelerometer(s) and/or gyroscope(s), use 95999)

Plain English Description

This test is performed using a miniaturized sensor embedded in a tonometer tip. The concave tonometer tip is designed in such a way that the cornea will take on the shape of the tonometer tip when positioned on the cornea. The tonometer tip is placed on the cornea and when a portion of the central cornea has conformed to the shape of the tip, the pressure sensor begins to take intraocular pressure (IOP) readings. The sensor can take up to 100 IOP readings per second. Measurement of ocular blood flow is obtained as the device generates a pulse wave that reflects heart rate and the mean difference between diastolic and systolic IOP. This measurement is called ocular pulse amplitude (OPA) and is a good indicator of the quality of ocular blood flow. This test is helpful in diagnosing normal tension glaucoma.

RVUs

Code	Work	PE	PE Non-Facility	MP	Total Non-Facility	Total Facility	Global
0198T	0.00	0.00	0.00	0.00	0.00	0.00	XXX

0207T

0207T Evacuation of meibomian glands, automated, using heat and intermittent pressure, unilateral

(For evacuation of meibomian glands using heat-delivered through wearable, open-eye eyelid treatment devices and manual gland expression, use 0563T. For evacuation of meibomian gland using manual gland expression only, use the appropriate evaluation and management code)

Plain English Description

The meibomian glands are located in the eyelids and secret the lipid layer of tear film that prevents rapid evaporation of tears. Dysfunction of meibomian glands is caused by blockage or thickening of the meibum. This can cause dry eye symptoms even in individuals who appear to produce adequate tearing. Using an automated device heat and intermittent pressure are applied unilaterally to the eyelid to relieve obstruction of the meibomian glands. The device consists of a compress and a sealed container that contains a heat source. Heat is released by an exothermic reaction. The compress remains on the eye and heat is applied for a predetermined length of time to help melt and liquefy the lipid secretions. Once the secretions have been liquefied, the device applies intermittent pressure to the eyelids to help express the lipid secretions.

RVUs

Code	Work	PE	PE Non-Facility	MP	Total Non-Facility	Total Facility	Global
0207T	0.00	0.00	0.00	0.00	0.00	0.00	XXX

0253T

0253T Insertion of anterior segment aqueous drainage device, without extraocular reservoir, internal approach, into the suprachoroidal space

(To report insertion of drainage device by external approach, use 66183)

(For arthrodesis, pre-sacral interbody technique, disc space preparation, discectomy, without instrumentation, with image guidance, includes bone graft when performed, L4-L5 interspace, L5-S1 interspace, use 22899)

Plain English Description

An anterior segment aqueous drainage device without an extraocular reservoir is inserted to treat chronic or progressive open angle glaucoma. The anterior chamber is accessed via a small, self-sealing incision in the cornea. The suprachoroidal space is accessed using a deep posterior scleral flap. A magnification lens such as a gonioscope is used to place and position the drainage device (shunt) at the angle of the anterior chamber. The drainage device traverses the sclera with the terminal end positioned in the suprachoroidal space.

RVUs

Code	Work	PE	PE Non-Facility	MP	Total Non-Facility	Total Facility	Global
0253T	0.00	0.00	0.00	0.00	0.00	0.00	YYY

0308T

0308T Insertion of ocular telescope prosthesis including removal of crystalline lens or intraocular lens prosthesis

(Do not report 0308T in conjunction with 65800-65815, 66020, 66030, 66600-66635, 66761, 66825, 66982-66986, 69990)

(For arthrodesis, pre-sacral interbody technique, including disc space preparation, discectomy, with posterior instrumentation, with image guidance, including bone graft, when performed, lumbar, L4-L5 interspace, use 22899)

(For motor function mapping using non-invasive navigated transcranial magnetic stimulation [nTMS] for therapeutic treatment planning, upper and lower extremity, use 64999)

Plain English Description

An ocular telescopic prosthesis is used to improve visual acuity in patients with end stage age-related macular degeneration (AMD). The wide angle micro optic telescope works in combination with optics of the cornea to create a telephoto system that can magnify objects 2.2-2.7 times their actual size. AMD typically causes a loss of vision in the central portion of the eye. When the telescopic lens is implanted into the cornea, incoming images are reflected onto the undamaged periphery of the retina. The procedure begins with a fairly large incision (12 mm) in the cornea or sclera, followed by removal of most of the crystalline lens or existing intraocular lens prosthesis, which is located behind the iris. The posterior capsule (elastic lens capsule) is left in place to help support the weight of the telescopic lens. The lens is secured to the posterior capsule with sutures brought through haptic loops on the lens. The patient will usually notice improved vision in the immediate post-operative period and will have the ability to focus on near and far objects using natural eye movements.

RVUs

Code	Work	PE	PE Non-Facility	MP	Total Non-Facility	Total Facility	Global
0308T	0.00	0.00	0.00	0.00	0.00	0.00	YYY

0329T

0329T Monitoring of intraocular pressure for 24 hours or longer, unilateral or bilateral, with interpretation and report

Plain English Description

A soft, hydrophilic, single use contact lens with an embedded pressure sensor is used to monitor intraocular pressure for a period of 24 hours or longer. The lens is inserted and the device activated during an outpatient visit with a physician/eye care professional. The pressure sensor in the contact lens detects circumferential changes (fluctuations in diameter) of the corneoscleral junction, which correlates to intraocular pressure (IOP). The readings are sent wirelessly to an antenna located in a circular adhesive worn around the eye. The antenna is connected to a portable recording unit where the data is saved and later downloaded to a computer program by the physician/eye care professional. The physician/eye care professional interprets the data collected, reports the results, and formulates an optimal treatment plan for the patient.

RVUs

Code	Work	PE	PE Non-Facility	MP	Total Non-Facility	Total Facility	Global
0329T	0.00	0.00	0.00	0.00	0.00	0.00	YYY

0330T

0330T Tear film imaging, unilateral or bilateral, with interpretation and report

Plain English Description

Ocular tear film is comprised of three layers, a lipid outer layer that helps retard tear evaporation, an aqueous middle layer and a mucus inner layer that anchors the tear film to the corneal epithelium. Tear film imaging is used to quantify the tear film by measuring the height of the tear meniscus, assess for instability of the tear film and identify dry spots. Tear film imaging can be accomplished using optical coherence tomography (OCT) or ellipsometry. OCT uses light waves to outline the anterior segment of the eye and the tear boundaries in a non-invasive, high resolution imaging technique. Ellipsometry measures the polarization states of light determined by the thickness and refractive index of the tear film lipid layer. Ellipsometry and OCT are often used together for multimodal tear film evaluation. These measurements aid in obtaining accurate refraction for fitting of corrective lenses and in successful outcome of cataract and refractive surgeries.

RVUs

Code	Work	PE	PE Non-Facility	MP	Total Non-Facility	Total Facility	Global
0330T	0.00	0.00	0.00	0.00	0.00	0.00	YYY

0333T

0333T Visual evoked potential, screening of visual acuity, automated, with report

(For visual evoked potential testing for glaucoma, use 0464T)

Plain English Description

Visual evoked potential (VEP) measures the functional integrity of the visual pathway (retina and optic nerve) to the visual cortex of the brain. Screening of visual acuity using an automated device is accomplished by placing the patient in front of a monitor, applying electrodes to the head/scalp, stimulating the visual field, and recording the brain's response. Automated visual stimuli can be in the form of strobe flash, flashing light-emitting diodes (LEDs), transient and steady state pattern reversal and pattern onset/offset (checkerboard). The test is useful for diagnosing amblyopia, refractive errors such as myopia (near-sightedness) and hyperopia (far-sightedness), astigmatism and strabismus in very young and/or non-verbal patients.

RVUs

Code	Work	PE	PE Non-Facility	MP	Total Non-Facility	Total Facility	Global
0333T	0.00	0.00	0.00	0.00	0.00	0.00	YYY

0378T-0379T

0378T Visual field assessment, with concurrent real time data analysis and accessible data storage with patient initiated data transmitted to a remote surveillance center for up to 30 days; review and interpretation with report by a physician or other qualified health care professional

0379T Visual field assessment, with concurrent real time data analysis and accessible data storage with patient initiated data transmitted to a remote surveillance center for up to 30 days; technical support and patient instructions, surveillance, analysis, and transmission of daily and emergent data reports as prescribed by a physician or other qualified health care professional

(For computer-aided animation and analysis of time series retinal images for the monitoring of disease progression, unilateral or bilateral, with interpretation and report, use 92499)

(0381T, 0382T, 0383T, 0384T, 0385T, 0386T have been deleted)

(For external heart rate and 3-axis accelerometer data recording up to 14 days to assess changes in heart rate and to monitor motion analysis for the purposes of diagnosing nocturnal epilepsy seizure events, including report, scanning analysis with report, review and interpretation by a physician or other qualified health care professional, use 95999)

Plain English Description

A non-invasive, at home procedure is performed by patients with age-related macular degeneration (AMD) to determine progression of disease using a tele-monitor and data management system. The patient performs a daily self test using a (ForeseeHome) AMD monitor to document surrogate markers of visual acuity over time. The data collected is transmitted via phoneline or modem to a (Notal Vision) Data Monitoring Center (DMC). The daily test is posted to a secure website accessible to both the patient and healthcare provider at any time. In the event of significant changes in the test, the DMC notifies the patient and healthcare provider to schedule an examination. Code 0378T is used by the physician or other qualified health care provider to bill for review and interpretation of the data with a written report. Code 0379T is used to bill for technical support and patient instruction related to the surveillance, analysis, and transmission of data associated with daily home use of the device.

RVUs

Code	Work	PE	PE Non-Facility	MP	Total Non-Facility	Total Facility	Global
0378T	0.00	0.00	0.00	0.00	0.00	0.00	XXX
0379T	0.00	0.00	0.00	0.00	0.00	0.00	XXX

0402T

0402T Collagen cross-linking of cornea, including removal of the corneal epithelium and intraoperative pachymetry, when performed (Report medication separately)

(Do not report 0402T in conjunction with 65435, 69990, 76514)

Plain English Description

A procedure is performed using riboflavin (Vitamin B2) and ultraviolet-A (UV-A) light to strengthen collagen bonds in the cornea. Collagen cross linking increases the number of fiber anchors that bond collagen together and is a first line treatment for keratoconus, pellucid marginal degeneration, and ectasia caused by LASIK. Collagen cross linking may also be used to treat corneal ulcers and infection, and to bond Intacs, tiny plastic discs, following surgical implantation within the cornea. With the patient reclining, a lid speculum is placed and anesthetic eye drops are instilled. Ultrasound pachymetry may be performed to measure the pre-treatment thickness of the cornea. A thin layer of epithelium may be removed for more rapid absorption of riboflavin, or the treatment may proceed with the epithelium in place as a transepithelial procedure. Riboflavin eye drops are instilled at measured intervals or until the riboflavin is detected in the anterior chamber of the eye using a blue filter on a slit lamp. The UV-A light is then applied to the corneal apex for a prescribed period of time. Ultrasound pachymetry may be performed to measure the post-treatment thickness of the cornea as well. Antibiotic eye drops are instilled and a bandage contact lens is applied following the treatment.

RVUs

Code	Work	PE	PE Non-Facility	MP	Total Non-Facility	Total Facility	Global
0402T	0.00	0.00	0.00	0.00	0.00	0.00	XXX

0444T-0445T

0444T Initial placement of a drug-eluting ocular insert under one or more eyelids, including fitting, training, and insertion, unilateral or bilateral

0445T Subsequent placement of a drug-eluting ocular insert under one or more eyelids, including re-training, and removal of existing insert, unilateral or bilateral

(For insertion and removal of drug-eluting implant into lacrimal canaliculus, use 68841)

Plain English Description

A procedure is performed to insert a drug eluting ocular insert under the eyelid. The drug-eluting ocular insert is a thin, sterile, multi-layered device comprised of an inner polymeric support with an outer layer impregnated with the drug/medication. The device sits under the eyelid and rests on the conjunctiva. Lacrimal fluid permeates the outer membrane and the drug is released by controlled diffusion. To insert the device, the intercanthal distance is measured and the appropriate size insert is selected. A topical ophthalmic anesthetic may be instilled in the eye. The upper eyelid is manually retracted and the insert is placed in the upper fornix. The lower eyelid is then retracted manually or with a scleral depressor and the bottom half of the insert is placed in the lower fornix. A portion of the insert should be visible in the medial canthus. The patient is instructed in proper care of the insert and how to manage it when slightly displaced. To remove the insert, the lower lid is retracted manually to expose the bottom half of the insert and the exposed ring is manually gripped and pulled from the eye. Code 0444T reports the initial fitting, training, and placement of a drug-eluting ocular insert under one or more eyelids, unilaterally or bilaterally. Code 0445T reports the removal of an existing insert, re-training, and replacement of a drug-eluting ocular insert, such as for continued medication dosing, either unilaterally or bilaterally.

RVUs

Code	Work	PE	PE Non-Facility	MP	Total Non-Facility	Total Facility	Global
0444T	0.00	0.00	0.00	0.00	0.00	0.00	YYY
0445T	0.00	0.00	0.00	0.00	0.00	0.00	YYY

0449T-0450T

0449T Insertion of aqueous drainage device, without extraocular reservoir, internal approach, into the subconjunctival space; initial device

✚ **0450T Insertion of aqueous drainage device, without extraocular reservoir, internal approach, into the subconjunctival space; each additional device (List separately in addition to code for primary procedure)**

(Use 0450T in conjunction with 0449T)

(For removal of aqueous drainage device without extraocular reservoir, placed into the subconjunctival space via internal approach, use 92499)

(For insertion of intraocular anterior segment drainage device into the trabecular meshwork without concomitant cataract removal with intraocular lens implant, use 0671T)

(For insertion or replacement of a permanently implantable aortic counterpulsation ventricular assist system, endovascular approach, and programming of sensing and therapeutic parameters, use 33999)

(For removal of permanently implantable aortic counterpulsation ventricular assist system, use 33999)

(For relocation of skin pocket with replacement of implanted aortic counterpulsation ventricular assist device, mechano-electrical skin interface and electrodes, use 33999)

(For repositioning of previously implanted aortic counterpulsation ventricular assist device, use 33999)

(For programming device evaluation [in person] with iterative adjustment of the implantable mechano-electrical skin interface and/or external driver, use 33999)

(For interrogation device evaluation [in person] with analysis, review, and report, use 33999)

Plain English Description

A procedure is performed to insert an aqueous drainage device into the subconjunctival space to lower intraocular pressure. Increased intraocular pressure can cause chronic, degenerative, optic nerve damage and lead to loss of vision. The angle is inspected using a gonioprism to locate the desired position to seat the drainage device. A gonioscope is placed on the surgical microscope to visualize the trabecular meshwork. A small, temporal, clear corneal (AB interno phaco) incision is made to access the anterior chamber, which is then filled with viscoelastic fluid. The anterior chamber is traversed to the pupillary margin with an inserter preloaded with the drainage device. The trabecular meshwork is again identified using the gonioprism and the device is released through the trabecular meshwork and into Schlemm's canal. The inserter is withdrawn and the anterior chamber is irrigated to remove viscoelastic fluid and blood. The anterior chamber is then filled with saline to achieve a normal physiologic pressure. Code 0449T reports the insertion of an initial aqueous drainage device, without an extraocular reservoir, through an internal approach into the subconjunctival space. Code 0450T reports the insertion of each additional device.

RVUs

Code	Work	PE	PE Non-Facility	MP	Total Non-Facility	Total Facility	Global
0449T	0.00	0.00	0.00	0.00	0.00	0.00	YYY
0450T	0.00	0.00	0.00	0.00	0.00	0.00	YYY

0464T

0464T Visual evoked potential, testing for glaucoma, with interpretation and report

(To report percutaneous/minimally invasive [indirect visualization] arthrodesis of the sacroiliac joint with image guidance, use 27279)

(For visual evoked potential screening of visual acuity, use 0333T)

Plain English Description

The visual evoked potential (VEP) test for glaucoma is used to assess the integrity of the afferent visual pathway by projecting a patterned stimulus (light flash or black/white pattern reversal) to generate a response that is captured by scalp electrodes along the occipital cortex. The VEP is displayed as a graph diagraming the speed and strength of the VEP as positive and negative waveforms. VEP may be indicated for non-verbal individuals or to confirm an intact visual pathway in patients complaining of vision loss without organic pathology.

RVUs

Code	Work	PE	PE Non-Facility	MP	Total Non-Facility	Total Facility	Global
0464T	0.00	0.00	0.00	0.00	0.00	0.00	YYY

0465T

0465T Suprachoroidal injection of a pharmacologic agent (does not include supply of medication)

(To report intravitreal injection/implantation, see 67025, 67027, 67028)

(For insertion, revision or replacement, or removal of chest wall respiratory sensor electrode or electrode array, see 64582, 64583, 64584)

Plain English Description

Suprachoroidal injection of a pharmacologic agent may be used to treat diseases of the posterior segment of the eye (retina, macula, optic nerve) including age-related macular degeneration, retinal vein occlusion, and diabetic macular edema. The suprachoroidal space is a narrow zone between the choroid and sclera extending from the limbus to the optic nerve. The suprachoroidal space includes a defined inner layer of the choroid (Brach's membrane) and a transition zone in the outer layer close to the sclera consisting of several fibrous lamellae of variable thickness. A hand held microinjector comprised of a syringe and very fine needle is used to inject the pharmacologic agent. The needle is inserted through the sclera and the fluid is injected into the posterior segment where it disperses around the globe and throughout the choroid and retina. Code 0465T reports the injection procedure. The pharmacologic agent is reported separately.

RVUs

Code	Work	PE	PE Non-Facility	MP	Total Non-Facility	Total Facility	Global
0465T	0.00	0.00	0.00	0.00	0.00	0.00	YYY

0469T

0469T Retinal polarization scan, ocular screening with on-site automated results, bilateral

(Do not report 0469T in conjunction with 92002, 92004, 92012, 92014)

(For ocular photoscreening, see 99174, 99177)

Plain English Description

A retinal polarization scan detects polarization changes generated by modulated polarized light as it passes through a unique pattern of nerve fibers in the fovea of the retina. The scan may be used to detect strabismus and other defocusing problems causing small angles of visual misalignment that may lead to amblyopia. The retina of each eye is scanned in a circular movement using a polarized near infrared light. Polarization-related changes from the light reflected back from the ocular fundus are then analyzed by the device and an automated report is generated.

RVUs

Code	Work	PE	PE Non-Facility	MP	Total Non-Facility	Total Facility	Global
0469T	0.00	0.00	0.00	0.00	0.00	0.00	XXX

0472T-0473T

0472T Device evaluation, interrogation, and initial programming of intraocular retinal electrode array (eg, retinal prosthesis), in person, with iterative adjustment of the implantable device to test functionality, select optimal permanent programmed values with analysis, including visual training, with review and report by a qualified health care professional

0473T Device evaluation and interrogation of intraocular retinal electrode array (eg, retinal prosthesis), in person, including reprogramming and visual training, when performed, with review and report by a qualified health care professional

(For implantation of intraocular electrode array, use 0100T)

(For reprogramming of implantable intraocular retinal electrode array device, use 0473T)

Plain English Description

A retinal prosthesis placed either epiretinally or subretinally delivers electrical impulses using a micro-photodiode array or micro-electrode array to treat profound vision loss by stimulating secondary nerve cells along the visual pathway. The device may be used in patients with vision loss caused by retinitis pigmentosa and age-related macular degeneration. These codes report in person device evaluation and interrogation, with review and report. Code 0472T includes initial programming, with iterative adjustment of the device for functionality testing and selection of optimal permanent programmed values with analysis, including visual training for the individual. Code 0473T reports reprogramming and visual training, when performed.

RVUs

Code	Work	PE	PE Non-Facility	MP	Total Non-Facility	Total Facility	Global
0472T	0.00	0.00	0.00	0.00	0.00	0.00	XXX
0473T	0.00	0.00	0.00	0.00	0.00	0.00	XXX

0474T

0474T Insertion of anterior segment aqueous drainage device, with creation of intraocular reservoir, internal approach, into the supraciliary space

Plain English Description

Insertion of an anterior segment aqueous drainage device with creation of an intraocular reservoir using internal approach into the supraciliary space may be performed to treat mild to moderate primary open angle glaucoma. The cylinder shaped fenestrated device rests in the supraciliary space between the sclera and ciliary body and creates a channel for aqueous fluid to flow out, reducing intraocular pressure. The device is loaded onto a guidewire attached to a hand held applier. Using microscope guidance, the applier is introduced through the paracentesis and guided across the anterior chamber to the implantation site. The guidewire is advanced into the supraciliary space with the device positioned just posterior to the scleral spur at the iris root. The device is delivered into the supraciliary space leaving only the most proximal retention ring of the device in the anterior chamber. The guidewire is then retracted and the applier and guidewire are removed from the anterior chamber.

RVUs

Code	Work	PE	PE Non-Facility	MP	Total Non-Facility	Total Facility	Global
0474T	0.00	0.00	0.00	0.00	0.00	0.00	XXX

0506T

0506T Macular pigment optical density measurement by heterochromatic flicker photometry, unilateral or bilateral, with interpretation and report

Plain English Description

Macular pigment optical density (MPOD) measurement using heterochromatic flicker photometry is a non-invasive test used to assess the thickness of a yellow pigment in the center (fovea) of the macula. This carotenoid pigment is comprised of lutein, meso-zeaxanthin and zeaxanthin. Low levels of macular pigment (MP) is associated with age-related macular degeneration (AMD). Meso-zeaxanthin and zeaxanthin are found in the cone cells of the fovea and lutein is found in the rod cells of the para-fovea. MP absorbs harmful blue light, protecting the photoreceptors in the eye from damage. Blue light is emitted from the sun, light bulbs, computer and tablet screens, television and cellphone displays. The density of MP varies naturally among individuals and may thin with aging, inherited genetic traits, dietary and lifestyle choices. Symptoms of MP thinning include loss of visual acuity, contrast sensitivity and glare recovery and photophobia. The eyes are assessed separately. With the patient positioned in front of the optical camera and the eye focused on a target inside, a monochromatic blue light with alternating and varying wavelengths and relative intensities is introduced and the responses are observed and downloaded into a computer software program. MPOD measurements ranges from 0-1 with low density identified as a range of 0-0.20, mid density 0.21-0.44 and high density 0.45-10. The lower the density score, the higher the risk for developing AMD. Code 0506T reports unilateral or bilateral MPOD measurement using heterochromatic photometry with computer software interpretation and report for comprehensive patient risk assessment and treatment plan.

RVUs

Code	Work	PE	PE Non-Facility	MP	Total Non-Facility	Total Facility	Global
0506T	0.00	0.00	0.00	0.00	0.00	0.00	XXX

0507T

0507T Near infrared dual imaging (ie, simultaneous reflective and transilluminated light) of meibomian glands, unilateral or bilateral, with interpretation and report

(For external ocular photography, use 92285)

(For tear film imaging, use 0330T)

Plain English Description

Near-infrared (NIR) dual imaging using simultaneous reflective and trans-illuminated light may be used to assess meibomian gland function. The meibomian glands (MG) are located along the margins of the upper and lower eyelids and secrete a lipid/protein fluid that helps to prevent tear film evaporation. These tiny glands number approximately 30 in the upper lid and 25 in the lower lid. Meibomian gland dysfunction (MGD) is characterized by obstruction of the MG orifices, lid margin hyperemia and telangiectasia, gland atrophy and compromise of the quality of tear film leading to functional dry eyes. MGD may be caused by infection, immune and autoimmune disease/disorders and hypersensitivity reaction. Symptoms include sandy/gritty discomfort, dryness, local irritation and blurred vision. Imaging is performed using a trans-illumination device to evert the eyelid with application of a NIR light source that images the lid. A camera captures and records high quality, high definition images of the MG. which are downloaded into a computer software program. Code 0507T reports unilateral or bilateral meibomian gland assessment using NIR dual imaging (simultaneous reflective and trans-illuminated light) with computer software interpretation and report for comprehensive patient risk assessment and treatment plan.

RVUs

Code	Work	PE	PE Non-Facility	MP	Total Non-Facility	Total Facility	Global
0507T	0.00	0.00	0.00	0.00	0.00	0.00	XXX

0509T

0509T Electroretinography (ERG) with interpretation and report, pattern (PERG)

(For full-field ERG, use 92273)

(For multifocal ERG, use 92274)

Plain English Description

Electroretinography (ERG) is performed to diagnose and evaluate conditions affecting the retina and optic nerve by measuring the electrical activity generated by retinal cells in response to light stimulus. Mydriatic drops are instilled to dilate the pupil. The patient is dark or light adapted for several minutes first, depending on the protocol. ERG electrodes are then placed on the surface of the eye using dim red illumination. There are several types of electrodes that can be used including contact lens electrodes placed over the cornea, or gold Mylar tape containing electrodes placed between the lower lid and the sclera or cornea. The electrodes are connected to a recording device. The head is kept stationary using head and chin supports. The eye is then stimulated by flashes of light from a bright light source such as LEDs, a strobe lamp, or a full-field dome with its own light source. The response to light flashes are first recorded in the dark and then with background lighting. The flash of light causes an electrical response in the retina that is captured by the electrodes, recorded, and represented digitally as a waveform. Pattern ERG (PERG) is a specialized type of electroretinography in which electrical responses are elicited from the retina by alternating checkerboard stimuli aimed at the central retina. Retinal responses to hundreds of stimuli are averaged to get a measurable signal. The test is then evaluated, which correlates to the health of the optic nerve and provides information about the ganglion cells and can serve as a test for early recognition of glaucoma. A written interpretation of findings is provided.

RVUs

Code	Work	PE	PE Non-Facility	MP	Total Non-Facility	Total Facility	Global
0509T	0.40	1.78	1.78	0.02	2.20	2.20	XXX

0514T

✚ **0514T Intraoperative visual axis identification using patient fixation (List separately in addition to code for primary procedure)**

(Use 0514T in conjunction with 66982, 66984)

Plain English Description

The use of an intraoperative visual axis identification device utilizing patient fixation can streamline the placement and anchoring of an intraocular lens (IOL) during cataract surgery. A transparent suction device is placed on the surface of the eye and the patient follows the surgeon's fixation instructions. Measurements are taken of the visual axis, a functional line connecting the fixation point with the nodal point of the eye, and translated into a reference landmark to guide the capsulotomy and placement of the IOL within the capsular bag surgically. Precise placement ensures better stability against IOL tilt and decentration to provide the best optical performance of an IOL, including increased visual quality and decreased night vision problems such as halo and glare. Report intraoperative visual axis identification separately, in addition to the primary procedure code.

RVUs

Code	Work	PE	PE Non-Facility	MP	Total Non-Facility	Total Facility	Global
0514T	0.00	0.00	0.00	0.00	0.00	0.00	ZZZ

0563T

0563T Evacuation of meibomian glands, using heat delivered through wearable, open-eye eyelid treatment devices and manual gland expression, bilateral

(For evacuation of meibomian gland using manual gland expression only, use the appropriate evaluation and management code)

Plain English Description

Meibomian glands, located in the eyelids, secrete oils on the surface of the eye to slow the evaporation of tears, which keeps the eyelids moist. There are between 25 and 40 meibomian glands in the upper eyelid and 20 to 30 glands in the lower lid. When meibomian glands become blocked, they stop secreting oil, causing tears to evaporate too rapidly. This condition is known as Meibomian Gland Dysfunction (MGD) and it is considered the primary pathology behind dry eye syndrome. In addition, blocked meibomian glands may also trigger blepharitis, or eyelid inflammation. Evacuation of meibomian glands uses a combination of heat and gentle manual pressure on the inner and outer eyelids to melt and then dissipate the waxy build-up clogging the meibomian glands. An anesthetic eye drop is delivered. A warming device is then slipped between the upper eyelid and the cornea to apply heat to the inside and outside surfaces of the eyelid to melt the waxy buildup clogging the glands. The clinician then applies manual compression to the outside of the eyelid to help remove the blockage. Care is taken to protect the cornea. The full procedure takes less than 10 minutes.

RVUs

Code	Work	PE	PE Non-Facility	MP	Total Non-Facility	Total Facility	Global
0563T	0.00	0.00	0.00	0.00	0.00	0.00	YYY

0604T-0606T

0604T Optical coherence tomography (OCT) of retina, remote, patient-initiated image capture and transmission to a remote surveillance center, unilateral or bilateral; initial device provision, set-up and patient education on use of equipment

0605T Optical coherence tomography (OCT) of retina, remote, patient-initiated image capture and transmission to a remote surveillance center, unilateral or bilateral; remote surveillance center technical support, data analyses and reports, with a minimum of 8 daily recordings, each 30 days

0606T Optical coherence tomography (OCT) of retina, remote, patient-initiated image capture and transmission to a remote surveillance center, unilateral or bilateral; review, interpretation and report by the prescribing physician or other qualified health care professional of remote surveillance center data analyses, each 30 days

(Do not report 0604T, 0605T, 0606T in conjunction with 99457, 99458)

Plain English Description

Remote, at home optical coherence tomography (OCT) is a diagnostic device for use in patients with neovascular retinal diseases leading to blindness such as exudative age-related macular degeneration. OCT allows visualization of retinal structures to assess treatment needs for eye diseases. Remote, home operated OCT is a light weight device that patients can use after a short tutorial to generate readable images without the need for a technician. The home device sits on a table like an upright computer monitor with a screen on top and built-in angled binoculars that the patient rests the eyes on while gripping the device at the base. After the diagnostic OCT test is done, a proprietary algorithm that uses AI machine learning performs an automated analysis of the data and generates a report, which is sent to the treating physician for review whenever a specified change in disease activity is noted. This technology allows for individualized retinal disease management without waiting for the next clinic visit or symptoms to appear. Home OCT can catch retinal fluid as it appears, map areas of intra-and subretinal fluid volume and thickness, and detect leakage and choroidal neovascularization early, thereby maintaining better vision. Report 0604T for initial device provision, set-up, and tutorial of image capture and data transmission. Report 0605T for data analyses and reports with remote surveillance center support on a minimum of 8 daily recordings, every 30 days. Use 0606T for the professional review, interpretation, and report of the remote surveillance center data analyses generated, every 30 days.

RVUs

Code	Work	PE	PE Non-Facility	MP	Total Non-Facility	Total Facility	Global
0604T	0.00	0.00	0.00	0.00	0.00	0.00	YYY
0605T	0.00	0.00	0.00	0.00	0.00	0.00	YYY
0606T	0.00	0.00	0.00	0.00	0.00	0.00	YYY

0616T-0618T

0616T Insertion of iris prosthesis, including suture fixation and repair or removal of iris, when performed; without removal of crystalline lens or intraocular lens, without insertion of intraocular lens

0617T Insertion of iris prosthesis, including suture fixation and repair or removal of iris, when performed; with removal of crystalline lens and insertion of intraocular lens

(Do not report 0617T in conjunction with 66982, 66983, 66984)

0618T Insertion of iris prosthesis, including suture fixation and repair or removal of iris, when performed; with secondary intraocular lens placement or intraocular lens exchange

(Do not report 0618T in conjunction with 66985, 66986)

(Do not report 0616T, 0617T, 0618T in conjunction with 66600, 66680, 66682)

Plain English Description

An iris prosthesis is a silicone disc used to treat a defective, missing, or damaged iris due to acquired defects or trauma, congenital aniridia, or albinism. The flexible disc is customized to the patient and colorized with a fixed diameter pupil to match the other eye. The back is a black surface that blocks light and allows it to pass only through the pupil. The outer diameter is cut to size with a trephine at the time of surgery to fit the patient and can be implanted into the capsular bag, the ciliary sulcus through a sclerocorneal approach or via 'open sky' approach during a concomitant penetrating keratoplasty. The disc is folded and inserted manually with forceps or an autoinjector. It can also be inserted with suture fixation, depending on the patient's anatomy and surgical needs, or fixed with sutures later if progressive zonulopathy causes displacement. Artificial iris placement should be done at the same time as an intraocular lens (IOL) placement for cataract patients who also need an iris prosthesis in order to avoid worsening vision with glare sensitivity when the cataract is treated first separately. Report 0616T for insertion of iris prosthesis alone and 0617T when done with removal of the crystalline lens and insertion of an IOL for cataract patients. Report 0618T for a prosthetic iris insertion with a secondary IOL placement or lens exchange.

RVUs

Code	Work	PE	PE Non-Facility	MP	Total Non-Facility	Total Facility	Global
0616T	0.00	0.00	0.00	0.00	0.00	0.00	YYY
0617T	0.00	0.00	0.00	0.00	0.00	0.00	YYY
0618T	0.00	0.00	0.00	0.00	0.00	0.00	YYY

0621T-0622T

0621T Trabeculostomy ab interno by laser

0622T Trabeculostomy ab interno by laser; with use of ophthalmic endoscope

(Do not report 0621T, 0622T in conjunction with 92020)

Plain English Description

To prevent glaucoma from progressing to blindness, it must be treated to reduce intraocular pressure (IOP). Trabeculostomy ab interno laser therapy is a treatment option known as micro-invasive glaucoma surgery (MIGS), which has minimal risk with a high safety rate. The ab interno approach decreases IOP by improving aqueous outflow through a direct opening created by multiple laser channels in the trabecular meshwork, made from within the anterior chamber. This opening communicates to the outer wall of Schlemm's canal and the collector channels. A probe of 500 µm diameter is used. A clear corneal incision of 0.8 mm minimum is made. The anterior chamber (AC) is filled with viscoelastic to prevent its collapse. The goniolens is then placed on the cornea, or an ophthalmic endoscope is used (0622T). The probe is advanced with the bevel up through the AC into direct contact with the trabecular meshwork. A foot pedal system allows the physician to apply the laser. Approximately 10 laser microchannels are then created over 90 degrees about 500 µm apart. Blood and microbubbles may appear as reflux from Schlemm's canal. This procedure is thought to produce an additional beneficial effect in the form of pneumatic canaloplasty that dilates Schlemm's canal. After the laser is applied and the photoablated tissue turns to gas, it is theorized that these microbubbles push against the outer wall of the canal and the adjacent collector channels, thereby opening the outflow tract even wider.

RVUs

Code	Work	PE	PE Non-Facility	MP	Total Non-Facility	Total Facility	Global
0621T	0.00	0.00	0.00	0.00	0.00	0.00	YYY
0622T	0.00	0.00	0.00	0.00	0.00	0.00	YYY

0660T-0661T

● **0660T Implantation of anterior segment intraocular nonbiodegradable drug-eluting system, internal approach**

(Report medication separately)

● **0661T Removal and reimplantation of anterior segment intraocular nonbiodegradable drug-eluting implant**

(Report medication separately)

Plain English Description

The insertion of drug-eluting implants provides targeted intraocular therapy for different ocular conditions and diseases. One such implantable, nonbiodegradable device provides long-term, continuous release of a proprietary formulation of glaucoma medication, travoprost, into the anterior chamber. The drug reduces intraocular pressure for significant treatment improvement, bypassing the corneal barrier and the need for patient compliance with an eyedrop regimen. The titanium implant is made up of a scleral anchor that affixes to the trabecular meshwork, the drug reservoir and a titrating elution membrane that facilitates the drug's release. A 2.4 mm incision is made in the eye and the anterior chamber angle is viewed via an ab interno approach. The scleral anchor is seated in the trabecular meshwork and securely attached by nudging it. The titanium implant is removed and replaced in a similar micro-invasive surgical procedure when depleted. Report 0660T for implantation of the nonbiodegradable drug-eluting system into the anterior segment via internal approach and 0661T for removal and reimplantation.

RVUs

Code	Work	PE	PE Non-Facility	MP	Total Non-Facility	Total Facility	Global
0660T	0.00	0.00	0.00	0.00	0.00	0.00	YYY
0661T	0.00	0.00	0.00	0.00	0.00	0.00	YYY

0671T

● **0671T Insertion of anterior segment aqueous drainage device into the trabecular meshwork, without external reservoir, and without concomitant cataract removal, one or more**

(Do not report 0671T in conjunction with 66989, 66991)

(For complex extracapsular cataract removal with intraocular lens implant without concomitant aqueous drainage device, use 66982)

(For extracapsular cataract removal with intraocular lens implant without concomitant aqueous drainage device, use 66984)

(For insertion of anterior segment drainage device into the subconjunctival space, use 0449T)

Plain English Description

An anterior segment aqueous drainage device(s) without an extraocular reservoir is inserted via an internal approach to treat chronic or progressive open angle glaucoma. A small, self-sealing incision is made in the cornea and the incision is deepened to access the anterior chamber. A magnification lens such as a gonioscope is used to place and position the drainage device (shunt) at the angle of the anterior chamber. The terminal end of the drainage device is positioned in the trabecular meshwork. It is not necessary to close the small corneal incision as it is so small that it will self-seal. The aqueous drainage device (one or more) is inserted independently and not in conjunction with cataract removal.

RVUs

Code	Work	PE	PE Non-Facility	MP	Total Non-Facility	Total Facility	Global
0671T	0.00	0.00	0.00	0.00	0.00	0.00	YYY

0699T

● **0699T Injection, posterior chamber of eye, medication**

Plain English Description

The posterior chamber lies between the iris and the lens and in front of the vitreous. The posterior chamber of the eye is involved in the production and circulation of aqueous humor. The clear, watery fluid is secreted by the ciliary body into the posterior chamber and then flows into the anterior chamber through the pupil. The aqueous humor helps maintain intraocular pressure, provides nutrients to the cornea and lens, and removes waste from the cornea and lens. For an injection of medication into the posterior chamber of the eye, the patient is positioned supine with head and neck supported. A topical ophthalmic anesthetic is applied and the eye is then cleansed with antiseptic. An eyelid speculum is placed and the injection site is marked. A fine needle with attached syringe is inserted through the cornea, across the anterior chamber and behind the iris toward the lens. The medication is then injected into the cavity. The needle is withdrawn, antibiotic eye drops are instilled and the eye may be patched.

RVUs

Code	Work	PE	PE Non-Facility	MP	Total Non-Facility	Total Facility	Global
0699T	0.00	0.00	0.00	0.00	0.00	0.00	YYY

0704T

● **0704T Remote treatment of amblyopia using an eye tracking device; device supply with initial set-up and patient education on use of equipment**

Plain English Description

An eye tracking device is a digital treatment device for amblyopia, or lazy eye, commonly treated by wearing a patch. Amblyopia occurs in early childhood when abnormal visual pathway development causes one eye to be favored while the other remains lazy and may wander inward or outward, not working in conjunction with the other eye. If not treated, it can remain present in later years and cause visual impairment. The eye tracking device replaces the patch and provides binocular treatment that helps the child develop stereotactic vision. Treatment is carried out while the child watches a choice of age-appropriate video content while at home under remote physician supervision and real-time monitoring from the cloud. The child wears a pair of proprietary shutter glasses that are connected to the system wirelessly, which controls eye occlusion and measures distance and tilt. While the childe watches the monitor, the optical image sensors track and record gaze position, presence and attention, taking samples 90 times every second to create a comprehensive eye movement pattern. All data collected is uploaded to the remote cloud platform and processed in real time to provide immediate analysis results to both caregivers and providers for treatment assessment. It can also help predict neurological conditions by detecting certain abnormal eye movement patterns. Report 0704T for provision of the device with initial set-up and patient education. Report 0705T for surveillance center technical support with data transmission and analysis, with a minimum of 18 training hours, each 30 days, and 0706T for the professional's interpretation and report, per calendar month.

RVUs

Code	Work	PE	PE Non-Facility	MP	Total Non-Facility	Total Facility	Global
0704T	0.00	0.00	0.00	0.00	0.00	0.00	XXX

0705T

● **0705T Remote treatment of amblyopia using an eye tracking device; surveillance center technical support including data transmission with analysis, with a minimum of 18 training hours, each 30 days**

Plain English Description

An eye tracking device is a digital treatment device for amblyopia, or lazy eye, commonly treated by wearing a patch. Amblyopia occurs in early childhood when abnormal visual pathway development causes one eye to be favored while the other remains lazy and may wander inward or outward, not working in conjunction with the other eye. If not treated, it can remain present in later years and cause visual impairment. The eye tracking device replaces the patch and provides binocular treatment that helps the child develop stereotactic vision. Treatment is carried out while the child watches a choice of age-appropriate video content while at home under remote physician supervision and real-time monitoring from the cloud. The child wears a pair of proprietary shutter glasses that are connected to the system wirelessly, which controls eye occlusion and measures distance and tilt. While the childe watches the monitor, the optical image sensors track and record gaze position, presence and attention, taking samples 90 times every second to create a comprehensive eye movement pattern. All data collected is uploaded to the remote cloud platform and processed in real time to provide immediate analysis results to both caregivers and providers for treatment assessment. It can also help predict neurological conditions by detecting certain abnormal eye movement patterns. Report 0704T for provision of the device with initial set-up and patient education. Report 0705T for surveillance center technical support with data transmission and analysis, with a minimum of 18 training hours, each 30 days, and 0706T for the professional's interpretation and report, per calendar month.

RVUs

Code	Work	PE	PE Non-Facility	MP	Total Non-Facility	Total Facility	Global
0705T	0.00	0.00	0.00	0.00	0.00	0.00	XXX

0706T

● **0706T Remote treatment of amblyopia using an eye tracking device; interpretation and report by physician or other qualified health care professional, per calendar month**

(Do not report 0704T, 0705T, 0706T in conjunction with 92065, when performed on the same day)

(Do not report 0704T, 0705T, 0706T in conjunction with 0687T, 0688T, when reported during the same period)

Plain English Description

An eye tracking device is a digital treatment device for amblyopia, or lazy eye, commonly treated by wearing a patch. Amblyopia occurs in early childhood when abnormal visual pathway development causes one eye to be favored while the other remains lazy and may wander inward or outward, not working in conjunction with the other eye. If not treated, it can remain present in later years and cause visual impairment. The eye tracking device replaces the patch and provides binocular treatment that helps the child develop stereotactic vision. Treatment is carried out while the child watches a choice of age-appropriate video content while at home under remote physician supervision and real-time monitoring from the cloud. The child wears a pair of proprietary shutter glasses that are connected to the system wirelessly, which controls eye occlusion and measures distance and tilt. While the childe watches the monitor, the optical image sensors track and record gaze position, presence and attention, taking samples 90 times every second to create a comprehensive eye movement pattern. All data collected is uploaded to the remote cloud platform and processed in real time to provide immediate analysis results to both caregivers and providers for treatment assessment. It can also help predict neurological conditions by detecting certain abnormal eye movement patterns. Report 0704T for provision of the device with initial set-up and patient education. Report 0705T for surveillance center technical support with data transmission and analysis, with a minimum of 18 training hours, each 30 days, and 0706T for the professional's interpretation and report, per calendar month.

RVUs

Code	Work	PE	PE Non-Facility	MP	Total Non-Facility	Total Facility	Global
0706T	0.00	0.00	0.00	0.00	0.00	0.00	XXX

G0117

G0117 Glaucoma screening for high risk patients furnished by an optometrist or ophthalmologist

RVUs

Global: XXX

	Work	PE	MP	Total
Facility	0.45	1.38	0.02	1.85
Non-facility	0.45	1.38	0.02	1.85

Modifiers (PAR)

Mod 50	Mod 51	Mod 62	Mod 80
0	0	0	0

Pub 100

G0117: Pub 100-02, 15, 280.1; 100-04, 18, 1.2, 70.1.1, 70.1.1.2

CCI Edits

Refer to Appendix A for CCI edits.

G0118

G0118 Glaucoma screening for high risk patient furnished under the direct supervision of an optometrist or ophthalmologist

RVUs

Global: XXX

	Work	PE	MP	Total
Facility	0.17	1.06	0.01	1.24
Non-facility	0.17	1.06	0.01	1.24

Modifiers (PAR)

Mod 50	Mod 51	Mod 62	Mod 80
0	0	0	0

Pub 100

G0118: Pub 100-02, 15, 280.1; 100-04, 18, 1.2, 70.1.1, 70.1.1.2

CCI Edits

Refer to Appendix A for CCI edits.

V2020

ⓘV2020 Frames, purchases

RVUs

Global: XXX

	Work	PE	MP	Total
Facility	0.00	0.00	0.00	0.00
Non-facility	0.00	0.00	0.00	0.00

Modifiers (PAR)

Mod 50	Mod 51	Mod 62	Mod 80
9	9	9	9

CCI Edits

Refer to Appendix A for CCI edits.

V2100

V2100 Sphere, single vision, plano to plus or minus 4.00, per lens

RVUs

Global: XXX

	Work	PE	MP	Total
Facility	0.00	0.00	0.00	0.00
Non-facility	0.00	0.00	0.00	0.00

Modifiers (PAR)

Mod 50	Mod 51	Mod 62	Mod 80
9	9	9	9

CCI Edits

Refer to Appendix A for CCI edits.

V2103

V2103 Spherocylinder, single vision, plano to plus or minus 4.00d sphere, .12 to 2.00d cylinder, per lens

RVUs

Global: XXX

	Work	PE	MP	Total
Facility	0.00	0.00	0.00	0.00
Non-facility	0.00	0.00	0.00	0.00

Modifiers (PAR)

Mod 50	Mod 51	Mod 62	Mod 80
9	9	9	9

CCI Edits

Refer to Appendix A for CCI edits.

V2200

V2200 Sphere, bifocal, plano to plus or minus 4.00d, per lens

RVUs

Global: XXX

	Work	PE	MP	Total
Facility	0.00	0.00	0.00	0.00
Non-facility	0.00	0.00	0.00	0.00

Modifiers (PAR)

Mod 50	Mod 51	Mod 62	Mod 80
9	9	9	9

CCI Edits

Refer to Appendix A for CCI edits.

V2203

V2203 Spherocylinder, bifocal, plano to plus or minus 4.00d sphere, .12 to 2.00d cylinder, per lens

RVUs Global: XXX

	Work	PE	MP	Total
Facility	0.00	0.00	0.00	0.00
Non-facility	0.00	0.00	0.00	0.00

Modifiers (PAR)

Mod 50	Mod 51	Mod 62	Mod 80
9	9	9	9

CCI Edits

Refer to Appendix A for CCI edits.

V2303

V2303 Spherocylinder, trifocal, plano to plus or minus 4.00d sphere, .12-2.00d cylinder, per lens

RVUs Global: XXX

	Work	PE	MP	Total
Facility	0.00	0.00	0.00	0.00
Non-facility	0.00	0.00	0.00	0.00

Modifiers (PAR)

Mod 50	Mod 51	Mod 62	Mod 80
9	9	9	9

CCI Edits

Refer to Appendix A for CCI edits.

V2744

ⓘV2744 Tint, photochromatic, per lens

RVUs Global: XXX

	Work	PE	MP	Total
Facility	0.00	0.00	0.00	0.00
Non-facility	0.00	0.00	0.00	0.00

Modifiers (PAR)

Mod 50	Mod 51	Mod 62	Mod 80
9	9	9	9

CCI Edits

Refer to Appendix A for CCI edits.

V2745

ⓘV2745 Addition to lens; tint, any color, solid, gradient or equal, excludes photochromatic, any lens material, per lens

RVUs Global: XXX

	Work	PE	MP	Total
Facility	0.00	0.00	0.00	0.00
Non-facility	0.00	0.00	0.00	0.00

Modifiers (PAR)

Mod 50	Mod 51	Mod 62	Mod 80
9	9	9	9

CCI Edits

Refer to Appendix A for CCI edits.

V2750

ⓘV2750 Anti-reflective coating, per lens

RVUs Global: XXX

	Work	PE	MP	Total
Facility	0.00	0.00	0.00	0.00
Non-facility	0.00	0.00	0.00	0.00

Modifiers (PAR)

Mod 50	Mod 51	Mod 62	Mod 80
9	9	9	9

CCI Edits

Refer to Appendix A for CCI edits.

V2755

ⓘV2755 U-v lens, per lens

RVUs Global: XXX

	Work	PE	MP	Total
Facility	0.00	0.00	0.00	0.00
Non-facility	0.00	0.00	0.00	0.00

Modifiers (PAR)

Mod 50	Mod 51	Mod 62	Mod 80
9	9	9	9

CCI Edits

Refer to Appendix A for CCI edits.

HCPCS Coding

V2760

V2760 Scratch resistant coating, per lens

RVUs

Global: XXX

	Work	PE	MP	Total
Facility	0.00	0.00	0.00	0.00
Non-facility	0.00	0.00	0.00	0.00

Modifiers (PAR)

Mod 50	Mod 51	Mod 62	Mod 80
9	9	9	9

CCI Edits

Refer to Appendix A for CCI edits.

V2782

ⓘV2782 Lens, index 1.54 to 1.65 plastic or 1.60 to 1.79 glass, excludes polycarbonate, per lens

RVUs

Global: XXX

	Work	PE	MP	Total
Facility	0.00	0.00	0.00	0.00
Non-facility	0.00	0.00	0.00	0.00

Modifiers (PAR)

Mod 50	Mod 51	Mod 62	Mod 80
9	9	9	9

CCI Edits

Refer to Appendix A for CCI edits.

V2784

ⓘV2784 Lens, polycarbonate or equal, any index, per lens

RVUs

Global: XXX

	Work	PE	MP	Total
Facility	0.00	0.00	0.00	0.00
Non-facility	0.00	0.00	0.00	0.00

Modifiers (PAR)

Mod 50	Mod 51	Mod 62	Mod 80
9	9	9	9

CCI Edits

Refer to Appendix A for CCI edits.

V2787

⊘V2787 Astigmatism correcting function of intraocular lens

RVUs

Global: XXX

	Work	PE	MP	Total
Facility	0.00	0.00	0.00	0.00
Non-facility	0.00	0.00	0.00	0.00

Modifiers (PAR)

Mod 50	Mod 51	Mod 62	Mod 80
9	9	9	9

Pub 100

V2787: Pub 100-04, 32, 120.1, 120.2

CCI Edits

Refer to Appendix A for CCI edits.

V2788

⊘V2788 Presbyopia correcting function of intraocular lens

RVUs

Global: XXX

	Work	PE	MP	Total
Facility	0.00	0.00	0.00	0.00
Non-facility	0.00	0.00	0.00	0.00

Modifiers (PAR)

Mod 50	Mod 51	Mod 62	Mod 80
9	9	9	9

Pub 100

V2788: Pub 100-04, 32, 120.1, 120.2

CCI Edits

Refer to Appendix A for CCI edits.

Modifiers

The CPT® code selected must be the one that most closely describes the service(s) and/or procedure(s) documented by the physician. However, sometimes certain services or procedures go above and beyond the definition of the assigned CPT code definition and require further clarification. For these and other reasons, modifiers were developed and implemented by the American Medical Association (AMA), the Centers for Medicare & Medicaid Services (CMS), and local Part B Medicare Administrative Contractors (MACs). These modifiers give health care providers a way to indicate that a service or procedure has been modified by some circumstance but still meets the code definition. Modifiers were designed to expand on the information already provided by the current CPT coding system and to assist in the prompt processing of claims. A CPT modifier is a two-digit numeric character reported with the appropriate CPT code, and is intended to transfer specific information regarding a certain procedure or service.

Modifiers are used to ensure payment accuracy, coding consistency, and editing under the outpatient prospective payment system (OPPS), and are also mandated for private practitioners (solo and multiple), ambulatory surgery centers (ASCs), and other outpatient hospital services.

Modifier Usage

Modifiers are indicated when:

- A service/procedure contains a professional and technical component but only one is applicable
- A service/procedure was performed by more than one physician and/or in more than one location
- The service reported was increased or decreased from that of the original definition
- Unusual events occurred during the service/procedure
- A service/procedure was performed more than once
- A bilateral procedure was performed
- Only part of a service was performed
- An adjunctive service was performed

If a modifier is to be utilized, the following must be documented in the patient's medical record:

- The special circumstances indicating the need to add that modifier
- All pertinent information and an adequate definition of the service/procedure performed supporting the use of the assigned modifier

CPT Modifiers

CPT modifiers are attached to the end of the appropriate CPT code. For professional services, modifiers will be reported as an attachment to the CPT code as reported on the CMS-1500 form, and for outpatient services, modifiers will be reported as an attachment to the CPT code as reported in the UB-04 form locator FL 44.

Some modifiers are strictly informational:

- Modifier 57, identifying a decision for surgery at the time of an evaluation and management service

Other modifiers are informational and indicate additional reimbursement may be warranted:

- Modifier 22, identifying an unusual service that is greater than what is typical for that code

Placement of a modifier after a CPT code does not always ensure additional reimbursement. A special report may be required if the service is rarely provided, unusual, variable, or new. The report should include pertinent information and an adequate definition or description of the nature, extent, and need for the service/procedure. It should also describe the complexity of the patient's symptoms, pertinent history and physical findings, diagnostic and therapeutic procedures, final diagnosis and associated conditions, and follow-up care.

Like CPT codes, the use of modifiers requires understanding of the purpose of each modifier. It is also important to identify when a modifier has been expanded or restricted by a payer prior to submission of a claim. There will also be times when the coding and modifier information issued by the CMS differs from that of CPT's coding guidelines on the usage of modifiers.

Note: For the purposes of this Modifier chapter, payer-specific information is indicated with the symbol ⓘ. It is good to check with individual payers to determine modifier acceptance.

The following is a list of CPT modifiers:

22 Increased Procedural Services

When the work required to provide a service is substantially greater than typically required, it may be identified by adding modifier 22 to the usual procedure code. Documentation must support the substantial additional work and the reason for the additional work (i.e., increased intensity, time, technical difficulty of procedure, severity of patient's condition, physical and mental effort required).

Note: This modifier should not be appended to an E/M service.

ⓘ Claims submitted to Medicare, Medicaid, and other payers containing modifier 22 for unusual procedural services that do not have attached supporting documentation that illustrates the unusual distinction of the services will be processed as if the procedure codes were not appended

Modifiers

with this modifier. Some payers might suspend the claims and request additional information from the provider, but this is the exception rather than the rule. For most payers, this modifier includes additional reimbursement to the provider for the additional work.

23 Unusual Anesthesia

Occasionally, a procedure, which usually requires either no anesthesia or local anesthesia, because of unusual circumstances must be done under general anesthesia. This circumstance may be reported by adding modifier 23 to the procedure code of the basic service.

24 Unrelated Evaluation and Management Service by the Same Physician or Other Qualified Health Care Professional During a Postoperative Period

The physician or other qualified health care professional may need to indicate that an evaluation and management service was performed during a postoperative period for a reason(s) unrelated to the original procedure. This circumstance may be reported by adding modifier 24 to the appropriate level of E/M service.

ⓘ By payer definition, a postoperative period is one that has been determined to be included in the payment for the procedure that was performed. During this time, the provider offers treatment for the procedure in follow-up visits, which is not reimbursed. Medicare has postoperative periods for procedures of 0, 10, or 90 days (number of days applicable for each procedure can be found in the Federal Register or Physician Fee Schedule (RBRVS) put out by CMS.) Commercial payers may vary the postoperative days; check with each to determine the appropriate number of days for a given procedure.

25 Significant, Separately Identifiable Evaluation and Management Service by the Same Physician or Other Qualified Health Care Professional on the Same Day of the Procedure or Other Service

It may be necessary to indicate that on the day a procedure or service identified by a CPT code was performed, the patient's condition required a significant, separately identifiable E/M service above and beyond the other service provided or beyond the usual preoperative or postoperative care associated with the procedure that was performed. A significant, separately identifiable E/M service is defined or substantiated by documentation that satisfies the relevant criteria for the respective E/M service to be reported (see **Evaluation and Management Services Guidelines** for instructions on determining level of E/M service). The E/M service may be prompted by the symptom or condition for which the procedure and/or service was provided. As such, different diagnoses are not required for reporting of the E/M service on the same date. This circumstance may be reported by adding modifier 25 to the appropriate level of E/M service.

Note: This modifier is not used to report an E/M service that resulted in a decision to perform surgery. See modifier 57. For significant, separately identifiable non-E/M services, see modifier 59.

ⓘ Modifier 25 Guidelines

1. Modifier 25 should be used only when a visit is separately payable when billed in addition to a minor surgical procedure (any surgery with a 0- or 10-day postoperative period per Medicare). Payment for pre- and postoperative work in minor procedures is included in the payment for the procedure. Where the decision to perform the minor procedure is typically made immediately before the service (e.g., sutures are needed to close a wound), it is considered to be a routine preoperative service and an E/M service should not be billed in addition to the minor procedure. In circumstances in which the physician provides an E/M service that is beyond the usual pre- and postoperative work for the service, the visit may be billed with a modifier 25. A modifier is not needed if the visit was performed the day before a minor surgery because the global period for minor procedures does not include the day prior to the surgery.
2. The global surgery policy does not apply to services of other physicians who may be rendering services during the pre- or postoperative period unless the physician is a member of the same group as the operating physician.
3. The provider must determine if the E/M service for which they are billing is clearly distinct from the surgical service. When the decision to perform the minor procedure is typically done immediately before the procedure is rendered, the visit should not be billed separately.

26 Professional Component

Certain procedures are a combination of a physician or other qualified health care professional component and a technical component. When the physician or other qualified health care professional component is reported separately, the service may be identified by adding modifier 26 to the usual procedure number.

ⓘ To determine which codes have both a professional and technical component for CMS, review the Federal Register and/or the Physician Fee Schedule for a breakdown. Usually commercial payers go along with CMS determinations of professional and technical components. Some CPT codes are already broken down into professional and technical components. Examples of these are:

93005 Electrocardiography, routine ECG with at least 12 leads; tracing only, without interpretation and report (technical component)

93010 Electrocardiography, routine ECG with at least 12 leads; interpretation and report only

Modifier 26 should not be appended to either of the codes because the nomenclature itself has determined that they are already technical or professional components.

32 Mandated Services

Services related to *mandated* consultation and/or related services (e.g., third-party payer, governmental, legislative, or regulatory requirement) may be identified by adding modifier 32 to the basic procedure.

33 Preventive Services

When the primary purpose of the service is the delivery of an evidence based service in accordance with the US Preventive Services Task Force A or B rating in effect and other preventive services identified in preventive services mandates (legislative or regulatory), the service may be identified by adding 33 to the procedure. For separately reported services specifically identified as preventive, the modifier should not be used.

47 Anesthesia by Surgeon

Regional or general anesthesia provided by the surgeon may be reported by adding modifier 47 to the basic service. (This does not include local anesthesia.)

Note: Modifier 47 would not be used as a modifier for the anesthesia procedures.

ⓘ This service is not covered by Medicare and many state Medicaid programs. Commercial payers and managed care organizations may cover this additional service.

50 Bilateral Procedure

Unless otherwise identified in the listings, bilateral procedures that are performed at the same session should be identified by adding modifier 50 to the appropriate 5-digit code.

Note: This modifier should not be appended to designated "add-on" codes (see Appendix D*).

ⓘ Reported as a one-line item for Medicare claims with modifier 50 appended to the end of the code. Some carriers or payers may request that bilateral procedures be reported with the LT and RT HCPCS Level II modifiers as two-line items.

51 Multiple Procedures

When multiple procedures, other than E/M Services, Physical Medicine and Rehabilitation services, or provision of supplies (e.g., vaccines), are performed at the same session by the same individual, the primary procedure or service may be reported as listed. The additional procedure(s) or service(s) may be identified by appending modifier 51 to the additional procedure or service code(s).

Note: This modifier should not be appended to designated "add-on" codes (see Appendix D*).

52 Reduced Services

Under certain circumstances a service or procedure is partially reduced or eliminated at the discretion of the physician or other qualified health care professional. Under these circumstances the service provided can be identified by its usual procedure number and the addition of modifier 52, signifying that the service is reduced. This provides a means of reporting reduced services without disturbing the identification of the basic service.

Note: For hospital outpatient reporting of a previously scheduled procedure/service that is partially reduced or cancelled as a result of extenuating circumstances or those that threaten the well-being of the patient prior to or after administration of anesthesia, see modifiers 73 and 74 (see modifiers approved for ASC hospital outpatient use).

ⓘ Procedures reported with modifier 52 are typically billed at a reduced amount. Most payers do not require documentation to support the use of modifier 52 and will reimburse the procedure at a reduced level.

53 Discontinued Procedure

Under certain circumstances, the physician or other qualified health care professional may elect to terminate a surgical or diagnostic procedure. Due to extenuating circumstances or those that threaten the well being of the patient, it may be necessary to indicate that a surgical or diagnostic procedure was started but discontinued. This circumstance may be reported by adding modifier 53 to the code reported by the individual for the discontinued procedure.

Note: This modifier is not used to report the elective cancellation of a procedure prior to the patient's anesthesia induction and/or surgical preparation in the operating suite. For outpatient hospital/ambulatory surgery center (ASC) reporting of a previously scheduled procedure/service that is partially reduced or cancelled as a result of extenuating circumstances or those that threaten the well being of the patient prior to or after administration of anesthesia, see modifiers 73 and 74 (see modifiers approved for ASC hospital outpatient use).

54 Surgical Care Only

When 1 physician or other qualified health care professional performs a surgical procedure and another provides preoperative and/or postoperative management, surgical services may be identified by adding modifier 54 to the usual procedure number.

ⓘ Both claims submitted by the surgeon and the other provider must report the date patient care was assumed and relinquished in block 19 of the CMS-1500 or electronic equivalent. Both the surgeon and the other provider must keep a copy of the written transfer agreement in the patient's medical record. Both providers will use the same CPT code, but they will use different modifiers that identify which portion of care they provided.

55 Postoperative Management Only

When 1 physician or other qualified health care professional performed the postoperative management and another performed the surgical procedure, the postoperative component may be identified by adding modifier 55 to the usual procedure number.

ⓘ Both providers will use the same CPT code, but they will use different modifiers that identify which portion of care they provided.

56 Preoperative Management Only

When 1 physician or other qualified health care professional performed the preoperative care and evaluation and another performed the surgical procedure, the preoperative component may be identified by adding modifier 56 to the usual procedure number.

ⓘ Both providers will use the same CPT code, but will they will use different modifiers that identify which portion of care they provided. Some payers do not allow modifier 56 as by their definition the pre-operative care is included in the surgical component.

57 Decision for Surgery

An evaluation and management service that resulted in the initial decision to perform the surgery may be identified by adding modifier 57 to the appropriate level of E/M service.

ⓘ Major Surgical Procedures

Major Surgery with a global period of 90 days (as defined by Medicare) include the day before and the day of surgery. For example, a visit the day before or the same day could be properly billed in addition to a cholecystotomy if the need for the surgery was found during the encounter. Modifier 57 should be added to the E/M code. Billing for a visit would not be appropriate if the physician was only discussing the upcoming surgical procedure.

Procedures with a 90 day global period are considered to be major surgery, as categorized by CMS. The RBRVS (Resource-Based Relative Value Scale) manual or Federal Register lists the global period for all procedure codes eligible for payment by Medicare.

ⓘ Minor Surgical Procedures

Procedures with a 0 or 10 day global period are considered to be minor or endoscopic surgeries, as categorized by CMS. E/M visits by the same physician on the same day as a minor surgery or endoscopy are included in the payment for the procedure, unless a significant, separately identifiable service is also performed.

58 Staged or Related Procedure or Service by the Same Physician or Other Qualified Health Care Professional During the Postoperative Period

It may be necessary to indicate that the performance of a procedure or service during the postoperative period was: (a) planned or anticipated (staged); (b) more extensive than the original procedure; or (c) for therapy following a diagnostic surgical procedure. This circumstance may be reported by adding modifier 58 to the staged or related procedure.

Note: For treatment of a problem that requires a return to the operating/procedure room (eg, unanticipated clinical condition), see modifier 78.

ⓘ Modifier 58 must be used for purposes of identifying procedures performed by the original physician during the postoperative period of the original procedure, within the constraints of the modifier's definition. These procedures cannot be repeat operations (unless the procedures are more extensive than the original procedure) and cannot be for the treatment of complications requiring a return trip to the operating room.

The existence of modifier 58 does not negate the global fee concept. Services that are included in CPT as multiple sessions or are defined as including multiple services or events may not be billed with this modifier. This modifier is designed to allow a method of reporting additional, related surgeries that are due to a progression of the disease and are not to be used to avoid global surgery edits applicable to staged procedures.

Modifier 58 should be used on surgical codes only and has no effect on the payment amount. It should not be used with the following codes because the codes are defined as "one or more sessions or stages":

66762	67031	67218
66821	67208	67220
66840	67210	67229

59 Distinct Procedural Service

Under certain circumstances, it may be necessary to indicate that a procedure or service was distinct or independent from other non-E/M services performed on the same day. Modifier 59 is used to identify procedures/services, other than E/M services, that are not normally reported together, but are appropriate under the circumstances. Documentation must support a different session, different procedure or surgery, different site or organ system, separate incision/excision, separate lesions, or separate injury (or area of injury in extensive injuries) not ordinarily encountered or performed on the same day by the same individual. However, when another already established modifier is more appropriate, it should be used rather than modifier 59. Only if no more descriptive modifier is available, and the use of modifier 59 best explains the circumstances, should modifier 59 be used.

Note: Modifier 59 should not be appended to an E/M service. To report a separate and distinct E/M service with a non-E/M service performed on the same date, see modifier 25.

ⓘ Modifier 59 was established to demonstrate that multiple, yet distinct, services were provided to a patient on the same date of service by the same provider. Because distinct procedures or services rendered on the same day by the same physician cannot be easily identified and properly adjudicated by simply listing the CPT procedure codes, modifier 59 assists the payer or Medicare carrier in applying the appropriate reimbursement protocol. If the modifier is not used in these circumstances, services may be denied, with the explanation of benefits stating that the payer does not reimburse for this service because it is part of another service that was performed at the same time.

62 Two Surgeons

When 2 surgeons work together as primary surgeons performing distinct part(s) of a procedure, each surgeon should report his/her distinct operative work by adding modifier 62 to the procedure code and any associated add-on code(s) for that procedure as long as both surgeons continue to work together as primary surgeons. Each surgeon should report the co-surgery once using the same procedure code. If additional procedure(s) (including add-on procedures[s]) are performed during the same surgical session, separate code(s) may also be reported with modifier 62 added.

Note: If a co-surgeon acts as an assistant in the performance of additional procedure(s), other than those reported with the modifier 62, during the same surgical session, those services may be reported using separate procedure code(s) with modifier 80 or modifier 82 added, as appropriate.

ⓘ According to Medicare, payment for the two physicians is based on the two physicians splitting 125% of the allowed charge(s). Check with other payers to determine payment based on this modifier. This modifier should not be confused with modifier 80 (assistant surgeon).

63 Procedure Performed on Infants Less Than 4 kg

Procedures performed on neonates and infants up to a present body weight of 4 kg may involve significantly increased complexity and physician or other qualified health care professional work commonly associated with these patients. This circumstance may be reported by adding modifier 63 to the procedure number.

Note: Unless otherwise designated, this modifier may only be appended to procedures/services listed in the 20100-69990 code series and 92920, 92928, 92953, 92960, 92986, 92987, 92990, 92997, 92998, 93312, 93313, 93314, 93315, 93316, 93317, 93318, 93452, 93505, 93563, 93564, 93568, 93580, 93582, 93590, 93591, 93592, 93593, 93594, 93595, 93596, 93597, 93598, 93615, 93616 from the Medicine/Cardiovascular section. Modifier 63 should not be appended to any CPT codes listed in the **Evaluation and Management Services, Anesthesia, Radiology, Pathology/Laboratory,** or **Medicine** sections (other than those identified above from the Medicine/Cardiovascular section).

66 Surgical Team

Under some circumstances, highly complex procedures (requiring the concomitant services of several physicians or other qualified health care professionals, often of different specialties, plus other highly skilled, specially trained personnel, various types of complex equipment) are carried out under the "surgical team" concept. Such circumstances may be identified by each participating individual with the addition of modifier 66 to the basic procedure number used for reporting services.

ⓘ Each surgeon that participates in the procedure would report the same CPT code with modifier 66. Only surgical CPT codes (10021-69990) should be used with modifier 66 unless otherwise stated by the payer.

76 Repeat Procedure or Service by Same Physician or Other Qualified Health Care Professional

It may be necessary to indicate that a procedure or service was repeated by the same physician or other qualified health care professional subsequent to the original procedure or service. This circumstance may be reported by adding modifier 76 to the repeated procedure or service.

Note: This modifier should not be appended to an E/M service.

77 Repeat Procedure or Service by Another Physician or Other Qualified Health Care Professional

It may be necessary to indicate that a basic procedure or service was repeated by another physician or other qualified health care professional subsequent to the original procedure or service. This circumstance may be reported by adding modifier 77 to the repeated procedure or service.

Note: This modifier should not be appended to an E/M service.

ⓘ Appending this modifier does not guarantee payment of the repeat procedure, but will assist in determining duplicate billings for the procedure.

78 Unplanned Return to the Operating/Procedure Room by the Same Physician or Other Qualified Health Care Professional Following Initial Procedure for a Related Procedure During the Postoperative Period

It may be necessary to indicate that another procedure was performed during the postoperative period of the initial procedure (unplanned procedure following initial procedure). When this procedure is related to the first, and requires the use of an operating/procedure room, it may be reported by adding modifier 78 to the related procedure. (For repeat procedures, see modifier 76.)

ⓘ Medicare includes specific medical and/or surgical care for postoperative complications within the global surgical package and does not allow additional payment. Included in the global surgical package are "additional medical and surgical services required of the surgeon during the postoperative period of the surgery because of complications which do not require additional trips to the operating room."

79 Unrelated Procedure or Service by the Same Physician or Other Qualified Health Care Professional During the Postoperative Period

The individual may need to indicate that the performance of a procedure or service during the postoperative period was unrelated to the original procedure. This circumstance may be reported by using modifier 79. (For repeat procedures on the same day, see modifier 76.)

ⓘ When billing for an unrelated procedure by the same physician during the postoperative period of an original procedure, a new postoperative period will begin with the subsequent procedure. A different ICD-10-CM diagnosis should be indicated on the claim.

80 Assistant Surgeon

Surgical assistant services may be identified by adding modifier 80 to the usual procedure number(s).

ⓘ Some surgical procedures are not eligible for this modifier; check the Medicare physician fee schedule or with other payers to determine payment eligibility

81 Minimum Assistant Surgeon

Minimum surgical assistant services are identified by adding modifier 81 to the usual procedure number.

ⓘ Check with payers to determine if payment is allowed for this modifier.

82 Assistant Surgeon (When Qualified Resident Surgeon Not Available)

The unavailability of a qualified resident surgeon is a prerequisite for use of modifier 82 appended to the usual procedure code number(s).

ⓘ In some hospitals with residency programs, Medicare pays through the medical program or graduate medical education (GME) program. Because of this, they will not reimburse for a resident when they are used as an assistant surgeon. Although under special circumstances, payment may be made if there is a emergent situation that is life-threatening.

90 Reference (Outside) Laboratory

When laboratory procedures are performed by a party other than the treating or reporting physician or other qualified health care professional, the procedure may be identified by adding modifier 90 to the usual procedure number.

ⓘ Check with payers to determine if the provider may bill for the laboratory procedure if not performed by the provider.

91 Repeat Clinical Diagnostic Laboratory Test

In the course of treatment of the patient, it may be necessary to repeat the same laboratory test on the same day to obtain subsequent (multiple) test results. Under these circumstances, the laboratory test performed can be identified by its usual procedure number and the addition of modifier 91.

Note: This modifier may not be used when tests are rerun to confirm initial results; due to testing problems with specimens or equipment; or for any other reason when a normal, one-time, reportable result is all that is required. This modifier may not be used when other code(s) describe a series of test results (eg, glucose tolerance tests, evocative/suppression testing). This modifier may only be used for laboratory test(s) performed more than once on the same day on the same patient.

92 Alternative Laboratory Platform Testing

When laboratory testing is performed using a kit or transportable instrument that wholly or in part consists of a single use, disposable analytical chamber, the service may be identified by adding modifier 92 to the usual laboratory procedure code (HIV testing 86701-86703, and 87389). The test does not require permanent dedicated space, hence by its design may be hand carried or transported to the vicinity of the patient for immediate testing at that site, although location of testing is not in itself determinative of the use of this modifier.

95 Synchronous Telemedicine Service Rendered Via a Real-Time Interactive Audio and Video Telecommunications System

Synchronous telemedicine service is defined as a real-time interaction between a physician or other qualified health care professional and a patient who is located at a distant site from the physician or other qualified health care professional. The totality of the communication of information exchanged between the physician or other qualified health care professional and the patient during the course of the synchronous telemedicine service must be of an amount and nature that would be sufficient to meet the key components and/or requirements of the same services when rendered via a face-to-face interaction. Modifier 95 may only be appended to the services listed in Appendix P*. Appendix P is the list of the CPT codes for services that are typically performed face-to-face, but may be rendered via a real-time (synchronous) interactive audio and video telecommunications system.

96 Habilitative Services

When a service or procedure that may be either habilitative or rehabilitative in nature is provided for habilitative purposes, the physician or other qualified health care professional may add modifier 96 to the service or procedure code to indicate that the service or procedure provided was a habilitative service. Habilitative services help an individual learn skills and functioning for daily living that the individual has not yet developed, and then keep and/or improve those learned skills. Habilitative services also help an individual keep, learn, or improve skills and functioning for daily living.

97 Rehabilitative Services

When a service or procedure that may be either habilitative or rehabilitative in nature is provided for rehabilitative purposes, the physician or other qualified health care professional may add modifier 97 to the service or procedure code to indicate that the service or procedure provided was a rehabilitative service. Rehabilitative services help an individual keep, get back, or improve skills and functioning for daily living that have been lost or impaired because the individual was sick, hurt, or disabled.

99 Multiple Modifiers

Under certain circumstances 2 or more modifiers may be necessary to completely delineate a service. In such situations modifier 99 should be added to the basic procedure, and other applicable modifiers may be listed as part of the description of the service.

ⓘ Check with payers to determine if this modifier is necessary when reporting multiple modifiers.

Modifiers Approved for Ambulatory Surgery Center (ASC) Hospital Outpatient Use

There are some differences in modifiers for professional and ASC hospital use. The following list consists of the only approved modifiers that can be used in an ASC/hospital setting:

*Pages in this section refer to the AMA *CPT® 2022 Professional Edition*

25 Significant, Separately Identifiable Evaluation and Management Service by the Same Physician or Other Qualified Health Care Professional on the Same Day of the Procedure or Other Service

It may be necessary to indicate that on the day a procedure or service identified by a CPT code was performed, the patient's condition required a significant, separately identifiable E/M service above and beyond the other service provided or beyond the usual preoperative and postoperative care associated with the procedure that was performed. A significant, separately identifiable E/M service is defined or substantiated by documentation that satisfies the relevant criteria for the respective E/M service to be reported (see **Evaluation and Management Services Guidelines** for instructions on determining level of E/M service). The E/M service may be prompted by the symptom or condition for which the procedure and/or service was provided. As such, different diagnoses are not required for reporting of the E/M services on the same date. This circumstance may be reported by adding modifier 25 to the appropriate level of E/M service.

Note: This modifier is not used to report an E/M service that resulted in a decision to perform surgery. See modifier 57. For significant, separately identifiable non-E/M services, see modifier 59.

ⓘ According to Medicare, modifier 25 may be appended to an Emergency Department Services E/M code (99281-99285) if provided on the same day as a diagnostic or therapeutic procedure.

27 Multiple Outpatient Hospital E/M Encounters on the Same Date

For hospital outpatient reporting purposes, utilization of hospital resources related to separate and distinct E/M encounters performed in multiple outpatient hospital settings on the same date may be reported by adding modifier 27 to each appropriate level outpatient and/or emergency department E/M code(s). This modifier provides a means of reporting circumstances involving evaluation and management services provided by physician(s) in more than one (multiple) outpatient hospital setting(s) (e.g., hospital emergency department, clinic).

Note: This modifier is not to be used for physician reporting of multiple E/M services performed by the same physician on the same date. For physician reporting of all outpatient E/M services provided by the same physician on the same date and performed in multiple outpatient setting(s) (eg, hospital emergency department, clinic), see **Evaluation and Management, Emergency Department**, or **Preventive Medicine Services** codes.

33 Preventive Services

When the primary purpose of the service is the delivery of an evidence based service in accordance with a US Preventive Services Task Force A or B rating in effect and other preventive services identified in preventive services mandates (legislative or regulatory), the services may be identified by adding 33 to the procedure. For separately reported services specifically identified as preventive, the modifier should not be used.

50 Bilateral Procedure

Unless otherwise identified in the listings, bilateral procedures that are performed at the same session should be identified by adding modifier 50 to the appropriate 5-digit code.

Note: This modifier should not be appended to designated "add-on" codes (see Appendix D*)

ⓘ Reported on procedures performed at the same operative session, this modifier should be reported only once as a one-line item for Medicare, with the modifier appended to the end of the code.

ⓘ Some payers may accept the bilateral procedures as two-line items, with HCPCS Level II modifiers LT and RT appended to the end of the codes.

52 Reduced Services

Under certain circumstances a service or procedure is partially reduced or eliminated at the discretion of the physician or other qualified health care professional. Under these circumstances the service provided can be identified by its usual procedure number and the addition of modifier 52, signifying that the service is reduced. This provides a means of reporting reduced services without disturbing the identification of the basic service.

Note: For hospital outpatient reporting of a previously scheduled procedure/service that is partially reduced or cancelled as a result of extenuating circumstances or those that threaten the well-being of the patient prior to or after administration of anesthesia, see modifiers 73 and 74. (see modifiers approved for ASC hospital outpatient use)

ⓘ Procedures reported with modifier 52 are typically billed at a reduced amount. Most payers do not require documentation to support the use of modifier 52 and will reimburse the procedure at a reduced level.

58 Staged or Related Procedure or Service by the Same Physician or Other Qualified Health Care Professional During the Postoperative Period

It may be necessary to indicate that the performance of a procedure or service during the postoperative period was: (a) planned or anticipated (staged); (b) more extensive than the original procedure; or (c) for therapy following a diagnostic surgical procedure. This circumstance may be reported by adding modifier 58 to the staged or related procedure.

Note: For treatment of a problem that requires a return to the operating/procedure room (e.g., unanticipated clinical condition), see modifier 78.

ⓘ Modifier 58 must be used for purposes of identifying procedures performed by the original physician during the postoperative period of the original procedure, within the constraints of the modifier's definition. These procedures cannot be repeat operations (unless the procedures are more extensive than the original procedure) and cannot be for the treatment of complications requiring a return trip to the operating room.

The existence of modifier 58 does not negate the global fee concept. Services that are included in CPT as multiple sessions or are defined as including multiple services or events may not be billed with this modifier. This modifier is designed to allow a method of reporting additional, related surgeries that are due to a progression of the disease and are not to be used to avoid global surgery edits applicable to staged procedures.

Modifier 58 should be used on surgical codes only and has no effect on the payment amount.

59 Distinct Procedural Service

Under certain circumstances, it may be necessary to indicate that a procedure or service was distinct or independent from other non-E/M services performed on the same day. Modifier 59 is used to identify procedures/services, other than E/M services, that are not normally reported together, but are appropriate under the circumstances. Documentation must support a different session, different procedure or surgery, different site or organ system, separate incision/excision, separate lesion, or separate injury (or area of injury in extensive injuries) not ordinarily encountered or performed on the same day by the same individual. However, when another already established modifier is appropriate it should be used rather than modifier 59. Only if no more descriptive modifier is available, and the use of modifier 59 best explains the circumstances, should modifier 59 be used.

*Pages in this section refer to the AMA *CPT® 2022 Professional Edition*

Note: Modifier 59 should not be appended to an E/M service. To report a separate and distinct E/M service with a non-E/M service performed on the same date, see modifier 25.

ⓘ Modifier 59 was established to demonstrate that multiple, yet distinct, services were provided to a patient on the same date of service by the same provider. Because distinct procedures or services rendered on the same day by the same physician cannot be easily identified and properly adjudicated by simply listing the CPT procedure codes, modifier 59 assists the payer or Medicare carrier in applying the appropriate reimbursement protocol. If the modifier is not used in these circumstances, services may be denied, with the explanation of benefits stating that the payer does not reimburse for this service because it is part of another service that was performed at the same time.

73 Discontinued Out-Patient Hospital/Ambulatory Surgery Center (ASC) Procedure Prior to Administration of Anesthesia

Due to extenuating circumstances or those that threaten the well being of the patient, the physician may cancel a surgical or diagnostic procedure subsequent to the patient's surgical preparation (including sedation when provided, and being taken to the room where the procedure is to be performed), but prior to the administration of anesthesia (local, regional block(s), or general). Under these circumstances, the intended service that is prepared for but cancelled can be reported by its usual procedure number and the addition of modifier 73.

Note: The elective cancellation of a service prior to the administration of anesthesia and/or surgical preparation of the patient should not be reported. For physician reporting of a discontinued procedure, see modifier 53.

74 Discontinued Out-Patient Hospital/Ambulatory Surgery Center (ASC) Procedure After Administration of Anesthesia

Due to extenuating circumstances or those that threaten the well being of the patient, the physician may terminate a surgical or diagnostic procedure after the administration of anesthesia (local, regional block(s), or general) or after the procedure was started (e.g., incision made, intubation started, scope inserted, etc.). Under these circumstances, the intended service that is prepared for but cancelled can be reported by its usual procedure number and the addition of modifier 74.

Note: The elective cancellation of a service prior to the administration of anesthesia and/or surgical preparation of the patient should not be reported. For physician reporting of a discontinued procedure, see modifier 53.

76 Repeat Procedure or Service by Same Physician or Other Qualified Health Care Professional

It may be necessary to indicate that a procedure or service was repeated subsequent to the original procedure or service. This circumstance may be reported by adding modifier 76 to the repeated procedure or service.

Note: This modifier should not be appended to an E/M service.

77 Repeat Procedure by Another Physician or Other Qualified Health Care Professional

It may be necessary to indicate that a basic procedure or service was repeated by another physician or other qualified health care professional subsequent to the original procedure or service. This circumstance may be reported by adding modifier 77 to the repeated procedure or service.

Note: This modifier should not be appended to an E/M service.

ⓘ Appending this modifier does not guarantee payment of the repeat procedure, but will assist in determining duplicate billings for the procedure.

78 Unplanned Return to the Operating/Procedure Room by the Same Physician or Other Qualified Health Care Professional Following Initial Procedure for a Related Procedure During the Postoperative Period

It may be necessary to indicate that another procedure was performed during the postoperative period of the initial procedure (unplanned procedure following initial procedure). When this procedure is related to the first, and requires the use of an operating/procedure room, it may be reported by adding modifier 78 to the related procedure. (For repeat procedures, see modifier 76.)

ⓘ Medicare includes specific medical and/or surgical care for postoperative complications within the global surgical package and does not allow additional payment. Included in the global surgical package are "additional medical and surgical services required of the surgeon during the postoperative period of the surgery because of complications which do not require additional trips to the operating room."

79 Unrelated Procedure or Service by the Same Physician or Other Qualified Health Care Professional During the Postoperative Period

The individual may need to indicate that the performance of a procedure or service during the postoperative period was unrelated to the original procedure. This circumstance may be reported by using modifier 79. (For repeat procedures on the same day, see modifier 76.)

ⓘ When billing for an unrelated procedure by the same physician during the postoperative period of an original procedure, a new postoperative period will begin with the subsequent procedure. A different diagnosis should be indicated on the claim to identify the unrelated procedure.

91 Repeat Clinical Diagnostic Laboratory Test

In the course of treatment of the patient, it may be necessary to repeat the same laboratory test on the same day to obtain subsequent (multiple) test results. Under these circumstances, the laboratory test performed can be identified by its usual procedure number and the addition of modifier 91.

Note: This modifier may not be used when tests are rerun to confirm initial results; due to testing problems with specimens or equipment; or for any other reason when a normal, one-time, reportable result is all that is required. This modifier may not be used when other code(s) describe a series of test results (e.g., glucose tolerance tests, evocative/suppression testing). This modifier may only be used for laboratory test(s) performed more than once on the same day on the same patient.

Category II Modifiers

The following performance measurement modifiers may be used for Category II codes to indicate that a service specified in the associated measure(s) was considered but, due to either medical, patient, or system circumstance(s) documented in the medical record, the service was not provided. These modifiers serve as denominator exclusions from the performance measure. The user should note that not all listed measures provide for exclusions (see Alphabetical Clinical Topics Listing for more discussion regarding exclusion criteria).

Category II modifiers should only be reported with Category II codes—they should not be reported with Category I or Category III codes. In addition, the modifiers in the Category II section should only be used where specified in the guidelines, reporting instructions, parenthetic notes, or code descriptor language listed in the Category II section (code listing and the Alphabetical Clinical Topics Listing).

1P Performance Measure Exclusion Modifier due to Medical Reasons

Reasons include:

- Not indicated (absence of organ/limb, already received/performed, other)
- Contraindicated (patient allergic history, potential adverse drug interaction, other)
- Other medical reasons

2P Performance Measure Exclusion Modifier due to Patient Reasons

Reasons include:

- Patient declined
- Economic, social, or religious reasons
- Other patient reasons

3P Performance Measure Exclusion Modifier due to System Reasons

Reasons include:

- Resources to perform the services not available
- Insurance coverage/payor-related limitations
- Other reasons attributable to health care delivery system

Modifier 8P is intended to be used as a "reporting modifier" to allow the reporting of circumstances when an action described in a measure's numerator is not performed and the reason is not otherwise specified.

8P Performance measure reporting modifier–action not performed, reason not otherwise specified

Level II (HCPCS/National) Modifiers

E1 Upper left, eyelid

E2 Lower left, eyelid

E3 Upper right, eyelid

E4 Lower right, eyelid

F1 Left hand, second digit

F2 Left hand, third digit

F3 Left hand, fourth digit

F4 Left hand, fifth digit

F5 Right hand, thumb

F6 Right hand, second digit

F7 Right hand, third digit

F8 Right hand, fourth digit

F9 Right hand, fifth digit

FA Left hand, thumb

GG Performance and payment of a screening mammogram and diagnostic mammogram on the same patient, same day

GH Diagnostic mammogram converted from screening mammogram on same day

LC Left circumflex coronary artery

LD Left anterior descending coronary artery

LM Left main coronary artery

LT Left side (used to identify procedures performed on the left side of the body)

QM Ambulance service provided under arrangement by a provider of services

QN Ambulance service furnished directly by a provider of services

RC Right coronary artery

RI Ramus intermedius coronary artery

RT Right side (used to identify procedures performed on the right side of the body)

T1 Left foot, second digit

T2 Left foot, third digit

T3 Left foot, fourth digit

T4 Left foot, fifth digit

T5 Right foot, great toe

T6 Right foot, second digit

T7 Right foot, third digit

T8 Right foot, fourth digit

T9 Right foot, fifth digit

TA Left foot, great toe

XE Separate Encounter *

XS Separate Structure *

XP Separate Practitioner *

XU Unusual Non-Overlapping Service *

(*HCPCS modifiers for selective identification of subsets of Distinct Procedural Services [59 modifier])

Modifier Rules

Mult Proc = Multiple Procedure (Modifier 51)

Indicates applicable payment-adjustment rule for multiple procedures:

0 No payment-adjustment rules for multiple procedures apply. If procedure is reported on the same day as another procedure, base the payment on the lower of (a) the actual charge, or (b) the fee-schedule amount for the procedure.

1 Standard payment-adjustment rules in effect before January 1, 1995 for multiple procedures apply. In the 1995 file, this indicator only applies to codes with a status code of "D." If procedure is reported on the same day as another procedure that has an indicator of 1, 2, or 3, rank the procedures by fee-schedule amount and apply the appropriate reduction to this code (100%, 50%, 25%, 25%, 25%, and by report). Base the payment on the lower of (a) the actual charge, or (b) the fee-schedule amount reduced by the appropriate percentage.

2 Standard payment-adjustment rules for multiple procedures apply. If procedure is reported on the same day as another procedure with an indicator of 1, 2, or 3, rank the procedures by fee-schedule amount and apply the appropriate reduction to this code (100%, 50%, 50%, 50%, 50% and by report). Base the payment on the lower of (a) the actual charge, or (b) the fee-schedule amount reduced by the appropriate percentage.

3 Special rules for multiple endoscopic procedures apply if procedure is billed with another endoscopy in the same family (i.e., another endoscopy that has the same base procedure). The base procedure for each code with this indicator is identified in the ENDO BASE field of this file. Apply the multiple endoscopy rules to a family before ranking the family

with the other procedures performed on the same day (for example, if multiple endoscopies in the same family are reported on the same day as endoscopies in another family or on the same day as a non-endoscopic procedure). If an endoscopic procedure is reported with only its base procedure, do not pay separately for the base procedure. Payment for the base procedure is included in the payment for the other endoscopy.

5 Subject to 20% of the practice expense component for certain therapy services (25% reduction for services rendered in an institutional setting - effective for services January 1, 2012 and after).

9 Concept does not apply.

Bilat Surg = Bilateral Surgery (Modifier 50)

Indicates services subject to payment adjustment.

0 150% payment adjustment for bilateral procedures does not apply. If procedure is reported with modifier 50 or with modifiers RT and LT, base the payment for the two sides on the lower of: (a) the total actual charge for both sides or (b) 100% of the fee-schedule amount for a single code. Example: The fee-schedule amount for code XXXXX is $125. The physician reports code XXXXX-LT with an actual charge of $100 and XXXXX-RT with an actual charge of $100. Payment should be based on the fee-schedule amount ($125) since it is lower than the total actual charges for the left and right sides ($200). The bilateral adjustment is inappropriate for codes in this category (a) because of physiology or anatomy, or (b) because the code description specifically states that it is a unilateral procedure and there is an existing code for the bilateral procedure.

1 150% payment adjustment for bilateral procedures applies. If the code is billed with the bilateral modifier or is reported twice on the same day by any other means (e.g., with RT and LT modifiers, or with a "2" in the units field), base the payment for these codes when reported as bilateral procedures on the lower of: (a) the total actual charge for both sides or (b) 150% of the fee-schedule amount for a single code. If the code is reported as a bilateral procedure and is reported with other procedure codes on the same day, apply the bilateral adjustment before applying any multiple procedure rules.

2 150% payment adjustment does not apply. RVUs are already based on the procedure being performed as a bilateral procedure. If the procedure is reported with modifier 50 or is reported twice on the same day by any other means (e.g., with RT and LT modifiers or with a "2" in the units field), base the payment for both sides on the lower of (a) the total actual charge by the physician for both sides, or (b) 100% of the fee-schedule for a single code. Example: The fee-schedule amount for code YYYYY is $125. The physician reports code YYYYY-LT with an actual charge of $100 and YYYYY-RT with an actual charge of $100. Payment should be based on the fee-schedule amount ($125) since it is lower than the total actual charges for the left and right sides ($200). The RVUs are based on a bilateral procedure because (a) the code descriptor specifically states that the procedure is bilateral, (b) the code descriptor states that the procedure may be performed either unilaterally or bilaterally, or (c) the procedure is usually performed as a bilateral procedure.

3 The usual payment adjustment for bilateral procedures does not apply. If the procedure is reported with modifier 50 or is reported for both sides on the same day by any other means (e.g., with RT and LT modifiers or with a "2" in the units field), base the payment for each side or organ or site of a paired organ on the lower of (a) the actual charge for each side or (b) 100% of the fee-schedule amount for each side. If the procedure is reported as a bilateral procedure and with other procedure codes on the same day, determine the fee-schedule amount for a bilateral procedure before applying any multiple procedure rules. Services in this category are generally radiology procedures or other diagnostic tests, which are not subject to the special payment rules for other bilateral surgeries.

9 Concept does not apply.

Asst Surg = Assistant at Surgery (Modifier 80)

Indicates services where an assistant at surgery is never paid for per Medicare Claims Manual.

0 Payment restriction for assistants at surgery applies to this procedure unless supporting documentation is submitted to establish medical necessity.

1 Statutory payment restriction for assistants at surgery applies to this procedure. Assistant at surgery may not be paid.

2 Payment restriction for assistants at surgery does not apply to this procedure. Assistant at surgery may be paid.

9 Concept does not apply.

Co Surg = Co-surgeons (Modifier 62)

Indicates services for which two surgeons, each in a different specialty, may be paid.

0 Co-surgeons not permitted for this procedure.

1 Co-surgeons could be paid, though supporting documentation is required to establish the medical necessity of two surgeons for the procedure.

2 Co-surgeons permitted and no documentation required if the two-specialty requirement is met.

9 Concept does not apply.

Team Surg = Team Surgery (Modifier 66)

Indicates services for which team surgeons may be paid.

0 Team surgeons not permitted for this procedure.

1 Team surgeons could be paid, though supporting documentation required to establish medical necessity of a team; pay by report.

2 Team surgeons permitted; pay by report.

9 Concept does not apply.

National Correct Coding Initiative

A. Introduction

The principles of correct coding apply to the CPT codes in the range 60000-69999. Several general guidelines are repeated in this Chapter.

Physicians should report the HCPCS/CPT code that describes the procedure performed to the greatest specificity possible. A HCPCS/CPT code should be reported only if all services described by the code are performed. A physician should not report multiple HCPCS/CPT codes if a single HCPCS/CPT code exists that describes the services. This type of unbundling is incorrect coding.

HCPCS/CPT codes include all services usually performed as part of the procedure as a standard of medical/surgical practice. A physician should not separately report these services simply because HCPCS/CPT codes exist for them.

Specific issues unique to this section of CPT are clarified in this chapter.

B. Evaluation and Management (E/M) Services

Medicare Global Surgery Rules define the rules for reporting evaluation and management (E/M) services with procedures covered by these rules. This section summarizes some of the rules.

All procedures on the Medicare Physician Fee Schedule are assigned a global period of 000, 010, 090, XXX, YYY, ZZZ, or MMM. The global concept does not apply to XXX procedures. The global period for YYY procedures is defined by the Carrier (A/B MAC processing practitioner service claims). All procedures with a global period of ZZZ are related to another procedure, and the applicable global period for the ZZZ code is determined by the related procedure. Procedures with a global period of MMM are maternity procedures. Since NCCI PTP edits are applied to same day services by the same provider to the same beneficiary, certain Global Surgery Rules are applicable to NCCI. An E/M service is separately reportable on the same date of service as a procedure with a global period of 000, 010, or 090 under limited circumstances.

If a procedure has a global period of 090 days, it is defined as a major surgical procedure. If an E/M is performed on the same date of service as a major surgical procedure for the purpose of deciding whether to perform this surgical procedure, the E/M service is separately reportable with modifier 57. Other preoperative E/M services on the same date of service as a major surgical procedure are included in the global payment for the procedure and are not separately reportable. NCCI does not contain edits based on this rule because Medicare Carriers (A/B MACs processing practitioner service claims) have separate edits. If a procedure has a global period of 000 or 010 days, it is defined as a minor surgical procedure. In general E/M services on the same date of service as the minor surgical procedure are included in the payment for the procedure. The decision to perform a minor surgical procedure is included in the payment for the minor surgical procedure and should not be reported separately as an E/M service. However, a significant and separately identifiable E/M service unrelated to the decision to perform the minor surgical procedure is separately reportable with modifier 25. The E/M service and minor surgical procedure do not require different diagnoses. If a minor surgical procedure is performed on a new patient, the same rules for reporting E/M services apply. The fact that the patient is "new" to the provider is not sufficient alone to justify reporting an E/M service on the same date of service as a minor surgical procedure. NCCI contains many, but not all, possible edits based on these principles.

Example: If a physician determines that a new patient with head trauma requires sutures, confirms the allergy and immunization status, obtains informed consent, and performs the repair, an E/M service is not separately reportable. However, if the physician also performs a medically reasonable and necessary full neurological examination, an E/M service may be separately reportable.

For major and minor surgical procedures, postoperative E/M services related to recovery from the surgical procedure during the postoperative period are included in the global surgical package as are E/M services related to complications of the surgery. Postoperative visits unrelated to the diagnosis for which the surgical procedure was performed unless related to a complication of surgery may be reported separately on the same day as a surgical procedure with modifier 24 ("Unrelated Evaluation and Management Service by the Same Physician or Other Qualified Health Care Professional During a Postoperative Period").

Procedures with a global surgery indicator of "XXX" are not covered by these rules. Many of these "XXX" procedures are performed by physicians and have inherent pre-procedure, intraprocedure, and post-procedure work usually performed each time the procedure is completed. This work should never be reported as a separate E/M code. Other "XXX" procedures are not usually performed by a physician and have no physician work relative value units associated with them. A physician should never report a separate E/M code with these procedures for the supervision of others performing the procedure or for the interpretation of the procedure. With most "XXX" procedures, the physician may, however, perform a significant and separately identifiable E/M service on the same date of service which may be reported by appending modifier 25 to the E/M code.

This E/M service may be related to the same diagnosis necessitating performance of the "XXX" procedure but cannot include any work inherent in the "XXX" procedure, supervision of others performing the "XXX" procedure, or time for interpreting the result of the "XXX" procedure. Appending modifier 25 to a significant, separately identifiable E/M service when performed on the same date of service as an "XXX" procedure is correct coding.

C. Surgery: Ophthalmology

1. When a subconjunctival injection (e.g., CPT code 68200) with local anesthetic is performed as part of a more extensive anesthetic procedure (e.g., peribulbar or retrobulbar block), the subconjunctival injection is not separately reportable. It is part of the anesthetic procedure and does not represent a separate service.

2. Iridectomy and/or anterior vitrectomy may be performed in conjunction with cataract extraction. If an iridectomy is performed in order to complete a cataract extraction, it is an integral part of the procedure and is not separately reportable. Similarly, the minimal vitreous loss occurring during routine cataract extraction does not represent a vitrectomy and is not separately reportable. If an iridectomy or vitrectomy that is separate and distinct from the cataract extraction is performed for an unrelated reason at the same patient encounter, the iridectomy and/or vitrectomy may be reported separately with an NCCI-associated modifier. The medical record must document the distinct medical necessity for each procedure. A trabeculectomy is separately reportable with a cataract extraction if performed for a purpose unrelated to the cataract extraction. For example, if a patient with glaucoma requires a cataract extraction and a trabeculectomy is the appropriate treatment for the glaucoma, the trabeculectomy may be separately reportable. However, performance of a trabeculectomy as a preventative service for an expected transient increase in intraocular pressure postoperatively, without other evidence for glaucoma, is not separately reportable.

3. CPT codes describing cataract extraction (66830-66984) are mutually exclusive of one another. Only one code from this CPT code range may be reported for an eye.

4. There are numerous CPT codes describing repair of retinal detachment (e.g., 67101-67113). These procedures are mutually exclusive and should not be reported separately for the ipsilateral eye on the same date of service. Some retinal detachment repair procedures include some vitreous procedures which are not separately reportable. For example, the procedure described by CPT code 67108 includes the procedures described by CPT codes 67015, 67025, 67028, 67031, 67036, 67039, and 67040.

5. The procedures described by CPT codes 68020-68200 (incision, drainage, biopsy, excision, or destruction of the conjunctiva) are included in all conjunctivoplasties (CPT codes 68320-68362). CPT codes 68020-68200 should not be reported separately with CPT codes 68320-68362 for the ipsilateral eye.

6. CPT code 67950 (canthoplasty) is included in repair procedures such as blepharoplasties (e.g., CPT codes 67917, 67924, 67961, 67966).

7. Correction of lid retraction (CPT code 67911) includes a full thickness graft (e.g., CPT code 15260) as part of the procedure. A full thickness graft code such as CPT code 15260 should not be reported separately with CPT code 67911 for the ipsilateral eye.

8. If it is medically reasonable and necessary to inject antisclerosing agents at the same patient encounter as surgery to correct glaucoma, the injection is included in the glaucoma procedure. CPT codes such as 67500, 67515, and 68200 for injection of anti-sclerosing agents (e.g., 5-FU, HCPCS code J9190) should not be reported separately with other pressure-reducing or glaucoma procedures.

9. Since visual field examination (CPT codes 92081-92083) would be performed prior to scheduling a patient for a blepharoplasty (CPT codes 15820-15823) or blepharoptosis (CPT codes 67901-67908) procedure, the visual field examination CPT codes should not be reported separately with the blepharoplasty or blepharoptosis procedure codes for the same date of service.

10. The CPT code descriptors for CPT code 67108 (repair of retinal detachment...) and 67113 (repair of complex retinal detachment...) include removal of lens if performed. CPT codes for removal of lens or cataract extraction (e.g., 66830- 66984) should not be reported separately.

11. Medicare Anesthesia Rules prohibit the physician performing an operative procedure from separately reporting anesthesia for that procedure except for moderate conscious sedation for some procedures. CPT codes describing ophthalmic injections (e.g., CPT codes 67500, 67515, 68200) should not be reported separately with other ophthalmic procedure codes when the injected substance is an anesthetic agent. Since Medicare Global Surgery Rules prohibit the separate reporting of postoperative pain management by the physician performing the procedure, the same CPT codes should not be reported separately by the physician performing the procedure for postoperative pain management.

12. CMS payment policy does not allow separate payment for a blepharoptosis procedure (CPT code 67901-67908) and blepharoplasty procedure (CPT codes 15822, 15823) on the ipsilateral upper eyelid.

13. CPT codes 65420 and 65426 describe excision of pterygium without and with graft respectively. Graft codes and the ocular surface reconstruction CPT codes 65780-65782 should not be reported separately with either of these codes for the ipsilateral eye.

14. CPT codes 92018 and 92019 (ophthalmological examination and evaluation, under general anesthesia...) are generally not separately reportable with ophthalmological surgical procedures. The examination and evaluation of an eye while a patient is under general anesthesia for another ophthalmological procedure is integral to the procedure. However, there are unusual circumstances when an adequate ophthalmological examination cannot be completed without anesthesia (e.g., uncooperative pediatric patient, severe eye trauma). In such situations CPT codes 92018 or 92019 may be separately reportable with appropriate documentation.

15. Procedures of the cornea should not be reported with anterior chamber "separate procedures" such as CPT codes 65800- 65815 and 66020. CMS payment policy does not allow separate payment for procedures including the "separate procedure" desig-

nation in their code descriptor when the "separate procedure" is performed with another procedure in an anatomically related area.

16. Repair of a surgical skin or mucous membrane incision (CPT codes 12001-13153) is generally included in the global surgical package. For procedures of the eye requiring a skin or mucous membrane incision (e.g., eyelid, orbitotomy, lacrimal system), simple, intermediate, and complex repair codes should not be reported separately.

17. Repair of an incision to perform an ophthalmic procedure is integral to completion of the procedure. It is a misuse of the repair of laceration codes (CPT codes 65270-65286) to separately report closure of a surgical incision of the conjunctiva, cornea, or sclera.

18. CPT codes 65280 and 65285 describe repair of laceration of the cornea and/or sclera. These codes should not be reported to describe repair of a surgical incision of the cornea and/or sclera which is integral to a surgical procedure (e.g., 65710- 65756).

19. Posterior segment ophthalmic surgical procedures (CPT codes 67005-67229) include extended ophthalmoscopy (CPT codes 92225, 92226), if performed during the operative procedure or post-operatively on the same date of service. Except when performed on an emergent basis, extended ophthalmoscopy would normally not be performed pre-operatively on the same date of service.

20. Injection of an antibiotic, steroid, and/or nonsteroidal anti-inflammatory drug during a cataract extraction procedure (e.g., CPT codes 66820-66986) or other ophthalmic procedure is not separately reportable. Physicians should not report CPT codes such as 66020, 66030, 67028, 67500, 67515, or 68200 for such injections.

21. CPT codes 67515 (injection into Tenon's capsule) and 68200 (subconjunctival injection) should not be reported with a paracentesis (e.g., CPT code 65800-65815) since the injections, if performed, are integral components of the paracentesis procedure.

22. Removal of corneal epithelium (e.g., CPT codes 65435, 65436) should not be reported with removal of corneal foreign body (e.g., CPT codes 65220, 65222) or repair of laceration of the cornea (e.g., CPT codes 65275-65285) for the ipsilateral eye.

23. Repair of entropion (CPT codes 67923, 67924) or repair of ectropion (CPT codes 67916, 67917) should not be reported with excision and repair of eyelid (CPT codes 67961, 67966) for the same eyelid. The latter codes include excision and repair of the eyelid involving lid margin, tarsus, conjunctiva, canthus, or full thickness and may include preparation for skin graft or pedicle flap with adjacent tissue transfer or rearrangement. A repair of entropion or repair of ectropion CPT code may be reported with an excision and repair of eyelid CPT code only if the procedures are performed on different eyelids. Modifiers E1, E2, E3, or E4 should be utilized to indicate that the procedures were performed on different eyelids.

24. CPT code 67028 (intravitreal injection of a pharmacologic agent (separate procedure)) should not be reported with CPT codes 65800-65815 (paracentesis of anterior chamber of the eye (separate procedure);...) when both procedures are performed on the same eye at the same patient encounter. Medicare policy does not allow two codes each defined as a "separate procedure" by its code descriptor to be reported together when performed in the same anatomic region at the same patient encounter.

25. CPT code 67028 describes intravitreal injection of a pharmacologic agent. CPT code 68200 (subconjunctival injection) performed on the ipsilateral side should not be reported separately with CPT code 67028.

D. Medicine: Ophthalmology

1. General ophthalmological services (CPT codes 92002- 92014) describe components of the ophthalmologic examination. When evaluation and management (E/M) codes are reported, these general ophthalmological service codes (e.g., CPT codes 92002-92014) should not be reported separately. The E/M service includes the general ophthalmological services.

2. Special ophthalmologic services represent specific services not included in a general or routine ophthalmological examination. Special ophthalmological services are recognized as significant, separately identifiable services and may be reported separately.

3. For procedures requiring intravenous injection of dye or other diagnostic agent, insertion of an intravenous catheter and dye injection are integral to the procedure and are not separately reportable. Therefore, CPT codes 36000 (introduction of a needle or catheter), 36410 (venipuncture), 96360-96368 (IV infusion), 96374-96376 (IV push injection), and selective vascular catheterization codes are not separately reportable with services requiring intravenous injection (e.g., CPT codes 92230, 92235, 92240, 92242, 92287).

4. CPT codes 92230 and 92235 (fluorescein angioscopy and angiography) include selective catheterization and injection procedures for angiography.

5. Fundus photography (CPT code 92250) and scanning ophthalmic computerized diagnostic imaging (e.g., CPT codes 92132, 92133, 92134) are generally mutually exclusive of one another in that a provider would use one technique or the other to evaluate fundal disease. However, there are a limited number of clinical conditions where both techniques are medically reasonable and necessary on the ipsilateral eye. In these situations, both CPT codes may be reported appending modifier 59 to CPT code 92250. (CPT code 92135 was deleted January 1, 2011.)

6. Posterior segment ophthalmic surgical procedures (CPT codes 67005-67229) include extended ophthalmoscopy (CPT codes 92225, 92226), if performed during the operative procedure or post-operatively on the same date of service. Except when performed on an emergent basis, extended ophthalmoscopy would normally not be performed pre-operatively on the same date of service.

7. CPT code 92071 (fitting of contact lens for treatment of ocular surface disease) should not be reported with a corneal procedure CPT code for a bandage contact lens applied after completion of a procedure on the cornea.

CCI Table Information

The CCI Modification indicator is noted with superscript letters and is also located in the footer of each page for reference purposes. The codes are suffixed as **0** or **1.**

- **0** indicates there is no circumstance in which a modifier would be allowed or appropriate, meaning services represented by the code combination will not be paid separately.
- **1** signifies a modifier is allowed in order to differentiate between the services provided.

Note: The responsibility for the content of this product is the Centers for Medicare and Medicaid Services (CMS) and no endorsement by the American Medical Association (AMA) is intended or should be implied. The AMA disclaims responsibility for any consequences or liability attributable to or related to any uses, non-use, or interpretation of information contained or not contained in this product.

The NCCI edits on the following tables represent only the codes contained in this book. There are NCCI edits for CPT codes not found in this guide. The edits herein represent all active edits as of 1/1/2022. NCCI edits are updated quarterly. To view all NCCI edits, as well as quarterly updates, visit www.cms.gov/nationalcorrectcodeinited/.

Code 1	Code 2
15820	0213T[0], 0216T[0], 0596T[1], 0597T[1], 11000[1], 11001[1], 11004[1], 11005[1], 11006[1], 11042[1], 11043[1], 11044[1], 11045[1], 11046[1], 11047[1], 11102[1], 11104[1], 11106[1], 12001[1], 12002[1], 12004[1], 12005[1], 12006[1], 12007[1], 12011[1], 12013[1], 12014[1], 12015[1], 12016[1], 12017[1], 12018[1], 12020[1], 12021[1], 12031[1], 12032[1], 12034[1], 12035[1], 12036[1], 12037[1], 12041[1], 12042[1], 12044[1], 12045[1], 12046[1], 12047[1], 12051[1], 12052[1], 12053[1], 12054[1], 12055[1], 12056[1], 12057[1], 13100[1], 13101[1], 13102[1], 13120[1], 13121[1], 13122[1], 13131[1], 13132[1], 13133[1], 13151[1], 13152[1], 13153[1], 36000[1], 36400[1], 36405[1], 36406[1], 36410[1], 36420[1], 36425[1], 36430[1], 36440[1], 36591[0], 36592[0], 36600[1], 36640[1], 43752[1], 51701[1], 51702[1], 51703[1], 62320[0], 62321[0], 62322[0], 62323[0], 62324[0], 62325[0], 62326[0], 62327[0], 64400[0], 64405[0], 64408[0], 64415[0], 64416[0], 64417[0], 64418[0], 64420[0], 64421[0], 64425[0], 64430[0], 64435[0], 64445[0], 64446[0], 64447[0], 64448[0], 64449[0], 64450[1], 64451[0], 64454[1], 64461[0], 64462[0], 64463[0], 64479[0], 64480[0], 64483[0], 64484[0], 64486[0], 64487[0], 64488[0], 64489[0], 64490[0], 64491[0], 64492[0], 64493[0], 64494[0], 64495[0], 64505[0], 64510[0], 64517[0], 64520[0], 64530[0], 69990[0], 92012[1], 92014[1], 92081[0], 92082[0], 92083[0], 92285[1], 93000[1], 93005[1], 93010[1], 93040[1], 93041[1], 93042[1], 93318[1], 93355[1], 94002[1], 94200[1], 94680[1], 94681[1], 94690[1], 95812[1], 95813[1], 95816[1], 95819[1], 95822[1], 95829[1], 95955[1], 96360[1], 96361[1], 96365[1], 96366[1], 96367[1], 96368[1], 96372[1], 96374[1], 96375[1], 96376[1], 96377[1], 96523[0], 97597[1], 97598[1], 97602[1], 99155[0], 99156[0], 99157[0], 99211[1], 99212[1], 99213[1], 99214[1], 99215[1], 99217[1], 99218[1], 99219[1], 99220[1], 99221[1], 99222[1], 99223[1], 99231[1], 99232[1], 99233[1], 99234[1], 99235[1], 99236[1], 99238[1], 99239[1], 99241[1], 99242[1], 99243[1], 99244[1], 99245[1], 99251[1], 99252[1], 99253[1], 99254[1], 99255[1], 99291[1], 99292[1], 99304[1], 99305[1], 99306[1], 99307[1], 99308[1], 99309[1], 99310[1], 99315[1], 99316[1], 99334[1], 99335[1], 99336[1], 99337[1], 99347[1], 99348[1], 99349[1], 99350[1], 99374[1], 99375[1], 99377[1], 99378[1], 99446[0], 99447[0], 99448[0], 99449[0], 99451[0], 99452[0], 99495[0], 99496[0], G0463[1], G0471[1], J0670[1], J2001[1]
15821	0213T[0], 0216T[0], 0596T[1], 0597T[1], 11000[1], 11001[1], 11004[1], 11005[1], 11006[1], 11042[1], 11043[1], 11044[1], 11045[1], 11046[1], 11047[1], 11102[1], 11104[1], 11106[1], 12001[1], 12002[1], 12004[1], 12005[1], 12006[1], 12007[1], 12011[1], 12013[1], 12014[1], 12015[1], 12016[1], 12017[1], 12018[1], 12020[1], 12021[1], 12031[1], 12032[1], 12034[1], 12035[1], 12036[1], 12037[1], 12041[1], 12042[1], 12044[1], 12045[1], 12046[1], 12047[1], 12051[1], 12052[1], 12053[1], 12054[1], 12055[1], 12056[1], 12057[1], 13100[1], 13101[1], 13102[1], 13120[1], 13121[1], 13122[1], 13131[1], 13132[1], 13133[1], 13151[1], 13152[1], 13153[1], 15820[1], 36000[1], 36400[1], 36405[1], 36406[1], 36410[1], 36420[1], 36425[1], 36430[1], 36440[1], 36591[0], 36592[0], 36600[1], 36640[1], 43752[1], 51701[1], 51702[1], 51703[1], 62320[0], 62321[0], 62322[0], 62323[0], 62324[0], 62325[0], 62326[0], 62327[0], 64400[0], 64405[0], 64408[0], 64415[0], 64416[0], 64417[0], 64418[0], 64420[0], 64421[0], 64425[0], 64430[0], 64435[0], 64445[0], 64446[0], 64447[0], 64448[0], 64449[0], 64450[1], 64451[0], 64454[1], 64461[0], 64462[0], 64463[0], 64479[0], 64480[0], 64483[0], 64484[0], 64486[0], 64487[0], 64488[0], 64489[0], 64490[0], 64491[0], 64492[0], 64493[0], 64494[0], 64495[0], 64505[0], 64510[0], 64517[0], 64520[0], 64530[0], 69990[0], 92012[1], 92014[1], 92081[0], 92082[0], 92083[0], 92285[1], 93000[1], 93005[1], 93010[1], 93040[1], 93041[1], 93042[1], 93318[1], 93355[1], 94002[1], 94200[1], 94680[1], 94681[1], 94690[1], 95812[1], 95813[1], 95816[1], 95819[1], 95822[1], 95829[1], 95955[1], 96360[1], 96361[1], 96365[1], 96366[1], 96367[1], 96368[1], 96372[1], 96374[1], 96375[1], 96376[1], 96377[1], 96523[0], 97597[1], 97598[1], 97602[1], 99155[0], 99156[0], 99157[0], 99211[1], 99212[1], 99213[1], 99214[1], 99215[1], 99217[1], 99218[1], 99219[1], 99220[1], 99221[1], 99222[1], 99223[1], 99231[1], 99232[1], 99233[1], 99234[1], 99235[1], 99236[1], 99238[1], 99239[1], 99241[1], 99242[1], 99243[1], 99244[1], 99245[1], 99251[1], 99252[1], 99253[1], 99254[1], 99255[1], 99291[1], 99292[1], 99304[1], 99305[1], 99306[1], 99307[1], 99308[1], 99309[1], 99310[1], 99315[1], 99316[1], 99334[1], 99335[1], 99336[1], 99337[1], 99347[1], 99348[1], 99349[1], 99350[1], 99374[1], 99375[1], 99377[1], 99378[1], 99446[0], 99447[0], 99448[0], 99449[0], 99451[0], 99452[0], 99495[0], 99496[0], G0463[1], G0471[1], J0670[1], J2001[1]
15822	0213T[0], 0216T[0], 0596T[1], 0597T[1], 11000[1], 11001[1], 11004[1], 11005[1], 11006[1], 11042[1], 11043[1], 11044[1], 11045[1], 11046[1], 11047[1], 11102[1], 11104[1], 11106[1], 12001[1], 12002[1], 12004[1], 12005[1], 12006[1], 12007[1], 12011[1], 12013[1], 12014[1], 12015[1], 12016[1], 12017[1], 12018[1], 12020[1], 12021[1], 12031[1], 12032[1], 12034[1], 12035[1], 12036[1], 12037[1], 12041[1], 12042[1], 12044[1], 12045[1], 12046[1], 12047[1], 12051[1], 12052[1], 12053[1], 12054[1], 12055[1], 12056[1], 12057[1], 13100[1], 13101[1], 13102[1], 13120[1], 13121[1], 13122[1], 13131[1], 13132[1], 13133[1], 13151[1], 13152[1], 13153[1], 36000[1], 36400[1], 36405[1], 36406[1], 36410[1], 36420[1], 36425[1], 36430[1], 36440[1], 36591[0], 36592[0], 36600[1], 36640[1], 43752[1], 51701[1], 51702[1], 51703[1], 62320[0], 62321[0], 62322[0], 62323[0], 62324[0], 62325[0], 62326[0], 62327[0], 64400[0], 64405[0], 64408[0], 64415[0], 64416[0], 64417[0], 64418[0], 64420[0], 64421[0], 64425[0], 64430[0], 64435[0], 64445[0], 64446[0], 64447[0], 64448[0], 64449[0], 64450[1], 64451[0], 64454[1], 64461[0], 64462[0], 64463[0], 64479[0], 64480[0], 64483[0], 64484[0], 64486[0], 64487[0], 64488[0], 64489[0], 64490[0], 64491[0], 64492[0], 64493[0], 64494[0], 64495[0], 64505[0], 64510[0], 64517[0], 64520[0], 64530[0], 69990[0], 92012[1], 92014[1], 92081[0], 92082[0], 92083[0], 92285[1], 93000[1], 93005[1], 93010[1], 93040[1], 93041[1], 93042[1], 93318[1], 93355[1], 94002[1], 94200[1], 94680[1], 94681[1], 94690[1], 95812[1], 95813[1], 95816[1], 95819[1], 95822[1], 95829[1], 95955[1], 96360[1], 96361[1], 96365[1], 96366[1], 96367[1], 96368[1], 96372[1], 96374[1], 96375[1], 96376[1], 96377[1], 96523[0], 97597[1], 97598[1], 97602[1], 99155[0], 99156[0], 99157[0], 99211[1], 99212[1], 99213[1], 99214[1], 99215[1], 99217[1], 99218[1], 99219[1], 99220[1], 99221[1], 99222[1], 99223[1], 99231[1], 99232[1], 99233[1], 99234[1], 99235[1], 99236[1], 99238[1], 99239[1], 99241[1], 99242[1], 99243[1], 99244[1], 99245[1], 99251[1], 99252[1], 99253[1], 99254[1], 99255[1], 99291[1], 99292[1], 99304[1], 99305[1], 99306[1], 99307[1], 99308[1], 99309[1], 99310[1], 99315[1], 99316[1], 99334[1], 99335[1], 99336[1], 99337[1], 99347[1], 99348[1], 99349[1], 99350[1], 99374[1], 99375[1], 99377[1], 99378[1], 99446[0], 99447[0], 99448[0], 99449[0], 99451[0], 99452[0], 99495[0], 99496[0], G0463[1], G0471[1], J0670[1], J2001[1]
15823	0213T[0], 0216T[0], 0596T[1], 0597T[1], 11000[1], 11001[1], 11004[1], 11005[1], 11006[1], 11042[1], 11043[1], 11044[1], 11045[1], 11046[1], 11047[1], 11102[1], 11104[1], 11106[1], 12001[1], 12002[1], 12004[1], 12005[1], 12006[1], 12007[1], 12011[1], 12013[1], 12014[1], 12015[1], 12016[1], 12017[1], 12018[1], 12020[1], 12021[1], 12031[1], 12032[1], 12034[1], 12035[1], 12036[1], 12037[1], 12041[1], 12042[1], 12044[1], 12045[1], 12046[1], 12047[1], 12051[1], 12052[1], 12053[1], 12054[1], 12055[1], 12056[1], 12057[1], 13100[1], 13101[1], 13102[1], 13120[1], 13121[1], 13122[1], 13131[1], 13132[1], 13133[1], 13151[1], 13152[1], 13153[1], 15822[1], 36000[1], 36400[1], 36405[1], 36406[1], 36410[1], 36420[1], 36425[1], 36430[1], 36440[1], 36591[0], 36592[0], 36600[1], 36640[1], 43752[1], 51701[1], 51702[1], 51703[1], 62320[0], 62321[0], 62322[0], 62323[0], 62324[0], 62325[0], 62326[0], 62327[0], 64400[0], 64405[0], 64408[0], 64415[0], 64416[0], 64417[0], 64418[0], 64420[0], 64421[0], 64425[0], 64430[0], 64435[0], 64445[0], 64446[0], 64447[0], 64448[0], 64449[0], 64450[1], 64451[0], 64454[1], 64461[0], 64462[0], 64463[0], 64479[0], 64480[0], 64483[0], 64484[0], 64486[0], 64487[0], 64488[0], 64489[0], 64490[0], 64491[0], 64492[0], 64493[0], 64494[0], 64495[0], 64505[0], 64510[0], 64517[0], 64520[0], 64530[0], 69990[0], 92012[1], 92014[1], 92081[0], 92082[0], 92083[0], 92285[1], 93000[1], 93005[1], 93010[1], 93040[1], 93041[1], 93042[1], 93318[1], 93355[1], 94002[1], 94200[1], 94680[1], 94681[1], 94690[1], 95812[1], 95813[1], 95816[1], 95819[1], 95822[1], 95829[1], 95955[1], 96360[1], 96361[1], 96365[1], 96366[1], 96367[1], 96368[1], 96372[1], 96374[1], 96375[1], 96376[1], 96377[1], 96523[0], 97597[1], 97598[1], 97602[1], 99155[0], 99156[0], 99157[0], 99211[1], 99212[1], 99213[1], 99214[1], 99215[1], 99217[1], 99218[1], 99219[1], 99220[1], 99221[1], 99222[1], 99223[1], 99231[1], 99232[1], 99233[1], 99234[1], 99235[1], 99236[1], 99238[1], 99239[1], 99241[1], 99242[1], 99243[1], 99244[1], 99245[1], 99251[1], 99252[1], 99253[1], 99254[1], 99255[1], 99291[1], 99292[1], 99304[1], 99305[1], 99306[1], 99307[1], 99308[1], 99309[1], 99310[1], 99315[1], 99316[1], 99334[1], 99335[1], 99336[1], 99337[1], 99347[1], 99348[1], 99349[1], 99350[1], 99374[1], 99375[1], 99377[1], 99378[1], 99446[0], 99447[0], 99448[0], 99449[0], 99451[0], 99452[0], 99495[0], 99496[0], G0463[1], G0471[1], J0670[1], J2001[1]
21385	0213T[0], 0216T[0], 0596T[1], 0597T[1], 0708T[1], 0709T[1], 12001[1], 12002[1], 12004[1], 12005[1], 12006[1], 12007[1], 12011[1], 12013[1], 12014[1], 12015[1], 12016[1], 12017[1], 12018[1], 12020[1], 12021[1], 12031[1], 12032[1], 12034[1], 12035[1], 12036[1], 12037[1], 12041[1], 12042[1], 12044[1], 12045[1], 12046[1], 12047[1], 12051[1], 12052[1], 12053[1], 12054[1], 12055[1], 12056[1], 12057[1], 13100[1], 13101[1], 13102[1], 13120[1], 13121[1], 13122[1], 13131[1], 13132[1], 13133[1], 13151[1], 13152[1], 13153[1], 21400[0], 21401[0], 36000[1], 36400[1], 36405[1], 36406[1], 36410[1], 36420[1], 36425[1], 36430[1], 36440[1], 36591[0], 36592[0], 36600[1], 36640[1], 43752[1], 51701[1], 51702[1], 51703[1], 62320[0], 62321[0], 62322[0], 62323[0], 62324[0], 62325[0], 62326[0], 62327[0], 64400[0], 64405[0], 64408[0], 64415[0], 64416[0], 64417[0], 64418[0], 64420[0], 64421[0], 64425[0], 64430[0], 64435[0], 64445[0], 64446[0], 64447[0], 64448[0], 64449[0], 64450[1], 64451[0], 64454[1], 64461[0], 64462[0], 64463[0], 64479[0], 64480[0], 64483[0], 64484[0], 64486[0], 64487[0], 64488[0], 64489[0], 64490[0], 64491[0], 64492[0], 64493[0], 64494[0], 64495[0], 64505[0], 64510[0], 64517[0], 64520[0], 64530[0], 67400[1], 67405[1], 67413[1], 67414[1], 67430[1], 67440[1], 67445[1], 67450[1], 69990[0], 92012[1], 92014[1], 93000[1], 93005[1], 93010[1], 93040[1], 93041[1], 93042[1], 93318[1], 93355[1], 94002[1], 94200[1], 94680[1], 94681[1], 94690[1], 95812[1], 95813[1], 95816[1], 95819[1], 95822[1], 95829[1], 95955[1], 96360[1], 96361[1], 96365[1], 96366[1], 96367[1], 96368[1], 96372[1], 96374[1], 96375[1], 96376[1], 96377[1], 96523[0], 97597[1], 97598[1], 97602[1], 97605[1], 97606[1], 97607[1], 97608[1], 99155[0], 99156[0], 99157[0], 99211[1], 99212[1], 99213[1], 99214[1], 99215[1], 99217[1], 99218[1], 99219[1], 99220[1], 99221[1], 99222[1], 99223[1], 99231[1], 99232[1], 99233[1], 99234[1], 99235[1], 99236[1], 99238[1], 99239[1], 99241[1], 99242[1], 99243[1], 99244[1], 99245[1], 99251[1], 99252[1], 99253[1], 99254[1], 99255[1], 99291[1], 99292[1], 99304[1], 99305[1], 99306[1], 99307[1], 99308[1], 99309[1], 99310[1], 99315[1], 99316[1], 99334[1], 99335[1], 99336[1], 99337[1], 99347[1], 99348[1], 99349[1], 99350[1], 99374[1], 99375[1], 99377[1], 99378[1], 99446[0], 99447[0], 99448[0], 99449[0], 99451[0], 99452[0], 99495[0], 99496[0], G0463[1], G0471[1]
21386	0213T[0], 0216T[0], 0596T[1], 0597T[1], 0708T[1], 0709T[1], 12001[1], 12002[1], 12004[1], 12005[1], 12006[1], 12007[1], 12011[1], 12013[1], 12014[1], 12015[1], 12016[1], 12017[1], 12018[1], 12020[1], 12021[1], 12031[1], 12032[1], 12034[1], 12035[1], 12036[1], 12037[1], 12041[1], 12042[1], 12044[1], 12045[1], 12046[1], 12047[1], 12051[1], 12052[1], 12053[1], 12054[1], 12055[1], 12056[1], 12057[1], 13100[1], 13101[1], 13102[1], 13120[1], 13121[1], 13122[1], 13131[1], 13132[1], 13133[1], 13151[1], 13152[1], 13153[1], 21400[0], 21401[0], 36000[1], 36400[1], 36405[1], 36406[1], 36410[1], 36420[1], 36425[1], 36430[1], 36440[1], 36591[0], 36592[0], 36600[1], 36640[1], 43752[1], 51701[1], 51702[1],

0 = Modifier usage not allowed or inappropriate 1 = Modifier usage allowed

Code 1	Code 2
	51703^1, 62320^0, 62321^0, 62322^0, 62323^0, 62324^0, 62325^0, 62326^0, 62327^0, 64400^0, 64405^0, 64408^0, 64415^0, 64416^0, 64417^0, 64418^0, 64420^0, 64421^0, 64425^0, 64430^0, 64435^0, 64445^0, 64446^0, 64447^0, 64448^0, 64449^0, 64450^1, 64451^0, 64454^1, 64461^0, 64462^0, 64463^0, 64479^0, 64480^0, 64483^0, 64484^0, 64486^0, 64487^0, 64488^0, 64489^0, 64490^0, 64491^0, 64492^0, 64493^0, 64494^0, 64495^0, 64505^0, 64510^0, 64517^0, 64520^0, 64530^0, 67400^1, 67405^1, 67413^1, 67414^1, 67430^1, 67440^1, 67445^1, 67450^1, 69990^0, 92012^1, 92014^1, 93000^1, 93005^1, 93010^1, 93040^1, 93041^1, 93042^1, 93318^1, 93355^1, 94002^1, 94200^1, 94680^1, 94681^1, 94690^1, 95812^1, 95813^1, 95816^1, 95819^1, 95822^1, 95829^1, 95955^1, 96360^1, 96361^1, 96365^1, 96366^1, 96367^1, 96368^1, 96372^1, 96374^1, 96375^1, 96376^1, 96377^1, 96523^0, 97597^1, 97598^1, 97602^1, 97605^1, 97606^1, 97607^1, 97608^1, 99155^0, 99156^0, 99157^0, 99211^1, 99212^1, 99213^1, 99214^1, 99215^1, 99217^1, 99218^1, 99219^1, 99220^1, 99221^1, 99222^1, 99223^1, 99231^1, 99232^1, 99233^1, 99234^1, 99235^1, 99236^1, 99238^1, 99239^1, 99241^1, 99242^1, 99243^1, 99244^1, 99245^1, 99251^1, 99252^1, 99253^1, 99254^1, 99255^1, 99291^1, 99292^1, 99304^1, 99305^1, 99306^1, 99307^1, 99308^1, 99309^1, 99310^1, 99315^1, 99316^1, 99334^1, 99335^1, 99336^1, 99337^1, 99347^1, 99348^1, 99349^1, 99350^1, 99374^1, 99375^1, 99377^1, 99378^1, 99446^0, 99447^0, 99448^0, 99449^0, 99451^0, 99452^0, 99495^0, 99496^0, G0463^1, G0471^1
21387	0213T^0, 0216T^0, 0596T^1, 0597T^1, 0708T^1, 0709T^1, 12001^1, 12002^1, 12004^1, 12005^1, 12006^1, 12007^1, 12011^1, 12013^1, 12014^1, 12015^1, 12016^1, 12017^1, 12018^1, 12020^1, 12021^1, 12031^1, 12032^1, 12034^1, 12035^1, 12036^1, 12037^1, 12041^1, 12042^1, 12044^1, 12045^1, 12046^1, 12047^1, 12051^1, 12052^1, 12053^1, 12054^1, 12055^1, 12056^1, 12057^1, 13100^1, 13101^1, 13102^1, 13120^1, 13121^1, 13122^1, 13131^1, 13132^1, 13133^1, 13151^1, 13152^1, 13153^1, 21400^0, 21401^0, 36000^1, 36400^1, 36405^1, 36406^1, 36410^1, 36420^1, 36425^1, 36430^1, 36440^1, 36591^0, 36592^0, 36600^1, 36640^1, 43752^1, 51701^1, 51702^1, 51703^1, 62320^0, 62321^0, 62322^0, 62323^0, 62324^0, 62325^0, 62326^0, 62327^0, 64400^0, 64405^0, 64408^0, 64415^0, 64416^0, 64417^0, 64418^0, 64420^0, 64421^0, 64425^0, 64430^0, 64435^0, 64445^0, 64446^0, 64447^0, 64448^0, 64449^0, 64450^1, 64451^0, 64454^1, 64461^0, 64462^0, 64463^0, 64479^0, 64480^0, 64483^0, 64484^0, 64486^0, 64487^0, 64488^0, 64489^0, 64490^0, 64491^0, 64492^0, 64493^0, 64494^0, 64495^0, 64505^0, 64510^0, 64517^0, 64520^0, 64530^0, 67400^1, 67405^1, 67413^1, 67414^1, 67430^1, 67440^1, 67445^1, 67450^1, 69990^0, 92012^1, 92014^1, 93000^1, 93005^1, 93010^1, 93040^1, 93041^1, 93042^1, 93318^1, 93355^1, 94002^1, 94200^1, 94680^1, 94681^1, 94690^1, 95812^1, 95813^1, 95816^1, 95819^1, 95822^1, 95829^1, 95955^1, 96360^1, 96361^1, 96365^1, 96366^1, 96367^1, 96368^1, 96372^1, 96374^1, 96375^1, 96376^1, 96377^1, 96523^0, 97597^1, 97598^1, 97602^1, 97605^1, 97606^1, 97607^1, 97608^1, 99155^0, 99156^0, 99157^0, 99211^1, 99212^1, 99213^1, 99214^1, 99215^1, 99217^1, 99218^1, 99219^1, 99220^1, 99221^1, 99222^1, 99223^1, 99231^1, 99232^1, 99233^1, 99234^1, 99235^1, 99236^1, 99238^1, 99239^1, 99241^1, 99242^1, 99243^1, 99244^1, 99245^1, 99251^1, 99252^1, 99253^1, 99254^1, 99255^1, 99291^1, 99292^1, 99304^1, 99305^1, 99306^1, 99307^1, 99308^1, 99309^1, 99310^1, 99315^1, 99316^1, 99334^1, 99335^1, 99336^1, 99337^1, 99347^1, 99348^1, 99349^1, 99350^1, 99374^1, 99375^1, 99377^1, 99378^1, 99446^0, 99447^0, 99448^0, 99449^0, 99451^0, 99452^0, 99495^0, 99496^0, G0463^1, G0471^1
21390	0213T^0, 0216T^0, 0596T^1, 0597T^1, 0708T^1, 0709T^1, 12001^1, 12002^1, 12004^1, 12005^1, 12006^1, 12007^1, 12011^1, 12013^1, 12014^1, 12015^1, 12016^1, 12017^1, 12018^1, 12020^1, 12021^1, 12031^1, 12032^1, 12034^1, 12035^1, 12036^1, 12037^1, 12041^1, 12042^1, 12044^1, 12045^1, 12046^1, 12047^1, 12051^1, 12052^1, 12053^1, 12054^1, 12055^1, 12056^1, 12057^1, 13100^1, 13101^1, 13102^1, 13120^1, 13121^1, 13122^1, 13131^1, 13132^1, 13133^1, 13151^1, 13152^1, 13153^1, 21400^0, 21401^0, 36000^1, 36400^1, 36405^1, 36406^1, 36410^1, 36420^1, 36425^1, 36430^1, 36440^1, 36591^0, 36592^0, 36600^1, 36640^1, 43752^1, 51701^1, 51702^1, 51703^1, 62320^0, 62321^0, 62322^0, 62323^0, 62324^0, 62325^0, 62326^0, 62327^0, 64400^0, 64405^0, 64408^0, 64415^0, 64416^0, 64417^0, 64418^0, 64420^0, 64421^0, 64425^0, 64430^0, 64435^0, 64445^0, 64446^0, 64447^0, 64448^0, 64449^0, 64450^1, 64451^0, 64454^1, 64461^0, 64462^0, 64463^0, 64479^0, 64480^0, 64483^0, 64484^0, 64486^0, 64487^0, 64488^0, 64489^0, 64490^0, 64491^0, 64492^0, 64493^0, 64494^0, 64495^0, 64505^0, 64510^0, 64517^0, 64520^0, 64530^0, 67400^1, 67405^1, 67413^1, 67414^1, 67430^1, 67440^1, 67445^1, 67450^1, 69990^0, 92012^1, 92014^1, 93000^1, 93005^1, 93010^1, 93040^1, 93041^1, 93042^1, 93318^1, 93355^1, 94002^1, 94200^1, 94680^1, 94681^1, 94690^1, 95812^1, 95813^1, 95816^1, 95819^1, 95822^1, 95829^1, 95955^1, 96360^1, 96361^1, 96365^1, 96366^1, 96367^1, 96368^1, 96372^1, 96374^1, 96375^1, 96376^1, 96377^1, 96523^0, 97597^1, 97598^1, 97602^1, 97605^1, 97606^1, 97607^1, 97608^1, 99155^0, 99156^0, 99157^0, 99211^1, 99212^1, 99213^1, 99214^1, 99215^1, 99217^1, 99218^1, 99219^1, 99220^1, 99221^1, 99222^1, 99223^1, 99231^1, 99232^1, 99233^1, 99234^1, 99235^1, 99236^1, 99238^1, 99239^1, 99241^1, 99242^1, 99243^1, 99244^1, 99245^1, 99251^1, 99252^1, 99253^1, 99254^1, 99255^1, 99291^1, 99292^1, 99304^1, 99305^1, 99306^1, 99307^1, 99308^1, 99309^1, 99310^1, 99315^1, 99316^1, 99334^1, 99335^1, 99336^1, 99337^1, 99347^1, 99348^1, 99349^1, 99350^1, 99374^1, 99375^1, 99377^1, 99378^1, 99446^0, 99447^0, 99448^0, 99449^0, 99451^0, 99452^0, 99495^0, 99496^0, G0463^1, G0471^1
21395	0213T^0, 0216T^0, 0596T^1, 0597T^1, 0708T^1, 0709T^1, 12001^1, 12002^1, 12004^1, 12005^1, 12006^1, 12007^1, 12011^1, 12013^1, 12014^1, 12015^1, 12016^1, 12017^1, 12018^1, 12020^1, 12021^1, 12031^1, 12032^1, 12034^1, 12035^1, 12036^1, 12037^1, 12041^1, 12042^1, 12044^1, 12045^1, 12046^1, 12047^1, 12051^1, 12052^1, 12053^1, 12054^1, 12055^1, 12056^1, 12057^1, 13100^1, 13101^1, 13102^1, 13120^1, 13121^1, 13122^1, 13131^1, 13132^1, 13133^1, 13151^1, 13152^1, 13153^1, 20900^1, 20902^1, 21400^0, 21401^0, 36000^1, 36400^1, 36405^1, 36406^1, 36410^1, 36420^1, 36425^1, 36430^1, 36440^1, 36591^0, 36592^0, 36600^1, 36640^1, 43752^1, 51701^1, 51702^1, 51703^1, 62320^0, 62321^0, 62322^0, 62323^0, 62324^0, 62325^0, 62326^0, 62327^0, 64400^0, 64405^0, 64408^0, 64415^0, 64416^0, 64417^0, 64418^0, 64420^0, 64421^0, 64425^0, 64430^0, 64435^0, 64445^0, 64446^0, 64447^0, 64448^0, 64449^0, 64450^1, 64451^0, 64454^1, 64461^0, 64462^0, 64463^0, 64479^0, 64480^0, 64483^0, 64484^0, 64486^0, 64487^0, 64488^0, 64489^0, 64490^0, 64491^0, 64492^0, 64493^0, 64494^0, 64495^0, 64505^0, 64510^0, 64517^0, 64520^0, 64530^0, 67400^1, 67405^1, 67413^1, 67414^1, 67430^1, 67440^1, 67445^1, 67450^1, 69990^0, 92012^1, 92014^1, 93000^1, 93005^1, 93010^1, 93040^1, 93041^1, 93042^1, 93318^1, 93355^1, 94002^1, 94200^1, 94680^1, 94681^1, 94690^1, 95812^1, 95813^1, 95816^1, 95819^1, 95822^1, 95829^1, 95955^1, 96360^1, 96361^1, 96365^1, 96366^1, 96367^1, 96368^1, 96372^1, 96374^1, 96375^1, 96376^1, 96377^1, 96523^0, 97597^1, 97598^1, 97602^1, 97605^1, 97606^1, 97607^1, 97608^1, 99155^0, 99156^0, 99157^0, 99211^1, 99212^1, 99213^1, 99214^1, 99215^1, 99217^1, 99218^1, 99219^1, 99220^1, 99221^1, 99222^1, 99223^1, 99231^1, 99232^1, 99233^1, 99234^1, 99235^1, 99236^1, 99238^1, 99239^1, 99241^1, 99242^1, 99243^1, 99244^1, 99245^1, 99251^1, 99252^1, 99253^1, 99254^1, 99255^1, 99291^1, 99292^1, 99304^1, 99305^1, 99306^1, 99307^1, 99308^1, 99309^1, 99310^1, 99315^1, 99316^1, 99334^1, 99335^1, 99336^1, 99337^1, 99347^1, 99348^1, 99349^1, 99350^1, 99374^1, 99375^1, 99377^1, 99378^1, 99446^0, 99447^0, 99448^0, 99449^0, 99451^0, 99452^0, 99495^0, 99496^0, G0463^1, G0471^1
21400	0213T^0, 0216T^0, 0596T^1, 0597T^1, 0708T^1, 0709T^1, 12001^1, 12002^1, 12004^1, 12005^1, 12006^1, 12007^1, 12011^1, 12013^1, 12014^1, 12015^1, 12016^1, 12017^1, 12018^1, 12020^1, 12021^1, 12031^1, 12032^1, 12034^1, 12035^1, 12036^1, 12037^1, 12041^1, 12042^1, 12044^1, 12045^1, 12046^1, 12047^1, 12051^1, 12052^1, 12053^1, 12054^1, 12055^1, 12056^1, 12057^1, 13100^1, 13101^1, 13102^1, 13120^1, 13121^1, 13122^1, 13131^1, 13132^1, 13133^1, 13151^1, 13152^1, 13153^1, 36000^1, 36400^1, 36405^1, 36406^1, 36410^1, 36420^1, 36425^1, 36430^1, 36440^1, 36591^0, 36592^0, 36600^1, 36640^1, 43752^1, 51701^1, 51702^1, 51703^1, 62320^0, 62321^0, 62322^0, 62323^0, 62324^0, 62325^0, 62326^0, 62327^0, 64400^0, 64405^0, 64408^0, 64415^0, 64416^0, 64417^0, 64418^0, 64420^0, 64421^0, 64425^0, 64430^0, 64435^0, 64445^0, 64446^0, 64447^0, 64448^0, 64449^0, 64450^1, 64451^0, 64454^1, 64461^0, 64462^0, 64463^0, 64479^0, 64480^0, 64483^0, 64484^0, 64486^0, 64487^0, 64488^0, 64489^0, 64490^0, 64491^0, 64492^0, 64493^0, 64494^0, 64495^0, 64505^0, 64510^0, 64517^0, 64520^0, 64530^0, 67400^1, 67405^1, 67413^1, 67414^1, 67430^1, 67440^1, 67445^1, 67450^1, 69990^0, 92012^1, 92014^1, 93000^1, 93005^1, 93010^1, 93040^1, 93041^1, 93042^1, 93318^1, 93355^1, 94002^1, 94200^1, 94680^1, 94681^1, 94690^1, 95812^1, 95813^1, 95816^1, 95819^1, 95822^1, 95829^1, 95955^1, 96360^1, 96361^1, 96365^1, 96366^1, 96367^1, 96368^1, 96372^1, 96374^1, 96375^1, 96376^1, 96377^1, 96523^0, 97597^1, 97598^1, 97602^1, 97605^1, 97606^1, 97607^1, 97608^1, 99155^0, 99156^0, 99157^0, 99211^1, 99212^1, 99213^1, 99214^1, 99215^1, 99217^1, 99218^1, 99219^1, 99220^1, 99221^1, 99222^1, 99223^1, 99231^1, 99232^1, 99233^1, 99234^1, 99235^1, 99236^1, 99238^1, 99239^1, 99241^1, 99242^1, 99243^1, 99244^1, 99245^1, 99251^1, 99252^1, 99253^1, 99254^1, 99255^1, 99291^1, 99292^1, 99304^1, 99305^1, 99306^1, 99307^1, 99308^1, 99309^1, 99310^1, 99315^1, 99316^1, 99334^1, 99335^1, 99336^1, 99337^1, 99347^1, 99348^1, 99349^1, 99350^1, 99374^1, 99375^1, 99377^1, 99378^1, 99446^0, 99447^0, 99448^0, 99449^0, 99451^0, 99452^0, 99495^0, 99496^0, G0463^1, G0471^1, J2001^1
21401	0213T^0, 0216T^0, 0596T^1, 0597T^1, 0708T^1, 0709T^1, 12001^1, 12002^1, 12004^1, 12005^1, 12006^1, 12007^1, 12011^1, 12013^1, 12014^1, 12015^1, 12016^1, 12017^1, 12018^1, 12020^1, 12021^1, 12031^1, 12032^1, 12034^1, 12035^1, 12036^1, 12037^1, 12041^1, 12042^1, 12044^1, 12045^1, 12046^1, 12047^1, 12051^1, 12052^1, 12053^1, 12054^1, 12055^1, 12056^1, 12057^1, 13100^1, 13101^1, 13102^1, 13120^1, 13121^1, 13122^1, 13131^1, 13132^1, 13133^1, 13151^1, 13152^1, 13153^1, 20650^1, 21400^1, 36000^1, 36400^1, 36405^1, 36406^1, 36410^1, 36420^1, 36425^1, 36430^1, 36440^1, 36591^0, 36592^0, 36600^1, 36640^1, 43752^1, 51701^1, 51702^1, 51703^1, 62320^0, 62321^0, 62322^0, 62323^0, 62324^0, 62325^0, 62326^0, 62327^0, 64400^0, 64405^0, 64408^0, 64415^0, 64416^0, 64417^0, 64418^0, 64420^0, 64421^0, 64425^0, 64430^0, 64435^0, 64445^0, 64446^0, 64447^0, 64448^0, 64449^0, 64450^1, 64451^0, 64454^1, 64461^0, 64462^0, 64463^0, 64479^0, 64480^0, 64483^0, 64484^0, 64486^0, 64487^0, 64488^0, 64489^0, 64490^0, 64491^0, 64492^0, 64493^0, 64494^0, 64495^0, 64505^0, 64510^0, 64517^0, 64520^0, 64530^0, 67400^1, 67405^1, 67413^1, 67414^1, 67430^1, 67440^1, 67445^1, 67450^1, 69990^0, 92012^1, 92014^1, 93000^1, 93005^1, 93010^1, 93040^1, 93041^1, 93042^1, 93318^1, 93355^1, 94002^1, 94200^1, 94680^1, 94681^1, 94690^1, 95812^1, 95813^1, 95816^1, 95819^1, 95822^1, 95829^1, 95955^1, 96360^1, 96361^1, 96365^1, 96366^1, 96367^1, 96368^1, 96372^1, 96374^1, 96375^1, 96376^1, 96377^1, 96523^0, 97597^1, 97598^1, 97602^1, 97605^1, 97606^1, 97607^1, 97608^1, 99155^0, 99156^0, 99157^0, 99211^1, 99212^1, 99213^1, 99214^1, 99215^1, 99217^1,

0 = Modifier usage not allowed or inappropriate 1 = Modifier usage allowed

Code 1	Code 2
	99218[1], 99219[1], 99220[1], 99221[1], 99222[1], 99223[1], 99231[1], 99232[1], 99233[1], 99234[1], 99235[1], 99236[1], 99238[1], 99239[1], 99241[1], 99242[1], 99243[1], 99244[1], 99245[1], 99251[1], 99252[1], 99253[1], 99254[1], 99255[1], 99291[1], 99292[1], 99304[1], 99305[1], 99306[1], 99307[1], 99308[1], 99309[1], 99310[1], 99315[1], 99316[1], 99334[1], 99335[1], 99336[1], 99337[1], 99347[1], 99348[1], 99349[1], 99350[1], 99374[1], 99375[1], 99377[1], 99378[1], 99446[0], 99447[0], 99448[0], 99449[0], 99451[0], 99452[0], 99495[0], 99496[0], G0463[1], G0471[1], J2001[1]
21406	0213T[0], 0216T[0], 0596T[1], 0597T[1], 0708T[1], 0709T[1], 12001[1], 12002[1], 12004[1], 12005[1], 12006[1], 12007[1], 12011[1], 12013[1], 12014[1], 12015[1], 12016[1], 12017[1], 12018[1], 12020[1], 12021[1], 12031[1], 12032[1], 12034[1], 12035[1], 12036[1], 12037[1], 12041[1], 12042[1], 12044[1], 12045[1], 12046[1], 12047[1], 12051[1], 12052[1], 12053[1], 12054[1], 12055[1], 12056[1], 12057[1], 13100[1], 13101[1], 13102[1], 13120[1], 13121[1], 13122[1], 13131[1], 13132[1], 13133[1], 13151[1], 13152[1], 13153[1], 20650[1], 21400[1], 21401[1], 36000[1], 36400[1], 36405[1], 36406[1], 36410[1], 36420[1], 36425[1], 36430[1], 36440[1], 36591[0], 36592[0], 36600[1], 36640[1], 43752[1], 51701[1], 51702[1], 51703[1], 62320[0], 62321[0], 62322[0], 62323[0], 62324[0], 62325[0], 62326[0], 62327[0], 64400[0], 64405[0], 64408[0], 64415[0], 64416[0], 64417[0], 64418[0], 64420[0], 64421[0], 64425[0], 64430[0], 64435[0], 64445[0], 64446[0], 64447[0], 64448[0], 64449[0], 64450[1], 64451[0], 64454[1], 64461[0], 64462[0], 64463[0], 64479[0], 64480[0], 64483[0], 64484[0], 64486[0], 64487[0], 64488[0], 64489[0], 64490[0], 64491[0], 64492[0], 64493[0], 64494[0], 64495[0], 64505[0], 64510[0], 64517[0], 64520[0], 64530[0], 67400[1], 67405[1], 67413[1], 67414[1], 67430[1], 67440[1], 67445[1], 67450[1], 69990[0], 92012[1], 92014[1], 93000[1], 93005[1], 93010[1], 93040[1], 93041[1], 93042[1], 93318[1], 93355[1], 94002[1], 94200[1], 94680[1], 94681[1], 94690[1], 95812[1], 95813[1], 95816[1], 95819[1], 95822[1], 95829[1], 95955[1], 96360[1], 96361[1], 96365[1], 96366[1], 96367[1], 96368[1], 96372[1], 96374[1], 96375[1], 96376[1], 96377[1], 96523[0], 97597[1], 97598[1], 97602[1], 97605[1], 97606[1], 97607[1], 97608[1], 99155[0], 99156[0], 99157[0], 99211[1], 99212[1], 99213[1], 99214[1], 99215[1], 99217[1], 99218[1], 99219[1], 99220[1], 99221[1], 99222[1], 99223[1], 99231[1], 99232[1], 99233[1], 99234[1], 99235[1], 99236[1], 99238[1], 99239[1], 99241[1], 99242[1], 99243[1], 99244[1], 99245[1], 99251[1], 99252[1], 99253[1], 99254[1], 99255[1], 99291[1], 99292[1], 99304[1], 99305[1], 99306[1], 99307[1], 99308[1], 99309[1], 99310[1], 99315[1], 99316[1], 99334[1], 99335[1], 99336[1], 99337[1], 99347[1], 99348[1], 99349[1], 99350[1], 99374[1], 99375[1], 99377[1], 99378[1], 99446[0], 99447[0], 99448[0], 99449[0], 99451[0], 99452[0], 99495[0], 99496[0], G0463[1], G0471[1]
21407	0213T[0], 0216T[0], 0596T[1], 0597T[1], 0708T[1], 0709T[1], 12001[1], 12002[1], 12004[1], 12005[1], 12006[1], 12007[1], 12011[1], 12013[1], 12014[1], 12015[1], 12016[1], 12017[1], 12018[1], 12020[1], 12021[1], 12031[1], 12032[1], 12034[1], 12035[1], 12036[1], 12037[1], 12041[1], 12042[1], 12044[1], 12045[1], 12046[1], 12047[1], 12051[1], 12052[1], 12053[1], 12054[1], 12055[1], 12056[1], 12057[1], 13100[1], 13101[1], 13102[1], 13120[1], 13121[1], 13122[1], 13131[1], 13132[1], 13133[1], 13151[1], 13152[1], 13153[1], 20650[1], 21400[1], 21401[1], 21406[1], 36000[1], 36400[1], 36405[1], 36406[1], 36410[1], 36420[1], 36425[1], 36430[1], 36440[1], 36591[0], 36592[0], 36600[1], 36640[1], 43752[1], 51701[1], 51702[1], 51703[1], 62320[0], 62321[0], 62322[0], 62323[0], 62324[0], 62325[0], 62326[0], 62327[0], 64400[0], 64405[0], 64408[0], 64415[0], 64416[0], 64417[0], 64418[0], 64420[0], 64421[0], 64425[0], 64430[0], 64435[0], 64445[0], 64446[0], 64447[0], 64448[0], 64449[0], 64450[1], 64451[0], 64454[1], 64461[0], 64462[0], 64463[0], 64479[0], 64480[0], 64483[0], 64484[0], 64486[0], 64487[0], 64488[0], 64489[0], 64490[0], 64491[0], 64492[0], 64493[0], 64494[0], 64495[0], 64505[0], 64510[0], 64517[0], 64520[0], 64530[0], 67400[1], 67405[1], 67413[1], 67414[1], 67430[1], 67440[1], 67445[1], 67450[1], 69990[0], 92012[1], 92014[1], 93000[1], 93005[1], 93010[1], 93040[1], 93041[1], 93042[1], 93318[1], 93355[1], 94002[1], 94200[1], 94680[1], 94681[1], 94690[1], 95812[1], 95813[1], 95816[1], 95819[1], 95822[1], 95829[1], 95955[1], 96360[1], 96361[1], 96365[1], 96366[1], 96367[1], 96368[1], 96372[1], 96374[1], 96375[1], 96376[1], 96377[1], 96523[0], 97597[1], 97598[1], 97602[1], 97605[1], 97606[1], 97607[1], 97608[1], 99155[0], 99156[0], 99157[0], 99211[1], 99212[1], 99213[1], 99214[1], 99215[1], 99217[1], 99218[1], 99219[1], 99220[1], 99221[1], 99222[1], 99223[1], 99231[1], 99232[1], 99233[1], 99234[1], 99235[1], 99236[1], 99238[1], 99239[1], 99241[1], 99242[1], 99243[1], 99244[1], 99245[1], 99251[1], 99252[1], 99253[1], 99254[1], 99255[1], 99291[1], 99292[1], 99304[1], 99305[1], 99306[1], 99307[1], 99308[1], 99309[1], 99310[1], 99315[1], 99316[1], 99334[1], 99335[1], 99336[1], 99337[1], 99347[1], 99348[1], 99349[1], 99350[1], 99374[1], 99375[1], 99377[1], 99378[1], 99446[0], 99447[0], 99448[0], 99449[0], 99451[0], 99452[0], 99495[0], 99496[0], G0463[1], G0471[1]
21408	0213T[0], 0216T[0], 0596T[1], 0597T[1], 0708T[1], 0709T[1], 12001[1], 12002[1], 12004[1], 12005[1], 12006[1], 12007[1], 12011[1], 12013[1], 12014[1], 12015[1], 12016[1], 12017[1], 12018[1], 12020[1], 12021[1], 12031[1], 12032[1], 12034[1], 12035[1], 12036[1], 12037[1], 12041[1], 12042[1], 12044[1], 12045[1], 12046[1], 12047[1], 12051[1], 12052[1], 12053[1], 12054[1], 12055[1], 12056[1], 12057[1], 13100[1], 13101[1], 13102[1], 13120[1], 13121[1], 13122[1], 13131[1], 13132[1], 13133[1], 13151[1], 13152[1], 13153[1], 20900[1], 20902[1], 21400[1], 21401[1], 36000[1], 36400[1], 36405[1], 36406[1], 36410[1], 36420[1], 36425[1], 36430[1], 36440[1], 36591[0], 36592[0], 36600[1], 36640[1], 43752[1], 51701[1], 51702[1], 51703[1], 62320[0], 62321[0], 62322[0], 62323[0], 62324[0], 62325[0], 62326[0], 62327[0], 64400[0], 64405[0], 64408[0], 64415[0], 64416[0], 64417[0], 64418[0], 64420[0], 64421[0], 64425[0], 64430[0], 64435[0], 64445[0], 64446[0], 64447[0], 64448[0], 64449[0], 64450[1], 64451[0], 64454[1], 64461[0], 64462[0], 64463[0], 64479[0], 64480[0], 64483[0], 64484[0], 64486[0], 64487[0], 64488[0], 64489[0], 64490[0], 64491[0], 64492[0], 64493[0], 64494[0], 64495[0], 64505[0], 64510[0], 64517[0], 64520[0], 64530[0], 67400[1], 67405[1], 67413[1], 67414[1], 67430[1], 67440[1], 67445[1], 67450[1], 69990[0], 92012[1], 92014[1], 93000[1], 93005[1], 93010[1], 93040[1], 93041[1], 93042[1], 93318[1], 93355[1], 94002[1], 94200[1], 94680[1], 94681[1], 94690[1], 95812[1], 95813[1], 95816[1], 95819[1], 95822[1], 95829[1], 95955[1], 96360[1], 96361[1], 96365[1], 96366[1], 96367[1], 96368[1], 96372[1], 96374[1], 96375[1], 96376[1], 96377[1], 96523[0], 97597[1], 97598[1], 97602[1], 97605[1], 97606[1], 97607[1], 97608[1], 99155[0], 99156[0], 99157[0], 99211[1], 99212[1], 99213[1], 99214[1], 99215[1], 99217[1], 99218[1], 99219[1], 99220[1], 99221[1], 99222[1], 99223[1], 99231[1], 99232[1], 99233[1], 99234[1], 99235[1], 99236[1], 99238[1], 99239[1], 99241[1], 99242[1], 99243[1], 99244[1], 99245[1], 99251[1], 99252[1], 99253[1], 99254[1], 99255[1], 99291[1], 99292[1], 99304[1], 99305[1], 99306[1], 99307[1], 99308[1], 99309[1], 99310[1], 99315[1], 99316[1], 99334[1], 99335[1], 99336[1], 99337[1], 99347[1], 99348[1], 99349[1], 99350[1], 99374[1], 99375[1], 99377[1], 99378[1], 99446[0], 99447[0], 99448[0], 99449[0], 99451[0], 99452[0], 99495[0], 99496[0], G0463[1], G0471[1]
65091	0213T[0], 0216T[0], 0596T[1], 0597T[1], 0708T[1], 0709T[1], 12001[1], 12002[1], 12004[1], 12005[1], 12006[1], 12007[1], 12011[1], 12013[1], 12014[1], 12015[1], 12016[1], 12017[1], 12018[1], 12020[1], 12021[1], 12031[1], 12032[1], 12034[1], 12035[1], 12036[1], 12037[1], 12041[1], 12042[1], 12044[1], 12045[1], 12046[1], 12047[1], 12051[1], 12052[1], 12053[1], 12054[1], 12055[1], 12056[1], 12057[1], 13100[1], 13101[1], 13102[1], 13120[1], 13121[1], 13122[1], 13131[1], 13132[1], 13133[1], 13151[1], 13152[1], 13153[1], 36000[1], 36400[1], 36405[1], 36406[1], 36410[1], 36420[1], 36425[1], 36430[1], 36440[1], 36591[0], 36592[0], 36600[1], 36640[1], 43752[1], 51701[1], 51702[1], 51703[1], 62320[0], 62321[0], 62322[0], 62323[0], 62324[0], 62325[0], 62326[0], 62327[0], 64400[0], 64405[0], 64408[0], 64415[0], 64416[0], 64417[0], 64418[0], 64420[0], 64421[0], 64425[0], 64430[0], 64435[0], 64445[0], 64446[0], 64447[0], 64448[0], 64449[0], 64450[0], 64451[0], 64454[0], 64461[0], 64462[0], 64463[0], 64479[0], 64480[0], 64483[0], 64484[0], 64486[0], 64487[0], 64488[0], 64489[0], 64490[0], 64491[0], 64492[0], 64493[0], 64494[0], 64495[0], 64505[0], 64510[0], 64517[0], 64520[0], 64530[0], 67500[1], 69990[0], 92012[1], 92014[1], 92018[1], 92019[1], 93000[1], 93005[1], 93010[1], 93040[1], 93041[1], 93042[1], 93318[1], 93355[1], 94002[1], 94200[1], 94680[1], 94681[1], 94690[1], 95812[1], 95813[1], 95816[1], 95819[1], 95822[1], 95829[1], 95955[1], 96360[1], 96361[1], 96365[1], 96366[1], 96367[1], 96368[1], 96372[1], 96374[1], 96375[1], 96376[1], 96377[1], 96523[0], 99155[0], 99156[0], 99157[0], 99211[1], 99212[1], 99213[1], 99214[1], 99215[1], 99217[1], 99218[1], 99219[1], 99220[1], 99221[1], 99222[1], 99223[1], 99231[1], 99232[1], 99233[1], 99234[1], 99235[1], 99236[1], 99238[1], 99239[1], 99241[1], 99242[1], 99243[1], 99244[1], 99245[1], 99251[1], 99252[1], 99253[1], 99254[1], 99255[1], 99291[1], 99292[1], 99304[1], 99305[1], 99306[1], 99307[1], 99308[1], 99309[1], 99310[1], 99315[1], 99316[1], 99334[1], 99335[1], 99336[1], 99337[1], 99347[1], 99348[1], 99349[1], 99350[1], 99374[1], 99375[1], 99377[1], 99378[1], 99446[0], 99447[0], 99448[0], 99449[0], 99451[0], 99452[0], 99495[0], 99496[0], G0463[1], G0471[1], J0670[1], J2001[1]
65093	0213T[0], 0216T[0], 0596T[1], 0597T[1], 0708T[1], 0709T[1], 12001[1], 12002[1], 12004[1], 12005[1], 12006[1], 12007[1], 12011[1], 12013[1], 12014[1], 12015[1], 12016[1], 12017[1], 12018[1], 12020[1], 12021[1], 12031[1], 12032[1], 12034[1], 12035[1], 12036[1], 12037[1], 12041[1], 12042[1], 12044[1], 12045[1], 12046[1], 12047[1], 12051[1], 12052[1], 12053[1], 12054[1], 12055[1], 12056[1], 12057[1], 13100[1], 13101[1], 13102[1], 13120[1], 13121[1], 13122[1], 13131[1], 13132[1], 13133[1], 13151[1], 13152[1], 13153[1], 36000[1], 36400[1], 36405[1], 36406[1], 36410[1], 36420[1], 36425[1], 36430[1], 36440[1], 36591[0], 36592[0], 36600[1], 36640[1], 43752[1], 51701[1], 51702[1], 51703[1], 62320[0], 62321[0], 62322[0], 62323[0], 62324[0], 62325[0], 62326[0], 62327[0], 64400[0], 64405[0], 64408[0], 64415[0], 64416[0], 64417[0], 64418[0], 64420[0], 64421[0], 64425[0], 64430[0], 64435[0], 64445[0], 64446[0], 64447[0], 64448[0], 64449[0], 64450[0], 64451[0], 64454[0], 64461[0], 64462[0], 64463[0], 64479[0], 64480[0], 64483[0], 64484[0], 64486[0], 64487[0], 64488[0], 64489[0], 64490[0], 64491[0], 64492[0], 64493[0], 64494[0], 64495[0], 64505[0], 64510[0], 64517[0], 64520[0], 64530[0], 65091[1], 65103[1], 65105[1], 65130[1], 67500[1], 69990[0], 92012[1], 92014[1], 92018[1], 92019[1], 93000[1], 93005[1], 93010[1], 93040[1], 93041[1], 93042[1], 93318[1], 93355[1], 94002[1], 94200[1], 94680[1], 94681[1], 94690[1], 95812[1], 95813[1], 95816[1], 95819[1], 95822[1], 95829[1], 95955[1], 96360[1], 96361[1], 96365[1], 96366[1], 96367[1], 96368[1], 96372[1], 96374[1], 96375[1], 96376[1], 96377[1], 96523[0], 99155[0], 99156[0], 99157[0], 99211[1], 99212[1], 99213[1], 99214[1], 99215[1], 99217[1], 99218[1], 99219[1], 99220[1], 99221[1], 99222[1], 99223[1], 99231[1], 99232[1], 99233[1], 99234[1], 99235[1], 99236[1], 99238[1], 99239[1], 99241[1], 99242[1], 99243[1], 99244[1], 99245[1], 99251[1], 99252[1], 99253[1], 99254[1], 99255[1], 99291[1], 99292[1], 99304[1], 99305[1], 99306[1], 99307[1], 99308[1], 99309[1], 99310[1], 99315[1], 99316[1], 99334[1], 99335[1], 99336[1], 99337[1], 99347[1], 99348[1], 99349[1], 99350[1], 99374[1], 99375[1], 99377[1], 99378[1], 99446[0], 99447[0], 99448[0], 99449[0], 99451[0], 99452[0], 99495[0], 99496[0], G0463[1], G0471[1], J0670[1], J2001[1]
65101	0213T[0], 0216T[0], 0596T[1], 0597T[1], 0708T[1], 0709T[1], 12001[1], 12002[1], 12004[1], 12005[1], 12006[1], 12007[1], 12011[1], 12013[1], 12014[1], 12015[1], 12016[1], 12017[1], 12018[1], 12020[1], 12021[1], 12031[1], 12032[1], 12034[1], 12035[1], 12036[1], 12037[1], 12041[1], 12042[1], 12044[1], 12045[1], 12046[1], 12047[1], 12051[1], 12052[1], 12053[1], 12054[1], 12055[1], 12056[1], 12057[1], 13100[1], 13101[1], 13102[1], 13120[1], 13121[1], 13122[1], 13131[1], 13132[1], 13133[1], 13151[1], 13152[1], 13153[1], 36000[1], 36400[1], 36405[1], 36406[1], 36410[1], 36420[1], 36425[1], 36430[1],

0 = Modifier usage not allowed or inappropriate 1 = Modifier usage allowed

Code 1	Code 2
	36440[1], 36591[0], 36592[0], 36600[1], 36640[1], 43752[1], 51701[1], 51702[1], 51703[1], 62320[0], 62321[0], 62322[0], 62323[0], 62324[0], 62325[0], 62326[0], 62327[0], 64400[0], 64405[0], 64408[0], 64415[0], 64416[0], 64417[0], 64418[0], 64420[0], 64421[0], 64425[0], 64430[0], 64435[0], 64445[0], 64446[0], 64447[0], 64448[0], 64449[0], 64450[0], 64451[0], 64454[0], 64461[0], 64462[0], 64463[0], 64479[0], 64480[0], 64483[0], 64484[0], 64486[0], 64487[0], 64488[0], 64489[0], 64490[0], 64491[0], 64492[0], 64493[0], 64494[0], 64495[0], 64505[0], 64510[0], 64517[0], 64520[0], 64530[0], 67500[1], 69990[0], 92012[1], 92014[1], 92018[1], 92019[1], 93000[1], 93005[1], 93010[1], 93040[1], 93041[1], 93042[1], 93318[1], 93355[1], 94002[1], 94200[1], 94680[1], 94681[1], 94690[1], 95812[1], 95813[1], 95816[1], 95819[1], 95822[1], 95829[1], 95955[1], 96360[1], 96361[1], 96365[1], 96366[1], 96367[1], 96368[1], 96372[1], 96374[1], 96375[1], 96376[1], 96377[1], 96523[0], 99155[0], 99156[0], 99157[0], 99211[1], 99212[1], 99213[1], 99214[1], 99215[1], 99217[1], 99218[1], 99219[1], 99220[1], 99221[1], 99222[1], 99223[1], 99231[1], 99232[1], 99233[1], 99234[1], 99235[1], 99236[1], 99238[1], 99239[1], 99241[1], 99242[1], 99243[1], 99244[1], 99245[1], 99251[1], 99252[1], 99253[1], 99254[1], 99255[1], 99291[1], 99292[1], 99304[1], 99305[1], 99306[1], 99307[1], 99308[1], 99309[1], 99310[1], 99315[1], 99316[1], 99334[1], 99335[1], 99336[1], 99337[1], 99347[1], 99348[1], 99349[1], 99350[1], 99374[1], 99375[1], 99377[1], 99378[1], 99446[0], 99447[0], 99448[0], 99449[0], 99451[0], 99452[0], 99495[0], 99496[0], G0463[1], G0471[1], J0670[1], J2001[1]
65103	0213T[0], 0216T[0], 0596T[1], 0597T[1], 0708T[1], 0709T[1], 12001[1], 12002[1], 12004[1], 12005[1], 12006[1], 12007[1], 12011[1], 12013[1], 12014[1], 12015[1], 12016[1], 12017[1], 12018[1], 12020[1], 12021[1], 12031[1], 12032[1], 12034[1], 12035[1], 12036[1], 12037[1], 12041[1], 12042[1], 12044[1], 12045[1], 12046[1], 12047[1], 12051[1], 12052[1], 12053[1], 12054[1], 12055[1], 12056[1], 12057[1], 13100[1], 13101[1], 13102[1], 13120[1], 13121[1], 13122[1], 13131[1], 13132[1], 13133[1], 13151[1], 13152[1], 13153[1], 36000[1], 36400[1], 36405[1], 36406[1], 36410[1], 36420[1], 36425[1], 36430[1], 36440[1], 36591[0], 36592[0], 36600[1], 36640[1], 43752[1], 51701[1], 51702[1], 51703[1], 62320[0], 62321[0], 62322[0], 62323[0], 62324[0], 62325[0], 62326[0], 62327[0], 64400[0], 64405[0], 64408[0], 64415[0], 64416[0], 64417[0], 64418[0], 64420[0], 64421[0], 64425[0], 64430[0], 64435[0], 64445[0], 64446[0], 64447[0], 64448[0], 64449[0], 64450[0], 64451[0], 64454[0], 64461[0], 64462[0], 64463[0], 64479[0], 64480[0], 64483[0], 64484[0], 64486[0], 64487[0], 64488[0], 64489[0], 64490[0], 64491[0], 64492[0], 64493[0], 64494[0], 64495[0], 64505[0], 64510[0], 64517[0], 64520[0], 64530[0], 65101[1], 65135[1], 67500[1], 69990[0], 92012[1], 92014[1], 92018[1], 92019[1], 93000[1], 93005[1], 93010[1], 93040[1], 93041[1], 93042[1], 93318[1], 93355[1], 94002[1], 94200[1], 94680[1], 94681[1], 94690[1], 95812[1], 95813[1], 95816[1], 95819[1], 95822[1], 95829[1], 95955[1], 96360[1], 96361[1], 96365[1], 96366[1], 96367[1], 96368[1], 96372[1], 96374[1], 96375[1], 96376[1], 96377[1], 96523[0], 99155[0], 99156[0], 99157[0], 99211[1], 99212[1], 99213[1], 99214[1], 99215[1], 99217[1], 99218[1], 99219[1], 99220[1], 99221[1], 99222[1], 99223[1], 99231[1], 99232[1], 99233[1], 99234[1], 99235[1], 99236[1], 99238[1], 99239[1], 99241[1], 99242[1], 99243[1], 99244[1], 99245[1], 99251[1], 99252[1], 99253[1], 99254[1], 99255[1], 99291[1], 99292[1], 99304[1], 99305[1], 99306[1], 99307[1], 99308[1], 99309[1], 99310[1], 99315[1], 99316[1], 99334[1], 99335[1], 99336[1], 99337[1], 99347[1], 99348[1], 99349[1], 99350[1], 99374[1], 99375[1], 99377[1], 99378[1], 99446[0], 99447[0], 99448[0], 99449[0], 99451[0], 99452[0], 99495[0], 99496[0], G0463[1], G0471[1], J0670[1], J2001[1]
65105	0213T[0], 0216T[0], 0596T[1], 0597T[1], 0708T[1], 0709T[1], 12001[1], 12002[1], 12004[1], 12005[1], 12006[1], 12007[1], 12011[1], 12013[1], 12014[1], 12015[1], 12016[1], 12017[1], 12018[1], 12020[1], 12021[1], 12031[1], 12032[1], 12034[1], 12035[1], 12036[1], 12037[1], 12041[1], 12042[1], 12044[1], 12045[1], 12046[1], 12047[1], 12051[1], 12052[1], 12053[1], 12054[1], 12055[1], 12056[1], 12057[1], 13100[1], 13101[1], 13102[1], 13120[1], 13121[1], 13122[1], 13131[1], 13132[1], 13133[1], 13151[1], 13152[1], 13153[1], 36000[1], 36400[1], 36405[1], 36406[1], 36410[1], 36420[1], 36425[1], 36430[1], 36440[1], 36591[0], 36592[0], 36600[1], 36640[1], 43752[1], 51701[1], 51702[1], 51703[1], 62320[0], 62321[0], 62322[0], 62323[0], 62324[0], 62325[0], 62326[0], 62327[0], 64400[0], 64405[0], 64408[0], 64415[0], 64416[0], 64417[0], 64418[0], 64420[0], 64421[0], 64425[0], 64430[0], 64435[0], 64445[0], 64446[0], 64447[0], 64448[0], 64449[0], 64450[0], 64451[0], 64454[0], 64461[0], 64462[0], 64463[0], 64479[0], 64480[0], 64483[0], 64484[0], 64486[0], 64487[0], 64488[0], 64489[0], 64490[0], 64491[0], 64492[0], 64493[0], 64494[0], 64495[0], 64505[0], 64510[0], 64517[0], 64520[0], 64530[0], 65101[1], 65103[1], 65140[1], 67500[1], 69990[0], 92012[1], 92014[1], 92018[1], 92019[1], 93000[1], 93005[1], 93010[1], 93040[1], 93041[1], 93042[1], 93318[1], 93355[1], 94002[1], 94200[1], 94680[1], 94681[1], 94690[1], 95812[1], 95813[1], 95816[1], 95819[1], 95822[1], 95829[1], 95955[1], 96360[1], 96361[1], 96365[1], 96366[1], 96367[1], 96368[1], 96372[1], 96374[1], 96375[1], 96376[1], 96377[1], 96523[0], 99155[0], 99156[0], 99157[0], 99211[1], 99212[1], 99213[1], 99214[1], 99215[1], 99217[1], 99218[1], 99219[1], 99220[1], 99221[1], 99222[1], 99223[1], 99231[1], 99232[1], 99233[1], 99234[1], 99235[1], 99236[1], 99238[1], 99239[1], 99241[1], 99242[1], 99243[1], 99244[1], 99245[1], 99251[1], 99252[1], 99253[1], 99254[1], 99255[1], 99291[1], 99292[1], 99304[1], 99305[1], 99306[1], 99307[1], 99308[1], 99309[1], 99310[1], 99315[1], 99316[1], 99334[1], 99335[1], 99336[1], 99337[1], 99347[1], 99348[1], 99349[1], 99350[1], 99374[1], 99375[1], 99377[1], 99378[1], 99446[0], 99447[0], 99448[0], 99449[0], 99451[0], 99452[0], 99495[0], 99496[0], G0463[1], G0471[1], J0670[1], J2001[1]
65110	0213T[0], 0216T[0], 0596T[1], 0597T[1], 0708T[1], 0709T[1], 11000[1], 11001[1], 11004[1], 11005[1], 11006[1], 11042[1], 11043[1], 11044[1], 11045[1], 11046[1], 11047[1], 12001[1], 12002[1], 12004[1], 12005[1], 12006[1], 12007[1], 12011[1], 12013[1], 12014[1], 12015[1], 12016[1], 12017[1], 12018[1], 12020[1], 12021[1], 12031[1], 12032[1], 12034[1], 12035[1], 12036[1], 12037[1], 12041[1], 12042[1], 12044[1], 12045[1], 12046[1], 12047[1], 12051[1], 12052[1], 12053[1], 12054[1], 12055[1], 12056[1], 12057[1], 13100[1], 13101[1], 13102[1], 13120[1], 13121[1], 13122[1], 13131[1], 13132[1], 13133[1], 13151[1], 13152[1], 13153[1], 31225[1], 36000[1], 36400[1], 36405[1], 36406[1], 36410[1], 36420[1], 36425[1], 36430[1], 36440[1], 36591[0], 36592[0], 36600[1], 36640[1], 43752[1], 51701[1], 51702[1], 51703[1], 62320[0], 62321[0], 62322[0], 62323[0], 62324[0], 62325[0], 62326[0], 62327[0], 64400[0], 64405[0], 64408[0], 64415[0], 64416[0], 64417[0], 64418[0], 64420[0], 64421[0], 64425[0], 64430[0], 64435[0], 64445[0], 64446[0], 64447[0], 64448[0], 64449[0], 64450[0], 64451[0], 64454[0], 64461[0], 64462[0], 64463[0], 64479[0], 64480[0], 64483[0], 64484[0], 64486[0], 64487[0], 64488[0], 64489[0], 64490[0], 64491[0], 64492[0], 64493[0], 64494[0], 64495[0], 64505[0], 64510[0], 64517[0], 64520[0], 64530[0], 65091[1], 65093[1], 65101[1], 65103[1], 65105[1], 67500[1], 69990[0], 92012[1], 92014[1], 92018[1], 92019[1], 93000[1], 93005[1], 93010[1], 93040[1], 93041[1], 93042[1], 93318[1], 93355[1], 94002[1], 94200[1], 94680[1], 94681[1], 94690[1], 95812[1], 95813[1], 95816[1], 95819[1], 95822[1], 95829[1], 95955[1], 96360[1], 96361[1], 96365[1], 96366[1], 96367[1], 96368[1], 96372[1], 96374[1], 96375[1], 96376[1], 96377[1], 96523[0], 97597[1], 97598[1], 97602[1], 99155[0], 99156[0], 99157[0], 99211[1], 99212[1], 99213[1], 99214[1], 99215[1], 99217[1], 99218[1], 99219[1], 99220[1], 99221[1], 99222[1], 99223[1], 99231[1], 99232[1], 99233[1], 99234[1], 99235[1], 99236[1], 99238[1], 99239[1], 99241[1], 99242[1], 99243[1], 99244[1], 99245[1], 99251[1], 99252[1], 99253[1], 99254[1], 99255[1], 99291[1], 99292[1], 99304[1], 99305[1], 99306[1], 99307[1], 99308[1], 99309[1], 99310[1], 99315[1], 99316[1], 99334[1], 99335[1], 99336[1], 99337[1], 99347[1], 99348[1], 99349[1], 99350[1], 99374[1], 99375[1], 99377[1], 99378[1], 99446[0], 99447[0], 99448[0], 99449[0], 99451[0], 99452[0], 99495[0], 99496[0], G0463[1], G0471[1], J0670[1], J2001[1]
65112	0213T[0], 0216T[0], 0596T[1], 0597T[1], 0708T[1], 0709T[1], 11000[1], 11001[1], 11004[1], 11005[1], 11006[1], 11042[1], 11043[1], 11044[1], 11045[1], 11046[1], 11047[1], 12001[1], 12002[1], 12004[1], 12005[1], 12006[1], 12007[1], 12011[1], 12013[1], 12014[1], 12015[1], 12016[1], 12017[1], 12018[1], 12020[1], 12021[1], 12031[1], 12032[1], 12034[1], 12035[1], 12036[1], 12037[1], 12041[1], 12042[1], 12044[1], 12045[1], 12046[1], 12047[1], 12051[1], 12052[1], 12053[1], 12054[1], 12055[1], 12056[1], 12057[1], 13100[1], 13101[1], 13102[1], 13120[1], 13121[1], 13122[1], 13131[1], 13132[1], 13133[1], 13151[1], 13152[1], 13153[1], 36000[1], 36400[1], 36405[1], 36406[1], 36410[1], 36420[1], 36425[1], 36430[1], 36440[1], 36591[0], 36592[0], 36600[1], 36640[1], 43752[1], 51701[1], 51702[1], 51703[1], 62320[0], 62321[0], 62322[0], 62323[0], 62324[0], 62325[0], 62326[0], 62327[0], 64400[0], 64405[0], 64408[0], 64415[0], 64416[0], 64417[0], 64418[0], 64420[0], 64421[0], 64425[0], 64430[0], 64435[0], 64445[0], 64446[0], 64447[0], 64448[0], 64449[0], 64450[0], 64451[0], 64454[0], 64461[0], 64462[0], 64463[0], 64479[0], 64480[0], 64483[0], 64484[0], 64486[0], 64487[0], 64488[0], 64489[0], 64490[0], 64491[0], 64492[0], 64493[0], 64494[0], 64495[0], 64505[0], 64510[0], 64517[0], 64520[0], 64530[0], 65091[1], 65093[1], 65101[1], 65103[1], 65105[1], 65110[1], 65114[1], 67500[1], 69990[0], 92012[1], 92014[1], 92018[1], 92019[1], 93000[1], 93005[1], 93010[1], 93040[1], 93041[1], 93042[1], 93318[1], 93355[1], 94002[1], 94200[1], 94680[1], 94681[1], 94690[1], 95812[1], 95813[1], 95816[1], 95819[1], 95822[1], 95829[1], 95955[1], 96360[1], 96361[1], 96365[1], 96366[1], 96367[1], 96368[1], 96372[1], 96374[1], 96375[1], 96376[1], 96377[1], 96523[0], 97597[1], 97598[1], 97602[1], 99155[0], 99156[0], 99157[0], 99211[1], 99212[1], 99213[1], 99214[1], 99215[1], 99217[1], 99218[1], 99219[1], 99220[1], 99221[1], 99222[1], 99223[1], 99231[1], 99232[1], 99233[1], 99234[1], 99235[1], 99236[1], 99238[1], 99239[1], 99241[1], 99242[1], 99243[1], 99244[1], 99245[1], 99251[1], 99252[1], 99253[1], 99254[1], 99255[1], 99291[1], 99292[1], 99304[1], 99305[1], 99306[1], 99307[1], 99308[1], 99309[1], 99310[1], 99315[1], 99316[1], 99334[1], 99335[1], 99336[1], 99337[1], 99347[1], 99348[1], 99349[1], 99350[1], 99374[1], 99375[1], 99377[1], 99378[1], 99446[0], 99447[0], 99448[0], 99449[0], 99451[0], 99452[0], 99495[0], 99496[0], G0463[1], G0471[1], J0670[1], J2001[1]
65114	0213T[0], 0216T[0], 0596T[1], 0597T[1], 0708T[1], 0709T[1], 11000[1], 11001[1], 11004[1], 11005[1], 11006[1], 11042[1], 11043[1], 11044[1], 11045[1], 11046[1], 11047[1], 12001[1], 12002[1], 12004[1], 12005[1], 12006[1], 12007[1], 12011[1], 12013[1], 12014[1], 12015[1], 12016[1], 12017[1], 12018[1], 12020[1], 12021[1], 12031[1], 12032[1], 12034[1], 12035[1], 12036[1], 12037[1], 12041[1], 12042[1], 12044[1], 12045[1], 12046[1], 12047[1], 12051[1], 12052[1], 12053[1], 12054[1], 12055[1], 12056[1], 12057[1], 13100[1], 13101[1], 13102[1], 13120[1], 13121[1], 13122[1], 13131[1], 13132[1], 13133[1], 13151[1], 13152[1], 13153[1], 14060[1], 14061[1], 15733[1], 36000[1], 36400[1], 36405[1], 36406[1], 36410[1], 36420[1], 36425[1], 36430[1], 36440[1], 36591[0], 36592[0], 36600[1], 36640[1], 43752[1], 51701[1], 51702[1], 51703[1], 62320[0], 62321[0], 62322[0], 62323[0], 62324[0], 62325[0], 62326[0], 62327[0], 64400[0], 64405[0], 64408[0], 64415[0], 64416[0], 64417[0], 64418[0], 64420[0], 64421[0], 64425[0], 64430[0], 64435[0], 64445[0], 64446[0], 64447[0], 64448[0], 64449[0], 64450[0], 64451[0], 64454[0], 64461[0], 64462[0], 64463[0], 64479[0], 64480[0], 64483[0], 64484[0], 64486[0], 64487[0], 64488[0], 64489[0], 64490[0], 64491[0], 64492[0], 64493[0], 64494[0], 64495[0], 64505[0], 64510[0], 64517[0], 64520[0], 64530[0], 65091[1], 65093[1], 65101[1], 65103[1], 65105[1], 65110[1], 67500[1], 69990[0], 92012[1], 92014[1], 92018[1], 92019[1], 93000[1], 93005[1], 93010[1], 93040[1], 93041[1], 93042[1], 93318[1], 93355[1], 94002[1], 94200[1], 94680[1], 94681[1], 94690[1], 95812[1], 95813[1], 95816[1], 95819[1], 95822[1], 95829[1], 95955[1], 96360[1], 96361[1], 96365[1], 96366[1], 96367[1], 96368[1], 96372[1], 96374[1], 96375[1], 96376[1], 96377[1], 96523[0], 97597[1], 97598[1], 97602[1],

0 = Modifier usage not allowed or inappropriate 1 = Modifier usage allowed

Code 1	Code 2
	99155[0], 99156[0], 99157[0], 99211[1], 99212[1], 99213[1], 99214[1], 99215[1], 99217[1], 99218[1], 99219[1], 99220[1], 99221[1], 99222[1], 99223[1], 99231[1], 99232[1], 99233[1], 99234[1], 99235[1], 99236[1], 99238[1], 99239[1], 99241[1], 99242[1], 99243[1], 99244[1], 99245[1], 99251[1], 99252[1], 99253[1], 99254[1], 99255[1], 99291[1], 99292[1], 99304[1], 99305[1], 99306[1], 99307[1], 99308[1], 99309[1], 99310[1], 99315[1], 99316[1], 99334[1], 99335[1], 99336[1], 99337[1], 99347[1], 99348[1], 99349[1], 99350[1], 99374[1], 99375[1], 99377[1], 99378[1], 99446[0], 99447[0], 99448[0], 99449[0], 99451[0], 99452[0], 99495[0], 99496[0], G0463[1], G0471[1], J0670[1], J2001[1]
65125	0213T[0], 0216T[0], 0596T[1], 0597T[1], 0708T[1], 0709T[1], 11000[1], 11001[1], 11004[1], 11005[1], 11006[1], 11042[1], 11043[1], 11044[1], 11045[1], 11046[1], 11047[1], 12001[1], 12002[1], 12004[1], 12005[1], 12006[1], 12007[1], 12011[1], 12013[1], 12014[1], 12015[1], 12016[1], 12017[1], 12018[1], 12020[1], 12021[1], 12031[1], 12032[1], 12034[1], 12035[1], 12036[1], 12037[1], 12041[1], 12042[1], 12044[1], 12045[1], 12046[1], 12047[1], 12051[1], 12052[1], 12053[1], 12054[1], 12055[1], 12056[1], 12057[1], 13100[1], 13101[1], 13102[1], 13120[1], 13121[1], 13122[1], 13131[1], 13132[1], 13133[1], 13151[1], 13152[1], 13153[1], 36000[1], 36400[1], 36405[1], 36406[1], 36410[1], 36420[1], 36425[1], 36430[1], 36440[1], 36591[0], 36592[0], 36600[1], 36640[1], 43752[1], 51701[1], 51702[1], 51703[1], 62320[0], 62321[0], 62322[0], 62323[0], 62324[0], 62325[0], 62326[0], 62327[0], 64400[0], 64405[0], 64408[0], 64415[0], 64416[0], 64417[0], 64418[0], 64420[0], 64421[0], 64425[0], 64430[0], 64435[0], 64445[0], 64446[0], 64447[0], 64448[0], 64449[0], 64450[0], 64451[0], 64454[0], 64461[0], 64462[0], 64463[0], 64479[0], 64480[0], 64483[0], 64484[0], 64486[0], 64487[0], 64488[0], 64489[0], 64490[0], 64491[0], 64492[0], 64493[0], 64494[0], 64495[0], 64505[0], 64510[0], 64517[0], 64520[0], 64530[0], 67500[1], 69990[0], 92012[1], 92014[1], 92018[1], 92019[1], 93000[1], 93005[1], 93010[1], 93040[1], 93041[1], 93042[1], 93318[1], 93355[1], 94002[1], 94200[1], 94680[1], 94681[1], 94690[1], 95812[1], 95813[1], 95816[1], 95819[1], 95822[1], 95829[1], 95955[1], 96360[1], 96361[1], 96365[1], 96366[1], 96367[1], 96368[1], 96372[1], 96374[1], 96375[1], 96376[1], 96377[1], 96523[0], 97597[1], 97598[1], 97602[1], 99155[0], 99156[0], 99157[0], 99211[1], 99212[1], 99213[1], 99214[1], 99215[1], 99217[1], 99218[1], 99219[1], 99220[1], 99221[1], 99222[1], 99223[1], 99231[1], 99232[1], 99233[1], 99234[1], 99235[1], 99236[1], 99238[1], 99239[1], 99241[1], 99242[1], 99243[1], 99244[1], 99245[1], 99251[1], 99252[1], 99253[1], 99254[1], 99255[1], 99291[1], 99292[1], 99304[1], 99305[1], 99306[1], 99307[1], 99308[1], 99309[1], 99310[1], 99315[1], 99316[1], 99334[1], 99335[1], 99336[1], 99337[1], 99347[1], 99348[1], 99349[1], 99350[1], 99374[1], 99375[1], 99377[1], 99378[1], 99446[0], 99447[0], 99448[0], 99449[0], 99451[0], 99452[0], 99495[0], 99496[0], G0463[1], G0471[1], J0670[1], J2001[1]
65130	0213T[0], 0216T[0], 0596T[1], 0597T[1], 0708T[1], 0709T[1], 11000[1], 11001[1], 11004[1], 11005[1], 11006[1], 11042[1], 11043[1], 11044[1], 11045[1], 11046[1], 11047[1], 12001[1], 12002[1], 12004[1], 12005[1], 12006[1], 12007[1], 12011[1], 12013[1], 12014[1], 12015[1], 12016[1], 12017[1], 12018[1], 12020[1], 12021[1], 12031[1], 12032[1], 12034[1], 12035[1], 12036[1], 12037[1], 12041[1], 12042[1], 12044[1], 12045[1], 12046[1], 12047[1], 12051[1], 12052[1], 12053[1], 12054[1], 12055[1], 12056[1], 12057[1], 13100[1], 13101[1], 13102[1], 13120[1], 13121[1], 13122[1], 13131[1], 13132[1], 13133[1], 13151[1], 13152[1], 13153[1], 36000[1], 36400[1], 36405[1], 36406[1], 36410[1], 36420[1], 36425[1], 36430[1], 36440[1], 36591[0], 36592[0], 36600[1], 36640[1], 43752[1], 51701[1], 51702[1], 51703[1], 62320[0], 62321[0], 62322[0], 62323[0], 62324[0], 62325[0], 62326[0], 62327[0], 64400[0], 64405[0], 64408[0], 64415[0], 64416[0], 64417[0], 64418[0], 64420[0], 64421[0], 64425[0], 64430[0], 64435[0], 64445[0], 64446[0], 64447[0], 64448[0], 64449[0], 64450[0], 64451[0], 64454[0], 64461[0], 64462[0], 64463[0], 64479[0], 64480[0], 64483[0], 64484[0], 64486[0], 64487[0], 64488[0], 64489[0], 64490[0], 64491[0], 64492[0], 64493[0], 64494[0], 64495[0], 64505[0], 64510[0], 64517[0], 64520[0], 64530[0], 65125[1], 65135[1], 65140[1], 67250[1], 67255[1], 67500[1], 69990[0], 92012[1], 92014[1], 92018[1], 92019[1], 93000[1], 93005[1], 93010[1], 93040[1], 93041[1], 93042[1], 93318[1], 93355[1], 94002[1], 94200[1], 94680[1], 94681[1], 94690[1], 95812[1], 95813[1], 95816[1], 95819[1], 95822[1], 95829[1], 95955[1], 96360[1], 96361[1], 96365[1], 96366[1], 96367[1], 96368[1], 96372[1], 96374[1], 96375[1], 96376[1], 96377[1], 96523[0], 97597[1], 97598[1], 97602[1], 99155[0], 99156[0], 99157[0], 99211[1], 99212[1], 99213[1], 99214[1], 99215[1], 99217[1], 99218[1], 99219[1], 99220[1], 99221[1], 99222[1], 99223[1], 99231[1], 99232[1], 99233[1], 99234[1], 99235[1], 99236[1], 99238[1], 99239[1], 99241[1], 99242[1], 99243[1], 99244[1], 99245[1], 99251[1], 99252[1], 99253[1], 99254[1], 99255[1], 99291[1], 99292[1], 99304[1], 99305[1], 99306[1], 99307[1], 99308[1], 99309[1], 99310[1], 99315[1], 99316[1], 99334[1], 99335[1], 99336[1], 99337[1], 99347[1], 99348[1], 99349[1], 99350[1], 99374[1], 99375[1], 99377[1], 99378[1], 99446[0], 99447[0], 99448[0], 99449[0], 99451[0], 99452[0], 99495[0], 99496[0], G0463[1], G0471[1], J0670[1], J2001[1]
65135	0213T[0], 0216T[0], 0596T[1], 0597T[1], 0708T[1], 0709T[1], 11000[1], 11001[1], 11004[1], 11005[1], 11006[1], 11042[1], 11043[1], 11044[1], 11045[1], 11046[1], 11047[1], 12001[1], 12002[1], 12004[1], 12005[1], 12006[1], 12007[1], 12011[1], 12013[1], 12014[1], 12015[1], 12016[1], 12017[1], 12018[1], 12020[1], 12021[1], 12031[1], 12032[1], 12034[1], 12035[1], 12036[1], 12037[1], 12041[1], 12042[1], 12044[1], 12045[1], 12046[1], 12047[1], 12051[1], 12052[1], 12053[1], 12054[1], 12055[1], 12056[1], 12057[1], 13100[1], 13101[1], 13102[1], 13120[1], 13121[1], 13122[1], 13131[1], 13132[1], 13133[1], 13151[1], 13152[1], 13153[1], 36000[1], 36400[1], 36405[1], 36406[1], 36410[1], 36420[1], 36425[1], 36430[1], 36440[1], 36591[0], 36592[0], 36600[1], 36640[1], 43752[1], 51701[1], 51702[1], 51703[1], 62320[0], 62321[0], 62322[0], 62323[0], 62324[0], 62325[0], 62326[0], 62327[0], 64400[0], 64405[0], 64408[0], 64415[0], 64416[0], 64417[0], 64418[0], 64420[0], 64421[0], 64425[0], 64430[0], 64435[0], 64445[0], 64446[0], 64447[0], 64448[0], 64449[0], 64450[0], 64451[0], 64454[0], 64461[0], 64462[0], 64463[0], 64479[0], 64480[0], 64483[0], 64484[0], 64486[0], 64487[0], 64488[0], 64489[0], 64490[0], 64491[0], 64492[0], 64493[0], 64494[0], 64495[0], 64505[0], 64510[0], 64517[0], 64520[0], 64530[0], 65125[1], 65140[1], 67250[1], 67500[1], 69990[0], 92012[1], 92014[1], 92018[1], 92019[1], 93000[1], 93005[1], 93010[1], 93040[1], 93041[1], 93042[1], 93318[1], 93355[1], 94002[1], 94200[1], 94680[1], 94681[1], 94690[1], 95812[1], 95813[1], 95816[1], 95819[1], 95822[1], 95829[1], 95955[1], 96360[1], 96361[1], 96365[1], 96366[1], 96367[1], 96368[1], 96372[1], 96374[1], 96375[1], 96376[1], 96377[1], 96523[0], 97597[1], 97598[1], 97602[1], 99155[0], 99156[0], 99157[0], 99211[1], 99212[1], 99213[1], 99214[1], 99215[1], 99217[1], 99218[1], 99219[1], 99220[1], 99221[1], 99222[1], 99223[1], 99231[1], 99232[1], 99233[1], 99234[1], 99235[1], 99236[1], 99238[1], 99239[1], 99241[1], 99242[1], 99243[1], 99244[1], 99245[1], 99251[1], 99252[1], 99253[1], 99254[1], 99255[1], 99291[1], 99292[1], 99304[1], 99305[1], 99306[1], 99307[1], 99308[1], 99309[1], 99310[1], 99315[1], 99316[1], 99334[1], 99335[1], 99336[1], 99337[1], 99347[1], 99348[1], 99349[1], 99350[1], 99374[1], 99375[1], 99377[1], 99378[1], 99446[0], 99447[0], 99448[0], 99449[0], 99451[0], 99452[0], 99495[0], 99496[0], G0463[1], G0471[1], J0670[1], J2001[1]
65140	0213T[0], 0216T[0], 0596T[1], 0597T[1], 0708T[1], 0709T[1], 11000[1], 11001[1], 11004[1], 11005[1], 11006[1], 11042[1], 11043[1], 11044[1], 11045[1], 11046[1], 11047[1], 12001[1], 12002[1], 12004[1], 12005[1], 12006[1], 12007[1], 12011[1], 12013[1], 12014[1], 12015[1], 12016[1], 12017[1], 12018[1], 12020[1], 12021[1], 12031[1], 12032[1], 12034[1], 12035[1], 12036[1], 12037[1], 12041[1], 12042[1], 12044[1], 12045[1], 12046[1], 12047[1], 12051[1], 12052[1], 12053[1], 12054[1], 12055[1], 12056[1], 12057[1], 13100[1], 13101[1], 13102[1], 13120[1], 13121[1], 13122[1], 13131[1], 13132[1], 13133[1], 13151[1], 13152[1], 13153[1], 36000[1], 36400[1], 36405[1], 36406[1], 36410[1], 36420[1], 36425[1], 36430[1], 36440[1], 36591[0], 36592[0], 36600[1], 36640[1], 43752[1], 51701[1], 51702[1], 51703[1], 62320[0], 62321[0], 62322[0], 62323[0], 62324[0], 62325[0], 62326[0], 62327[0], 64400[0], 64405[0], 64408[0], 64415[0], 64416[0], 64417[0], 64418[0], 64420[0], 64421[0], 64425[0], 64430[0], 64435[0], 64445[0], 64446[0], 64447[0], 64448[0], 64449[0], 64450[0], 64451[0], 64454[0], 64461[0], 64462[0], 64463[0], 64479[0], 64480[0], 64483[0], 64484[0], 64486[0], 64487[0], 64488[0], 64489[0], 64490[0], 64491[0], 64492[0], 64493[0], 64494[0], 64495[0], 64505[0], 64510[0], 64517[0], 64520[0], 64530[0], 65125[1], 67250[1], 67500[1], 69990[0], 92012[1], 92014[1], 92018[1], 92019[1], 93000[1], 93005[1], 93010[1], 93040[1], 93041[1], 93042[1], 93318[1], 93355[1], 94002[1], 94200[1], 94680[1], 94681[1], 94690[1], 95812[1], 95813[1], 95816[1], 95819[1], 95822[1], 95829[1], 95955[1], 96360[1], 96361[1], 96365[1], 96366[1], 96367[1], 96368[1], 96372[1], 96374[1], 96375[1], 96376[1], 96377[1], 96523[0], 97597[1], 97598[1], 97602[1], 99155[0], 99156[0], 99157[0], 99211[1], 99212[1], 99213[1], 99214[1], 99215[1], 99217[1], 99218[1], 99219[1], 99220[1], 99221[1], 99222[1], 99223[1], 99231[1], 99232[1], 99233[1], 99234[1], 99235[1], 99236[1], 99238[1], 99239[1], 99241[1], 99242[1], 99243[1], 99244[1], 99245[1], 99251[1], 99252[1], 99253[1], 99254[1], 99255[1], 99291[1], 99292[1], 99304[1], 99305[1], 99306[1], 99307[1], 99308[1], 99309[1], 99310[1], 99315[1], 99316[1], 99334[1], 99335[1], 99336[1], 99337[1], 99347[1], 99348[1], 99349[1], 99350[1], 99374[1], 99375[1], 99377[1], 99378[1], 99446[0], 99447[0], 99448[0], 99449[0], 99451[0], 99452[0], 99495[0], 99496[0], G0463[1], G0471[1], J0670[1], J2001[1]
65150	0213T[0], 0216T[0], 0596T[1], 0597T[1], 0708T[1], 0709T[1], 11000[1], 11001[1], 11004[1], 11005[1], 11006[1], 11042[1], 11043[1], 11044[1], 11045[1], 11046[1], 11047[1], 12001[1], 12002[1], 12004[1], 12005[1], 12006[1], 12007[1], 12011[1], 12013[1], 12014[1], 12015[1], 12016[1], 12017[1], 12018[1], 12020[1], 12021[1], 12031[1], 12032[1], 12034[1], 12035[1], 12036[1], 12037[1], 12041[1], 12042[1], 12044[1], 12045[1], 12046[1], 12047[1], 12051[1], 12052[1], 12053[1], 12054[1], 12055[1], 12056[1], 12057[1], 13100[1], 13101[1], 13102[1], 13120[1], 13121[1], 13122[1], 13131[1], 13132[1], 13133[1], 13151[1], 13152[1], 13153[1], 36000[1], 36400[1], 36405[1], 36406[1], 36410[1], 36420[1], 36425[1], 36430[1], 36440[1], 36591[0], 36592[0], 36600[1], 36640[1], 43752[1], 51701[1], 51702[1], 51703[1], 62320[0], 62321[0], 62322[0], 62323[0], 62324[0], 62325[0], 62326[0], 62327[0], 64400[0], 64405[0], 64408[0], 64415[0], 64416[0], 64417[0], 64418[0], 64420[0], 64421[0], 64425[0], 64430[0], 64435[0], 64445[0], 64446[0], 64447[0], 64448[0], 64449[0], 64450[0], 64451[0], 64454[0], 64461[0], 64462[0], 64463[0], 64479[0], 64480[0], 64483[0], 64484[0], 64486[0], 64487[0], 64488[0], 64489[0], 64490[0], 64491[0], 64492[0], 64493[0], 64494[0], 64495[0], 64505[0], 64510[0], 64517[0], 64520[0], 64530[0], 65125[1], 65155[1], 65175[1], 67250[1], 67500[1], 69990[0], 92012[1], 92014[1], 92018[1], 92019[1], 93000[1], 93005[1], 93010[1], 93040[1], 93041[1], 93042[1], 93318[1], 93355[1], 94002[1], 94200[1], 94680[1], 94681[1], 94690[1], 95812[1], 95813[1], 95816[1], 95819[1], 95822[1], 95829[1], 95955[1], 96360[1], 96361[1], 96365[1], 96366[1], 96367[1], 96368[1], 96372[1], 96374[1], 96375[1], 96376[1], 96377[1], 96523[0], 97597[1], 97598[1], 97602[1], 99155[0], 99156[0], 99157[0], 99211[1], 99212[1], 99213[1], 99214[1], 99215[1], 99217[1], 99218[1], 99219[1], 99220[1], 99221[1], 99222[1], 99223[1], 99231[1], 99232[1], 99233[1], 99234[1], 99235[1], 99236[1], 99238[1], 99239[1], 99241[1], 99242[1], 99243[1], 99244[1], 99245[1], 99251[1], 99252[1], 99253[1], 99254[1], 99255[1], 99291[1], 99292[1], 99304[1], 99305[1], 99306[1], 99307[1], 99308[1], 99309[1], 99310[1], 99315[1], 99316[1], 99334[1], 99335[1], 99336[1], 99337[1], 99347[1], 99348[1], 99349[1], 99350[1], 99374[1], 99375[1], 99377[1], 99378[1], 99446[0], 99447[0], 99448[0], 99449[0], 99451[0], 99452[0], 99495[0], 99496[0], G0463[1], G0471[1], J0670[1], J2001[1]

0 = Modifier usage not allowed or inappropriate 1 = Modifier usage allowed

Code 1	Code 2
65155	0213T[0], 0216T[0], 0596T[1], 0597T[1], 0708T[1], 0709T[1], 11000[1], 11001[1], 11004[1], 11005[1], 11006[1], 11042[1], 11043[1], 11044[1], 11045[1], 11046[1], 11047[1], 12001[1], 12002[1], 12004[1], 12005[1], 12006[1], 12007[1], 12011[1], 12013[1], 12014[1], 12015[1], 12016[1], 12017[1], 12018[1], 12020[1], 12021[1], 12031[1], 12032[1], 12034[1], 12035[1], 12036[1], 12037[1], 12041[1], 12042[1], 12044[1], 12045[1], 12046[1], 12047[1], 12051[1], 12052[1], 12053[1], 12054[1], 12055[1], 12056[1], 12057[1], 13100[1], 13101[1], 13102[1], 13120[1], 13121[1], 13122[1], 13131[1], 13132[1], 13133[1], 13151[1], 13152[1], 13153[1], 36000[1], 36400[1], 36405[1], 36406[1], 36410[1], 36420[1], 36425[1], 36430[1], 36440[1], 36591[0], 36592[0], 36600[1], 36640[1], 43752[1], 51701[1], 51702[1], 51703[1], 62320[0], 62321[0], 62322[0], 62323[0], 62324[0], 62325[0], 62326[0], 62327[0], 64400[0], 64405[0], 64408[0], 64415[0], 64416[0], 64417[0], 64418[0], 64420[0], 64421[0], 64425[0], 64430[0], 64435[0], 64445[0], 64446[0], 64447[0], 64448[0], 64449[0], 64450[0], 64451[0], 64454[0], 64461[0], 64462[0], 64463[0], 64479[0], 64480[0], 64483[0], 64484[0], 64486[0], 64487[0], 64488[0], 64489[0], 64490[0], 64491[0], 64492[0], 64493[0], 64494[0], 64495[0], 64505[0], 64510[0], 64517[0], 64520[0], 64530[0], 65125[1], 65175[1], 67250[1], 67500[1], 69990[0], 92012[1], 92014[1], 92018[1], 92019[1], 93000[1], 93005[1], 93010[1], 93040[1], 93041[1], 93042[1], 93318[1], 93355[1], 94002[1], 94200[1], 94680[1], 94681[1], 94690[1], 95812[1], 95813[1], 95816[1], 95819[1], 95822[1], 95829[1], 95955[1], 96360[1], 96361[1], 96365[1], 96366[1], 96367[1], 96368[1], 96372[1], 96374[1], 96375[1], 96376[1], 96377[1], 96523[0], 97597[1], 97598[1], 97602[1], 99155[0], 99156[0], 99157[0], 99211[1], 99212[1], 99213[1], 99214[1], 99215[1], 99217[1], 99218[1], 99219[1], 99220[1], 99221[1], 99222[1], 99223[1], 99231[1], 99232[1], 99233[1], 99234[1], 99235[1], 99236[1], 99238[1], 99239[1], 99241[1], 99242[1], 99243[1], 99244[1], 99245[1], 99251[1], 99252[1], 99253[1], 99254[1], 99255[1], 99291[1], 99292[1], 99304[1], 99305[1], 99306[1], 99307[1], 99308[1], 99309[1], 99310[1], 99315[1], 99316[1], 99334[1], 99335[1], 99336[1], 99337[1], 99347[1], 99348[1], 99349[1], 99350[1], 99374[1], 99375[1], 99377[1], 99378[1], 99446[0], 99447[0], 99448[0], 99449[0], 99451[0], 99452[0], 99495[0], 99496[0], G0463[1], G0471[1], J0670[1], J2001[1]
65175	0213T[0], 0216T[0], 0596T[1], 0597T[1], 0708T[1], 0709T[1], 11000[1], 11001[1], 11004[1], 11005[1], 11006[1], 11042[1], 11043[1], 11044[1], 11045[1], 11046[1], 11047[1], 12001[1], 12002[1], 12004[1], 12005[1], 12006[1], 12007[1], 12011[1], 12013[1], 12014[1], 12015[1], 12016[1], 12017[1], 12018[1], 12020[1], 12021[1], 12031[1], 12032[1], 12034[1], 12035[1], 12036[1], 12037[1], 12041[1], 12042[1], 12044[1], 12045[1], 12046[1], 12047[1], 12051[1], 12052[1], 12053[1], 12054[1], 12055[1], 12056[1], 12057[1], 13100[1], 13101[1], 13102[1], 13120[1], 13121[1], 13122[1], 13131[1], 13132[1], 13133[1], 13151[1], 13152[1], 13153[1], 36000[1], 36400[1], 36405[1], 36406[1], 36410[1], 36420[1], 36425[1], 36430[1], 36440[1], 36591[0], 36592[0], 36600[1], 36640[1], 43752[1], 51701[1], 51702[1], 51703[1], 62320[0], 62321[0], 62322[0], 62323[0], 62324[0], 62325[0], 62326[0], 62327[0], 64400[0], 64405[0], 64408[0], 64415[0], 64416[0], 64417[0], 64418[0], 64420[0], 64421[0], 64425[0], 64430[0], 64435[0], 64445[0], 64446[0], 64447[0], 64448[0], 64449[0], 64450[0], 64451[0], 64454[0], 64461[0], 64462[0], 64463[0], 64479[0], 64480[0], 64483[0], 64484[0], 64486[0], 64487[0], 64488[0], 64489[0], 64490[0], 64491[0], 64492[0], 64493[0], 64494[0], 64495[0], 64505[0], 64510[0], 64517[0], 64520[0], 64530[0], 65125[1], 65900[1], 67250[1], 67500[1], 69990[0], 92012[1], 92014[1], 92018[1], 92019[1], 93000[1], 93005[1], 93010[1], 93040[1], 93041[1], 93042[1], 93318[1], 93355[1], 94002[1], 94200[1], 94680[1], 94681[1], 94690[1], 95812[1], 95813[1], 95816[1], 95819[1], 95822[1], 95829[1], 95955[1], 96360[1], 96361[1], 96365[1], 96366[1], 96367[1], 96368[1], 96372[1], 96374[1], 96375[1], 96376[1], 96377[1], 96523[0], 97597[1], 97598[1], 97602[1], 99155[0], 99156[0], 99157[0], 99211[1], 99212[1], 99213[1], 99214[1], 99215[1], 99217[1], 99218[1], 99219[1], 99220[1], 99221[1], 99222[1], 99223[1], 99231[1], 99232[1], 99233[1], 99234[1], 99235[1], 99236[1], 99238[1], 99239[1], 99241[1], 99242[1], 99243[1], 99244[1], 99245[1], 99251[1], 99252[1], 99253[1], 99254[1], 99255[1], 99291[1], 99292[1], 99304[1], 99305[1], 99306[1], 99307[1], 99308[1], 99309[1], 99310[1], 99315[1], 99316[1], 99334[1], 99335[1], 99336[1], 99337[1], 99347[1], 99348[1], 99349[1], 99350[1], 99374[1], 99375[1], 99377[1], 99378[1], 99446[0], 99447[0], 99448[0], 99449[0], 99451[0], 99452[0], 99495[0], 99496[0], G0463[1], G0471[1], J0670[1], J2001[1]
65205	0213T[0], 0216T[0], 0596T[1], 0597T[1], 0708T[1], 0709T[1], 11000[1], 11001[1], 11004[1], 11005[1], 11006[1], 11042[1], 11043[1], 11044[1], 11045[1], 11046[1], 11047[1], 12001[1], 12002[1], 12004[1], 12005[1], 12006[1], 12007[1], 12011[1], 12013[1], 12014[1], 12015[1], 12016[1], 12017[1], 12018[1], 12020[1], 12021[1], 12031[1], 12032[1], 12034[1], 12035[1], 12036[1], 12037[1], 12041[1], 12042[1], 12044[1], 12045[1], 12046[1], 12047[1], 12051[1], 12052[1], 12053[1], 12054[1], 12055[1], 12056[1], 12057[1], 13100[1], 13101[1], 13102[1], 13120[1], 13121[1], 13122[1], 13131[1], 13132[1], 13133[1], 13151[1], 13152[1], 13153[1], 36000[1], 36400[1], 36405[1], 36406[1], 36410[1], 36420[1], 36425[1], 36430[1], 36440[1], 36591[0], 36592[0], 36600[1], 36640[1], 43752[1], 51701[1], 51702[1], 51703[1], 62320[0], 62321[0], 62322[0], 62323[0], 62324[0], 62325[0], 62326[0], 62327[0], 64400[0], 64405[0], 64408[0], 64415[0], 64416[0], 64417[0], 64418[0], 64420[0], 64421[0], 64425[0], 64430[0], 64435[0], 64445[0], 64446[0], 64447[0], 64448[0], 64449[0], 64450[0], 64451[0], 64454[0], 64461[0], 64462[0], 64463[0], 64479[0], 64480[0], 64483[0], 64484[0], 64486[0], 64487[0], 64488[0], 64489[0], 64490[0], 64491[0], 64492[0], 64493[0], 64494[0], 64495[0], 64505[0], 64510[0], 64517[0], 64520[0], 64530[0], 67250[1], 67500[1], 69990[0], 92012[1], 92014[1], 92018[1], 92019[1], 93000[1], 93005[1], 93010[1], 93040[1], 93041[1], 93042[1], 93318[1], 93355[1], 94002[1], 94200[1], 94680[1], 94681[1], 94690[1], 95812[1], 95813[1], 95816[1], 95819[1], 95822[1], 95829[1], 95955[1], 96360[1], 96361[1], 96365[1], 96366[1], 96367[1], 96368[1], 96372[1], 96374[1], 96375[1], 96376[1], 96377[1], 96523[0], 97597[1], 97598[1], 97602[1], 99155[0], 99156[0], 99157[0], 99211[1], 99212[1], 99213[1], 99214[1], 99215[1], 99217[1], 99218[1], 99219[1], 99220[1], 99221[1], 99222[1], 99223[1], 99231[1], 99232[1], 99233[1], 99234[1], 99235[1], 99236[1], 99238[1], 99239[1], 99241[1], 99242[1], 99243[1], 99244[1], 99245[1], 99251[1], 99252[1], 99253[1], 99254[1], 99255[1], 99291[1], 99292[1], 99304[1], 99305[1], 99306[1], 99307[1], 99308[1], 99309[1], 99310[1], 99315[1], 99316[1], 99334[1], 99335[1], 99336[1], 99337[1], 99347[1], 99348[1], 99349[1], 99350[1], 99374[1], 99375[1], 99377[1], 99378[1], 99446[0], 99447[0], 99448[0], 99449[0], 99451[0], 99452[0], 99495[1], 99496[1], G0463[1], G0471[1]
65210	0213T[0], 0216T[0], 0596T[1], 0597T[1], 0708T[1], 0709T[1], 11000[1], 11001[1], 11004[1], 11005[1], 11006[1], 11042[1], 11043[1], 11044[1], 11045[1], 11046[1], 11047[1], 12001[1], 12002[1], 12004[1], 12005[1], 12006[1], 12007[1], 12011[1], 12013[1], 12014[1], 12015[1], 12016[1], 12017[1], 12018[1], 12020[1], 12021[1], 12031[1], 12032[1], 12034[1], 12035[1], 12036[1], 12037[1], 12041[1], 12042[1], 12044[1], 12045[1], 12046[1], 12047[1], 12051[1], 12052[1], 12053[1], 12054[1], 12055[1], 12056[1], 12057[1], 13100[1], 13101[1], 13102[1], 13120[1], 13121[1], 13122[1], 13131[1], 13132[1], 13133[1], 13151[1], 13152[1], 13153[1], 36000[1], 36400[1], 36405[1], 36406[1], 36410[1], 36420[1], 36425[1], 36430[1], 36440[1], 36591[0], 36592[0], 36600[1], 36640[1], 43752[1], 51701[1], 51702[1], 51703[1], 62320[0], 62321[0], 62322[0], 62323[0], 62324[0], 62325[0], 62326[0], 62327[0], 64400[0], 64405[0], 64408[0], 64415[0], 64416[0], 64417[0], 64418[0], 64420[0], 64421[0], 64425[0], 64430[0], 64435[0], 64445[0], 64446[0], 64447[0], 64448[0], 64449[0], 64450[0], 64451[0], 64454[0], 64461[0], 64462[0], 64463[0], 64479[0], 64480[0], 64483[0], 64484[0], 64486[0], 64487[0], 64488[0], 64489[0], 64490[0], 64491[0], 64492[0], 64493[0], 64494[0], 64495[0], 64505[0], 64510[0], 64517[0], 64520[0], 64530[0], 65205[1], 67250[1], 67500[1], 69990[0], 92012[1], 92014[1], 92018[1], 92019[1], 93000[1], 93005[1], 93010[1], 93040[1], 93041[1], 93042[1], 93318[1], 93355[1], 94002[1], 94200[1], 94680[1], 94681[1], 94690[1], 95812[1], 95813[1], 95816[1], 95819[1], 95822[1], 95829[1], 95955[1], 96360[1], 96361[1], 96365[1], 96366[1], 96367[1], 96368[1], 96372[1], 96374[1], 96375[1], 96376[1], 96377[1], 96523[0], 97597[1], 97598[1], 97602[1], 99155[0], 99156[0], 99157[0], 99211[1], 99212[1], 99213[1], 99214[1], 99215[1], 99217[1], 99218[1], 99219[1], 99220[1], 99221[1], 99222[1], 99223[1], 99231[1], 99232[1], 99233[1], 99234[1], 99235[1], 99236[1], 99238[1], 99239[1], 99241[1], 99242[1], 99243[1], 99244[1], 99245[1], 99251[1], 99252[1], 99253[1], 99254[1], 99255[1], 99291[1], 99292[1], 99304[1], 99305[1], 99306[1], 99307[1], 99308[1], 99309[1], 99310[1], 99315[1], 99316[1], 99334[1], 99335[1], 99336[1], 99337[1], 99347[1], 99348[1], 99349[1], 99350[1], 99374[1], 99375[1], 99377[1], 99378[1], 99446[0], 99447[0], 99448[0], 99449[0], 99451[0], 99452[0], 99495[1], 99496[1], G0463[1], G0471[1], J2001[1]
65220	0213T[0], 0216T[0], 0402T[1], 0596T[1], 0597T[1], 0708T[1], 0709T[1], 11000[1], 11001[1], 11004[1], 11005[1], 11006[1], 11042[1], 11043[1], 11044[1], 11045[1], 11046[1], 11047[1], 12001[1], 12002[1], 12004[1], 12005[1], 12006[1], 12007[1], 12011[1], 12013[1], 12014[1], 12015[1], 12016[1], 12017[1], 12018[1], 12020[1], 12021[1], 12031[1], 12032[1], 12034[1], 12035[1], 12036[1], 12037[1], 12041[1], 12042[1], 12044[1], 12045[1], 12046[1], 12047[1], 12051[1], 12052[1], 12053[1], 12054[1], 12055[1], 12056[1], 12057[1], 13100[1], 13101[1], 13102[1], 13120[1], 13121[1], 13122[1], 13131[1], 13132[1], 13133[1], 13151[1], 13152[1], 13153[1], 36000[1], 36400[1], 36405[1], 36406[1], 36410[1], 36420[1], 36425[1], 36430[1], 36440[1], 36591[0], 36592[0], 36600[1], 36640[1], 43752[1], 51701[1], 51702[1], 51703[1], 62320[0], 62321[0], 62322[0], 62323[0], 62324[0], 62325[0], 62326[0], 62327[0], 64400[0], 64405[0], 64408[0], 64415[0], 64416[0], 64417[0], 64418[0], 64420[0], 64421[0], 64425[0], 64430[0], 64435[0], 64445[0], 64446[0], 64447[0], 64448[0], 64449[0], 64450[0], 64451[0], 64454[0], 64461[0], 64462[0], 64463[0], 64479[0], 64480[0], 64483[0], 64484[0], 64486[0], 64487[0], 64488[0], 64489[0], 64490[0], 64491[0], 64492[0], 64493[0], 64494[0], 64495[0], 64505[0], 64510[0], 64517[0], 64520[0], 64530[0], 65430[1], 65435[1], 65436[1], 67250[1], 67500[1], 69990[0], 92012[1], 92014[1], 92018[1], 92019[1], 92071[1], 93000[1], 93005[1], 93010[1], 93040[1], 93041[1], 93042[1], 93318[1], 93355[1], 94002[1], 94200[1], 94680[1], 94681[1], 94690[1], 95812[1], 95813[1], 95816[1], 95819[1], 95822[1], 95829[1], 95955[1], 96360[1], 96361[1], 96365[1], 96366[1], 96367[1], 96368[1], 96372[1], 96374[1], 96375[1], 96376[1], 96377[1], 96523[0], 97597[1], 97598[1], 97602[1], 99155[0], 99156[0], 99157[0], 99211[1], 99212[1], 99213[1], 99214[1], 99215[1], 99217[1], 99218[1], 99219[1], 99220[1], 99221[1], 99222[1], 99223[1], 99231[1], 99232[1], 99233[1], 99234[1], 99235[1], 99236[1], 99238[1], 99239[1], 99241[1], 99242[1], 99243[1], 99244[1], 99245[1], 99251[1], 99252[1], 99253[1], 99254[1], 99255[1], 99291[1], 99292[1], 99304[1], 99305[1], 99306[1], 99307[1], 99308[1], 99309[1], 99310[1], 99315[1], 99316[1], 99334[1], 99335[1], 99336[1], 99337[1], 99347[1], 99348[1], 99349[1], 99350[1], 99374[1], 99375[1], 99377[1], 99378[1], 99446[0], 99447[0], 99448[0], 99449[0], 99451[0], 99452[0], 99495[1], 99496[1], G0463[1], G0471[1], J2001[1]
65222	0213T[0], 0216T[0], 0402T[1], 0596T[1], 0597T[1], 0708T[1], 0709T[1], 11000[1], 11001[1], 11004[1], 11005[1], 11006[1], 11042[1], 11043[1], 11044[1], 11045[1], 11046[1], 11047[1], 12001[1], 12002[1], 12004[1], 12005[1], 12006[1], 12007[1], 12011[1], 12013[1], 12014[1], 12015[1], 12016[1], 12017[1], 12018[1], 12020[1], 12021[1], 12031[1], 12032[1], 12034[1], 12035[1], 12036[1], 12037[1], 12041[1], 12042[1], 12044[1], 12045[1], 12046[1], 12047[1], 12051[1], 12052[1], 12053[1], 12054[1], 12055[1], 12056[1], 12057[1], 13100[1], 13101[1], 13102[1], 13120[1], 13121[1], 13122[1], 13131[1], 13132[1], 13133[1], 13151[1], 13152[1], 13153[1], 36000[1], 36400[1], 36405[1], 36406[1], 36410[1], 36420[1], 36425[1], 36430[1], 36440[1], 36591[0], 36592[0], 36600[1], 36640[1], 43752[1], 51701[1], 51702[1],

0 = Modifier usage not allowed or inappropriate 1 = Modifier usage allowed

Code 1	Code 2
	51703[1], 62320[0], 62321[0], 62322[0], 62323[0], 62324[0], 62325[0], 62326[0], 62327[0], 64400[0], 64405[0], 64408[0], 64415[0], 64416[0], 64417[0], 64418[0], 64420[0], 64421[0], 64425[0], 64430[0], 64435[0], 64445[0], 64446[0], 64447[0], 64448[0], 64449[0], 64450[0], 64451[0], 64454[0], 64461[0], 64462[0], 64463[0], 64479[0], 64480[0], 64483[0], 64484[0], 64486[0], 64487[0], 64488[0], 64489[0], 64490[0], 64491[0], 64492[0], 64493[0], 64494[0], 64495[0], 64505[0], 64510[0], 64517[0], 64520[0], 64530[0], 65220[1], 65435[1], 65436[1], 67250[1], 67500[1], 69990[0], 92012[1], 92014[1], 92018[1], 92019[1], 92071[1], 93000[1], 93005[1], 93010[1], 93040[1], 93041[1], 93042[1], 93318[1], 93355[1], 94002[1], 94200[1], 94680[1], 94681[1], 94690[1], 95812[1], 95813[1], 95816[1], 95819[1], 95822[1], 95829[1], 95955[1], 96360[1], 96361[1], 96365[1], 96366[1], 96367[1], 96368[1], 96372[1], 96374[1], 96375[1], 96376[1], 96377[1], 96523[0], 97597[1], 97598[1], 97602[1], 99155[0], 99156[0], 99157[0], 99211[1], 99212[1], 99213[1], 99214[1], 99215[1], 99217[1], 99218[1], 99219[1], 99220[1], 99221[1], 99222[1], 99223[1], 99231[1], 99232[1], 99233[1], 99234[1], 99235[1], 99236[1], 99238[1], 99239[1], 99241[1], 99242[1], 99243[1], 99244[1], 99245[1], 99251[1], 99252[1], 99253[1], 99254[1], 99255[1], 99291[1], 99292[1], 99304[1], 99305[1], 99306[1], 99307[1], 99308[1], 99309[1], 99310[1], 99315[1], 99316[1], 99334[1], 99335[1], 99336[1], 99337[1], 99347[1], 99348[1], 99349[1], 99350[1], 99374[1], 99375[1], 99377[1], 99378[1], 99446[0], 99447[0], 99448[0], 99449[0], 99451[0], 99452[0], 99495[1], 99496[1], G0463[1], G0471[1], J2001[1]
65235	0213T[0], 0216T[0], 0596T[1], 0597T[1], 0708T[1], 0709T[1], 11000[1], 11001[1], 11004[1], 11005[1], 11006[1], 11042[1], 11043[1], 11044[1], 11045[1], 11046[1], 11047[1], 12001[1], 12002[1], 12004[1], 12005[1], 12006[1], 12007[1], 12011[1], 12013[1], 12014[1], 12015[1], 12016[1], 12017[1], 12018[1], 12020[1], 12021[1], 12031[1], 12032[1], 12034[1], 12035[1], 12036[1], 12037[1], 12041[1], 12042[1], 12044[1], 12045[1], 12046[1], 12047[1], 12051[1], 12052[1], 12053[1], 12054[1], 12055[1], 12056[1], 12057[1], 13100[1], 13101[1], 13102[1], 13120[1], 13121[1], 13122[1], 13131[1], 13132[1], 13133[1], 13151[1], 13152[1], 13153[1], 36000[1], 36400[1], 36405[1], 36406[1], 36410[1], 36420[1], 36425[1], 36430[1], 36440[1], 36591[0], 36592[0], 36600[1], 36640[1], 43752[1], 51701[1], 51702[1], 51703[1], 62320[0], 62321[0], 62322[0], 62323[0], 62324[0], 62325[0], 62326[0], 62327[0], 64400[0], 64405[0], 64408[0], 64415[0], 64416[0], 64417[0], 64418[0], 64420[0], 64421[0], 64425[0], 64430[0], 64435[0], 64445[0], 64446[0], 64447[0], 64448[0], 64449[0], 64450[0], 64451[0], 64454[0], 64461[0], 64462[0], 64463[0], 64479[0], 64480[0], 64483[0], 64484[0], 64486[0], 64487[0], 64488[0], 64489[0], 64490[0], 64491[0], 64492[0], 64493[0], 64494[0], 64495[0], 64505[0], 64510[0], 64517[0], 64520[0], 64530[0], 67250[1], 67500[1], 69990[0], 92012[1], 92014[1], 92018[1], 92019[1], 93000[1], 93005[1], 93010[1], 93040[1], 93041[1], 93042[1], 93318[1], 93355[1], 94002[1], 94200[1], 94680[1], 94681[1], 94690[1], 95812[1], 95813[1], 95816[1], 95819[1], 95822[1], 95829[1], 95955[1], 96360[1], 96361[1], 96365[1], 96366[1], 96367[1], 96368[1], 96372[1], 96374[1], 96375[1], 96376[1], 96377[1], 96523[0], 97597[1], 97598[1], 97602[1], 99155[0], 99156[0], 99157[0], 99211[1], 99212[1], 99213[1], 99214[1], 99215[1], 99217[1], 99218[1], 99219[1], 99220[1], 99221[1], 99222[1], 99223[1], 99231[1], 99232[1], 99233[1], 99234[1], 99235[1], 99236[1], 99238[1], 99239[1], 99241[1], 99242[1], 99243[1], 99244[1], 99245[1], 99251[1], 99252[1], 99253[1], 99254[1], 99255[1], 99291[1], 99292[1], 99304[1], 99305[1], 99306[1], 99307[1], 99308[1], 99309[1], 99310[1], 99315[1], 99316[1], 99334[1], 99335[1], 99336[1], 99337[1], 99347[1], 99348[1], 99349[1], 99350[1], 99374[1], 99375[1], 99377[1], 99378[1], 99446[0], 99447[0], 99448[0], 99449[0], 99451[0], 99452[0], 99495[0], 99496[0], G0463[1], G0471[1]
65260	0213T[0], 0216T[0], 0596T[1], 0597T[1], 0708T[1], 0709T[1], 11000[1], 11001[1], 11004[1], 11005[1], 11006[1], 11042[1], 11043[1], 11044[1], 11045[1], 11046[1], 11047[1], 12001[1], 12002[1], 12004[1], 12005[1], 12006[1], 12007[1], 12011[1], 12013[1], 12014[1], 12015[1], 12016[1], 12017[1], 12018[1], 12020[1], 12021[1], 12031[1], 12032[1], 12034[1], 12035[1], 12036[1], 12037[1], 12041[1], 12042[1], 12044[1], 12045[1], 12046[1], 12047[1], 12051[1], 12052[1], 12053[1], 12054[1], 12055[1], 12056[1], 12057[1], 13100[1], 13101[1], 13102[1], 13120[1], 13121[1], 13122[1], 13131[1], 13132[1], 13133[1], 13151[1], 13152[1], 13153[1], 36000[1], 36400[1], 36405[1], 36406[1], 36410[1], 36420[1], 36425[1], 36430[1], 36440[1], 36591[0], 36592[0], 36600[1], 36640[1], 43752[1], 51701[1], 51702[1], 51703[1], 62320[0], 62321[0], 62322[0], 62323[0], 62324[0], 62325[0], 62326[0], 62327[0], 64400[0], 64405[0], 64408[0], 64415[0], 64416[0], 64417[0], 64418[0], 64420[0], 64421[0], 64425[0], 64430[0], 64435[0], 64445[0], 64446[0], 64447[0], 64448[0], 64449[0], 64450[0], 64451[0], 64454[0], 64461[0], 64462[0], 64463[0], 64479[0], 64480[0], 64483[0], 64484[0], 64486[0], 64487[0], 64488[0], 64489[0], 64490[0], 64491[0], 64492[0], 64493[0], 64494[0], 64495[0], 64505[0], 64510[0], 64517[0], 64520[0], 64530[0], 67250[1], 67500[1], 69990[0], 92012[1], 92014[1], 92018[1], 92019[1], 93000[1], 93005[1], 93010[1], 93040[1], 93041[1], 93042[1], 93318[1], 93355[1], 94002[1], 94200[1], 94680[1], 94681[1], 94690[1], 95812[1], 95813[1], 95816[1], 95819[1], 95822[1], 95829[1], 95955[1], 96360[1], 96361[1], 96365[1], 96366[1], 96367[1], 96368[1], 96372[1], 96374[1], 96375[1], 96376[1], 96377[1], 96523[0], 97597[1], 97598[1], 97602[1], 99155[0], 99156[0], 99157[0], 99211[1], 99212[1], 99213[1], 99214[1], 99215[1], 99217[1], 99218[1], 99219[1], 99220[1], 99221[1], 99222[1], 99223[1], 99231[1], 99232[1], 99233[1], 99234[1], 99235[1], 99236[1], 99238[1], 99239[1], 99241[1], 99242[1], 99243[1], 99244[1], 99245[1], 99251[1], 99252[1], 99253[1], 99254[1], 99255[1], 99291[1], 99292[1], 99304[1], 99305[1], 99306[1], 99307[1], 99308[1], 99309[1], 99310[1], 99315[1], 99316[1], 99334[1], 99335[1], 99336[1], 99337[1], 99347[1], 99348[1], 99349[1], 99350[1], 99374[1], 99375[1], 99377[1], 99378[1], 99446[0], 99447[0], 99448[0], 99449[0], 99451[0], 99452[0], 99495[0], 99496[0], G0463[1], G0471[1], J0670[1], J2001[1]
65265	0213T[0], 0216T[0], 0596T[1], 0597T[1], 0708T[1], 0709T[1], 11000[1], 11001[1], 11004[1], 11005[1], 11006[1], 11042[1], 11043[1], 11044[1], 11045[1], 11046[1], 11047[1], 12001[1], 12002[1], 12004[1], 12005[1], 12006[1], 12007[1], 12011[1], 12013[1], 12014[1], 12015[1], 12016[1], 12017[1], 12018[1], 12020[1], 12021[1], 12031[1], 12032[1], 12034[1], 12035[1], 12036[1], 12037[1], 12041[1], 12042[1], 12044[1], 12045[1], 12046[1], 12047[1], 12051[1], 12052[1], 12053[1], 12054[1], 12055[1], 12056[1], 12057[1], 13100[1], 13101[1], 13102[1], 13120[1], 13121[1], 13122[1], 13131[1], 13132[1], 13133[1], 13151[1], 13152[1], 13153[1], 36000[1], 36400[1], 36405[1], 36406[1], 36410[1], 36420[1], 36425[1], 36430[1], 36440[1], 36591[0], 36592[0], 36600[1], 36640[1], 43752[1], 51701[1], 51702[1], 51703[1], 62320[0], 62321[0], 62322[0], 62323[0], 62324[0], 62325[0], 62326[0], 62327[0], 64400[0], 64405[0], 64408[0], 64415[0], 64416[0], 64417[0], 64418[0], 64420[0], 64421[0], 64425[0], 64430[0], 64435[0], 64445[0], 64446[0], 64447[0], 64448[0], 64449[0], 64450[0], 64451[0], 64454[0], 64461[0], 64462[0], 64463[0], 64479[0], 64480[0], 64483[0], 64484[0], 64486[0], 64487[0], 64488[0], 64489[0], 64490[0], 64491[0], 64492[0], 64493[0], 64494[0], 64495[0], 64505[0], 64510[0], 64517[0], 64520[0], 64530[0], 65260[1], 67036[1], 67250[1], 67500[1], 69990[0], 92012[1], 92014[1], 92018[1], 92019[1], 93000[1], 93005[1], 93010[1], 93040[1], 93041[1], 93042[1], 93318[1], 93355[1], 94002[1], 94200[1], 94680[1], 94681[1], 94690[1], 95812[1], 95813[1], 95816[1], 95819[1], 95822[1], 95829[1], 95955[1], 96360[1], 96361[1], 96365[1], 96366[1], 96367[1], 96368[1], 96372[1], 96374[1], 96375[1], 96376[1], 96377[1], 96523[0], 97597[1], 97598[1], 97602[1], 99155[0], 99156[0], 99157[0], 99211[1], 99212[1], 99213[1], 99214[1], 99215[1], 99217[1], 99218[1], 99219[1], 99220[1], 99221[1], 99222[1], 99223[1], 99231[1], 99232[1], 99233[1], 99234[1], 99235[1], 99236[1], 99238[1], 99239[1], 99241[1], 99242[1], 99243[1], 99244[1], 99245[1], 99251[1], 99252[1], 99253[1], 99254[1], 99255[1], 99291[1], 99292[1], 99304[1], 99305[1], 99306[1], 99307[1], 99308[1], 99309[1], 99310[1], 99315[1], 99316[1], 99334[1], 99335[1], 99336[1], 99337[1], 99347[1], 99348[1], 99349[1], 99350[1], 99374[1], 99375[1], 99377[1], 99378[1], 99446[0], 99447[0], 99448[0], 99449[0], 99451[0], 99452[0], 99495[0], 99496[0], G0463[1], G0471[1], J0670[1], J2001[1]
65270	0213T[0], 0216T[0], 0596T[1], 0597T[1], 0708T[1], 0709T[1], 11000[1], 11001[1], 11004[1], 11005[1], 11006[1], 11042[1], 11043[1], 11044[1], 11045[1], 11046[1], 11047[1], 12001[1], 12002[1], 12004[1], 12005[1], 12006[1], 12007[1], 12011[1], 12013[1], 12014[1], 12015[1], 12016[1], 12017[1], 12018[1], 12020[1], 12021[1], 12031[1], 12032[1], 12034[1], 12035[1], 12036[1], 12037[1], 12041[1], 12042[1], 12044[1], 12045[1], 12046[1], 12047[1], 12051[1], 12052[1], 12053[1], 12054[1], 12055[1], 12056[1], 12057[1], 13100[1], 13101[1], 13102[1], 13120[1], 13121[1], 13122[1], 13131[1], 13132[1], 13133[1], 13151[1], 13152[1], 13153[1], 36000[1], 36400[1], 36405[1], 36406[1], 36410[1], 36420[1], 36425[1], 36430[1], 36440[1], 36591[0], 36592[0], 36600[1], 36640[1], 43752[1], 51701[1], 51702[1], 51703[1], 62320[0], 62321[0], 62322[0], 62323[0], 62324[0], 62325[0], 62326[0], 62327[0], 64400[0], 64405[0], 64408[0], 64415[0], 64416[0], 64417[0], 64418[0], 64420[0], 64421[0], 64425[0], 64430[0], 64435[0], 64445[0], 64446[0], 64447[0], 64448[0], 64449[0], 64450[0], 64451[0], 64454[0], 64461[0], 64462[0], 64463[0], 64479[0], 64480[0], 64483[0], 64484[0], 64486[0], 64487[0], 64488[0], 64489[0], 64490[0], 64491[0], 64492[0], 64493[0], 64494[0], 64495[0], 64505[0], 64510[0], 64517[0], 64520[0], 64530[0], 67250[1], 67500[1], 69990[0], 92012[1], 92014[1], 92018[1], 92019[1], 93000[1], 93005[1], 93010[1], 93040[1], 93041[1], 93042[1], 93318[1], 93355[1], 94002[1], 94200[1], 94680[1], 94681[1], 94690[1], 95812[1], 95813[1], 95816[1], 95819[1], 95822[1], 95829[1], 95955[1], 96360[1], 96361[1], 96365[1], 96366[1], 96367[1], 96368[1], 96372[1], 96374[1], 96375[1], 96376[1], 96377[1], 96523[0], 97597[1], 97598[1], 97602[1], 99155[0], 99156[0], 99157[0], 99211[1], 99212[1], 99213[1], 99214[1], 99215[1], 99217[1], 99218[1], 99219[1], 99220[1], 99221[1], 99222[1], 99223[1], 99231[1], 99232[1], 99233[1], 99234[1], 99235[1], 99236[1], 99238[1], 99239[1], 99241[1], 99242[1], 99243[1], 99244[1], 99245[1], 99251[1], 99252[1], 99253[1], 99254[1], 99255[1], 99291[1], 99292[1], 99304[1], 99305[1], 99306[1], 99307[1], 99308[1], 99309[1], 99310[1], 99315[1], 99316[1], 99334[1], 99335[1], 99336[1], 99337[1], 99347[1], 99348[1], 99349[1], 99350[1], 99374[1], 99375[1], 99377[1], 99378[1], 99446[0], 99447[0], 99448[0], 99449[0], 99451[0], 99452[0], 99495[0], 99496[0], G0463[1], G0471[1], J2001[1]
65272	0213T[0], 0216T[0], 0596T[1], 0597T[1], 0708T[1], 0709T[1], 12001[1], 12002[1], 12004[1], 12005[1], 12006[1], 12007[1], 12011[1], 12013[1], 12014[1], 12015[1], 12016[1], 12017[1], 12018[1], 12020[1], 12021[1], 12031[1], 12032[1], 12034[1], 12035[1], 12036[1], 12037[1], 12041[1], 12042[1], 12044[1], 12045[1], 12046[1], 12047[1], 12051[1], 12052[1], 12053[1], 12054[1], 12055[1], 12056[1], 12057[1], 13100[1], 13101[1], 13102[1], 13120[1], 13121[1], 13122[1], 13131[1], 13132[1], 13133[1], 13151[1], 13152[1], 13153[1], 36000[1], 36400[1], 36405[1], 36406[1], 36410[1], 36420[1], 36425[1], 36430[1], 36440[1], 36591[0], 36592[0], 36600[1], 36640[1], 43752[1], 51701[1], 51702[1], 51703[1], 62320[0], 62321[0], 62322[0], 62323[0], 62324[0], 62325[0], 62326[0], 62327[0], 64400[0], 64405[0], 64408[0], 64415[0], 64416[0], 64417[0], 64418[0], 64420[0], 64421[0], 64425[0], 64430[0], 64435[0], 64445[0], 64446[0], 64447[0], 64448[0], 64449[0], 64450[0], 64451[0], 64454[0], 64461[0], 64462[0], 64463[0], 64479[0], 64480[0], 64483[0], 64484[0], 64486[0], 64487[0], 64488[0], 64489[0], 64490[0], 64491[0], 64492[0], 64493[0], 64494[0], 64495[0], 64505[0], 64510[0], 64517[0], 64520[0], 64530[0], 65270[1], 67250[1], 67500[1], 69990[0], 92012[1], 92014[1], 92018[1], 92019[1], 93000[1], 93005[1], 93010[1], 93040[1], 93041[1], 93042[1], 93318[1], 93355[1], 94002[1], 94200[1], 94680[1], 94681[1], 94690[1], 95812[1], 95813[1], 95816[1], 95819[1], 95822[1], 95829[1], 95955[1], 96360[1], 96361[1], 96365[1], 96366[1], 96367[1], 96368[1], 96372[1], 96374[1], 96375[1], 96376[1], 96377[1], 96523[0], 99155[0], 99156[0], 99157[0], 99211[1], 99212[1], 99213[1], 99214[1], 99215[1], 99217[1], 99218[1], 99219[1],

Appendix A: NCCI - CPT Codes

0 = Modifier usage not allowed or inappropriate 1 = Modifier usage allowed

Code 1	Code 2
	99220[1], 99221[1], 99222[1], 99223[1], 99231[1], 99232[1], 99233[1], 99234[1], 99235[1], 99236[1], 99238[1], 99239[1], 99241[1], 99242[1], 99243[1], 99244[1], 99245[1], 99251[1], 99252[1], 99253[1], 99254[1], 99255[1], 99291[1], 99292[1], 99304[1], 99305[1], 99306[1], 99307[1], 99308[1], 99309[1], 99310[1], 99315[1], 99316[1], 99334[1], 99335[1], 99336[1], 99337[1], 99347[1], 99348[1], 99349[1], 99350[1], 99374[1], 99375[1], 99377[1], 99378[1], 99446[0], 99447[0], 99448[0], 99449[0], 99451[0], 99452[0], 99495[0], 99496[0], G0463[1], G0471[1], J0670[1], J2001[1]
65273	0213T[0], 0216T[0], 0596T[1], 0597T[1], 0708T[1], 0709T[1], 12001[1], 12002[1], 12004[1], 12005[1], 12006[1], 12007[1], 12011[1], 12013[1], 12014[1], 12015[1], 12016[1], 12017[1], 12018[1], 12020[1], 12021[1], 12031[1], 12032[1], 12034[1], 12035[1], 12036[1], 12037[1], 12041[1], 12042[1], 12044[1], 12045[1], 12046[1], 12047[1], 12051[1], 12052[1], 12053[1], 12054[1], 12055[1], 12056[1], 12057[1], 13100[1], 13101[1], 13102[1], 13120[1], 13121[1], 13122[1], 13131[1], 13132[1], 13133[1], 13151[1], 13152[1], 13153[1], 36000[1], 36400[1], 36405[1], 36406[1], 36410[1], 36420[1], 36425[1], 36430[1], 36440[1], 36591[0], 36592[0], 36600[1], 36640[1], 43752[1], 51701[1], 51702[1], 51703[1], 62320[0], 62321[0], 62322[0], 62323[0], 62324[0], 62325[0], 62326[0], 62327[0], 64400[0], 64405[0], 64408[0], 64415[0], 64416[0], 64417[0], 64418[0], 64420[0], 64421[0], 64425[0], 64430[0], 64435[0], 64445[0], 64446[0], 64447[0], 64448[0], 64449[0], 64450[0], 64451[0], 64454[0], 64461[0], 64462[0], 64463[0], 64479[0], 64480[0], 64483[0], 64484[0], 64486[0], 64487[0], 64488[0], 64489[0], 64490[0], 64491[0], 64492[0], 64493[0], 64494[0], 64495[0], 64505[0], 64510[0], 64517[0], 64520[0], 64530[0], 65270[1], 65272[1], 67250[1], 67500[1], 69990[0], 92012[1], 92014[1], 92018[1], 92019[1], 93000[1], 93005[1], 93010[1], 93040[1], 93041[1], 93042[1], 93318[1], 93355[1], 94002[1], 94200[1], 94680[1], 94681[1], 94690[1], 95812[1], 95813[1], 95816[1], 95819[1], 95822[1], 95829[1], 95955[1], 96360[1], 96361[1], 96365[1], 96366[1], 96367[1], 96368[1], 96372[1], 96374[1], 96375[1], 96376[1], 96377[1], 96523[0], 99155[0], 99156[0], 99157[0], 99211[1], 99212[1], 99213[1], 99214[1], 99215[1], 99217[1], 99218[1], 99219[1], 99220[1], 99221[1], 99222[1], 99223[1], 99231[1], 99232[1], 99233[1], 99234[1], 99235[1], 99236[1], 99238[1], 99239[1], 99241[1], 99242[1], 99243[1], 99244[1], 99245[1], 99251[1], 99252[1], 99253[1], 99254[1], 99255[1], 99291[1], 99292[1], 99304[1], 99305[1], 99306[1], 99307[1], 99308[1], 99309[1], 99310[1], 99315[1], 99316[1], 99334[1], 99335[1], 99336[1], 99337[1], 99347[1], 99348[1], 99349[1], 99350[1], 99374[1], 99375[1], 99377[1], 99378[1], 99446[0], 99447[0], 99448[0], 99449[0], 99451[0], 99452[0], 99495[0], 99496[0], G0463[1], G0471[1], J2001[1]
65275	0213T[0], 0216T[0], 0596T[1], 0597T[1], 0708T[1], 0709T[1], 11000[1], 11001[1], 11004[1], 11005[1], 11006[1], 11042[1], 11043[1], 11044[1], 11045[1], 11046[1], 11047[1], 12001[1], 12002[1], 12004[1], 12005[1], 12006[1], 12007[1], 12011[1], 12013[1], 12014[1], 12015[1], 12016[1], 12017[1], 12018[1], 12020[1], 12021[1], 12031[1], 12032[1], 12034[1], 12035[1], 12036[1], 12037[1], 12041[1], 12042[1], 12044[1], 12045[1], 12046[1], 12047[1], 12051[1], 12052[1], 12053[1], 12054[1], 12055[1], 12056[1], 12057[1], 13100[1], 13101[1], 13102[1], 13120[1], 13121[1], 13122[1], 13131[1], 13132[1], 13133[1], 13151[1], 13152[1], 13153[1], 36000[1], 36400[1], 36405[1], 36406[1], 36410[1], 36420[1], 36425[1], 36430[1], 36440[1], 36591[0], 36592[0], 36600[1], 36640[1], 43752[1], 51701[1], 51702[1], 51703[1], 62320[0], 62321[0], 62322[0], 62323[0], 62324[0], 62325[0], 62326[0], 62327[0], 64400[0], 64405[0], 64408[0], 64415[0], 64416[0], 64417[0], 64418[0], 64420[0], 64421[0], 64425[0], 64430[0], 64435[0], 64445[0], 64446[0], 64447[0], 64448[0], 64449[0], 64450[0], 64451[0], 64454[0], 64461[0], 64462[0], 64463[0], 64479[0], 64480[0], 64483[0], 64484[0], 64486[0], 64487[0], 64488[0], 64489[0], 64490[0], 64491[0], 64492[0], 64493[0], 64494[0], 64495[0], 64505[0], 64510[0], 64517[0], 64520[0], 64530[0], 65220[1], 65222[1], 65270[1], 65272[1], 65273[1], 65430[1], 67250[1], 67500[1], 69990[0], 92012[1], 92014[1], 92018[1], 92019[1], 92071[1], 93000[1], 93005[1], 93010[1], 93040[1], 93041[1], 93042[1], 93318[1], 93355[1], 94002[1], 94200[1], 94680[1], 94681[1], 94690[1], 95812[1], 95813[1], 95816[1], 95819[1], 95822[1], 95829[1], 95955[1], 96360[1], 96361[1], 96365[1], 96366[1], 96367[1], 96368[1], 96372[1], 96374[1], 96375[1], 96376[1], 96377[1], 96523[0], 97597[1], 97598[1], 97602[1], 99155[0], 99156[0], 99157[0], 99211[1], 99212[1], 99213[1], 99214[1], 99215[1], 99217[1], 99218[1], 99219[1], 99220[1], 99221[1], 99222[1], 99223[1], 99231[1], 99232[1], 99233[1], 99234[1], 99235[1], 99236[1], 99238[1], 99239[1], 99241[1], 99242[1], 99243[1], 99244[1], 99245[1], 99251[1], 99252[1], 99253[1], 99254[1], 99255[1], 99291[1], 99292[1], 99304[1], 99305[1], 99306[1], 99307[1], 99308[1], 99309[1], 99310[1], 99315[1], 99316[1], 99334[1], 99335[1], 99336[1], 99337[1], 99347[1], 99348[1], 99349[1], 99350[1], 99374[1], 99375[1], 99377[1], 99378[1], 99446[0], 99447[0], 99448[0], 99449[0], 99451[0], 99452[0], 99495[0], 99496[0], G0463[1], G0471[1], J2001[1]
65280	0213T[0], 0216T[0], 0596T[1], 0597T[1], 0708T[1], 0709T[1], 12001[1], 12002[1], 12004[1], 12005[1], 12006[1], 12007[1], 12011[1], 12013[1], 12014[1], 12015[1], 12016[1], 12017[1], 12018[1], 12020[1], 12021[1], 12031[1], 12032[1], 12034[1], 12035[1], 12036[1], 12037[1], 12041[1], 12042[1], 12044[1], 12045[1], 12046[1], 12047[1], 12051[1], 12052[1], 12053[1], 12054[1], 12055[1], 12056[1], 12057[1], 13100[1], 13101[1], 13102[1], 13120[1], 13121[1], 13122[1], 13131[1], 13132[1], 13133[1], 13151[1], 13152[1], 13153[1], 36000[1], 36400[1], 36405[1], 36406[1], 36410[1], 36420[1], 36425[1], 36430[1], 36440[1], 36591[0], 36592[0], 36600[1], 36640[1], 43752[1], 51701[1], 51702[1], 51703[1], 62320[0], 62321[0], 62322[0], 62323[0], 62324[0], 62325[0], 62326[0], 62327[0], 64400[0], 64405[0], 64408[0], 64415[0], 64416[0], 64417[0], 64418[0], 64420[0], 64421[0], 64425[0], 64430[0], 64435[0], 64445[0], 64446[0], 64447[0], 64448[0], 64449[0], 64450[0], 64451[0], 64454[0], 64461[0], 64462[0], 64463[0], 64479[0], 64480[0], 64483[0], 64484[0], 64486[0], 64487[0], 64488[0], 64489[0], 64490[0], 64491[0], 64492[0], 64493[0], 64494[0], 64495[0], 64505[0], 64510[0], 64517[0], 64520[0], 64530[0], 65270[1], 65272[1], 65273[1], 65275[1], 65430[1], 67250[1], 67500[1], 69990[0], 92012[1], 92014[1], 92018[1], 92019[1], 92071[1], 93000[1], 93005[1], 93010[1], 93040[1], 93041[1], 93042[1], 93318[1], 93355[1], 94002[1], 94200[1], 94680[1], 94681[1], 94690[1], 95812[1], 95813[1], 95816[1], 95819[1], 95822[1], 95829[1], 95955[1], 96360[1], 96361[1], 96365[1], 96366[1], 96367[1], 96368[1], 96372[1], 96374[1], 96375[1], 96376[1], 96377[1], 96523[0], 99155[0], 99156[0], 99157[0], 99211[1], 99212[1], 99213[1], 99214[1], 99215[1], 99217[1], 99218[1], 99219[1], 99220[1], 99221[1], 99222[1], 99223[1], 99231[1], 99232[1], 99233[1], 99234[1], 99235[1], 99236[1], 99238[1], 99239[1], 99241[1], 99242[1], 99243[1], 99244[1], 99245[1], 99251[1], 99252[1], 99253[1], 99254[1], 99255[1], 99291[1], 99292[1], 99304[1], 99305[1], 99306[1], 99307[1], 99308[1], 99309[1], 99310[1], 99315[1], 99316[1], 99334[1], 99335[1], 99336[1], 99337[1], 99347[1], 99348[1], 99349[1], 99350[1], 99374[1], 99375[1], 99377[1], 99378[1], 99446[0], 99447[0], 99448[0], 99449[0], 99451[0], 99452[0], 99495[0], 99496[0], G0463[1], G0471[1], J2001[1]
65285	0213T[0], 0216T[0], 0596T[1], 0597T[1], 0708T[1], 0709T[1], 11000[1], 11001[1], 11004[1], 11005[1], 11006[1], 11042[1], 11043[1], 11044[1], 11045[1], 11046[1], 11047[1], 12001[1], 12002[1], 12004[1], 12005[1], 12006[1], 12007[1], 12011[1], 12013[1], 12014[1], 12015[1], 12016[1], 12017[1], 12018[1], 12020[1], 12021[1], 12031[1], 12032[1], 12034[1], 12035[1], 12036[1], 12037[1], 12041[1], 12042[1], 12044[1], 12045[1], 12046[1], 12047[1], 12051[1], 12052[1], 12053[1], 12054[1], 12055[1], 12056[1], 12057[1], 13100[1], 13101[1], 13102[1], 13120[1], 13121[1], 13122[1], 13131[1], 13132[1], 13133[1], 13151[1], 13152[1], 13153[1], 36000[1], 36400[1], 36405[1], 36406[1], 36410[1], 36420[1], 36425[1], 36430[1], 36440[1], 36591[0], 36592[0], 36600[1], 36640[1], 43752[1], 51701[1], 51702[1], 51703[1], 62320[0], 62321[0], 62322[0], 62323[0], 62324[0], 62325[0], 62326[0], 62327[0], 64400[0], 64405[0], 64408[0], 64415[0], 64416[0], 64417[0], 64418[0], 64420[0], 64421[0], 64425[0], 64430[0], 64435[0], 64445[0], 64446[0], 64447[0], 64448[0], 64449[0], 64450[0], 64451[0], 64454[0], 64461[0], 64462[0], 64463[0], 64479[0], 64480[0], 64483[0], 64484[0], 64486[0], 64487[0], 64488[0], 64489[0], 64490[0], 64491[0], 64492[0], 64493[0], 64494[0], 64495[0], 64505[0], 64510[0], 64517[0], 64520[0], 64530[0], 65270[1], 65272[1], 65273[1], 65275[1], 65280[1], 65430[1], 65930[1], 67250[1], 67500[1], 69990[0], 92012[1], 92014[1], 92018[1], 92019[1], 93000[1], 93005[1], 93010[1], 93040[1], 93041[1], 93042[1], 93318[1], 93355[1], 94002[1], 94200[1], 94680[1], 94681[1], 94690[1], 95812[1], 95813[1], 95816[1], 95819[1], 95822[1], 95829[1], 95955[1], 96360[1], 96361[1], 96365[1], 96366[1], 96367[1], 96368[1], 96372[1], 96374[1], 96375[1], 96376[1], 96377[1], 96523[0], 97597[1], 97598[1], 97602[1], 99155[0], 99156[0], 99157[0], 99211[1], 99212[1], 99213[1], 99214[1], 99215[1], 99217[1], 99218[1], 99219[1], 99220[1], 99221[1], 99222[1], 99223[1], 99231[1], 99232[1], 99233[1], 99234[1], 99235[1], 99236[1], 99238[1], 99239[1], 99241[1], 99242[1], 99243[1], 99244[1], 99245[1], 99251[1], 99252[1], 99253[1], 99254[1], 99255[1], 99291[1], 99292[1], 99304[1], 99305[1], 99306[1], 99307[1], 99308[1], 99309[1], 99310[1], 99315[1], 99316[1], 99334[1], 99335[1], 99336[1], 99337[1], 99347[1], 99348[1], 99349[1], 99350[1], 99374[1], 99375[1], 99377[1], 99378[1], 99446[0], 99447[0], 99448[0], 99449[0], 99451[0], 99452[0], 99495[0], 99496[0], G0463[1], G0471[1]
65286	0213T[0], 0216T[0], 0596T[1], 0597T[1], 0708T[1], 0709T[1], 12001[1], 12002[1], 12004[1], 12005[1], 12006[1], 12007[1], 12011[1], 12013[1], 12014[1], 12015[1], 12016[1], 12017[1], 12018[1], 12020[1], 12021[1], 12031[1], 12032[1], 12034[1], 12035[1], 12036[1], 12037[1], 12041[1], 12042[1], 12044[1], 12045[1], 12046[1], 12047[1], 12051[1], 12052[1], 12053[1], 12054[1], 12055[1], 12056[1], 12057[1], 13100[1], 13101[1], 13102[1], 13120[1], 13121[1], 13122[1], 13131[1], 13132[1], 13133[1], 13151[1], 13152[1], 13153[1], 36000[1], 36400[1], 36405[1], 36406[1], 36410[1], 36420[1], 36425[1], 36430[1], 36440[1], 36591[0], 36592[0], 36600[1], 36640[1], 43752[1], 51701[1], 51702[1], 51703[1], 62320[0], 62321[0], 62322[0], 62323[0], 62324[0], 62325[0], 62326[0], 62327[0], 64400[0], 64405[0], 64408[0], 64415[0], 64416[0], 64417[0], 64418[0], 64420[0], 64421[0], 64425[0], 64430[0], 64435[0], 64445[0], 64446[0], 64447[0], 64448[0], 64449[0], 64450[0], 64451[0], 64454[0], 64461[0], 64462[0], 64463[0], 64479[0], 64480[0], 64483[0], 64484[0], 64486[0], 64487[0], 64488[0], 64489[0], 64490[0], 64491[0], 64492[0], 64493[0], 64494[0], 64495[0], 64505[0], 64510[0], 64517[0], 64520[0], 64530[0], 67250[1], 67500[1], 69990[0], 92012[1], 92014[1], 92018[1], 92019[1], 92071[1], 93000[1], 93005[1], 93010[1], 93040[1], 93041[1], 93042[1], 93318[1], 93355[1], 94002[1], 94200[1], 94680[1], 94681[1], 94690[1], 95812[1], 95813[1], 95816[1], 95819[1], 95822[1], 95829[1], 95955[1], 96360[1], 96361[1], 96365[1], 96366[1], 96367[1], 96368[1], 96372[1], 96374[1], 96375[1], 96376[1], 96377[1], 96523[0], 99155[0], 99156[0], 99157[0], 99211[1], 99212[1], 99213[1], 99214[1], 99215[1], 99217[1], 99218[1], 99219[1], 99220[1], 99221[1], 99222[1], 99223[1], 99231[1], 99232[1], 99233[1], 99234[1], 99235[1], 99236[1], 99238[1], 99239[1], 99241[1], 99242[1], 99243[1], 99244[1], 99245[1], 99251[1], 99252[1], 99253[1], 99254[1], 99255[1], 99291[1], 99292[1], 99304[1], 99305[1], 99306[1], 99307[1], 99308[1], 99309[1], 99310[1], 99315[1], 99316[1], 99334[1], 99335[1], 99336[1], 99337[1], 99347[1], 99348[1], 99349[1], 99350[1], 99374[1], 99375[1], 99377[1], 99378[1], 99446[0], 99447[0], 99448[0], 99449[0], 99451[0], 99452[0], 99495[0], 99496[0], G0463[1], G0471[1], J2001[1]
65290	0213T[0], 0216T[0], 0596T[1], 0597T[1], 0708T[1], 0709T[1], 12001[1], 12002[1], 12004[1], 12005[1], 12006[1], 12007[1], 12011[1], 12013[1], 12014[1], 12015[1], 12016[1], 12017[1], 12018[1], 12020[1], 12021[1], 12031[1], 12032[1], 12034[1], 12035[1], 12036[1], 12037[1], 12041[1], 12042[1], 12044[1], 12045[1], 12046[1], 12047[1], 12051[1], 12052[1], 12053[1], 12054[1], 12055[1], 12056[1], 12057[1],

0 = Modifier usage not allowed or inappropriate   1 = Modifier usage allowed

Code 1	Code 2
	13100[1], 13101[1], 13102[1], 13120[1], 13121[1], 13122[1], 13131[1], 13132[1], 13133[1], 13151[1], 13152[1], 13153[1], 36000[1], 36400[1], 36405[1], 36406[1], 36410[1], 36420[1], 36425[1], 36430[1], 36440[1], 36591[0], 36592[0], 36600[1], 36640[1], 43752[1], 51701[1], 51702[1], 51703[1], 62320[0], 62321[0], 62322[0], 62323[0], 62324[0], 62325[0], 62326[0], 62327[0], 64400[0], 64405[0], 64408[0], 64415[0], 64416[0], 64417[0], 64418[0], 64420[0], 64421[0], 64425[0], 64430[0], 64435[0], 64445[0], 64446[0], 64447[0], 64448[0], 64449[0], 64450[0], 64451[0], 64454[0], 64461[0], 64462[0], 64463[0], 64479[0], 64480[0], 64483[0], 64484[0], 64486[0], 64487[0], 64488[0], 64489[0], 64490[0], 64491[0], 64492[0], 64493[0], 64494[0], 64495[0], 64505[0], 64510[0], 64517[0], 64520[0], 64530[0], 67250[1], 67500[1], 69990[0], 92012[1], 92014[1], 92018[1], 92019[1], 93000[1], 93005[1], 93010[1], 93040[1], 93041[1], 93042[1], 93318[1], 93355[1], 94002[1], 94200[1], 94680[1], 94681[1], 94690[1], 95812[1], 95813[1], 95816[1], 95819[1], 95822[1], 95829[1], 95955[1], 96360[1], 96361[1], 96365[1], 96366[1], 96367[1], 96368[1], 96372[1], 96374[1], 96375[1], 96376[1], 96377[1], 96523[0], 99155[0], 99156[0], 99157[0], 99211[1], 99212[1], 99213[1], 99214[1], 99215[1], 99217[1], 99218[1], 99219[1], 99220[1], 99221[1], 99222[1], 99223[1], 99231[1], 99232[1], 99233[1], 99234[1], 99235[1], 99236[1], 99238[1], 99239[1], 99241[1], 99242[1], 99243[1], 99244[1], 99245[1], 99251[1], 99252[1], 99253[1], 99254[1], 99255[1], 99291[1], 99292[1], 99304[1], 99305[1], 99306[1], 99307[1], 99308[1], 99309[1], 99310[1], 99315[1], 99316[1], 99334[1], 99335[1], 99336[1], 99337[1], 99347[1], 99348[1], 99349[1], 99350[1], 99374[1], 99375[1], 99377[1], 99378[1], 99446[0], 99447[0], 99448[0], 99449[0], 99451[0], 99452[0], 99495[0], 99496[0], G0463[1], G0471[1]
65400	0213T[0], 0216T[0], 0596T[1], 0597T[1], 0708T[1], 0709T[1], 11000[1], 11001[1], 11004[1], 11005[1], 11006[1], 11042[1], 11043[1], 11044[1], 11045[1], 11046[1], 11047[1], 12001[1], 12002[1], 12004[1], 12005[1], 12006[1], 12007[1], 12011[1], 12013[1], 12014[1], 12015[1], 12016[1], 12017[1], 12018[1], 12020[1], 12021[1], 12031[1], 12032[1], 12034[1], 12035[1], 12036[1], 12037[1], 12041[1], 12042[1], 12044[1], 12045[1], 12046[1], 12047[1], 12051[1], 12052[1], 12053[1], 12054[1], 12055[1], 12056[1], 12057[1], 13100[1], 13101[1], 13102[1], 13120[1], 13121[1], 13122[1], 13131[1], 13132[1], 13133[1], 13151[1], 13152[1], 13153[1], 36000[1], 36400[1], 36405[1], 36406[1], 36410[1], 36420[1], 36425[1], 36430[1], 36440[1], 36591[0], 36592[0], 36600[1], 36640[1], 43752[1], 51701[1], 51702[1], 51703[1], 62320[0], 62321[0], 62322[0], 62323[0], 62324[0], 62325[0], 62326[0], 62327[0], 64400[0], 64405[0], 64408[0], 64415[0], 64416[0], 64417[0], 64418[0], 64420[0], 64421[0], 64425[0], 64430[0], 64435[0], 64445[0], 64446[0], 64447[0], 64448[0], 64449[0], 64450[0], 64451[0], 64454[0], 64461[0], 64462[0], 64463[0], 64479[0], 64480[0], 64483[0], 64484[0], 64486[0], 64487[0], 64488[0], 64489[0], 64490[0], 64491[0], 64492[0], 64493[0], 64494[0], 64495[0], 64505[0], 64510[0], 64517[0], 64520[0], 64530[0], 65410[1], 67250[1], 67500[1], 68371[1], 69990[0], 92012[1], 92014[1], 92018[1], 92019[1], 92071[1], 93000[1], 93005[1], 93010[1], 93040[1], 93041[1], 93042[1], 93318[1], 93355[1], 94002[1], 94200[1], 94680[1], 94681[1], 94690[1], 95812[1], 95813[1], 95816[1], 95819[1], 95822[1], 95829[1], 95955[1], 96360[1], 96361[1], 96365[1], 96366[1], 96367[1], 96368[1], 96372[1], 96374[1], 96375[1], 96376[1], 96377[1], 96523[0], 97597[1], 97598[1], 97602[1], 99155[0], 99156[0], 99157[0], 99211[1], 99212[1], 99213[1], 99214[1], 99215[1], 99217[1], 99218[1], 99219[1], 99220[1], 99221[1], 99222[1], 99223[1], 99231[1], 99232[1], 99233[1], 99234[1], 99235[1], 99236[1], 99238[1], 99239[1], 99241[1], 99242[1], 99243[1], 99244[1], 99245[1], 99251[1], 99252[1], 99253[1], 99254[1], 99255[1], 99291[1], 99292[1], 99304[1], 99305[1], 99306[1], 99307[1], 99308[1], 99309[1], 99310[1], 99315[1], 99316[1], 99334[1], 99335[1], 99336[1], 99337[1], 99347[1], 99348[1], 99349[1], 99350[1], 99374[1], 99375[1], 99377[1], 99378[1], 99446[0], 99447[0], 99448[0], 99449[0], 99451[0], 99452[0], 99495[0], 99496[0], G0463[1], G0471[1], J0670[1], J2001[1]
65410	0213T[0], 0216T[0], 0596T[1], 0597T[1], 0708T[1], 0709T[1], 10005[1], 10007[1], 10009[1], 10011[1], 10021[1], 12001[1], 12002[1], 12004[1], 12005[1], 12006[1], 12007[1], 12011[1], 12013[1], 12014[1], 12015[1], 12016[1], 12017[1], 12018[1], 12020[1], 12021[1], 12031[1], 12032[1], 12034[1], 12035[1], 12036[1], 12037[1], 12041[1], 12042[1], 12044[1], 12045[1], 12046[1], 12047[1], 12051[1], 12052[1], 12053[1], 12054[1], 12055[1], 12056[1], 12057[1], 13100[1], 13101[1], 13102[1], 13120[1], 13121[1], 13122[1], 13131[1], 13132[1], 13133[1], 13151[1], 13152[1], 13153[1], 36000[1], 36400[1], 36405[1], 36406[1], 36410[1], 36420[1], 36425[1], 36430[1], 36440[1], 36591[0], 36592[0], 36600[1], 36640[1], 43752[1], 51701[1], 51702[1], 51703[1], 62320[0], 62321[0], 62322[0], 62323[0], 62324[0], 62325[0], 62326[0], 62327[0], 64400[0], 64405[0], 64408[0], 64415[0], 64416[0], 64417[0], 64418[0], 64420[0], 64421[0], 64425[0], 64430[0], 64435[0], 64445[0], 64446[0], 64447[0], 64448[0], 64449[0], 64450[0], 64451[0], 64454[0], 64461[0], 64462[0], 64463[0], 64479[0], 64480[0], 64483[0], 64484[0], 64486[0], 64487[0], 64488[0], 64489[0], 64490[0], 64491[0], 64492[0], 64493[0], 64494[0], 64495[0], 64505[0], 64510[0], 64517[0], 64520[0], 64530[0], 67250[1], 67500[1], 69990[0], 92012[1], 92014[1], 92018[1], 92019[1], 92071[1], 93000[1], 93005[1], 93010[1], 93040[1], 93041[1], 93042[1], 93318[1], 93355[1], 94002[1], 94200[1], 94680[1], 94681[1], 94690[1], 95812[1], 95813[1], 95816[1], 95819[1], 95822[1], 95829[1], 95955[1], 96360[1], 96361[1], 96365[1], 96366[1], 96367[1], 96368[1], 96372[1], 96374[1], 96375[1], 96376[1], 96377[1], 96523[0], 99155[0], 99156[0], 99157[0], 99211[1], 99212[1], 99213[1], 99214[1], 99215[1], 99217[1], 99218[1], 99219[1], 99220[1], 99221[1], 99222[1], 99223[1], 99231[1], 99232[1], 99233[1], 99234[1], 99235[1], 99236[1], 99238[1], 99239[1], 99241[1], 99242[1], 99243[1], 99244[1], 99245[1], 99251[1], 99252[1], 99253[1], 99254[1], 99255[1], 99291[1], 99292[1], 99304[1], 99305[1], 99306[1], 99307[1], 99308[1], 99309[1], 99310[1], 99315[1], 99316[1], 99334[1], 99335[1], 99336[1], 99337[1], 99347[1], 99348[1], 99349[1], 99350[1], 99374[1], 99375[1], 99377[1], 99378[1], 99446[0], 99447[0], 99448[0], 99449[0], 99451[0], 99452[0], 99495[1], 99496[1], G0463[1], G0471[1]
65420	0213T[0], 0216T[0], 0596T[1], 0597T[1], 0708T[1], 0709T[1], 11000[1], 11001[1], 11004[1], 11005[1], 11006[1], 11042[1], 11043[1], 11044[1], 11045[1], 11046[1], 11047[1], 12001[1], 12002[1], 12004[1], 12005[1], 12006[1], 12007[1], 12011[1], 12013[1], 12014[1], 12015[1], 12016[1], 12017[1], 12018[1], 12020[1], 12021[1], 12031[1], 12032[1], 12034[1], 12035[1], 12036[1], 12037[1], 12041[1], 12042[1], 12044[1], 12045[1], 12046[1], 12047[1], 12051[1], 12052[1], 12053[1], 12054[1], 12055[1], 12056[1], 12057[1], 13100[1], 13101[1], 13102[1], 13120[1], 13121[1], 13122[1], 13131[1], 13132[1], 13133[1], 13151[1], 13152[1], 13153[1], 36000[1], 36400[1], 36405[1], 36406[1], 36410[1], 36420[1], 36425[1], 36430[1], 36440[1], 36591[0], 36592[0], 36600[1], 36640[1], 43752[1], 51701[1], 51702[1], 51703[1], 62320[0], 62321[0], 62322[0], 62323[0], 62324[0], 62325[0], 62326[0], 62327[0], 64400[0], 64405[0], 64408[0], 64415[0], 64416[0], 64417[0], 64418[0], 64420[0], 64421[0], 64425[0], 64430[0], 64435[0], 64445[0], 64446[0], 64447[0], 64448[0], 64449[0], 64450[0], 64451[0], 64454[0], 64461[0], 64462[0], 64463[0], 64479[0], 64480[0], 64483[0], 64484[0], 64486[0], 64487[0], 64488[0], 64489[0], 64490[0], 64491[0], 64492[0], 64493[0], 64494[0], 64495[0], 64505[0], 64510[0], 64517[0], 64520[0], 64530[0], 65400[1], 65778[1], 65779[1], 65780[1], 65781[1], 65782[1], 67250[1], 67500[1], 68320[1], 69990[0], 92012[1], 92014[1], 92018[1], 92019[1], 92071[1], 93000[1], 93005[1], 93010[1], 93040[1], 93041[1], 93042[1], 93318[1], 93355[1], 94002[1], 94200[1], 94680[1], 94681[1], 94690[1], 95812[1], 95813[1], 95816[1], 95819[1], 95822[1], 95829[1], 95955[1], 96360[1], 96361[1], 96365[1], 96366[1], 96367[1], 96368[1], 96372[1], 96374[1], 96375[1], 96376[1], 96377[1], 96523[0], 97597[1], 97598[1], 97602[1], 99155[0], 99156[0], 99157[0], 99211[1], 99212[1], 99213[1], 99214[1], 99215[1], 99217[1], 99218[1], 99219[1], 99220[1], 99221[1], 99222[1], 99223[1], 99231[1], 99232[1], 99233[1], 99234[1], 99235[1], 99236[1], 99238[1], 99239[1], 99241[1], 99242[1], 99243[1], 99244[1], 99245[1], 99251[1], 99252[1], 99253[1], 99254[1], 99255[1], 99291[1], 99292[1], 99304[1], 99305[1], 99306[1], 99307[1], 99308[1], 99309[1], 99310[1], 99315[1], 99316[1], 99334[1], 99335[1], 99336[1], 99337[1], 99347[1], 99348[1], 99349[1], 99350[1], 99374[1], 99375[1], 99377[1], 99378[1], 99446[0], 99447[0], 99448[0], 99449[0], 99451[0], 99452[0], 99495[0], 99496[0], G0463[1], G0471[1], J0670[1], J2001[1]
65426	0213T[0], 0216T[0], 0596T[1], 0597T[1], 0708T[1], 0709T[1], 11000[1], 11001[1], 11004[1], 11005[1], 11006[1], 11042[1], 11043[1], 11044[1], 11045[1], 11046[1], 11047[1], 12001[1], 12002[1], 12004[1], 12005[1], 12006[1], 12007[1], 12011[1], 12013[1], 12014[1], 12015[1], 12016[1], 12017[1], 12018[1], 12020[1], 12021[1], 12031[1], 12032[1], 12034[1], 12035[1], 12036[1], 12037[1], 12041[1], 12042[1], 12044[1], 12045[1], 12046[1], 12047[1], 12051[1], 12052[1], 12053[1], 12054[1], 12055[1], 12056[1], 12057[1], 13100[1], 13101[1], 13102[1], 13120[1], 13121[1], 13122[1], 13131[1], 13132[1], 13133[1], 13151[1], 13152[1], 13153[1], 36000[1], 36400[1], 36405[1], 36406[1], 36410[1], 36420[1], 36425[1], 36430[1], 36440[1], 36591[0], 36592[0], 36600[1], 36640[1], 43752[1], 51701[1], 51702[1], 51703[1], 62320[0], 62321[0], 62322[0], 62323[0], 62324[0], 62325[0], 62326[0], 62327[0], 64400[0], 64405[0], 64408[0], 64415[0], 64416[0], 64417[0], 64418[0], 64420[0], 64421[0], 64425[0], 64430[0], 64435[0], 64445[0], 64446[0], 64447[0], 64448[0], 64449[0], 64450[0], 64451[0], 64454[0], 64461[0], 64462[0], 64463[0], 64479[0], 64480[0], 64483[0], 64484[0], 64486[0], 64487[0], 64488[0], 64489[0], 64490[0], 64491[0], 64492[0], 64493[0], 64494[0], 64495[0], 64505[0], 64510[0], 64517[0], 64520[0], 64530[0], 65400[1], 65420[1], 65778[1], 65779[1], 65780[1], 65781[1], 65782[1], 67250[1], 67500[1], 68320[1], 68371[1], 69990[0], 92012[1], 92014[1], 92018[1], 92019[1], 92071[1], 93000[1], 93005[1], 93010[1], 93040[1], 93041[1], 93042[1], 93318[1], 93355[1], 94002[1], 94200[1], 94680[1], 94681[1], 94690[1], 95812[1], 95813[1], 95816[1], 95819[1], 95822[1], 95829[1], 95955[1], 96360[1], 96361[1], 96365[1], 96366[1], 96367[1], 96368[1], 96372[1], 96374[1], 96375[1], 96376[1], 96377[1], 96523[0], 97597[1], 97598[1], 97602[1], 99155[0], 99156[0], 99157[0], 99211[1], 99212[1], 99213[1], 99214[1], 99215[1], 99217[1], 99218[1], 99219[1], 99220[1], 99221[1], 99222[1], 99223[1], 99231[1], 99232[1], 99233[1], 99234[1], 99235[1], 99236[1], 99238[1], 99239[1], 99241[1], 99242[1], 99243[1], 99244[1], 99245[1], 99251[1], 99252[1], 99253[1], 99254[1], 99255[1], 99291[1], 99292[1], 99304[1], 99305[1], 99306[1], 99307[1], 99308[1], 99309[1], 99310[1], 99315[1], 99316[1], 99334[1], 99335[1], 99336[1], 99337[1], 99347[1], 99348[1], 99349[1], 99350[1], 99374[1], 99375[1], 99377[1], 99378[1], 99446[0], 99447[0], 99448[0], 99449[0], 99451[0], 99452[0], 99495[0], 99496[0], G0463[1], G0471[1], J0670[1], J2001[1]
65430	0213T[0], 0216T[0], 0596T[1], 0597T[1], 0708T[1], 0709T[1], 12001[1], 12002[1], 12004[1], 12005[1], 12006[1], 12007[1], 12011[1], 12013[1], 12014[1], 12015[1], 12016[1], 12017[1], 12018[1], 12020[1], 12021[1], 12031[1], 12032[1], 12034[1], 12035[1], 12036[1], 12037[1], 12041[1], 12042[1], 12044[1], 12045[1], 12046[1], 12047[1], 12051[1], 12052[1], 12053[1], 12054[1], 12055[1], 12056[1], 12057[1], 13100[1], 13101[1], 13102[1], 13120[1], 13121[1], 13122[1], 13131[1], 13132[1], 13133[1], 13151[1], 13152[1], 13153[1], 36000[1], 36400[1], 36405[1], 36406[1], 36410[1], 36420[1], 36425[1], 36430[1], 36440[1], 36591[0], 36592[0], 36600[1], 36640[1], 43752[1], 51701[1], 51702[1], 51703[1], 62320[0], 62321[0], 62322[0], 62323[0], 62324[0], 62325[0], 62326[0], 62327[0], 64400[0], 64405[0], 64408[0], 64415[0], 64416[0], 64417[0], 64418[0], 64420[0], 64421[0], 64425[0], 64430[0], 64435[0], 64445[0], 64446[0], 64447[0], 64448[0], 64449[0], 64450[0], 64451[0], 64454[0], 64461[0], 64462[0], 64463[0], 64479[0], 64480[0], 64483[0], 64484[0], 64486[0], 64487[0], 64488[0], 64489[0], 64490[0], 64491[0], 64492[0], 64493[0], 64494[0], 64495[0], 64505[0], 64510[0], 64517[0], 64520[0], 64530[0], 65778[1], 67250[1], 67500[1], 69990[0], 92012[1], 92014[1], 92018[1], 92019[1], 92071[1], 93000[1], 93005[1],

0 = Modifier usage not allowed or inappropriate 1 = Modifier usage allowed

Appendix A: NCCI - CPT Codes

Code 1	Code 2
	93010[1], 93040[1], 93041[1], 93042[1], 93318[1], 93355[1], 94002[1], 94200[1], 94680[1], 94681[1], 94690[1], 95812[1], 95813[1], 95816[1], 95819[1], 95822[1], 95829[1], 95955[1], 96360[1], 96361[1], 96365[1], 96366[1], 96367[1], 96368[1], 96372[1], 96374[1], 96375[1], 96376[1], 96377[1], 96523[0], 99155[0], 99156[0], 99157[0], 99211[1], 99212[1], 99213[1], 99214[1], 99215[1], 99217[1], 99218[1], 99219[1], 99220[1], 99221[1], 99222[1], 99223[1], 99231[1], 99232[1], 99233[1], 99234[1], 99235[1], 99236[1], 99238[1], 99239[1], 99241[1], 99242[1], 99243[1], 99244[1], 99245[1], 99251[1], 99252[1], 99253[1], 99254[1], 99255[1], 99291[1], 99292[1], 99304[1], 99305[1], 99306[1], 99307[1], 99308[1], 99309[1], 99310[1], 99315[1], 99316[1], 99334[1], 99335[1], 99336[1], 99337[1], 99347[1], 99348[1], 99349[1], 99350[1], 99374[1], 99375[1], 99377[1], 99378[1], 99446[0], 99447[0], 99448[0], 99449[0], 99451[0], 99452[0], 99495[1], 99496[1], G0463[1], G0471[1], J2001[1]
65435	0213T[0], 0216T[0], 0402T[1], 0596T[1], 0597T[1], 0708T[1], 0709T[1], 11000[1], 11001[1], 11004[1], 11005[1], 11006[1], 11042[1], 11043[1], 11044[1], 11045[1], 11046[1], 11047[1], 12001[1], 12002[1], 12004[1], 12005[1], 12006[1], 12007[1], 12011[1], 12013[1], 12014[1], 12015[1], 12016[1], 12017[1], 12018[1], 12020[1], 12021[1], 12031[1], 12032[1], 12034[1], 12035[1], 12036[1], 12037[1], 12041[1], 12042[1], 12044[1], 12045[1], 12046[1], 12047[1], 12051[1], 12052[1], 12053[1], 12054[1], 12055[1], 12056[1], 12057[1], 13100[1], 13101[1], 13102[1], 13120[1], 13121[1], 13122[1], 13131[1], 13132[1], 13133[1], 13151[1], 13152[1], 13153[1], 36000[1], 36400[1], 36405[1], 36406[1], 36410[1], 36420[1], 36425[1], 36430[1], 36440[1], 36591[0], 36592[0], 36600[1], 36640[1], 43752[1], 51701[1], 51702[1], 51703[1], 62320[0], 62321[0], 62322[0], 62323[0], 62324[0], 62325[0], 62326[0], 62327[0], 64400[0], 64405[0], 64408[0], 64415[0], 64416[0], 64417[0], 64418[0], 64420[0], 64421[0], 64425[0], 64430[0], 64435[0], 64445[0], 64446[0], 64447[0], 64448[0], 64449[0], 64450[0], 64451[0], 64454[0], 64461[0], 64462[0], 64463[0], 64479[0], 64480[0], 64483[0], 64484[0], 64486[0], 64487[0], 64488[0], 64489[0], 64490[0], 64491[0], 64492[0], 64493[0], 64494[0], 64495[0], 64505[0], 64510[0], 64517[0], 64520[0], 64530[0], 65275[1], 65280[1], 65285[1], 65430[1], 67250[1], 67500[1], 69990[0], 92012[1], 92014[1], 92018[1], 92019[1], 92071[1], 93000[1], 93005[1], 93010[1], 93040[1], 93041[1], 93042[1], 93318[1], 93355[1], 94002[1], 94200[1], 94680[1], 94681[1], 94690[1], 95812[1], 95813[1], 95816[1], 95819[1], 95822[1], 95829[1], 95955[1], 96360[1], 96361[1], 96365[1], 96366[1], 96367[1], 96368[1], 96372[1], 96374[1], 96375[1], 96376[1], 96377[1], 96523[0], 97597[1], 97598[1], 97602[1], 99155[0], 99156[0], 99157[0], 99211[1], 99212[1], 99213[1], 99214[1], 99215[1], 99217[1], 99218[1], 99219[1], 99220[1], 99221[1], 99222[1], 99223[1], 99231[1], 99232[1], 99233[1], 99234[1], 99235[1], 99236[1], 99238[1], 99239[1], 99241[1], 99242[1], 99243[1], 99244[1], 99245[1], 99251[1], 99252[1], 99253[1], 99254[1], 99255[1], 99291[1], 99292[1], 99304[1], 99305[1], 99306[1], 99307[1], 99308[1], 99309[1], 99310[1], 99315[1], 99316[1], 99334[1], 99335[1], 99336[1], 99337[1], 99347[1], 99348[1], 99349[1], 99350[1], 99374[1], 99375[1], 99377[1], 99378[1], 99446[0], 99447[0], 99448[0], 99449[0], 99451[0], 99452[0], 99495[1], 99496[1], G0463[1], G0471[1]
65436	0213T[0], 0216T[0], 0402T[1], 0596T[1], 0597T[1], 0708T[1], 0709T[1], 11000[1], 11001[1], 11004[1], 11005[1], 11006[1], 11042[1], 11043[1], 11044[1], 11045[1], 11046[1], 11047[1], 12001[1], 12002[1], 12004[1], 12005[1], 12006[1], 12007[1], 12011[1], 12013[1], 12014[1], 12015[1], 12016[1], 12017[1], 12018[1], 12020[1], 12021[1], 12031[1], 12032[1], 12034[1], 12035[1], 12036[1], 12037[1], 12041[1], 12042[1], 12044[1], 12045[1], 12046[1], 12047[1], 12051[1], 12052[1], 12053[1], 12054[1], 12055[1], 12056[1], 12057[1], 13100[1], 13101[1], 13102[1], 13120[1], 13121[1], 13122[1], 13131[1], 13132[1], 13133[1], 13151[1], 13152[1], 13153[1], 36000[1], 36400[1], 36405[1], 36406[1], 36410[1], 36420[1], 36425[1], 36430[1], 36440[1], 36591[0], 36592[0], 36600[1], 36640[1], 43752[1], 51701[1], 51702[1], 51703[1], 62320[0], 62321[0], 62322[0], 62323[0], 62324[0], 62325[0], 62326[0], 62327[0], 64400[0], 64405[0], 64408[0], 64415[0], 64416[0], 64417[0], 64418[0], 64420[0], 64421[0], 64425[0], 64430[0], 64435[0], 64445[0], 64446[0], 64447[0], 64448[0], 64449[0], 64450[0], 64451[0], 64454[0], 64461[0], 64462[0], 64463[0], 64479[0], 64480[0], 64483[0], 64484[0], 64486[0], 64487[0], 64488[0], 64489[0], 64490[0], 64491[0], 64492[0], 64493[0], 64494[0], 64495[0], 64505[0], 64510[0], 64517[0], 64520[0], 64530[0], 65275[1], 65280[1], 65285[1], 65430[1], 65435[1], 67250[1], 67500[1], 69990[0], 92012[1], 92014[1], 92018[1], 92019[1], 92071[1], 93000[1], 93005[1], 93010[1], 93040[1], 93041[1], 93042[1], 93318[1], 93355[1], 94002[1], 94200[1], 94680[1], 94681[1], 94690[1], 95812[1], 95813[1], 95816[1], 95819[1], 95822[1], 95829[1], 95955[1], 96360[1], 96361[1], 96365[1], 96366[1], 96367[1], 96368[1], 96372[1], 96374[1], 96375[1], 96376[1], 96377[1], 96523[0], 97597[1], 97598[1], 97602[1], 99155[0], 99156[0], 99157[0], 99211[1], 99212[1], 99213[1], 99214[1], 99215[1], 99217[1], 99218[1], 99219[1], 99220[1], 99221[1], 99222[1], 99223[1], 99231[1], 99232[1], 99233[1], 99234[1], 99235[1], 99236[1], 99238[1], 99239[1], 99241[1], 99242[1], 99243[1], 99244[1], 99245[1], 99251[1], 99252[1], 99253[1], 99254[1], 99255[1], 99291[1], 99292[1], 99304[1], 99305[1], 99306[1], 99307[1], 99308[1], 99309[1], 99310[1], 99315[1], 99316[1], 99334[1], 99335[1], 99336[1], 99337[1], 99347[1], 99348[1], 99349[1], 99350[1], 99374[1], 99375[1], 99377[1], 99378[1], 99446[0], 99447[0], 99448[0], 99449[0], 99451[0], 99452[0], 99495[0], 99496[0], G0463[1], G0471[1], J2001[1]
65450	0213T[0], 0216T[0], 0596T[1], 0597T[1], 0708T[1], 0709T[1], 12001[1], 12002[1], 12004[1], 12005[1], 12006[1], 12007[1], 12011[1], 12013[1], 12014[1], 12015[1], 12016[1], 12017[1], 12018[1], 12020[1], 12021[1], 12031[1], 12032[1], 12034[1], 12035[1], 12036[1], 12037[1], 12041[1], 12042[1], 12044[1], 12045[1], 12046[1], 12047[1], 12051[1], 12052[1], 12053[1], 12054[1], 12055[1], 12056[1], 12057[1], 13100[1], 13101[1], 13102[1], 13120[1], 13121[1], 13122[1], 13131[1], 13132[1], 13133[1], 13151[1], 13152[1], 13153[1], 36000[1], 36400[1], 36405[1], 36406[1], 36410[1], 36420[1], 36425[1], 36430[1], 36440[1], 36591[0], 36592[0], 36600[1], 36640[1], 43752[1], 51701[1], 51702[1], 51703[1], 62320[0], 62321[0], 62322[0], 62323[0], 62324[0], 62325[0], 62326[0], 62327[0], 64400[0], 64405[0], 64408[0], 64415[0], 64416[0], 64417[0], 64418[0], 64420[0], 64421[0], 64425[0], 64430[0], 64435[0], 64445[0], 64446[0], 64447[0], 64448[0], 64449[0], 64450[0], 64451[0], 64454[0], 64461[0], 64462[0], 64463[0], 64479[0], 64480[0], 64483[0], 64484[0], 64486[0], 64487[0], 64488[0], 64489[0], 64490[0], 64491[0], 64492[0], 64493[0], 64494[0], 64495[0], 64505[0], 64510[0], 64517[0], 64520[0], 64530[0], 67250[1], 67500[1], 69990[0], 92012[1], 92014[1], 92018[1], 92019[1], 92071[1], 93000[1], 93005[1], 93010[1], 93040[1], 93041[1], 93042[1], 93318[1], 93355[1], 94002[1], 94200[1], 94680[1], 94681[1], 94690[1], 95812[1], 95813[1], 95816[1], 95819[1], 95822[1], 95829[1], 95955[1], 96360[1], 96361[1], 96365[1], 96366[1], 96367[1], 96368[1], 96372[1], 96374[1], 96375[1], 96376[1], 96377[1], 96523[0], 99155[0], 99156[0], 99157[0], 99211[1], 99212[1], 99213[1], 99214[1], 99215[1], 99217[1], 99218[1], 99219[1], 99220[1], 99221[1], 99222[1], 99223[1], 99231[1], 99232[1], 99233[1], 99234[1], 99235[1], 99236[1], 99238[1], 99239[1], 99241[1], 99242[1], 99243[1], 99244[1], 99245[1], 99251[1], 99252[1], 99253[1], 99254[1], 99255[1], 99291[1], 99292[1], 99304[1], 99305[1], 99306[1], 99307[1], 99308[1], 99309[1], 99310[1], 99315[1], 99316[1], 99334[1], 99335[1], 99336[1], 99337[1], 99347[1], 99348[1], 99349[1], 99350[1], 99374[1], 99375[1], 99377[1], 99378[1], 99446[0], 99447[0], 99448[0], 99449[0], 99451[0], 99452[0], 99495[0], 99496[0], G0463[1], G0471[1], J2001[1]
65600	0213T[0], 0216T[0], 0596T[1], 0597T[1], 0708T[1], 0709T[1], 12001[1], 12002[1], 12004[1], 12005[1], 12006[1], 12007[1], 12011[1], 12013[1], 12014[1], 12015[1], 12016[1], 12017[1], 12018[1], 12020[1], 12021[1], 12031[1], 12032[1], 12034[1], 12035[1], 12036[1], 12037[1], 12041[1], 12042[1], 12044[1], 12045[1], 12046[1], 12047[1], 12051[1], 12052[1], 12053[1], 12054[1], 12055[1], 12056[1], 12057[1], 13100[1], 13101[1], 13102[1], 13120[1], 13121[1], 13122[1], 13131[1], 13132[1], 13133[1], 13151[1], 13152[1], 13153[1], 36000[1], 36400[1], 36405[1], 36406[1], 36410[1], 36420[1], 36425[1], 36430[1], 36440[1], 36591[0], 36592[0], 36600[1], 36640[1], 43752[1], 51701[1], 51702[1], 51703[1], 62320[0], 62321[0], 62322[0], 62323[0], 62324[0], 62325[0], 62326[0], 62327[0], 64400[0], 64405[0], 64408[0], 64415[0], 64416[0], 64417[0], 64418[0], 64420[0], 64421[0], 64425[0], 64430[0], 64435[0], 64445[0], 64446[0], 64447[0], 64448[0], 64449[0], 64450[0], 64451[0], 64454[0], 64461[0], 64462[0], 64463[0], 64479[0], 64480[0], 64483[0], 64484[0], 64486[0], 64487[0], 64488[0], 64489[0], 64490[0], 64491[0], 64492[0], 64493[0], 64494[0], 64495[0], 64505[0], 64510[0], 64517[0], 64520[0], 64530[0], 67250[1], 67500[1], 69990[0], 92012[1], 92014[1], 92018[1], 92019[1], 92071[1], 93000[1], 93005[1], 93010[1], 93040[1], 93041[1], 93042[1], 93318[1], 93355[1], 94002[1], 94200[1], 94680[1], 94681[1], 94690[1], 95812[1], 95813[1], 95816[1], 95819[1], 95822[1], 95829[1], 95955[1], 96360[1], 96361[1], 96365[1], 96366[1], 96367[1], 96368[1], 96372[1], 96374[1], 96375[1], 96376[1], 96377[1], 96523[0], 99155[0], 99156[0], 99157[0], 99211[1], 99212[1], 99213[1], 99214[1], 99215[1], 99217[1], 99218[1], 99219[1], 99220[1], 99221[1], 99222[1], 99223[1], 99231[1], 99232[1], 99233[1], 99234[1], 99235[1], 99236[1], 99238[1], 99239[1], 99241[1], 99242[1], 99243[1], 99244[1], 99245[1], 99251[1], 99252[1], 99253[1], 99254[1], 99255[1], 99291[1], 99292[1], 99304[1], 99305[1], 99306[1], 99307[1], 99308[1], 99309[1], 99310[1], 99315[1], 99316[1], 99334[1], 99335[1], 99336[1], 99337[1], 99347[1], 99348[1], 99349[1], 99350[1], 99374[1], 99375[1], 99377[1], 99378[1], 99446[0], 99447[0], 99448[0], 99449[0], 99451[0], 99452[0], 99495[0], 99496[0], G0463[1], G0471[1], J0670[1], J2001[1]
65710	0213T[0], 0216T[0], 0402T[1], 0596T[1], 0597T[1], 0708T[1], 0709T[1], 11000[1], 11001[1], 11004[1], 11005[1], 11006[1], 11042[1], 11043[1], 11044[1], 11045[1], 11046[1], 11047[1], 12001[1], 12002[1], 12004[1], 12005[1], 12006[1], 12007[1], 12011[1], 12013[1], 12014[1], 12015[1], 12016[1], 12017[1], 12018[1], 12020[1], 12021[1], 12031[1], 12032[1], 12034[1], 12035[1], 12036[1], 12037[1], 12041[1], 12042[1], 12044[1], 12045[1], 12046[1], 12047[1], 12051[1], 12052[1], 12053[1], 12054[1], 12055[1], 12056[1], 12057[1], 13100[1], 13101[1], 13102[1], 13120[1], 13121[1], 13122[1], 13131[1], 13132[1], 13133[1], 13151[1], 13152[1], 13153[1], 36000[1], 36400[1], 36405[1], 36406[1], 36410[1], 36420[1], 36425[1], 36430[1], 36440[1], 36591[0], 36592[0], 36600[1], 36640[1], 43752[1], 51701[1], 51702[1], 51703[1], 62320[0], 62321[0], 62322[0], 62323[0], 62324[0], 62325[0], 62326[0], 62327[0], 64400[0], 64405[0], 64408[0], 64415[0], 64416[0], 64417[0], 64418[0], 64420[0], 64421[0], 64425[0], 64430[0], 64435[0], 64445[0], 64446[0], 64447[0], 64448[0], 64449[0], 64450[0], 64451[0], 64454[0], 64461[0], 64462[0], 64463[0], 64479[0], 64480[0], 64483[0], 64484[0], 64486[0], 64487[0], 64488[0], 64489[0], 64490[0], 64491[0], 64492[0], 64493[0], 64494[0], 64495[0], 64505[0], 64510[0], 64517[0], 64520[0], 64530[0], 65280[1], 65286[1], 65400[1], 65410[1], 65420[1], 65426[1], 65435[1], 65436[1], 65450[1], 65730[1], 65750[1], 65755[1], 65772[1], 65775[1], 65778[1], 65779[1], 65780[1], 65800[1], 65815[1], 66020[1], 67250[1], 67500[1], 69990[0], 92012[1], 92014[1], 92018[1], 92019[1], 92025[1], 92071[1], 93000[1], 93005[1], 93010[1], 93040[1], 93041[1], 93042[1], 93318[1], 93355[1], 94002[1], 94200[1], 94680[1], 94681[1], 94690[1], 95812[1], 95813[1], 95816[1], 95819[1], 95822[1], 95829[1], 95955[1], 96360[1], 96361[1], 96365[1], 96366[1], 96367[1], 96368[1], 96372[1], 96374[1], 96375[1], 96376[1], 96377[1], 96523[0], 97597[1], 97598[1], 97602[1], 99155[0], 99156[0], 99157[0], 99211[1], 99212[1], 99213[1], 99214[1], 99215[1], 99217[1], 99218[1], 99219[1], 99220[1], 99221[1], 99222[1], 99223[1], 99231[1], 99232[1], 99233[1], 99234[1], 99235[1], 99236[1], 99238[1], 99239[1], 99241[1], 99242[1], 99243[1], 99244[1], 99245[1], 99251[1], 99252[1], 99253[1], 99254[1], 99255[1], 99291[1], 99292[1], 99304[1], 99305[1], 99306[1], 99307[1], 99308[1], 99309[1], 99310[1], 99315[1], 99316[1], 99334[1], 99335[1], 99336[1], 99337[1], 99347[1], 99348[1], 99349[1], 99350[1], 99374[1], 99375[1], 99377[1],

0 = Modifier usage not allowed or inappropriate 1 = Modifier usage allowed

Appendix A: NCCI - CPT Codes

Code 1	Code 2
	99378[1], 99446[0], 99447[0], 99448[0], 99449[0], 99451[0], 99452[0], 99495[0], 99496[0], G0463[1], G0471[1]
65730	0213T[0], 0216T[0], 0402T[1], 0596T[1], 0597T[1], 0616T[1], 0617T[1], 0618T[1], 0699T[1], 0708T[1], 0709T[1], 11000[1], 11001[1], 11004[1], 11005[1], 11006[1], 11042[1], 11043[1], 11044[1], 11045[1], 11046[1], 11047[1], 12001[1], 12002[1], 12004[1], 12005[1], 12006[1], 12007[1], 12011[1], 12013[1], 12014[1], 12015[1], 12016[1], 12017[1], 12018[1], 12020[1], 12021[1], 12031[1], 12032[1], 12034[1], 12035[1], 12036[1], 12037[1], 12041[1], 12042[1], 12044[1], 12045[1], 12046[1], 12047[1], 12051[1], 12052[1], 12053[1], 12054[1], 12055[1], 12056[1], 12057[1], 13100[1], 13101[1], 13102[1], 13120[1], 13121[1], 13122[1], 13131[1], 13132[1], 13133[1], 13151[1], 13152[1], 13153[1], 36000[1], 36400[1], 36405[1], 36406[1], 36410[1], 36420[1], 36425[1], 36430[1], 36440[1], 36591[0], 36592[0], 36600[1], 36640[1], 43752[1], 51701[1], 51702[1], 51703[1], 62320[0], 62321[0], 62322[0], 62323[0], 62324[0], 62325[0], 62326[0], 62327[0], 64400[0], 64405[0], 64408[0], 64415[0], 64416[0], 64417[0], 64418[0], 64420[0], 64421[0], 64425[0], 64430[0], 64435[0], 64445[0], 64446[0], 64447[0], 64448[0], 64449[0], 64450[0], 64451[0], 64454[0], 64461[0], 64462[0], 64463[0], 64479[0], 64480[0], 64483[0], 64484[0], 64486[0], 64487[0], 64488[0], 64489[0], 64490[0], 64491[0], 64492[0], 64493[0], 64494[0], 64495[0], 64505[0], 64510[0], 64517[0], 64520[0], 64530[0], 65280[1], 65286[1], 65400[1], 65410[1], 65420[1], 65426[1], 65435[1], 65436[1], 65450[1], 65750[1], 65755[1], 65772[1], 65775[1], 65778[1], 65779[1], 65780[1], 65800[1], 65815[1], 65920[1], 65930[1], 66020[1], 66030[1], 66680[1], 67005[1], 67010[1], 67250[1], 67500[1], 67515[1], 67875[1], 69990[0], 92012[1], 92014[1], 92018[1], 92019[1], 92025[1], 92071[1], 92504[1], 93000[1], 93005[1], 93010[1], 93040[1], 93041[1], 93042[1], 93318[1], 93355[1], 94002[1], 94200[1], 94680[1], 94681[1], 94690[1], 95812[1], 95813[1], 95816[1], 95819[1], 95822[1], 95829[1], 95955[1], 96360[1], 96361[1], 96365[1], 96366[1], 96367[1], 96368[1], 96372[1], 96374[1], 96375[1], 96376[1], 96377[1], 96523[0], 97597[1], 97598[1], 97602[1], 99155[0], 99156[0], 99157[0], 99211[1], 99212[1], 99213[1], 99214[1], 99215[1], 99217[1], 99218[1], 99219[1], 99220[1], 99221[1], 99222[1], 99223[1], 99231[1], 99232[1], 99233[1], 99234[1], 99235[1], 99236[1], 99238[1], 99239[1], 99241[1], 99242[1], 99243[1], 99244[1], 99245[1], 99251[1], 99252[1], 99253[1], 99254[1], 99255[1], 99291[1], 99292[1], 99304[1], 99305[1], 99306[1], 99307[1], 99308[1], 99309[1], 99310[1], 99315[1], 99316[1], 99334[1], 99335[1], 99336[1], 99337[1], 99347[1], 99348[1], 99349[1], 99350[1], 99374[1], 99375[1], 99377[1], 99378[1], 99446[0], 99447[0], 99448[0], 99449[0], 99451[0], 99452[0], 99495[0], 99496[0], G0463[1], G0471[1]
65750	0213T[0], 0216T[0], 0402T[1], 0596T[1], 0597T[1], 0616T[1], 0618T[1], 0699T[1], 0708T[1], 0709T[1], 11000[1], 11001[1], 11004[1], 11005[1], 11006[1], 11042[1], 11043[1], 11044[1], 11045[1], 11046[1], 11047[1], 12001[1], 12002[1], 12004[1], 12005[1], 12006[1], 12007[1], 12011[1], 12013[1], 12014[1], 12015[1], 12016[1], 12017[1], 12018[1], 12020[1], 12021[1], 12031[1], 12032[1], 12034[1], 12035[1], 12036[1], 12037[1], 12041[1], 12042[1], 12044[1], 12045[1], 12046[1], 12047[1], 12051[1], 12052[1], 12053[1], 12054[1], 12055[1], 12056[1], 12057[1], 13100[1], 13101[1], 13102[1], 13120[1], 13121[1], 13122[1], 13131[1], 13132[1], 13133[1], 13151[1], 13152[1], 13153[1], 36000[1], 36400[1], 36405[1], 36406[1], 36410[1], 36420[1], 36425[1], 36430[1], 36440[1], 36591[0], 36592[0], 36600[1], 36640[1], 43752[1], 51701[1], 51702[1], 51703[1], 62320[0], 62321[0], 62322[0], 62323[0], 62324[0], 62325[0], 62326[0], 62327[0], 64400[0], 64405[0], 64408[0], 64415[0], 64416[0], 64417[0], 64418[0], 64420[0], 64421[0], 64425[0], 64430[0], 64435[0], 64445[0], 64446[0], 64447[0], 64448[0], 64449[0], 64450[0], 64451[0], 64454[0], 64461[0], 64462[0], 64463[0], 64479[0], 64480[0], 64483[0], 64484[0], 64486[0], 64487[0], 64488[0], 64489[0], 64490[0], 64491[0], 64492[0], 64493[0], 64494[0], 64495[0], 64505[0], 64510[0], 64517[0], 64520[0], 64530[0], 65280[1], 65286[1], 65400[1], 65410[1], 65420[1], 65426[1], 65435[1], 65436[1], 65450[1], 65756[1], 65772[1], 65775[1], 65778[1], 65779[1], 65780[1], 65782[1], 65800[1], 65815[1], 65920[1], 65930[1], 66020[1], 66030[1], 66680[1], 67005[1], 67010[1], 67250[1], 67500[1], 67875[1], 69990[0], 92012[1], 92014[1], 92018[1], 92019[1], 92025[1], 92071[1], 92504[1], 93000[1], 93005[1], 93010[1], 93040[1], 93041[1], 93042[1], 93318[1], 93355[1], 94002[1], 94200[1], 94680[1], 94681[1], 94690[1], 95812[1], 95813[1], 95816[1], 95819[1], 95822[1], 95829[1], 95955[1], 96360[1], 96361[1], 96365[1], 96366[1], 96367[1], 96368[1], 96372[1], 96374[1], 96375[1], 96376[1], 96377[1], 96523[0], 97597[1], 97598[1], 97602[1], 99155[0], 99156[0], 99157[0], 99211[1], 99212[1], 99213[1], 99214[1], 99215[1], 99217[1], 99218[1], 99219[1], 99220[1], 99221[1], 99222[1], 99223[1], 99231[1], 99232[1], 99233[1], 99234[1], 99235[1], 99236[1], 99238[1], 99239[1], 99241[1], 99242[1], 99243[1], 99244[1], 99245[1], 99251[1], 99252[1], 99253[1], 99254[1], 99255[1], 99291[1], 99292[1], 99304[1], 99305[1], 99306[1], 99307[1], 99308[1], 99309[1], 99310[1], 99315[1], 99316[1], 99334[1], 99335[1], 99336[1], 99337[1], 99347[1], 99348[1], 99349[1], 99350[1], 99374[1], 99375[1], 99377[1], 99378[1], 99446[0], 99447[0], 99448[0], 99449[0], 99451[0], 99452[0], 99495[0], 99496[0], G0463[1], G0471[1]
65755	0213T[0], 0216T[0], 0402T[1], 0596T[1], 0597T[1], 0616T[1], 0618T[1], 0699T[1], 0708T[1], 0709T[1], 11000[1], 11001[1], 11004[1], 11005[1], 11006[1], 11042[1], 11043[1], 11044[1], 11045[1], 11046[1], 11047[1], 12001[1], 12002[1], 12004[1], 12005[1], 12006[1], 12007[1], 12011[1], 12013[1], 12014[1], 12015[1], 12016[1], 12017[1], 12018[1], 12020[1], 12021[1], 12031[1], 12032[1], 12034[1], 12035[1], 12036[1], 12037[1], 12041[1], 12042[1], 12044[1], 12045[1], 12046[1], 12047[1], 12051[1], 12052[1], 12053[1], 12054[1], 12055[1], 12056[1], 12057[1], 13100[1], 13101[1], 13102[1], 13120[1], 13121[1], 13122[1], 13131[1], 13132[1], 13133[1], 13151[1], 13152[1], 13153[1], 36000[1], 36400[1], 36405[1], 36406[1], 36410[1], 36420[1], 36425[1], 36430[1], 36440[1], 36591[0], 36592[0], 36600[1], 36640[1], 43752[1], 51701[1], 51702[1], 51703[1], 62320[0], 62321[0], 62322[0], 62323[0], 62324[0], 62325[0], 62326[0], 62327[0], 64400[0], 64405[0], 64408[0], 64415[0], 64416[0], 64417[0], 64418[0], 64420[0], 64421[0], 64425[0], 64430[0], 64435[0], 64445[0], 64446[0], 64447[0], 64448[0], 64449[0], 64450[0], 64451[0], 64454[0], 64461[0], 64462[0], 64463[0], 64479[0], 64480[0], 64483[0], 64484[0], 64486[0], 64487[0], 64488[0], 64489[0], 64490[0], 64491[0], 64492[0], 64493[0], 64494[0], 64495[0], 64505[0], 64510[0], 64517[0], 64520[0], 64530[0], 65280[1], 65286[1], 65400[1], 65410[1], 65420[1], 65426[1], 65435[1], 65436[1], 65450[1], 65750[1], 65772[1], 65775[1], 65778[1], 65779[1], 65780[1], 65782[1], 65800[1], 65815[1], 65930[1], 66020[1], 66030[1], 66680[1], 67005[1], 67010[1], 67250[1], 67500[1], 67515[1], 67875[1], 69990[0], 92012[1], 92014[1], 92018[1], 92019[1], 92025[1], 92071[1], 92504[1], 93000[1], 93005[1], 93010[1], 93040[1], 93041[1], 93042[1], 93318[1], 93355[1], 94002[1], 94200[1], 94680[1], 94681[1], 94690[1], 95812[1], 95813[1], 95816[1], 95819[1], 95822[1], 95829[1], 95955[1], 96360[1], 96361[1], 96365[1], 96366[1], 96367[1], 96368[1], 96372[1], 96374[1], 96375[1], 96376[1], 96377[1], 96523[0], 97597[1], 97598[1], 97602[1], 99155[0], 99156[0], 99157[0], 99211[1], 99212[1], 99213[1], 99214[1], 99215[1], 99217[1], 99218[1], 99219[1], 99220[1], 99221[1], 99222[1], 99223[1], 99231[1], 99232[1], 99233[1], 99234[1], 99235[1], 99236[1], 99238[1], 99239[1], 99241[1], 99242[1], 99243[1], 99244[1], 99245[1], 99251[1], 99252[1], 99253[1], 99254[1], 99255[1], 99291[1], 99292[1], 99304[1], 99305[1], 99306[1], 99307[1], 99308[1], 99309[1], 99310[1], 99315[1], 99316[1], 99334[1], 99335[1], 99336[1], 99337[1], 99347[1], 99348[1], 99349[1], 99350[1], 99374[1], 99375[1], 99377[1], 99378[1], 99446[0], 99447[0], 99448[0], 99449[0], 99451[0], 99452[0], 99495[0], 99496[0], G0463[1], G0471[1]
65756	0213T[1], 0216T[1], 0596T[1], 0597T[1], 0708T[1], 0709T[1], 11000[1], 11001[1], 11004[1], 11005[1], 11006[1], 11042[1], 11043[1], 11044[1], 11045[1], 11046[1], 11047[1], 12001[1], 12002[1], 12004[1], 12005[1], 12006[1], 12007[1], 12011[1], 12013[1], 12014[1], 12015[1], 12016[1], 12017[1], 12018[1], 12020[1], 12021[1], 12031[1], 12032[1], 12034[1], 12035[1], 12036[1], 12037[1], 12041[1], 12042[1], 12044[1], 12045[1], 12046[1], 12047[1], 12051[1], 12052[1], 12053[1], 12054[1], 12055[1], 12056[1], 12057[1], 13100[1], 13101[1], 13102[1], 13120[1], 13121[1], 13122[1], 13131[1], 13132[1], 13133[1], 13151[1], 13152[1], 13153[1], 36000[1], 36400[1], 36405[1], 36406[1], 36410[1], 36420[1], 36425[1], 36430[1], 36440[1], 36591[0], 36592[0], 36600[1], 36640[1], 43752[1], 51701[1], 51702[1], 51703[1], 62320[0], 62321[0], 62322[0], 62323[0], 62324[1], 62325[1], 62326[1], 62327[1], 64400[0], 64405[0], 64408[0], 64415[1], 64416[1], 64417[1], 64418[0], 64420[0], 64421[0], 64425[0], 64430[0], 64435[0], 64445[0], 64446[0], 64447[0], 64448[0], 64449[0], 64450[1], 64451[0], 64454[1], 64461[0], 64462[0], 64463[0], 64479[0], 64480[0], 64483[0], 64484[0], 64486[0], 64487[0], 64488[0], 64489[0], 64490[1], 64491[0], 64492[0], 64493[1], 64494[0], 64495[0], 64505[0], 64510[0], 64517[0], 64520[0], 64530[0], 65235[1], 65280[1], 65286[1], 65400[1], 65410[1], 65710[1], 65730[1], 65755[1], 65778[1], 65779[1], 65780[1], 65782[1], 65800[1], 65815[1], 66020[1], 67250[1], 67500[1], 69990[0], 92012[1], 92014[1], 92018[1], 92019[1], 92025[1], 92071[1], 93000[1], 93005[1], 93010[1], 93040[1], 93041[1], 93042[1], 93318[1], 93355[1], 94002[1], 94200[1], 94680[1], 94681[1], 94690[1], 95812[1], 95813[1], 95816[1], 95819[1], 95822[1], 95829[1], 95955[1], 96360[1], 96361[1], 96365[1], 96366[1], 96367[1], 96368[1], 96372[1], 96374[1], 96375[1], 96376[1], 96377[1], 96523[0], 97597[1], 97598[1], 97602[1], 99155[0], 99156[0], 99157[0], 99211[1], 99212[1], 99213[1], 99214[1], 99215[1], 99217[1], 99218[1], 99219[1], 99220[1], 99221[1], 99222[1], 99223[1], 99231[1], 99232[1], 99233[1], 99234[1], 99235[1], 99236[1], 99238[1], 99239[1], 99241[1], 99242[1], 99243[1], 99244[1], 99245[1], 99251[1], 99252[1], 99253[1], 99254[1], 99255[1], 99291[1], 99292[1], 99304[1], 99305[1], 99306[1], 99307[1], 99308[1], 99309[1], 99310[1], 99315[1], 99316[1], 99334[1], 99335[1], 99336[1], 99337[1], 99347[1], 99348[1], 99349[1], 99350[1], 99374[1], 99375[1], 99377[1], 99378[1], 99446[0], 99447[0], 99448[0], 99449[0], 99451[0], 99452[0], 99495[0], 99496[0], G0463[1], G0471[1]
65757	36591[0], 36592[0], 69990[0], 92071[1], 96523[0]
65760	36591[0], 36592[0], 69990[0], 92071[1], 96523[0]
65765	36591[0], 36592[0], 69990[0], 92071[1], 96523[0]
65767	11000[1], 11001[1], 11004[1], 11005[1], 11006[1], 11042[1], 11043[1], 11044[1], 11045[1], 11046[1], 11047[1], 36591[0], 36592[0], 69990[0], 92071[1], 96523[0], 97597[1], 97598[1], 97602[1]
65770	0213T[0], 0216T[0], 0596T[1], 0597T[1], 0708T[1], 0709T[1], 12001[1], 12002[1], 12004[1], 12005[1], 12006[1], 12007[1], 12011[1], 12013[1], 12014[1], 12015[1], 12016[1], 12017[1], 12018[1], 12020[1], 12021[1], 12031[1], 12032[1], 12034[1], 12035[1], 12036[1], 12037[1], 12041[1], 12042[1], 12044[1], 12045[1], 12046[1], 12047[1], 12051[1], 12052[1], 12053[1], 12054[1], 12055[1], 12056[1], 12057[1], 13100[1], 13101[1], 13102[1], 13120[1], 13121[1], 13122[1], 13131[1], 13132[1], 13133[1], 13151[1], 13152[1], 13153[1], 36000[1], 36400[1], 36405[1], 36406[1], 36410[1], 36420[1], 36425[1], 36430[1], 36440[1], 36591[0], 36592[0], 36600[1], 36640[1], 43752[1], 51701[1], 51702[1], 51703[1], 62320[0], 62321[0], 62322[0], 62323[0], 62324[0], 62325[0], 62326[0], 62327[0], 64400[0], 64405[0], 64408[0], 64415[0], 64416[0], 64417[0], 64418[0], 64420[0], 64421[0], 64425[0], 64430[0], 64435[0], 64445[0], 64446[0], 64447[0], 64448[0], 64449[0], 64450[0], 64451[0], 64454[0], 64461[0], 64462[0], 64463[0], 64479[0], 64480[0], 64483[0], 64484[0], 64486[0], 64487[0], 64488[0], 64489[0], 64490[0], 64491[0], 64492[0], 64493[0], 64494[0], 64495[0], 64505[0], 64510[0], 64517[0], 64520[0], 64530[0], 67250[1], 67500[1], 69990[0], 92012[1], 92014[1], 92018[1], 92019[1], 92025[1], 92071[1], 93000[1], 93005[1],

0 = Modifier usage not allowed or inappropriate 1 = Modifier usage allowed

Appendix A: NCCI - CPT Codes

Code 1	Code 2
	93010[1], 93040[1], 93041[1], 93042[1], 93318[1], 93355[1], 94002[1], 94200[1], 94680[1], 94681[1], 94690[1], 95812[1], 95813[1], 95816[1], 95819[1], 95822[1], 95829[1], 95955[1], 96360[1], 96361[1], 96365[1], 96366[1], 96367[1], 96368[1], 96372[1], 96374[1], 96375[1], 96376[1], 96377[1], 96523[0], 99155[0], 99156[0], 99157[0], 99211[1], 99212[1], 99213[1], 99214[1], 99215[1], 99217[1], 99218[1], 99219[1], 99220[1], 99221[1], 99222[1], 99223[1], 99231[1], 99232[1], 99233[1], 99234[1], 99235[1], 99236[1], 99238[1], 99239[1], 99241[1], 99242[1], 99243[1], 99244[1], 99245[1], 99251[1], 99252[1], 99253[1], 99254[1], 99255[1], 99291[1], 99292[1], 99304[1], 99305[1], 99306[1], 99307[1], 99308[1], 99309[1], 99310[1], 99315[1], 99316[1], 99334[1], 99335[1], 99336[1], 99337[1], 99347[1], 99348[1], 99349[1], 99350[1], 99374[1], 99375[1], 99377[1], 99378[1], 99446[0], 99447[0], 99448[0], 99449[0], 99451[0], 99452[0], 99495[0], 99496[0], G0463[1], G0471[1], J0670[1], J2001[1]
65771	11000[1], 11001[1], 11004[1], 11005[1], 11006[1], 11042[1], 11043[1], 11044[1], 11045[1], 11046[1], 11047[1], 36591[0], 36592[0], 69990[0], 92071[1], 96523[0], 97597[1], 97598[1], 97602[1]
65772	0213T[0], 0216T[0], 0596T[1], 0597T[1], 0708T[1], 0709T[1], 12001[1], 12002[1], 12004[1], 12005[1], 12006[1], 12007[1], 12011[1], 12013[1], 12014[1], 12015[1], 12016[1], 12017[1], 12018[1], 12020[1], 12021[1], 12031[1], 12032[1], 12034[1], 12035[1], 12036[1], 12037[1], 12041[1], 12042[1], 12044[1], 12045[1], 12046[1], 12047[1], 12051[1], 12052[1], 12053[1], 12054[1], 12055[1], 12056[1], 12057[1], 13100[1], 13101[1], 13102[1], 13120[1], 13121[1], 13122[1], 13131[1], 13132[1], 13133[1], 13151[1], 13152[1], 13153[1], 36000[1], 36400[1], 36405[1], 36406[1], 36410[1], 36420[1], 36425[1], 36430[1], 36440[1], 36591[0], 36592[0], 36600[1], 36640[1], 43752[1], 51701[1], 51702[1], 51703[1], 62320[0], 62321[0], 62322[0], 62323[0], 62324[0], 62325[0], 62326[0], 62327[0], 64400[0], 64405[0], 64408[0], 64415[0], 64416[0], 64417[0], 64418[0], 64420[0], 64421[0], 64425[0], 64430[0], 64435[0], 64445[0], 64446[0], 64447[0], 64448[0], 64449[0], 64450[0], 64451[0], 64454[0], 64461[0], 64462[0], 64463[0], 64479[0], 64480[0], 64483[0], 64484[0], 64486[0], 64487[0], 64488[0], 64489[0], 64490[0], 64491[0], 64492[0], 64493[0], 64494[0], 64495[0], 64505[0], 64510[0], 64517[0], 64520[0], 64530[0], 65280[1], 65286[1], 65400[1], 65410[1], 65785[1], 65800[1], 66020[1], 66250[1], 67250[1], 67500[1], 69990[0], 92012[1], 92014[1], 92018[1], 92019[1], 92071[1], 93000[1], 93005[1], 93010[1], 93040[1], 93041[1], 93042[1], 93318[1], 93355[1], 94002[1], 94200[1], 94680[1], 94681[1], 94690[1], 95812[1], 95813[1], 95816[1], 95819[1], 95822[1], 95829[1], 95955[1], 96360[1], 96361[1], 96365[1], 96366[1], 96367[1], 96368[1], 96372[1], 96374[1], 96375[1], 96376[1], 96377[1], 96523[0], 99155[0], 99156[0], 99157[0], 99211[1], 99212[1], 99213[1], 99214[1], 99215[1], 99217[1], 99218[1], 99219[1], 99220[1], 99221[1], 99222[1], 99223[1], 99231[1], 99232[1], 99233[1], 99234[1], 99235[1], 99236[1], 99238[1], 99239[1], 99241[1], 99242[1], 99243[1], 99244[1], 99245[1], 99251[1], 99252[1], 99253[1], 99254[1], 99255[1], 99291[1], 99292[1], 99304[1], 99305[1], 99306[1], 99307[1], 99308[1], 99309[1], 99310[1], 99315[1], 99316[1], 99334[1], 99335[1], 99336[1], 99337[1], 99347[1], 99348[1], 99349[1], 99350[1], 99374[1], 99375[1], 99377[1], 99378[1], 99446[0], 99447[0], 99448[0], 99449[0], 99451[0], 99452[0], 99495[0], 99496[0], G0463[1], G0471[1], J0670[1], J2001[1]
65775	0213T[0], 0216T[0], 0596T[1], 0597T[1], 0708T[1], 0709T[1], 11000[1], 11001[1], 11004[1], 11005[1], 11006[1], 11042[1], 11043[1], 11044[1], 11045[1], 11046[1], 11047[1], 12001[1], 12002[1], 12004[1], 12005[1], 12006[1], 12007[1], 12011[1], 12013[1], 12014[1], 12015[1], 12016[1], 12017[1], 12018[1], 12020[1], 12021[1], 12031[1], 12032[1], 12034[1], 12035[1], 12036[1], 12037[1], 12041[1], 12042[1], 12044[1], 12045[1], 12046[1], 12047[1], 12051[1], 12052[1], 12053[1], 12054[1], 12055[1], 12056[1], 12057[1], 13100[1], 13101[1], 13102[1], 13120[1], 13121[1], 13122[1], 13131[1], 13132[1], 13133[1], 13151[1], 13152[1], 13153[1], 36000[1], 36400[1], 36405[1], 36406[1], 36410[1], 36420[1], 36425[1], 36430[1], 36440[1], 36591[0], 36592[0], 36600[1], 36640[1], 43752[1], 51701[1], 51702[1], 51703[1], 62320[0], 62321[0], 62322[0], 62323[0], 62324[0], 62325[0], 62326[0], 62327[0], 64400[0], 64405[0], 64408[0], 64415[0], 64416[0], 64417[0], 64418[0], 64420[0], 64421[0], 64425[0], 64430[0], 64435[0], 64445[0], 64446[0], 64447[0], 64448[0], 64449[0], 64450[0], 64451[0], 64454[0], 64461[0], 64462[0], 64463[0], 64479[0], 64480[0], 64483[0], 64484[0], 64486[0], 64487[0], 64488[0], 64489[0], 64490[0], 64491[0], 64492[0], 64493[0], 64494[0], 64495[0], 64505[0], 64510[0], 64517[0], 64520[0], 64530[0], 65280[1], 65286[1], 65400[1], 65410[1], 65772[1], 65785[1], 65800[1], 66020[1], 66250[1], 67250[1], 67500[1], 69990[0], 92012[1], 92014[1], 92018[1], 92019[1], 92071[1], 93000[1], 93005[1], 93010[1], 93040[1], 93041[1], 93042[1], 93318[1], 93355[1], 94002[1], 94200[1], 94680[1], 94681[1], 94690[1], 95812[1], 95813[1], 95816[1], 95819[1], 95822[1], 95829[1], 95955[1], 96360[1], 96361[1], 96365[1], 96366[1], 96367[1], 96368[1], 96372[1], 96374[1], 96375[1], 96376[1], 96377[1], 96523[0], 97597[1], 97598[1], 97602[1], 99155[0], 99156[0], 99157[0], 99211[1], 99212[1], 99213[1], 99214[1], 99215[1], 99217[1], 99218[1], 99219[1], 99220[1], 99221[1], 99222[1], 99223[1], 99231[1], 99232[1], 99233[1], 99234[1], 99235[1], 99236[1], 99238[1], 99239[1], 99241[1], 99242[1], 99243[1], 99244[1], 99245[1], 99251[1], 99252[1], 99253[1], 99254[1], 99255[1], 99291[1], 99292[1], 99304[1], 99305[1], 99306[1], 99307[1], 99308[1], 99309[1], 99310[1], 99315[1], 99316[1], 99334[1], 99335[1], 99336[1], 99337[1], 99347[1], 99348[1], 99349[1], 99350[1], 99374[1], 99375[1], 99377[1], 99378[1], 99446[0], 99447[0], 99448[0], 99449[0], 99451[0], 99452[0], 99495[0], 99496[0], G0463[1], G0471[1]
65778	0596T[1], 0597T[1], 0708T[1], 0709T[1], 12001[1], 12002[1], 12004[1], 12005[1], 12006[1], 12007[1], 12011[1], 12013[1], 12014[1], 12015[1], 12016[1], 12017[1], 12018[1], 12020[1], 12021[1], 12031[1], 12032[1], 12034[1], 12035[1], 12036[1], 12037[1], 12041[1], 12042[1], 12044[1], 12045[1], 12046[1], 12047[1], 12051[1], 12052[1], 12053[1], 12054[1], 12055[1], 12056[1], 12057[1], 13100[1], 13101[1], 13102[1], 13120[1], 13121[1], 13122[1], 13131[1], 13132[1], 13133[1], 13151[1], 13152[1], 13153[1], 36000[1], 36400[1], 36405[1], 36406[1], 36410[1], 36420[1], 36425[1], 36430[1], 36440[1], 36591[0], 36592[0], 36600[1], 36640[1], 43752[1], 51701[1], 51702[1], 51703[1], 62320[0], 62321[0], 62322[0], 62323[0], 62324[0], 62325[0], 62326[0], 62327[0], 64400[0], 64405[0], 64408[0], 64415[0], 64416[0], 64417[0], 64418[0], 64420[0], 64421[0], 64425[0], 64430[0], 64435[0], 64445[0], 64446[0], 64447[0], 64448[0], 64449[0], 64450[0], 64451[0], 64454[0], 64461[0], 64462[0], 64463[0], 64479[0], 64480[0], 64483[0], 64484[0], 64486[0], 64487[0], 64488[0], 64489[0], 64490[0], 64491[0], 64492[0], 64493[0], 64494[0], 64495[0], 64505[0], 64510[0], 64517[0], 64520[0], 64530[0], 65280[1], 65286[1], 65400[1], 65410[1], 65435[1], 65781[1], 65782[1], 66020[1], 67250[1], 67500[1], 69990[0], 92012[1], 92014[1], 92018[1], 92019[1], 92071[1], 93000[1], 93005[1], 93010[1], 93040[1], 93041[1], 93042[1], 93318[1], 93355[1], 94002[1], 94200[1], 94680[1], 94681[1], 94690[1], 95812[1], 95813[1], 95816[1], 95819[1], 95822[1], 95829[1], 95955[1], 96360[1], 96361[1], 96365[1], 96366[1], 96367[1], 96368[1], 96372[1], 96374[1], 96375[1], 96376[1], 96377[1], 96523[0], 99155[0], 99156[0], 99157[0], 99211[1], 99212[1], 99213[1], 99214[1], 99215[1], 99217[1], 99218[1], 99219[1], 99220[1], 99221[1], 99222[1], 99223[1], 99231[1], 99232[1], 99233[1], 99234[1], 99235[1], 99236[1], 99238[1], 99239[1], 99241[1], 99242[1], 99243[1], 99244[1], 99245[1], 99251[1], 99252[1], 99253[1], 99254[1], 99255[1], 99291[1], 99292[1], 99304[1], 99305[1], 99306[1], 99307[1], 99308[1], 99309[1], 99310[1], 99315[1], 99316[1], 99334[1], 99335[1], 99336[1], 99337[1], 99347[1], 99348[1], 99349[1], 99350[1], 99374[1], 99375[1], 99377[1], 99378[1], 99446[0], 99447[0], 99448[0], 99449[0], 99451[0], 99452[0], 99495[0], 99496[0], G0463[1], G0471[1], V2790[0]
65779	0596T[1], 0597T[1], 0708T[1], 0709T[1], 12001[1], 12002[1], 12004[1], 12005[1], 12006[1], 12007[1], 12011[1], 12013[1], 12014[1], 12015[1], 12016[1], 12017[1], 12018[1], 12020[1], 12021[1], 12031[1], 12032[1], 12034[1], 12035[1], 12036[1], 12037[1], 12041[1], 12042[1], 12044[1], 12045[1], 12046[1], 12047[1], 12051[1], 12052[1], 12053[1], 12054[1], 12055[1], 12056[1], 12057[1], 13100[1], 13101[1], 13102[1], 13120[1], 13121[1], 13122[1], 13131[1], 13132[1], 13133[1], 13151[1], 13152[1], 13153[1], 36000[1], 36400[1], 36405[1], 36406[1], 36410[1], 36420[1], 36425[1], 36430[1], 36440[1], 36591[0], 36592[0], 36600[1], 36640[1], 43752[1], 51701[1], 51702[1], 51703[1], 62320[0], 62321[0], 62322[0], 62323[0], 62324[0], 62325[0], 62326[0], 62327[0], 64400[0], 64405[0], 64408[0], 64415[0], 64416[0], 64417[0], 64418[0], 64420[0], 64421[0], 64425[0], 64430[0], 64435[0], 64445[0], 64446[0], 64447[0], 64448[0], 64449[0], 64450[0], 64451[0], 64454[0], 64461[0], 64462[0], 64463[0], 64479[0], 64480[0], 64483[0], 64484[0], 64486[0], 64487[0], 64488[0], 64489[0], 64490[0], 64491[0], 64492[0], 64493[0], 64494[0], 64495[0], 64505[0], 64510[0], 64517[0], 64520[0], 64530[0], 65280[1], 65286[1], 65400[1], 65410[1], 65430[1], 65435[1], 65778[1], 65780[1], 65782[1], 66020[1], 67250[1], 67500[1], 69990[0], 92012[1], 92014[1], 92018[1], 92019[1], 92071[1], 93000[1], 93005[1], 93010[1], 93040[1], 93041[1], 93042[1], 93318[1], 93355[1], 94002[1], 94200[1], 94680[1], 94681[1], 94690[1], 95812[1], 95813[1], 95816[1], 95819[1], 95822[1], 95829[1], 95955[1], 96360[1], 96361[1], 96365[1], 96366[1], 96367[1], 96368[1], 96372[1], 96374[1], 96375[1], 96376[1], 96377[1], 96523[0], 99155[0], 99156[0], 99157[0], 99211[1], 99212[1], 99213[1], 99214[1], 99215[1], 99217[1], 99218[1], 99219[1], 99220[1], 99221[1], 99222[1], 99223[1], 99231[1], 99232[1], 99233[1], 99234[1], 99235[1], 99236[1], 99238[1], 99239[1], 99241[1], 99242[1], 99243[1], 99244[1], 99245[1], 99251[1], 99252[1], 99253[1], 99254[1], 99255[1], 99291[1], 99292[1], 99304[1], 99305[1], 99306[1], 99307[1], 99308[1], 99309[1], 99310[1], 99315[1], 99316[1], 99334[1], 99335[1], 99336[1], 99337[1], 99347[1], 99348[1], 99349[1], 99350[1], 99374[1], 99375[1], 99377[1], 99378[1], 99446[0], 99447[0], 99448[0], 99449[0], 99451[0], 99452[0], 99495[0], 99496[0], G0463[1], G0471[1], J0670[1], J2001[1], V2790[0]
65780	0213T[0], 0216T[0], 0596T[1], 0597T[1], 0708T[1], 0709T[1], 12001[1], 12002[1], 12004[1], 12005[1], 12006[1], 12007[1], 12011[1], 12013[1], 12014[1], 12015[1], 12016[1], 12017[1], 12018[1], 12020[1], 12021[1], 12031[1], 12032[1], 12034[1], 12035[1], 12036[1], 12037[1], 12041[1], 12042[1], 12044[1], 12045[1], 12046[1], 12047[1], 12051[1], 12052[1], 12053[1], 12054[1], 12055[1], 12056[1], 12057[1], 13100[1], 13101[1], 13102[1], 13120[1], 13121[1], 13122[1], 13131[1], 13132[1], 13133[1], 13151[1], 13152[1], 13153[1], 36000[1], 36400[1], 36405[1], 36406[1], 36410[1], 36420[1], 36425[1], 36430[1], 36440[1], 36591[0], 36592[0], 36600[1], 36640[1], 43752[1], 51701[1], 51702[1], 51703[1], 62320[0], 62321[0], 62322[0], 62323[0], 62324[0], 62325[0], 62326[0], 62327[0], 64400[0], 64405[0], 64408[0], 64415[0], 64416[0], 64417[0], 64418[0], 64420[0], 64421[0], 64425[0], 64430[0], 64435[0], 64445[0], 64446[0], 64447[0], 64448[0], 64449[0], 64450[0], 64451[0], 64454[0], 64461[0], 64462[0], 64463[0], 64479[0], 64480[0], 64483[0], 64484[0], 64486[0], 64487[0], 64488[0], 64489[0], 64490[0], 64491[0], 64492[0], 64493[0], 64494[0], 64495[0], 64505[0], 64510[0], 64517[0], 64520[0], 64530[0], 65280[1], 65286[1], 65400[1], 65410[1], 65778[1], 65800[1], 66020[1], 67250[1], 67500[1], 69990[0], 92012[1], 92014[1], 92018[1], 92019[1], 92071[1], 92504[1], 93000[1], 93005[1], 93010[1], 93040[1], 93041[1], 93042[1], 93318[1], 93355[1], 94002[1], 94200[1], 94680[1], 94681[1], 94690[1], 95812[1], 95813[1], 95816[1], 95819[1], 95822[1], 95829[1], 95955[1], 96360[1], 96361[1], 96365[1], 96366[1], 96367[1], 96368[1], 96372[1], 96374[1], 96375[1], 96376[1], 96377[1], 96523[0], 99155[0], 99156[0], 99157[0], 99211[1], 99212[1], 99213[1], 99214[1], 99215[1], 99217[1], 99218[1], 99219[1], 99220[1], 99221[1], 99222[1], 99223[1], 99231[1], 99232[1], 99233[1], 99234[1], 99235[1], 99236[1], 99238[1], 99239[1], 99241[1], 99242[1], 99243[1], 99244[1], 99245[1], 99251[1], 99252[1], 99253[1], 99254[1], 99255[1], 99291[1], 99292[1], 99304[1], 99305[1], 99306[1], 99307[1], 99308[1], 99309[1], 99310[1], 99315[1], 99316[1], 99334[1], 99335[1], 99336[1], 99337[1], 99347[1], 99348[1], 99349[1], 99350[1], 99374[1],

0 = Modifier usage not allowed or inappropriate 1 = Modifier usage allowed

Code 1	Code 2
	99375[1], 99377[1], 99378[1], 99446[0], 99447[0], 99448[0], 99449[0], 99451[0], 99452[0], 99495[0], 99496[0], G0463[1], G0471[1]
65781	0213T[0], 0216T[0], 0596T[1], 0597T[1], 0708T[1], 0709T[1], 12001[1], 12002[1], 12004[1], 12005[1], 12006[1], 12007[1], 12011[1], 12013[1], 12014[1], 12015[1], 12016[1], 12017[1], 12018[1], 12020[1], 12021[1], 12031[1], 12032[1], 12034[1], 12035[1], 12036[1], 12037[1], 12041[1], 12042[1], 12044[1], 12045[1], 12046[1], 12047[1], 12051[1], 12052[1], 12053[1], 12054[1], 12055[1], 12056[1], 12057[1], 13100[1], 13101[1], 13102[1], 13120[1], 13121[1], 13122[1], 13131[1], 13132[1], 13133[1], 13151[1], 13152[1], 13153[1], 36000[1], 36400[1], 36405[1], 36406[1], 36410[1], 36420[1], 36425[1], 36430[1], 36440[1], 36591[0], 36592[0], 36600[1], 36640[1], 43752[1], 51701[1], 51702[1], 51703[1], 62320[0], 62321[0], 62322[0], 62323[0], 62324[0], 62325[0], 62326[0], 62327[0], 64400[0], 64405[0], 64408[0], 64415[0], 64416[0], 64417[0], 64418[0], 64420[0], 64421[0], 64425[0], 64430[0], 64435[0], 64445[0], 64446[0], 64447[0], 64448[0], 64449[0], 64450[0], 64451[0], 64454[0], 64461[0], 64462[0], 64463[0], 64479[0], 64480[0], 64483[0], 64484[0], 64486[0], 64487[0], 64488[0], 64489[0], 64490[0], 64491[0], 64492[0], 64493[0], 64494[0], 64495[0], 64505[0], 64510[0], 64517[0], 64520[0], 64530[0], 65280[1], 65286[1], 65400[1], 65410[1], 65710[1], 65730[1], 65750[1], 65755[1], 65756[1], 65779[1], 65780[1], 65782[1], 65800[1], 66020[1], 67250[1], 67500[1], 69990[0], 92012[1], 92014[1], 92018[1], 92019[1], 92071[1], 92504[1], 93000[1], 93005[1], 93010[1], 93040[1], 93041[1], 93042[1], 93318[1], 93355[1], 94002[1], 94200[1], 94680[1], 94681[1], 94690[1], 95812[1], 95813[1], 95816[1], 95819[1], 95822[1], 95829[1], 95955[1], 96360[1], 96361[1], 96365[1], 96366[1], 96367[1], 96368[1], 96372[1], 96374[1], 96375[1], 96376[1], 96377[1], 96523[0], 99155[0], 99156[0], 99157[0], 99211[1], 99212[1], 99213[1], 99214[1], 99215[1], 99217[1], 99218[1], 99219[1], 99220[1], 99221[1], 99222[1], 99223[1], 99231[1], 99232[1], 99233[1], 99234[1], 99235[1], 99236[1], 99238[1], 99239[1], 99241[1], 99242[1], 99243[1], 99244[1], 99245[1], 99251[1], 99252[1], 99253[1], 99254[1], 99255[1], 99291[1], 99292[1], 99304[1], 99305[1], 99306[1], 99307[1], 99308[1], 99309[1], 99310[1], 99315[1], 99316[1], 99334[1], 99335[1], 99336[1], 99337[1], 99347[1], 99348[1], 99349[1], 99350[1], 99374[1], 99375[1], 99377[1], 99378[1], 99446[0], 99447[0], 99448[0], 99449[0], 99451[0], 99452[0], 99495[0], 99496[0], G0463[1], G0471[1]
65782	0213T[0], 0216T[0], 0596T[1], 0597T[1], 0708T[1], 0709T[1], 12001[1], 12002[1], 12004[1], 12005[1], 12006[1], 12007[1], 12011[1], 12013[1], 12014[1], 12015[1], 12016[1], 12017[1], 12018[1], 12020[1], 12021[1], 12031[1], 12032[1], 12034[1], 12035[1], 12036[1], 12037[1], 12041[1], 12042[1], 12044[1], 12045[1], 12046[1], 12047[1], 12051[1], 12052[1], 12053[1], 12054[1], 12055[1], 12056[1], 12057[1], 13100[1], 13101[1], 13102[1], 13120[1], 13121[1], 13122[1], 13131[1], 13132[1], 13133[1], 13151[1], 13152[1], 13153[1], 36000[1], 36400[1], 36405[1], 36406[1], 36410[1], 36420[1], 36425[1], 36430[1], 36440[1], 36591[0], 36592[0], 36600[1], 36640[1], 43752[1], 51701[1], 51702[1], 51703[1], 62320[0], 62321[0], 62322[0], 62323[0], 62324[0], 62325[0], 62326[0], 62327[0], 64400[0], 64405[0], 64408[0], 64415[0], 64416[0], 64417[0], 64418[0], 64420[0], 64421[0], 64425[0], 64430[0], 64435[0], 64445[0], 64446[0], 64447[0], 64448[0], 64449[0], 64450[0], 64451[0], 64454[0], 64461[0], 64462[0], 64463[0], 64479[0], 64480[0], 64483[0], 64484[0], 64486[0], 64487[0], 64488[0], 64489[0], 64490[0], 64491[0], 64492[0], 64493[0], 64494[0], 64495[0], 64505[0], 64510[0], 64517[0], 64520[0], 64530[0], 65280[1], 65286[1], 65400[1], 65410[1], 65710[1], 65730[1], 65780[1], 65800[1], 66020[1], 67250[1], 67500[1], 69990[0], 92012[1], 92014[1], 92018[1], 92019[1], 92071[1], 92504[1], 93000[1], 93005[1], 93010[1], 93040[1], 93041[1], 93042[1], 93318[1], 93355[1], 94002[1], 94200[1], 94680[1], 94681[1], 94690[1], 95812[1], 95813[1], 95816[1], 95819[1], 95822[1], 95829[1], 95955[1], 96360[1], 96361[1], 96365[1], 96366[1], 96367[1], 96368[1], 96372[1], 96374[1], 96375[1], 96376[1], 96377[1], 96523[0], 99155[0], 99156[0], 99157[0], 99211[1], 99212[1], 99213[1], 99214[1], 99215[1], 99217[1], 99218[1], 99219[1], 99220[1], 99221[1], 99222[1], 99223[1], 99231[1], 99232[1], 99233[1], 99234[1], 99235[1], 99236[1], 99238[1], 99239[1], 99241[1], 99242[1], 99243[1], 99244[1], 99245[1], 99251[1], 99252[1], 99253[1], 99254[1], 99255[1], 99291[1], 99292[1], 99304[1], 99305[1], 99306[1], 99307[1], 99308[1], 99309[1], 99310[1], 99315[1], 99316[1], 99334[1], 99335[1], 99336[1], 99337[1], 99347[1], 99348[1], 99349[1], 99350[1], 99374[1], 99375[1], 99377[1], 99378[1], 99446[0], 99447[0], 99448[0], 99449[0], 99451[0], 99452[0], 99495[0], 99496[0], G0463[1], G0471[1]
65785	00140[0], 00144[0], 0213T[0], 0216T[0], 0596T[1], 0597T[1], 0708T[1], 0709T[1], 12001[0], 12002[1], 12004[1], 12005[1], 12006[1], 12007[1], 12011[1], 12013[1], 12014[1], 12015[1], 12016[1], 12017[1], 12018[1], 12020[1], 12021[1], 12031[1], 12032[1], 12034[1], 12035[1], 12036[1], 12037[1], 12041[1], 12042[1], 12044[1], 12045[1], 12046[1], 12047[1], 12051[1], 12052[1], 12053[1], 12054[1], 12055[1], 12056[1], 12057[1], 13100[1], 13101[1], 13102[1], 13120[1], 13121[1], 13122[1], 13131[1], 13132[1], 13133[1], 13151[1], 13152[1], 13153[1], 36000[1], 36400[1], 36405[1], 36406[1], 36410[1], 36420[1], 36425[1], 36430[1], 36440[1], 36591[0], 36592[0], 36600[1], 36640[1], 43752[1], 51701[1], 51702[1], 51703[1], 62320[0], 62321[0], 62322[0], 62323[0], 62324[0], 62325[0], 62326[0], 62327[0], 64400[0], 64405[0], 64408[0], 64415[0], 64416[0], 64417[0], 64418[0], 64420[0], 64421[0], 64425[0], 64430[0], 64435[0], 64445[0], 64446[0], 64447[0], 64448[0], 64449[0], 64450[0], 64451[0], 64454[0], 64461[0], 64462[0], 64463[0], 64479[0], 64480[0], 64483[0], 64484[0], 64486[0], 64487[0], 64488[0], 64489[0], 64490[0], 64491[0], 64492[0], 64493[0], 64494[0], 64495[0], 64505[0], 64510[0], 64517[0], 64520[0], 64530[0], 67500[1], 68200[1], 69990[0], 92012[1], 92014[1], 93000[1], 93005[1], 93010[1], 93040[1], 93041[1], 93042[1], 93318[1], 94002[1], 94200[1], 94680[1], 94681[1], 94690[1], 95812[1], 95813[1], 95816[1], 95819[1], 95822[1], 95829[1], 95955[1], 96360[1], 96361[1], 96365[1], 96366[1], 96367[1], 96368[1], 96372[1], 96374[1], 96375[1], 96376[1], 96377[1], 96523[0], 99155[0], 99156[0], 99157[0], 99211[1], 99212[1], 99213[1], 99214[1], 99215[1], 99217[1], 99218[1], 99219[1], 99220[1], 99221[1], 99222[1], 99223[1], 99231[1], 99232[1], 99233[1], 99234[1], 99235[1], 99236[1], 99238[1], 99239[1], 99241[1], 99242[1], 99243[1], 99244[1], 99245[1], 99251[1], 99252[1], 99253[1], 99254[1], 99255[1], 99291[1], 99292[1], 99304[1], 99305[1], 99306[1], 99307[1], 99308[1], 99309[1], 99310[1], 99315[1], 99316[1], 99334[1], 99335[1], 99336[1], 99337[1], 99347[1], 99348[1], 99349[1], 99350[1], 99374[1], 99375[1], 99377[1], 99378[1], 99446[0], 99447[0], 99448[0], 99449[0], 99451[0], 99452[0], J0670[1], J2001[1]
65800	0213T[0], 0216T[0], 0465T[1], 0596T[1], 0597T[1], 0699T[1], 0708T[1], 0709T[1], 11000[1], 11001[1], 11004[1], 11005[1], 11006[1], 11042[1], 11043[1], 11044[1], 11045[1], 11046[1], 11047[1], 12001[1], 12002[1], 12004[1], 12005[1], 12006[1], 12007[1], 12011[1], 12013[1], 12014[1], 12015[1], 12016[1], 12017[1], 12018[1], 12020[1], 12021[1], 12031[1], 12032[1], 12034[1], 12035[1], 12036[1], 12037[1], 12041[1], 12042[1], 12044[1], 12045[1], 12046[1], 12047[1], 12051[1], 12052[1], 12053[1], 12054[1], 12055[1], 12056[1], 12057[1], 13100[1], 13101[1], 13102[1], 13120[1], 13121[1], 13122[1], 13131[1], 13132[1], 13133[1], 13151[1], 13152[1], 13153[1], 36000[1], 36400[1], 36405[1], 36406[1], 36410[1], 36420[1], 36425[1], 36430[1], 36440[1], 36591[0], 36592[0], 36600[1], 36640[1], 43752[1], 51701[1], 51702[1], 51703[1], 62320[0], 62321[0], 62322[0], 62323[0], 62324[0], 62325[0], 62326[0], 62327[0], 64400[0], 64405[0], 64408[0], 64415[0], 64416[0], 64417[0], 64418[0], 64420[0], 64421[0], 64425[0], 64430[0], 64435[0], 64445[0], 64446[0], 64447[0], 64448[0], 64449[0], 64450[0], 64451[0], 64454[0], 64461[0], 64462[0], 64463[0], 64479[0], 64480[0], 64483[0], 64484[0], 64486[0], 64487[0], 64488[0], 64489[0], 64490[0], 64491[0], 64492[0], 64493[0], 64494[0], 64495[0], 64505[0], 64510[0], 64517[0], 64520[0], 64530[0], 65810[1], 65815[1], 66020[1], 66030[1], 67028[1], 67250[1], 67500[1], 67515[1], 68200[1], 69990[0], 92012[1], 92014[1], 92018[1], 92019[1], 93000[1], 93005[1], 93010[1], 93040[1], 93041[1], 93042[1], 93318[1], 93355[1], 94002[1], 94200[1], 94680[1], 94681[1], 94690[1], 95812[1], 95813[1], 95816[1], 95819[1], 95822[1], 95829[1], 95955[1], 96360[1], 96361[1], 96365[1], 96366[1], 96367[1], 96368[1], 96372[1], 96374[1], 96375[1], 96376[1], 96377[1], 96523[0], 97597[1], 97598[1], 97602[1], 99155[0], 99156[0], 99157[0], 99211[1], 99212[1], 99213[1], 99214[1], 99215[1], 99217[1], 99218[1], 99219[1], 99220[1], 99221[1], 99222[1], 99223[1], 99231[1], 99232[1], 99233[1], 99234[1], 99235[1], 99236[1], 99238[1], 99239[1], 99241[1], 99242[1], 99243[1], 99244[1], 99245[1], 99251[1], 99252[1], 99253[1], 99254[1], 99255[1], 99291[1], 99292[1], 99304[1], 99305[1], 99306[1], 99307[1], 99308[1], 99309[1], 99310[1], 99315[1], 99316[1], 99334[1], 99335[1], 99336[1], 99337[1], 99347[1], 99348[1], 99349[1], 99350[1], 99374[1], 99375[1], 99377[1], 99378[1], 99446[0], 99447[0], 99448[0], 99449[0], 99451[0], 99452[0], 99495[1], 99496[1], G0463[1], G0471[1]
65810	0213T[0], 0216T[0], 0465T[1], 0596T[1], 0597T[1], 0699T[1], 0708T[1], 0709T[1], 11000[1], 11001[1], 11004[1], 11005[1], 11006[1], 11042[1], 11043[1], 11044[1], 11045[1], 11046[1], 11047[1], 12001[1], 12002[1], 12004[1], 12005[1], 12006[1], 12007[1], 12011[1], 12013[1], 12014[1], 12015[1], 12016[1], 12017[1], 12018[1], 12020[1], 12021[1], 12031[1], 12032[1], 12034[1], 12035[1], 12036[1], 12037[1], 12041[1], 12042[1], 12044[1], 12045[1], 12046[1], 12047[1], 12051[1], 12052[1], 12053[1], 12054[1], 12055[1], 12056[1], 12057[1], 13100[1], 13101[1], 13102[1], 13120[1], 13121[1], 13122[1], 13131[1], 13132[1], 13133[1], 13151[1], 13152[1], 13153[1], 36000[1], 36400[1], 36405[1], 36406[1], 36410[1], 36420[1], 36425[1], 36430[1], 36440[1], 36591[0], 36592[0], 36600[1], 36640[1], 43752[1], 51701[1], 51702[1], 51703[1], 62320[0], 62321[0], 62322[0], 62323[0], 62324[0], 62325[0], 62326[0], 62327[0], 64400[0], 64405[0], 64408[0], 64415[0], 64416[0], 64417[0], 64418[0], 64420[0], 64421[0], 64425[0], 64430[0], 64435[0], 64445[0], 64446[0], 64447[0], 64448[0], 64449[0], 64450[0], 64451[0], 64454[0], 64461[0], 64462[0], 64463[0], 64479[0], 64480[0], 64483[0], 64484[0], 64486[0], 64487[0], 64488[0], 64489[0], 64490[0], 64491[0], 64492[0], 64493[0], 64494[0], 64495[0], 64505[0], 64510[0], 64517[0], 64520[0], 64530[0], 65815[1], 66020[1], 66030[1], 67028[1], 67250[1], 67500[1], 67515[1], 68200[1], 69990[0], 92012[1], 92014[1], 92018[1], 92019[1], 93000[1], 93005[1], 93010[1], 93040[1], 93041[1], 93042[1], 93318[1], 93355[1], 94002[1], 94200[1], 94680[1], 94681[1], 94690[1], 95812[1], 95813[1], 95816[1], 95819[1], 95822[1], 95829[1], 95955[1], 96360[1], 96361[1], 96365[1], 96366[1], 96367[1], 96368[1], 96372[1], 96374[1], 96375[1], 96376[1], 96377[1], 96523[0], 97597[1], 97598[1], 97602[1], 99155[0], 99156[0], 99157[0], 99211[1], 99212[1], 99213[1], 99214[1], 99215[1], 99217[1], 99218[1], 99219[1], 99220[1], 99221[1], 99222[1], 99223[1], 99231[1], 99232[1], 99233[1], 99234[1], 99235[1], 99236[1], 99238[1], 99239[1], 99241[1], 99242[1], 99243[1], 99244[1], 99245[1], 99251[1], 99252[1], 99253[1], 99254[1], 99255[1], 99291[1], 99292[1], 99304[1], 99305[1], 99306[1], 99307[1], 99308[1], 99309[1], 99310[1], 99315[1], 99316[1], 99334[1], 99335[1], 99336[1], 99337[1], 99347[1], 99348[1], 99349[1], 99350[1], 99374[1], 99375[1], 99377[1], 99378[1], 99446[0], 99447[0], 99448[0], 99449[0], 99451[0], 99452[0], 99495[0], 99496[0], G0463[1], G0471[1], J2001[1]
65815	0213T[0], 0216T[0], 0465T[1], 0596T[1], 0597T[1], 0699T[1], 0708T[1], 0709T[1], 11000[1], 11001[1], 11004[1], 11005[1], 11006[1], 11042[1], 11043[1], 11044[1], 11045[1], 11046[1], 11047[1], 12001[1], 12002[1], 12004[1], 12005[1], 12006[1], 12007[1], 12011[1], 12013[1], 12014[1], 12015[1], 12016[1], 12017[1], 12018[1], 12020[1], 12021[1], 12031[1], 12032[1], 12034[1], 12035[1], 12036[1], 12037[1], 12041[1], 12042[1], 12044[1], 12045[1], 12046[1], 12047[1], 12051[1], 12052[1], 12053[1], 12054[1], 12055[1], 12056[1], 12057[1], 13100[1], 13101[1], 13102[1], 13120[1], 13121[1], 13122[1], 13131[1], 13132[1], 13133[1], 13151[1], 13152[1], 13153[1], 36000[1], 36400[1], 36405[1], 36406[1], 36410[1],

Appendix A: NCCI - CPT Codes

0 = Modifier usage not allowed or inappropriate 1 = Modifier usage allowed

Code 1	Code 2
	36420[1], 36425[1], 36430[1], 36440[1], 36591[0], 36592[0], 36600[1], 36640[1], 43752[1], 51701[1], 51702[1], 51703[1], 62320[0], 62321[0], 62322[0], 62323[0], 62324[0], 62325[0], 62326[0], 62327[0], 64400[0], 64405[0], 64408[0], 64415[0], 64416[0], 64417[0], 64418[0], 64420[0], 64421[0], 64425[0], 64430[0], 64435[0], 64445[0], 64446[0], 64447[0], 64448[0], 64449[0], 64450[0], 64451[0], 64454[0], 64461[0], 64462[0], 64463[0], 64479[0], 64480[0], 64483[0], 64484[0], 64486[0], 64487[0], 64488[0], 64489[0], 64490[0], 64491[0], 64492[0], 64493[0], 64494[0], 64495[0], 64505[0], 64510[0], 64517[0], 64520[0], 64530[0], 66020[1], 66030[1], 67028[1], 67250[1], 67500[1], 67515[1], 68200[1], 69990[0], 92012[1], 92014[1], 92018[1], 92019[1], 93000[1], 93005[1], 93010[1], 93040[1], 93041[1], 93042[1], 93318[1], 93355[1], 94002[1], 94200[1], 94680[1], 94681[1], 94690[1], 95812[1], 95813[1], 95816[1], 95819[1], 95822[1], 95829[1], 95955[1], 96360[1], 96361[1], 96365[1], 96366[1], 96367[1], 96368[1], 96372[1], 96374[1], 96375[1], 96376[1], 96377[1], 96523[0], 97597[1], 97598[1], 97602[1], 99155[0], 99156[0], 99157[0], 99211[1], 99212[1], 99213[1], 99214[1], 99215[1], 99217[1], 99218[1], 99219[1], 99220[1], 99221[1], 99222[1], 99223[1], 99231[1], 99232[1], 99233[1], 99234[1], 99235[1], 99236[1], 99238[1], 99239[1], 99241[1], 99242[1], 99243[1], 99244[1], 99245[1], 99251[1], 99252[1], 99253[1], 99254[1], 99255[1], 99291[1], 99292[1], 99304[1], 99305[1], 99306[1], 99307[1], 99308[1], 99309[1], 99310[1], 99315[1], 99316[1], 99334[1], 99335[1], 99336[1], 99337[1], 99347[1], 99348[1], 99349[1], 99350[1], 99374[1], 99375[1], 99377[1], 99378[1], 99446[0], 99447[0], 99448[0], 99449[0], 99451[0], 99452[0], 99495[0], 99496[0], G0463[1], G0471[1], J0670[1], J2001[1]
65820	0213T[0], 0216T[0], 0596T[1], 0597T[1], 0699T[1], 0708T[1], 0709T[1], 11000[1], 11001[1], 11004[1], 11005[1], 11006[1], 11042[1], 11043[1], 11044[1], 11045[1], 11046[1], 11047[1], 12001[1], 12002[1], 12004[1], 12005[1], 12006[1], 12007[1], 12011[1], 12013[1], 12014[1], 12015[1], 12016[1], 12017[1], 12018[1], 12020[1], 12021[1], 12031[1], 12032[1], 12034[1], 12035[1], 12036[1], 12037[1], 12041[1], 12042[1], 12044[1], 12045[1], 12046[1], 12047[1], 12051[1], 12052[1], 12053[1], 12054[1], 12055[1], 12056[1], 12057[1], 13100[1], 13101[1], 13102[1], 13120[1], 13121[1], 13122[1], 13131[1], 13132[1], 13133[1], 13151[1], 13152[1], 13153[1], 36000[1], 36400[1], 36405[1], 36406[1], 36410[1], 36420[1], 36425[1], 36430[1], 36440[1], 36591[0], 36592[0], 36600[1], 36640[1], 43752[1], 51701[1], 51702[1], 51703[1], 62320[0], 62321[0], 62322[0], 62323[0], 62324[0], 62325[0], 62326[0], 62327[0], 64400[0], 64405[0], 64408[0], 64415[0], 64416[0], 64417[0], 64418[0], 64420[0], 64421[0], 64425[0], 64430[0], 64435[0], 64445[0], 64446[0], 64447[0], 64448[0], 64449[0], 64450[0], 64451[0], 64454[0], 64461[0], 64462[0], 64463[0], 64479[0], 64480[0], 64483[0], 64484[0], 64486[0], 64487[0], 64488[0], 64489[0], 64490[0], 64491[0], 64492[0], 64493[0], 64494[0], 64495[0], 64505[0], 64510[0], 64517[0], 64520[0], 64530[0], 65800[1], 65810[1], 65815[1], 66020[1], 66030[1], 66625[1], 66630[1], 67250[1], 67500[1], 69990[0], 92012[1], 92014[1], 92018[1], 92019[1], 93000[1], 93005[1], 93010[1], 93040[1], 93041[1], 93042[1], 93318[1], 93355[1], 94002[1], 94200[1], 94680[1], 94681[1], 94690[1], 95812[1], 95813[1], 95816[1], 95819[1], 95822[1], 95829[1], 95955[1], 96360[1], 96361[1], 96365[1], 96366[1], 96367[1], 96368[1], 96372[1], 96374[1], 96375[1], 96376[1], 96377[1], 96523[0], 97597[1], 97598[1], 97602[1], 99155[0], 99156[0], 99157[0], 99211[1], 99212[1], 99213[1], 99214[1], 99215[1], 99217[1], 99218[1], 99219[1], 99220[1], 99221[1], 99222[1], 99223[1], 99231[1], 99232[1], 99233[1], 99234[1], 99235[1], 99236[1], 99238[1], 99239[1], 99241[1], 99242[1], 99243[1], 99244[1], 99245[1], 99251[1], 99252[1], 99253[1], 99254[1], 99255[1], 99291[1], 99292[1], 99304[1], 99305[1], 99306[1], 99307[1], 99308[1], 99309[1], 99310[1], 99315[1], 99316[1], 99334[1], 99335[1], 99336[1], 99337[1], 99347[1], 99348[1], 99349[1], 99350[1], 99374[1], 99375[1], 99377[1], 99378[1], 99446[0], 99447[0], 99448[0], 99449[0], 99451[0], 99452[0], 99495[0], 99496[0], G0463[1], G0471[1], J0670[1], J2001[1]
65850	0213T[0], 0216T[0], 0596T[1], 0597T[1], 0699T[1], 0708T[1], 0709T[1], 11000[1], 11001[1], 11004[1], 11005[1], 11006[1], 11042[1], 11043[1], 11044[1], 11045[1], 11046[1], 11047[1], 12001[1], 12002[1], 12004[1], 12005[1], 12006[1], 12007[1], 12011[1], 12013[1], 12014[1], 12015[1], 12016[1], 12017[1], 12018[1], 12020[1], 12021[1], 12031[1], 12032[1], 12034[1], 12035[1], 12036[1], 12037[1], 12041[1], 12042[1], 12044[1], 12045[1], 12046[1], 12047[1], 12051[1], 12052[1], 12053[1], 12054[1], 12055[1], 12056[1], 12057[1], 13100[1], 13101[1], 13102[1], 13120[1], 13121[1], 13122[1], 13131[1], 13132[1], 13133[1], 13151[1], 13152[1], 13153[1], 36000[1], 36400[1], 36405[1], 36406[1], 36410[1], 36420[1], 36425[1], 36430[1], 36440[1], 36591[0], 36592[0], 36600[1], 36640[1], 43752[1], 51701[1], 51702[1], 51703[1], 62320[0], 62321[0], 62322[0], 62323[0], 62324[0], 62325[0], 62326[0], 62327[0], 64400[0], 64405[0], 64408[0], 64415[0], 64416[0], 64417[0], 64418[0], 64420[0], 64421[0], 64425[0], 64430[0], 64435[0], 64445[0], 64446[0], 64447[0], 64448[0], 64449[0], 64450[0], 64451[0], 64454[0], 64461[0], 64462[0], 64463[0], 64479[0], 64480[0], 64483[0], 64484[0], 64486[0], 64487[0], 64488[0], 64489[0], 64490[0], 64491[0], 64492[0], 64493[0], 64494[0], 64495[0], 64505[0], 64510[0], 64517[0], 64520[0], 64530[0], 65800[1], 65810[1], 65815[1], 65820[1], 66020[1], 66030[1], 66170[1], 67250[1], 67500[1], 69990[0], 92012[1], 92014[1], 92018[1], 92019[1], 93000[1], 93005[1], 93010[1], 93040[1], 93041[1], 93042[1], 93318[1], 93355[1], 94002[1], 94200[1], 94680[1], 94681[1], 94690[1], 95812[1], 95813[1], 95816[1], 95819[1], 95822[1], 95829[1], 95955[1], 96360[1], 96361[1], 96365[1], 96366[1], 96367[1], 96368[1], 96372[1], 96374[1], 96375[1], 96376[1], 96377[1], 96523[0], 97597[1], 97598[1], 97602[1], 99155[0], 99156[0], 99157[0], 99211[1], 99212[1], 99213[1], 99214[1], 99215[1], 99217[1], 99218[1], 99219[1], 99220[1], 99221[1], 99222[1], 99223[1], 99231[1], 99232[1], 99233[1], 99234[1], 99235[1], 99236[1], 99238[1], 99239[1], 99241[1], 99242[1], 99243[1], 99244[1], 99245[1], 99251[1], 99252[1], 99253[1], 99254[1], 99255[1], 99291[1], 99292[1], 99304[1], 99305[1], 99306[1], 99307[1], 99308[1], 99309[1], 99310[1], 99315[1], 99316[1], 99334[1], 99335[1], 99336[1], 99337[1], 99347[1], 99348[1], 99349[1], 99350[1], 99374[1], 99375[1], 99377[1], 99378[1], 99446[0], 99447[0], 99448[0], 99449[0], 99451[0], 99452[0], 99495[0], 99496[0], G0463[1], G0471[1], J0670[1], J2001[1]
65855	0213T[0], 0216T[0], 0596T[1], 0597T[1], 0708T[1], 0709T[1], 11000[1], 11001[1], 11004[1], 11005[1], 11006[1], 11042[1], 11043[1], 11044[1], 11045[1], 11046[1], 11047[1], 12001[1], 12002[1], 12004[1], 12005[1], 12006[1], 12007[1], 12011[1], 12013[1], 12014[1], 12015[1], 12016[1], 12017[1], 12018[1], 12020[1], 12021[1], 12031[1], 12032[1], 12034[1], 12035[1], 12036[1], 12037[1], 12041[1], 12042[1], 12044[1], 12045[1], 12046[1], 12047[1], 12051[1], 12052[1], 12053[1], 12054[1], 12055[1], 12056[1], 12057[1], 13100[1], 13101[1], 13102[1], 13120[1], 13121[1], 13122[1], 13131[1], 13132[1], 13133[1], 13151[1], 13152[1], 13153[1], 36000[1], 36400[1], 36405[1], 36406[1], 36410[1], 36420[1], 36425[1], 36430[1], 36440[1], 36591[0], 36592[0], 36600[1], 36640[1], 43752[1], 51701[1], 51702[1], 51703[1], 62320[0], 62321[0], 62322[0], 62323[0], 62324[0], 62325[0], 62326[0], 62327[0], 64400[0], 64405[0], 64408[0], 64415[0], 64416[0], 64417[0], 64418[0], 64420[0], 64421[0], 64425[0], 64430[0], 64435[0], 64445[0], 64446[0], 64447[0], 64448[0], 64449[0], 64450[0], 64451[0], 64454[0], 64461[0], 64462[0], 64463[0], 64479[0], 64480[0], 64483[0], 64484[0], 64486[0], 64487[0], 64488[0], 64489[0], 64490[0], 64491[0], 64492[0], 64493[0], 64494[0], 64495[0], 64505[0], 64510[0], 64517[0], 64520[0], 64530[0], 65820[1], 65850[1], 66170[1], 67250[1], 67500[1], 69990[0], 92012[1], 92014[1], 92018[1], 92019[1], 92020[1], 92504[1], 93000[1], 93005[1], 93010[1], 93040[1], 93041[1], 93042[1], 93318[1], 93355[1], 94002[1], 94200[1], 94680[1], 94681[1], 94690[1], 95812[1], 95813[1], 95816[1], 95819[1], 95822[1], 95829[1], 95955[1], 96360[1], 96361[1], 96365[1], 96366[1], 96367[1], 96368[1], 96372[1], 96374[1], 96375[1], 96376[1], 96377[1], 96523[0], 97597[1], 97598[1], 97602[1], 99155[0], 99156[0], 99157[0], 99211[1], 99212[1], 99213[1], 99214[1], 99215[1], 99217[1], 99218[1], 99219[1], 99220[1], 99221[1], 99222[1], 99223[1], 99231[1], 99232[1], 99233[1], 99234[1], 99235[1], 99236[1], 99238[1], 99239[1], 99241[1], 99242[1], 99243[1], 99244[1], 99245[1], 99251[1], 99252[1], 99253[1], 99254[1], 99255[1], 99291[1], 99292[1], 99304[1], 99305[1], 99306[1], 99307[1], 99308[1], 99309[1], 99310[1], 99315[1], 99316[1], 99334[1], 99335[1], 99336[1], 99337[1], 99347[1], 99348[1], 99349[1], 99350[1], 99374[1], 99375[1], 99377[1], 99378[1], 99446[0], 99447[0], 99448[0], 99449[0], 99451[0], 99452[0], 99495[0], 99496[0], G0463[1], G0471[1]
65860	0213T[0], 0216T[0], 0596T[1], 0597T[1], 0621T[1], 0622T[1], 0708T[1], 0709T[1], 12001[1], 12002[1], 12004[1], 12005[1], 12006[1], 12007[1], 12011[1], 12013[1], 12014[1], 12015[1], 12016[1], 12017[1], 12018[1], 12020[1], 12021[1], 12031[1], 12032[1], 12034[1], 12035[1], 12036[1], 12037[1], 12041[1], 12042[1], 12044[1], 12045[1], 12046[1], 12047[1], 12051[1], 12052[1], 12053[1], 12054[1], 12055[1], 12056[1], 12057[1], 13100[1], 13101[1], 13102[1], 13120[1], 13121[1], 13122[1], 13131[1], 13132[1], 13133[1], 13151[1], 13152[1], 13153[1], 36000[1], 36400[1], 36405[1], 36406[1], 36410[1], 36420[1], 36425[1], 36430[1], 36440[1], 36591[0], 36592[0], 36600[1], 36640[1], 43752[1], 51701[1], 51702[1], 51703[1], 62320[0], 62321[0], 62322[0], 62323[0], 62324[0], 62325[0], 62326[0], 62327[0], 64400[0], 64405[0], 64408[0], 64415[0], 64416[0], 64417[0], 64418[0], 64420[0], 64421[0], 64425[0], 64430[0], 64435[0], 64445[0], 64446[0], 64447[0], 64448[0], 64449[0], 64450[0], 64451[0], 64454[0], 64461[0], 64462[0], 64463[0], 64479[0], 64480[0], 64483[0], 64484[0], 64486[0], 64487[0], 64488[0], 64489[0], 64490[0], 64491[0], 64492[0], 64493[0], 64494[0], 64495[0], 64505[0], 64510[0], 64517[0], 64520[0], 64530[0], 65855[1], 67250[1], 67500[1], 69990[0], 92012[1], 92014[1], 92018[1], 92019[1], 93000[1], 93005[1], 93010[1], 93040[1], 93041[1], 93042[1], 93318[1], 93355[1], 94002[1], 94200[1], 94680[1], 94681[1], 94690[1], 95812[1], 95813[1], 95816[1], 95819[1], 95822[1], 95829[1], 95955[1], 96360[1], 96361[1], 96365[1], 96366[1], 96367[1], 96368[1], 96372[1], 96374[1], 96375[1], 96376[1], 96377[1], 96523[0], 99155[0], 99156[0], 99157[0], 99211[1], 99212[1], 99213[1], 99214[1], 99215[1], 99217[1], 99218[1], 99219[1], 99220[1], 99221[1], 99222[1], 99223[1], 99231[1], 99232[1], 99233[1], 99234[1], 99235[1], 99236[1], 99238[1], 99239[1], 99241[1], 99242[1], 99243[1], 99244[1], 99245[1], 99251[1], 99252[1], 99253[1], 99254[1], 99255[1], 99291[1], 99292[1], 99304[1], 99305[1], 99306[1], 99307[1], 99308[1], 99309[1], 99310[1], 99315[1], 99316[1], 99334[1], 99335[1], 99336[1], 99337[1], 99347[1], 99348[1], 99349[1], 99350[1], 99374[1], 99375[1], 99377[1], 99378[1], 99446[0], 99447[0], 99448[0], 99449[0], 99451[0], 99452[0], 99495[0], 99496[0], G0463[1], G0471[1]
65865	0213T[0], 0216T[0], 0596T[1], 0597T[1], 0621T[1], 0622T[1], 0708T[1], 0709T[1], 12001[1], 12002[1], 12004[1], 12005[1], 12006[1], 12007[1], 12011[1], 12013[1], 12014[1], 12015[1], 12016[1], 12017[1], 12018[1], 12020[1], 12021[1], 12031[1], 12032[1], 12034[1], 12035[1], 12036[1], 12037[1], 12041[1], 12042[1], 12044[1], 12045[1], 12046[1], 12047[1], 12051[1], 12052[1], 12053[1], 12054[1], 12055[1], 12056[1], 12057[1], 13100[1], 13101[1], 13102[1], 13120[1], 13121[1], 13122[1], 13131[1], 13132[1], 13133[1], 13151[1], 13152[1], 13153[1], 36000[1], 36400[1], 36405[1], 36406[1], 36410[1], 36420[1], 36425[1], 36430[1], 36440[1], 36591[0], 36592[0], 36600[1], 36640[1], 43752[1], 51701[1], 51702[1], 51703[1], 62320[0], 62321[0], 62322[0], 62323[0], 62324[0], 62325[0], 62326[0], 62327[0], 64400[0], 64405[0], 64408[0], 64415[0], 64416[0], 64417[0], 64418[0], 64420[0], 64421[0], 64425[0], 64430[0], 64435[0], 64445[0], 64446[0], 64447[0], 64448[0], 64449[0], 64450[0], 64451[0], 64454[0], 64461[0], 64462[0], 64463[0], 64479[0], 64480[0], 64483[0], 64484[0], 64486[0], 64487[0], 64488[0], 64489[0], 64490[0], 64491[0], 64492[0], 64493[0], 64494[0], 64495[0], 64505[0], 64510[0], 64517[0], 64520[0], 64530[0], 65855[1], 65860[1], 65870[1], 67250[1], 67500[1], 69990[0], 92012[1], 92014[1], 92018[1], 92019[1], 93000[1], 93005[1], 93010[1], 93040[1], 93041[1], 93042[1], 93318[1], 93355[1], 94002[1], 94200[1], 94680[1], 94681[1], 94690[1], 95812[1], 95813[1], 95816[1], 95819[1], 95822[1], 95829[1],

Code 1	Code 2
	95955[1], 96360[1], 96361[1], 96365[1], 96366[1], 96367[1], 96368[1], 96372[1], 96374[1], 96375[1], 96376[1], 96377[1], 96523[0], 99155[0], 99156[0], 99157[0], 99211[1], 99212[1], 99213[1], 99214[1], 99215[1], 99217[1], 99218[1], 99219[1], 99220[1], 99221[1], 99222[1], 99223[1], 99231[1], 99232[1], 99233[1], 99234[1], 99235[1], 99236[1], 99238[1], 99239[1], 99241[1], 99242[1], 99243[1], 99244[1], 99245[1], 99251[1], 99252[1], 99253[1], 99254[1], 99255[1], 99291[1], 99292[1], 99304[1], 99305[1], 99306[1], 99307[1], 99308[1], 99309[1], 99310[1], 99315[1], 99316[1], 99334[1], 99335[1], 99336[1], 99337[1], 99347[1], 99348[1], 99349[1], 99350[1], 99374[1], 99375[1], 99377[1], 99378[1], 99446[0], 99447[0], 99448[0], 99449[0], 99451[0], 99452[0], 99495[0], 99496[0], G0463[1], G0471[1], J0670[1], J2001[1]
65870	0213T[0], 0216T[0], 0596T[1], 0597T[1], 0621T[1], 0622T[1], 0708T[1], 0709T[1], 12001[1], 12002[1], 12004[1], 12005[1], 12006[1], 12007[1], 12011[1], 12013[1], 12014[1], 12015[1], 12016[1], 12017[1], 12018[1], 12020[1], 12021[1], 12031[1], 12032[1], 12034[1], 12035[1], 12036[1], 12037[1], 12041[1], 12042[1], 12044[1], 12045[1], 12046[1], 12047[1], 12051[1], 12052[1], 12053[1], 12054[1], 12055[1], 12056[1], 12057[1], 13100[1], 13101[1], 13102[1], 13120[1], 13121[1], 13122[1], 13131[1], 13132[1], 13133[1], 13151[1], 13152[1], 13153[1], 36000[1], 36400[1], 36405[1], 36406[1], 36410[1], 36420[1], 36425[1], 36430[1], 36440[1], 36591[0], 36592[0], 36600[1], 36640[1], 43752[1], 51701[1], 51702[1], 51703[1], 62320[0], 62321[0], 62322[0], 62323[0], 62324[0], 62325[0], 62326[0], 62327[0], 64400[0], 64405[0], 64408[0], 64415[0], 64416[0], 64417[0], 64418[0], 64420[0], 64421[0], 64425[0], 64430[0], 64435[0], 64445[0], 64446[0], 64447[0], 64448[0], 64449[0], 64450[0], 64451[0], 64454[0], 64461[0], 64462[0], 64463[0], 64479[0], 64480[0], 64483[0], 64484[0], 64486[0], 64487[0], 64488[0], 64489[0], 64490[0], 64491[0], 64492[0], 64493[0], 64494[0], 64495[0], 64505[0], 64510[0], 64517[0], 64520[0], 64530[0], 65855[1], 65860[1], 67250[1], 67500[1], 69990[0], 92012[1], 92014[1], 92018[1], 92019[1], 93000[1], 93005[1], 93010[1], 93040[1], 93041[1], 93042[1], 93318[1], 93355[1], 94002[1], 94200[1], 94680[1], 94681[1], 94690[1], 95812[1], 95813[1], 95816[1], 95819[1], 95822[1], 95829[1], 95955[1], 96360[1], 96361[1], 96365[1], 96366[1], 96367[1], 96368[1], 96372[1], 96374[1], 96375[1], 96376[1], 96377[1], 96523[0], 99155[0], 99156[0], 99157[0], 99211[1], 99212[1], 99213[1], 99214[1], 99215[1], 99217[1], 99218[1], 99219[1], 99220[1], 99221[1], 99222[1], 99223[1], 99231[1], 99232[1], 99233[1], 99234[1], 99235[1], 99236[1], 99238[1], 99239[1], 99241[1], 99242[1], 99243[1], 99244[1], 99245[1], 99251[1], 99252[1], 99253[1], 99254[1], 99255[1], 99291[1], 99292[1], 99304[1], 99305[1], 99306[1], 99307[1], 99308[1], 99309[1], 99310[1], 99315[1], 99316[1], 99334[1], 99335[1], 99336[1], 99337[1], 99347[1], 99348[1], 99349[1], 99350[1], 99374[1], 99375[1], 99377[1], 99378[1], 99446[0], 99447[0], 99448[0], 99449[0], 99451[0], 99452[0], 99495[0], 99496[0], G0463[1], G0471[1], J0670[1], J2001[1]
65875	0213T[0], 0216T[0], 0596T[1], 0597T[1], 0621T[1], 0622T[1], 0708T[1], 0709T[1], 12001[1], 12002[1], 12004[1], 12005[1], 12006[1], 12007[1], 12011[1], 12013[1], 12014[1], 12015[1], 12016[1], 12017[1], 12018[1], 12020[1], 12021[1], 12031[1], 12032[1], 12034[1], 12035[1], 12036[1], 12037[1], 12041[1], 12042[1], 12044[1], 12045[1], 12046[1], 12047[1], 12051[1], 12052[1], 12053[1], 12054[1], 12055[1], 12056[1], 12057[1], 13100[1], 13101[1], 13102[1], 13120[1], 13121[1], 13122[1], 13131[1], 13132[1], 13133[1], 13151[1], 13152[1], 13153[1], 36000[1], 36400[1], 36405[1], 36406[1], 36410[1], 36420[1], 36425[1], 36430[1], 36440[1], 36591[0], 36592[0], 36600[1], 36640[1], 43752[1], 51701[1], 51702[1], 51703[1], 62320[0], 62321[0], 62322[0], 62323[0], 62324[0], 62325[0], 62326[0], 62327[0], 64400[0], 64405[0], 64408[0], 64415[0], 64416[0], 64417[0], 64418[0], 64420[0], 64421[0], 64425[0], 64430[0], 64435[0], 64445[0], 64446[0], 64447[0], 64448[0], 64449[0], 64450[0], 64451[0], 64454[0], 64461[0], 64462[0], 64463[0], 64479[0], 64480[0], 64483[0], 64484[0], 64486[0], 64487[0], 64488[0], 64489[0], 64490[0], 64491[0], 64492[0], 64493[0], 64494[0], 64495[0], 64505[0], 64510[0], 64517[0], 64520[0], 64530[0], 65855[1], 65860[1], 65865[1], 65870[1], 67250[1], 67500[1], 69990[0], 92012[1], 92014[1], 92018[1], 92019[1], 93000[1], 93005[1], 93010[1], 93040[1], 93041[1], 93042[1], 93318[1], 93355[1], 94002[1], 94200[1], 94680[1], 94681[1], 94690[1], 95812[1], 95813[1], 95816[1], 95819[1], 95822[1], 95829[1], 95955[1], 96360[1], 96361[1], 96365[1], 96366[1], 96367[1], 96368[1], 96372[1], 96374[1], 96375[1], 96376[1], 96377[1], 96523[0], 99155[0], 99156[0], 99157[0], 99211[1], 99212[1], 99213[1], 99214[1], 99215[1], 99217[1], 99218[1], 99219[1], 99220[1], 99221[1], 99222[1], 99223[1], 99231[1], 99232[1], 99233[1], 99234[1], 99235[1], 99236[1], 99238[1], 99239[1], 99241[1], 99242[1], 99243[1], 99244[1], 99245[1], 99251[1], 99252[1], 99253[1], 99254[1], 99255[1], 99291[1], 99292[1], 99304[1], 99305[1], 99306[1], 99307[1], 99308[1], 99309[1], 99310[1], 99315[1], 99316[1], 99334[1], 99335[1], 99336[1], 99337[1], 99347[1], 99348[1], 99349[1], 99350[1], 99374[1], 99375[1], 99377[1], 99378[1], 99446[0], 99447[0], 99448[0], 99449[0], 99451[0], 99452[0], 99495[0], 99496[0], G0463[1], G0471[1], J0670[1], J2001[1]
65880	0213T[0], 0216T[0], 0596T[1], 0597T[1], 0621T[1], 0622T[1], 0708T[1], 0709T[1], 12001[1], 12002[1], 12004[1], 12005[1], 12006[1], 12007[1], 12011[1], 12013[1], 12014[1], 12015[1], 12016[1], 12017[1], 12018[1], 12020[1], 12021[1], 12031[1], 12032[1], 12034[1], 12035[1], 12036[1], 12037[1], 12041[1], 12042[1], 12044[1], 12045[1], 12046[1], 12047[1], 12051[1], 12052[1], 12053[1], 12054[1], 12055[1], 12056[1], 12057[1], 13100[1], 13101[1], 13102[1], 13120[1], 13121[1], 13122[1], 13131[1], 13132[1], 13133[1], 13151[1], 13152[1], 13153[1], 36000[1], 36400[1], 36405[1], 36406[1], 36410[1], 36420[1], 36425[1], 36430[1], 36440[1], 36591[0], 36592[0], 36600[1], 36640[1], 43752[1], 51701[1], 51702[1], 51703[1], 62320[0], 62321[0], 62322[0], 62323[0], 62324[0], 62325[0], 62326[0], 62327[0], 64400[0], 64405[0], 64408[0], 64415[0], 64416[0], 64417[0], 64418[0], 64420[0], 64421[0], 64425[0], 64430[0], 64435[0], 64445[0], 64446[0], 64447[0], 64448[0], 64449[0], 64450[0], 64451[0], 64454[0], 64461[0], 64462[0], 64463[0], 64479[0], 64480[0], 64483[0], 64484[0], 64486[0], 64487[0], 64488[0], 64489[0], 64490[0], 64491[0], 64492[0], 64493[0], 64494[0], 64495[0], 64505[0], 64510[0], 64517[0], 64520[0], 64530[0], 65855[1], 65860[1], 65865[1], 65870[1], 65875[1], 67250[1], 67500[1], 69990[0], 92012[1], 92014[1], 92018[1], 92019[1], 93000[1], 93005[1], 93010[1], 93040[1], 93041[1], 93042[1], 93318[1], 93355[1], 94002[1], 94200[1], 94680[1], 94681[1], 94690[1], 95812[1], 95813[1], 95816[1], 95819[1], 95822[1], 95829[1], 95955[1], 96360[1], 96361[1], 96365[1], 96366[1], 96367[1], 96368[1], 96372[1], 96374[1], 96375[1], 96376[1], 96377[1], 96523[0], 99155[0], 99156[0], 99157[0], 99211[1], 99212[1], 99213[1], 99214[1], 99215[1], 99217[1], 99218[1], 99219[1], 99220[1], 99221[1], 99222[1], 99223[1], 99231[1], 99232[1], 99233[1], 99234[1], 99235[1], 99236[1], 99238[1], 99239[1], 99241[1], 99242[1], 99243[1], 99244[1], 99245[1], 99251[1], 99252[1], 99253[1], 99254[1], 99255[1], 99291[1], 99292[1], 99304[1], 99305[1], 99306[1], 99307[1], 99308[1], 99309[1], 99310[1], 99315[1], 99316[1], 99334[1], 99335[1], 99336[1], 99337[1], 99347[1], 99348[1], 99349[1], 99350[1], 99374[1], 99375[1], 99377[1], 99378[1], 99446[0], 99447[0], 99448[0], 99449[0], 99451[0], 99452[0], 99495[0], 99496[0], G0463[1], G0471[1], J0670[1], J2001[1]
65900	0213T[0], 0216T[0], 0596T[1], 0597T[1], 0708T[1], 0709T[1], 11000[1], 11001[1], 11004[1], 11005[1], 11006[1], 11042[1], 11043[1], 11044[1], 11045[1], 11046[1], 11047[1], 12001[1], 12002[1], 12004[1], 12005[1], 12006[1], 12007[1], 12011[1], 12013[1], 12014[1], 12015[1], 12016[1], 12017[1], 12018[1], 12020[1], 12021[1], 12031[1], 12032[1], 12034[1], 12035[1], 12036[1], 12037[1], 12041[1], 12042[1], 12044[1], 12045[1], 12046[1], 12047[1], 12051[1], 12052[1], 12053[1], 12054[1], 12055[1], 12056[1], 12057[1], 13100[1], 13101[1], 13102[1], 13120[1], 13121[1], 13122[1], 13131[1], 13132[1], 13133[1], 13151[1], 13152[1], 13153[1], 36000[1], 36400[1], 36405[1], 36406[1], 36410[1], 36420[1], 36425[1], 36430[1], 36440[1], 36591[0], 36592[0], 36600[1], 36640[1], 43752[1], 51701[1], 51702[1], 51703[1], 62320[0], 62321[0], 62322[0], 62323[0], 62324[0], 62325[0], 62326[0], 62327[0], 64400[0], 64405[0], 64408[0], 64415[0], 64416[0], 64417[0], 64418[0], 64420[0], 64421[0], 64425[0], 64430[0], 64435[0], 64445[0], 64446[0], 64447[0], 64448[0], 64449[0], 64450[0], 64451[0], 64454[0], 64461[0], 64462[0], 64463[0], 64479[0], 64480[0], 64483[0], 64484[0], 64486[0], 64487[0], 64488[0], 64489[0], 64490[0], 64491[0], 64492[0], 64493[0], 64494[0], 64495[0], 64505[0], 64510[0], 64517[0], 64520[0], 64530[0], 65800[1], 65865[1], 65870[1], 65875[1], 67250[1], 67500[1], 69990[0], 92012[1], 92014[1], 92018[1], 92019[1], 93000[1], 93005[1], 93010[1], 93040[1], 93041[1], 93042[1], 93318[1], 93355[1], 94002[1], 94200[1], 94680[1], 94681[1], 94690[1], 95812[1], 95813[1], 95816[1], 95819[1], 95822[1], 95829[1], 95955[1], 96360[1], 96361[1], 96365[1], 96366[1], 96367[1], 96368[1], 96372[1], 96374[1], 96375[1], 96376[1], 96377[1], 96523[0], 97597[1], 97598[1], 97602[1], 99155[0], 99156[0], 99157[0], 99211[1], 99212[1], 99213[1], 99214[1], 99215[1], 99217[1], 99218[1], 99219[1], 99220[1], 99221[1], 99222[1], 99223[1], 99231[1], 99232[1], 99233[1], 99234[1], 99235[1], 99236[1], 99238[1], 99239[1], 99241[1], 99242[1], 99243[1], 99244[1], 99245[1], 99251[1], 99252[1], 99253[1], 99254[1], 99255[1], 99291[1], 99292[1], 99304[1], 99305[1], 99306[1], 99307[1], 99308[1], 99309[1], 99310[1], 99315[1], 99316[1], 99334[1], 99335[1], 99336[1], 99337[1], 99347[1], 99348[1], 99349[1], 99350[1], 99374[1], 99375[1], 99377[1], 99378[1], 99446[0], 99447[0], 99448[0], 99449[0], 99451[0], 99452[0], 99495[0], 99496[0], G0463[1], G0471[1], J0670[1], J2001[1]
65920	0213T[0], 0216T[0], 0596T[1], 0597T[1], 0708T[1], 0709T[1], 11000[1], 11001[1], 11004[1], 11005[1], 11006[1], 11042[1], 11043[1], 11044[1], 11045[1], 11046[1], 11047[1], 12001[1], 12002[1], 12004[1], 12005[1], 12006[1], 12007[1], 12011[1], 12013[1], 12014[1], 12015[1], 12016[1], 12017[1], 12018[1], 12020[1], 12021[1], 12031[1], 12032[1], 12034[1], 12035[1], 12036[1], 12037[1], 12041[1], 12042[1], 12044[1], 12045[1], 12046[1], 12047[1], 12051[1], 12052[1], 12053[1], 12054[1], 12055[1], 12056[1], 12057[1], 13100[1], 13101[1], 13102[1], 13120[1], 13121[1], 13122[1], 13131[1], 13132[1], 13133[1], 13151[1], 13152[1], 13153[1], 36000[1], 36400[1], 36405[1], 36406[1], 36410[1], 36420[1], 36425[1], 36430[1], 36440[1], 36591[0], 36592[0], 36600[1], 36640[1], 43752[1], 51701[1], 51702[1], 51703[1], 62320[0], 62321[0], 62322[0], 62323[0], 62324[0], 62325[0], 62326[0], 62327[0], 64400[0], 64405[0], 64408[0], 64415[0], 64416[0], 64417[0], 64418[0], 64420[0], 64421[0], 64425[0], 64430[0], 64435[0], 64445[0], 64446[0], 64447[0], 64448[0], 64449[0], 64450[0], 64451[0], 64454[0], 64461[0], 64462[0], 64463[0], 64479[0], 64480[0], 64483[0], 64484[0], 64486[0], 64487[0], 64488[0], 64489[0], 64490[0], 64491[0], 64492[0], 64493[0], 64494[0], 64495[0], 64505[0], 64510[0], 64517[0], 64520[0], 64530[0], 65865[1], 65870[1], 65875[1], 67005[1], 67010[1], 67250[1], 67500[1], 69990[0], 92012[1], 92014[1], 92018[1], 92019[1], 93000[1], 93005[1], 93010[1], 93040[1], 93041[1], 93042[1], 93318[1], 93355[1], 94002[1], 94200[1], 94680[1], 94681[1], 94690[1], 95812[1], 95813[1], 95816[1], 95819[1], 95822[1], 95829[1], 95955[1], 96360[1], 96361[1], 96365[1], 96366[1], 96367[1], 96368[1], 96372[1], 96374[1], 96375[1], 96376[1], 96377[1], 96523[0], 97597[1], 97598[1], 97602[1], 99155[0], 99156[0], 99157[0], 99211[1], 99212[1], 99213[1], 99214[1], 99215[1], 99217[1], 99218[1], 99219[1], 99220[1], 99221[1], 99222[1], 99223[1], 99231[1], 99232[1], 99233[1], 99234[1], 99235[1], 99236[1], 99238[1], 99239[1], 99241[1], 99242[1], 99243[1], 99244[1], 99245[1], 99251[1], 99252[1], 99253[1], 99254[1], 99255[1], 99291[1], 99292[1], 99304[1], 99305[1], 99306[1], 99307[1], 99308[1], 99309[1], 99310[1], 99315[1], 99316[1], 99334[1], 99335[1], 99336[1], 99337[1], 99347[1], 99348[1], 99349[1], 99350[1], 99374[1], 99375[1], 99377[1], 99378[1], 99446[0], 99447[0], 99448[0], 99449[0], 99451[0], 99452[0], 99495[0], 99496[0], G0463[1], G0471[1], J0670[1], J2001[1]

0 = Modifier usage not allowed or inappropriate 1 = Modifier usage allowed

Code 1	Code 2
65930	0213T[0], 0216T[0], 0596T[1], 0597T[1], 0708T[1], 0709T[1], 11000[1], 11001[1], 11004[1], 11005[1], 11006[1], 11042[1], 11043[1], 11044[1], 11045[1], 11046[1], 11047[1], 12001[1], 12002[1], 12004[1], 12005[1], 12006[1], 12007[1], 12011[1], 12013[1], 12014[1], 12015[1], 12016[1], 12017[1], 12018[1], 12020[1], 12021[1], 12031[1], 12032[1], 12034[1], 12035[1], 12036[1], 12037[1], 12041[1], 12042[1], 12044[1], 12045[1], 12046[1], 12047[1], 12051[1], 12052[1], 12053[1], 12054[1], 12055[1], 12056[1], 12057[1], 13100[1], 13101[1], 13102[1], 13120[1], 13121[1], 13122[1], 13131[1], 13132[1], 13133[1], 13151[1], 13152[1], 13153[1], 36000[1], 36400[1], 36405[1], 36406[1], 36410[1], 36420[1], 36425[1], 36430[1], 36440[1], 36591[0], 36592[0], 36600[1], 36640[1], 43752[1], 51701[1], 51702[1], 51703[1], 62320[0], 62321[0], 62322[0], 62323[0], 62324[0], 62325[0], 62326[0], 62327[0], 64400[0], 64405[0], 64408[0], 64415[0], 64416[0], 64417[0], 64418[0], 64420[0], 64421[0], 64425[0], 64430[0], 64435[0], 64445[0], 64446[0], 64447[0], 64448[0], 64449[0], 64450[0], 64451[0], 64454[0], 64461[0], 64462[0], 64463[0], 64479[0], 64480[0], 64483[0], 64484[0], 64486[0], 64487[0], 64488[0], 64489[0], 64490[0], 64491[0], 64492[0], 64493[0], 64494[0], 64495[0], 64505[0], 64510[0], 64517[0], 64520[0], 64530[0], 65800[1], 65865[1], 65870[1], 65875[1], 67500[1], 69990[0], 92012[1], 92014[1], 92018[1], 92019[1], 93000[1], 93005[1], 93010[1], 93040[1], 93041[1], 93042[1], 93318[1], 93355[1], 94002[1], 94200[1], 94680[1], 94681[1], 94690[1], 95812[1], 95813[1], 95816[1], 95819[1], 95822[1], 95829[1], 95955[1], 96360[1], 96361[1], 96365[1], 96366[1], 96367[1], 96368[1], 96372[1], 96374[1], 96375[1], 96376[1], 96377[1], 96523[0], 97597[1], 97598[1], 97602[1], 99155[0], 99156[0], 99157[0], 99211[1], 99212[1], 99213[1], 99214[1], 99215[1], 99217[1], 99218[1], 99219[1], 99220[1], 99221[1], 99222[1], 99223[1], 99231[1], 99232[1], 99233[1], 99234[1], 99235[1], 99236[1], 99238[1], 99239[1], 99241[1], 99242[1], 99243[1], 99244[1], 99245[1], 99251[1], 99252[1], 99253[1], 99254[1], 99255[1], 99291[1], 99292[1], 99304[1], 99305[1], 99306[1], 99307[1], 99308[1], 99309[1], 99310[1], 99315[1], 99316[1], 99334[1], 99335[1], 99336[1], 99337[1], 99347[1], 99348[1], 99349[1], 99350[1], 99374[1], 99375[1], 99377[1], 99378[1], 99446[0], 99447[0], 99448[0], 99449[0], 99451[0], 99452[0], 99495[0], 99496[0], G0463[1], G0471[1], J0670[1], J2001[1]
66020	0213T[0], 0216T[0], 0596T[1], 0597T[1], 0708T[1], 0709T[1], 12001[1], 12002[1], 12004[1], 12005[1], 12006[1], 12007[1], 12011[1], 12013[1], 12014[1], 12015[1], 12016[1], 12017[1], 12018[1], 12020[1], 12021[1], 12031[1], 12032[1], 12034[1], 12035[1], 12036[1], 12037[1], 12041[1], 12042[1], 12044[1], 12045[1], 12046[1], 12047[1], 12051[1], 12052[1], 12053[1], 12054[1], 12055[1], 12056[1], 12057[1], 13100[1], 13101[1], 13102[1], 13120[1], 13121[1], 13122[1], 13131[1], 13132[1], 13133[1], 13151[1], 13152[1], 13153[1], 36000[1], 36400[1], 36405[1], 36406[1], 36410[1], 36420[1], 36425[1], 36430[1], 36440[1], 36591[0], 36592[0], 36600[1], 36640[1], 43752[1], 51701[1], 51702[1], 51703[1], 62320[0], 62321[0], 62322[0], 62323[0], 62324[0], 62325[0], 62326[0], 62327[0], 64400[0], 64405[0], 64408[0], 64415[0], 64416[0], 64417[0], 64418[0], 64420[0], 64421[0], 64425[0], 64430[0], 64435[0], 64445[0], 64446[0], 64447[0], 64448[0], 64449[0], 64450[0], 64451[0], 64454[0], 64461[0], 64462[0], 64463[0], 64479[0], 64480[0], 64483[0], 64484[0], 64486[0], 64487[0], 64488[0], 64489[0], 64490[0], 64491[0], 64492[0], 64493[0], 64494[0], 64495[0], 64505[0], 64510[0], 64517[0], 64520[0], 64530[0], 67500[1], 69990[0], 92012[1], 92014[1], 92018[1], 92019[1], 93000[1], 93005[1], 93010[1], 93040[1], 93041[1], 93042[1], 93318[1], 93355[1], 94002[1], 94200[1], 94680[1], 94681[1], 94690[1], 95812[1], 95813[1], 95816[1], 95819[1], 95822[1], 95829[1], 95955[1], 96360[1], 96361[1], 96365[1], 96366[1], 96367[1], 96368[1], 96372[1], 96374[1], 96375[1], 96376[1], 96377[1], 96523[0], 99155[0], 99156[0], 99157[0], 99211[1], 99212[1], 99213[1], 99214[1], 99215[1], 99217[1], 99218[1], 99219[1], 99220[1], 99221[1], 99222[1], 99223[1], 99231[1], 99232[1], 99233[1], 99234[1], 99235[1], 99236[1], 99238[1], 99239[1], 99241[1], 99242[1], 99243[1], 99244[1], 99245[1], 99251[1], 99252[1], 99253[1], 99254[1], 99255[1], 99291[1], 99292[1], 99304[1], 99305[1], 99306[1], 99307[1], 99308[1], 99309[1], 99310[1], 99315[1], 99316[1], 99334[1], 99335[1], 99336[1], 99337[1], 99347[1], 99348[1], 99349[1], 99350[1], 99374[1], 99375[1], 99377[1], 99378[1], 99446[0], 99447[0], 99448[0], 99449[0], 99451[0], 99452[0], 99495[0], 99496[0], G0463[1], G0471[1]
66030	0213T[0], 0216T[0], 0596T[1], 0597T[1], 0708T[1], 0709T[1], 12001[1], 12002[1], 12004[1], 12005[1], 12006[1], 12007[1], 12011[1], 12013[1], 12014[1], 12015[1], 12016[1], 12017[1], 12018[1], 12020[1], 12021[1], 12031[1], 12032[1], 12034[1], 12035[1], 12036[1], 12037[1], 12041[1], 12042[1], 12044[1], 12045[1], 12046[1], 12047[1], 12051[1], 12052[1], 12053[1], 12054[1], 12055[1], 12056[1], 12057[1], 13100[1], 13101[1], 13102[1], 13120[1], 13121[1], 13122[1], 13131[1], 13132[1], 13133[1], 13151[1], 13152[1], 13153[1], 36000[1], 36400[1], 36405[1], 36406[1], 36410[1], 36420[1], 36425[1], 36430[1], 36440[1], 36591[0], 36592[0], 36600[1], 36640[1], 43752[1], 51701[1], 51702[1], 51703[1], 62320[0], 62321[0], 62322[0], 62323[0], 62324[0], 62325[0], 62326[0], 62327[0], 64400[0], 64405[0], 64408[0], 64415[0], 64416[0], 64417[0], 64418[0], 64420[0], 64421[0], 64425[0], 64430[0], 64435[0], 64445[0], 64446[0], 64447[0], 64448[0], 64449[0], 64450[0], 64451[0], 64454[0], 64461[0], 64462[0], 64463[0], 64479[0], 64480[0], 64483[0], 64484[0], 64486[0], 64487[0], 64488[0], 64489[0], 64490[0], 64491[0], 64492[0], 64493[0], 64494[0], 64495[0], 64505[0], 64510[0], 64517[0], 64520[0], 64530[0], 67250[1], 67500[1], 69990[0], 92012[1], 92014[1], 92018[1], 92019[1], 93000[1], 93005[1], 93010[1], 93040[1], 93041[1], 93042[1], 93318[1], 93355[1], 94002[1], 94200[1], 94680[1], 94681[1], 94690[1], 95812[1], 95813[1], 95816[1], 95819[1], 95822[1], 95829[1], 95955[1], 96360[1], 96361[1], 96365[1], 96366[1], 96367[1], 96368[1], 96372[1], 96374[1], 96375[1], 96376[1], 96377[1], 96523[0], 99155[0], 99156[0], 99157[0], 99211[1], 99212[1], 99213[1], 99214[1], 99215[1], 99217[1], 99218[1], 99219[1], 99220[1], 99221[1], 99222[1], 99223[1], 99231[1], 99232[1], 99233[1], 99234[1], 99235[1], 99236[1], 99238[1], 99239[1], 99241[1], 99242[1], 99243[1], 99244[1], 99245[1], 99251[1], 99252[1], 99253[1], 99254[1], 99255[1], 99291[1], 99292[1], 99304[1], 99305[1], 99306[1], 99307[1], 99308[1], 99309[1], 99310[1], 99315[1], 99316[1], 99334[1], 99335[1], 99336[1], 99337[1], 99347[1], 99348[1], 99349[1], 99350[1], 99374[1], 99375[1], 99377[1], 99378[1], 99446[0], 99447[0], 99448[0], 99449[0], 99451[0], 99452[0], 99495[0], 99496[0], G0463[1], G0471[1]
66130	0213T[0], 0216T[0], 0596T[1], 0597T[1], 0708T[1], 0709T[1], 11000[1], 11001[1], 11004[1], 11005[1], 11006[1], 11042[1], 11043[1], 11044[1], 11045[1], 11046[1], 11047[1], 12001[1], 12002[1], 12004[1], 12005[1], 12006[1], 12007[1], 12011[1], 12013[1], 12014[1], 12015[1], 12016[1], 12017[1], 12018[1], 12020[1], 12021[1], 12031[1], 12032[1], 12034[1], 12035[1], 12036[1], 12037[1], 12041[1], 12042[1], 12044[1], 12045[1], 12046[1], 12047[1], 12051[1], 12052[1], 12053[1], 12054[1], 12055[1], 12056[1], 12057[1], 13100[1], 13101[1], 13102[1], 13120[1], 13121[1], 13122[1], 13131[1], 13132[1], 13133[1], 13151[1], 13152[1], 13153[1], 36000[1], 36400[1], 36405[1], 36406[1], 36410[1], 36420[1], 36425[1], 36430[1], 36440[1], 36591[0], 36592[0], 36600[1], 36640[1], 43752[1], 51701[1], 51702[1], 51703[1], 62320[0], 62321[0], 62322[0], 62323[0], 62324[0], 62325[0], 62326[0], 62327[0], 64400[0], 64405[0], 64408[0], 64415[0], 64416[0], 64417[0], 64418[0], 64420[0], 64421[0], 64425[0], 64430[0], 64435[0], 64445[0], 64446[0], 64447[0], 64448[0], 64449[0], 64450[0], 64451[0], 64454[0], 64461[0], 64462[0], 64463[0], 64479[0], 64480[0], 64483[0], 64484[0], 64486[0], 64487[0], 64488[0], 64489[0], 64490[0], 64491[0], 64492[0], 64493[0], 64494[0], 64495[0], 64505[0], 64510[0], 64517[0], 64520[0], 64530[0], 67250[1], 67255[1], 67500[1], 69990[0], 92012[1], 92014[1], 92018[1], 92019[1], 93000[1], 93005[1], 93010[1], 93040[1], 93041[1], 93042[1], 93318[1], 93355[1], 94002[1], 94200[1], 94680[1], 94681[1], 94690[1], 95812[1], 95813[1], 95816[1], 95819[1], 95822[1], 95829[1], 95955[1], 96360[1], 96361[1], 96365[1], 96366[1], 96367[1], 96368[1], 96372[1], 96374[1], 96375[1], 96376[1], 96377[1], 96523[0], 97597[1], 97598[1], 97602[1], 99155[0], 99156[0], 99157[0], 99211[1], 99212[1], 99213[1], 99214[1], 99215[1], 99217[1], 99218[1], 99219[1], 99220[1], 99221[1], 99222[1], 99223[1], 99231[1], 99232[1], 99233[1], 99234[1], 99235[1], 99236[1], 99238[1], 99239[1], 99241[1], 99242[1], 99243[1], 99244[1], 99245[1], 99251[1], 99252[1], 99253[1], 99254[1], 99255[1], 99291[1], 99292[1], 99304[1], 99305[1], 99306[1], 99307[1], 99308[1], 99309[1], 99310[1], 99315[1], 99316[1], 99334[1], 99335[1], 99336[1], 99337[1], 99347[1], 99348[1], 99349[1], 99350[1], 99374[1], 99375[1], 99377[1], 99378[1], 99446[0], 99447[0], 99448[0], 99449[0], 99451[0], 99452[0], 99495[0], 99496[0], G0463[1], G0471[1], J0670[1], J2001[1]
66150	0213T[0], 0216T[0], 0596T[1], 0597T[1], 0708T[1], 0709T[1], 11000[1], 11001[1], 11004[1], 11005[1], 11006[1], 11042[1], 11043[1], 11044[1], 11045[1], 11046[1], 11047[1], 12001[1], 12002[1], 12004[1], 12005[1], 12006[1], 12007[1], 12011[1], 12013[1], 12014[1], 12015[1], 12016[1], 12017[1], 12018[1], 12020[1], 12021[1], 12031[1], 12032[1], 12034[1], 12035[1], 12036[1], 12037[1], 12041[1], 12042[1], 12044[1], 12045[1], 12046[1], 12047[1], 12051[1], 12052[1], 12053[1], 12054[1], 12055[1], 12056[1], 12057[1], 13100[1], 13101[1], 13102[1], 13120[1], 13121[1], 13122[1], 13131[1], 13132[1], 13133[1], 13151[1], 13152[1], 13153[1], 36000[1], 36400[1], 36405[1], 36406[1], 36410[1], 36420[1], 36425[1], 36430[1], 36440[1], 36591[0], 36592[0], 36600[1], 36640[1], 43752[1], 51701[1], 51702[1], 51703[1], 62320[0], 62321[0], 62322[0], 62323[0], 62324[0], 62325[0], 62326[0], 62327[0], 64400[0], 64405[0], 64408[0], 64415[0], 64416[0], 64417[0], 64418[0], 64420[0], 64421[0], 64425[0], 64430[0], 64435[0], 64445[0], 64446[0], 64447[0], 64448[0], 64449[0], 64450[0], 64451[0], 64454[0], 64461[0], 64462[0], 64463[0], 64479[0], 64480[0], 64483[0], 64484[0], 64486[0], 64487[0], 64488[0], 64489[0], 64490[0], 64491[0], 64492[0], 64493[0], 64494[0], 64495[0], 64505[0], 64510[0], 64517[0], 64520[0], 64530[0], 65820[1], 66160[1], 66170[1], 66172[1], 66625[1], 67255[1], 67500[1], 68200[1], 69990[0], 92012[1], 92014[1], 92018[1], 92019[1], 93000[1], 93005[1], 93010[1], 93040[1], 93041[1], 93042[1], 93318[1], 93355[1], 94002[1], 94200[1], 94680[1], 94681[1], 94690[1], 95812[1], 95813[1], 95816[1], 95819[1], 95822[1], 95829[1], 95955[1], 96360[1], 96361[1], 96365[1], 96366[1], 96367[1], 96368[1], 96372[1], 96374[1], 96375[1], 96376[1], 96377[1], 96523[0], 97597[1], 97598[1], 97602[1], 99155[0], 99156[0], 99157[0], 99211[1], 99212[1], 99213[1], 99214[1], 99215[1], 99217[1], 99218[1], 99219[1], 99220[1], 99221[1], 99222[1], 99223[1], 99231[1], 99232[1], 99233[1], 99234[1], 99235[1], 99236[1], 99238[1], 99239[1], 99241[1], 99242[1], 99243[1], 99244[1], 99245[1], 99251[1], 99252[1], 99253[1], 99254[1], 99255[1], 99291[1], 99292[1], 99304[1], 99305[1], 99306[1], 99307[1], 99308[1], 99309[1], 99310[1], 99315[1], 99316[1], 99334[1], 99335[1], 99336[1], 99337[1], 99347[1], 99348[1], 99349[1], 99350[1], 99374[1], 99375[1], 99377[1], 99378[1], 99446[0], 99447[0], 99448[0], 99449[0], 99451[0], 99452[0], 99495[0], 99496[0], G0463[1], G0471[1], J0670[1], J2001[1]
66155	0213T[0], 0216T[0], 0596T[1], 0597T[1], 0708T[1], 0709T[1], 11000[1], 11001[1], 11004[1], 11005[1], 11006[1], 11042[1], 11043[1], 11044[1], 11045[1], 11046[1], 11047[1], 12001[1], 12002[1], 12004[1], 12005[1], 12006[1], 12007[1], 12011[1], 12013[1], 12014[1], 12015[1], 12016[1], 12017[1], 12018[1], 12020[1], 12021[1], 12031[1], 12032[1], 12034[1], 12035[1], 12036[1], 12037[1], 12041[1], 12042[1], 12044[1], 12045[1], 12046[1], 12047[1], 12051[1], 12052[1], 12053[1], 12054[1], 12055[1], 12056[1], 12057[1], 13100[1], 13101[1], 13102[1], 13120[1], 13121[1], 13122[1], 13131[1], 13132[1], 13133[1], 13151[1], 13152[1], 13153[1], 36000[1], 36400[1], 36405[1], 36406[1], 36410[1], 36420[1], 36425[1], 36430[1], 36440[1], 36591[0], 36592[0], 36600[1], 36640[1], 43752[1], 51701[1], 51702[1], 51703[1], 62320[0], 62321[0], 62322[0], 62323[0], 62324[0], 62325[0], 62326[0], 62327[0], 64400[0], 64405[0], 64408[0], 64415[0], 64416[0], 64417[0], 64418[0], 64420[0], 64421[0], 64425[0], 64430[0], 64435[0],

0 = Modifier usage not allowed or inappropriate 1 = Modifier usage allowed

Code 1	Code 2
	64445[0], 64446[0], 64447[0], 64448[0], 64449[0], 64450[0], 64451[0], 64454[0], 64461[0], 64462[0], 64463[0], 64479[0], 64480[0], 64483[0], 64484[0], 64486[0], 64487[0], 64488[0], 64489[0], 64490[0], 64491[0], 64492[0], 64493[0], 64494[0], 64495[0], 64505[0], 64510[0], 64517[0], 64520[0], 64530[0], 65820[1], 66150[1], 66160[1], 66170[1], 66172[1], 66625[1], 67255[1], 67500[1], 69990[0], 92012[1], 92014[1], 92018[1], 92019[1], 93000[1], 93005[1], 93010[1], 93040[1], 93041[1], 93042[1], 93318[1], 93355[1], 94002[1], 94200[1], 94680[1], 94681[1], 94690[1], 95812[1], 95813[1], 95816[1], 95819[1], 95822[1], 95829[1], 95955[1], 96360[1], 96361[1], 96365[1], 96366[1], 96367[1], 96368[1], 96372[1], 96374[1], 96375[1], 96376[1], 96377[1], 96523[0], 97597[1], 97598[1], 97602[1], 99155[0], 99156[0], 99157[0], 99211[1], 99212[1], 99213[1], 99214[1], 99215[1], 99217[1], 99218[1], 99219[1], 99220[1], 99221[1], 99222[1], 99223[1], 99231[1], 99232[1], 99233[1], 99234[1], 99235[1], 99236[1], 99238[1], 99239[1], 99241[1], 99242[1], 99243[1], 99244[1], 99245[1], 99251[1], 99252[1], 99253[1], 99254[1], 99255[1], 99291[1], 99292[1], 99304[1], 99305[1], 99306[1], 99307[1], 99308[1], 99309[1], 99310[1], 99315[1], 99316[1], 99334[1], 99335[1], 99336[1], 99337[1], 99347[1], 99348[1], 99349[1], 99350[1], 99374[1], 99375[1], 99377[1], 99378[1], 99446[0], 99447[0], 99448[0], 99449[0], 99451[0], 99452[0], 99495[0], 99496[0], G0463[1], G0471[1], J0670[1], J2001[1]
66160	0213T[0], 0216T[0], 0596T[1], 0597T[1], 0708T[1], 0709T[1], 11000[1], 11001[1], 11004[1], 11005[1], 11006[1], 11042[1], 11043[1], 11044[1], 11045[1], 11046[1], 11047[1], 12001[1], 12002[1], 12004[1], 12005[1], 12006[1], 12007[1], 12011[1], 12013[1], 12014[1], 12015[1], 12016[1], 12017[1], 12018[1], 12020[1], 12021[1], 12031[1], 12032[1], 12034[1], 12035[1], 12036[1], 12037[1], 12041[1], 12042[1], 12044[1], 12045[1], 12046[1], 12047[1], 12051[1], 12052[1], 12053[1], 12054[1], 12055[1], 12056[1], 12057[1], 13100[1], 13101[1], 13102[1], 13120[1], 13121[1], 13122[1], 13131[1], 13132[1], 13133[1], 13151[1], 13152[1], 13153[1], 36000[1], 36400[1], 36405[1], 36406[1], 36410[1], 36420[1], 36425[1], 36430[1], 36440[1], 36591[0], 36592[0], 36600[1], 36640[1], 43752[1], 51701[1], 51702[1], 51703[1], 62320[0], 62321[0], 62322[0], 62323[0], 62324[0], 62325[0], 62326[0], 62327[0], 64400[0], 64405[0], 64408[0], 64415[0], 64416[0], 64417[0], 64418[0], 64420[0], 64421[0], 64425[0], 64430[0], 64435[0], 64445[0], 64446[0], 64447[0], 64448[0], 64449[0], 64450[0], 64451[0], 64454[0], 64461[0], 64462[0], 64463[0], 64479[0], 64480[0], 64483[0], 64484[0], 64486[0], 64487[0], 64488[0], 64489[0], 64490[0], 64491[0], 64492[0], 64493[0], 64494[0], 64495[0], 64505[0], 64510[0], 64517[0], 64520[0], 64530[0], 65820[1], 66170[1], 66172[1], 66625[1], 67255[1], 67500[1], 69990[0], 92012[1], 92014[1], 92018[1], 92019[1], 93000[1], 93005[1], 93010[1], 93040[1], 93041[1], 93042[1], 93318[1], 93355[1], 94002[1], 94200[1], 94680[1], 94681[1], 94690[1], 95812[1], 95813[1], 95816[1], 95819[1], 95822[1], 95829[1], 95955[1], 96360[1], 96361[1], 96365[1], 96366[1], 96367[1], 96368[1], 96372[1], 96374[1], 96375[1], 96376[1], 96377[1], 96523[0], 97597[1], 97598[1], 97602[1], 99155[0], 99156[0], 99157[0], 99211[1], 99212[1], 99213[1], 99214[1], 99215[1], 99217[1], 99218[1], 99219[1], 99220[1], 99221[1], 99222[1], 99223[1], 99231[1], 99232[1], 99233[1], 99234[1], 99235[1], 99236[1], 99238[1], 99239[1], 99241[1], 99242[1], 99243[1], 99244[1], 99245[1], 99251[1], 99252[1], 99253[1], 99254[1], 99255[1], 99291[1], 99292[1], 99304[1], 99305[1], 99306[1], 99307[1], 99308[1], 99309[1], 99310[1], 99315[1], 99316[1], 99334[1], 99335[1], 99336[1], 99337[1], 99347[1], 99348[1], 99349[1], 99350[1], 99374[1], 99375[1], 99377[1], 99378[1], 99446[0], 99447[0], 99448[0], 99449[0], 99451[0], 99452[0], 99495[0], 99496[0], G0463[1], G0471[1], J0670[1], J2001[1]
66170	0213T[0], 0216T[0], 0253T[1], 0449T[1], 0474T[1], 0596T[1], 0597T[1], 0616T[1], 0617T[1], 0618T[1], 0671T[1], 0699T[1], 0708T[1], 0709T[1], 11000[1], 11001[1], 11004[1], 11005[1], 11006[1], 11042[1], 11043[1], 11044[1], 11045[1], 11046[1], 11047[1], 12001[1], 12002[1], 12004[1], 12005[1], 12006[1], 12007[1], 12011[1], 12013[1], 12014[1], 12015[1], 12016[1], 12017[1], 12018[1], 12020[1], 12021[1], 12031[1], 12032[1], 12034[1], 12035[1], 12036[1], 12037[1], 12041[1], 12042[1], 12044[1], 12045[1], 12046[1], 12047[1], 12051[1], 12052[1], 12053[1], 12054[1], 12055[1], 12056[1], 12057[1], 13100[1], 13101[1], 13102[1], 13120[1], 13121[1], 13122[1], 13131[1], 13132[1], 13133[1], 13151[1], 13152[1], 13153[1], 36000[1], 36400[1], 36405[1], 36406[1], 36410[1], 36420[1], 36425[1], 36430[1], 36440[1], 36591[0], 36592[0], 36600[1], 36640[1], 43752[1], 51701[1], 51702[1], 51703[1], 62320[0], 62321[0], 62322[0], 62323[0], 62324[0], 62325[0], 62326[0], 62327[0], 64400[0], 64405[0], 64408[0], 64415[0], 64416[0], 64417[0], 64418[0], 64420[0], 64421[0], 64425[0], 64430[0], 64435[0], 64445[0], 64446[0], 64447[0], 64448[0], 64449[0], 64450[0], 64451[0], 64454[0], 64461[0], 64462[0], 64463[0], 64479[0], 64480[0], 64483[0], 64484[0], 64486[0], 64487[0], 64488[0], 64489[0], 64490[0], 64491[0], 64492[0], 64493[0], 64494[0], 64495[0], 64505[0], 64510[0], 64517[0], 64520[0], 64530[0], 65820[1], 66030[1], 66172[1], 66183[1], 66625[1], 66680[1], 66740[1], 66989[1], 66991[1], 67005[1], 67255[1], 67500[1], 68130[1], 68200[1], 69990[0], 92012[1], 92014[1], 92018[1], 92019[1], 92504[1], 93000[1], 93005[1], 93010[1], 93040[1], 93041[1], 93042[1], 93318[1], 93355[1], 94002[1], 94200[1], 94680[1], 94681[1], 94690[1], 95812[1], 95813[1], 95816[1], 95819[1], 95822[1], 95829[1], 95955[1], 96360[1], 96361[1], 96365[1], 96366[1], 96367[1], 96368[1], 96372[1], 96374[1], 96375[1], 96376[1], 96377[1], 96523[0], 97597[1], 97598[1], 97602[1], 99155[0], 99156[0], 99157[0], 99211[1], 99212[1], 99213[1], 99214[1], 99215[1], 99217[1], 99218[1], 99219[1], 99220[1], 99221[1], 99222[1], 99223[1], 99231[1], 99232[1], 99233[1], 99234[1], 99235[1], 99236[1], 99238[1], 99239[1], 99241[1], 99242[1], 99243[1], 99244[1], 99245[1], 99251[1], 99252[1], 99253[1], 99254[1], 99255[1], 99291[1], 99292[1], 99304[1], 99305[1], 99306[1], 99307[1], 99308[1], 99309[1], 99310[1], 99315[1], 99316[1], 99334[1], 99335[1], 99336[1], 99337[1], 99347[1], 99348[1], 99349[1], 99350[1], 99374[1], 99375[1], 99377[1], 99378[1], 99446[0], 99447[0], 99448[0], 99449[0], 99451[0], 99452[0], 99495[0], 99496[0], G0463[1], G0471[1], J0670[1], J2001[1]
66172	0213T[0], 0216T[0], 0253T[1], 0449T[1], 0474T[1], 0596T[1], 0597T[1], 0616T[1], 0617T[1], 0618T[1], 0621T[1], 0622T[1], 0671T[1], 0708T[1], 0709T[1], 11000[1], 11001[1], 11004[1], 11005[1], 11006[1], 11042[1], 11043[1], 11044[1], 11045[1], 11046[1], 11047[1], 12001[1], 12002[1], 12004[1], 12005[1], 12006[1], 12007[1], 12011[1], 12013[1], 12014[1], 12015[1], 12016[1], 12017[1], 12018[1], 12020[1], 12021[1], 12031[1], 12032[1], 12034[1], 12035[1], 12036[1], 12037[1], 12041[1], 12042[1], 12044[1], 12045[1], 12046[1], 12047[1], 12051[1], 12052[1], 12053[1], 12054[1], 12055[1], 12056[1], 12057[1], 13100[1], 13101[1], 13102[1], 13120[1], 13121[1], 13122[1], 13131[1], 13132[1], 13133[1], 13151[1], 13152[1], 13153[1], 36000[1], 36400[1], 36405[1], 36406[1], 36410[1], 36420[1], 36425[1], 36430[1], 36440[1], 36591[0], 36592[0], 36600[1], 36640[1], 43752[1], 51701[1], 51702[1], 51703[1], 62320[0], 62321[0], 62322[0], 62323[0], 62324[0], 62325[0], 62326[0], 62327[0], 64400[0], 64405[0], 64408[0], 64415[0], 64416[0], 64417[0], 64418[0], 64420[0], 64421[0], 64425[0], 64430[0], 64435[0], 64445[0], 64446[0], 64447[0], 64448[0], 64449[0], 64450[0], 64451[0], 64454[0], 64461[0], 64462[0], 64463[0], 64479[0], 64480[0], 64483[0], 64484[0], 64486[0], 64487[0], 64488[0], 64489[0], 64490[0], 64491[0], 64492[0], 64493[0], 64494[0], 64495[0], 64505[0], 64510[0], 64517[0], 64520[0], 64530[0], 65820[1], 65850[1], 66183[1], 66250[1], 66625[1], 66680[1], 66740[1], 66989[1], 66991[1], 67005[1], 67015[1], 67250[1], 67255[1], 67500[1], 68130[1], 68200[1], 69990[0], 92012[1], 92014[1], 92018[1], 92019[1], 93000[1], 93005[1], 93010[1], 93040[1], 93041[1], 93042[1], 93318[1], 93355[1], 94002[1], 94200[1], 94680[1], 94681[1], 94690[1], 95812[1], 95813[1], 95816[1], 95819[1], 95822[1], 95829[1], 95955[1], 96360[1], 96361[1], 96365[1], 96366[1], 96367[1], 96368[1], 96372[1], 96374[1], 96375[1], 96376[1], 96377[1], 96523[0], 97597[1], 97598[1], 97602[1], 99155[0], 99156[0], 99157[0], 99211[1], 99212[1], 99213[1], 99214[1], 99215[1], 99217[1], 99218[1], 99219[1], 99220[1], 99221[1], 99222[1], 99223[1], 99231[1], 99232[1], 99233[1], 99234[1], 99235[1], 99236[1], 99238[1], 99239[1], 99241[1], 99242[1], 99243[1], 99244[1], 99245[1], 99251[1], 99252[1], 99253[1], 99254[1], 99255[1], 99291[1], 99292[1], 99304[1], 99305[1], 99306[1], 99307[1], 99308[1], 99309[1], 99310[1], 99315[1], 99316[1], 99334[1], 99335[1], 99336[1], 99337[1], 99347[1], 99348[1], 99349[1], 99350[1], 99374[1], 99375[1], 99377[1], 99378[1], 99446[0], 99447[0], 99448[0], 99449[0], 99451[0], 99452[0], 99495[0], 99496[0], G0463[1], G0471[1], J0670[1], J2001[1]
66174	00140[0], 0596T[1], 0597T[1], 0616T[1], 0617T[1], 0618T[1], 0699T[1], 0708T[1], 0709T[1], 12001[1], 12002[1], 12004[1], 12005[1], 12006[1], 12007[1], 12011[1], 12013[1], 12014[1], 12015[1], 12016[1], 12017[1], 12018[1], 12020[1], 12021[1], 12031[1], 12032[1], 12034[1], 12035[1], 12036[1], 12037[1], 12041[1], 12042[1], 12044[1], 12045[1], 12046[1], 12047[1], 12051[1], 12052[1], 12053[1], 12054[1], 12055[1], 12056[1], 12057[1], 13100[1], 13101[1], 13102[1], 13120[1], 13121[1], 13122[1], 13131[1], 13132[1], 13133[1], 13151[1], 13152[1], 13153[1], 36000[1], 36400[1], 36405[1], 36406[1], 36410[1], 36420[1], 36425[1], 36430[1], 36440[1], 36591[0], 36592[0], 36600[1], 36640[1], 43752[1], 51701[1], 51702[1], 51703[1], 62320[0], 62321[0], 62322[0], 62323[0], 62324[0], 62325[0], 62326[0], 62327[0], 64400[0], 64405[0], 64408[0], 64415[0], 64416[0], 64417[0], 64418[0], 64420[0], 64421[0], 64425[0], 64430[0], 64435[0], 64445[0], 64446[0], 64447[0], 64448[0], 64449[0], 64450[0], 64451[0], 64454[0], 64461[0], 64462[0], 64463[0], 64479[0], 64480[0], 64483[0], 64484[0], 64486[0], 64487[0], 64488[0], 64489[0], 64490[0], 64491[0], 64492[0], 64493[0], 64494[0], 64495[0], 64505[0], 64510[0], 64517[0], 64520[0], 64530[0], 65800[1], 65810[1], 65815[1], 65820[1], 65860[1], 66020[1], 66030[1], 66500[1], 66505[1], 66625[1], 66630[1], 66635[1], 66682[1], 67250[1], 67255[1], 67500[1], 67515[1], 68200[1], 69990[0], 92012[1], 92014[1], 92018[1], 92019[1], 93000[1], 93005[1], 93010[1], 93040[1], 93041[1], 93042[1], 93318[1], 93355[1], 94002[1], 94200[1], 94680[1], 94681[1], 94690[1], 95812[1], 95813[1], 95816[1], 95819[1], 95822[1], 95829[1], 95955[1], 96360[1], 96361[1], 96365[1], 96366[1], 96367[1], 96368[1], 96372[1], 96374[1], 96375[1], 96376[1], 96377[1], 96523[0], 99155[0], 99156[0], 99157[0], 99211[1], 99212[1], 99213[1], 99214[1], 99215[1], 99217[1], 99218[1], 99219[1], 99220[1], 99221[1], 99222[1], 99223[1], 99231[1], 99232[1], 99233[1], 99234[1], 99235[1], 99236[1], 99238[1], 99239[1], 99241[1], 99242[1], 99243[1], 99244[1], 99245[1], 99251[1], 99252[1], 99253[1], 99254[1], 99255[1], 99291[1], 99292[1], 99304[1], 99305[1], 99306[1], 99307[1], 99308[1], 99309[1], 99310[1], 99315[1], 99316[1], 99334[1], 99335[1], 99336[1], 99337[1], 99347[1], 99348[1], 99349[1], 99350[1], 99374[1], 99375[1], 99377[1], 99378[1], 99446[0], 99447[0], 99448[0], 99449[0], 99451[0], 99452[0], 99495[0], 99496[0], G0463[1], G0471[1]
66175	00140[0], 0596T[1], 0597T[1], 0616T[1], 0617T[1], 0618T[1], 0699T[1], 0708T[1], 0709T[1], 12001[1], 12002[1], 12004[1], 12005[1], 12006[1], 12007[1], 12011[1], 12013[1], 12014[1], 12015[1], 12016[1], 12017[1], 12018[1], 12020[1], 12021[1], 12031[1], 12032[1], 12034[1], 12035[1], 12036[1], 12037[1], 12041[1], 12042[1], 12044[1], 12045[1], 12046[1], 12047[1], 12051[1], 12052[1], 12053[1], 12054[1], 12055[1], 12056[1], 12057[1], 13100[1], 13101[1], 13102[1], 13120[1], 13121[1], 13122[1], 13131[1], 13132[1], 13133[1], 13151[1], 13152[1], 13153[1], 36000[1], 36400[1], 36405[1], 36406[1], 36410[1], 36420[1], 36425[1], 36430[1], 36440[1], 36591[0], 36592[0], 36600[1], 36640[1], 43752[1], 51701[1], 51702[1], 51703[1], 62320[0], 62321[0], 62322[0], 62323[0], 62324[0], 62325[0], 62326[0], 62327[0], 64400[0], 64405[0], 64408[0], 64415[0], 64416[0], 64417[0], 64418[0], 64420[0], 64421[0], 64425[0], 64430[0], 64435[0], 64445[0], 64446[0], 64447[0], 64448[0], 64449[0], 64450[0], 64451[0], 64454[0], 64461[0], 64462[0], 64463[0], 64479[0], 64480[0], 64483[0], 64484[0], 64486[0], 64487[0], 64488[0],

0 = Modifier usage not allowed or inappropriate 1 = Modifier usage allowed

Code 1	Code 2
	64489[0], 64490[0], 64491[0], 64492[0], 64493[0], 64494[0], 64495[0], 64505[0], 64510[0], 64517[0], 64520[0], 64530[0], 65800[1], 65810[1], 65815[1], 65820[1], 65860[1], 66020[1], 66030[1], 66174[1], 66500[1], 66505[1], 66625[1], 66630[1], 66635[1], 66682[1], 67250[1], 67255[1], 67500[1], 67515[1], 68200[1], 69990[0], 92012[1], 92014[1], 92018[1], 92019[1], 93000[1], 93005[1], 93010[1], 93040[1], 93041[1], 93042[1], 93318[1], 93355[1], 94002[1], 94200[1], 94680[1], 94681[1], 94690[1], 95812[1], 95813[1], 95816[1], 95819[1], 95822[1], 95829[1], 95955[1], 96360[1], 96361[1], 96365[1], 96366[1], 96367[1], 96368[1], 96372[1], 96374[1], 96375[1], 96376[1], 96377[1], 96523[0], 99155[0], 99156[0], 99157[0], 99211[1], 99212[1], 99213[1], 99214[1], 99215[1], 99217[1], 99218[1], 99219[1], 99220[1], 99221[1], 99222[1], 99223[1], 99231[1], 99232[1], 99233[1], 99234[1], 99235[1], 99236[1], 99238[1], 99239[1], 99241[1], 99242[1], 99243[1], 99244[1], 99245[1], 99251[1], 99252[1], 99253[1], 99254[1], 99255[1], 99291[1], 99292[1], 99304[1], 99305[1], 99306[1], 99307[1], 99308[1], 99309[1], 99310[1], 99315[1], 99316[1], 99334[1], 99335[1], 99336[1], 99337[1], 99347[1], 99348[1], 99349[1], 99350[1], 99374[1], 99375[1], 99377[1], 99378[1], 99446[0], 99447[0], 99448[0], 99449[0], 99451[0], 99452[0], 99495[0], 99496[0], G0463[1], G0471[1]
66179	0213T[0], 0216T[0], 0253T[1], 0449T[1], 0450T[1], 0474T[1], 0596T[1], 0597T[1], 0671T[1], 0708T[1], 0709T[1], 12001[1], 12002[1], 12004[1], 12005[1], 12006[1], 12007[1], 12011[1], 12013[1], 12014[1], 12015[1], 12016[1], 12017[1], 12018[1], 12020[1], 12021[1], 12031[1], 12032[1], 12034[1], 12035[1], 12036[1], 12037[1], 12041[1], 12042[1], 12044[1], 12045[1], 12046[1], 12047[1], 12051[1], 12052[1], 12053[1], 12054[1], 12055[1], 12056[1], 12057[1], 13100[1], 13101[1], 13102[1], 13120[1], 13121[1], 13122[1], 13131[1], 13132[1], 13133[1], 13151[1], 13152[1], 13153[1], 36000[1], 36400[1], 36405[1], 36406[1], 36410[1], 36420[1], 36425[1], 36430[1], 36440[1], 36591[0], 36592[0], 36600[1], 36640[1], 43752[1], 51701[1], 51702[1], 51703[1], 62320[0], 62321[0], 62322[0], 62323[0], 62324[0], 62325[0], 62326[0], 62327[0], 64400[0], 64405[0], 64408[0], 64415[0], 64416[0], 64417[0], 64418[0], 64420[0], 64421[0], 64425[0], 64430[0], 64435[0], 64445[0], 64446[0], 64447[0], 64448[0], 64449[0], 64450[0], 64451[0], 64454[0], 64461[0], 64462[0], 64463[0], 64479[0], 64480[0], 64483[0], 64484[0], 64486[0], 64487[0], 64488[0], 64489[0], 64490[0], 64491[0], 64492[0], 64493[0], 64494[0], 64495[0], 64505[0], 64510[0], 64517[0], 64520[0], 64530[0], 66183[1], 66184[1], 66185[1], 66989[1], 66991[1], 67250[1], 67255[1], 67500[1], 69990[0], 92012[1], 92014[1], 92018[1], 92019[1], 93000[1], 93005[1], 93010[1], 93040[1], 93041[1], 93042[1], 93318[1], 93355[1], 94002[1], 94200[1], 94680[1], 94681[1], 94690[1], 95812[1], 95813[1], 95816[1], 95819[1], 95822[1], 95829[1], 95955[1], 96360[1], 96361[1], 96365[1], 96366[1], 96367[1], 96368[1], 96372[1], 96374[1], 96375[1], 96376[1], 96377[1], 96523[0], 99155[0], 99156[0], 99157[0], 99211[1], 99212[1], 99213[1], 99214[1], 99215[1], 99217[1], 99218[1], 99219[1], 99220[1], 99221[1], 99222[1], 99223[1], 99231[1], 99232[1], 99233[1], 99234[1], 99235[1], 99236[1], 99238[1], 99239[1], 99241[1], 99242[1], 99243[1], 99244[1], 99245[1], 99251[1], 99252[1], 99253[1], 99254[1], 99255[1], 99291[1], 99292[1], 99304[1], 99305[1], 99306[1], 99307[1], 99308[1], 99309[1], 99310[1], 99315[1], 99316[1], 99334[1], 99335[1], 99336[1], 99337[1], 99347[1], 99348[1], 99349[1], 99350[1], 99374[1], 99375[1], 99377[1], 99378[1], 99446[0], 99447[0], 99448[0], 99449[0], 99451[0], 99452[0], 99495[0], 99496[0], G0463[1], G0471[1]
66180	0213T[0], 0216T[0], 0253T[1], 0449T[1], 0450T[1], 0474T[1], 0596T[1], 0597T[1], 0671T[1], 0708T[1], 0709T[1], 12001[1], 12002[1], 12004[1], 12005[1], 12006[1], 12007[1], 12011[1], 12013[1], 12014[1], 12015[1], 12016[1], 12017[1], 12018[1], 12020[1], 12021[1], 12031[1], 12032[1], 12034[1], 12035[1], 12036[1], 12037[1], 12041[1], 12042[1], 12044[1], 12045[1], 12046[1], 12047[1], 12051[1], 12052[1], 12053[1], 12054[1], 12055[1], 12056[1], 12057[1], 13100[1], 13101[1], 13102[1], 13120[1], 13121[1], 13122[1], 13131[1], 13132[1], 13133[1], 13151[1], 13152[1], 13153[1], 36000[1], 36400[1], 36405[1], 36406[1], 36410[1], 36420[1], 36425[1], 36430[1], 36440[1], 36591[0], 36592[0], 36600[1], 36640[1], 43752[1], 51701[1], 51702[1], 51703[1], 62320[0], 62321[0], 62322[0], 62323[0], 62324[0], 62325[0], 62326[0], 62327[0], 64400[0], 64405[0], 64408[0], 64415[0], 64416[0], 64417[0], 64418[0], 64420[0], 64421[0], 64425[0], 64430[0], 64435[0], 64445[0], 64446[0], 64447[0], 64448[0], 64449[0], 64450[0], 64451[0], 64454[0], 64461[0], 64462[0], 64463[0], 64479[0], 64480[0], 64483[0], 64484[0], 64486[0], 64487[0], 64488[0], 64489[0], 64490[0], 64491[0], 64492[0], 64493[0], 64494[0], 64495[0], 64505[0], 64510[0], 64517[0], 64520[0], 64530[0], 66179[1], 66183[1], 66184[1], 66185[1], 66989[1], 66991[1], 67250[1], 67255[1], 67500[1], 68320[1], 69990[0], 92012[1], 92014[1], 92018[1], 92019[1], 93000[1], 93005[1], 93010[1], 93040[1], 93041[1], 93042[1], 93318[1], 93355[1], 94002[1], 94200[1], 94680[1], 94681[1], 94690[1], 95812[1], 95813[1], 95816[1], 95819[1], 95822[1], 95829[1], 95955[1], 96360[1], 96361[1], 96365[1], 96366[1], 96367[1], 96368[1], 96372[1], 96374[1], 96375[1], 96376[1], 96377[1], 96523[0], 99155[0], 99156[0], 99157[0], 99211[1], 99212[1], 99213[1], 99214[1], 99215[1], 99217[1], 99218[1], 99219[1], 99220[1], 99221[1], 99222[1], 99223[1], 99231[1], 99232[1], 99233[1], 99234[1], 99235[1], 99236[1], 99238[1], 99239[1], 99241[1], 99242[1], 99243[1], 99244[1], 99245[1], 99251[1], 99252[1], 99253[1], 99254[1], 99255[1], 99291[1], 99292[1], 99304[1], 99305[1], 99306[1], 99307[1], 99308[1], 99309[1], 99310[1], 99315[1], 99316[1], 99334[1], 99335[1], 99336[1], 99337[1], 99347[1], 99348[1], 99349[1], 99350[1], 99374[1], 99375[1], 99377[1], 99378[1], 99446[0], 99447[0], 99448[0], 99449[0], 99451[0], 99452[0], 99495[0], 99496[0], G0463[1], G0471[1]
66183	00140[0], 0213T[0], 0216T[0], 0253T[1], 0449T[1], 0450T[1], 0474T[1], 0596T[1], 0597T[1], 0671T[1], 0699T[1], 0708T[1], 0709T[1], 11000[1], 11001[1], 11004[1], 11005[1], 11006[1], 11042[1], 11043[1], 11044[1], 11045[1], 11046[1], 11047[1], 12001[1], 12002[1], 12004[1], 12005[1], 12006[1], 12007[1], 12011[1], 12013[1], 12014[1], 12015[1], 12016[1], 12017[1], 12018[1], 12020[1], 12021[1], 12031[1], 12032[1], 12034[1], 12035[1], 12036[1], 12037[1], 12041[1], 12042[1], 12044[1], 12045[1], 12046[1], 12047[1], 12051[1], 12052[1], 12053[1], 12054[1], 12055[1], 12056[1], 12057[1], 13100[1], 13101[1], 13102[1], 13120[1], 13121[1], 13122[1], 13131[1], 13132[1], 13133[1], 13151[1], 13152[1], 13153[1], 36000[1], 36400[1], 36405[1], 36406[1], 36410[1], 36420[1], 36425[1], 36430[1], 36440[1], 36591[0], 36592[0], 36600[1], 36640[1], 43752[1], 51701[1], 51702[1], 51703[1], 62320[0], 62321[0], 62322[0], 62323[0], 62324[0], 62325[0], 62326[0], 62327[0], 64400[0], 64405[0], 64408[0], 64415[0], 64416[0], 64417[0], 64418[0], 64420[0], 64421[0], 64425[0], 64430[0], 64435[0], 64445[0], 64446[0], 64447[0], 64448[0], 64449[0], 64450[0], 64451[0], 64454[0], 64461[0], 64462[0], 64463[0], 64479[0], 64480[0], 64483[0], 64484[0], 64486[0], 64487[0], 64488[0], 64489[0], 64490[0], 64491[0], 64492[0], 64493[0], 64494[0], 64495[0], 64505[0], 64510[0], 64517[0], 64520[0], 64530[0], 65800[1], 65810[1], 65815[1], 66020[1], 66030[1], 66184[1], 66185[1], 66989[1], 66991[1], 67500[1], 67515[1], 69990[0], 92012[1], 92014[1], 92018[1], 92019[1], 93000[1], 93005[1], 93010[1], 93040[1], 93041[1], 93042[1], 93318[1], 93355[1], 94002[1], 94200[1], 94680[1], 94681[1], 94690[1], 95812[1], 95813[1], 95816[1], 95819[1], 95822[1], 95829[1], 95955[1], 96360[1], 96361[1], 96365[1], 96366[1], 96367[1], 96368[1], 96372[1], 96374[1], 96375[1], 96376[1], 96377[1], 96523[0], 97597[1], 97598[1], 97602[1], 99155[0], 99156[0], 99157[0], 99211[1], 99212[1], 99213[1], 99214[1], 99215[1], 99217[1], 99218[1], 99219[1], 99220[1], 99221[1], 99222[1], 99223[1], 99231[1], 99232[1], 99233[1], 99234[1], 99235[1], 99236[1], 99238[1], 99239[1], 99241[1], 99242[1], 99243[1], 99244[1], 99245[1], 99251[1], 99252[1], 99253[1], 99254[1], 99255[1], 99291[1], 99292[1], 99304[1], 99305[1], 99306[1], 99307[1], 99308[1], 99309[1], 99310[1], 99315[1], 99316[1], 99334[1], 99335[1], 99336[1], 99337[1], 99347[1], 99348[1], 99349[1], 99350[1], 99374[1], 99375[1], 99377[1], 99378[1], 99446[0], 99447[0], 99448[0], 99449[0], 99451[0], 99452[0], G0463[1], G0471[1]
66184	0213T[0], 0216T[0], 0449T[1], 0450T[1], 0474T[1], 0596T[1], 0597T[1], 0671T[1], 0708T[1], 0709T[1], 11000[1], 11001[1], 11004[1], 11005[1], 11006[1], 11042[1], 11043[1], 11044[1], 11045[1], 11046[1], 11047[1], 12001[1], 12002[1], 12004[1], 12005[1], 12006[1], 12007[1], 12011[1], 12013[1], 12014[1], 12015[1], 12016[1], 12017[1], 12018[1], 12020[1], 12021[1], 12031[1], 12032[1], 12034[1], 12035[1], 12036[1], 12037[1], 12041[1], 12042[1], 12044[1], 12045[1], 12046[1], 12047[1], 12051[1], 12052[1], 12053[1], 12054[1], 12055[1], 12056[1], 12057[1], 13100[1], 13101[1], 13102[1], 13120[1], 13121[1], 13122[1], 13131[1], 13132[1], 13133[1], 13151[1], 13152[1], 13153[1], 36000[1], 36400[1], 36405[1], 36406[1], 36410[1], 36420[1], 36425[1], 36430[1], 36440[1], 36591[0], 36592[0], 36600[1], 36640[1], 43752[1], 51701[1], 51702[1], 51703[1], 62320[0], 62321[0], 62322[0], 62323[0], 62324[0], 62325[0], 62326[0], 62327[0], 64400[0], 64405[0], 64408[0], 64415[0], 64416[0], 64417[0], 64418[0], 64420[0], 64421[0], 64425[0], 64430[0], 64435[0], 64445[0], 64446[0], 64447[0], 64448[0], 64449[0], 64450[0], 64451[0], 64454[0], 64461[0], 64462[0], 64463[0], 64479[0], 64480[0], 64483[0], 64484[0], 64486[0], 64487[0], 64488[0], 64489[0], 64490[0], 64491[0], 64492[0], 64493[0], 64494[0], 64495[0], 64505[0], 64510[0], 64517[0], 64520[0], 64530[0], 65820[1], 66989[1], 66991[1], 67250[1], 67255[1], 67500[1], 69990[0], 92012[1], 92014[1], 92018[1], 92019[1], 93000[1], 93005[1], 93010[1], 93040[1], 93041[1], 93042[1], 93318[1], 93355[1], 94002[1], 94200[1], 94680[1], 94681[1], 94690[1], 95812[1], 95813[1], 95816[1], 95819[1], 95822[1], 95829[1], 95955[1], 96360[1], 96361[1], 96365[1], 96366[1], 96367[1], 96368[1], 96372[1], 96374[1], 96375[1], 96376[1], 96377[1], 96523[0], 97597[1], 97598[1], 97602[1], 99155[0], 99156[0], 99157[0], 99211[1], 99212[1], 99213[1], 99214[1], 99215[1], 99217[1], 99218[1], 99219[1], 99220[1], 99221[1], 99222[1], 99223[1], 99231[1], 99232[1], 99233[1], 99234[1], 99235[1], 99236[1], 99238[1], 99239[1], 99241[1], 99242[1], 99243[1], 99244[1], 99245[1], 99251[1], 99252[1], 99253[1], 99254[1], 99255[1], 99291[1], 99292[1], 99304[1], 99305[1], 99306[1], 99307[1], 99308[1], 99309[1], 99310[1], 99315[1], 99316[1], 99334[1], 99335[1], 99336[1], 99337[1], 99347[1], 99348[1], 99349[1], 99350[1], 99374[1], 99375[1], 99377[1], 99378[1], 99446[0], 99447[0], 99448[0], 99449[0], 99451[0], 99452[0], 99495[0], 99496[0], G0463[1], G0471[1], J0670[1], J2001[1]
66185	0213T[0], 0216T[0], 0449T[1], 0450T[1], 0474T[1], 0596T[1], 0597T[1], 0671T[1], 0708T[1], 0709T[1], 11000[1], 11001[1], 11004[1], 11005[1], 11006[1], 11042[1], 11043[1], 11044[1], 11045[1], 11046[1], 11047[1], 12001[1], 12002[1], 12004[1], 12005[1], 12006[1], 12007[1], 12011[1], 12013[1], 12014[1], 12015[1], 12016[1], 12017[1], 12018[1], 12020[1], 12021[1], 12031[1], 12032[1], 12034[1], 12035[1], 12036[1], 12037[1], 12041[1], 12042[1], 12044[1], 12045[1], 12046[1], 12047[1], 12051[1], 12052[1], 12053[1], 12054[1], 12055[1], 12056[1], 12057[1], 13100[1], 13101[1], 13102[1], 13120[1], 13121[1], 13122[1], 13131[1], 13132[1], 13133[1], 13151[1], 13152[1], 13153[1], 36000[1], 36400[1], 36405[1], 36406[1], 36410[1], 36420[1], 36425[1], 36430[1], 36440[1], 36591[0], 36592[0], 36600[1], 36640[1], 43752[1], 51701[1], 51702[1], 51703[1], 62320[0], 62321[0], 62322[0], 62323[0], 62324[0], 62325[0], 62326[0], 62327[0], 64400[0], 64405[0], 64408[0], 64415[0], 64416[0], 64417[0], 64418[0], 64420[0], 64421[0], 64425[0], 64430[0], 64435[0], 64445[0], 64446[0], 64447[0], 64448[0], 64449[0], 64450[0], 64451[0], 64454[0], 64461[0], 64462[0], 64463[0], 64479[0], 64480[0], 64483[0], 64484[0], 64486[0], 64487[0], 64488[0], 64489[0], 64490[0], 64491[0], 64492[0], 64493[0], 64494[0], 64495[0], 64505[0], 64510[0], 64517[0], 64520[0], 64530[0], 65820[1], 66184[1], 66991[1], 67250[1], 67255[1], 67500[1], 69990[0], 92012[1], 92014[1], 92018[1], 92019[1], 93000[1], 93005[1], 93010[1], 93040[1], 93041[1], 93042[1], 93318[1], 93355[1], 94002[1], 94200[1], 94680[1], 94681[1], 94690[1], 95812[1], 95813[1], 95816[1], 95819[1], 95822[1], 95829[1], 95955[1], 96360[1], 96361[1], 96365[1], 96366[1], 96367[1], 96368[1], 96372[1], 96374[1], 96375[1], 96376[1], 96377[1], 96523[0], 97597[1], 97598[1], 97602[1],

0 = Modifier usage not allowed or inappropriate 1 = Modifier usage allowed

Code 1	Code 2
	99155[0], 99156[0], 99157[0], 99211[1], 99212[1], 99213[1], 99214[1], 99215[1], 99217[1], 99218[1], 99219[1], 99220[1], 99221[1], 99222[1], 99223[1], 99231[1], 99232[1], 99233[1], 99234[1], 99235[1], 99236[1], 99238[1], 99239[1], 99241[1], 99242[1], 99243[1], 99244[1], 99245[1], 99251[1], 99252[1], 99253[1], 99254[1], 99255[1], 99291[1], 99292[1], 99304[1], 99305[1], 99306[1], 99307[1], 99308[1], 99309[1], 99310[1], 99315[1], 99316[1], 99334[1], 99335[1], 99336[1], 99337[1], 99347[1], 99348[1], 99349[1], 99350[1], 99374[1], 99375[1], 99377[1], 99378[1], 99446[0], 99447[0], 99448[0], 99449[0], 99451[0], 99452[0], 99495[0], 99496[0], G0463[1], G0471[1], J0670[1], J2001[1]
66225	0213T[0], 0216T[0], 0596T[1], 0597T[1], 0708T[1], 0709T[1], 12001[1], 12002[1], 12004[1], 12005[1], 12006[1], 12007[1], 12011[1], 12013[1], 12014[1], 12015[1], 12016[1], 12017[1], 12018[1], 12020[1], 12021[1], 12031[1], 12032[1], 12034[1], 12035[1], 12036[1], 12037[1], 12041[1], 12042[1], 12044[1], 12045[1], 12046[1], 12047[1], 12051[1], 12052[1], 12053[1], 12054[1], 12055[1], 12056[1], 12057[1], 13100[1], 13101[1], 13102[1], 13120[1], 13121[1], 13122[1], 13131[1], 13132[1], 13133[1], 13151[1], 13152[1], 13153[1], 36000[1], 36400[1], 36405[1], 36406[1], 36410[1], 36420[1], 36425[1], 36430[1], 36440[1], 36591[0], 36592[0], 36600[1], 36640[1], 43752[1], 51701[1], 51702[1], 51703[1], 62320[0], 62321[0], 62322[0], 62323[0], 62324[0], 62325[0], 62326[0], 62327[0], 64400[0], 64405[0], 64408[0], 64415[0], 64416[0], 64417[0], 64418[0], 64420[0], 64421[0], 64425[0], 64430[0], 64435[0], 64445[0], 64446[0], 64447[0], 64448[0], 64449[0], 64450[0], 64451[0], 64454[0], 64461[0], 64462[0], 64463[0], 64479[0], 64480[0], 64483[0], 64484[0], 64486[0], 64487[0], 64488[0], 64489[0], 64490[0], 64491[0], 64492[0], 64493[0], 64494[0], 64495[0], 64505[0], 64510[0], 64517[0], 64520[0], 64530[0], 66130[1], 67500[1], 69990[0], 92012[1], 92014[1], 92018[1], 92019[1], 93000[1], 93005[1], 93010[1], 93040[1], 93041[1], 93042[1], 93318[1], 93355[1], 94002[1], 94200[1], 94680[1], 94681[1], 94690[1], 95812[1], 95813[1], 95816[1], 95819[1], 95822[1], 95829[1], 95955[1], 96360[1], 96361[1], 96365[1], 96366[1], 96367[1], 96368[1], 96372[1], 96374[1], 96375[1], 96376[1], 96377[1], 96523[0], 99155[0], 99156[0], 99157[0], 99211[1], 99212[1], 99213[1], 99214[1], 99215[1], 99217[1], 99218[1], 99219[1], 99220[1], 99221[1], 99222[1], 99223[1], 99231[1], 99232[1], 99233[1], 99234[1], 99235[1], 99236[1], 99238[1], 99239[1], 99241[1], 99242[1], 99243[1], 99244[1], 99245[1], 99251[1], 99252[1], 99253[1], 99254[1], 99255[1], 99291[1], 99292[1], 99304[1], 99305[1], 99306[1], 99307[1], 99308[1], 99309[1], 99310[1], 99315[1], 99316[1], 99334[1], 99335[1], 99336[1], 99337[1], 99347[1], 99348[1], 99349[1], 99350[1], 99374[1], 99375[1], 99377[1], 99378[1], 99446[0], 99447[0], 99448[0], 99449[0], 99451[0], 99452[0], 99495[0], 99496[0], G0463[1], G0471[1]
66250	0213T[0], 0216T[0], 0596T[1], 0597T[1], 0708T[1], 0709T[1], 11000[1], 11001[1], 11004[1], 11005[1], 11006[1], 11042[1], 11043[1], 11044[1], 11045[1], 11046[1], 11047[1], 12001[1], 12002[1], 12004[1], 12005[1], 12006[1], 12007[1], 12011[1], 12013[1], 12014[1], 12015[1], 12016[1], 12017[1], 12018[1], 12020[1], 12021[1], 12031[1], 12032[1], 12034[1], 12035[1], 12036[1], 12037[1], 12041[1], 12042[1], 12044[1], 12045[1], 12046[1], 12047[1], 12051[1], 12052[1], 12053[1], 12054[1], 12055[1], 12056[1], 12057[1], 13100[1], 13101[1], 13102[1], 13120[1], 13121[1], 13122[1], 13131[1], 13132[1], 13133[1], 13151[1], 13152[1], 13153[1], 36000[1], 36400[1], 36405[1], 36406[1], 36410[1], 36420[1], 36425[1], 36430[1], 36440[1], 36591[0], 36592[0], 36600[1], 36640[1], 43752[1], 51701[1], 51702[1], 51703[1], 62320[0], 62321[0], 62322[0], 62323[0], 62324[0], 62325[0], 62326[0], 62327[0], 64400[0], 64405[0], 64408[0], 64415[0], 64416[0], 64417[0], 64418[0], 64420[0], 64421[0], 64425[0], 64430[0], 64435[0], 64445[0], 64446[0], 64447[0], 64448[0], 64449[0], 64450[0], 64451[0], 64454[0], 64461[0], 64462[0], 64463[0], 64479[0], 64480[0], 64483[0], 64484[0], 64486[0], 64487[0], 64488[0], 64489[0], 64490[0], 64491[0], 64492[0], 64493[0], 64494[0], 64495[0], 64505[0], 64510[0], 64517[0], 64520[0], 64530[0], 67500[1], 67515[1], 69990[0], 92012[1], 92014[1], 92018[1], 92019[1], 93000[1], 93005[1], 93010[1], 93040[1], 93041[1], 93042[1], 93318[1], 93355[1], 94002[1], 94200[1], 94680[1], 94681[1], 94690[1], 95812[1], 95813[1], 95816[1], 95819[1], 95822[1], 95829[1], 95955[1], 96360[1], 96361[1], 96365[1], 96366[1], 96367[1], 96368[1], 96372[1], 96374[1], 96375[1], 96376[1], 96377[1], 96523[0], 97597[1], 97598[1], 97602[1], 99155[0], 99156[0], 99157[0], 99211[1], 99212[1], 99213[1], 99214[1], 99215[1], 99217[1], 99218[1], 99219[1], 99220[1], 99221[1], 99222[1], 99223[1], 99231[1], 99232[1], 99233[1], 99234[1], 99235[1], 99236[1], 99238[1], 99239[1], 99241[1], 99242[1], 99243[1], 99244[1], 99245[1], 99251[1], 99252[1], 99253[1], 99254[1], 99255[1], 99291[1], 99292[1], 99304[1], 99305[1], 99306[1], 99307[1], 99308[1], 99309[1], 99310[1], 99315[1], 99316[1], 99334[1], 99335[1], 99336[1], 99337[1], 99347[1], 99348[1], 99349[1], 99350[1], 99374[1], 99375[1], 99377[1], 99378[1], 99446[0], 99447[0], 99448[0], 99449[0], 99451[0], 99452[0], 99495[0], 99496[0], G0463[1], G0471[1], J0670[1], J2001[1]
66500	0213T[0], 0216T[0], 0596T[1], 0597T[1], 0708T[1], 0709T[1], 11000[1], 11001[1], 11004[1], 11005[1], 11006[1], 11042[1], 11043[1], 11044[1], 11045[1], 11046[1], 11047[1], 12001[1], 12002[1], 12004[1], 12005[1], 12006[1], 12007[1], 12011[1], 12013[1], 12014[1], 12015[1], 12016[1], 12017[1], 12018[1], 12020[1], 12021[1], 12031[1], 12032[1], 12034[1], 12035[1], 12036[1], 12037[1], 12041[1], 12042[1], 12044[1], 12045[1], 12046[1], 12047[1], 12051[1], 12052[1], 12053[1], 12054[1], 12055[1], 12056[1], 12057[1], 13100[1], 13101[1], 13102[1], 13120[1], 13121[1], 13122[1], 13131[1], 13132[1], 13133[1], 13151[1], 13152[1], 13153[1], 36000[1], 36400[1], 36405[1], 36406[1], 36410[1], 36420[1], 36425[1], 36430[1], 36440[1], 36591[0], 36592[0], 36600[1], 36640[1], 43752[1], 51701[1], 51702[1], 51703[1], 62320[0], 62321[0], 62322[0], 62323[0], 62324[0], 62325[0], 62326[0], 62327[0], 64400[0], 64405[0], 64408[0], 64415[0], 64416[0], 64417[0], 64418[0], 64420[0], 64421[0], 64425[0], 64430[0], 64435[0], 64445[0], 64446[0], 64447[0], 64448[0], 64449[0], 64450[0], 64451[0], 64454[0], 64461[0], 64462[0], 64463[0], 64479[0], 64480[0], 64483[0], 64484[0], 64486[0], 64487[0], 64488[0], 64489[0], 64490[0], 64491[0], 64492[0], 64493[0], 64494[0], 64495[0], 64505[0], 64510[0], 64517[0], 64520[0], 64530[0], 66250[1], 67500[1], 69990[0], 92012[1], 92014[1], 92018[1], 92019[1], 93000[1], 93005[1], 93010[1], 93040[1], 93041[1], 93042[1], 93318[1], 93355[1], 94002[1], 94200[1], 94680[1], 94681[1], 94690[1], 95812[1], 95813[1], 95816[1], 95819[1], 95822[1], 95829[1], 95955[1], 96360[1], 96361[1], 96365[1], 96366[1], 96367[1], 96368[1], 96372[1], 96374[1], 96375[1], 96376[1], 96377[1], 96523[0], 97597[1], 97598[1], 97602[1], 99155[0], 99156[0], 99157[0], 99211[1], 99212[1], 99213[1], 99214[1], 99215[1], 99217[1], 99218[1], 99219[1], 99220[1], 99221[1], 99222[1], 99223[1], 99231[1], 99232[1], 99233[1], 99234[1], 99235[1], 99236[1], 99238[1], 99239[1], 99241[1], 99242[1], 99243[1], 99244[1], 99245[1], 99251[1], 99252[1], 99253[1], 99254[1], 99255[1], 99291[1], 99292[1], 99304[1], 99305[1], 99306[1], 99307[1], 99308[1], 99309[1], 99310[1], 99315[1], 99316[1], 99334[1], 99335[1], 99336[1], 99337[1], 99347[1], 99348[1], 99349[1], 99350[1], 99374[1], 99375[1], 99377[1], 99378[1], 99446[0], 99447[0], 99448[0], 99449[0], 99451[0], 99452[0], 99495[0], 99496[0], G0463[1], G0471[1], J0670[1], J2001[1]
66505	0213T[0], 0216T[0], 0596T[1], 0597T[1], 0708T[1], 0709T[1], 11000[1], 11001[1], 11004[1], 11005[1], 11006[1], 11042[1], 11043[1], 11044[1], 11045[1], 11046[1], 11047[1], 12001[1], 12002[1], 12004[1], 12005[1], 12006[1], 12007[1], 12011[1], 12013[1], 12014[1], 12015[1], 12016[1], 12017[1], 12018[1], 12020[1], 12021[1], 12031[1], 12032[1], 12034[1], 12035[1], 12036[1], 12037[1], 12041[1], 12042[1], 12044[1], 12045[1], 12046[1], 12047[1], 12051[1], 12052[1], 12053[1], 12054[1], 12055[1], 12056[1], 12057[1], 13100[1], 13101[1], 13102[1], 13120[1], 13121[1], 13122[1], 13131[1], 13132[1], 13133[1], 13151[1], 13152[1], 13153[1], 36000[1], 36400[1], 36405[1], 36406[1], 36410[1], 36420[1], 36425[1], 36430[1], 36440[1], 36591[0], 36592[0], 36600[1], 36640[1], 43752[1], 51701[1], 51702[1], 51703[1], 62320[0], 62321[0], 62322[0], 62323[0], 62324[0], 62325[0], 62326[0], 62327[0], 64400[0], 64405[0], 64408[0], 64415[0], 64416[0], 64417[0], 64418[0], 64420[0], 64421[0], 64425[0], 64430[0], 64435[0], 64445[0], 64446[0], 64447[0], 64448[0], 64449[0], 64450[0], 64451[0], 64454[0], 64461[0], 64462[0], 64463[0], 64479[0], 64480[0], 64483[0], 64484[0], 64486[0], 64487[0], 64488[0], 64489[0], 64490[0], 64491[0], 64492[0], 64493[0], 64494[0], 64495[0], 64505[0], 64510[0], 64517[0], 64520[0], 64530[0], 66250[1], 67500[1], 69990[0], 92012[1], 92014[1], 92018[1], 92019[1], 93000[1], 93005[1], 93010[1], 93040[1], 93041[1], 93042[1], 93318[1], 93355[1], 94002[1], 94200[1], 94680[1], 94681[1], 94690[1], 95812[1], 95813[1], 95816[1], 95819[1], 95822[1], 95829[1], 95955[1], 96360[1], 96361[1], 96365[1], 96366[1], 96367[1], 96368[1], 96372[1], 96374[1], 96375[1], 96376[1], 96377[1], 96523[0], 97597[1], 97598[1], 97602[1], 99155[0], 99156[0], 99157[0], 99211[1], 99212[1], 99213[1], 99214[1], 99215[1], 99217[1], 99218[1], 99219[1], 99220[1], 99221[1], 99222[1], 99223[1], 99231[1], 99232[1], 99233[1], 99234[1], 99235[1], 99236[1], 99238[1], 99239[1], 99241[1], 99242[1], 99243[1], 99244[1], 99245[1], 99251[1], 99252[1], 99253[1], 99254[1], 99255[1], 99291[1], 99292[1], 99304[1], 99305[1], 99306[1], 99307[1], 99308[1], 99309[1], 99310[1], 99315[1], 99316[1], 99334[1], 99335[1], 99336[1], 99337[1], 99347[1], 99348[1], 99349[1], 99350[1], 99374[1], 99375[1], 99377[1], 99378[1], 99446[0], 99447[0], 99448[0], 99449[0], 99451[0], 99452[0], 99495[0], 99496[0], G0463[1], G0471[1], J0670[1], J2001[1]
66600	0213T[0], 0216T[0], 0596T[1], 0597T[1], 0708T[1], 0709T[1], 11000[1], 11001[1], 11004[1], 11005[1], 11006[1], 11042[1], 11043[1], 11044[1], 11045[1], 11046[1], 11047[1], 12001[1], 12002[1], 12004[1], 12005[1], 12006[1], 12007[1], 12011[1], 12013[1], 12014[1], 12015[1], 12016[1], 12017[1], 12018[1], 12020[1], 12021[1], 12031[1], 12032[1], 12034[1], 12035[1], 12036[1], 12037[1], 12041[1], 12042[1], 12044[1], 12045[1], 12046[1], 12047[1], 12051[1], 12052[1], 12053[1], 12054[1], 12055[1], 12056[1], 12057[1], 13100[1], 13101[1], 13102[1], 13120[1], 13121[1], 13122[1], 13131[1], 13132[1], 13133[1], 13151[1], 13152[1], 13153[1], 36000[1], 36400[1], 36405[1], 36406[1], 36410[1], 36420[1], 36425[1], 36430[1], 36440[1], 36591[0], 36592[0], 36600[1], 36640[1], 43752[1], 51701[1], 51702[1], 51703[1], 62320[0], 62321[0], 62322[0], 62323[0], 62324[0], 62325[0], 62326[0], 62327[0], 64400[0], 64405[0], 64408[0], 64415[0], 64416[0], 64417[0], 64418[0], 64420[0], 64421[0], 64425[0], 64430[0], 64435[0], 64445[0], 64446[0], 64447[0], 64448[0], 64449[0], 64450[0], 64451[0], 64454[0], 64461[0], 64462[0], 64463[0], 64479[0], 64480[0], 64483[0], 64484[0], 64486[0], 64487[0], 64488[0], 64489[0], 64490[0], 64491[0], 64492[0], 64493[0], 64494[0], 64495[0], 64505[0], 64510[0], 64517[0], 64520[0], 64530[0], 66250[1], 66500[1], 66505[1], 66625[1], 66630[1], 66635[1], 66680[1], 66761[1], 66762[1], 66770[1], 67500[1], 69990[0], 92012[1], 92014[1], 92018[1], 92019[1], 93000[1], 93005[1], 93010[1], 93040[1], 93041[1], 93042[1], 93318[1], 93355[1], 94002[1], 94200[1], 94680[1], 94681[1], 94690[1], 95812[1], 95813[1], 95816[1], 95819[1], 95822[1], 95829[1], 95955[1], 96360[1], 96361[1], 96365[1], 96366[1], 96367[1], 96368[1], 96372[1], 96374[1], 96375[1], 96376[1], 96377[1], 96523[0], 97597[1], 97598[1], 97602[1], 99155[0], 99156[0], 99157[0], 99211[1], 99212[1], 99213[1], 99214[1], 99215[1], 99217[1], 99218[1], 99219[1], 99220[1], 99221[1], 99222[1], 99223[1], 99231[1], 99232[1], 99233[1], 99234[1], 99235[1], 99236[1], 99238[1], 99239[1], 99241[1], 99242[1], 99243[1], 99244[1], 99245[1], 99251[1], 99252[1], 99253[1], 99254[1], 99255[1], 99291[1], 99292[1], 99304[1], 99305[1], 99306[1], 99307[1], 99308[1], 99309[1], 99310[1], 99315[1], 99316[1], 99334[1], 99335[1], 99336[1], 99337[1], 99347[1], 99348[1], 99349[1], 99350[1], 99374[1], 99375[1], 99377[1], 99378[1], 99446[0], 99447[0], 99448[0], 99449[0], 99451[0], 99452[0], 99495[0], 99496[0], G0463[1], G0471[1], J0670[1], J2001[1]
66605	0213T[0], 0216T[0], 0596T[1], 0597T[1], 0616T[1], 0618T[1], 0708T[1], 0709T[1], 11000[1], 11001[1], 11004[1], 11005[1], 11006[1], 11042[1], 11043[1], 11044[1], 11045[1], 11046[1], 11047[1], 12001[1], 12002[1], 12004[1], 12005[1], 12006[1], 12007[1], 12011[1], 12013[1], 12014[1], 12015[1], 12016[1],

0 = Modifier usage not allowed or inappropriate 1 = Modifier usage allowed

Code 1	Code 2
	12017[1], 12018[1], 12020[1], 12021[1], 12031[1], 12032[1], 12034[1], 12035[1], 12036[1], 12037[1], 12041[1], 12042[1], 12044[1], 12045[1], 12046[1], 12047[1], 12051[1], 12052[1], 12053[1], 12054[1], 12055[1], 12056[1], 12057[1], 13100[1], 13101[1], 13102[1], 13120[1], 13121[1], 13122[1], 13131[1], 13132[1], 13133[1], 13151[1], 13152[1], 13153[1], 36000[1], 36400[1], 36405[1], 36406[1], 36410[1], 36420[1], 36425[1], 36430[1], 36440[1], 36591[0], 36592[0], 36600[1], 36640[1], 43752[1], 51701[1], 51702[1], 51703[1], 62320[0], 62321[0], 62322[0], 62323[0], 62324[0], 62325[0], 62326[0], 62327[0], 64400[0], 64405[0], 64408[0], 64415[0], 64416[0], 64417[0], 64418[0], 64420[0], 64421[0], 64425[0], 64430[0], 64435[0], 64445[0], 64446[0], 64447[0], 64448[0], 64449[0], 64450[0], 64451[0], 64454[0], 64461[0], 64462[0], 64463[0], 64479[0], 64480[0], 64483[0], 64484[0], 64486[0], 64487[0], 64488[0], 64489[0], 64490[0], 64491[0], 64492[0], 64493[0], 64494[0], 64495[0], 64505[0], 64510[0], 64517[0], 64520[0], 64530[0], 66250[1], 66500[1], 66505[1], 66600[1], 66625[1], 66630[1], 66635[1], 66680[1], 66761[1], 66762[1], 66770[1], 67500[1], 69990[0], 92012[1], 92014[1], 92018[1], 92019[1], 93000[1], 93005[1], 93010[1], 93040[1], 93041[1], 93042[1], 93318[1], 93355[1], 94002[1], 94200[1], 94680[1], 94681[1], 94690[1], 95812[1], 95813[1], 95816[1], 95819[1], 95822[1], 95829[1], 95955[1], 96360[1], 96361[1], 96365[1], 96366[1], 96367[1], 96368[1], 96372[1], 96374[1], 96375[1], 96376[1], 96377[1], 96523[0], 97597[1], 97598[1], 97602[1], 99155[0], 99156[0], 99157[0], 99211[1], 99212[1], 99213[1], 99214[1], 99215[1], 99217[1], 99218[1], 99219[1], 99220[1], 99221[1], 99222[1], 99223[1], 99231[1], 99232[1], 99233[1], 99234[1], 99235[1], 99236[1], 99238[1], 99239[1], 99241[1], 99242[1], 99243[1], 99244[1], 99245[1], 99251[1], 99252[1], 99253[1], 99254[1], 99255[1], 99291[1], 99292[1], 99304[1], 99305[1], 99306[1], 99307[1], 99308[1], 99309[1], 99310[1], 99315[1], 99316[1], 99334[1], 99335[1], 99336[1], 99337[1], 99347[1], 99348[1], 99349[1], 99350[1], 99374[1], 99375[1], 99377[1], 99378[1], 99446[0], 99447[0], 99448[0], 99449[0], 99451[0], 99452[0], 99495[0], 99496[0], G0463[1], G0471[1], J0670[1], J2001[1]
66625	0213T[0], 0216T[0], 0596T[1], 0597T[1], 0708T[1], 0709T[1], 11000[1], 11001[1], 11004[1], 11005[1], 11006[1], 11042[1], 11043[1], 11044[1], 11045[1], 11046[1], 11047[1], 12001[1], 12002[1], 12004[1], 12005[1], 12006[1], 12007[1], 12011[1], 12013[1], 12014[1], 12015[1], 12016[1], 12017[1], 12018[1], 12020[1], 12021[1], 12031[1], 12032[1], 12034[1], 12035[1], 12036[1], 12037[1], 12041[1], 12042[1], 12044[1], 12045[1], 12046[1], 12047[1], 12051[1], 12052[1], 12053[1], 12054[1], 12055[1], 12056[1], 12057[1], 13100[1], 13101[1], 13102[1], 13120[1], 13121[1], 13122[1], 13131[1], 13132[1], 13133[1], 13151[1], 13152[1], 13153[1], 36000[1], 36400[1], 36405[1], 36406[1], 36410[1], 36420[1], 36425[1], 36430[1], 36440[1], 36591[0], 36592[0], 36600[1], 36640[1], 43752[1], 51701[1], 51702[1], 51703[1], 62320[0], 62321[0], 62322[0], 62323[0], 62324[0], 62325[0], 62326[0], 62327[0], 64400[0], 64405[0], 64408[0], 64415[0], 64416[0], 64417[0], 64418[0], 64420[0], 64421[0], 64425[0], 64430[0], 64435[0], 64445[0], 64446[0], 64447[0], 64448[0], 64449[0], 64450[0], 64451[0], 64454[0], 64461[0], 64462[0], 64463[0], 64479[0], 64480[0], 64483[0], 64484[0], 64486[0], 64487[0], 64488[0], 64489[0], 64490[0], 64491[0], 64492[0], 64493[0], 64494[0], 64495[0], 64505[0], 64510[0], 64517[0], 64520[0], 64530[0], 66250[1], 66500[1], 66505[1], 67500[1], 69990[0], 92012[1], 92014[1], 92018[1], 92019[1], 93000[1], 93005[1], 93010[1], 93040[1], 93041[1], 93042[1], 93318[1], 93355[1], 94002[1], 94200[1], 94680[1], 94681[1], 94690[1], 95812[1], 95813[1], 95816[1], 95819[1], 95822[1], 95829[1], 95955[1], 96360[1], 96361[1], 96365[1], 96366[1], 96367[1], 96368[1], 96372[1], 96374[1], 96375[1], 96376[1], 96377[1], 96523[0], 97597[1], 97598[1], 97602[1], 99155[0], 99156[0], 99157[0], 99211[1], 99212[1], 99213[1], 99214[1], 99215[1], 99217[1], 99218[1], 99219[1], 99220[1], 99221[1], 99222[1], 99223[1], 99231[1], 99232[1], 99233[1], 99234[1], 99235[1], 99236[1], 99238[1], 99239[1], 99241[1], 99242[1], 99243[1], 99244[1], 99245[1], 99251[1], 99252[1], 99253[1], 99254[1], 99255[1], 99291[1], 99292[1], 99304[1], 99305[1], 99306[1], 99307[1], 99308[1], 99309[1], 99310[1], 99315[1], 99316[1], 99334[1], 99335[1], 99336[1], 99337[1], 99347[1], 99348[1], 99349[1], 99350[1], 99374[1], 99375[1], 99377[1], 99378[1], 99446[0], 99447[0], 99448[0], 99449[0], 99451[0], 99452[0], 99495[0], 99496[0], G0463[1], G0471[1], J2001[1]
66630	0213T[0], 0216T[0], 0596T[1], 0597T[1], 0708T[1], 0709T[1], 11000[1], 11001[1], 11004[1], 11005[1], 11006[1], 11042[1], 11043[1], 11044[1], 11045[1], 11046[1], 11047[1], 12001[1], 12002[1], 12004[1], 12005[1], 12006[1], 12007[1], 12011[1], 12013[1], 12014[1], 12015[1], 12016[1], 12017[1], 12018[1], 12020[1], 12021[1], 12031[1], 12032[1], 12034[1], 12035[1], 12036[1], 12037[1], 12041[1], 12042[1], 12044[1], 12045[1], 12046[1], 12047[1], 12051[1], 12052[1], 12053[1], 12054[1], 12055[1], 12056[1], 12057[1], 13100[1], 13101[1], 13102[1], 13120[1], 13121[1], 13122[1], 13131[1], 13132[1], 13133[1], 13151[1], 13152[1], 13153[1], 36000[1], 36400[1], 36405[1], 36406[1], 36410[1], 36420[1], 36425[1], 36430[1], 36440[1], 36591[0], 36592[0], 36600[1], 36640[1], 43752[1], 51701[1], 51702[1], 51703[1], 62320[0], 62321[0], 62322[0], 62323[0], 62324[0], 62325[0], 62326[0], 62327[0], 64400[0], 64405[0], 64408[0], 64415[0], 64416[0], 64417[0], 64418[0], 64420[0], 64421[0], 64425[0], 64430[0], 64435[0], 64445[0], 64446[0], 64447[0], 64448[0], 64449[0], 64450[0], 64451[0], 64454[0], 64461[0], 64462[0], 64463[0], 64479[0], 64480[0], 64483[0], 64484[0], 64486[0], 64487[0], 64488[0], 64489[0], 64490[0], 64491[0], 64492[0], 64493[0], 64494[0], 64495[0], 64505[0], 64510[0], 64517[0], 64520[0], 64530[0], 66250[1], 66500[1], 66505[1], 66625[1], 67500[1], 69990[0], 92012[1], 92014[1], 92018[1], 92019[1], 93000[1], 93005[1], 93010[1], 93040[1], 93041[1], 93042[1], 93318[1], 93355[1], 94002[1], 94200[1], 94680[1], 94681[1], 94690[1], 95812[1], 95813[1], 95816[1], 95819[1], 95822[1], 95829[1], 95955[1], 96360[1], 96361[1], 96365[1], 96366[1], 96367[1], 96368[1], 96372[1], 96374[1], 96375[1], 96376[1], 96377[1], 96523[0], 97597[1], 97598[1], 97602[1], 99155[0], 99156[0], 99157[0], 99211[1], 99212[1], 99213[1], 99214[1], 99215[1], 99217[1], 99218[1], 99219[1], 99220[1], 99221[1], 99222[1], 99223[1], 99231[1], 99232[1], 99233[1], 99234[1], 99235[1], 99236[1], 99238[1], 99239[1], 99241[1], 99242[1], 99243[1], 99244[1], 99245[1], 99251[1], 99252[1], 99253[1], 99254[1], 99255[1], 99291[1], 99292[1], 99304[1], 99305[1], 99306[1], 99307[1], 99308[1], 99309[1], 99310[1], 99315[1], 99316[1], 99334[1], 99335[1], 99336[1], 99337[1], 99347[1], 99348[1], 99349[1], 99350[1], 99374[1], 99375[1], 99377[1], 99378[1], 99446[0], 99447[0], 99448[0], 99449[0], 99451[0], 99452[0], 99495[0], 99496[0], G0463[1], G0471[1], J2001[1]
66635	0213T[0], 0216T[0], 0596T[1], 0597T[1], 0708T[1], 0709T[1], 11000[1], 11001[1], 11004[1], 11005[1], 11006[1], 11042[1], 11043[1], 11044[1], 11045[1], 11046[1], 11047[1], 12001[1], 12002[1], 12004[1], 12005[1], 12006[1], 12007[1], 12011[1], 12013[1], 12014[1], 12015[1], 12016[1], 12017[1], 12018[1], 12020[1], 12021[1], 12031[1], 12032[1], 12034[1], 12035[1], 12036[1], 12037[1], 12041[1], 12042[1], 12044[1], 12045[1], 12046[1], 12047[1], 12051[1], 12052[1], 12053[1], 12054[1], 12055[1], 12056[1], 12057[1], 13100[1], 13101[1], 13102[1], 13120[1], 13121[1], 13122[1], 13131[1], 13132[1], 13133[1], 13151[1], 13152[1], 13153[1], 36000[1], 36400[1], 36405[1], 36406[1], 36410[1], 36420[1], 36425[1], 36430[1], 36440[1], 36591[0], 36592[0], 36600[1], 36640[1], 43752[1], 51701[1], 51702[1], 51703[1], 62320[0], 62321[0], 62322[0], 62323[0], 62324[0], 62325[0], 62326[0], 62327[0], 64400[0], 64405[0], 64408[0], 64415[0], 64416[0], 64417[0], 64418[0], 64420[0], 64421[0], 64425[0], 64430[0], 64435[0], 64445[0], 64446[0], 64447[0], 64448[0], 64449[0], 64450[0], 64451[0], 64454[0], 64461[0], 64462[0], 64463[0], 64479[0], 64480[0], 64483[0], 64484[0], 64486[0], 64487[0], 64488[0], 64489[0], 64490[0], 64491[0], 64492[0], 64493[0], 64494[0], 64495[0], 64505[0], 64510[0], 64517[0], 64520[0], 64530[0], 66250[1], 66500[1], 66505[1], 66625[1], 66630[1], 67500[1], 69990[0], 92012[1], 92014[1], 92018[1], 92019[1], 93000[1], 93005[1], 93010[1], 93040[1], 93041[1], 93042[1], 93318[1], 93355[1], 94002[1], 94200[1], 94680[1], 94681[1], 94690[1], 95812[1], 95813[1], 95816[1], 95819[1], 95822[1], 95829[1], 95955[1], 96360[1], 96361[1], 96365[1], 96366[1], 96367[1], 96368[1], 96372[1], 96374[1], 96375[1], 96376[1], 96377[1], 96523[0], 97597[1], 97598[1], 97602[1], 99155[0], 99156[0], 99157[0], 99211[1], 99212[1], 99213[1], 99214[1], 99215[1], 99217[1], 99218[1], 99219[1], 99220[1], 99221[1], 99222[1], 99223[1], 99231[1], 99232[1], 99233[1], 99234[1], 99235[1], 99236[1], 99238[1], 99239[1], 99241[1], 99242[1], 99243[1], 99244[1], 99245[1], 99251[1], 99252[1], 99253[1], 99254[1], 99255[1], 99291[1], 99292[1], 99304[1], 99305[1], 99306[1], 99307[1], 99308[1], 99309[1], 99310[1], 99315[1], 99316[1], 99334[1], 99335[1], 99336[1], 99337[1], 99347[1], 99348[1], 99349[1], 99350[1], 99374[1], 99375[1], 99377[1], 99378[1], 99446[0], 99447[0], 99448[0], 99449[0], 99451[0], 99452[0], 99495[0], 99496[0], G0463[1], G0471[1], J2001[1]
66680	0213T[0], 0216T[0], 0596T[1], 0597T[1], 0708T[1], 0709T[1], 12001[1], 12002[1], 12004[1], 12005[1], 12006[1], 12007[1], 12011[1], 12013[1], 12014[1], 12015[1], 12016[1], 12017[1], 12018[1], 12020[1], 12021[1], 12031[1], 12032[1], 12034[1], 12035[1], 12036[1], 12037[1], 12041[1], 12042[1], 12044[1], 12045[1], 12046[1], 12047[1], 12051[1], 12052[1], 12053[1], 12054[1], 12055[1], 12056[1], 12057[1], 13100[1], 13101[1], 13102[1], 13120[1], 13121[1], 13122[1], 13131[1], 13132[1], 13133[1], 13151[1], 13152[1], 13153[1], 36000[1], 36400[1], 36405[1], 36406[1], 36410[1], 36420[1], 36425[1], 36430[1], 36440[1], 36591[0], 36592[0], 36600[1], 36640[1], 43752[1], 51701[1], 51702[1], 51703[1], 62320[0], 62321[0], 62322[0], 62323[0], 62324[0], 62325[0], 62326[0], 62327[0], 64400[0], 64405[0], 64408[0], 64415[0], 64416[0], 64417[0], 64418[0], 64420[0], 64421[0], 64425[0], 64430[0], 64435[0], 64445[0], 64446[0], 64447[0], 64448[0], 64449[0], 64450[0], 64451[0], 64454[0], 64461[0], 64462[0], 64463[0], 64479[0], 64480[0], 64483[0], 64484[0], 64486[0], 64487[0], 64488[0], 64489[0], 64490[0], 64491[0], 64492[0], 64493[0], 64494[0], 64495[0], 64505[0], 64510[0], 64517[0], 64520[0], 64530[0], 66500[1], 66505[1], 66625[1], 66630[1], 66635[1], 67500[1], 69990[0], 92012[1], 92014[1], 92018[1], 92019[1], 93000[1], 93005[1], 93010[1], 93040[1], 93041[1], 93042[1], 93318[1], 93355[1], 94002[1], 94200[1], 94680[1], 94681[1], 94690[1], 95812[1], 95813[1], 95816[1], 95819[1], 95822[1], 95829[1], 95955[1], 96360[1], 96361[1], 96365[1], 96366[1], 96367[1], 96368[1], 96372[1], 96374[1], 96375[1], 96376[1], 96377[1], 96523[0], 99155[0], 99156[0], 99157[0], 99211[1], 99212[1], 99213[1], 99214[1], 99215[1], 99217[1], 99218[1], 99219[1], 99220[1], 99221[1], 99222[1], 99223[1], 99231[1], 99232[1], 99233[1], 99234[1], 99235[1], 99236[1], 99238[1], 99239[1], 99241[1], 99242[1], 99243[1], 99244[1], 99245[1], 99251[1], 99252[1], 99253[1], 99254[1], 99255[1], 99291[1], 99292[1], 99304[1], 99305[1], 99306[1], 99307[1], 99308[1], 99309[1], 99310[1], 99315[1], 99316[1], 99334[1], 99335[1], 99336[1], 99337[1], 99347[1], 99348[1], 99349[1], 99350[1], 99374[1], 99375[1], 99377[1], 99378[1], 99446[0], 99447[0], 99448[0], 99449[0], 99451[0], 99452[0], 99495[0], 99496[0], G0463[1], G0471[1], J0670[1], J2001[1]
66682	0213T[0], 0216T[0], 0596T[1], 0597T[1], 0708T[1], 0709T[1], 12001[1], 12002[1], 12004[1], 12005[1], 12006[1], 12007[1], 12011[1], 12013[1], 12014[1], 12015[1], 12016[1], 12017[1], 12018[1], 12020[1], 12021[1], 12031[1], 12032[1], 12034[1], 12035[1], 12036[1], 12037[1], 12041[1], 12042[1], 12044[1], 12045[1], 12046[1], 12047[1], 12051[1], 12052[1], 12053[1], 12054[1], 12055[1], 12056[1], 12057[1], 13100[1], 13101[1], 13102[1], 13120[1], 13121[1], 13122[1], 13131[1], 13132[1], 13133[1], 13151[1], 13152[1], 13153[1], 36000[1], 36400[1], 36405[1], 36406[1], 36410[1], 36420[1], 36425[1], 36430[1], 36440[1], 36591[0], 36592[0], 36600[1], 36640[1], 43752[1], 51701[1], 51702[1], 51703[1], 62320[0], 62321[0], 62322[0], 62323[0], 62324[0], 62325[0], 62326[0], 62327[0], 64400[0], 64405[0], 64408[0], 64415[0], 64416[0], 64417[0], 64418[0], 64420[0], 64421[0], 64425[0], 64430[0], 64435[0], 64445[0], 64446[0], 64447[0], 64448[0], 64449[0], 64450[0], 64451[0], 64454[0], 64461[0], 64462[0], 64463[0],

0 = Modifier usage not allowed or inappropriate 1 = Modifier usage allowed

Code 1	Code 2
	64479[0], 64480[0], 64483[0], 64484[0], 64486[0], 64487[0], 64488[0], 64489[0], 64490[0], 64491[0], 64492[0], 64493[0], 64494[0], 64495[0], 64505[0], 64510[0], 64517[0], 64520[0], 64530[0], 66250[1], 66500[1], 66505[1], 66625[1], 66630[1], 66635[1], 67500[1], 69990[0], 92012[1], 92014[1], 92018[1], 92019[1], 93000[1], 93005[1], 93010[1], 93040[1], 93041[1], 93042[1], 93318[1], 93355[1], 94002[1], 94200[1], 94680[1], 94681[1], 94690[1], 95812[1], 95813[1], 95816[1], 95819[1], 95822[1], 95829[1], 95955[1], 96360[1], 96361[1], 96365[1], 96366[1], 96367[1], 96368[1], 96372[1], 96374[1], 96375[1], 96376[1], 96377[1], 96523[0], 99155[0], 99156[0], 99157[0], 99211[1], 99212[1], 99213[1], 99214[1], 99215[1], 99217[1], 99218[1], 99219[1], 99220[1], 99221[1], 99222[1], 99223[1], 99231[1], 99232[1], 99233[1], 99234[1], 99235[1], 99236[1], 99238[1], 99239[1], 99241[1], 99242[1], 99243[1], 99244[1], 99245[1], 99251[1], 99252[1], 99253[1], 99254[1], 99255[1], 99291[1], 99292[1], 99304[1], 99305[1], 99306[1], 99307[1], 99308[1], 99309[1], 99310[1], 99315[1], 99316[1], 99334[1], 99335[1], 99336[1], 99337[1], 99347[1], 99348[1], 99349[1], 99350[1], 99374[1], 99375[1], 99377[1], 99378[1], 99446[0], 99447[0], 99448[0], 99449[0], 99451[0], 99452[0], 99495[0], 99496[0], G0463[1], G0471[1], J0670[1], J2001[1]
66700	0213T[0], 0216T[0], 0596T[1], 0597T[1], 0708T[1], 0709T[1], 12001[1], 12002[1], 12004[1], 12005[1], 12006[1], 12007[1], 12011[1], 12013[1], 12014[1], 12015[1], 12016[1], 12017[1], 12018[1], 12020[1], 12021[1], 12031[1], 12032[1], 12034[1], 12035[1], 12036[1], 12037[1], 12041[1], 12042[1], 12044[1], 12045[1], 12046[1], 12047[1], 12051[1], 12052[1], 12053[1], 12054[1], 12055[1], 12056[1], 12057[1], 13100[1], 13101[1], 13102[1], 13120[1], 13121[1], 13122[1], 13131[1], 13132[1], 13133[1], 13151[1], 13152[1], 13153[1], 36000[1], 36400[1], 36405[1], 36406[1], 36410[1], 36420[1], 36425[1], 36430[1], 36440[1], 36591[0], 36592[0], 36600[1], 36640[1], 43752[1], 51701[1], 51702[1], 51703[1], 62320[0], 62321[0], 62322[0], 62323[0], 62324[0], 62325[0], 62326[0], 62327[0], 64400[0], 64405[0], 64408[0], 64415[0], 64416[0], 64417[0], 64418[0], 64420[0], 64421[0], 64425[0], 64430[0], 64435[0], 64445[0], 64446[0], 64447[0], 64448[0], 64449[0], 64450[0], 64451[0], 64454[0], 64461[0], 64462[0], 64463[0], 64479[0], 64480[0], 64483[0], 64484[0], 64486[0], 64487[0], 64488[0], 64489[0], 64490[0], 64491[0], 64492[0], 64493[0], 64494[0], 64495[0], 64505[0], 64510[0], 64517[0], 64520[0], 64530[0], 66250[1], 66500[1], 66505[1], 66625[1], 66630[1], 66635[1], 66770[1], 67500[1], 69990[0], 92012[1], 92014[1], 92018[1], 92019[1], 93000[1], 93005[1], 93010[1], 93040[1], 93041[1], 93042[1], 93318[1], 93355[1], 94002[1], 94200[1], 94680[1], 94681[1], 94690[1], 95812[1], 95813[1], 95816[1], 95819[1], 95822[1], 95829[1], 95955[1], 96360[1], 96361[1], 96365[1], 96366[1], 96367[1], 96368[1], 96372[1], 96374[1], 96375[1], 96376[1], 96377[1], 96523[0], 99155[0], 99156[0], 99157[0], 99211[1], 99212[1], 99213[1], 99214[1], 99215[1], 99217[1], 99218[1], 99219[1], 99220[1], 99221[1], 99222[1], 99223[1], 99231[1], 99232[1], 99233[1], 99234[1], 99235[1], 99236[1], 99238[1], 99239[1], 99241[1], 99242[1], 99243[1], 99244[1], 99245[1], 99251[1], 99252[1], 99253[1], 99254[1], 99255[1], 99291[1], 99292[1], 99304[1], 99305[1], 99306[1], 99307[1], 99308[1], 99309[1], 99310[1], 99315[1], 99316[1], 99334[1], 99335[1], 99336[1], 99337[1], 99347[1], 99348[1], 99349[1], 99350[1], 99374[1], 99375[1], 99377[1], 99378[1], 99446[0], 99447[0], 99448[0], 99449[0], 99451[0], 99452[0], 99495[0], 99496[0], G0463[1], G0471[1], J0670[1], J2001[1]
66710	0213T[0], 0216T[0], 0596T[1], 0597T[1], 0708T[1], 0709T[1], 12001[1], 12002[1], 12004[1], 12005[1], 12006[1], 12007[1], 12011[1], 12013[1], 12014[1], 12015[1], 12016[1], 12017[1], 12018[1], 12020[1], 12021[1], 12031[1], 12032[1], 12034[1], 12035[1], 12036[1], 12037[1], 12041[1], 12042[1], 12044[1], 12045[1], 12046[1], 12047[1], 12051[1], 12052[1], 12053[1], 12054[1], 12055[1], 12056[1], 12057[1], 13100[1], 13101[1], 13102[1], 13120[1], 13121[1], 13122[1], 13131[1], 13132[1], 13133[1], 13151[1], 13152[1], 13153[1], 36000[1], 36400[1], 36405[1], 36406[1], 36410[1], 36420[1], 36425[1], 36430[1], 36440[1], 36591[0], 36592[0], 36600[1], 36640[1], 43752[1], 51701[1], 51702[1], 51703[1], 62320[0], 62321[0], 62322[0], 62323[0], 62324[0], 62325[0], 62326[0], 62327[0], 64400[0], 64405[0], 64408[0], 64415[0], 64416[0], 64417[0], 64418[0], 64420[0], 64421[0], 64425[0], 64430[0], 64435[0], 64445[0], 64446[0], 64447[0], 64448[0], 64449[0], 64450[0], 64451[0], 64454[0], 64461[0], 64462[0], 64463[0], 64479[0], 64480[0], 64483[0], 64484[0], 64486[0], 64487[0], 64488[0], 64489[0], 64490[0], 64491[0], 64492[0], 64493[0], 64494[0], 64495[0], 64505[0], 64510[0], 64517[0], 64520[0], 64530[0], 65820[1], 66250[1], 66500[1], 66505[1], 66625[1], 66630[1], 66635[1], 66700[1], 66770[1], 67500[1], 69990[0], 92012[1], 92014[1], 92018[1], 92019[1], 93000[1], 93005[1], 93010[1], 93040[1], 93041[1], 93042[1], 93318[1], 93355[1], 94002[1], 94200[1], 94680[1], 94681[1], 94690[1], 95812[1], 95813[1], 95816[1], 95819[1], 95822[1], 95829[1], 95955[1], 96360[1], 96361[1], 96365[1], 96366[1], 96367[1], 96368[1], 96372[1], 96374[1], 96375[1], 96376[1], 96377[1], 96523[0], 99155[0], 99156[0], 99157[0], 99211[1], 99212[1], 99213[1], 99214[1], 99215[1], 99217[1], 99218[1], 99219[1], 99220[1], 99221[1], 99222[1], 99223[1], 99231[1], 99232[1], 99233[1], 99234[1], 99235[1], 99236[1], 99238[1], 99239[1], 99241[1], 99242[1], 99243[1], 99244[1], 99245[1], 99251[1], 99252[1], 99253[1], 99254[1], 99255[1], 99291[1], 99292[1], 99304[1], 99305[1], 99306[1], 99307[1], 99308[1], 99309[1], 99310[1], 99315[1], 99316[1], 99334[1], 99335[1], 99336[1], 99337[1], 99347[1], 99348[1], 99349[1], 99350[1], 99374[1], 99375[1], 99377[1], 99378[1], 99446[0], 99447[0], 99448[0], 99449[0], 99451[0], 99452[0], 99495[0], 99496[0], G0463[1], G0471[1], J0670[1], J2001[1]
66711	0213T[0], 0216T[0], 0596T[1], 0597T[1], 0621T[1], 0622T[1], 0699T[1], 0708T[1], 0709T[1], 12001[1], 12002[1], 12004[1], 12005[1], 12006[1], 12007[1], 12011[1], 12013[1], 12014[1], 12015[1], 12016[1], 12017[1], 12018[1], 12020[1], 12021[1], 12031[1], 12032[1], 12034[1], 12035[1], 12036[1], 12037[1], 12041[1], 12042[1], 12044[1], 12045[1], 12046[1], 12047[1], 12051[1], 12052[1], 12053[1], 12054[1], 12055[1], 12056[1], 12057[1], 13100[1], 13101[1], 13102[1], 13120[1], 13121[1], 13122[1], 13131[1], 13132[1], 13133[1], 13151[1], 13152[1], 13153[1], 36000[1], 36400[1], 36405[1], 36406[1], 36410[1], 36420[1], 36425[1], 36430[1], 36440[1], 36591[0], 36592[0], 36600[1], 36640[1], 43752[1], 51701[1], 51702[1], 51703[1], 62320[0], 62321[0], 62322[0], 62323[0], 62324[0], 62325[0], 62326[0], 62327[0], 64400[0], 64405[0], 64408[0], 64415[0], 64416[0], 64417[0], 64418[0], 64420[0], 64421[0], 64425[0], 64430[0], 64435[0], 64445[0], 64446[0], 64447[0], 64448[0], 64449[0], 64450[0], 64451[0], 64454[0], 64461[0], 64462[0], 64463[0], 64479[0], 64480[0], 64483[0], 64484[0], 64486[0], 64487[0], 64488[0], 64489[0], 64490[0], 64491[0], 64492[0], 64493[0], 64494[0], 64495[0], 64505[0], 64510[0], 64517[0], 64520[0], 64530[0], 65800[1], 65815[1], 65820[1], 65850[1], 65855[1], 65860[1], 65865[1], 65870[1], 65875[1], 65880[1], 66020[1], 66030[1], 66500[1], 66505[1], 66625[1], 66630[1], 66635[1], 66700[1], 66710[1], 66720[1], 66740[1], 66770[1], 66987[1], 66988[1], 66990[1], 67500[1], 69990[0], 92012[1], 92014[1], 92018[1], 92019[1], 93000[1], 93005[1], 93010[1], 93040[1], 93041[1], 93042[1], 93318[1], 93355[1], 94002[1], 94200[1], 94680[1], 94681[1], 94690[1], 95812[1], 95813[1], 95816[1], 95819[1], 95822[1], 95829[1], 95955[1], 96360[1], 96361[1], 96365[1], 96366[1], 96367[1], 96368[1], 96372[1], 96374[1], 96375[1], 96376[1], 96377[1], 96523[0], 99155[0], 99156[0], 99157[0], 99211[1], 99212[1], 99213[1], 99214[1], 99215[1], 99217[1], 99218[1], 99219[1], 99220[1], 99221[1], 99222[1], 99223[1], 99231[1], 99232[1], 99233[1], 99234[1], 99235[1], 99236[1], 99238[1], 99239[1], 99241[1], 99242[1], 99243[1], 99244[1], 99245[1], 99251[1], 99252[1], 99253[1], 99254[1], 99255[1], 99291[1], 99292[1], 99304[1], 99305[1], 99306[1], 99307[1], 99308[1], 99309[1], 99310[1], 99315[1], 99316[1], 99334[1], 99335[1], 99336[1], 99337[1], 99347[1], 99348[1], 99349[1], 99350[1], 99374[1], 99375[1], 99377[1], 99378[1], 99446[0], 99447[0], 99448[0], 99449[0], 99451[0], 99452[0], 99495[0], 99496[0], G0463[1], G0471[1]
66720	0213T[0], 0216T[0], 0596T[1], 0597T[1], 0708T[1], 0709T[1], 12001[1], 12002[1], 12004[1], 12005[1], 12006[1], 12007[1], 12011[1], 12013[1], 12014[1], 12015[1], 12016[1], 12017[1], 12018[1], 12020[1], 12021[1], 12031[1], 12032[1], 12034[1], 12035[1], 12036[1], 12037[1], 12041[1], 12042[1], 12044[1], 12045[1], 12046[1], 12047[1], 12051[1], 12052[1], 12053[1], 12054[1], 12055[1], 12056[1], 12057[1], 13100[1], 13101[1], 13102[1], 13120[1], 13121[1], 13122[1], 13131[1], 13132[1], 13133[1], 13151[1], 13152[1], 13153[1], 36000[1], 36400[1], 36405[1], 36406[1], 36410[1], 36420[1], 36425[1], 36430[1], 36440[1], 36591[0], 36592[0], 36600[1], 36640[1], 43752[1], 51701[1], 51702[1], 51703[1], 62320[0], 62321[0], 62322[0], 62323[0], 62324[0], 62325[0], 62326[0], 62327[0], 64400[0], 64405[0], 64408[0], 64415[0], 64416[0], 64417[0], 64418[0], 64420[0], 64421[0], 64425[0], 64430[0], 64435[0], 64445[0], 64446[0], 64447[0], 64448[0], 64449[0], 64450[0], 64451[0], 64454[0], 64461[0], 64462[0], 64463[0], 64479[0], 64480[0], 64483[0], 64484[0], 64486[0], 64487[0], 64488[0], 64489[0], 64490[0], 64491[0], 64492[0], 64493[0], 64494[0], 64495[0], 64505[0], 64510[0], 64517[0], 64520[0], 64530[0], 66250[1], 66500[1], 66505[1], 66625[1], 66630[1], 66635[1], 66700[1], 66710[1], 66770[1], 67500[1], 69990[0], 92012[1], 92014[1], 92018[1], 92019[1], 93000[1], 93005[1], 93010[1], 93040[1], 93041[1], 93042[1], 93318[1], 93355[1], 94002[1], 94200[1], 94680[1], 94681[1], 94690[1], 95812[1], 95813[1], 95816[1], 95819[1], 95822[1], 95829[1], 95955[1], 96360[1], 96361[1], 96365[1], 96366[1], 96367[1], 96368[1], 96372[1], 96374[1], 96375[1], 96376[1], 96377[1], 96523[0], 99155[0], 99156[0], 99157[0], 99211[1], 99212[1], 99213[1], 99214[1], 99215[1], 99217[1], 99218[1], 99219[1], 99220[1], 99221[1], 99222[1], 99223[1], 99231[1], 99232[1], 99233[1], 99234[1], 99235[1], 99236[1], 99238[1], 99239[1], 99241[1], 99242[1], 99243[1], 99244[1], 99245[1], 99251[1], 99252[1], 99253[1], 99254[1], 99255[1], 99291[1], 99292[1], 99304[1], 99305[1], 99306[1], 99307[1], 99308[1], 99309[1], 99310[1], 99315[1], 99316[1], 99334[1], 99335[1], 99336[1], 99337[1], 99347[1], 99348[1], 99349[1], 99350[1], 99374[1], 99375[1], 99377[1], 99378[1], 99446[0], 99447[0], 99448[0], 99449[0], 99451[0], 99452[0], 99495[0], 99496[0], G0463[1], G0471[1], J0670[1], J2001[1]
66740	0213T[0], 0216T[0], 0596T[1], 0597T[1], 0708T[1], 0709T[1], 12001[1], 12002[1], 12004[1], 12005[1], 12006[1], 12007[1], 12011[1], 12013[1], 12014[1], 12015[1], 12016[1], 12017[1], 12018[1], 12020[1], 12021[1], 12031[1], 12032[1], 12034[1], 12035[1], 12036[1], 12037[1], 12041[1], 12042[1], 12044[1], 12045[1], 12046[1], 12047[1], 12051[1], 12052[1], 12053[1], 12054[1], 12055[1], 12056[1], 12057[1], 13100[1], 13101[1], 13102[1], 13120[1], 13121[1], 13122[1], 13131[1], 13132[1], 13133[1], 13151[1], 13152[1], 13153[1], 36000[1], 36400[1], 36405[1], 36406[1], 36410[1], 36420[1], 36425[1], 36430[1], 36440[1], 36591[0], 36592[0], 36600[1], 36640[1], 43752[1], 51701[1], 51702[1], 51703[1], 62320[0], 62321[0], 62322[0], 62323[0], 62324[0], 62325[0], 62326[0], 62327[0], 64400[0], 64405[0], 64408[0], 64415[0], 64416[0], 64417[0], 64418[0], 64420[0], 64421[0], 64425[0], 64430[0], 64435[0], 64445[0], 64446[0], 64447[0], 64448[0], 64449[0], 64450[0], 64451[0], 64454[0], 64461[0], 64462[0], 64463[0], 64479[0], 64480[0], 64483[0], 64484[0], 64486[0], 64487[0], 64488[0], 64489[0], 64490[0], 64491[0], 64492[0], 64493[0], 64494[0], 64495[0], 64505[0], 64510[0], 64517[0], 64520[0], 64530[0], 66250[1], 66500[1], 66505[1], 66625[1], 66630[1], 66635[1], 66700[1], 66710[1], 66720[1], 66770[1], 67500[1], 69990[0], 92012[1], 92014[1], 92018[1], 92019[1], 93000[1], 93005[1], 93010[1], 93040[1], 93041[1], 93042[1], 93318[1], 93355[1], 94002[1], 94200[1], 94680[1], 94681[1], 94690[1], 95812[1], 95813[1], 95816[1], 95819[1], 95822[1], 95829[1], 95955[1], 96360[1], 96361[1], 96365[1], 96366[1], 96367[1], 96368[1], 96372[1], 96374[1], 96375[1], 96376[1], 96377[1], 96523[0], 99155[0], 99156[0], 99157[0], 99211[1], 99212[1], 99213[1], 99214[1], 99215[1], 99217[1], 99218[1], 99219[1], 99220[1], 99221[1], 99222[1], 99223[1], 99231[1], 99232[1], 99233[1], 99234[1], 99235[1], 99236[1], 99238[1], 99239[1],

0 = Modifier usage not allowed or inappropriate 1 = Modifier usage allowed

Code 1	Code 2
	99241[1], 99242[1], 99243[1], 99244[1], 99245[1], 99251[1], 99252[1], 99253[1], 99254[1], 99255[1], 99291[1], 99292[1], 99304[1], 99305[1], 99306[1], 99307[1], 99308[1], 99309[1], 99310[1], 99315[1], 99316[1], 99334[1], 99335[1], 99336[1], 99337[1], 99347[1], 99348[1], 99349[1], 99350[1], 99374[1], 99375[1], 99377[1], 99378[1], 99446[0], 99447[0], 99448[0], 99449[0], 99451[0], 99452[0], 99495[0], 99496[0], G0463[1], G0471[1], J0670[1], J2001[1]
66761	0213T[0], 0216T[0], 0596T[1], 0597T[1], 0621T[1], 0622T[1], 0708T[1], 0709T[1], 11000[1], 11001[1], 11004[1], 11005[1], 11006[1], 11042[1], 11043[1], 11044[1], 11045[1], 11046[1], 11047[1], 12001[1], 12002[1], 12004[1], 12005[1], 12006[1], 12007[1], 12011[1], 12013[1], 12014[1], 12015[1], 12016[1], 12017[1], 12018[1], 12020[1], 12021[1], 12031[1], 12032[1], 12034[1], 12035[1], 12036[1], 12037[1], 12041[1], 12042[1], 12044[1], 12045[1], 12046[1], 12047[1], 12051[1], 12052[1], 12053[1], 12054[1], 12055[1], 12056[1], 12057[1], 13100[1], 13101[1], 13102[1], 13120[1], 13121[1], 13122[1], 13131[1], 13132[1], 13133[1], 13151[1], 13152[1], 13153[1], 36000[1], 36400[1], 36405[1], 36406[1], 36410[1], 36420[1], 36425[1], 36430[1], 36440[1], 36591[0], 36592[0], 36600[1], 36640[1], 43752[1], 51701[1], 51702[1], 51703[1], 62320[0], 62321[0], 62322[0], 62323[0], 62324[0], 62325[0], 62326[0], 62327[0], 64400[0], 64405[0], 64408[0], 64415[0], 64416[0], 64417[0], 64418[0], 64420[0], 64421[0], 64425[0], 64430[0], 64435[0], 64445[0], 64446[0], 64447[0], 64448[0], 64449[0], 64450[0], 64451[0], 64454[0], 64461[0], 64462[0], 64463[0], 64479[0], 64480[0], 64483[0], 64484[0], 64486[0], 64487[0], 64488[0], 64489[0], 64490[0], 64491[0], 64492[0], 64493[0], 64494[0], 64495[0], 64505[0], 64510[0], 64517[0], 64520[0], 64530[0], 65855[1], 66250[1], 66762[1], 66770[1], 66984[1], 66988[1], 66991[1], 67500[1], 69990[0], 92012[1], 92014[1], 92018[1], 92019[1], 92504[1], 93000[1], 93005[1], 93010[1], 93040[1], 93041[1], 93042[1], 93318[1], 93355[1], 94002[1], 94200[1], 94680[1], 94681[1], 94690[1], 95812[1], 95813[1], 95816[1], 95819[1], 95822[1], 95829[1], 95955[1], 96360[1], 96361[1], 96365[1], 96366[1], 96367[1], 96368[1], 96372[1], 96374[1], 96375[1], 96376[1], 96377[1], 96523[0], 97597[1], 97598[1], 97602[1], 99155[0], 99156[0], 99157[0], 99211[1], 99212[1], 99213[1], 99214[1], 99215[1], 99217[1], 99218[1], 99219[1], 99220[1], 99221[1], 99222[1], 99223[1], 99231[1], 99232[1], 99233[1], 99234[1], 99235[1], 99236[1], 99238[1], 99239[1], 99241[1], 99242[1], 99243[1], 99244[1], 99245[1], 99251[1], 99252[1], 99253[1], 99254[1], 99255[1], 99291[1], 99292[1], 99304[1], 99305[1], 99306[1], 99307[1], 99308[1], 99309[1], 99310[1], 99315[1], 99316[1], 99334[1], 99335[1], 99336[1], 99337[1], 99347[1], 99348[1], 99349[1], 99350[1], 99374[1], 99375[1], 99377[1], 99378[1], 99446[0], 99447[0], 99448[0], 99449[0], 99451[0], 99452[0], 99495[0], 99496[0], G0463[1], G0471[1]
66762	0213T[0], 0216T[0], 0596T[1], 0597T[1], 0708T[1], 0709T[1], 11000[1], 11001[1], 11004[1], 11005[1], 11006[1], 11042[1], 11043[1], 11044[1], 11045[1], 11046[1], 11047[1], 12001[1], 12002[1], 12004[1], 12005[1], 12006[1], 12007[1], 12011[1], 12013[1], 12014[1], 12015[1], 12016[1], 12017[1], 12018[1], 12020[1], 12021[1], 12031[1], 12032[1], 12034[1], 12035[1], 12036[1], 12037[1], 12041[1], 12042[1], 12044[1], 12045[1], 12046[1], 12047[1], 12051[1], 12052[1], 12053[1], 12054[1], 12055[1], 12056[1], 12057[1], 13100[1], 13101[1], 13102[1], 13120[1], 13121[1], 13122[1], 13131[1], 13132[1], 13133[1], 13151[1], 13152[1], 13153[1], 36000[1], 36400[1], 36405[1], 36406[1], 36410[1], 36420[1], 36425[1], 36430[1], 36440[1], 36591[0], 36592[0], 36600[1], 36640[1], 43752[1], 51701[1], 51702[1], 51703[1], 62320[0], 62321[0], 62322[0], 62323[0], 62324[0], 62325[0], 62326[0], 62327[0], 64400[0], 64405[0], 64408[0], 64415[0], 64416[0], 64417[0], 64418[0], 64420[0], 64421[0], 64425[0], 64430[0], 64435[0], 64445[0], 64446[0], 64447[0], 64448[0], 64449[0], 64450[0], 64451[0], 64454[0], 64461[0], 64462[0], 64463[0], 64479[0], 64480[0], 64483[0], 64484[0], 64486[0], 64487[0], 64488[0], 64489[0], 64490[0], 64491[0], 64492[0], 64493[0], 64494[0], 64495[0], 64505[0], 64510[0], 64517[0], 64520[0], 64530[0], 65820[1], 66250[1], 66770[1], 67500[1], 69990[0], 92012[1], 92014[1], 92018[1], 92019[1], 93000[1], 93005[1], 93010[1], 93040[1], 93041[1], 93042[1], 93318[1], 93355[1], 94002[1], 94200[1], 94680[1], 94681[1], 94690[1], 95812[1], 95813[1], 95816[1], 95819[1], 95822[1], 95829[1], 95955[1], 96360[1], 96361[1], 96365[1], 96366[1], 96367[1], 96368[1], 96372[1], 96374[1], 96375[1], 96376[1], 96377[1], 96523[0], 97597[1], 97598[1], 97602[1], 99155[0], 99156[0], 99157[0], 99211[1], 99212[1], 99213[1], 99214[1], 99215[1], 99217[1], 99218[1], 99219[1], 99220[1], 99221[1], 99222[1], 99223[1], 99231[1], 99232[1], 99233[1], 99234[1], 99235[1], 99236[1], 99238[1], 99239[1], 99241[1], 99242[1], 99243[1], 99244[1], 99245[1], 99251[1], 99252[1], 99253[1], 99254[1], 99255[1], 99291[1], 99292[1], 99304[1], 99305[1], 99306[1], 99307[1], 99308[1], 99309[1], 99310[1], 99315[1], 99316[1], 99334[1], 99335[1], 99336[1], 99337[1], 99347[1], 99348[1], 99349[1], 99350[1], 99374[1], 99375[1], 99377[1], 99378[1], 99446[0], 99447[0], 99448[0], 99449[0], 99451[0], 99452[0], 99495[0], 99496[0], G0463[1], G0471[1]
66770	0213T[0], 0216T[0], 0596T[1], 0597T[1], 0708T[1], 0709T[1], 11000[1], 11001[1], 11004[1], 11005[1], 11006[1], 11042[1], 11043[1], 11044[1], 11045[1], 11046[1], 11047[1], 12001[1], 12002[1], 12004[1], 12005[1], 12006[1], 12007[1], 12011[1], 12013[1], 12014[1], 12015[1], 12016[1], 12017[1], 12018[1], 12020[1], 12021[1], 12031[1], 12032[1], 12034[1], 12035[1], 12036[1], 12037[1], 12041[1], 12042[1], 12044[1], 12045[1], 12046[1], 12047[1], 12051[1], 12052[1], 12053[1], 12054[1], 12055[1], 12056[1], 12057[1], 13100[1], 13101[1], 13102[1], 13120[1], 13121[1], 13122[1], 13131[1], 13132[1], 13133[1], 13151[1], 13152[1], 13153[1], 36000[1], 36400[1], 36405[1], 36406[1], 36410[1], 36420[1], 36425[1], 36430[1], 36440[1], 36591[0], 36592[0], 36600[1], 36640[1], 43752[1], 51701[1], 51702[1], 51703[1], 62320[0], 62321[0], 62322[0], 62323[0], 62324[0], 62325[0], 62326[0], 62327[0], 64400[0], 64405[0], 64408[0], 64415[0], 64416[0], 64417[0], 64418[0], 64420[0], 64421[0], 64425[0], 64430[0], 64435[0], 64445[0], 64446[0], 64447[0], 64448[0], 64449[0], 64450[0], 64451[0], 64454[0], 64461[0], 64462[0], 64463[0], 64479[0], 64480[0], 64483[0], 64484[0], 64486[0], 64487[0], 64488[0], 64489[0], 64490[0], 64491[0], 64492[0], 64493[0], 64494[0], 64495[0], 64505[0], 64510[0], 64517[0], 64520[0], 64530[0], 66250[1], 67500[1], 68200[1], 69990[0], 92012[1], 92014[1], 92018[1], 92019[1], 93000[1], 93005[1], 93010[1], 93040[1], 93041[1], 93042[1], 93318[1], 93355[1], 94002[1], 94200[1], 94680[1], 94681[1], 94690[1], 95812[1], 95813[1], 95816[1], 95819[1], 95822[1], 95829[1], 95955[1], 96360[1], 96361[1], 96365[1], 96366[1], 96367[1], 96368[1], 96372[1], 96374[1], 96375[1], 96376[1], 96377[1], 96523[0], 97597[1], 97598[1], 97602[1], 99155[0], 99156[0], 99157[0], 99211[1], 99212[1], 99213[1], 99214[1], 99215[1], 99217[1], 99218[1], 99219[1], 99220[1], 99221[1], 99222[1], 99223[1], 99231[1], 99232[1], 99233[1], 99234[1], 99235[1], 99236[1], 99238[1], 99239[1], 99241[1], 99242[1], 99243[1], 99244[1], 99245[1], 99251[1], 99252[1], 99253[1], 99254[1], 99255[1], 99291[1], 99292[1], 99304[1], 99305[1], 99306[1], 99307[1], 99308[1], 99309[1], 99310[1], 99315[1], 99316[1], 99334[1], 99335[1], 99336[1], 99337[1], 99347[1], 99348[1], 99349[1], 99350[1], 99374[1], 99375[1], 99377[1], 99378[1], 99446[0], 99447[0], 99448[0], 99449[0], 99451[0], 99452[0], 99495[0], 99496[0], G0463[1], G0471[1], J0670[1], J2001[1]
66820	0213T[0], 0216T[0], 0465T[1], 0596T[1], 0597T[1], 0616T[1], 0699T[1], 0708T[1], 0709T[1], 12001[1], 12002[1], 12004[1], 12005[1], 12006[1], 12007[1], 12011[1], 12013[1], 12014[1], 12015[1], 12016[1], 12017[1], 12018[1], 12020[1], 12021[1], 12031[1], 12032[1], 12034[1], 12035[1], 12036[1], 12037[1], 12041[1], 12042[1], 12044[1], 12045[1], 12046[1], 12047[1], 12051[1], 12052[1], 12053[1], 12054[1], 12055[1], 12056[1], 12057[1], 13100[1], 13101[1], 13102[1], 13120[1], 13121[1], 13122[1], 13131[1], 13132[1], 13133[1], 13151[1], 13152[1], 13153[1], 36000[1], 36400[1], 36405[1], 36406[1], 36410[1], 36420[1], 36425[1], 36430[1], 36440[1], 36591[0], 36592[0], 36600[1], 36640[1], 43752[1], 51701[1], 51702[1], 51703[1], 62320[0], 62321[0], 62322[0], 62323[0], 62324[0], 62325[0], 62326[0], 62327[0], 64400[0], 64405[0], 64408[0], 64415[0], 64416[0], 64417[0], 64418[0], 64420[0], 64421[0], 64425[0], 64430[0], 64435[0], 64445[0], 64446[0], 64447[0], 64448[0], 64449[0], 64450[0], 64451[0], 64454[0], 64461[0], 64462[0], 64463[0], 64479[0], 64480[0], 64483[0], 64484[0], 64486[0], 64487[0], 64488[0], 64489[0], 64490[0], 64491[0], 64492[0], 64493[0], 64494[0], 64495[0], 64505[0], 64510[0], 64517[0], 64520[0], 64530[0], 66030[1], 66250[1], 66500[1], 66505[1], 66600[1], 66605[1], 66625[1], 66630[1], 66635[1], 66680[1], 66682[1], 67028[1], 67500[1], 68200[1], 69990[0], 92012[1], 92014[1], 92018[1], 92019[1], 93000[1], 93005[1], 93010[1], 93040[1], 93041[1], 93042[1], 93318[1], 93355[1], 94002[1], 94200[1], 94680[1], 94681[1], 94690[1], 95812[1], 95813[1], 95816[1], 95819[1], 95822[1], 95829[1], 95955[1], 96360[1], 96361[1], 96365[1], 96366[1], 96367[1], 96368[1], 96372[1], 96374[1], 96375[1], 96376[1], 96377[1], 96523[0], 99155[0], 99156[0], 99157[0], 99211[1], 99212[1], 99213[1], 99214[1], 99215[1], 99217[1], 99218[1], 99219[1], 99220[1], 99221[1], 99222[1], 99223[1], 99231[1], 99232[1], 99233[1], 99234[1], 99235[1], 99236[1], 99238[1], 99239[1], 99241[1], 99242[1], 99243[1], 99244[1], 99245[1], 99251[1], 99252[1], 99253[1], 99254[1], 99255[1], 99291[1], 99292[1], 99304[1], 99305[1], 99306[1], 99307[1], 99308[1], 99309[1], 99310[1], 99315[1], 99316[1], 99334[1], 99335[1], 99336[1], 99337[1], 99347[1], 99348[1], 99349[1], 99350[1], 99374[1], 99375[1], 99377[1], 99378[1], 99446[0], 99447[0], 99448[0], 99449[0], 99451[0], 99452[0], 99495[0], 99496[0], G0463[1], G0471[1], J0670[1], J2001[1]
66821	0213T[0], 0216T[0], 0465T[1], 0596T[1], 0597T[1], 0616T[1], 0699T[1], 0708T[1], 0709T[1], 12001[1], 12002[1], 12004[1], 12005[1], 12006[1], 12007[1], 12011[1], 12013[1], 12014[1], 12015[1], 12016[1], 12017[1], 12018[1], 12020[1], 12021[1], 12031[1], 12032[1], 12034[1], 12035[1], 12036[1], 12037[1], 12041[1], 12042[1], 12044[1], 12045[1], 12046[1], 12047[1], 12051[1], 12052[1], 12053[1], 12054[1], 12055[1], 12056[1], 12057[1], 13100[1], 13101[1], 13102[1], 13120[1], 13121[1], 13122[1], 13131[1], 13132[1], 13133[1], 13151[1], 13152[1], 13153[1], 36000[1], 36400[1], 36405[1], 36406[1], 36410[1], 36420[1], 36425[1], 36430[1], 36440[1], 36591[0], 36592[0], 36600[1], 36640[1], 43752[1], 51701[1], 51702[1], 51703[1], 62320[0], 62321[0], 62322[0], 62323[0], 62324[0], 62325[0], 62326[0], 62327[0], 64400[0], 64405[0], 64408[0], 64415[0], 64416[0], 64417[0], 64418[0], 64420[0], 64421[0], 64425[0], 64430[0], 64435[0], 64445[0], 64446[0], 64447[0], 64448[0], 64449[0], 64450[0], 64451[0], 64454[0], 64461[0], 64462[0], 64463[0], 64479[0], 64480[0], 64483[0], 64484[0], 64486[0], 64487[0], 64488[0], 64489[0], 64490[0], 64491[0], 64492[0], 64493[0], 64494[0], 64495[0], 64505[0], 64510[0], 64517[0], 64520[0], 64530[0], 66030[1], 66250[1], 66500[1], 66505[1], 66600[1], 66605[1], 66625[1], 66630[1], 66635[1], 66680[1], 66682[1], 66820[1], 67028[1], 67036[1], 67500[1], 68200[1], 69990[0], 92012[1], 92014[1], 92018[1], 92019[1], 93000[1], 93005[1], 93010[1], 93040[1], 93041[1], 93042[1], 93318[1], 93355[1], 94002[1], 94200[1], 94680[1], 94681[1], 94690[1], 95812[1], 95813[1], 95816[1], 95819[1], 95822[1], 95829[1], 95955[1], 96360[1], 96361[1], 96365[1], 96366[1], 96367[1], 96368[1], 96372[1], 96374[1], 96375[1], 96376[1], 96377[1], 96523[0], 99155[0], 99156[0], 99157[0], 99211[1], 99212[1], 99213[1], 99214[1], 99215[1], 99217[1], 99218[1], 99219[1], 99220[1], 99221[1], 99222[1], 99223[1], 99231[1], 99232[1], 99233[1], 99234[1], 99235[1], 99236[1], 99238[1], 99239[1], 99241[1], 99242[1], 99243[1], 99244[1], 99245[1], 99251[1], 99252[1], 99253[1], 99254[1], 99255[1], 99291[1], 99292[1], 99304[1], 99305[1], 99306[1], 99307[1], 99308[1], 99309[1], 99310[1], 99315[1], 99316[1], 99334[1], 99335[1], 99336[1], 99337[1], 99347[1], 99348[1], 99349[1], 99350[1], 99374[1], 99375[1], 99377[1], 99378[1], 99446[0], 99447[0], 99448[0], 99449[0], 99451[0], 99452[0], 99495[0], 99496[0], G0463[1], G0471[1]

0 = Modifier usage not allowed or inappropriate   1 = Modifier usage allowed

Appendix A: NCCI - CPT Codes

Code 1	Code 2
66825	0213T[0], 0216T[0], 0465T[1], 0596T[1], 0597T[1], 0616T[1], 0699T[1], 0708T[1], 0709T[1], 12001[1], 12002[1], 12004[1], 12005[1], 12006[1], 12007[1], 12011[1], 12013[1], 12014[1], 12015[1], 12016[1], 12017[1], 12018[1], 12020[1], 12021[1], 12031[1], 12032[1], 12034[1], 12035[1], 12036[1], 12037[1], 12041[1], 12042[1], 12044[1], 12045[1], 12046[1], 12047[1], 12051[1], 12052[1], 12053[1], 12054[1], 12055[1], 12056[1], 12057[1], 13100[1], 13101[1], 13102[1], 13120[1], 13121[1], 13122[1], 13131[1], 13132[1], 13133[1], 13151[1], 13152[1], 13153[1], 36000[1], 36400[1], 36405[1], 36406[1], 36410[1], 36420[1], 36425[1], 36430[1], 36440[1], 36591[0], 36592[0], 36600[1], 36640[1], 43752[1], 51701[1], 51702[1], 51703[1], 62320[0], 62321[0], 62322[0], 62323[0], 62324[0], 62325[0], 62326[0], 62327[0], 64400[0], 64405[0], 64408[0], 64415[0], 64416[0], 64417[0], 64418[0], 64420[0], 64421[0], 64425[0], 64430[0], 64435[0], 64445[0], 64446[0], 64447[0], 64448[0], 64449[0], 64450[0], 64451[0], 64454[0], 64461[0], 64462[0], 64463[0], 64479[0], 64480[0], 64483[0], 64484[0], 64486[0], 64487[0], 64488[0], 64489[0], 64490[0], 64491[0], 64492[0], 64493[0], 64494[0], 64495[0], 64505[0], 64510[0], 64517[0], 64520[0], 64530[0], 66030[1], 66250[1], 66500[1], 66505[1], 66600[1], 66605[1], 66625[1], 66630[1], 66635[1], 66680[1], 66682[1], 67028[1], 67500[1], 68200[1], 69990[0], 92012[1], 92014[1], 92018[1], 92019[1], 93000[1], 93005[1], 93010[1], 93040[1], 93041[1], 93042[1], 93318[1], 93355[1], 94002[1], 94200[1], 94680[1], 94681[1], 94690[1], 95812[1], 95813[1], 95816[1], 95819[1], 95822[1], 95829[1], 95955[1], 96360[1], 96361[1], 96365[1], 96366[1], 96367[1], 96368[1], 96372[1], 96374[1], 96375[1], 96376[1], 96377[1], 96523[0], 99155[0], 99156[0], 99157[0], 99211[1], 99212[1], 99213[1], 99214[1], 99215[1], 99217[1], 99218[1], 99219[1], 99220[1], 99221[1], 99222[1], 99223[1], 99231[1], 99232[1], 99233[1], 99234[1], 99235[1], 99236[1], 99238[1], 99239[1], 99241[1], 99242[1], 99243[1], 99244[1], 99245[1], 99251[1], 99252[1], 99253[1], 99254[1], 99255[1], 99291[1], 99292[1], 99304[1], 99305[1], 99306[1], 99307[1], 99308[1], 99309[1], 99310[1], 99315[1], 99316[1], 99334[1], 99335[1], 99336[1], 99337[1], 99347[1], 99348[1], 99349[1], 99350[1], 99374[1], 99375[1], 99377[1], 99378[1], 99446[0], 99447[0], 99448[0], 99449[0], 99451[0], 99452[0], 99495[0], 99496[0], G0463[1], G0471[1], J0670[1], J2001[1]
66830	0213T[0], 0216T[0], 0465T[1], 0596T[1], 0597T[1], 0616T[1], 0618T[1], 0699T[1], 0708T[1], 0709T[1], 11000[1], 11001[1], 11004[1], 11005[1], 11006[1], 11042[1], 11043[1], 11044[1], 11045[1], 11046[1], 11047[1], 12001[1], 12002[1], 12004[1], 12005[1], 12006[1], 12007[1], 12011[1], 12013[1], 12014[1], 12015[1], 12016[1], 12017[1], 12018[1], 12020[1], 12021[1], 12031[1], 12032[1], 12034[1], 12035[1], 12036[1], 12037[1], 12041[1], 12042[1], 12044[1], 12045[1], 12046[1], 12047[1], 12051[1], 12052[1], 12053[1], 12054[1], 12055[1], 12056[1], 12057[1], 13100[1], 13101[1], 13102[1], 13120[1], 13121[1], 13122[1], 13131[1], 13132[1], 13133[1], 13151[1], 13152[1], 13153[1], 36000[1], 36400[1], 36405[1], 36406[1], 36410[1], 36420[1], 36425[1], 36430[1], 36440[1], 36591[0], 36592[0], 36600[1], 36640[1], 43752[1], 51701[1], 51702[1], 51703[1], 62320[0], 62321[0], 62322[0], 62323[0], 62324[0], 62325[0], 62326[0], 62327[0], 64400[0], 64405[0], 64408[0], 64415[0], 64416[0], 64417[0], 64418[0], 64420[0], 64421[0], 64425[0], 64430[0], 64435[0], 64445[0], 64446[0], 64447[0], 64448[0], 64449[0], 64450[0], 64451[0], 64454[0], 64461[0], 64462[0], 64463[0], 64479[0], 64480[0], 64483[0], 64484[0], 64486[0], 64487[0], 64488[0], 64489[0], 64490[0], 64491[0], 64492[0], 64493[0], 64494[0], 64495[0], 64505[0], 64510[0], 64517[0], 64520[0], 64530[0], 65772[1], 65775[1], 66030[1], 66250[1], 66500[1], 66505[1], 66600[1], 66605[1], 66625[1], 66630[1], 66635[1], 66820[1], 66821[1], 66825[1], 67005[1], 67028[1], 67500[1], 67715[1], 68200[1], 69990[0], 92012[1], 92014[1], 92018[1], 92019[1], 93000[1], 93005[1], 93010[1], 93040[1], 93041[1], 93042[1], 93318[1], 93355[1], 94002[1], 94200[1], 94680[1], 94681[1], 94690[1], 95812[1], 95813[1], 95816[1], 95819[1], 95822[1], 95829[1], 95955[1], 96360[1], 96361[1], 96365[1], 96366[1], 96367[1], 96368[1], 96372[1], 96374[1], 96375[1], 96376[1], 96377[1], 96523[0], 97597[1], 97598[1], 97602[1], 99155[0], 99156[0], 99157[0], 99211[1], 99212[1], 99213[1], 99214[1], 99215[1], 99217[1], 99218[1], 99219[1], 99220[1], 99221[1], 99222[1], 99223[1], 99231[1], 99232[1], 99233[1], 99234[1], 99235[1], 99236[1], 99238[1], 99239[1], 99241[1], 99242[1], 99243[1], 99244[1], 99245[1], 99251[1], 99252[1], 99253[1], 99254[1], 99255[1], 99291[1], 99292[1], 99304[1], 99305[1], 99306[1], 99307[1], 99308[1], 99309[1], 99310[1], 99315[1], 99316[1], 99334[1], 99335[1], 99336[1], 99337[1], 99347[1], 99348[1], 99349[1], 99350[1], 99374[1], 99375[1], 99377[1], 99378[1], 99446[0], 99447[0], 99448[0], 99449[0], 99451[0], 99452[0], 99495[0], 99496[0], G0463[1], G0471[1]
66840	0213T[0], 0216T[0], 0465T[1], 0596T[1], 0597T[1], 0616T[1], 0618T[1], 0699T[1], 0708T[1], 0709T[1], 11000[1], 11001[1], 11004[1], 11005[1], 11006[1], 11042[1], 11043[1], 11044[1], 11045[1], 11046[1], 11047[1], 12001[1], 12002[1], 12004[1], 12005[1], 12006[1], 12007[1], 12011[1], 12013[1], 12014[1], 12015[1], 12016[1], 12017[1], 12018[1], 12020[1], 12021[1], 12031[1], 12032[1], 12034[1], 12035[1], 12036[1], 12037[1], 12041[1], 12042[1], 12044[1], 12045[1], 12046[1], 12047[1], 12051[1], 12052[1], 12053[1], 12054[1], 12055[1], 12056[1], 12057[1], 13100[1], 13101[1], 13102[1], 13120[1], 13121[1], 13122[1], 13131[1], 13132[1], 13133[1], 13151[1], 13152[1], 13153[1], 36000[1], 36400[1], 36405[1], 36406[1], 36410[1], 36420[1], 36425[1], 36430[1], 36440[1], 36591[0], 36592[0], 36600[1], 36640[1], 43752[1], 51701[1], 51702[1], 51703[1], 62320[0], 62321[0], 62322[0], 62323[0], 62324[0], 62325[0], 62326[0], 62327[0], 64400[0], 64405[0], 64408[0], 64415[0], 64416[0], 64417[0], 64418[0], 64420[0], 64421[0], 64425[0], 64430[0], 64435[0], 64445[0], 64446[0], 64447[0], 64448[0], 64449[0], 64450[0], 64451[0], 64454[0], 64461[0], 64462[0], 64463[0], 64479[0], 64480[0], 64483[0], 64484[0], 64486[0], 64487[0], 64488[0], 64489[0], 64490[0], 64491[0], 64492[0], 64493[0], 64494[0], 64495[0], 64505[0], 64510[0], 64517[0], 64520[0], 64530[0], 65772[1], 65775[1], 66030[1], 66250[1], 66500[1], 66505[1], 66600[1], 66605[1], 66625[1], 66630[1], 66635[1], 66820[1], 66821[1], 66825[1], 66830[1], 67028[1], 67500[1], 67715[1], 68200[1], 69990[0], 92012[1], 92014[1], 92018[1], 92019[1], 93000[1], 93005[1], 93010[1], 93040[1], 93041[1], 93042[1], 93318[1], 93355[1], 94002[1], 94200[1], 94680[1], 94681[1], 94690[1], 95812[1], 95813[1], 95816[1], 95819[1], 95822[1], 95829[1], 95955[1], 96360[1], 96361[1], 96365[1], 96366[1], 96367[1], 96368[1], 96372[1], 96374[1], 96375[1], 96376[1], 96377[1], 96523[0], 97597[1], 97598[1], 97602[1], 99155[0], 99156[0], 99157[0], 99211[1], 99212[1], 99213[1], 99214[1], 99215[1], 99217[1], 99218[1], 99219[1], 99220[1], 99221[1], 99222[1], 99223[1], 99231[1], 99232[1], 99233[1], 99234[1], 99235[1], 99236[1], 99238[1], 99239[1], 99241[1], 99242[1], 99243[1], 99244[1], 99245[1], 99251[1], 99252[1], 99253[1], 99254[1], 99255[1], 99291[1], 99292[1], 99304[1], 99305[1], 99306[1], 99307[1], 99308[1], 99309[1], 99310[1], 99315[1], 99316[1], 99334[1], 99335[1], 99336[1], 99337[1], 99347[1], 99348[1], 99349[1], 99350[1], 99374[1], 99375[1], 99377[1], 99378[1], 99446[0], 99447[0], 99448[0], 99449[0], 99451[0], 99452[0], 99495[0], 99496[0], G0463[1], G0471[1]
66850	0213T[0], 0216T[0], 0465T[1], 0596T[1], 0597T[1], 0616T[1], 0699T[1], 0708T[1], 0709T[1], 11000[1], 11001[1], 11004[1], 11005[1], 11006[1], 11042[1], 11043[1], 11044[1], 11045[1], 11046[1], 11047[1], 12001[1], 12002[1], 12004[1], 12005[1], 12006[1], 12007[1], 12011[1], 12013[1], 12014[1], 12015[1], 12016[1], 12017[1], 12018[1], 12020[1], 12021[1], 12031[1], 12032[1], 12034[1], 12035[1], 12036[1], 12037[1], 12041[1], 12042[1], 12044[1], 12045[1], 12046[1], 12047[1], 12051[1], 12052[1], 12053[1], 12054[1], 12055[1], 12056[1], 12057[1], 13100[1], 13101[1], 13102[1], 13120[1], 13121[1], 13122[1], 13131[1], 13132[1], 13133[1], 13151[1], 13152[1], 13153[1], 36000[1], 36400[1], 36405[1], 36406[1], 36410[1], 36420[1], 36425[1], 36430[1], 36440[1], 36591[0], 36592[0], 36600[1], 36640[1], 43752[1], 51701[1], 51702[1], 51703[1], 62320[0], 62321[0], 62322[0], 62323[0], 62324[0], 62325[0], 62326[0], 62327[0], 64400[0], 64405[0], 64408[0], 64415[0], 64416[0], 64417[0], 64418[0], 64420[0], 64421[0], 64425[0], 64430[0], 64435[0], 64445[0], 64446[0], 64447[0], 64448[0], 64449[0], 64450[0], 64451[0], 64454[0], 64461[0], 64462[0], 64463[0], 64479[0], 64480[0], 64483[0], 64484[0], 64486[0], 64487[0], 64488[0], 64489[0], 64490[0], 64491[0], 64492[0], 64493[0], 64494[0], 64495[0], 64505[0], 64510[0], 64517[0], 64520[0], 64530[0], 65772[1], 65775[1], 66030[1], 66250[1], 66500[1], 66505[1], 66600[1], 66605[1], 66625[1], 66630[1], 66635[1], 66820[1], 66821[1], 66825[1], 66830[1], 66840[1], 66920[1], 66940[1], 66983[1], 66984[1], 66988[1], 66991[1], 67028[1], 67500[1], 67715[1], 68200[1], 69990[0], 92012[1], 92014[1], 92018[1], 92019[1], 93000[1], 93005[1], 93010[1], 93040[1], 93041[1], 93042[1], 93318[1], 93355[1], 94002[1], 94200[1], 94680[1], 94681[1], 94690[1], 95812[1], 95813[1], 95816[1], 95819[1], 95822[1], 95829[1], 95955[1], 96360[1], 96361[1], 96365[1], 96366[1], 96367[1], 96368[1], 96372[1], 96374[1], 96375[1], 96376[1], 96377[1], 96523[0], 97597[1], 97598[1], 97602[1], 99155[0], 99156[0], 99157[0], 99211[1], 99212[1], 99213[1], 99214[1], 99215[1], 99217[1], 99218[1], 99219[1], 99220[1], 99221[1], 99222[1], 99223[1], 99231[1], 99232[1], 99233[1], 99234[1], 99235[1], 99236[1], 99238[1], 99239[1], 99241[1], 99242[1], 99243[1], 99244[1], 99245[1], 99251[1], 99252[1], 99253[1], 99254[1], 99255[1], 99291[1], 99292[1], 99304[1], 99305[1], 99306[1], 99307[1], 99308[1], 99309[1], 99310[1], 99315[1], 99316[1], 99334[1], 99335[1], 99336[1], 99337[1], 99347[1], 99348[1], 99349[1], 99350[1], 99374[1], 99375[1], 99377[1], 99378[1], 99446[0], 99447[0], 99448[0], 99449[0], 99451[0], 99452[0], 99495[0], 99496[0], G0463[1], G0471[1]
66852	0213T[0], 0216T[0], 0465T[1], 0596T[1], 0597T[1], 0616T[1], 0618T[1], 0699T[1], 0708T[1], 0709T[1], 11000[1], 11001[1], 11004[1], 11005[1], 11006[1], 11042[1], 11043[1], 11044[1], 11045[1], 11046[1], 11047[1], 12001[1], 12002[1], 12004[1], 12005[1], 12006[1], 12007[1], 12011[1], 12013[1], 12014[1], 12015[1], 12016[1], 12017[1], 12018[1], 12020[1], 12021[1], 12031[1], 12032[1], 12034[1], 12035[1], 12036[1], 12037[1], 12041[1], 12042[1], 12044[1], 12045[1], 12046[1], 12047[1], 12051[1], 12052[1], 12053[1], 12054[1], 12055[1], 12056[1], 12057[1], 13100[1], 13101[1], 13102[1], 13120[1], 13121[1], 13122[1], 13131[1], 13132[1], 13133[1], 13151[1], 13152[1], 13153[1], 36000[1], 36400[1], 36405[1], 36406[1], 36410[1], 36420[1], 36425[1], 36430[1], 36440[1], 36591[0], 36592[0], 36600[1], 36640[1], 43752[1], 51701[1], 51702[1], 51703[1], 62320[0], 62321[0], 62322[0], 62323[0], 62324[0], 62325[0], 62326[0], 62327[0], 64400[0], 64405[0], 64408[0], 64415[0], 64416[0], 64417[0], 64418[0], 64420[0], 64421[0], 64425[0], 64430[0], 64435[0], 64445[0], 64446[0], 64447[0], 64448[0], 64449[0], 64450[0], 64451[0], 64454[0], 64461[0], 64462[0], 64463[0], 64479[0], 64480[0], 64483[0], 64484[0], 64486[0], 64487[0], 64488[0], 64489[0], 64490[0], 64491[0], 64492[0], 64493[0], 64494[0], 64495[0], 64505[0], 64510[0], 64517[0], 64520[0], 64530[0], 65235[1], 65772[1], 65775[1], 66030[1], 66500[1], 66505[1], 66600[1], 66605[1], 66625[1], 66630[1], 66635[1], 66820[1], 66821[1], 66825[1], 66830[1], 66840[1], 66850[1], 66920[1], 66930[1], 66940[1], 66983[1], 66984[1], 66988[1], 66991[1], 67028[1], 67036[1], 67500[1], 67715[1], 68200[1], 69990[0], 92012[1], 92014[1], 92018[1], 92019[1], 93000[1], 93005[1], 93010[1], 93040[1], 93041[1], 93042[1], 93318[1], 93355[1], 94002[1], 94200[1], 94680[1], 94681[1], 94690[1], 95812[1], 95813[1], 95816[1], 95819[1], 95822[1], 95829[1], 95955[1], 96360[1], 96361[1], 96365[1], 96366[1], 96367[1], 96368[1], 96372[1], 96374[1], 96375[1], 96376[1], 96377[1], 96523[0], 97597[1], 97598[1], 97602[1], 99155[0], 99156[0], 99157[0], 99211[1], 99212[1], 99213[1], 99214[1], 99215[1], 99217[1], 99218[1], 99219[1], 99220[1], 99221[1], 99222[1], 99223[1], 99231[1], 99232[1], 99233[1], 99234[1], 99235[1], 99236[1], 99238[1], 99239[1], 99241[1], 99242[1], 99243[1], 99244[1], 99245[1], 99251[1], 99252[1], 99253[1], 99254[1], 99255[1], 99291[1], 99292[1], 99304[1], 99305[1], 99306[1], 99307[1], 99308[1], 99309[1], 99310[1], 99315[1], 99316[1], 99334[1], 99335[1], 99336[1], 99337[1], 99347[1], 99348[1], 99349[1], 99350[1], 99374[1], 99375[1], 99377[1], 99378[1], 99446[0], 99447[0], 99448[0], 99449[0], 99451[0], 99452[0], 99495[0], 99496[0], G0463[1], G0471[1]

0 = Modifier usage not allowed or inappropriate 1 = Modifier usage allowed

Code 1	Code 2
66920	0213T[0], 0216T[0], 0465T[1], 0596T[1], 0597T[1], 0616T[1], 0618T[1], 0699T[1], 0708T[1], 0709T[1], 11000[1], 11001[1], 11004[1], 11005[1], 11006[1], 11042[1], 11043[1], 11044[1], 11045[1], 11046[1], 11047[1], 12001[1], 12002[1], 12004[1], 12005[1], 12006[1], 12007[1], 12011[1], 12013[1], 12014[1], 12015[1], 12016[1], 12017[1], 12018[1], 12020[1], 12021[1], 12031[1], 12032[1], 12034[1], 12035[1], 12036[1], 12037[1], 12041[1], 12042[1], 12044[1], 12045[1], 12046[1], 12047[1], 12051[1], 12052[1], 12053[1], 12054[1], 12055[1], 12056[1], 12057[1], 13100[1], 13101[1], 13102[1], 13120[1], 13121[1], 13122[1], 13131[1], 13132[1], 13133[1], 13151[1], 13152[1], 13153[1], 36000[1], 36400[1], 36405[1], 36406[1], 36410[1], 36420[1], 36425[1], 36430[1], 36440[1], 36591[0], 36592[0], 36600[1], 36640[1], 43752[1], 51701[1], 51702[1], 51703[1], 62320[0], 62321[0], 62322[0], 62323[0], 62324[0], 62325[0], 62326[0], 62327[0], 64400[0], 64405[0], 64408[0], 64415[0], 64416[0], 64417[0], 64418[0], 64420[0], 64421[0], 64425[0], 64430[0], 64435[0], 64445[0], 64446[0], 64447[0], 64448[0], 64449[0], 64450[0], 64451[0], 64454[0], 64461[0], 64462[0], 64463[0], 64479[0], 64480[0], 64483[0], 64484[0], 64486[0], 64487[0], 64488[0], 64489[0], 64490[0], 64491[0], 64492[0], 64493[0], 64494[0], 64495[0], 64505[0], 64510[0], 64517[0], 64520[0], 64530[0], 65772[1], 65775[1], 66030[1], 66250[1], 66500[1], 66505[1], 66600[1], 66605[1], 66625[1], 66630[1], 66635[1], 66820[1], 66821[1], 66825[1], 66830[1], 66840[1], 66983[1], 67005[1], 67028[1], 67500[1], 67715[1], 68200[1], 69990[0], 92012[1], 92014[1], 92018[1], 92019[1], 93000[1], 93005[1], 93010[1], 93040[1], 93041[1], 93042[1], 93318[1], 93355[1], 94002[1], 94200[1], 94680[1], 94681[1], 94690[1], 95812[1], 95813[1], 95816[1], 95819[1], 95822[1], 95829[1], 95955[1], 96360[1], 96361[1], 96365[1], 96366[1], 96367[1], 96368[1], 96372[1], 96374[1], 96375[1], 96376[1], 96377[1], 96523[0], 97597[1], 97598[1], 97602[1], 99155[0], 99156[0], 99157[0], 99211[1], 99212[1], 99213[1], 99214[1], 99215[1], 99217[1], 99218[1], 99219[1], 99220[1], 99221[1], 99222[1], 99223[1], 99231[1], 99232[1], 99233[1], 99234[1], 99235[1], 99236[1], 99238[1], 99239[1], 99241[1], 99242[1], 99243[1], 99244[1], 99245[1], 99251[1], 99252[1], 99253[1], 99254[1], 99255[1], 99291[1], 99292[1], 99304[1], 99305[1], 99306[1], 99307[1], 99308[1], 99309[1], 99310[1], 99315[1], 99316[1], 99334[1], 99335[1], 99336[1], 99337[1], 99347[1], 99348[1], 99349[1], 99350[1], 99374[1], 99375[1], 99377[1], 99378[1], 99446[0], 99447[0], 99448[0], 99449[0], 99451[0], 99452[0], 99495[0], 99496[0], G0463[1], G0471[1]
66930	0213T[0], 0216T[0], 0465T[1], 0596T[1], 0597T[1], 0616T[1], 0618T[1], 0699T[1], 0708T[1], 0709T[1], 11000[1], 11001[1], 11004[1], 11005[1], 11006[1], 11042[1], 11043[1], 11044[1], 11045[1], 11046[1], 11047[1], 12001[1], 12002[1], 12004[1], 12005[1], 12006[1], 12007[1], 12011[1], 12013[1], 12014[1], 12015[1], 12016[1], 12017[1], 12018[1], 12020[1], 12021[1], 12031[1], 12032[1], 12034[1], 12035[1], 12036[1], 12037[1], 12041[1], 12042[1], 12044[1], 12045[1], 12046[1], 12047[1], 12051[1], 12052[1], 12053[1], 12054[1], 12055[1], 12056[1], 12057[1], 13100[1], 13101[1], 13102[1], 13120[1], 13121[1], 13122[1], 13131[1], 13132[1], 13133[1], 13151[1], 13152[1], 13153[1], 36000[1], 36400[1], 36405[1], 36406[1], 36410[1], 36420[1], 36425[1], 36430[1], 36440[1], 36591[0], 36592[0], 36600[1], 36640[1], 43752[1], 51701[1], 51702[1], 51703[1], 62320[0], 62321[0], 62322[0], 62323[0], 62324[0], 62325[0], 62326[0], 62327[0], 64400[0], 64405[0], 64408[0], 64415[0], 64416[0], 64417[0], 64418[0], 64420[0], 64421[0], 64425[0], 64430[0], 64435[0], 64445[0], 64446[0], 64447[0], 64448[0], 64449[0], 64450[0], 64451[0], 64454[0], 64461[0], 64462[0], 64463[0], 64479[0], 64480[0], 64483[0], 64484[0], 64486[0], 64487[0], 64488[0], 64489[0], 64490[0], 64491[0], 64492[0], 64493[0], 64494[0], 64495[0], 64505[0], 64510[0], 64517[0], 64520[0], 64530[0], 65235[1], 65772[1], 65775[1], 66030[1], 66250[1], 66500[1], 66505[1], 66600[1], 66605[1], 66625[1], 66630[1], 66635[1], 66820[1], 66821[1], 66825[1], 66830[1], 66840[1], 66850[1], 66920[1], 66940[1], 66983[1], 66984[1], 66988[1], 66991[1], 67028[1], 67500[1], 67715[1], 68200[1], 69990[0], 92012[1], 92014[1], 92018[1], 92019[1], 93000[1], 93005[1], 93010[1], 93040[1], 93041[1], 93042[1], 93318[1], 93355[1], 94002[1], 94200[1], 94680[1], 94681[1], 94690[1], 95812[1], 95813[1], 95816[1], 95819[1], 95822[1], 95829[1], 95955[1], 96360[1], 96361[1], 96365[1], 96366[1], 96367[1], 96368[1], 96372[1], 96374[1], 96375[1], 96376[1], 96377[1], 96523[0], 97597[1], 97598[1], 97602[1], 99155[0], 99156[0], 99157[0], 99211[1], 99212[1], 99213[1], 99214[1], 99215[1], 99217[1], 99218[1], 99219[1], 99220[1], 99221[1], 99222[1], 99223[1], 99231[1], 99232[1], 99233[1], 99234[1], 99235[1], 99236[1], 99238[1], 99239[1], 99241[1], 99242[1], 99243[1], 99244[1], 99245[1], 99251[1], 99252[1], 99253[1], 99254[1], 99255[1], 99291[1], 99292[1], 99304[1], 99305[1], 99306[1], 99307[1], 99308[1], 99309[1], 99310[1], 99315[1], 99316[1], 99334[1], 99335[1], 99336[1], 99337[1], 99347[1], 99348[1], 99349[1], 99350[1], 99374[1], 99375[1], 99377[1], 99378[1], 99446[0], 99447[0], 99448[0], 99449[0], 99451[0], 99452[0], 99495[0], 99496[0], G0463[1], G0471[1]
66940	0213T[0], 0216T[0], 0465T[1], 0596T[1], 0597T[1], 0616T[1], 0618T[1], 0699T[1], 0708T[1], 0709T[1], 11000[1], 11001[1], 11004[1], 11005[1], 11006[1], 11042[1], 11043[1], 11044[1], 11045[1], 11046[1], 11047[1], 12001[1], 12002[1], 12004[1], 12005[1], 12006[1], 12007[1], 12011[1], 12013[1], 12014[1], 12015[1], 12016[1], 12017[1], 12018[1], 12020[1], 12021[1], 12031[1], 12032[1], 12034[1], 12035[1], 12036[1], 12037[1], 12041[1], 12042[1], 12044[1], 12045[1], 12046[1], 12047[1], 12051[1], 12052[1], 12053[1], 12054[1], 12055[1], 12056[1], 12057[1], 13100[1], 13101[1], 13102[1], 13120[1], 13121[1], 13122[1], 13131[1], 13132[1], 13133[1], 13151[1], 13152[1], 13153[1], 36000[1], 36400[1], 36405[1], 36406[1], 36410[1], 36420[1], 36425[1], 36430[1], 36440[1], 36591[0], 36592[0], 36600[1], 36640[1], 43752[1], 51701[1], 51702[1], 51703[1], 62320[0], 62321[0], 62322[0], 62323[0], 62324[0], 62325[0], 62326[0], 62327[0], 64400[0], 64405[0], 64408[0], 64415[0], 64416[0], 64417[0], 64418[0], 64420[0], 64421[0], 64425[0], 64430[0], 64435[0], 64445[0], 64446[0], 64447[0], 64448[0], 64449[0], 64450[0], 64451[0], 64454[0], 64461[0], 64462[0], 64463[0], 64479[0], 64480[0], 64483[0], 64484[0], 64486[0], 64487[0], 64488[0], 64489[0], 64490[0], 64491[0], 64492[0], 64493[0], 64494[0], 64495[0], 64505[0], 64510[0], 64517[0], 64520[0], 64530[0], 65772[1], 65775[1], 66030[1], 66500[1], 66505[1], 66600[1], 66605[1], 66625[1], 66630[1], 66635[1], 66820[1], 66821[1], 66825[1], 66830[1], 66840[1], 66920[1], 66983[1], 66984[1], 66988[1], 66991[1], 67028[1], 67500[1], 67715[1], 68200[1], 69990[0], 92012[1], 92014[1], 92018[1], 92019[1], 93000[1], 93005[1], 93010[1], 93040[1], 93041[1], 93042[1], 93318[1], 93355[1], 94002[1], 94200[1], 94680[1], 94681[1], 94690[1], 95812[1], 95813[1], 95816[1], 95819[1], 95822[1], 95829[1], 95955[1], 96360[1], 96361[1], 96365[1], 96366[1], 96367[1], 96368[1], 96372[1], 96374[1], 96375[1], 96376[1], 96377[1], 96523[0], 97597[1], 97598[1], 97602[1], 99155[0], 99156[0], 99157[0], 99211[1], 99212[1], 99213[1], 99214[1], 99215[1], 99217[1], 99218[1], 99219[1], 99220[1], 99221[1], 99222[1], 99223[1], 99231[1], 99232[1], 99233[1], 99234[1], 99235[1], 99236[1], 99238[1], 99239[1], 99241[1], 99242[1], 99243[1], 99244[1], 99245[1], 99251[1], 99252[1], 99253[1], 99254[1], 99255[1], 99291[1], 99292[1], 99304[1], 99305[1], 99306[1], 99307[1], 99308[1], 99309[1], 99310[1], 99315[1], 99316[1], 99334[1], 99335[1], 99336[1], 99337[1], 99347[1], 99348[1], 99349[1], 99350[1], 99374[1], 99375[1], 99377[1], 99378[1], 99446[0], 99447[0], 99448[0], 99449[0], 99451[0], 99452[0], 99495[0], 99496[0], G0463[1], G0471[1]
66982	00142[0], 0213T[0], 0216T[0], 0308T[1], 0465T[1], 0596T[1], 0597T[1], 0616T[1], 0618T[1], 0671T[1], 0699T[1], 0708T[1], 0709T[1], 11000[1], 11001[1], 11004[1], 11005[1], 11006[1], 11042[1], 11043[1], 11044[1], 11045[1], 11046[1], 11047[1], 12001[1], 12002[1], 12004[1], 12005[1], 12006[1], 12007[1], 12011[1], 12013[1], 12014[1], 12015[1], 12016[1], 12017[1], 12018[1], 12020[1], 12021[1], 12031[1], 12032[1], 12034[1], 12035[1], 12036[1], 12037[1], 12041[1], 12042[1], 12044[1], 12045[1], 12046[1], 12047[1], 12051[1], 12052[1], 12053[1], 12054[1], 12055[1], 12056[1], 12057[1], 13100[1], 13101[1], 13102[1], 13120[1], 13121[1], 13122[1], 13131[1], 13132[1], 13133[1], 13151[1], 13152[1], 13153[1], 36000[1], 36400[1], 36405[1], 36406[1], 36410[1], 36420[1], 36425[1], 36430[1], 36440[1], 36591[0], 36592[0], 36600[1], 36640[1], 43752[1], 51701[1], 51702[1], 51703[1], 62320[0], 62321[0], 62322[0], 62323[0], 62324[0], 62325[0], 62326[0], 62327[0], 64405[0], 64408[0], 64415[0], 64416[0], 64417[0], 64418[0], 64420[0], 64421[0], 64425[0], 64430[0], 64435[0], 64445[0], 64446[0], 64447[0], 64448[0], 64449[0], 64450[0], 64451[0], 64454[0], 64461[0], 64462[0], 64463[0], 64479[0], 64480[0], 64483[0], 64484[0], 64486[0], 64487[0], 64488[0], 64489[0], 64490[0], 64491[0], 64492[0], 64493[0], 64494[0], 64495[0], 64505[0], 64510[0], 64517[0], 64520[0], 64530[0], 65426[1], 65750[1], 65755[1], 65772[1], 65775[1], 65810[1], 65860[1], 65865[1], 65870[1], 65875[1], 65880[1], 66020[1], 66030[1], 66250[1], 66500[1], 66505[1], 66600[1], 66605[1], 66625[1], 66630[1], 66635[1], 66680[1], 66711[1], 66761[1], 66820[1], 66821[1], 66825[1], 66830[1], 66840[1], 66850[1], 66852[1], 66920[1], 66930[1], 66940[1], 66983[1], 66984[1], 66985[1], 66986[1], 66987[1], 66988[1], 66991[1], 67005[1], 67010[1], 67028[1], 67500[1], 67505[1], 67515[1], 67715[1], 68200[1], 69990[0], 92012[1], 92014[1], 92018[1], 92019[1], 93000[1], 93005[1], 93010[1], 93040[1], 93041[1], 93042[1], 93318[1], 93355[1], 94002[1], 94200[1], 94680[1], 94681[1], 94690[1], 95812[1], 95813[1], 95816[1], 95819[1], 95822[1], 95829[1], 95955[1], 96360[1], 96361[1], 96365[1], 96366[1], 96367[1], 96368[1], 96372[1], 96374[1], 96375[1], 96376[1], 96377[1], 96523[0], 97597[1], 97598[1], 97602[1], 99155[0], 99156[0], 99157[0], 99211[1], 99212[1], 99213[1], 99214[1], 99215[1], 99217[1], 99218[1], 99219[1], 99220[1], 99221[1], 99222[1], 99223[1], 99231[1], 99232[1], 99233[1], 99234[1], 99235[1], 99236[1], 99238[1], 99239[1], 99241[1], 99242[1], 99243[1], 99244[1], 99245[1], 99251[1], 99252[1], 99253[1], 99254[1], 99255[1], 99291[1], 99292[1], 99304[1], 99305[1], 99306[1], 99307[1], 99308[1], 99309[1], 99310[1], 99315[1], 99316[1], 99334[1], 99335[1], 99336[1], 99337[1], 99347[1], 99348[1], 99349[1], 99350[1], 99374[1], 99375[1], 99377[1], 99378[1], 99446[0], 99447[0], 99448[0], 99449[0], 99451[0], 99452[0], 99495[0], 99496[0], G0463[1], G0471[1]
66983	0213T[0], 0216T[0], 0308T[1], 0465T[1], 0596T[1], 0597T[1], 0616T[1], 0699T[1], 0708T[1], 0709T[1], 11000[1], 11001[1], 11004[1], 11005[1], 11006[1], 11042[1], 11043[1], 11044[1], 11045[1], 11046[1], 11047[1], 12001[1], 12002[1], 12004[1], 12005[1], 12006[1], 12007[1], 12011[1], 12013[1], 12014[1], 12015[1], 12016[1], 12017[1], 12018[1], 12020[1], 12021[1], 12031[1], 12032[1], 12034[1], 12035[1], 12036[1], 12037[1], 12041[1], 12042[1], 12044[1], 12045[1], 12046[1], 12047[1], 12051[1], 12052[1], 12053[1], 12054[1], 12055[1], 12056[1], 12057[1], 13100[1], 13101[1], 13102[1], 13120[1], 13121[1], 13122[1], 13131[1], 13132[1], 13133[1], 13151[1], 13152[1], 13153[1], 36000[1], 36400[1], 36405[1], 36406[1], 36410[1], 36420[1], 36425[1], 36430[1], 36440[1], 36591[0], 36592[0], 36600[1], 36640[1], 43752[1], 51701[1], 51702[1], 51703[1], 62320[0], 62321[0], 62322[0], 62323[0], 62324[0], 62325[0], 62326[0], 62327[0], 64400[0], 64405[0], 64408[0], 64415[0], 64416[0], 64417[0], 64418[0], 64420[0], 64421[0], 64425[0], 64430[0], 64435[0], 64445[0], 64446[0], 64447[0], 64448[0], 64449[0], 64450[0], 64451[0], 64454[0], 64461[0], 64462[0], 64463[0], 64479[0], 64480[0], 64483[0], 64484[0], 64486[0], 64487[0], 64488[0], 64489[0], 64490[0], 64491[0], 64492[0], 64493[0], 64494[0], 64495[0], 64505[0], 64510[0], 64517[0], 64520[0], 64530[0], 65235[1], 65260[1], 65265[1], 65772[1], 65775[1], 66030[1], 66250[1], 66500[1], 66505[1], 66600[1], 66605[1], 66625[1], 66630[1], 66635[1], 66820[1], 66821[1], 66825[1], 66830[1], 66840[1], 67005[1], 67028[1], 67500[1], 67715[1], 68200[1], 69990[0], 92012[1], 92014[1], 92018[1], 92019[1], 93000[1], 93005[1], 93010[1], 93040[1], 93041[1], 93042[1], 93318[1], 93355[1], 94002[1], 94200[1], 94680[1], 94681[1], 94690[1], 95812[1], 95813[1], 95816[1], 95819[1], 95822[1], 95829[1], 95955[1], 96360[1], 96361[1], 96365[1], 96366[1], 96367[1], 96368[1], 96372[1], 96374[1], 96375[1], 96376[1], 96377[1], 96523[0], 97597[1], 97598[1], 97602[1], 99155[0], 99156[0], 99157[0], 99211[1], 99212[1], 99213[1], 99214[1], 99215[1], 99217[1], 99218[1], 99219[1], 99220[1],

0 = Modifier usage not allowed or inappropriate 1 = Modifier usage allowed

Code 1	Code 2
	99221[1], 99222[1], 99223[1], 99231[1], 99232[1], 99233[1], 99234[1], 99235[1], 99236[1], 99238[1], 99239[1], 99241[1], 99242[1], 99243[1], 99244[1], 99245[1], 99251[1], 99252[1], 99253[1], 99254[1], 99255[1], 99291[1], 99292[1], 99304[1], 99305[1], 99306[1], 99307[1], 99308[1], 99309[1], 99310[1], 99315[1], 99316[1], 99334[1], 99335[1], 99336[1], 99337[1], 99347[1], 99348[1], 99349[1], 99350[1], 99374[1], 99375[1], 99377[1], 99378[1], 99446[0], 99447[0], 99448[0], 99449[0], 99451[0], 99452[0], 99495[0], 99496[0], G0463[1], G0471[1]
66984	00142[0], 00144[0], 0213T[0], 0216T[0], 0308T[1], 0465T[1], 0596T[1], 0597T[1], 0616T[1], 0671T[1], 0699T[1], 0708T[1], 0709T[1], 11000[1], 11001[1], 11004[1], 11005[1], 11006[1], 11042[1], 11043[1], 11044[1], 11045[1], 11046[1], 11047[1], 12001[1], 12002[1], 12004[1], 12005[1], 12006[1], 12007[1], 12011[1], 12013[1], 12014[1], 12015[1], 12016[1], 12017[1], 12018[1], 12020[1], 12021[1], 12031[1], 12032[1], 12034[1], 12035[1], 12036[1], 12037[1], 12041[1], 12042[1], 12044[1], 12045[1], 12046[1], 12047[1], 12051[1], 12052[1], 12053[1], 12054[1], 12055[1], 12056[1], 12057[1], 13100[1], 13101[1], 13102[1], 13120[1], 13121[1], 13122[1], 13131[1], 13132[1], 13133[1], 13151[1], 13152[1], 13153[1], 36000[1], 36400[1], 36405[1], 36406[1], 36410[1], 36420[1], 36425[1], 36430[1], 36440[1], 36591[0], 36592[0], 36600[1], 36640[1], 43752[1], 51701[1], 51702[1], 51703[1], 62320[0], 62321[0], 62322[0], 62323[0], 62324[0], 62325[0], 62326[0], 62327[0], 64405[0], 64408[0], 64415[0], 64416[0], 64417[0], 64418[0], 64420[0], 64421[0], 64425[0], 64430[0], 64435[0], 64445[0], 64446[0], 64447[0], 64448[0], 64449[0], 64450[0], 64451[0], 64454[0], 64461[0], 64462[0], 64463[0], 64479[0], 64480[0], 64483[0], 64484[0], 64486[0], 64487[0], 64488[0], 64489[0], 64490[0], 64491[0], 64492[0], 64493[0], 64494[0], 64495[0], 64505[0], 64510[0], 64517[0], 64520[0], 64530[0], 65426[1], 65750[1], 65755[1], 65772[1], 65775[1], 65810[1], 65860[1], 65865[1], 65870[1], 65875[1], 65880[1], 66020[1], 66030[1], 66250[1], 66500[1], 66505[1], 66600[1], 66605[1], 66625[1], 66630[1], 66635[1], 66680[1], 66711[1], 66820[1], 66821[1], 66825[1], 66830[1], 66840[1], 66920[1], 66983[1], 66988[1], 67005[1], 67010[1], 67028[1], 67500[1], 67505[1], 67515[1], 67715[1], 68200[1], 69990[0], 92012[1], 92014[1], 92018[1], 92019[1], 93000[1], 93005[1], 93010[1], 93040[1], 93041[1], 93042[1], 93318[1], 93355[1], 94002[1], 94200[1], 94680[1], 94681[1], 94690[1], 95812[1], 95813[1], 95816[1], 95819[1], 95822[1], 95829[1], 95955[1], 96360[1], 96361[1], 96365[1], 96366[1], 96367[1], 96368[1], 96372[1], 96374[1], 96375[1], 96376[1], 96377[1], 96523[0], 97597[1], 97598[1], 97602[1], 99155[0], 99156[0], 99157[0], 99211[1], 99212[1], 99213[1], 99214[1], 99215[1], 99217[1], 99218[1], 99219[1], 99220[1], 99221[1], 99222[1], 99223[1], 99231[1], 99232[1], 99233[1], 99234[1], 99235[1], 99236[1], 99238[1], 99239[1], 99241[1], 99242[1], 99243[1], 99244[1], 99245[1], 99251[1], 99252[1], 99253[1], 99254[1], 99255[1], 99291[1], 99292[1], 99304[1], 99305[1], 99306[1], 99307[1], 99308[1], 99309[1], 99310[1], 99315[1], 99316[1], 99334[1], 99335[1], 99336[1], 99337[1], 99347[1], 99348[1], 99349[1], 99350[1], 99374[1], 99375[1], 99377[1], 99378[1], 99446[0], 99447[0], 99448[0], 99449[0], 99451[0], 99452[0], 99495[0], 99496[0], G0463[1], G0471[1]
66985	0213T[0], 0216T[0], 0308T[1], 0465T[1], 0596T[1], 0597T[1], 0699T[1], 0708T[1], 0709T[1], 11000[1], 11001[1], 11004[1], 11005[1], 11006[1], 11042[1], 11043[1], 11044[1], 11045[1], 11046[1], 11047[1], 12001[1], 12002[1], 12004[1], 12005[1], 12006[1], 12007[1], 12011[1], 12013[1], 12014[1], 12015[1], 12016[1], 12017[1], 12018[1], 12020[1], 12021[1], 12031[1], 12032[1], 12034[1], 12035[1], 12036[1], 12037[1], 12041[1], 12042[1], 12044[1], 12045[1], 12046[1], 12047[1], 12051[1], 12052[1], 12053[1], 12054[1], 12055[1], 12056[1], 12057[1], 13100[1], 13101[1], 13102[1], 13120[1], 13121[1], 13122[1], 13131[1], 13132[1], 13133[1], 13151[1], 13152[1], 13153[1], 36000[1], 36400[1], 36405[1], 36406[1], 36410[1], 36420[1], 36425[1], 36430[1], 36440[1], 36591[0], 36592[0], 36600[1], 36640[1], 43752[1], 51701[1], 51702[1], 51703[1], 62320[0], 62321[0], 62322[0], 62323[0], 62324[0], 62325[0], 62326[0], 62327[0], 64400[0], 64405[0], 64408[0], 64415[0], 64416[0], 64417[0], 64418[0], 64420[0], 64421[0], 64425[0], 64430[0], 64435[0], 64445[0], 64446[0], 64447[0], 64448[0], 64449[0], 64450[0], 64451[0], 64454[0], 64461[0], 64462[0], 64463[0], 64479[0], 64480[0], 64483[0], 64484[0], 64486[0], 64487[0], 64488[0], 64489[0], 64490[0], 64491[0], 64492[0], 64493[0], 64494[0], 64495[0], 64505[0], 64510[0], 64517[0], 64520[0], 64530[0], 65920[1], 66030[1], 66250[1], 66500[1], 66625[1], 66820[1], 66821[1], 66825[1], 66850[1], 66983[1], 66984[1], 66988[1], 66991[1], 67028[1], 67500[1], 68200[1], 69990[0], 92012[1], 92014[1], 92018[1], 92019[1], 93000[1], 93005[1], 93010[1], 93040[1], 93041[1], 93042[1], 93318[1], 93355[1], 94002[1], 94200[1], 94680[1], 94681[1], 94690[1], 95812[1], 95813[1], 95816[1], 95819[1], 95822[1], 95829[1], 95955[1], 96360[1], 96361[1], 96365[1], 96366[1], 96367[1], 96368[1], 96372[1], 96374[1], 96375[1], 96376[1], 96377[1], 96523[0], 97597[1], 97598[1], 97602[1], 99155[0], 99156[0], 99157[0], 99211[1], 99212[1], 99213[1], 99214[1], 99215[1], 99217[1], 99218[1], 99219[1], 99220[1], 99221[1], 99222[1], 99223[1], 99231[1], 99232[1], 99233[1], 99234[1], 99235[1], 99236[1], 99238[1], 99239[1], 99241[1], 99242[1], 99243[1], 99244[1], 99245[1], 99251[1], 99252[1], 99253[1], 99254[1], 99255[1], 99291[1], 99292[1], 99304[1], 99305[1], 99306[1], 99307[1], 99308[1], 99309[1], 99310[1], 99315[1], 99316[1], 99334[1], 99335[1], 99336[1], 99337[1], 99347[1], 99348[1], 99349[1], 99350[1], 99374[1], 99375[1], 99377[1], 99378[1], 99446[0], 99447[0], 99448[0], 99449[0], 99451[0], 99452[0], 99495[0], 99496[0], G0463[1], G0471[1]
66986	0213T[0], 0216T[0], 0308T[1], 0465T[1], 0596T[1], 0597T[1], 0699T[1], 0708T[1], 0709T[1], 12001[1], 12002[1], 12004[1], 12005[1], 12006[1], 12007[1], 12011[1], 12013[1], 12014[1], 12015[1], 12016[1], 12017[1], 12018[1], 12020[1], 12021[1], 12031[1], 12032[1], 12034[1], 12035[1], 12036[1], 12037[1], 12041[1], 12042[1], 12044[1], 12045[1], 12046[1], 12047[1], 12051[1], 12052[1], 12053[1], 12054[1], 12055[1], 12056[1], 12057[1], 13100[1], 13101[1], 13102[1], 13120[1], 13121[1], 13122[1], 13131[1], 13132[1], 13133[1], 13151[1], 13152[1], 13153[1], 36000[1], 36400[1], 36405[1], 36406[1], 36410[1], 36420[1], 36425[1], 36430[1], 36440[1], 36591[0], 36592[0], 36600[1], 36640[1], 43752[1], 51701[1], 51702[1], 51703[1], 62320[0], 62321[0], 62322[0], 62323[0], 62324[0], 62325[0], 62326[0], 62327[0], 64400[0], 64405[0], 64408[0], 64415[0], 64416[0], 64417[0], 64418[0], 64420[0], 64421[0], 64425[0], 64430[0], 64435[0], 64445[0], 64446[0], 64447[0], 64448[0], 64449[0], 64450[0], 64451[0], 64454[0], 64461[0], 64462[0], 64463[0], 64479[0], 64480[0], 64483[0], 64484[0], 64486[0], 64487[0], 64488[0], 64489[0], 64490[0], 64491[0], 64492[0], 64493[0], 64494[0], 64495[0], 64505[0], 64510[0], 64517[0], 64520[0], 64530[0], 65920[1], 66030[1], 66250[1], 66500[1], 66820[1], 66821[1], 66825[1], 66985[1], 67028[1], 67500[1], 68200[1], 69990[0], 92012[1], 92014[1], 92018[1], 92019[1], 93000[1], 93005[1], 93010[1], 93040[1], 93041[1], 93042[1], 93318[1], 93355[1], 94002[1], 94200[1], 94680[1], 94681[1], 94690[1], 95812[1], 95813[1], 95816[1], 95819[1], 95822[1], 95829[1], 95955[1], 96360[1], 96361[1], 96365[1], 96366[1], 96367[1], 96368[1], 96372[1], 96374[1], 96375[1], 96376[1], 96377[1], 96523[0], 99155[0], 99156[0], 99157[0], 99211[1], 99212[1], 99213[1], 99214[1], 99215[1], 99217[1], 99218[1], 99219[1], 99220[1], 99221[1], 99222[1], 99223[1], 99231[1], 99232[1], 99233[1], 99234[1], 99235[1], 99236[1], 99238[1], 99239[1], 99241[1], 99242[1], 99243[1], 99244[1], 99245[1], 99251[1], 99252[1], 99253[1], 99254[1], 99255[1], 99291[1], 99292[1], 99304[1], 99305[1], 99306[1], 99307[1], 99308[1], 99309[1], 99310[1], 99315[1], 99316[1], 99334[1], 99335[1], 99336[1], 99337[1], 99347[1], 99348[1], 99349[1], 99350[1], 99374[1], 99375[1], 99377[1], 99378[1], 99446[0], 99447[0], 99448[0], 99449[0], 99451[0], 99452[0], 99495[0], 99496[0], G0463[1], G0471[1]
66987	00142[0], 0213T[0], 0216T[0], 0308T[1], 0465T[1], 0616T[1], 0618T[1], 0621T[1], 0622T[1], 0699T[1], 11000[1], 11001[1], 36591[0], 36592[0], 64450[0], 65426[1], 65750[1], 65755[1], 65772[1], 65775[1], 65800[1], 65810[1], 65815[1], 65820[1], 65850[1], 65855[1], 65860[1], 65865[1], 65870[1], 65875[1], 65880[1], 66020[1], 66030[1], 66250[1], 66500[1], 66505[1], 66600[1], 66605[1], 66625[1], 66630[1], 66635[1], 66680[1], 66700[1], 66710[1], 66720[1], 66740[1], 66761[1], 66770[1], 66820[1], 66821[1], 66825[1], 66830[1], 66840[1], 66850[1], 66852[1], 66920[1], 66930[1], 66940[1], 66983[1], 66984[1], 66985[1], 66986[1], 66990[1], 66991[1], 67005[1], 67010[1], 67028[1], 67500[1], 67505[1], 67515[1], 67715[1], 68200[1], 92018[1], 92019[1], 93355[1], 96523[0], 99211[1], 99212[1], 99213[1], 99214[1], 99215[1], 99217[1], 99218[1], 99219[1], 99220[1], 99221[1], 99222[1], 99223[1], 99231[1], 99232[1], 99233[1], 99234[1], 99235[1], 99236[1], 99238[1], 99239[1], 99241[1], 99242[1], 99243[1], 99244[1], 99245[1], 99251[1], 99252[1], 99253[1], 99254[1], 99255[1], 99291[1], 99292[1], 99304[1], 99305[1], 99306[1], 99307[1], 99308[1], 99309[1], 99310[1], 99315[1], 99316[1], 99334[1], 99335[1], 99336[1], 99337[1], 99347[1], 99348[1], 99349[1], 99350[1], 99374[1], 99375[1], 99377[1], 99378[1], 99446[0], 99447[0], 99448[0], 99449[0], 99451[0], 99452[0], 99495[0], 99496[0], G0463[1], G0471[1]
66988	00142[0], 00144[0], 0213T[0], 0216T[0], 0308T[1], 0465T[1], 0616T[1], 0621T[1], 0622T[1], 0671T[1], 0699T[1], 36591[0], 36592[0], 64450[0], 65426[1], 65750[1], 65755[1], 65772[1], 65775[1], 65800[1], 65810[1], 65815[1], 65820[1], 65850[1], 65855[1], 65860[1], 65865[1], 65870[1], 65875[1], 65880[1], 66020[1], 66030[1], 66250[1], 66500[1], 66505[1], 66600[1], 66605[1], 66625[1], 66630[1], 66635[1], 66680[1], 66700[1], 66710[1], 66720[1], 66740[1], 66770[1], 66820[1], 66821[1], 66825[1], 66830[1], 66840[1], 66920[1], 66983[1], 66990[1], 67005[1], 67010[1], 67028[1], 67500[1], 67505[1], 67515[1], 67715[1], 68200[1], 92018[1], 92019[1], 93318[1], 93355[1], 96376[1], 96523[0], 97602[1], 99211[1], 99212[1], 99213[1], 99214[1], 99215[1], 99217[1], 99218[1], 99219[1], 99220[1], 99221[1], 99222[1], 99223[1], 99231[1], 99232[1], 99233[1], 99234[1], 99235[1], 99236[1], 99238[1], 99239[1], 99241[1], 99242[1], 99243[1], 99244[1], 99245[1], 99251[1], 99252[1], 99253[1], 99254[1], 99255[1], 99291[1], 99292[1], 99304[1], 99305[1], 99306[1], 99307[1], 99308[1], 99309[1], 99310[1], 99315[1], 99316[1], 99334[1], 99335[1], 99336[1], 99337[1], 99347[1], 99348[1], 99349[1], 99350[1], 99374[1], 99375[1], 99377[1], 99378[1], 99446[0], 99447[0], 99448[0], 99449[0], 99451[0], 99452[0], 99495[0], 99496[0], G0463[1], G0471[1]
66989	00142[0], 0213T[0], 0216T[0], 0253T[1], 0308T[1], 0449T[1], 0450T[1], 0465T[1], 0474T[1], 0596T[1], 0597T[1], 0616T[1], 0618T[1], 0671T[1], 11000[1], 11001[1], 11004[1], 11005[1], 11006[1], 11042[1], 11043[1], 11044[1], 11045[1], 11046[1], 11047[1], 12001[1], 12002[1], 12004[1], 12005[1], 12006[1], 12007[1], 12011[1], 12013[1], 12014[1], 12015[1], 12016[1], 12017[1], 12018[1], 12020[1], 12021[1], 12031[1], 12032[1], 12034[1], 12035[1], 12036[1], 12037[1], 12041[1], 12042[1], 12044[1], 12045[1], 12046[1], 12047[1], 12051[1], 12052[1], 12053[1], 12054[1], 12055[1], 12056[1], 12057[1], 13100[1], 13101[1], 13102[1], 13120[1], 13121[1], 13122[1], 13131[1], 13132[1], 13133[1], 13151[1], 13152[1], 13153[1], 36000[1], 36400[1], 36405[1], 36406[1], 36410[1], 36420[1], 36425[1], 36430[1], 36440[1], 36591[0], 36592[0], 36600[1], 36640[1], 43752[1], 51701[1], 51702[1], 51703[1], 61650[1], 62320[0], 62321[0], 62322[0], 62323[0], 62324[0], 62325[0], 62326[0], 62327[0], 64400[0], 64405[0], 64408[0], 64415[0], 64416[0], 64417[0], 64418[0], 64420[0], 64421[0], 64425[0], 64430[0], 64435[0], 64445[0], 64446[0], 64447[0], 64448[0], 64449[0], 64450[0], 64451[0], 64454[0], 64461[0], 64462[0], 64463[0], 64479[0], 64480[0], 64483[0], 64484[0], 64486[0], 64487[0], 64488[0], 64489[0], 64490[0], 64491[0], 64492[0], 64493[0], 64494[0], 64495[0], 64505[0], 64510[0], 64517[0], 64520[0], 64530[0], 65426[1], 65750[1], 65755[1], 65772[1], 65775[1], 65800[1], 65810[1], 65815[1], 65860[1], 65865[1], 65870[1], 65875[1], 65880[1], 66020[1], 66030[1], 66250[1], 66500[1], 66505[1], 66600[1], 66605[1], 66625[1], 66630[1], 66635[1], 66680[1], 66711[1], 66761[1], 66820[1], 66821[1], 66825[1], 66830[1], 66840[1],

Appendix A: NCCI - CPT Codes

0 = Modifier usage not allowed or inappropriate 1 = Modifier usage allowed

Code 1	Code 2
	66850^1, 66852^1, 66920^1, 66930^1, 66940^1, 66982^1, 66983^1, 66984^1, 66985^1, 66986^1, 66987^1, 66988^1, 66991^1, 67005^1, 67010^1, 67028^1, 67500^1, 67505^1, 67515^1, 67715^1, 68200^1, 69990^0, 92012^1, 92014^1, 92018^1, 92019^1, 93000^1, 93005^1, 93010^1, 93040^1, 93041^1, 93042^1, 93318^1, 93355^1, 94002^1, 94200^1, 94680^1, 94681^1, 94690^1, 95812^1, 95813^1, 95816^1, 95819^1, 95822^1, 95829^1, 95955^1, 96360^1, 96361^1, 96365^1, 96366^1, 96367^1, 96368^1, 96372^1, 96374^1, 96375^1, 96376^1, 96377^1, 96523^0, 97597^1, 97598^1, 97602^1, 99155^0, 99156^0, 99157^0, 99211^1, 99212^1, 99213^1, 99214^1, 99215^1, 99217^1, 99218^1, 99219^1, 99220^1, 99221^1, 99222^1, 99223^1, 99231^1, 99232^1, 99233^1, 99234^1, 99235^1, 99236^1, 99238^1, 99239^1, 99241^1, 99242^1, 99243^1, 99244^1, 99245^1, 99251^1, 99252^1, 99253^1, 99254^1, 99255^1, 99291^1, 99292^1, 99304^1, 99305^1, 99306^1, 99307^1, 99308^1, 99309^1, 99310^1, 99315^1, 99316^1, 99334^1, 99335^1, 99336^1, 99347^1, 99348^1, 99349^1, 99350^1, 99374^1, 99375^1, 99377^1, 99378^1, 99446^0, 99447^0, 99448^0, 99449^0, 99451^0, 99452^0, 99495^0, 99496^0, G0463^1, G0471^1
66990	0213T^1, 0216T^1, 36000^1, 36410^1, 36591^0, 36592^0, 61650^1, 62324^1, 62325^1, 62326^1, 62327^1, 64415^1, 64417^1, 64450^1, 64454^1, 64486^1, 64487^1, 64488^1, 64489^1, 64490^1, 64493^1, 67500^1, 69990^0, 96360^1, 96365^1, 96523^0
66991	00142^0, 00144^0, 0213T^0, 0216T^0, 0253T^1, 0308T^1, 0449T^1, 0450T^1, 0465T^1, 0474T^1, 0596T^1, 0597T^1, 0616T^1, 0671T^1, 11000^1, 11001^1, 11004^1, 11005^1, 11006^1, 11042^1, 11043^1, 11044^1, 11045^1, 11046^1, 11047^1, 12001^1, 12002^1, 12004^1, 12005^1, 12006^1, 12007^1, 12011^1, 12013^1, 12014^1, 12015^1, 12016^1, 12017^1, 12018^1, 12020^1, 12021^1, 12031^1, 12032^1, 12034^1, 12035^1, 12036^1, 12037^1, 12041^1, 12042^1, 12044^1, 12045^1, 12046^1, 12047^1, 12051^1, 12052^1, 12053^1, 12054^1, 12055^1, 12056^1, 12057^1, 13100^1, 13101^1, 13102^1, 13120^1, 13121^1, 13122^1, 13131^1, 13132^1, 13133^1, 13151^1, 13152^1, 13153^1, 36000^1, 36400^1, 36405^1, 36406^1, 36410^1, 36420^1, 36425^1, 36430^1, 36440^1, 36591^0, 36592^0, 36600^1, 36640^1, 43752^1, 51701^1, 51702^1, 51703^1, 61650^1, 62320^0, 62321^0, 62322^0, 62323^0, 62324^0, 62325^0, 62326^0, 62327^0, 64400^0, 64405^0, 64408^0, 64415^0, 64416^0, 64417^0, 64418^0, 64420^0, 64421^0, 64425^0, 64430^0, 64435^0, 64445^0, 64446^0, 64447^0, 64448^0, 64449^0, 64450^0, 64451^0, 64454^0, 64461^0, 64462^0, 64463^0, 64479^0, 64480^0, 64483^0, 64484^0, 64486^0, 64487^0, 64488^0, 64489^0, 64490^0, 64491^0, 64492^0, 64493^0, 64494^0, 64495^0, 64505^0, 64510^0, 64517^0, 64520^0, 64530^0, 65235^1, 65260^1, 65265^1, 65400^1, 65420^1, 65426^1, 65730^1, 65750^1, 65755^1, 65772^1, 65775^1, 65800^1, 65810^1, 65815^1, 65850^1, 65855^1, 65860^1, 65865^1, 65870^1, 65875^1, 65880^1, 66020^1, 66030^1, 66250^1, 66500^1, 66505^1, 66600^1, 66605^1, 66625^1, 66630^1, 66635^1, 66680^1, 66711^1, 66762^1, 66820^1, 66821^1, 66825^1, 66830^1, 66840^1, 66920^1, 66983^1, 66984^1, 66988^1, 67005^1, 67010^1, 67015^1, 67028^1, 67500^1, 67505^1, 67515^1, 67715^1, 68200^1, 69990^0, 92012^1, 92014^1, 92018^1, 92019^1, 93000^1, 93005^1, 93010^1, 93040^1, 93041^1, 93042^1, 93318^1, 93355^1, 94002^1, 94200^1, 94680^1, 94681^1, 94690^1, 95812^1, 95813^1, 95816^1, 95819^1, 95822^1, 95829^1, 95955^1, 96360^1, 96361^1, 96365^1, 96366^1, 96367^1, 96368^1, 96372^1, 96374^1, 96375^1, 96376^1, 96377^1, 96523^0, 97597^1, 97598^1, 97602^1, 99155^0, 99156^0, 99157^0, 99211^1, 99212^1, 99213^1, 99214^1, 99215^1, 99217^1, 99218^1, 99219^1, 99220^1, 99221^1, 99222^1, 99223^1, 99231^1, 99232^1, 99233^1, 99234^1, 99235^1, 99236^1, 99238^1, 99239^1, 99241^1, 99242^1, 99243^1, 99244^1, 99245^1, 99251^1, 99252^1, 99253^1, 99254^1, 99255^1, 99291^1, 99292^1, 99304^1, 99305^1, 99306^1, 99307^1, 99308^1, 99309^1, 99310^1, 99315^1, 99316^1, 99334^1, 99335^1, 99336^1, 99337^1, 99347^1, 99348^1, 99349^1, 99350^1, 99374^1, 99375^1, 99377^1, 99378^1, 99446^0, 99447^0, 99448^0, 99449^0, 99451^0, 99452^0, 99495^0, 99496^0, G0463^1, G0471^1
67005	0213T^0, 0216T^0, 0465T^1, 0596T^1, 0597T^1, 0699T^1, 0708T^1, 0709T^1, 11000^1, 11001^1, 11004^1, 11005^1, 11006^1, 11042^1, 11043^1, 11044^1, 11045^1, 11046^1, 11047^1, 12001^1, 12002^1, 12004^1, 12005^1, 12006^1, 12007^1, 12011^1, 12013^1, 12014^1, 12015^1, 12016^1, 12017^1, 12018^1, 12020^1, 12021^1, 12031^1, 12032^1, 12034^1, 12035^1, 12036^1, 12037^1, 12041^1, 12042^1, 12044^1, 12045^1, 12046^1, 12047^1, 12051^1, 12052^1, 12053^1, 12054^1, 12055^1, 12056^1, 12057^1, 13100^1, 13101^1, 13102^1, 13120^1, 13121^1, 13122^1, 13131^1, 13132^1, 13133^1, 13151^1, 13152^1, 13153^1, 36000^1, 36400^1, 36405^1, 36406^1, 36410^1, 36420^1, 36425^1, 36430^1, 36440^1, 36591^0, 36592^0, 36600^1, 36640^1, 43752^1, 51701^1, 51702^1, 51703^1, 62320^0, 62321^0, 62322^0, 62323^0, 62324^0, 62325^0, 62326^0, 62327^0, 64400^0, 64405^0, 64408^0, 64415^0, 64416^0, 64417^0, 64418^0, 64420^0, 64421^0, 64425^0, 64430^0, 64435^0, 64445^0, 64446^0, 64447^0, 64448^0, 64449^0, 64450^0, 64451^0, 64454^0, 64461^0, 64462^0, 64463^0, 64479^0, 64480^0, 64483^0, 64484^0, 64486^0, 64487^0, 64488^0, 64489^0, 64490^0, 64491^0, 64492^0, 64493^0, 64494^0, 64495^0, 64505^0, 64510^0, 64517^0, 64520^0, 64530^0, 66030^1, 67025^1, 67028^1, 67141^1, 67145^1, 67500^1, 69990^0, 92012^1, 92014^1, 92018^1, 92019^1, 92201^1, 92202^1, 93000^1, 93005^1, 93010^1, 93040^1, 93041^1, 93042^1, 93318^1, 93355^1, 94002^1, 94200^1, 94680^1, 94681^1, 94690^1, 95812^1, 95813^1, 95816^1, 95819^1, 95822^1, 95829^1, 95955^1, 96360^1, 96361^1, 96365^1, 96366^1, 96367^1, 96368^1, 96372^1, 96374^1, 96375^1, 96376^1, 96377^1, 96523^0, 97597^1, 97598^1, 97602^1, 99155^0, 99156^0, 99157^0, 99211^1, 99212^1, 99213^1, 99214^1, 99215^1, 99217^1, 99218^1, 99219^1, 99220^1, 99221^1, 99222^1, 99223^1, 99231^1, 99232^1, 99233^1, 99234^1, 99235^1, 99236^1, 99238^1, 99239^1, 99241^1, 99242^1, 99243^1, 99244^1, 99245^1, 99251^1, 99252^1, 99253^1, 99254^1, 99255^1, 99291^1, 99292^1, 99304^1, 99305^1, 99306^1, 99307^1, 99308^1, 99309^1, 99310^1, 99315^1, 99316^1, 99334^1, 99335^1, 99336^1, 99337^1, 99347^1, 99348^1, 99349^1, 99350^1, 99374^1, 99375^1, 99377^1, 99378^1, 99446^0, 99447^0, 99448^0, 99449^0, 99451^0, 99452^0, 99495^0, 99496^0, G0463^1, G0471^1
67010	0213T^0, 0216T^0, 0465T^1, 0596T^1, 0597T^1, 0699T^1, 0708T^1, 0709T^1, 11000^1, 11001^1, 11004^1, 11005^1, 11006^1, 11042^1, 11043^1, 11044^1, 11045^1, 11046^1, 11047^1, 12001^1, 12002^1, 12004^1, 12005^1, 12006^1, 12007^1, 12011^1, 12013^1, 12014^1, 12015^1, 12016^1, 12017^1, 12018^1, 12020^1, 12021^1, 12031^1, 12032^1, 12034^1, 12035^1, 12036^1, 12037^1, 12041^1, 12042^1, 12044^1, 12045^1, 12046^1, 12047^1, 12051^1, 12052^1, 12053^1, 12054^1, 12055^1, 12056^1, 12057^1, 13100^1, 13101^1, 13102^1, 13120^1, 13121^1, 13122^1, 13131^1, 13132^1, 13133^1, 13151^1, 13152^1, 13153^1, 36000^1, 36400^1, 36405^1, 36406^1, 36410^1, 36420^1, 36425^1, 36430^1, 36440^1, 36591^0, 36592^0, 36600^1, 36640^1, 43752^1, 51701^1, 51702^1, 51703^1, 62320^0, 62321^0, 62322^0, 62323^0, 62324^0, 62325^0, 62326^0, 62327^0, 64400^0, 64405^0, 64408^0, 64415^0, 64416^0, 64417^0, 64418^0, 64420^0, 64421^0, 64425^0, 64430^0, 64435^0, 64445^0, 64446^0, 64447^0, 64448^0, 64449^0, 64450^0, 64451^0, 64454^0, 64461^0, 64462^0, 64463^0, 64479^0, 64480^0, 64483^0, 64484^0, 64486^0, 64487^0, 64488^0, 64489^0, 64490^0, 64491^0, 64492^0, 64493^0, 64494^0, 64495^0, 64505^0, 64510^0, 64517^0, 64520^0, 64530^0, 66030^1, 67005^1, 67025^1, 67028^1, 67141^1, 67145^1, 67500^1, 69990^0, 92012^1, 92014^1, 92018^1, 92019^1, 92201^1, 92202^1, 93000^1, 93005^1, 93010^1, 93040^1, 93041^1, 93042^1, 93318^1, 93355^1, 94002^1, 94200^1, 94680^1, 94681^1, 94690^1, 95812^1, 95813^1, 95816^1, 95819^1, 95822^1, 95829^1, 95955^1, 96360^1, 96361^1, 96365^1, 96366^1, 96367^1, 96368^1, 96372^1, 96374^1, 96375^1, 96376^1, 96377^1, 96523^0, 97597^1, 97598^1, 97602^1, 99155^0, 99156^0, 99157^0, 99211^1, 99212^1, 99213^1, 99214^1, 99215^1, 99217^1, 99218^1, 99219^1, 99220^1, 99221^1, 99222^1, 99223^1, 99231^1, 99232^1, 99233^1, 99234^1, 99235^1, 99236^1, 99238^1, 99239^1, 99241^1, 99242^1, 99243^1, 99244^1, 99245^1, 99251^1, 99252^1, 99253^1, 99254^1, 99255^1, 99291^1, 99292^1, 99304^1, 99305^1, 99306^1, 99307^1, 99308^1, 99309^1, 99310^1, 99315^1, 99316^1, 99334^1, 99335^1, 99336^1, 99337^1, 99347^1, 99348^1, 99349^1, 99350^1, 99374^1, 99375^1, 99377^1, 99378^1, 99446^0, 99447^0, 99448^0, 99449^0, 99451^0, 99452^0, 99495^0, 99496^0, G0463^1, G0471^1
67015	0213T^0, 0216T^0, 0465T^1, 0596T^1, 0597T^1, 0708T^1, 0709T^1, 11000^1, 11001^1, 11004^1, 11005^1, 11006^1, 11042^1, 11043^1, 11044^1, 11045^1, 11046^1, 11047^1, 12001^1, 12002^1, 12004^1, 12005^1, 12006^1, 12007^1, 12011^1, 12013^1, 12014^1, 12015^1, 12016^1, 12017^1, 12018^1, 12020^1, 12021^1, 12031^1, 12032^1, 12034^1, 12035^1, 12036^1, 12037^1, 12041^1, 12042^1, 12044^1, 12045^1, 12046^1, 12047^1, 12051^1, 12052^1, 12053^1, 12054^1, 12055^1, 12056^1, 12057^1, 13100^1, 13101^1, 13102^1, 13120^1, 13121^1, 13122^1, 13131^1, 13132^1, 13133^1, 13151^1, 13152^1, 13153^1, 36000^1, 36400^1, 36405^1, 36406^1, 36410^1, 36420^1, 36425^1, 36430^1, 36440^1, 36591^0, 36592^0, 36600^1, 36640^1, 43752^1, 51701^1, 51702^1, 51703^1, 62320^0, 62321^0, 62322^0, 62323^0, 62324^0, 62325^0, 62326^0, 62327^0, 64400^0, 64405^0, 64408^0, 64415^0, 64416^0, 64417^0, 64418^0, 64420^0, 64421^0, 64425^0, 64430^0, 64435^0, 64445^0, 64446^0, 64447^0, 64448^0, 64449^0, 64450^0, 64451^0, 64454^0, 64461^0, 64462^0, 64463^0, 64479^0, 64480^0, 64483^0, 64484^0, 64486^0, 64487^0, 64488^0, 64489^0, 64490^0, 64491^0, 64492^0, 64493^0, 64494^0, 64495^0, 64505^0, 64510^0, 64517^0, 64520^0, 64530^0, 67005^1, 67010^1, 67025^1, 67028^1, 67141^1, 67145^1, 67500^1, 69990^0, 92012^1, 92014^1, 92018^1, 92019^1, 92201^1, 92202^1, 93000^1, 93005^1, 93010^1, 93040^1, 93041^1, 93042^1, 93318^1, 93355^1, 94002^1, 94200^1, 94680^1, 94681^1, 94690^1, 95812^1, 95813^1, 95816^1, 95819^1, 95822^1, 95829^1, 95955^1, 96360^1, 96361^1, 96365^1, 96366^1, 96367^1, 96368^1, 96372^1, 96374^1, 96375^1, 96376^1, 96377^1, 96523^0, 97597^1, 97598^1, 97602^1, 99155^0, 99156^0, 99157^0, 99211^1, 99212^1, 99213^1, 99214^1, 99215^1, 99217^1, 99218^1, 99219^1, 99220^1, 99221^1, 99222^1, 99223^1, 99231^1, 99232^1, 99233^1, 99234^1, 99235^1, 99236^1, 99238^1, 99239^1, 99241^1, 99242^1, 99243^1, 99244^1, 99245^1, 99251^1, 99252^1, 99253^1, 99254^1, 99255^1, 99291^1, 99292^1, 99304^1, 99305^1, 99306^1, 99307^1, 99308^1, 99309^1, 99310^1, 99315^1, 99316^1, 99334^1, 99335^1, 99336^1, 99337^1, 99347^1, 99348^1, 99349^1, 99350^1, 99374^1, 99375^1, 99377^1, 99378^1, 99446^0, 99447^0, 99448^0, 99449^0, 99451^0, 99452^0, 99495^0, 99496^0, G0463^1, G0471^1, J0670^1, J2001^1
67025	0213T^0, 0216T^0, 0465T^1, 0596T^1, 0597T^1, 0708T^1, 0709T^1, 12001^1, 12002^1, 12004^1, 12005^1, 12006^1, 12007^1, 12011^1, 12013^1, 12014^1, 12015^1, 12016^1, 12017^1, 12018^1, 12020^1, 12021^1, 12031^1, 12032^1, 12034^1, 12035^1, 12036^1, 12037^1, 12041^1, 12042^1, 12044^1, 12045^1, 12046^1, 12047^1, 12051^1, 12052^1, 12053^1, 12054^1, 12055^1, 12056^1, 12057^1, 13100^1, 13101^1, 13102^1, 13120^1, 13121^1, 13122^1, 13131^1, 13132^1, 13133^1, 13151^1, 13152^1, 13153^1, 36000^1, 36400^1, 36405^1, 36406^1, 36410^1, 36420^1, 36425^1, 36430^1, 36440^1, 36591^0, 36592^0, 36600^1, 36640^1, 43752^1, 51701^1, 51702^1, 51703^1, 62320^0, 62321^0, 62322^0, 62323^0, 62324^0, 62325^0, 62326^0, 62327^0, 64400^0, 64405^0, 64408^0, 64415^0, 64416^0, 64417^0, 64418^0, 64420^0, 64421^0, 64425^0, 64430^0, 64435^0,

0 = Modifier usage not allowed or inappropriate 1 = Modifier usage allowed

Appendix A: NCCI - CPT Codes

Code 1	Code 2
	64445[0], 64446[0], 64447[0], 64448[0], 64449[0], 64450[0], 64451[0], 64454[0], 64461[0], 64462[0], 64463[0], 64479[0], 64480[0], 64483[0], 64484[0], 64486[0], 64487[0], 64488[0], 64489[0], 64490[0], 64491[0], 64492[0], 64493[0], 64494[0], 64495[0], 64505[0], 64510[0], 64517[0], 64520[0], 64530[0], 67028[1], 67141[1], 67145[1], 67500[1], 69990[0], 92012[1], 92014[1], 92018[1], 92019[1], 92201[1], 92202[1], 93000[1], 93005[1], 93010[1], 93040[1], 93041[1], 93042[1], 93318[1], 93355[1], 94002[1], 94200[1], 94680[1], 94681[1], 94690[1], 95812[1], 95813[1], 95816[1], 95819[1], 95822[1], 95829[1], 95955[1], 96360[1], 96361[1], 96365[1], 96366[1], 96367[1], 96368[1], 96372[1], 96374[1], 96375[1], 96376[1], 96377[1], 96523[0], 99155[0], 99156[0], 99157[0], 99211[1], 99212[1], 99213[1], 99214[1], 99215[1], 99217[1], 99218[1], 99219[1], 99220[1], 99221[1], 99222[1], 99223[1], 99231[1], 99232[1], 99233[1], 99234[1], 99235[1], 99236[1], 99238[1], 99239[1], 99241[1], 99242[1], 99243[1], 99244[1], 99245[1], 99251[1], 99252[1], 99253[1], 99254[1], 99255[1], 99291[1], 99292[1], 99304[1], 99305[1], 99306[1], 99307[1], 99308[1], 99309[1], 99310[1], 99315[1], 99316[1], 99334[1], 99335[1], 99336[1], 99337[1], 99347[1], 99348[1], 99349[1], 99350[1], 99374[1], 99375[1], 99377[1], 99378[1], 99446[0], 99447[0], 99448[0], 99449[0], 99451[0], 99452[0], 99495[0], 99496[0], G0463[1], G0471[1], J0670[1], J2001[1]
67027	0213T[0], 0216T[0], 0465T[1], 0596T[1], 0597T[1], 0708T[1], 0709T[1], 11000[1], 11001[1], 11004[1], 11005[1], 11006[1], 11042[1], 11043[1], 11044[1], 11045[1], 11046[1], 11047[1], 12001[1], 12002[1], 12004[1], 12005[1], 12006[1], 12007[1], 12011[1], 12013[1], 12014[1], 12015[1], 12016[1], 12017[1], 12018[1], 12020[1], 12021[1], 12031[1], 12032[1], 12034[1], 12035[1], 12036[1], 12037[1], 12041[1], 12042[1], 12044[1], 12045[1], 12046[1], 12047[1], 12051[1], 12052[1], 12053[1], 12054[1], 12055[1], 12056[1], 12057[1], 13100[1], 13101[1], 13102[1], 13120[1], 13121[1], 13122[1], 13131[1], 13132[1], 13133[1], 13151[1], 13152[1], 13153[1], 36000[1], 36400[1], 36405[1], 36406[1], 36410[1], 36420[1], 36425[1], 36430[1], 36440[1], 36591[0], 36592[0], 36600[1], 36640[1], 43752[1], 51701[1], 51702[1], 51703[1], 62320[0], 62321[0], 62322[0], 62323[0], 62324[0], 62325[0], 62326[0], 62327[0], 64400[0], 64405[0], 64408[0], 64415[0], 64416[0], 64417[0], 64418[0], 64420[0], 64421[0], 64425[0], 64430[0], 64435[0], 64445[0], 64446[0], 64447[0], 64448[0], 64449[0], 64450[0], 64451[0], 64454[0], 64461[0], 64462[0], 64463[0], 64479[0], 64480[0], 64483[0], 64484[0], 64486[0], 64487[0], 64488[0], 64489[0], 64490[0], 64491[0], 64492[0], 64493[0], 64494[0], 64495[0], 64505[0], 64510[0], 64517[0], 64520[0], 64530[0], 67005[1], 67010[1], 67015[1], 67025[1], 67028[1], 67036[1], 67121[1], 67500[1], 69990[0], 92012[1], 92014[1], 92018[1], 92019[1], 92201[1], 92202[1], 93000[1], 93005[1], 93010[1], 93040[1], 93041[1], 93042[1], 93318[1], 93355[1], 94002[1], 94200[1], 94680[1], 94681[1], 94690[1], 95812[1], 95813[1], 95816[1], 95819[1], 95822[1], 95829[1], 95955[1], 96360[1], 96361[1], 96365[1], 96366[1], 96367[1], 96368[1], 96372[1], 96374[1], 96375[1], 96376[1], 96377[1], 96523[0], 97597[1], 97598[1], 97602[1], 99155[0], 99156[0], 99157[0], 99211[1], 99212[1], 99213[1], 99214[1], 99215[1], 99217[1], 99218[1], 99219[1], 99220[1], 99221[1], 99222[1], 99223[1], 99231[1], 99232[1], 99233[1], 99234[1], 99235[1], 99236[1], 99238[1], 99239[1], 99241[1], 99242[1], 99243[1], 99244[1], 99245[1], 99251[1], 99252[1], 99253[1], 99254[1], 99255[1], 99291[1], 99292[1], 99304[1], 99305[1], 99306[1], 99307[1], 99308[1], 99309[1], 99310[1], 99315[1], 99316[1], 99334[1], 99335[1], 99336[1], 99337[1], 99347[1], 99348[1], 99349[1], 99350[1], 99374[1], 99375[1], 99377[1], 99378[1], 99446[0], 99447[0], 99448[0], 99449[0], 99451[0], 99452[0], 99495[0], 99496[0], G0463[1], G0471[1], J2001[1]
67028	0213T[0], 0216T[0], 0596T[1], 0597T[1], 0708T[1], 0709T[1], 12001[1], 12002[1], 12004[1], 12005[1], 12006[1], 12007[1], 12011[1], 12013[1], 12014[1], 12015[1], 12016[1], 12017[1], 12018[1], 12020[1], 12021[1], 12031[1], 12032[1], 12034[1], 12035[1], 12036[1], 12037[1], 12041[1], 12042[1], 12044[1], 12045[1], 12046[1], 12047[1], 12051[1], 12052[1], 12053[1], 12054[1], 12055[1], 12056[1], 12057[1], 13100[1], 13101[1], 13102[1], 13120[1], 13121[1], 13122[1], 13131[1], 13132[1], 13133[1], 13151[1], 13152[1], 13153[1], 36000[1], 36400[1], 36405[1], 36406[1], 36410[1], 36420[1], 36425[1], 36430[1], 36440[1], 36591[0], 36592[0], 36600[1], 36640[1], 43752[1], 51701[1], 51702[1], 51703[1], 62320[0], 62321[0], 62322[0], 62323[0], 62324[0], 62325[0], 62326[0], 62327[0], 64400[0], 64405[0], 64408[0], 64415[0], 64416[0], 64417[0], 64418[0], 64420[0], 64421[0], 64425[0], 64430[0], 64435[0], 64445[0], 64446[0], 64447[0], 64448[0], 64449[0], 64450[0], 64451[0], 64454[0], 64461[0], 64462[0], 64463[0], 64479[0], 64480[0], 64483[0], 64484[0], 64486[0], 64487[0], 64488[0], 64489[0], 64490[0], 64491[0], 64492[0], 64493[0], 64494[0], 64495[0], 64505[0], 64510[0], 64517[0], 64520[0], 64530[0], 67500[1], 68200[1], 69990[0], 92018[1], 92019[1], 92201[1], 92202[1], 93000[1], 93005[1], 93010[1], 93040[1], 93041[1], 93042[1], 93318[1], 93355[1], 94002[1], 94200[1], 94680[1], 94681[1], 94690[1], 95812[1], 95813[1], 95816[1], 95819[1], 95822[1], 95829[1], 95955[1], 96360[1], 96361[1], 96365[1], 96366[1], 96367[1], 96368[1], 96372[1], 96374[1], 96375[1], 96376[1], 96377[1], 96523[0], 99155[0], 99156[0], 99157[0], 99211[1], 99212[1], 99213[1], 99214[1], 99215[1], 99217[1], 99218[1], 99219[1], 99220[1], 99221[1], 99222[1], 99223[1], 99231[1], 99232[1], 99233[1], 99234[1], 99235[1], 99236[1], 99238[1], 99239[1], 99241[1], 99242[1], 99243[1], 99244[1], 99245[1], 99251[1], 99252[1], 99253[1], 99254[1], 99255[1], 99291[1], 99292[1], 99304[1], 99305[1], 99306[1], 99307[1], 99308[1], 99309[1], 99310[1], 99315[1], 99316[1], 99334[1], 99335[1], 99336[1], 99337[1], 99347[1], 99348[1], 99349[1], 99350[1], 99374[1], 99375[1], 99377[1], 99378[1], 99446[0], 99447[0], 99448[0], 99449[0], 99451[0], 99452[0], 99495[1], 99496[1], G0463[1], G0471[1], J0670[1], J2001[1]
67030	0213T[0], 0216T[0], 0465T[1], 0596T[1], 0597T[1], 0708T[1], 0709T[1], 11000[1], 11001[1], 11004[1], 11005[1], 11006[1], 11042[1], 11043[1], 11044[1], 11045[1], 11046[1], 11047[1], 12001[1], 12002[1], 12004[1], 12005[1], 12006[1], 12007[1], 12011[1], 12013[1], 12014[1], 12015[1], 12016[1], 12017[1], 12018[1], 12020[1], 12021[1], 12031[1], 12032[1], 12034[1], 12035[1], 12036[1], 12037[1], 12041[1], 12042[1], 12044[1], 12045[1], 12046[1], 12047[1], 12051[1], 12052[1], 12053[1], 12054[1], 12055[1], 12056[1], 12057[1], 13100[1], 13101[1], 13102[1], 13120[1], 13121[1], 13122[1], 13131[1], 13132[1], 13133[1], 13151[1], 13152[1], 13153[1], 36000[1], 36400[1], 36405[1], 36406[1], 36410[1], 36420[1], 36425[1], 36430[1], 36440[1], 36591[0], 36592[0], 36600[1], 36640[1], 43752[1], 51701[1], 51702[1], 51703[1], 62320[0], 62321[0], 62322[0], 62323[0], 62324[0], 62325[0], 62326[0], 62327[0], 64400[0], 64405[0], 64408[0], 64415[0], 64416[0], 64417[0], 64418[0], 64420[0], 64421[0], 64425[0], 64430[0], 64435[0], 64445[0], 64446[0], 64447[0], 64448[0], 64449[0], 64450[0], 64451[0], 64454[0], 64461[0], 64462[0], 64463[0], 64479[0], 64480[0], 64483[0], 64484[0], 64486[0], 64487[0], 64488[0], 64489[0], 64490[0], 64491[0], 64492[0], 64493[0], 64494[0], 64495[0], 64505[0], 64510[0], 64517[0], 64520[0], 64530[0], 67005[1], 67010[1], 67015[1], 67025[1], 67028[1], 67039[1], 67040[1], 67500[1], 69990[0], 92012[1], 92014[1], 92018[1], 92019[1], 92201[1], 92202[1], 93000[1], 93005[1], 93010[1], 93040[1], 93041[1], 93042[1], 93318[1], 93355[1], 94002[1], 94200[1], 94680[1], 94681[1], 94690[1], 95812[1], 95813[1], 95816[1], 95819[1], 95822[1], 95829[1], 95955[1], 96360[1], 96361[1], 96365[1], 96366[1], 96367[1], 96368[1], 96372[1], 96374[1], 96375[1], 96376[1], 96377[1], 96523[0], 97597[1], 97598[1], 97602[1], 99155[0], 99156[0], 99157[0], 99211[1], 99212[1], 99213[1], 99214[1], 99215[1], 99217[1], 99218[1], 99219[1], 99220[1], 99221[1], 99222[1], 99223[1], 99231[1], 99232[1], 99233[1], 99234[1], 99235[1], 99236[1], 99238[1], 99239[1], 99241[1], 99242[1], 99243[1], 99244[1], 99245[1], 99251[1], 99252[1], 99253[1], 99254[1], 99255[1], 99291[1], 99292[1], 99304[1], 99305[1], 99306[1], 99307[1], 99308[1], 99309[1], 99310[1], 99315[1], 99316[1], 99334[1], 99335[1], 99336[1], 99337[1], 99347[1], 99348[1], 99349[1], 99350[1], 99374[1], 99375[1], 99377[1], 99378[1], 99446[0], 99447[0], 99448[0], 99449[0], 99451[0], 99452[0], 99495[0], 99496[0], G0463[1], G0471[1], J0670[1], J2001[1]
67031	0213T[0], 0216T[0], 0465T[1], 0596T[1], 0597T[1], 0708T[1], 0709T[1], 12001[1], 12002[1], 12004[1], 12005[1], 12006[1], 12007[1], 12011[1], 12013[1], 12014[1], 12015[1], 12016[1], 12017[1], 12018[1], 12020[1], 12021[1], 12031[1], 12032[1], 12034[1], 12035[1], 12036[1], 12037[1], 12041[1], 12042[1], 12044[1], 12045[1], 12046[1], 12047[1], 12051[1], 12052[1], 12053[1], 12054[1], 12055[1], 12056[1], 12057[1], 13100[1], 13101[1], 13102[1], 13120[1], 13121[1], 13122[1], 13131[1], 13132[1], 13133[1], 13151[1], 13152[1], 13153[1], 36000[1], 36400[1], 36405[1], 36406[1], 36410[1], 36420[1], 36425[1], 36430[1], 36440[1], 36591[0], 36592[0], 36600[1], 36640[1], 43752[1], 51701[1], 51702[1], 51703[1], 62320[0], 62321[0], 62322[0], 62323[0], 62324[0], 62325[0], 62326[0], 62327[0], 64400[0], 64405[0], 64408[0], 64415[0], 64416[0], 64417[0], 64418[0], 64420[0], 64421[0], 64425[0], 64430[0], 64435[0], 64445[0], 64446[0], 64447[0], 64448[0], 64449[0], 64450[0], 64451[0], 64454[0], 64461[0], 64462[0], 64463[0], 64479[0], 64480[0], 64483[0], 64484[0], 64486[0], 64487[0], 64488[0], 64489[0], 64490[0], 64491[0], 64492[0], 64493[0], 64494[0], 64495[0], 64505[0], 64510[0], 64517[0], 64520[0], 64530[0], 66821[1], 67005[1], 67010[1], 67025[1], 67028[1], 67030[1], 67039[1], 67040[1], 67500[1], 69990[0], 92012[1], 92014[1], 92018[1], 92019[1], 92201[1], 92202[1], 93000[1], 93005[1], 93010[1], 93040[1], 93041[1], 93042[1], 93318[1], 93355[1], 94002[1], 94200[1], 94680[1], 94681[1], 94690[1], 95812[1], 95813[1], 95816[1], 95819[1], 95822[1], 95829[1], 95955[1], 96360[1], 96361[1], 96365[1], 96366[1], 96367[1], 96368[1], 96372[1], 96374[1], 96375[1], 96376[1], 96377[1], 96523[0], 99155[0], 99156[0], 99157[0], 99211[1], 99212[1], 99213[1], 99214[1], 99215[1], 99217[1], 99218[1], 99219[1], 99220[1], 99221[1], 99222[1], 99223[1], 99231[1], 99232[1], 99233[1], 99234[1], 99235[1], 99236[1], 99238[1], 99239[1], 99241[1], 99242[1], 99243[1], 99244[1], 99245[1], 99251[1], 99252[1], 99253[1], 99254[1], 99255[1], 99291[1], 99292[1], 99304[1], 99305[1], 99306[1], 99307[1], 99308[1], 99309[1], 99310[1], 99315[1], 99316[1], 99334[1], 99335[1], 99336[1], 99337[1], 99347[1], 99348[1], 99349[1], 99350[1], 99374[1], 99375[1], 99377[1], 99378[1], 99446[0], 99447[0], 99448[0], 99449[0], 99451[0], 99452[0], 99495[0], 99496[0], G0463[1], G0471[1]
67036	0213T[0], 0216T[0], 0465T[1], 0596T[1], 0597T[1], 0708T[1], 0709T[1], 11000[1], 11001[1], 11004[1], 11005[1], 11006[1], 11042[1], 11043[1], 11044[1], 11045[1], 11046[1], 11047[1], 12001[1], 12002[1], 12004[1], 12005[1], 12006[1], 12007[1], 12011[1], 12013[1], 12014[1], 12015[1], 12016[1], 12017[1], 12018[1], 12020[1], 12021[1], 12031[1], 12032[1], 12034[1], 12035[1], 12036[1], 12037[1], 12041[1], 12042[1], 12044[1], 12045[1], 12046[1], 12047[1], 12051[1], 12052[1], 12053[1], 12054[1], 12055[1], 12056[1], 12057[1], 13100[1], 13101[1], 13102[1], 13120[1], 13121[1], 13122[1], 13131[1], 13132[1], 13133[1], 13151[1], 13152[1], 13153[1], 36000[1], 36400[1], 36405[1], 36406[1], 36410[1], 36420[1], 36425[1], 36430[1], 36440[1], 36591[0], 36592[0], 36600[1], 36640[1], 43752[1], 51701[1], 51702[1], 51703[1], 62320[0], 62321[0], 62322[0], 62323[0], 62324[0], 62325[0], 62326[0], 62327[0], 64400[0], 64405[0], 64408[0], 64415[0], 64416[0], 64417[0], 64418[0], 64420[0], 64421[0], 64425[0], 64430[0], 64435[0], 64445[0], 64446[0], 64447[0], 64448[0], 64449[0], 64450[0], 64451[0], 64454[0], 64461[0], 64462[0], 64463[0], 64479[0], 64480[0], 64483[0], 64484[0], 64486[0], 64487[0], 64488[0], 64489[0], 64490[0], 64491[0], 64492[0], 64493[0], 64494[0], 64495[0], 64505[0], 64510[0], 64517[0], 64520[0], 64530[0], 65800[1], 65810[1], 65815[1], 66820[1], 66830[1], 66840[1], 66920[1], 66930[1], 66940[1], 67005[1], 67010[1], 67015[1], 67025[1], 67028[1], 67030[1], 67031[1], 67101[1], 67105[1], 67110[1], 67141[1], 67145[1], 67210[1], 67220[1], 67221[1], 67500[1], 67515[1], 68200[1], 69990[0], 92012[1], 92014[1], 92018[1], 92019[1], 92201[1], 92202[1], 93000[1], 93005[1], 93010[1], 93040[1], 93041[1], 93042[1], 93318[1], 93355[1], 94002[1], 94200[1], 94680[1], 94681[1], 94690[1], 95812[1], 95813[1], 95816[1], 95819[1], 95822[1], 95829[1], 95955[1], 96360[1], 96361[1], 96365[1], 96366[1], 96367[1],

0 = Modifier usage not allowed or inappropriate 1 = Modifier usage allowed

Code 1	Code 2
	96368[1], 96372[1], 96374[1], 96375[1], 96376[1], 96377[1], 96523[0], 97597[1], 97598[1], 97602[1], 99155[0], 99156[0], 99157[0], 99211[1], 99212[1], 99213[1], 99214[1], 99215[1], 99217[1], 99218[1], 99219[1], 99220[1], 99221[1], 99222[1], 99223[1], 99231[1], 99232[1], 99233[1], 99234[1], 99235[1], 99236[1], 99238[1], 99239[1], 99241[1], 99242[1], 99243[1], 99244[1], 99245[1], 99251[1], 99252[1], 99253[1], 99254[1], 99255[1], 99291[1], 99292[1], 99304[1], 99305[1], 99306[1], 99307[1], 99308[1], 99309[1], 99310[1], 99315[1], 99316[1], 99334[1], 99335[1], 99336[1], 99337[1], 99347[1], 99348[1], 99349[1], 99350[1], 99374[1], 99375[1], 99377[1], 99378[1], 99446[0], 99447[0], 99448[0], 99449[0], 99451[0], 99452[0], 99495[0], 99496[0], G0463[1], G0471[1]
67039	0213T[0], 0216T[0], 0465T[1], 0596T[1], 0597T[1], 0708T[1], 0709T[1], 11000[1], 11001[1], 11004[1], 11005[1], 11006[1], 11042[1], 11043[1], 11044[1], 11045[1], 11046[1], 11047[1], 12001[1], 12002[1], 12004[1], 12005[1], 12006[1], 12007[1], 12011[1], 12013[1], 12014[1], 12015[1], 12016[1], 12017[1], 12018[1], 12020[1], 12021[1], 12031[1], 12032[1], 12034[1], 12035[1], 12036[1], 12037[1], 12041[1], 12042[1], 12044[1], 12045[1], 12046[1], 12047[1], 12051[1], 12052[1], 12053[1], 12054[1], 12055[1], 12056[1], 12057[1], 13100[1], 13101[1], 13102[1], 13120[1], 13121[1], 13122[1], 13131[1], 13132[1], 13133[1], 13151[1], 13152[1], 13153[1], 36000[1], 36400[1], 36405[1], 36406[1], 36410[1], 36420[1], 36425[1], 36430[1], 36440[1], 36591[0], 36592[0], 36600[1], 36640[1], 43752[1], 51701[1], 51702[1], 51703[1], 62320[0], 62321[0], 62322[0], 62323[0], 62324[0], 62325[0], 62326[0], 62327[0], 64400[0], 64405[0], 64408[0], 64415[0], 64416[0], 64417[0], 64418[0], 64420[0], 64421[0], 64425[0], 64430[0], 64435[0], 64445[0], 64446[0], 64447[0], 64448[0], 64449[0], 64450[0], 64451[0], 64454[0], 64461[0], 64462[0], 64463[0], 64479[0], 64480[0], 64483[0], 64484[0], 64486[0], 64487[0], 64488[0], 64489[0], 64490[0], 64491[0], 64492[0], 64493[0], 64494[0], 64495[0], 64505[0], 64510[0], 64517[0], 64520[0], 64530[0], 65800[1], 65810[1], 65815[1], 66830[1], 66840[1], 66852[1], 66920[1], 66930[1], 66940[1], 67005[1], 67010[1], 67015[1], 67025[1], 67027[1], 67028[1], 67036[1], 67101[1], 67105[1], 67107[1], 67110[1], 67141[1], 67145[1], 67210[1], 67220[1], 67221[1], 67225[1], 67229[1], 67500[1], 67515[1], 68200[1], 69990[0], 92012[1], 92014[1], 92018[1], 92019[1], 92201[1], 92202[1], 93000[1], 93005[1], 93010[1], 93040[1], 93041[1], 93042[1], 93318[1], 93355[1], 94002[1], 94200[1], 94680[1], 94681[1], 94690[1], 95812[1], 95813[1], 95816[1], 95819[1], 95822[1], 95829[1], 95955[1], 96360[1], 96361[1], 96365[1], 96366[1], 96367[1], 96368[1], 96372[1], 96374[1], 96375[1], 96376[1], 96377[1], 96523[0], 97597[1], 97598[1], 97602[1], 99155[0], 99156[0], 99157[0], 99211[1], 99212[1], 99213[1], 99214[1], 99215[1], 99217[1], 99218[1], 99219[1], 99220[1], 99221[1], 99222[1], 99223[1], 99231[1], 99232[1], 99233[1], 99234[1], 99235[1], 99236[1], 99238[1], 99239[1], 99241[1], 99242[1], 99243[1], 99244[1], 99245[1], 99251[1], 99252[1], 99253[1], 99254[1], 99255[1], 99291[1], 99292[1], 99304[1], 99305[1], 99306[1], 99307[1], 99308[1], 99309[1], 99310[1], 99315[1], 99316[1], 99334[1], 99335[1], 99336[1], 99337[1], 99347[1], 99348[1], 99349[1], 99350[1], 99374[1], 99375[1], 99377[1], 99378[1], 99446[0], 99447[0], 99448[0], 99449[0], 99451[0], 99452[0], 99495[0], 99496[0], G0186[1], G0463[1], G0471[1]
67040	0213T[0], 0216T[0], 0465T[1], 0596T[1], 0597T[1], 0708T[1], 0709T[1], 11000[1], 11001[1], 11004[1], 11005[1], 11006[1], 11042[1], 11043[1], 11044[1], 11045[1], 11046[1], 11047[1], 12001[1], 12002[1], 12004[1], 12005[1], 12006[1], 12007[1], 12011[1], 12013[1], 12014[1], 12015[1], 12016[1], 12017[1], 12018[1], 12020[1], 12021[1], 12031[1], 12032[1], 12034[1], 12035[1], 12036[1], 12037[1], 12041[1], 12042[1], 12044[1], 12045[1], 12046[1], 12047[1], 12051[1], 12052[1], 12053[1], 12054[1], 12055[1], 12056[1], 12057[1], 13100[1], 13101[1], 13102[1], 13120[1], 13121[1], 13122[1], 13131[1], 13132[1], 13133[1], 13151[1], 13152[1], 13153[1], 36000[1], 36400[1], 36405[1], 36406[1], 36410[1], 36420[1], 36425[1], 36430[1], 36440[1], 36591[0], 36592[0], 36600[1], 36640[1], 43752[1], 51701[1], 51702[1], 51703[1], 62320[0], 62321[0], 62322[0], 62323[0], 62324[0], 62325[0], 62326[0], 62327[0], 64400[0], 64405[0], 64408[0], 64415[0], 64416[0], 64417[0], 64418[0], 64420[0], 64421[0], 64425[0], 64430[0], 64435[0], 64445[0], 64446[0], 64447[0], 64448[0], 64449[0], 64450[0], 64451[0], 64454[0], 64461[0], 64462[0], 64463[0], 64479[0], 64480[0], 64483[0], 64484[0], 64486[0], 64487[0], 64488[0], 64489[0], 64490[0], 64491[0], 64492[0], 64493[0], 64494[0], 64495[0], 64505[0], 64510[0], 64517[0], 64520[0], 64530[0], 65800[1], 65810[1], 65815[1], 66830[1], 66840[1], 66852[1], 66920[1], 66930[1], 66940[1], 67005[1], 67010[1], 67015[1], 67025[1], 67027[1], 67028[1], 67036[1], 67039[1], 67041[1], 67101[1], 67105[1], 67107[1], 67110[1], 67141[1], 67145[1], 67210[1], 67220[1], 67221[1], 67225[1], 67229[1], 67500[1], 67515[1], 68200[1], 69990[0], 92012[1], 92014[1], 92018[1], 92019[1], 92201[1], 92202[1], 93000[1], 93005[1], 93010[1], 93040[1], 93041[1], 93042[1], 93318[1], 93355[1], 94002[1], 94200[1], 94680[1], 94681[1], 94690[1], 95812[1], 95813[1], 95816[1], 95819[1], 95822[1], 95829[1], 95955[1], 96360[1], 96361[1], 96365[1], 96366[1], 96367[1], 96368[1], 96372[1], 96374[1], 96375[1], 96376[1], 96377[1], 96523[0], 97597[1], 97598[1], 97602[1], 99155[0], 99156[0], 99157[0], 99211[1], 99212[1], 99213[1], 99214[1], 99215[1], 99217[1], 99218[1], 99219[1], 99220[1], 99221[1], 99222[1], 99223[1], 99231[1], 99232[1], 99233[1], 99234[1], 99235[1], 99236[1], 99238[1], 99239[1], 99241[1], 99242[1], 99243[1], 99244[1], 99245[1], 99251[1], 99252[1], 99253[1], 99254[1], 99255[1], 99291[1], 99292[1], 99304[1], 99305[1], 99306[1], 99307[1], 99308[1], 99309[1], 99310[1], 99315[1], 99316[1], 99334[1], 99335[1], 99336[1], 99337[1], 99347[1], 99348[1], 99349[1], 99350[1], 99374[1], 99375[1], 99377[1], 99378[1], 99446[0], 99447[0], 99448[0], 99449[0], 99451[0], 99452[0], 99495[0], 99496[0], G0186[1], G0463[1], G0471[1]
67041	0213T[0], 0216T[0], 0465T[1], 0708T[1], 0709T[1], 11000[1], 11001[1], 11004[1], 11005[1], 11006[1], 11042[1], 11043[1], 11044[1], 11045[1], 11046[1], 11047[1], 12001[1], 12002[1], 12004[1], 12005[1], 12006[1], 12007[1], 12011[1], 12013[1], 12014[1], 12015[1], 12016[1], 12017[1], 12018[1], 12020[1], 12021[1], 12031[1], 12032[1], 12034[1], 12035[1], 12036[1], 12037[1], 12041[1], 12042[1], 12044[1], 12045[1], 12046[1], 12047[1], 12051[1], 12052[1], 12053[1], 12054[1], 12055[1], 12056[1], 12057[1], 13100[1], 13101[1], 13102[1], 13120[1], 13121[1], 13122[1], 13131[1], 13132[1], 13133[1], 13151[1], 13152[1], 13153[1], 36000[1], 36400[1], 36405[1], 36406[1], 36410[1], 36420[1], 36425[1], 36430[1], 36440[1], 36591[0], 36592[0], 36600[1], 36640[1], 43752[1], 62320[0], 62321[0], 62322[0], 62323[0], 62324[0], 62325[0], 62326[0], 62327[0], 64400[0], 64405[0], 64408[0], 64415[0], 64416[0], 64417[0], 64418[0], 64420[0], 64421[0], 64425[0], 64430[0], 64435[0], 64445[0], 64446[0], 64447[0], 64448[0], 64449[0], 64450[0], 64451[0], 64454[0], 64461[0], 64462[0], 64463[0], 64479[0], 64480[0], 64483[0], 64484[0], 64486[0], 64487[0], 64488[0], 64489[0], 64490[0], 64491[0], 64492[0], 64493[0], 64494[0], 64495[0], 64505[0], 64510[0], 64517[0], 64520[0], 64530[0], 65800[1], 65810[1], 65815[1], 66830[1], 66840[1], 66852[1], 66920[1], 66930[1], 66940[1], 67005[1], 67010[1], 67015[1], 67025[1], 67027[1], 67028[1], 67030[1], 67031[1], 67036[1], 67039[1], 67101[1], 67105[1], 67107[1], 67110[1], 67120[1], 67121[1], 67141[1], 67145[1], 67208[1], 67210[1], 67220[1], 67221[1], 67227[1], 67228[1], 67500[1], 67515[1], 68200[1], 69990[0], 92012[1], 92014[1], 92018[1], 92019[1], 92201[1], 92202[1], 93000[1], 93005[1], 93010[1], 93040[1], 93041[1], 93042[1], 93318[1], 93355[1], 94002[1], 94200[1], 94680[1], 94681[1], 94690[1], 95812[1], 95813[1], 95816[1], 95819[1], 95822[1], 95829[1], 95955[1], 96360[1], 96361[1], 96365[1], 96366[1], 96367[1], 96368[1], 96372[1], 96374[1], 96375[1], 96376[1], 96377[1], 96523[0], 97597[1], 97598[1], 97602[1], 99155[0], 99156[0], 99157[0], 99211[1], 99212[1], 99213[1], 99214[1], 99215[1], 99217[1], 99218[1], 99219[1], 99220[1], 99221[1], 99222[1], 99223[1], 99231[1], 99232[1], 99233[1], 99234[1], 99235[1], 99236[1], 99238[1], 99239[1], 99241[1], 99242[1], 99243[1], 99244[1], 99245[1], 99251[1], 99252[1], 99253[1], 99254[1], 99255[1], 99291[1], 99292[1], 99304[1], 99305[1], 99306[1], 99307[1], 99308[1], 99309[1], 99310[1], 99315[1], 99316[1], 99334[1], 99335[1], 99336[1], 99337[1], 99347[1], 99348[1], 99349[1], 99350[1], 99374[1], 99375[1], 99377[1], 99378[1], 99446[0], 99447[0], 99448[0], 99449[0], 99451[0], 99452[0], 99495[0], 99496[0], G0463[1]
67042	0213T[0], 0216T[0], 0465T[1], 0708T[1], 0709T[1], 11000[1], 11001[1], 11004[1], 11005[1], 11006[1], 11042[1], 11043[1], 11044[1], 11045[1], 11046[1], 11047[1], 12001[1], 12002[1], 12004[1], 12005[1], 12006[1], 12007[1], 12011[1], 12013[1], 12014[1], 12015[1], 12016[1], 12017[1], 12018[1], 12020[1], 12021[1], 12031[1], 12032[1], 12034[1], 12035[1], 12036[1], 12037[1], 12041[1], 12042[1], 12044[1], 12045[1], 12046[1], 12047[1], 12051[1], 12052[1], 12053[1], 12054[1], 12055[1], 12056[1], 12057[1], 13100[1], 13101[1], 13102[1], 13120[1], 13121[1], 13122[1], 13131[1], 13132[1], 13133[1], 13151[1], 13152[1], 13153[1], 36000[1], 36400[1], 36405[1], 36406[1], 36410[1], 36420[1], 36425[1], 36430[1], 36440[1], 36591[0], 36592[0], 36600[1], 36640[1], 43752[1], 62320[0], 62321[0], 62322[0], 62323[0], 62324[0], 62325[0], 62326[0], 62327[0], 64400[0], 64405[0], 64408[0], 64415[0], 64416[0], 64417[0], 64418[0], 64420[0], 64421[0], 64425[0], 64430[0], 64435[0], 64445[0], 64446[0], 64447[0], 64448[0], 64449[0], 64450[0], 64451[0], 64454[0], 64461[0], 64462[0], 64463[0], 64479[0], 64480[0], 64483[0], 64484[0], 64486[0], 64487[0], 64488[0], 64489[0], 64490[0], 64491[0], 64492[0], 64493[0], 64494[0], 64495[0], 64505[0], 64510[0], 64517[0], 64520[0], 64530[0], 65800[1], 65810[1], 65815[1], 66830[1], 66840[1], 66852[1], 66920[1], 66930[1], 66940[1], 67005[1], 67010[1], 67015[1], 67025[1], 67027[1], 67028[1], 67030[1], 67031[1], 67036[1], 67039[1], 67040[1], 67041[1], 67101[1], 67105[1], 67107[1], 67110[1], 67141[1], 67145[1], 67208[1], 67210[1], 67218[1], 67220[1], 67221[1], 67227[1], 67228[1], 67500[1], 67515[1], 68200[1], 69990[0], 92012[1], 92014[1], 92018[1], 92019[1], 92201[1], 92202[1], 93000[1], 93005[1], 93010[1], 93040[1], 93041[1], 93042[1], 93318[1], 93355[1], 94002[1], 94200[1], 94680[1], 94681[1], 94690[1], 95812[1], 95813[1], 95816[1], 95819[1], 95822[1], 95829[1], 95955[1], 96360[1], 96361[1], 96365[1], 96366[1], 96367[1], 96368[1], 96372[1], 96374[1], 96375[1], 96376[1], 96377[1], 96523[0], 97597[1], 97598[1], 97602[1], 99155[0], 99156[0], 99157[0], 99211[1], 99212[1], 99213[1], 99214[1], 99215[1], 99217[1], 99218[1], 99219[1], 99220[1], 99221[1], 99222[1], 99223[1], 99231[1], 99232[1], 99233[1], 99234[1], 99235[1], 99236[1], 99238[1], 99239[1], 99241[1], 99242[1], 99243[1], 99244[1], 99245[1], 99251[1], 99252[1], 99253[1], 99254[1], 99255[1], 99291[1], 99292[1], 99304[1], 99305[1], 99306[1], 99307[1], 99308[1], 99309[1], 99310[1], 99315[1], 99316[1], 99334[1], 99335[1], 99336[1], 99337[1], 99347[1], 99348[1], 99349[1], 99350[1], 99374[1], 99375[1], 99377[1], 99378[1], 99446[0], 99447[0], 99448[0], 99449[0], 99451[0], 99452[0], 99495[0], 99496[0], G0463[1]
67043	0213T[0], 0216T[0], 0465T[1], 0708T[1], 0709T[1], 11000[1], 11001[1], 11004[1], 11005[1], 11006[1], 11042[1], 11043[1], 11044[1], 11045[1], 11046[1], 11047[1], 12001[1], 12002[1], 12004[1], 12005[1], 12006[1], 12007[1], 12011[1], 12013[1], 12014[1], 12015[1], 12016[1], 12017[1], 12018[1], 12020[1], 12021[1], 12031[1], 12032[1], 12034[1], 12035[1], 12036[1], 12037[1], 12041[1], 12042[1], 12044[1], 12045[1], 12046[1], 12047[1], 12051[1], 12052[1], 12053[1], 12054[1], 12055[1], 12056[1], 12057[1], 13100[1], 13101[1], 13102[1], 13120[1], 13121[1], 13122[1], 13131[1], 13132[1], 13133[1], 13151[1], 13152[1], 13153[1], 36000[1], 36400[1], 36405[1], 36406[1], 36410[1], 36420[1], 36425[1], 36430[1], 36440[1], 36591[0], 36592[0], 36600[1], 36640[1], 43752[1], 62320[0], 62321[0], 62322[0], 62323[0], 62324[0], 62325[0], 62326[0], 62327[0], 64400[0], 64405[0], 64408[0], 64415[0], 64416[0], 64417[0], 64418[0], 64420[0], 64421[0], 64425[0], 64430[0], 64435[0], 64445[0], 64446[0], 64447[0], 64448[0], 64449[0], 64450[0], 64451[0], 64454[0], 64461[0], 64462[0], 64463[0], 64479[0], 64480[0], 64483[0], 64484[0], 64486[0], 64487[0], 64488[0], 64489[0], 64490[0], 64491[0], 64492[0], 64493[0], 64494[0], 64495[0], 64505[0], 64510[0], 64517[0], 64520[0], 64530[0], 65800[1], 65810[1], 65815[1], 66830[1], 66840[1], 66852[1], 66920[1], 66930[1], 66940[1], 67005[1], 67010[1], 67015[1], 67025[1], 67027[1],

0 = Modifier usage not allowed or inappropriate 1 = Modifier usage allowed

Appendix A: NCCI - CPT Codes

Code 1	Code 2
	67028[1], 67030[1], 67031[1], 67036[1], 67039[1], 67040[1], 67041[1], 67042[1], 67101[1], 67105[1], 67107[1], 67108[1], 67110[1], 67141[1], 67145[1], 67208[1], 67210[1], 67218[1], 67220[1], 67221[1], 67227[1], 67228[1], 67229[1], 67500[1], 67515[1], 68200[1], 69990[0], 92012[1], 92014[1], 92018[1], 92019[1], 92201[1], 92202[1], 93000[1], 93005[1], 93010[1], 93040[1], 93041[1], 93042[1], 93318[1], 93355[1], 94002[1], 94200[1], 94680[1], 94681[1], 94690[1], 95812[1], 95813[1], 95816[1], 95819[1], 95822[1], 95829[1], 95955[1], 96360[1], 96361[1], 96365[1], 96366[1], 96367[1], 96368[1], 96372[1], 96374[1], 96375[1], 96376[1], 96377[1], 96523[0], 97597[1], 97598[1], 97602[1], 99155[0], 99156[0], 99157[0], 99211[1], 99212[1], 99213[1], 99214[1], 99215[1], 99217[1], 99218[1], 99219[1], 99220[1], 99221[1], 99222[1], 99223[1], 99231[1], 99232[1], 99233[1], 99234[1], 99235[1], 99236[1], 99238[1], 99239[1], 99241[1], 99242[1], 99243[1], 99244[1], 99245[1], 99251[1], 99252[1], 99253[1], 99254[1], 99255[1], 99291[1], 99292[1], 99304[1], 99305[1], 99306[1], 99307[1], 99308[1], 99309[1], 99310[1], 99315[1], 99316[1], 99334[1], 99335[1], 99336[1], 99337[1], 99347[1], 99348[1], 99349[1], 99350[1], 99374[1], 99375[1], 99377[1], 99378[1], 99446[0], 99447[0], 99448[0], 99449[0], 99451[0], 99452[0], 99495[0], 99496[0], G0463[1]
67101	0213T[0], 0216T[0], 0465T[1], 0596T[1], 0597T[1], 0708T[1], 0709T[1], 12001[1], 12002[1], 12004[1], 12005[1], 12006[1], 12007[1], 12011[1], 12013[1], 12014[1], 12015[1], 12016[1], 12017[1], 12018[1], 12020[1], 12021[1], 12031[1], 12032[1], 12034[1], 12035[1], 12036[1], 12037[1], 12041[1], 12042[1], 12044[1], 12045[1], 12046[1], 12047[1], 12051[1], 12052[1], 12053[1], 12054[1], 12055[1], 12056[1], 12057[1], 13100[1], 13101[1], 13102[1], 13120[1], 13121[1], 13122[1], 13131[1], 13132[1], 13133[1], 13151[1], 13152[1], 13153[1], 36000[1], 36400[1], 36405[1], 36406[1], 36410[1], 36420[1], 36425[1], 36430[1], 36440[1], 36591[0], 36592[0], 36600[1], 36640[1], 43752[1], 51701[1], 51702[1], 51703[1], 62320[0], 62321[0], 62322[0], 62323[0], 62324[0], 62325[0], 62326[0], 62327[0], 64400[0], 64405[0], 64408[0], 64415[0], 64416[0], 64417[0], 64418[0], 64420[0], 64421[0], 64425[0], 64430[0], 64435[0], 64445[0], 64446[0], 64447[0], 64448[0], 64449[0], 64450[0], 64451[0], 64454[0], 64461[0], 64462[0], 64463[0], 64479[0], 64480[0], 64483[0], 64484[0], 64486[0], 64487[0], 64488[0], 64489[0], 64490[0], 64491[0], 64492[0], 64493[0], 64494[0], 64495[0], 64505[0], 64510[0], 64517[0], 64520[0], 64530[0], 67005[1], 67010[1], 67015[1], 67025[1], 67028[1], 67105[1], 67107[1], 67141[1], 67145[1], 67208[1], 67227[1], 67228[1], 67500[1], 69990[0], 92012[1], 92014[1], 92018[1], 92019[1], 92201[1], 92202[1], 93000[1], 93005[1], 93010[1], 93040[1], 93041[1], 93042[1], 93318[1], 93355[1], 94002[1], 94200[1], 94680[1], 94681[1], 94690[1], 95812[1], 95813[1], 95816[1], 95819[1], 95822[1], 95829[1], 95955[1], 96360[1], 96361[1], 96365[1], 96366[1], 96367[1], 96368[1], 96372[1], 96374[1], 96375[1], 96376[1], 96377[1], 96523[0], 99155[0], 99156[0], 99157[0], 99211[1], 99212[1], 99213[1], 99214[1], 99215[1], 99217[1], 99218[1], 99219[1], 99220[1], 99221[1], 99222[1], 99223[1], 99231[1], 99232[1], 99233[1], 99234[1], 99235[1], 99236[1], 99238[1], 99239[1], 99241[1], 99242[1], 99243[1], 99244[1], 99245[1], 99251[1], 99252[1], 99253[1], 99254[1], 99255[1], 99291[1], 99292[1], 99304[1], 99305[1], 99306[1], 99307[1], 99308[1], 99309[1], 99310[1], 99315[1], 99316[1], 99334[1], 99335[1], 99336[1], 99337[1], 99347[1], 99348[1], 99349[1], 99350[1], 99374[1], 99375[1], 99377[1], 99378[1], 99446[0], 99447[0], 99448[0], 99449[0], 99451[0], 99452[0], 99495[0], 99496[0], G0463[1], G0471[1], J0670[1], J2001[1]
67105	0213T[0], 0216T[0], 0465T[1], 0596T[1], 0597T[1], 0708T[1], 0709T[1], 12001[1], 12002[1], 12004[1], 12005[1], 12006[1], 12007[1], 12011[1], 12013[1], 12014[1], 12015[1], 12016[1], 12017[1], 12018[1], 12020[1], 12021[1], 12031[1], 12032[1], 12034[1], 12035[1], 12036[1], 12037[1], 12041[1], 12042[1], 12044[1], 12045[1], 12046[1], 12047[1], 12051[1], 12052[1], 12053[1], 12054[1], 12055[1], 12056[1], 12057[1], 13100[1], 13101[1], 13102[1], 13120[1], 13121[1], 13122[1], 13131[1], 13132[1], 13133[1], 13151[1], 13152[1], 13153[1], 36000[1], 36400[1], 36405[1], 36406[1], 36410[1], 36420[1], 36425[1], 36430[1], 36440[1], 36591[0], 36592[0], 36600[1], 36640[1], 43752[1], 51701[1], 51702[1], 51703[1], 62320[0], 62321[0], 62322[0], 62323[0], 62324[0], 62325[0], 62326[0], 62327[0], 64400[0], 64405[0], 64408[0], 64415[0], 64416[0], 64417[0], 64418[0], 64420[0], 64421[0], 64425[0], 64430[0], 64435[0], 64445[0], 64446[0], 64447[0], 64448[0], 64449[0], 64450[0], 64451[0], 64454[0], 64461[0], 64462[0], 64463[0], 64479[0], 64480[0], 64483[0], 64484[0], 64486[0], 64487[0], 64488[0], 64489[0], 64490[0], 64491[0], 64492[0], 64493[0], 64494[0], 64495[0], 64505[0], 64510[0], 64517[0], 64520[0], 64530[0], 67010[1], 67015[1], 67028[1], 67141[1], 67145[1], 67208[1], 67210[1], 67220[1], 67221[1], 67225[1], 67227[1], 67228[1], 67500[1], 69990[0], 92012[1], 92014[1], 92018[1], 92019[1], 92201[1], 92202[1], 93000[1], 93005[1], 93010[1], 93040[1], 93041[1], 93042[1], 93318[1], 93355[1], 94002[1], 94200[1], 94680[1], 94681[1], 94690[1], 95812[1], 95813[1], 95816[1], 95819[1], 95822[1], 95829[1], 95955[1], 96360[1], 96361[1], 96365[1], 96366[1], 96367[1], 96368[1], 96372[1], 96374[1], 96375[1], 96376[1], 96377[1], 96523[0], 99155[0], 99156[0], 99157[0], 99211[1], 99212[1], 99213[1], 99214[1], 99215[1], 99217[1], 99218[1], 99219[1], 99220[1], 99221[1], 99222[1], 99223[1], 99231[1], 99232[1], 99233[1], 99234[1], 99235[1], 99236[1], 99238[1], 99239[1], 99241[1], 99242[1], 99243[1], 99244[1], 99245[1], 99251[1], 99252[1], 99253[1], 99254[1], 99255[1], 99291[1], 99292[1], 99304[1], 99305[1], 99306[1], 99307[1], 99308[1], 99309[1], 99310[1], 99315[1], 99316[1], 99334[1], 99335[1], 99336[1], 99337[1], 99347[1], 99348[1], 99349[1], 99350[1], 99374[1], 99375[1], 99377[1], 99378[1], 99446[0], 99447[0], 99448[0], 99449[0], 99451[0], 99452[0], 99495[0], 99496[0], G0186[1], G0463[1], G0471[1], J0670[1], J2001[1]
67107	0213T[0], 0216T[0], 0465T[1], 0596T[1], 0597T[1], 0708T[1], 0709T[1], 12001[1], 12002[1], 12004[1], 12005[1], 12006[1], 12007[1], 12011[1], 12013[1], 12014[1], 12015[1], 12016[1], 12017[1], 12018[1], 12020[1], 12021[1], 12031[1], 12032[1], 12034[1], 12035[1], 12036[1], 12037[1], 12041[1], 12042[1], 12044[1], 12045[1], 12046[1], 12047[1], 12051[1], 12052[1], 12053[1], 12054[1], 12055[1], 12056[1], 12057[1], 13100[1], 13101[1], 13102[1], 13120[1], 13121[1], 13122[1], 13131[1], 13132[1], 13133[1], 13151[1], 13152[1], 13153[1], 36000[1], 36400[1], 36405[1], 36406[1], 36410[1], 36420[1], 36425[1], 36430[1], 36440[1], 36591[0], 36592[0], 36600[1], 36640[1], 43752[1], 51701[1], 51702[1], 51703[1], 62320[0], 62321[0], 62322[0], 62323[0], 62324[0], 62325[0], 62326[0], 62327[0], 64400[0], 64405[0], 64408[0], 64415[0], 64416[0], 64417[0], 64418[0], 64420[0], 64421[0], 64425[0], 64430[0], 64435[0], 64445[0], 64446[0], 64447[0], 64448[0], 64449[0], 64450[0], 64451[0], 64454[0], 64461[0], 64462[0], 64463[0], 64479[0], 64480[0], 64483[0], 64484[0], 64486[0], 64487[0], 64488[0], 64489[0], 64490[0], 64491[0], 64492[0], 64493[0], 64494[0], 64495[0], 64505[0], 64510[0], 64517[0], 64520[0], 64530[0], 67005[1], 67010[1], 67015[1], 67028[1], 67036[1], 67105[1], 67141[1], 67145[1], 67208[1], 67210[1], 67220[1], 67221[1], 67225[1], 67228[1], 67229[1], 67500[1], 69990[0], 92012[1], 92014[1], 92018[1], 92019[1], 92201[1], 92202[1], 93000[1], 93005[1], 93010[1], 93040[1], 93041[1], 93042[1], 93318[1], 93355[1], 94002[1], 94200[1], 94680[1], 94681[1], 94690[1], 95812[1], 95813[1], 95816[1], 95819[1], 95822[1], 95829[1], 95955[1], 96360[1], 96361[1], 96365[1], 96366[1], 96367[1], 96368[1], 96372[1], 96374[1], 96375[1], 96376[1], 96377[1], 96523[0], 99155[0], 99156[0], 99157[0], 99211[1], 99212[1], 99213[1], 99214[1], 99215[1], 99217[1], 99218[1], 99219[1], 99220[1], 99221[1], 99222[1], 99223[1], 99231[1], 99232[1], 99233[1], 99234[1], 99235[1], 99236[1], 99238[1], 99239[1], 99241[1], 99242[1], 99243[1], 99244[1], 99245[1], 99251[1], 99252[1], 99253[1], 99254[1], 99255[1], 99291[1], 99292[1], 99304[1], 99305[1], 99306[1], 99307[1], 99308[1], 99309[1], 99310[1], 99315[1], 99316[1], 99334[1], 99335[1], 99336[1], 99337[1], 99347[1], 99348[1], 99349[1], 99350[1], 99374[1], 99375[1], 99377[1], 99378[1], 99446[0], 99447[0], 99448[0], 99449[0], 99451[0], 99452[0], 99495[0], 99496[0], G0186[1], G0463[1], G0471[1]
67108	0213T[0], 0216T[0], 0308T[1], 0465T[1], 0596T[1], 0597T[1], 0617T[1], 0708T[1], 0709T[1], 11000[1], 11001[1], 11004[1], 11005[1], 11006[1], 11042[1], 11043[1], 11044[1], 11045[1], 11046[1], 11047[1], 12001[1], 12002[1], 12004[1], 12005[1], 12006[1], 12007[1], 12011[1], 12013[1], 12014[1], 12015[1], 12016[1], 12017[1], 12018[1], 12020[1], 12021[1], 12031[1], 12032[1], 12034[1], 12035[1], 12036[1], 12037[1], 12041[1], 12042[1], 12044[1], 12045[1], 12046[1], 12047[1], 12051[1], 12052[1], 12053[1], 12054[1], 12055[1], 12056[1], 12057[1], 13100[1], 13101[1], 13102[1], 13120[1], 13121[1], 13122[1], 13131[1], 13132[1], 13133[1], 13151[1], 13152[1], 13153[1], 36000[1], 36400[1], 36405[1], 36406[1], 36410[1], 36420[1], 36425[1], 36430[1], 36440[1], 36591[0], 36592[0], 36600[1], 36640[1], 43752[1], 51701[1], 51702[1], 51703[1], 62320[0], 62321[0], 62322[0], 62323[0], 62324[0], 62325[0], 62326[0], 62327[0], 64400[0], 64405[0], 64408[0], 64415[0], 64416[0], 64417[0], 64418[0], 64420[0], 64421[0], 64425[0], 64430[0], 64435[0], 64445[0], 64446[0], 64447[0], 64448[0], 64449[0], 64450[0], 64451[0], 64454[0], 64461[0], 64462[0], 64463[0], 64479[0], 64480[0], 64483[0], 64484[0], 64486[0], 64487[0], 64488[0], 64489[0], 64490[0], 64491[0], 64492[0], 64493[0], 64494[0], 64495[0], 64505[0], 64510[0], 64517[0], 64520[0], 64530[0], 66840[1], 66850[1], 66852[1], 66920[1], 66930[1], 66940[1], 66982[1], 66983[1], 66984[1], 66987[1], 66988[1], 66989[1], 66991[1], 67015[1], 67025[1], 67028[1], 67031[1], 67036[1], 67039[1], 67040[1], 67041[1], 67042[1], 67101[1], 67105[1], 67107[1], 67121[1], 67141[1], 67145[1], 67208[1], 67210[1], 67220[1], 67221[1], 67225[1], 67227[1], 67228[1], 67229[1], 67500[1], 68200[1], 69990[0], 92012[1], 92014[1], 92018[1], 92019[1], 92201[1], 92202[1], 93000[1], 93005[1], 93010[1], 93040[1], 93041[1], 93042[1], 93318[1], 93355[1], 94002[1], 94200[1], 94680[1], 94681[1], 94690[1], 95812[1], 95813[1], 95816[1], 95819[1], 95822[1], 95829[1], 95955[1], 96360[1], 96361[1], 96365[1], 96366[1], 96367[1], 96368[1], 96372[1], 96374[1], 96375[1], 96376[1], 96377[1], 96523[0], 97597[1], 97598[1], 97602[1], 99155[0], 99156[0], 99157[0], 99211[1], 99212[1], 99213[1], 99214[1], 99215[1], 99217[1], 99218[1], 99219[1], 99220[1], 99221[1], 99222[1], 99223[1], 99231[1], 99232[1], 99233[1], 99234[1], 99235[1], 99236[1], 99238[1], 99239[1], 99241[1], 99242[1], 99243[1], 99244[1], 99245[1], 99251[1], 99252[1], 99253[1], 99254[1], 99255[1], 99291[1], 99292[1], 99304[1], 99305[1], 99306[1], 99307[1], 99308[1], 99309[1], 99310[1], 99315[1], 99316[1], 99334[1], 99335[1], 99336[1], 99337[1], 99347[1], 99348[1], 99349[1], 99350[1], 99374[1], 99375[1], 99377[1], 99378[1], 99446[0], 99447[0], 99448[0], 99449[0], 99451[0], 99452[0], 99495[0], 99496[0], G0186[1], G0463[1], G0471[1], J2001[1]
67110	0213T[0], 0216T[0], 0465T[1], 0596T[1], 0597T[1], 0708T[1], 0709T[1], 12001[1], 12002[1], 12004[1], 12005[1], 12006[1], 12007[1], 12011[1], 12013[1], 12014[1], 12015[1], 12016[1], 12017[1], 12018[1], 12020[1], 12021[1], 12031[1], 12032[1], 12034[1], 12035[1], 12036[1], 12037[1], 12041[1], 12042[1], 12044[1], 12045[1], 12046[1], 12047[1], 12051[1], 12052[1], 12053[1], 12054[1], 12055[1], 12056[1], 12057[1], 13100[1], 13101[1], 13102[1], 13120[1], 13121[1], 13122[1], 13131[1], 13132[1], 13133[1], 13151[1], 13152[1], 13153[1], 36000[1], 36400[1], 36405[1], 36406[1], 36410[1], 36420[1], 36425[1], 36430[1], 36440[1], 36591[0], 36592[0], 36600[1], 36640[1], 43752[1], 51701[1], 51702[1], 51703[1], 62320[0], 62321[0], 62322[0], 62323[0], 62324[0], 62325[0], 62326[0], 62327[0], 64400[0], 64405[0], 64408[0], 64415[0], 64416[0], 64417[0], 64418[0], 64420[0], 64421[0], 64425[0], 64430[0], 64435[0], 64445[0], 64446[0], 64447[0], 64448[0], 64449[0], 64450[0], 64451[0], 64454[0], 64461[0], 64462[0], 64463[0], 64479[0], 64480[0], 64483[0], 64484[0], 64486[0], 64487[0], 64488[0], 64489[0], 64490[0], 64491[0], 64492[0], 64493[0], 64494[0], 64495[0], 64505[0], 64510[0], 64517[0], 64520[0], 64530[0], 67005[1], 67010[1], 67015[1], 67025[1], 67028[1], 67030[1], 67031[1], 67101[1], 67105[1], 67107[1], 67108[1], 67141[1], 67145[1], 67500[1], 69990[0], 92012[1], 92014[1], 92018[1], 92019[1], 92201[1],

0 = Modifier usage not allowed or inappropriate 1 = Modifier usage allowed

Code 1	Code 2
	92202[1], 93000[1], 93005[1], 93010[1], 93040[1], 93041[1], 93042[1], 93318[1], 93355[1], 94002[1], 94200[1], 94680[1], 94681[1], 94690[1], 95812[1], 95813[1], 95816[1], 95819[1], 95822[1], 95829[1], 95955[1], 96360[1], 96361[1], 96365[1], 96366[1], 96367[1], 96368[1], 96372[1], 96374[1], 96375[1], 96376[1], 96377[1], 96523[0], 99155[0], 99156[0], 99157[0], 99211[1], 99212[1], 99213[1], 99214[1], 99215[1], 99217[1], 99218[1], 99219[1], 99220[1], 99221[1], 99222[1], 99223[1], 99231[1], 99232[1], 99233[1], 99234[1], 99235[1], 99236[1], 99238[1], 99239[1], 99241[1], 99242[1], 99243[1], 99244[1], 99245[1], 99251[1], 99252[1], 99253[1], 99254[1], 99255[1], 99291[1], 99292[1], 99304[1], 99305[1], 99306[1], 99307[1], 99308[1], 99309[1], 99310[1], 99315[1], 99316[1], 99334[1], 99335[1], 99336[1], 99337[1], 99347[1], 99348[1], 99349[1], 99350[1], 99374[1], 99375[1], 99377[1], 99378[1], 99446[0], 99447[0], 99448[0], 99449[0], 99451[0], 99452[0], 99495[0], 99496[0], G0463[1], G0471[1], J0670[1], J2001[1]
67113	0213T[0], 0216T[0], 0308T[1], 0465T[1], 0617T[1], 0708T[1], 0709T[1], 11000[1], 11001[1], 11004[1], 11005[1], 11006[1], 11042[1], 11043[1], 11044[1], 11045[1], 11046[1], 11047[1], 12001[1], 12002[1], 12004[1], 12005[1], 12006[1], 12007[1], 12011[1], 12013[1], 12014[1], 12015[1], 12016[1], 12017[1], 12018[1], 12020[1], 12021[1], 12031[1], 12032[1], 12034[1], 12035[1], 12036[1], 12037[1], 12041[1], 12042[1], 12044[1], 12045[1], 12046[1], 12047[1], 12051[1], 12052[1], 12053[1], 12054[1], 12055[1], 12056[1], 12057[1], 13100[1], 13101[1], 13102[1], 13120[1], 13121[1], 13122[1], 13131[1], 13132[1], 13133[1], 13151[1], 13152[1], 13153[1], 36000[1], 36400[1], 36405[1], 36406[1], 36410[1], 36420[1], 36425[1], 36430[1], 36440[1], 36591[0], 36592[0], 36600[1], 36640[1], 43752[1], 62320[0], 62321[0], 62322[0], 62323[0], 62324[0], 62325[0], 62326[0], 62327[0], 64408[0], 64415[0], 64416[0], 64417[0], 64418[0], 64420[0], 64421[0], 64425[0], 64430[0], 64435[0], 64445[0], 64446[0], 64447[0], 64448[0], 64449[0], 64450[0], 64451[0], 64454[0], 64461[0], 64462[0], 64463[0], 64479[0], 64480[0], 64483[0], 64484[0], 64486[0], 64487[0], 64488[0], 64489[0], 64490[0], 64491[0], 64492[0], 64493[0], 64494[0], 64495[0], 64505[0], 64510[0], 64517[0], 64520[0], 64530[0], 66830[1], 66840[1], 66850[1], 66852[1], 66920[1], 66930[1], 66940[1], 66982[1], 66983[1], 66984[1], 66987[1], 66988[1], 66989[1], 66991[1], 67005[1], 67010[1], 67015[1], 67025[1], 67028[1], 67030[1], 67031[1], 67036[1], 67039[1], 67040[1], 67041[1], 67042[1], 67043[1], 67101[1], 67105[1], 67107[1], 67108[1], 67110[1], 67141[1], 67145[1], 67208[1], 67210[1], 67218[1], 67220[1], 67221[1], 67227[1], 67228[1], 67500[1], 67515[1], 68200[1], 69990[0], 92012[1], 92014[1], 92018[1], 92019[1], 92201[1], 92202[1], 93000[1], 93005[1], 93010[1], 93040[1], 93041[1], 93042[1], 93318[1], 93355[1], 94002[1], 94200[1], 94680[1], 94681[1], 94690[1], 95812[1], 95813[1], 95816[1], 95819[1], 95822[1], 95829[1], 95955[1], 96360[1], 96361[1], 96365[1], 96366[1], 96367[1], 96368[1], 96372[1], 96374[1], 96375[1], 96376[1], 96377[1], 96523[0], 97597[1], 97598[1], 97602[1], 99155[0], 99156[0], 99157[0], 99211[1], 99212[1], 99213[1], 99214[1], 99215[1], 99217[1], 99218[1], 99219[1], 99220[1], 99221[1], 99222[1], 99223[1], 99231[1], 99232[1], 99233[1], 99234[1], 99235[1], 99236[1], 99238[1], 99239[1], 99241[1], 99242[1], 99243[1], 99244[1], 99245[1], 99251[1], 99252[1], 99253[1], 99254[1], 99255[1], 99291[1], 99292[1], 99304[1], 99305[1], 99306[1], 99307[1], 99308[1], 99309[1], 99310[1], 99315[1], 99316[1], 99334[1], 99335[1], 99336[1], 99337[1], 99347[1], 99348[1], 99349[1], 99350[1], 99374[1], 99375[1], 99377[1], 99378[1], 99446[0], 99447[0], 99448[0], 99449[0], 99451[0], 99452[0], 99495[0], 99496[0], G0186[1], G0463[1]
67115	0213T[0], 0216T[0], 0465T[1], 0596T[1], 0597T[1], 0708T[1], 0709T[1], 12001[1], 12002[1], 12004[1], 12005[1], 12006[1], 12007[1], 12011[1], 12013[1], 12014[1], 12015[1], 12016[1], 12017[1], 12018[1], 12020[1], 12021[1], 12031[1], 12032[1], 12034[1], 12035[1], 12036[1], 12037[1], 12041[1], 12042[1], 12044[1], 12045[1], 12046[1], 12047[1], 12051[1], 12052[1], 12053[1], 12054[1], 12055[1], 12056[1], 12057[1], 13100[1], 13101[1], 13102[1], 13120[1], 13121[1], 13122[1], 13131[1], 13132[1], 13133[1], 13151[1], 13152[1], 13153[1], 36000[1], 36400[1], 36405[1], 36406[1], 36410[1], 36420[1], 36425[1], 36430[1], 36440[1], 36591[0], 36592[0], 36600[1], 36640[1], 43752[1], 51701[1], 51702[1], 51703[1], 62320[0], 62321[0], 62322[0], 62323[0], 62324[0], 62325[0], 62326[0], 62327[0], 64400[0], 64405[0], 64408[0], 64415[0], 64416[0], 64417[0], 64418[0], 64420[0], 64421[0], 64425[0], 64430[0], 64435[0], 64445[0], 64446[0], 64447[0], 64448[0], 64449[0], 64450[0], 64451[0], 64454[0], 64461[0], 64462[0], 64463[0], 64479[0], 64480[0], 64483[0], 64484[0], 64486[0], 64487[0], 64488[0], 64489[0], 64490[0], 64491[0], 64492[0], 64493[0], 64494[0], 64495[0], 64505[0], 64510[0], 64517[0], 64520[0], 64530[0], 67028[1], 67500[1], 69990[0], 92012[1], 92014[1], 92018[1], 92019[1], 92201[1], 92202[1], 93000[1], 93005[1], 93010[1], 93040[1], 93041[1], 93042[1], 93318[1], 93355[1], 94002[1], 94200[1], 94680[1], 94681[1], 94690[1], 95812[1], 95813[1], 95816[1], 95819[1], 95822[1], 95829[1], 95955[1], 96360[1], 96361[1], 96365[1], 96366[1], 96367[1], 96368[1], 96372[1], 96374[1], 96375[1], 96376[1], 96377[1], 96523[0], 99155[0], 99156[0], 99157[0], 99211[1], 99212[1], 99213[1], 99214[1], 99215[1], 99217[1], 99218[1], 99219[1], 99220[1], 99221[1], 99222[1], 99223[1], 99231[1], 99232[1], 99233[1], 99234[1], 99235[1], 99236[1], 99238[1], 99239[1], 99241[1], 99242[1], 99243[1], 99244[1], 99245[1], 99251[1], 99252[1], 99253[1], 99254[1], 99255[1], 99291[1], 99292[1], 99304[1], 99305[1], 99306[1], 99307[1], 99308[1], 99309[1], 99310[1], 99315[1], 99316[1], 99334[1], 99335[1], 99336[1], 99337[1], 99347[1], 99348[1], 99349[1], 99350[1], 99374[1], 99375[1], 99377[1], 99378[1], 99446[0], 99447[0], 99448[0], 99449[0], 99451[0], 99452[0], 99495[0], 99496[0], G0463[1], G0471[1], J2001[1]
67120	0213T[0], 0216T[0], 0465T[1], 0596T[1], 0597T[1], 0708T[1], 0709T[1], 11000[1], 11001[1], 11004[1], 11005[1], 11006[1], 11042[1], 11043[1], 11044[1], 11045[1], 11046[1], 11047[1], 12001[1], 12002[1], 12004[1], 12005[1], 12006[1], 12007[1], 12011[1], 12013[1], 12014[1], 12015[1], 12016[1], 12017[1], 12018[1], 12020[1], 12021[1], 12031[1], 12032[1], 12034[1], 12035[1], 12036[1], 12037[1], 12041[1], 12042[1], 12044[1], 12045[1], 12046[1], 12047[1], 12051[1], 12052[1], 12053[1], 12054[1], 12055[1], 12056[1], 12057[1], 13100[1], 13101[1], 13102[1], 13120[1], 13121[1], 13122[1], 13131[1], 13132[1], 13133[1], 13151[1], 13152[1], 13153[1], 36000[1], 36400[1], 36405[1], 36406[1], 36410[1], 36420[1], 36425[1], 36430[1], 36440[1], 36591[0], 36592[0], 36600[1], 36640[1], 43752[1], 51701[1], 51702[1], 51703[1], 62320[0], 62321[0], 62322[0], 62323[0], 62324[0], 62325[0], 62326[0], 62327[0], 64400[0], 64405[0], 64408[0], 64415[0], 64416[0], 64417[0], 64418[0], 64420[0], 64421[0], 64425[0], 64430[0], 64435[0], 64445[0], 64446[0], 64447[0], 64448[0], 64449[0], 64450[0], 64451[0], 64454[0], 64461[0], 64462[0], 64463[0], 64479[0], 64480[0], 64483[0], 64484[0], 64486[0], 64487[0], 64488[0], 64489[0], 64490[0], 64491[0], 64492[0], 64493[0], 64494[0], 64495[0], 64505[0], 64510[0], 64517[0], 64520[0], 64530[0], 65175[1], 65260[1], 65265[1], 67005[1], 67010[1], 67015[1], 67025[1], 67028[1], 67030[1], 67031[1], 67036[1], 67039[1], 67040[1], 67500[1], 69990[0], 92012[1], 92014[1], 92018[1], 92019[1], 92201[1], 92202[1], 93000[1], 93005[1], 93010[1], 93040[1], 93041[1], 93042[1], 93318[1], 93355[1], 94002[1], 94200[1], 94680[1], 94681[1], 94690[1], 95812[1], 95813[1], 95816[1], 95819[1], 95822[1], 95829[1], 95955[1], 96360[1], 96361[1], 96365[1], 96366[1], 96367[1], 96368[1], 96372[1], 96374[1], 96375[1], 96376[1], 96377[1], 96523[0], 97597[1], 97598[1], 97602[1], 99155[0], 99156[0], 99157[0], 99211[1], 99212[1], 99213[1], 99214[1], 99215[1], 99217[1], 99218[1], 99219[1], 99220[1], 99221[1], 99222[1], 99223[1], 99231[1], 99232[1], 99233[1], 99234[1], 99235[1], 99236[1], 99238[1], 99239[1], 99241[1], 99242[1], 99243[1], 99244[1], 99245[1], 99251[1], 99252[1], 99253[1], 99254[1], 99255[1], 99291[1], 99292[1], 99304[1], 99305[1], 99306[1], 99307[1], 99308[1], 99309[1], 99310[1], 99315[1], 99316[1], 99334[1], 99335[1], 99336[1], 99337[1], 99347[1], 99348[1], 99349[1], 99350[1], 99374[1], 99375[1], 99377[1], 99378[1], 99446[0], 99447[0], 99448[0], 99449[0], 99451[0], 99452[0], 99495[0], 99496[0], G0463[1], G0471[1], J0670[1], J2001[1]
67121	0213T[0], 0216T[0], 0465T[1], 0596T[1], 0597T[1], 0708T[1], 0709T[1], 11000[1], 11001[1], 11004[1], 11005[1], 11006[1], 11042[1], 11043[1], 11044[1], 11045[1], 11046[1], 11047[1], 12001[1], 12002[1], 12004[1], 12005[1], 12006[1], 12007[1], 12011[1], 12013[1], 12014[1], 12015[1], 12016[1], 12017[1], 12018[1], 12020[1], 12021[1], 12031[1], 12032[1], 12034[1], 12035[1], 12036[1], 12037[1], 12041[1], 12042[1], 12044[1], 12045[1], 12046[1], 12047[1], 12051[1], 12052[1], 12053[1], 12054[1], 12055[1], 12056[1], 12057[1], 13100[1], 13101[1], 13102[1], 13120[1], 13121[1], 13122[1], 13131[1], 13132[1], 13133[1], 13151[1], 13152[1], 13153[1], 36000[1], 36400[1], 36405[1], 36406[1], 36410[1], 36420[1], 36425[1], 36430[1], 36440[1], 36591[0], 36592[0], 36600[1], 36640[1], 43752[1], 51701[1], 51702[1], 51703[1], 62320[0], 62321[0], 62322[0], 62323[0], 62324[0], 62325[0], 62326[0], 62327[0], 64400[0], 64405[0], 64408[0], 64415[0], 64416[0], 64417[0], 64418[0], 64420[0], 64421[0], 64425[0], 64430[0], 64435[0], 64445[0], 64446[0], 64447[0], 64448[0], 64449[0], 64450[0], 64451[0], 64454[0], 64461[0], 64462[0], 64463[0], 64479[0], 64480[0], 64483[0], 64484[0], 64486[0], 64487[0], 64488[0], 64489[0], 64490[0], 64491[0], 64492[0], 64493[0], 64494[0], 64495[0], 64505[0], 64510[0], 64517[0], 64520[0], 64530[0], 65260[1], 65265[1], 67005[1], 67010[1], 67015[1], 67025[1], 67028[1], 67030[1], 67031[1], 67036[1], 67039[1], 67040[1], 67120[1], 67500[1], 69990[0], 92012[1], 92014[1], 92018[1], 92019[1], 92201[1], 92202[1], 93000[1], 93005[1], 93010[1], 93040[1], 93041[1], 93042[1], 93318[1], 93355[1], 94002[1], 94200[1], 94680[1], 94681[1], 94690[1], 95812[1], 95813[1], 95816[1], 95819[1], 95822[1], 95829[1], 95955[1], 96360[1], 96361[1], 96365[1], 96366[1], 96367[1], 96368[1], 96372[1], 96374[1], 96375[1], 96376[1], 96377[1], 96523[0], 97597[1], 97598[1], 97602[1], 99155[0], 99156[0], 99157[0], 99211[1], 99212[1], 99213[1], 99214[1], 99215[1], 99217[1], 99218[1], 99219[1], 99220[1], 99221[1], 99222[1], 99223[1], 99231[1], 99232[1], 99233[1], 99234[1], 99235[1], 99236[1], 99238[1], 99239[1], 99241[1], 99242[1], 99243[1], 99244[1], 99245[1], 99251[1], 99252[1], 99253[1], 99254[1], 99255[1], 99291[1], 99292[1], 99304[1], 99305[1], 99306[1], 99307[1], 99308[1], 99309[1], 99310[1], 99315[1], 99316[1], 99334[1], 99335[1], 99336[1], 99337[1], 99347[1], 99348[1], 99349[1], 99350[1], 99374[1], 99375[1], 99377[1], 99378[1], 99446[0], 99447[0], 99448[0], 99449[0], 99451[0], 99452[0], 99495[0], 99496[0], G0463[1], G0471[1], J2001[1]
67141	0213T[0], 0216T[0], 0596T[1], 0597T[1], 0708T[1], 0709T[1], 12001[1], 12002[1], 12004[1], 12005[1], 12006[1], 12007[1], 12011[1], 12013[1], 12014[1], 12015[1], 12016[1], 12017[1], 12018[1], 12020[1], 12021[1], 12031[1], 12032[1], 12034[1], 12035[1], 12036[1], 12037[1], 12041[1], 12042[1], 12044[1], 12045[1], 12046[1], 12047[1], 12051[1], 12052[1], 12053[1], 12054[1], 12055[1], 12056[1], 12057[1], 13100[1], 13101[1], 13102[1], 13120[1], 13121[1], 13122[1], 13131[1], 13132[1], 13133[1], 13151[1], 13152[1], 13153[1], 36000[1], 36400[1], 36405[1], 36406[1], 36410[1], 36420[1], 36425[1], 36430[1], 36440[1], 36591[0], 36592[0], 36600[1], 36640[1], 43752[1], 51701[1], 51702[1], 51703[1], 62320[0], 62321[0], 62322[0], 62323[0], 62324[0], 62325[0], 62326[0], 62327[0], 64400[0], 64405[0], 64408[0], 64415[0], 64416[0], 64417[0], 64418[0], 64420[0], 64421[0], 64425[0], 64430[0], 64435[0], 64445[0], 64446[0], 64447[0], 64448[0], 64449[0], 64450[0], 64451[0], 64454[0], 64461[0], 64462[0], 64463[0], 64479[0], 64480[0], 64483[0], 64484[0], 64486[0], 64487[0], 64488[0], 64489[0], 64490[0], 64491[0], 64492[0], 64493[0], 64494[0], 64495[0], 64505[0], 64510[0], 64517[0], 64520[0], 64530[0], 67145[1], 67500[1], 69990[0], 92012[1], 92014[1], 92018[1], 92019[1], 92201[1], 92202[1], 93000[1], 93005[1], 93010[1], 93040[1], 93041[1], 93042[1], 93318[1], 93355[1], 94002[1], 94200[1], 94680[1], 94681[1], 94690[1], 95812[1], 95813[1], 95816[1], 95819[1], 95822[1], 95829[1], 95955[1], 96360[1], 96361[1], 96365[1], 96366[1], 96367[1], 96368[1], 96372[1], 96374[1], 96375[1], 96376[1], 96377[1], 96523[0], 99155[0], 99156[0], 99157[0], 99211[1], 99212[1], 99213[1], 99214[1], 99215[1], 99217[1], 99218[1],

0 = Modifier usage not allowed or inappropriate 1 = Modifier usage allowed

Code 1	Code 2
	99219[1], 99220[1], 99221[1], 99222[1], 99223[1], 99231[1], 99232[1], 99233[1], 99234[1], 99235[1], 99236[1], 99238[1], 99239[1], 99241[1], 99242[1], 99243[1], 99244[1], 99245[1], 99251[1], 99252[1], 99253[1], 99254[1], 99255[1], 99291[1], 99292[1], 99304[1], 99305[1], 99306[1], 99307[1], 99308[1], 99309[1], 99310[1], 99315[1], 99316[1], 99334[1], 99335[1], 99336[1], 99337[1], 99347[1], 99348[1], 99349[1], 99350[1], 99374[1], 99375[1], 99377[1], 99378[1], 99446[0], 99447[0], 99448[0], 99449[0], 99451[0], 99452[0], 99495[0], 99496[0], G0463[1], G0471[1], J0670[1], J2001[1]
67145	0213T[0], 0216T[0], 0596T[1], 0597T[1], 0708T[1], 0709T[1], 12001[1], 12002[1], 12004[1], 12005[1], 12006[1], 12007[1], 12011[1], 12013[1], 12014[1], 12015[1], 12016[1], 12017[1], 12018[1], 12020[1], 12021[1], 12031[1], 12032[1], 12034[1], 12035[1], 12036[1], 12037[1], 12041[1], 12042[1], 12044[1], 12045[1], 12046[1], 12047[1], 12051[1], 12052[1], 12053[1], 12054[1], 12055[1], 12056[1], 12057[1], 13100[1], 13101[1], 13102[1], 13120[1], 13121[1], 13122[1], 13131[1], 13132[1], 13133[1], 13151[1], 13152[1], 13153[1], 36000[1], 36400[1], 36405[1], 36406[1], 36410[1], 36420[1], 36425[1], 36430[1], 36440[1], 36591[0], 36592[0], 36600[1], 36640[1], 43752[1], 51701[1], 51702[1], 51703[1], 62320[0], 62321[0], 62322[0], 62323[0], 62324[0], 62325[0], 62326[0], 62327[0], 64400[0], 64405[0], 64408[0], 64415[0], 64416[0], 64417[0], 64418[0], 64420[0], 64421[0], 64425[0], 64430[0], 64435[0], 64445[0], 64446[0], 64447[0], 64448[0], 64449[0], 64450[0], 64451[0], 64454[0], 64461[0], 64462[0], 64463[0], 64479[0], 64480[0], 64483[0], 64484[0], 64486[0], 64487[0], 64488[0], 64489[0], 64490[0], 64491[0], 64492[0], 64493[0], 64494[0], 64495[0], 64505[0], 64510[0], 64517[0], 64520[0], 64530[0], 67500[1], 69990[0], 92012[1], 92014[1], 92018[1], 92019[1], 92201[1], 92202[1], 93000[1], 93005[1], 93010[1], 93040[1], 93041[1], 93042[1], 93318[1], 93355[1], 94002[1], 94200[1], 94680[1], 94681[1], 94690[1], 95812[1], 95813[1], 95816[1], 95819[1], 95822[1], 95829[1], 95955[1], 96360[1], 96361[1], 96365[1], 96366[1], 96367[1], 96368[1], 96372[1], 96374[1], 96375[1], 96376[1], 96377[1], 96523[0], 99155[0], 99156[0], 99157[0], 99211[1], 99212[1], 99213[1], 99214[1], 99215[1], 99217[1], 99218[1], 99219[1], 99220[1], 99221[1], 99222[1], 99223[1], 99231[1], 99232[1], 99233[1], 99234[1], 99235[1], 99236[1], 99238[1], 99239[1], 99241[1], 99242[1], 99243[1], 99244[1], 99245[1], 99251[1], 99252[1], 99253[1], 99254[1], 99255[1], 99291[1], 99292[1], 99304[1], 99305[1], 99306[1], 99307[1], 99308[1], 99309[1], 99310[1], 99315[1], 99316[1], 99334[1], 99335[1], 99336[1], 99337[1], 99347[1], 99348[1], 99349[1], 99350[1], 99374[1], 99375[1], 99377[1], 99378[1], 99446[0], 99447[0], 99448[0], 99449[0], 99451[0], 99452[0], 99495[0], 99496[0], G0463[1], G0471[1], J0670[1], J2001[1]
67208	0213T[0], 0216T[0], 0465T[1], 0596T[1], 0597T[1], 0708T[1], 0709T[1], 12001[1], 12002[1], 12004[1], 12005[1], 12006[1], 12007[1], 12011[1], 12013[1], 12014[1], 12015[1], 12016[1], 12017[1], 12018[1], 12020[1], 12021[1], 12031[1], 12032[1], 12034[1], 12035[1], 12036[1], 12037[1], 12041[1], 12042[1], 12044[1], 12045[1], 12046[1], 12047[1], 12051[1], 12052[1], 12053[1], 12054[1], 12055[1], 12056[1], 12057[1], 13100[1], 13101[1], 13102[1], 13120[1], 13121[1], 13122[1], 13131[1], 13132[1], 13133[1], 13151[1], 13152[1], 13153[1], 36000[1], 36400[1], 36405[1], 36406[1], 36410[1], 36420[1], 36425[1], 36430[1], 36440[1], 36591[0], 36592[0], 36600[1], 36640[1], 43752[1], 51701[1], 51702[1], 51703[1], 62320[0], 62321[0], 62322[0], 62323[0], 62324[0], 62325[0], 62326[0], 62327[0], 64400[0], 64405[0], 64408[0], 64415[0], 64416[0], 64417[0], 64418[0], 64420[0], 64421[0], 64425[0], 64430[0], 64435[0], 64445[0], 64446[0], 64447[0], 64448[0], 64449[0], 64450[0], 64451[0], 64454[0], 64461[0], 64462[0], 64463[0], 64479[0], 64480[0], 64483[0], 64484[0], 64486[0], 64487[0], 64488[0], 64489[0], 64490[0], 64491[0], 64492[0], 64493[0], 64494[0], 64495[0], 64505[0], 64510[0], 64517[0], 64520[0], 64530[0], 67015[1], 67025[1], 67028[1], 67030[1], 67031[1], 67036[1], 67039[1], 67040[1], 67141[1], 67210[1], 67500[1], 69990[0], 92012[1], 92014[1], 92018[1], 92019[1], 92201[1], 92202[1], 93000[1], 93005[1], 93010[1], 93040[1], 93041[1], 93042[1], 93318[1], 93355[1], 94002[1], 94200[1], 94680[1], 94681[1], 94690[1], 95812[1], 95813[1], 95816[1], 95819[1], 95822[1], 95829[1], 95955[1], 96360[1], 96361[1], 96365[1], 96366[1], 96367[1], 96368[1], 96372[1], 96374[1], 96375[1], 96376[1], 96377[1], 96523[0], 99155[0], 99156[0], 99157[0], 99211[1], 99212[1], 99213[1], 99214[1], 99215[1], 99217[1], 99218[1], 99219[1], 99220[1], 99221[1], 99222[1], 99223[1], 99231[1], 99232[1], 99233[1], 99234[1], 99235[1], 99236[1], 99238[1], 99239[1], 99241[1], 99242[1], 99243[1], 99244[1], 99245[1], 99251[1], 99252[1], 99253[1], 99254[1], 99255[1], 99291[1], 99292[1], 99304[1], 99305[1], 99306[1], 99307[1], 99308[1], 99309[1], 99310[1], 99315[1], 99316[1], 99334[1], 99335[1], 99336[1], 99337[1], 99347[1], 99348[1], 99349[1], 99350[1], 99374[1], 99375[1], 99377[1], 99378[1], 99446[0], 99447[0], 99448[0], 99449[0], 99451[0], 99452[0], 99495[0], 99496[0], G0463[1], G0471[1], J0670[1], J2001[1]
67210	0213T[0], 0216T[0], 0596T[1], 0597T[1], 0708T[1], 0709T[1], 12001[1], 12002[1], 12004[1], 12005[1], 12006[1], 12007[1], 12011[1], 12013[1], 12014[1], 12015[1], 12016[1], 12017[1], 12018[1], 12020[1], 12021[1], 12031[1], 12032[1], 12034[1], 12035[1], 12036[1], 12037[1], 12041[1], 12042[1], 12044[1], 12045[1], 12046[1], 12047[1], 12051[1], 12052[1], 12053[1], 12054[1], 12055[1], 12056[1], 12057[1], 13100[1], 13101[1], 13102[1], 13120[1], 13121[1], 13122[1], 13131[1], 13132[1], 13133[1], 13151[1], 13152[1], 13153[1], 36000[1], 36400[1], 36405[1], 36406[1], 36410[1], 36420[1], 36425[1], 36430[1], 36440[1], 36591[0], 36592[0], 36600[1], 36640[1], 43752[1], 51701[1], 51702[1], 51703[1], 62320[0], 62321[0], 62322[0], 62323[0], 62324[0], 62325[0], 62326[0], 62327[0], 64400[0], 64405[0], 64408[0], 64415[0], 64416[0], 64417[0], 64418[0], 64420[0], 64421[0], 64425[0], 64430[0], 64435[0], 64445[0], 64446[0], 64447[0], 64448[0], 64449[0], 64450[0], 64451[0], 64454[0], 64461[0], 64462[0], 64463[0], 64479[0], 64480[0], 64483[0], 64484[0], 64486[0], 64487[0], 64488[0], 64489[0], 64490[0], 64491[0], 64492[0], 64493[0], 64494[0], 64495[0], 64505[0], 64510[0], 64517[0], 64520[0], 64530[0], 67005[1], 67010[1], 67015[1], 67145[1], 67220[1], 67221[1], 67228[1], 67500[1], 69990[0], 92012[1], 92014[1], 92018[1], 92019[1], 92201[1], 92202[1], 93000[1], 93005[1], 93010[1], 93040[1], 93041[1], 93042[1], 93318[1], 93355[1], 94002[1], 94200[1], 94680[1], 94681[1], 94690[1], 95812[1], 95813[1], 95816[1], 95819[1], 95822[1], 95829[1], 95955[1], 96360[1], 96361[1], 96365[1], 96366[1], 96367[1], 96368[1], 96372[1], 96374[1], 96375[1], 96376[1], 96377[1], 96523[0], 99155[0], 99156[0], 99157[0], 99211[1], 99212[1], 99213[1], 99214[1], 99215[1], 99217[1], 99218[1], 99219[1], 99220[1], 99221[1], 99222[1], 99223[1], 99231[1], 99232[1], 99233[1], 99234[1], 99235[1], 99236[1], 99238[1], 99239[1], 99241[1], 99242[1], 99243[1], 99244[1], 99245[1], 99251[1], 99252[1], 99253[1], 99254[1], 99255[1], 99291[1], 99292[1], 99304[1], 99305[1], 99306[1], 99307[1], 99308[1], 99309[1], 99310[1], 99315[1], 99316[1], 99334[1], 99335[1], 99336[1], 99337[1], 99347[1], 99348[1], 99349[1], 99350[1], 99374[1], 99375[1], 99377[1], 99378[1], 99446[0], 99447[0], 99448[0], 99449[0], 99451[0], 99452[0], 99495[0], 99496[0], G0463[1], G0471[1], J0670[1], J2001[1]
67218	0213T[0], 0216T[0], 0465T[1], 0596T[1], 0597T[1], 0708T[1], 0709T[1], 11000[1], 11001[1], 11004[1], 11005[1], 11006[1], 11042[1], 11043[1], 11044[1], 11045[1], 11046[1], 11047[1], 12001[1], 12002[1], 12004[1], 12005[1], 12006[1], 12007[1], 12011[1], 12013[1], 12014[1], 12015[1], 12016[1], 12017[1], 12018[1], 12020[1], 12021[1], 12031[1], 12032[1], 12034[1], 12035[1], 12036[1], 12037[1], 12041[1], 12042[1], 12044[1], 12045[1], 12046[1], 12047[1], 12051[1], 12052[1], 12053[1], 12054[1], 12055[1], 12056[1], 12057[1], 13100[1], 13101[1], 13102[1], 13120[1], 13121[1], 13122[1], 13131[1], 13132[1], 13133[1], 13151[1], 13152[1], 13153[1], 36000[1], 36400[1], 36405[1], 36406[1], 36410[1], 36420[1], 36425[1], 36430[1], 36440[1], 36591[0], 36592[0], 36600[1], 36640[1], 43752[1], 51701[1], 51702[1], 51703[1], 62320[0], 62321[0], 62322[0], 62323[0], 62324[0], 62325[0], 62326[0], 62327[0], 64400[0], 64405[0], 64408[0], 64415[0], 64416[0], 64417[0], 64418[0], 64420[0], 64421[0], 64425[0], 64430[0], 64435[0], 64445[0], 64446[0], 64447[0], 64448[0], 64449[0], 64450[0], 64451[0], 64454[0], 64461[0], 64462[0], 64463[0], 64479[0], 64480[0], 64483[0], 64484[0], 64486[0], 64487[0], 64488[0], 64489[0], 64490[0], 64491[0], 64492[0], 64493[0], 64494[0], 64495[0], 64505[0], 64510[0], 64517[0], 64520[0], 64530[0], 67005[1], 67010[1], 67015[1], 67025[1], 67028[1], 67030[1], 67031[1], 67036[1], 67039[1], 67040[1], 67041[1], 67500[1], 69990[0], 92012[1], 92014[1], 92018[1], 92019[1], 92201[1], 92202[1], 93000[1], 93005[1], 93010[1], 93040[1], 93041[1], 93042[1], 93318[1], 93355[1], 94002[1], 94200[1], 94680[1], 94681[1], 94690[1], 95812[1], 95813[1], 95816[1], 95819[1], 95822[1], 95829[1], 95955[1], 96360[1], 96361[1], 96365[1], 96366[1], 96367[1], 96368[1], 96372[1], 96374[1], 96375[1], 96376[1], 96377[1], 96523[0], 97597[1], 97598[1], 97602[1], 99155[0], 99156[0], 99157[0], 99211[1], 99212[1], 99213[1], 99214[1], 99215[1], 99217[1], 99218[1], 99219[1], 99220[1], 99221[1], 99222[1], 99223[1], 99231[1], 99232[1], 99233[1], 99234[1], 99235[1], 99236[1], 99238[1], 99239[1], 99241[1], 99242[1], 99243[1], 99244[1], 99245[1], 99251[1], 99252[1], 99253[1], 99254[1], 99255[1], 99291[1], 99292[1], 99304[1], 99305[1], 99306[1], 99307[1], 99308[1], 99309[1], 99310[1], 99315[1], 99316[1], 99334[1], 99335[1], 99336[1], 99337[1], 99347[1], 99348[1], 99349[1], 99350[1], 99374[1], 99375[1], 99377[1], 99378[1], 99446[0], 99447[0], 99448[0], 99449[0], 99451[0], 99452[0], 99495[0], 99496[0], G0463[1], G0471[1], J0670[1], J2001[1]
67220	0213T[0], 0216T[0], 0596T[1], 0597T[1], 0708T[1], 0709T[1], 12001[1], 12002[1], 12004[1], 12005[1], 12006[1], 12007[1], 12011[1], 12013[1], 12014[1], 12015[1], 12016[1], 12017[1], 12018[1], 12020[1], 12021[1], 12031[1], 12032[1], 12034[1], 12035[1], 12036[1], 12037[1], 12041[1], 12042[1], 12044[1], 12045[1], 12046[1], 12047[1], 12051[1], 12052[1], 12053[1], 12054[1], 12055[1], 12056[1], 12057[1], 13100[1], 13101[1], 13102[1], 13120[1], 13121[1], 13122[1], 13131[1], 13132[1], 13133[1], 13151[1], 13152[1], 13153[1], 36000[1], 36400[1], 36405[1], 36406[1], 36410[1], 36420[1], 36425[1], 36430[1], 36440[1], 36591[0], 36592[0], 36600[1], 36640[1], 43752[1], 51701[1], 51702[1], 51703[1], 62320[0], 62321[0], 62322[0], 62323[0], 62324[0], 62325[0], 62326[0], 62327[0], 64400[0], 64405[0], 64408[0], 64415[0], 64416[0], 64417[0], 64418[0], 64420[0], 64421[0], 64425[0], 64430[0], 64435[0], 64445[0], 64446[0], 64447[0], 64448[0], 64449[0], 64450[0], 64451[0], 64454[0], 64461[0], 64462[0], 64463[0], 64479[0], 64480[0], 64483[0], 64484[0], 64486[0], 64487[0], 64488[0], 64489[0], 64490[0], 64491[0], 64492[0], 64493[0], 64494[0], 64495[0], 64505[0], 64510[0], 64517[0], 64520[0], 64530[0], 67005[1], 67010[1], 67015[1], 67145[1], 67221[1], 67500[1], 69990[0], 92012[1], 92014[1], 92018[1], 92019[1], 92201[1], 92202[1], 93000[1], 93005[1], 93010[1], 93040[1], 93041[1], 93042[1], 93318[1], 93355[1], 94002[1], 94200[1], 94680[1], 94681[1], 94690[1], 95812[1], 95813[1], 95816[1], 95819[1], 95822[1], 95829[1], 95955[1], 96360[1], 96361[1], 96365[1], 96366[1], 96367[1], 96368[1], 96372[1], 96374[1], 96375[1], 96376[1], 96377[1], 96523[0], 99155[0], 99156[0], 99157[0], 99211[1], 99212[1], 99213[1], 99214[1], 99215[1], 99217[1], 99218[1], 99219[1], 99220[1], 99221[1], 99222[1], 99223[1], 99231[1], 99232[1], 99233[1], 99234[1], 99235[1], 99236[1], 99238[1], 99239[1], 99241[1], 99242[1], 99243[1], 99244[1], 99245[1], 99251[1], 99252[1], 99253[1], 99254[1], 99255[1], 99291[1], 99292[1], 99304[1], 99305[1], 99306[1], 99307[1], 99308[1], 99309[1], 99310[1], 99315[1], 99316[1], 99334[1], 99335[1], 99336[1], 99337[1], 99347[1], 99348[1], 99349[1], 99350[1], 99374[1], 99375[1], 99377[1], 99378[1], 99446[0], 99447[0], 99448[0], 99449[0], 99451[0], 99452[0], 99495[0], 99496[0], G0463[1], G0471[1], J0670[1], J2001[1]
67221	0213T[0], 0216T[0], 0596T[1], 0597T[1], 0708T[1], 0709T[1], 12001[1], 12002[1], 12004[1], 12005[1], 12006[1], 12007[1], 12011[1], 12013[1], 12014[1], 12015[1], 12016[1], 12017[1], 12018[1], 12020[1], 12021[1], 12031[1], 12032[1], 12034[1], 12035[1], 12036[1], 12037[1], 12041[1], 12042[1], 12044[1],

Appendix A: NCCI - CPT Codes

Code 1	Code 2
	12045[1], 12046[1], 12047[1], 12051[1], 12052[1], 12053[1], 12054[1], 12055[1], 12056[1], 12057[1], 13100[1], 13101[1], 13102[1], 13120[1], 13121[1], 13122[1], 13131[1], 13132[1], 13133[1], 13151[1], 13152[1], 13153[1], 36000[1], 36400[1], 36405[1], 36406[1], 36410[1], 36420[1], 36425[1], 36430[1], 36440[1], 36591[0], 36592[0], 36600[1], 36640[1], 43752[1], 51701[1], 51702[1], 51703[1], 62320[0], 62321[0], 62322[0], 62323[0], 62324[0], 62325[0], 62326[0], 62327[0], 64400[0], 64405[0], 64408[0], 64415[0], 64416[0], 64417[0], 64418[0], 64420[0], 64421[0], 64425[0], 64430[0], 64435[0], 64445[0], 64446[0], 64447[0], 64448[0], 64449[0], 64450[0], 64451[0], 64454[0], 64461[0], 64462[0], 64463[0], 64479[0], 64480[0], 64483[0], 64484[0], 64486[0], 64487[0], 64488[0], 64489[0], 64490[0], 64491[0], 64492[0], 64493[0], 64494[0], 64495[0], 64505[0], 64510[0], 64517[0], 64520[0], 64530[0], 67005[1], 67010[1], 67015[1], 67145[1], 67500[1], 69990[0], 92012[1], 92014[1], 92018[1], 92019[1], 92201[1], 92202[1], 93000[1], 93005[1], 93010[1], 93040[1], 93041[1], 93042[1], 93318[1], 93355[1], 94002[1], 94200[1], 94680[1], 94681[1], 94690[1], 95812[1], 95813[1], 95816[1], 95819[1], 95822[1], 95829[1], 95955[1], 96360[0], 96361[1], 96365[0], 96366[1], 96367[1], 96368[1], 96372[1], 96374[1], 96375[1], 96376[1], 96377[1], 96523[0], 96570[1], 96571[1], 99155[0], 99156[0], 99157[0], 99211[1], 99212[1], 99213[1], 99214[1], 99215[1], 99217[1], 99218[1], 99219[1], 99220[1], 99221[1], 99222[1], 99223[1], 99231[1], 99232[1], 99233[1], 99234[1], 99235[1], 99236[1], 99238[1], 99239[1], 99241[1], 99242[1], 99243[1], 99244[1], 99245[1], 99251[1], 99252[1], 99253[1], 99254[1], 99255[1], 99291[1], 99292[1], 99304[1], 99305[1], 99306[1], 99307[1], 99308[1], 99309[1], 99310[1], 99315[1], 99316[1], 99334[1], 99335[1], 99336[1], 99337[1], 99347[1], 99348[1], 99349[1], 99350[1], 99374[1], 99375[1], 99377[1], 99378[1], 99446[0], 99447[0], 99448[0], 99449[0], 99451[0], 99452[0], 99495[1], 99496[1], G0463[1], G0471[1]
67225	0213T[1], 0216T[1], 36000[1], 36400[1], 36410[1], 36425[1], 36591[0], 36592[0], 61650[1], 62324[1], 62325[1], 62326[1], 62327[1], 64415[1], 64416[1], 64417[1], 64450[1], 64454[1], 64486[1], 64487[1], 64488[1], 64489[1], 64490[1], 64493[1], 67005[1], 67010[1], 67015[1], 67145[1], 67210[1], 67500[1], 69990[0], 92201[1], 92202[1], 96523[0]
67227	0213T[0], 0216T[0], 0596T[1], 0597T[1], 0708T[1], 0709T[1], 12001[1], 12002[1], 12004[1], 12005[1], 12006[1], 12007[1], 12011[1], 12013[1], 12014[1], 12015[1], 12016[1], 12017[1], 12018[1], 12020[1], 12021[1], 12031[1], 12032[1], 12034[1], 12035[1], 12036[1], 12037[1], 12041[1], 12042[1], 12044[1], 12045[1], 12046[1], 12047[1], 12051[1], 12052[1], 12053[1], 12054[1], 12055[1], 12056[1], 12057[1], 13100[1], 13101[1], 13102[1], 13120[1], 13121[1], 13122[1], 13131[1], 13132[1], 13133[1], 13151[1], 13152[1], 13153[1], 36000[1], 36400[1], 36405[1], 36406[1], 36410[1], 36420[1], 36425[1], 36430[1], 36440[1], 36591[0], 36592[0], 36600[1], 36640[1], 43752[1], 51701[1], 51702[1], 51703[1], 62320[0], 62321[0], 62322[0], 62323[0], 62324[0], 62325[0], 62326[0], 62327[0], 64400[0], 64405[0], 64408[0], 64415[0], 64416[0], 64417[0], 64418[0], 64420[0], 64421[0], 64425[0], 64430[0], 64435[0], 64445[0], 64446[0], 64447[0], 64448[0], 64449[0], 64450[0], 64451[0], 64454[0], 64461[0], 64462[0], 64463[0], 64479[0], 64480[0], 64483[0], 64484[0], 64486[0], 64487[0], 64488[0], 64489[0], 64490[0], 64491[0], 64492[0], 64493[0], 64494[0], 64495[0], 64505[0], 64510[0], 64517[0], 64520[0], 64530[0], 66700[1], 66720[1], 67005[1], 67010[1], 67015[1], 67031[1], 67036[1], 67039[1], 67040[1], 67141[1], 67145[1], 67208[1], 67210[1], 67228[1], 67500[1], 69990[0], 92012[1], 92014[1], 92018[1], 92019[1], 92201[1], 92202[1], 93000[1], 93005[1], 93010[1], 93040[1], 93041[1], 93042[1], 93318[1], 93355[1], 94002[1], 94200[1], 94680[1], 94681[1], 94690[1], 95812[1], 95813[1], 95816[1], 95819[1], 95822[1], 95829[1], 95955[1], 96360[1], 96361[1], 96365[1], 96366[1], 96367[1], 96368[1], 96372[1], 96374[1], 96375[1], 96376[1], 96377[1], 96523[0], 99155[0], 99156[0], 99157[0], 99211[1], 99212[1], 99213[1], 99214[1], 99215[1], 99217[1], 99218[1], 99219[1], 99220[1], 99221[1], 99222[1], 99223[1], 99231[1], 99232[1], 99233[1], 99234[1], 99235[1], 99236[1], 99238[1], 99239[1], 99241[1], 99242[1], 99243[1], 99244[1], 99245[1], 99251[1], 99252[1], 99253[1], 99254[1], 99255[1], 99291[1], 99292[1], 99304[1], 99305[1], 99306[1], 99307[1], 99308[1], 99309[1], 99310[1], 99315[1], 99316[1], 99334[1], 99335[1], 99336[1], 99337[1], 99347[1], 99348[1], 99349[1], 99350[1], 99374[1], 99375[1], 99377[1], 99378[1], 99446[0], 99447[0], 99448[0], 99449[0], 99451[0], 99452[0], 99495[0], 99496[0], G0463[1], G0471[1], J0670[1], J2001[1]
67228	0213T[0], 0216T[0], 0596T[1], 0597T[1], 0708T[1], 0709T[1], 12001[1], 12002[1], 12004[1], 12005[1], 12006[1], 12007[1], 12011[1], 12013[1], 12014[1], 12015[1], 12016[1], 12017[1], 12018[1], 12020[1], 12021[1], 12031[1], 12032[1], 12034[1], 12035[1], 12036[1], 12037[1], 12041[1], 12042[1], 12044[1], 12045[1], 12046[1], 12047[1], 12051[1], 12052[1], 12053[1], 12054[1], 12055[1], 12056[1], 12057[1], 13100[1], 13101[1], 13102[1], 13120[1], 13121[1], 13122[1], 13131[1], 13132[1], 13133[1], 13151[1], 13152[1], 13153[1], 36000[1], 36400[1], 36405[1], 36406[1], 36410[1], 36420[1], 36425[1], 36430[1], 36440[1], 36591[0], 36592[0], 36600[1], 36640[1], 43752[1], 51701[1], 51702[1], 51703[1], 62320[0], 62321[0], 62322[0], 62323[0], 62324[0], 62325[0], 62326[0], 62327[0], 64400[0], 64405[0], 64408[0], 64415[0], 64416[0], 64417[0], 64418[0], 64420[0], 64421[0], 64425[0], 64430[0], 64435[0], 64445[0], 64446[0], 64447[0], 64448[0], 64449[0], 64450[0], 64451[0], 64454[0], 64461[0], 64462[0], 64463[0], 64479[0], 64480[0], 64483[0], 64484[0], 64486[0], 64487[0], 64488[0], 64489[0], 64490[0], 64491[0], 64492[0], 64493[0], 64494[0], 64495[0], 64505[0], 64510[0], 64517[0], 64520[0], 64530[0], 66821[1], 67005[1], 67010[1], 67015[1], 67030[1], 67031[1], 67036[1], 67039[1], 67040[1], 67141[1], 67145[1], 67208[1], 67220[1], 67221[1], 67225[1], 67500[1], 67515[1], 69990[0], 92012[1], 92014[1], 92018[1], 92019[1], 92201[1], 92202[1], 93000[1], 93005[1], 93010[1], 93040[1], 93041[1], 93042[1], 93318[1], 93355[1], 94002[1], 94200[1], 94680[1], 94681[1], 94690[1], 95812[1], 95813[1], 95816[1], 95819[1], 95822[1], 95829[1], 95955[1], 96360[1], 96361[1], 96365[1], 96366[1], 96367[1], 96368[1], 96372[1], 96374[1], 96375[1], 96376[1], 96377[1], 96523[0], 99155[0], 99156[0], 99157[0], 99211[1], 99212[1], 99213[1], 99214[1], 99215[1], 99217[1], 99218[1], 99219[1], 99220[1], 99221[1], 99222[1], 99223[1], 99231[1], 99232[1], 99233[1], 99234[1], 99235[1], 99236[1], 99238[1], 99239[1], 99241[1], 99242[1], 99243[1], 99244[1], 99245[1], 99251[1], 99252[1], 99253[1], 99254[1], 99255[1], 99291[1], 99292[1], 99304[1], 99305[1], 99306[1], 99307[1], 99308[1], 99309[1], 99310[1], 99315[1], 99316[1], 99334[1], 99335[1], 99336[1], 99337[1], 99347[1], 99348[1], 99349[1], 99350[1], 99374[1], 99375[1], 99377[1], 99378[1], 99446[0], 99447[0], 99448[0], 99449[0], 99451[0], 99452[0], 99495[0], 99496[0], G0463[1], G0471[1], J0670[1], J2001[1]
67229	0213T[0], 0216T[0], 0708T[1], 0709T[1], 12001[1], 12002[1], 12004[1], 12005[1], 12006[1], 12007[1], 12011[1], 12013[1], 12014[1], 12015[1], 12016[1], 12017[1], 12018[1], 12020[1], 12021[1], 12031[1], 12032[1], 12034[1], 12035[1], 12036[1], 12037[1], 12041[1], 12042[1], 12044[1], 12045[1], 12046[1], 12047[1], 12051[1], 12052[1], 12053[1], 12054[1], 12055[1], 12056[1], 12057[1], 13100[1], 13101[1], 13102[1], 13120[1], 13121[1], 13122[1], 13131[1], 13132[1], 13133[1], 13151[1], 13152[1], 13153[1], 36000[1], 36400[1], 36405[1], 36406[1], 36410[1], 36420[1], 36425[1], 36430[1], 36440[1], 36591[0], 36592[0], 36600[1], 36640[1], 43752[1], 62320[0], 62321[0], 62322[0], 62323[0], 62324[0], 62325[0], 62326[0], 62327[0], 64400[0], 64405[0], 64408[0], 64415[0], 64416[0], 64417[0], 64418[0], 64420[0], 64421[0], 64425[0], 64430[0], 64435[0], 64445[0], 64446[0], 64447[0], 64448[0], 64449[0], 64450[0], 64451[0], 64454[0], 64461[0], 64462[0], 64463[0], 64479[0], 64480[0], 64483[0], 64484[0], 64486[0], 64487[0], 64488[0], 64489[0], 64490[0], 64491[0], 64492[0], 64493[0], 64494[0], 64495[0], 64505[0], 64510[0], 64517[0], 64520[0], 64530[0], 66720[1], 66821[1], 67101[1], 67105[1], 67141[1], 67145[1], 67208[1], 67210[1], 67220[1], 67227[1], 67228[1], 67500[1], 67515[1], 69990[0], 92012[1], 92014[1], 92018[1], 92019[1], 92201[1], 92202[1], 93000[1], 93005[1], 93010[1], 93040[1], 93041[1], 93042[1], 93318[1], 93355[1], 94002[1], 94200[1], 94680[1], 94681[1], 94690[1], 95812[1], 95813[1], 95816[1], 95819[1], 95822[1], 95829[1], 95955[1], 96360[1], 96361[1], 96365[1], 96366[1], 96367[1], 96368[1], 96372[1], 96374[1], 96375[1], 96376[1], 96377[1], 96523[0], 99155[0], 99156[0], 99157[0], 99211[1], 99212[1], 99213[1], 99214[1], 99215[1], 99217[1], 99218[1], 99219[1], 99220[1], 99221[1], 99222[1], 99223[1], 99231[1], 99232[1], 99233[1], 99234[1], 99235[1], 99236[1], 99238[1], 99239[1], 99241[1], 99242[1], 99243[1], 99244[1], 99245[1], 99251[1], 99252[1], 99253[1], 99254[1], 99255[1], 99291[1], 99292[1], 99304[1], 99305[1], 99306[1], 99307[1], 99308[1], 99309[1], 99310[1], 99315[1], 99316[1], 99334[1], 99335[1], 99336[1], 99337[1], 99347[1], 99348[1], 99349[1], 99350[1], 99374[1], 99375[1], 99377[1], 99378[1], 99446[0], 99447[0], 99448[0], 99449[0], 99451[0], 99452[0], 99495[0], 99496[0], G0186[1], G0463[1]
67250	0213T[0], 0216T[0], 0596T[1], 0597T[1], 0708T[1], 0709T[1], 12001[1], 12002[1], 12004[1], 12005[1], 12006[1], 12007[1], 12011[1], 12013[1], 12014[1], 12015[1], 12016[1], 12017[1], 12018[1], 12020[1], 12021[1], 12031[1], 12032[1], 12034[1], 12035[1], 12036[1], 12037[1], 12041[1], 12042[1], 12044[1], 12045[1], 12046[1], 12047[1], 12051[1], 12052[1], 12053[1], 12054[1], 12055[1], 12056[1], 12057[1], 13100[1], 13101[1], 13102[1], 13120[1], 13121[1], 13122[1], 13131[1], 13132[1], 13133[1], 13151[1], 13152[1], 13153[1], 36000[1], 36400[1], 36405[1], 36406[1], 36410[1], 36420[1], 36425[1], 36430[1], 36440[1], 36591[0], 36592[0], 36600[1], 36640[1], 43752[1], 51701[1], 51702[1], 51703[1], 62320[0], 62321[0], 62322[0], 62323[0], 62324[0], 62325[0], 62326[0], 62327[0], 64400[0], 64405[0], 64408[0], 64415[0], 64416[0], 64417[0], 64418[0], 64420[0], 64421[0], 64425[0], 64430[0], 64435[0], 64445[0], 64446[0], 64447[0], 64448[0], 64449[0], 64450[0], 64451[0], 64454[0], 64461[0], 64462[0], 64463[0], 64479[0], 64480[0], 64483[0], 64484[0], 64486[0], 64487[0], 64488[0], 64489[0], 64490[0], 64491[0], 64492[0], 64493[0], 64494[0], 64495[0], 64505[0], 64510[0], 64517[0], 64520[0], 64530[0], 67500[1], 69990[0], 92012[1], 92014[1], 92018[1], 92019[1], 93000[1], 93005[1], 93010[1], 93040[1], 93041[1], 93042[1], 93318[1], 93355[1], 94002[1], 94200[1], 94680[1], 94681[1], 94690[1], 95812[1], 95813[1], 95816[1], 95819[1], 95822[1], 95829[1], 95955[1], 96360[1], 96361[1], 96365[1], 96366[1], 96367[1], 96368[1], 96372[1], 96374[1], 96375[1], 96376[1], 96377[1], 96523[0], 99155[0], 99156[0], 99157[0], 99211[1], 99212[1], 99213[1], 99214[1], 99215[1], 99217[1], 99218[1], 99219[1], 99220[1], 99221[1], 99222[1], 99223[1], 99231[1], 99232[1], 99233[1], 99234[1], 99235[1], 99236[1], 99238[1], 99239[1], 99241[1], 99242[1], 99243[1], 99244[1], 99245[1], 99251[1], 99252[1], 99253[1], 99254[1], 99255[1], 99291[1], 99292[1], 99304[1], 99305[1], 99306[1], 99307[1], 99308[1], 99309[1], 99310[1], 99315[1], 99316[1], 99334[1], 99335[1], 99336[1], 99337[1], 99347[1], 99348[1], 99349[1], 99350[1], 99374[1], 99375[1], 99377[1], 99378[1], 99446[0], 99447[0], 99448[0], 99449[0], 99451[0], 99452[0], 99495[0], 99496[0], G0463[1], G0471[1], J0670[1], J2001[1]
67255	0213T[0], 0216T[0], 0596T[1], 0597T[1], 0708T[1], 0709T[1], 12001[1], 12002[1], 12004[1], 12005[1], 12006[1], 12007[1], 12011[1], 12013[1], 12014[1], 12015[1], 12016[1], 12017[1], 12018[1], 12020[1], 12021[1], 12031[1], 12032[1], 12034[1], 12035[1], 12036[1], 12037[1], 12041[1], 12042[1], 12044[1], 12045[1], 12046[1], 12047[1], 12051[1], 12052[1], 12053[1], 12054[1], 12055[1], 12056[1], 12057[1], 13100[1], 13101[1], 13102[1], 13120[1], 13121[1], 13122[1], 13131[1], 13132[1], 13133[1], 13151[1], 13152[1], 13153[1], 36000[1], 36400[1], 36405[1], 36406[1], 36410[1], 36420[1], 36425[1], 36430[1], 36440[1], 36591[0], 36592[0], 36600[1], 36640[1], 43752[1], 51701[1], 51702[1], 51703[1], 62320[0], 62321[0], 62322[0], 62323[0], 62324[0], 62325[0], 62326[0], 62327[0], 64400[0], 64405[0], 64408[0],

0 = Modifier usage not allowed or inappropriate 1 = Modifier usage allowed

Code 1	Code 2
	64415[0], 64416[0], 64417[0], 64418[0], 64420[0], 64421[0], 64425[0], 64430[0], 64435[0], 64445[0], 64446[0], 64447[0], 64448[0], 64449[0], 64450[0], 64451[0], 64454[0], 64461[0], 64462[0], 64463[0], 64479[0], 64480[0], 64483[0], 64484[0], 64486[0], 64487[0], 64488[0], 64489[0], 64490[0], 64491[0], 64492[0], 64493[0], 64494[0], 64495[0], 64505[0], 64510[0], 64517[0], 64520[0], 64530[0], 67250[1], 67500[1], 69990[0], 92012[1], 92014[1], 92018[1], 92019[1], 93000[1], 93005[1], 93010[1], 93040[1], 93041[1], 93042[1], 93318[1], 93355[1], 94002[1], 94200[1], 94680[1], 94681[1], 94690[1], 95812[1], 95813[1], 95816[1], 95819[1], 95822[1], 95829[1], 95955[1], 96360[1], 96361[1], 96365[1], 96366[1], 96367[1], 96368[1], 96372[1], 96374[1], 96375[1], 96376[1], 96377[1], 96523[0], 99155[0], 99156[0], 99157[0], 99211[1], 99212[1], 99213[1], 99214[1], 99215[1], 99217[1], 99218[1], 99219[1], 99220[1], 99221[1], 99222[1], 99223[1], 99231[1], 99232[1], 99233[1], 99234[1], 99235[1], 99236[1], 99238[1], 99239[1], 99241[1], 99242[1], 99243[1], 99244[1], 99245[1], 99251[1], 99252[1], 99253[1], 99254[1], 99255[1], 99291[1], 99292[1], 99304[1], 99305[1], 99306[1], 99307[1], 99308[1], 99309[1], 99310[1], 99315[1], 99316[1], 99334[1], 99335[1], 99336[1], 99337[1], 99347[1], 99348[1], 99349[1], 99350[1], 99374[1], 99375[1], 99377[1], 99378[1], 99446[0], 99447[0], 99448[0], 99449[0], 99451[0], 99452[0], 99495[0], 99496[0], G0463[1], G0471[1], J0670[1], J2001[1]
67311	0213T[0], 0216T[0], 0596T[1], 0597T[1], 0708T[1], 0709T[1], 11000[1], 11001[1], 11004[1], 11005[1], 11006[1], 11042[1], 11043[1], 11044[1], 11045[1], 11046[1], 11047[1], 12001[1], 12002[1], 12004[1], 12005[1], 12006[1], 12007[1], 12011[1], 12013[1], 12014[1], 12015[1], 12016[1], 12017[1], 12018[1], 12020[1], 12021[1], 12031[1], 12032[1], 12034[1], 12035[1], 12036[1], 12037[1], 12041[1], 12042[1], 12044[1], 12045[1], 12046[1], 12047[1], 12051[1], 12052[1], 12053[1], 12054[1], 12055[1], 12056[1], 12057[1], 13100[1], 13101[1], 13102[1], 13120[1], 13121[1], 13122[1], 13131[1], 13132[1], 13133[1], 13151[1], 13152[1], 13153[1], 36000[1], 36400[1], 36405[1], 36406[1], 36410[1], 36420[1], 36425[1], 36430[1], 36440[1], 36591[0], 36592[0], 36600[1], 36640[1], 43752[1], 51701[1], 51702[1], 51703[1], 62320[0], 62321[0], 62322[0], 62323[0], 62324[0], 62325[0], 62326[0], 62327[0], 64400[0], 64405[0], 64408[0], 64415[0], 64416[0], 64417[0], 64418[0], 64420[0], 64421[0], 64425[0], 64430[0], 64435[0], 64445[0], 64446[0], 64447[0], 64448[0], 64449[0], 64450[0], 64451[0], 64454[0], 64461[0], 64462[0], 64463[0], 64479[0], 64480[0], 64483[0], 64484[0], 64486[0], 64487[0], 64488[0], 64489[0], 64490[0], 64491[0], 64492[0], 64493[0], 64494[0], 64495[0], 64505[0], 64510[0], 64517[0], 64520[0], 64530[0], 67343[1], 67500[1], 69990[0], 92012[1], 92014[1], 92018[1], 92019[1], 93000[1], 93005[1], 93010[1], 93040[1], 93041[1], 93042[1], 93318[1], 93355[1], 94002[1], 94200[1], 94680[1], 94681[1], 94690[1], 95812[1], 95813[1], 95816[1], 95819[1], 95822[1], 95829[1], 95955[1], 96360[1], 96361[1], 96365[1], 96366[1], 96367[1], 96368[1], 96372[1], 96374[1], 96375[1], 96376[1], 96377[1], 96523[0], 97597[1], 97598[1], 97602[1], 99155[0], 99156[0], 99157[0], 99211[1], 99212[1], 99213[1], 99214[1], 99215[1], 99217[1], 99218[1], 99219[1], 99220[1], 99221[1], 99222[1], 99223[1], 99231[1], 99232[1], 99233[1], 99234[1], 99235[1], 99236[1], 99238[1], 99239[1], 99241[1], 99242[1], 99243[1], 99244[1], 99245[1], 99251[1], 99252[1], 99253[1], 99254[1], 99255[1], 99291[1], 99292[1], 99304[1], 99305[1], 99306[1], 99307[1], 99308[1], 99309[1], 99310[1], 99315[1], 99316[1], 99334[1], 99335[1], 99336[1], 99337[1], 99347[1], 99348[1], 99349[1], 99350[1], 99374[1], 99375[1], 99377[1], 99378[1], 99446[0], 99447[0], 99448[0], 99449[0], 99451[0], 99452[0], 99495[0], 99496[0], G0463[1], G0471[1]
67312	0213T[0], 0216T[0], 0596T[1], 0597T[1], 0708T[1], 0709T[1], 11000[1], 11001[1], 11004[1], 11005[1], 11006[1], 11042[1], 11043[1], 11044[1], 11045[1], 11046[1], 11047[1], 12001[1], 12002[1], 12004[1], 12005[1], 12006[1], 12007[1], 12011[1], 12013[1], 12014[1], 12015[1], 12016[1], 12017[1], 12018[1], 12020[1], 12021[1], 12031[1], 12032[1], 12034[1], 12035[1], 12036[1], 12037[1], 12041[1], 12042[1], 12044[1], 12045[1], 12046[1], 12047[1], 12051[1], 12052[1], 12053[1], 12054[1], 12055[1], 12056[1], 12057[1], 13100[1], 13101[1], 13102[1], 13120[1], 13121[1], 13122[1], 13131[1], 13132[1], 13133[1], 13151[1], 13152[1], 13153[1], 36000[1], 36400[1], 36405[1], 36406[1], 36410[1], 36420[1], 36425[1], 36430[1], 36440[1], 36591[0], 36592[0], 36600[1], 36640[1], 43752[1], 51701[1], 51702[1], 51703[1], 62320[0], 62321[0], 62322[0], 62323[0], 62324[0], 62325[0], 62326[0], 62327[0], 64400[0], 64405[0], 64408[0], 64415[0], 64416[0], 64417[0], 64418[0], 64420[0], 64421[0], 64425[0], 64430[0], 64435[0], 64445[0], 64446[0], 64447[0], 64448[0], 64449[0], 64450[0], 64451[0], 64454[0], 64461[0], 64462[0], 64463[0], 64479[0], 64480[0], 64483[0], 64484[0], 64486[0], 64487[0], 64488[0], 64489[0], 64490[0], 64491[0], 64492[0], 64493[0], 64494[0], 64495[0], 64505[0], 64510[0], 64517[0], 64520[0], 64530[0], 67311[1], 67343[1], 67500[1], 69990[0], 92012[1], 92014[1], 92018[1], 92019[1], 93000[1], 93005[1], 93010[1], 93040[1], 93041[1], 93042[1], 93318[1], 93355[1], 94002[1], 94200[1], 94680[1], 94681[1], 94690[1], 95812[1], 95813[1], 95816[1], 95819[1], 95822[1], 95829[1], 95955[1], 96360[1], 96361[1], 96365[1], 96366[1], 96367[1], 96368[1], 96372[1], 96374[1], 96375[1], 96376[1], 96377[1], 96523[0], 97597[1], 97598[1], 97602[1], 99155[0], 99156[0], 99157[0], 99211[1], 99212[1], 99213[1], 99214[1], 99215[1], 99217[1], 99218[1], 99219[1], 99220[1], 99221[1], 99222[1], 99223[1], 99231[1], 99232[1], 99233[1], 99234[1], 99235[1], 99236[1], 99238[1], 99239[1], 99241[1], 99242[1], 99243[1], 99244[1], 99245[1], 99251[1], 99252[1], 99253[1], 99254[1], 99255[1], 99291[1], 99292[1], 99304[1], 99305[1], 99306[1], 99307[1], 99308[1], 99309[1], 99310[1], 99315[1], 99316[1], 99334[1], 99335[1], 99336[1], 99337[1], 99347[1], 99348[1], 99349[1], 99350[1], 99374[1], 99375[1], 99377[1], 99378[1], 99446[0], 99447[0], 99448[0], 99449[0], 99451[0], 99452[0], 99495[0], 99496[0], G0463[1], G0471[1]
67314	0213T[0], 0216T[0], 0596T[1], 0597T[1], 0708T[1], 0709T[1], 11000[1], 11001[1], 11004[1], 11005[1], 11006[1], 11042[1], 11043[1], 11044[1], 11045[1], 11046[1], 11047[1], 12001[1], 12002[1], 12004[1], 12005[1], 12006[1], 12007[1], 12011[1], 12013[1], 12014[1], 12015[1], 12016[1], 12017[1], 12018[1], 12020[1], 12021[1], 12031[1], 12032[1], 12034[1], 12035[1], 12036[1], 12037[1], 12041[1], 12042[1], 12044[1], 12045[1], 12046[1], 12047[1], 12051[1], 12052[1], 12053[1], 12054[1], 12055[1], 12056[1], 12057[1], 13100[1], 13101[1], 13102[1], 13120[1], 13121[1], 13122[1], 13131[1], 13132[1], 13133[1], 13151[1], 13152[1], 13153[1], 36000[1], 36400[1], 36405[1], 36406[1], 36410[1], 36420[1], 36425[1], 36430[1], 36440[1], 36591[0], 36592[0], 36600[1], 36640[1], 43752[1], 51701[1], 51702[1], 51703[1], 62320[0], 62321[0], 62322[0], 62323[0], 62324[0], 62325[0], 62326[0], 62327[0], 64400[0], 64405[0], 64408[0], 64415[0], 64416[0], 64417[0], 64418[0], 64420[0], 64421[0], 64425[0], 64430[0], 64435[0], 64445[0], 64446[0], 64447[0], 64448[0], 64449[0], 64450[0], 64451[0], 64454[0], 64461[0], 64462[0], 64463[0], 64479[0], 64480[0], 64483[0], 64484[0], 64486[0], 64487[0], 64488[0], 64489[0], 64490[0], 64491[0], 64492[0], 64493[0], 64494[0], 64495[0], 64505[0], 64510[0], 64517[0], 64520[0], 64530[0], 67343[1], 67500[1], 69990[0], 92012[1], 92014[1], 92018[1], 92019[1], 93000[1], 93005[1], 93010[1], 93040[1], 93041[1], 93042[1], 93318[1], 93355[1], 94002[1], 94200[1], 94680[1], 94681[1], 94690[1], 95812[1], 95813[1], 95816[1], 95819[1], 95822[1], 95829[1], 95955[1], 96360[1], 96361[1], 96365[1], 96366[1], 96367[1], 96368[1], 96372[1], 96374[1], 96375[1], 96376[1], 96377[1], 96523[0], 97597[1], 97598[1], 97602[1], 99155[0], 99156[0], 99157[0], 99211[1], 99212[1], 99213[1], 99214[1], 99215[1], 99217[1], 99218[1], 99219[1], 99220[1], 99221[1], 99222[1], 99223[1], 99231[1], 99232[1], 99233[1], 99234[1], 99235[1], 99236[1], 99238[1], 99239[1], 99241[1], 99242[1], 99243[1], 99244[1], 99245[1], 99251[1], 99252[1], 99253[1], 99254[1], 99255[1], 99291[1], 99292[1], 99304[1], 99305[1], 99306[1], 99307[1], 99308[1], 99309[1], 99310[1], 99315[1], 99316[1], 99334[1], 99335[1], 99336[1], 99337[1], 99347[1], 99348[1], 99349[1], 99350[1], 99374[1], 99375[1], 99377[1], 99378[1], 99446[0], 99447[0], 99448[0], 99449[0], 99451[0], 99452[0], 99495[0], 99496[0], G0463[1], G0471[1]
67316	0213T[0], 0216T[0], 0596T[1], 0597T[1], 0708T[1], 0709T[1], 11000[1], 11001[1], 11004[1], 11005[1], 11006[1], 11042[1], 11043[1], 11044[1], 11045[1], 11046[1], 11047[1], 12001[1], 12002[1], 12004[1], 12005[1], 12006[1], 12007[1], 12011[1], 12013[1], 12014[1], 12015[1], 12016[1], 12017[1], 12018[1], 12020[1], 12021[1], 12031[1], 12032[1], 12034[1], 12035[1], 12036[1], 12037[1], 12041[1], 12042[1], 12044[1], 12045[1], 12046[1], 12047[1], 12051[1], 12052[1], 12053[1], 12054[1], 12055[1], 12056[1], 12057[1], 13100[1], 13101[1], 13102[1], 13120[1], 13121[1], 13122[1], 13131[1], 13132[1], 13133[1], 13151[1], 13152[1], 13153[1], 36000[1], 36400[1], 36405[1], 36406[1], 36410[1], 36420[1], 36425[1], 36430[1], 36440[1], 36591[0], 36592[0], 36600[1], 36640[1], 43752[1], 51701[1], 51702[1], 51703[1], 62320[0], 62321[0], 62322[0], 62323[0], 62324[0], 62325[0], 62326[0], 62327[0], 64400[0], 64405[0], 64408[0], 64415[0], 64416[0], 64417[0], 64418[0], 64420[0], 64421[0], 64425[0], 64430[0], 64435[0], 64445[0], 64446[0], 64447[0], 64448[0], 64449[0], 64450[0], 64451[0], 64454[0], 64461[0], 64462[0], 64463[0], 64479[0], 64480[0], 64483[0], 64484[0], 64486[0], 64487[0], 64488[0], 64489[0], 64490[0], 64491[0], 64492[0], 64493[0], 64494[0], 64495[0], 64505[0], 64510[0], 64517[0], 64520[0], 64530[0], 67314[1], 67343[1], 67500[1], 69990[0], 92012[1], 92014[1], 92018[1], 92019[1], 93000[1], 93005[1], 93010[1], 93040[1], 93041[1], 93042[1], 93318[1], 93355[1], 94002[1], 94200[1], 94680[1], 94681[1], 94690[1], 95812[1], 95813[1], 95816[1], 95819[1], 95822[1], 95829[1], 95955[1], 96360[1], 96361[1], 96365[1], 96366[1], 96367[1], 96368[1], 96372[1], 96374[1], 96375[1], 96376[1], 96377[1], 96523[0], 97597[1], 97598[1], 97602[1], 99155[0], 99156[0], 99157[0], 99211[1], 99212[1], 99213[1], 99214[1], 99215[1], 99217[1], 99218[1], 99219[1], 99220[1], 99221[1], 99222[1], 99223[1], 99231[1], 99232[1], 99233[1], 99234[1], 99235[1], 99236[1], 99238[1], 99239[1], 99241[1], 99242[1], 99243[1], 99244[1], 99245[1], 99251[1], 99252[1], 99253[1], 99254[1], 99255[1], 99291[1], 99292[1], 99304[1], 99305[1], 99306[1], 99307[1], 99308[1], 99309[1], 99310[1], 99315[1], 99316[1], 99334[1], 99335[1], 99336[1], 99337[1], 99347[1], 99348[1], 99349[1], 99350[1], 99374[1], 99375[1], 99377[1], 99378[1], 99446[0], 99447[0], 99448[0], 99449[0], 99451[0], 99452[0], 99495[0], 99496[0], G0463[1], G0471[1]
67318	0213T[0], 0216T[0], 0596T[1], 0597T[1], 0708T[1], 0709T[1], 12001[1], 12002[1], 12004[1], 12005[1], 12006[1], 12007[1], 12011[1], 12013[1], 12014[1], 12015[1], 12016[1], 12017[1], 12018[1], 12020[1], 12021[1], 12031[1], 12032[1], 12034[1], 12035[1], 12036[1], 12037[1], 12041[1], 12042[1], 12044[1], 12045[1], 12046[1], 12047[1], 12051[1], 12052[1], 12053[1], 12054[1], 12055[1], 12056[1], 12057[1], 13100[1], 13101[1], 13102[1], 13120[1], 13121[1], 13122[1], 13131[1], 13132[1], 13133[1], 13151[1], 13152[1], 13153[1], 36000[1], 36400[1], 36405[1], 36406[1], 36410[1], 36420[1], 36425[1], 36430[1], 36440[1], 36591[0], 36592[0], 36600[1], 36640[1], 43752[1], 51701[1], 51702[1], 51703[1], 62320[0], 62321[0], 62322[0], 62323[0], 62324[0], 62325[0], 62326[0], 62327[0], 64400[0], 64405[0], 64408[0], 64415[0], 64416[0], 64417[0], 64418[0], 64420[0], 64421[0], 64425[0], 64430[0], 64435[0], 64445[0], 64446[0], 64447[0], 64448[0], 64449[0], 64450[0], 64451[0], 64454[0], 64461[0], 64462[0], 64463[0], 64479[0], 64480[0], 64483[0], 64484[0], 64486[0], 64487[0], 64488[0], 64489[0], 64490[0], 64491[0], 64492[0], 64493[0], 64494[0], 64495[0], 64505[0], 64510[0], 64517[0], 64520[0], 64530[0], 67343[1], 67500[1], 69990[0], 92012[1], 92014[1], 92018[1], 92019[1], 93000[1], 93005[1], 93010[1], 93040[1], 93041[1], 93042[1], 93318[1], 93355[1], 94002[1], 94200[1], 94680[1], 94681[1], 94690[1], 95812[1], 95813[1], 95816[1], 95819[1], 95822[1], 95829[1], 95955[1], 96360[1], 96361[1], 96365[1], 96366[1], 96367[1], 96368[1], 96372[1], 96374[1], 96375[1], 96376[1], 96377[1], 96523[0], 99155[0], 99156[0], 99157[0], 99211[1], 99212[1], 99213[1], 99214[1], 99215[1], 99217[1], 99218[1], 99219[1], 99220[1], 99221[1], 99222[1], 99223[1], 99231[1], 99232[1], 99233[1], 99234[1], 99235[1], 99236[1], 99238[1], 99239[1], 99241[1], 99242[1], 99243[1], 99244[1], 99245[1], 99251[1], 99252[1], 99253[1], 99254[1], 99255[1], 99291[1], 99292[1], 99304[1], 99305[1], 99306[1], 99307[1], 99308[1], 99309[1], 99310[1],

0 = Modifier usage not allowed or inappropriate 1 = Modifier usage allowed

Code 1	Code 2
	99315[1], 99316[1], 99334[1], 99335[1], 99336[1], 99337[1], 99347[1], 99348[1], 99349[1], 99350[1], 99374[1], 99375[1], 99377[1], 99378[1], 99446[0], 99447[0], 99448[0], 99449[0], 99451[0], 99452[0], 99495[0], 99496[0], G0463[1], G0471[1]
67320	36591[0], 36592[0], 67343[1], 69990[0], 96523[0]
67331	36591[0], 36592[0], 67332[1], 67343[1], 69990[0], 96523[0]
67332	36591[0], 36592[0], 67343[1], 69990[0], 96523[0]
67334	36591[0], 36592[0], 67343[1], 69990[0], 96523[0]
67335	36591[0], 36592[0], 69990[0], 96523[0]
67340	36591[0], 36592[0], 67343[1], 69990[0], 96523[0]
67343	0213T[0], 0216T[0], 0596T[1], 0597T[1], 0708T[1], 0709T[1], 12001[1], 12002[1], 12004[1], 12005[1], 12006[1], 12007[1], 12011[1], 12013[1], 12014[1], 12015[1], 12016[1], 12017[1], 12018[1], 12020[1], 12021[1], 12031[1], 12032[1], 12034[1], 12035[1], 12036[1], 12037[1], 12041[1], 12042[1], 12044[1], 12045[1], 12046[1], 12047[1], 12051[1], 12052[1], 12053[1], 12054[1], 12055[1], 12056[1], 12057[1], 13100[1], 13101[1], 13102[1], 13120[1], 13121[1], 13122[1], 13131[1], 13132[1], 13133[1], 13151[1], 13152[1], 13153[1], 36000[1], 36400[1], 36405[1], 36406[1], 36410[1], 36420[1], 36425[1], 36430[1], 36440[1], 36591[0], 36592[0], 36600[1], 36640[1], 43752[1], 51701[1], 51702[1], 51703[1], 62320[0], 62321[0], 62322[0], 62323[0], 62324[0], 62325[0], 62326[0], 62327[0], 64400[0], 64405[0], 64408[0], 64415[0], 64416[0], 64417[0], 64418[0], 64420[0], 64421[0], 64425[0], 64430[0], 64435[0], 64445[0], 64446[0], 64447[0], 64448[0], 64449[0], 64450[0], 64451[0], 64454[0], 64461[0], 64462[0], 64463[0], 64479[0], 64480[0], 64483[0], 64484[0], 64486[0], 64487[0], 64488[0], 64489[0], 64490[0], 64491[0], 64492[0], 64493[0], 64494[0], 64495[0], 64505[0], 64510[0], 64517[0], 64520[0], 64530[0], 67500[1], 69990[0], 92012[1], 92014[1], 92018[1], 92019[1], 93000[1], 93005[1], 93010[1], 93040[1], 93041[1], 93042[1], 93318[1], 93355[1], 94002[1], 94200[1], 94680[1], 94681[1], 94690[1], 95812[1], 95813[1], 95816[1], 95819[1], 95822[1], 95829[1], 95955[1], 96360[1], 96361[1], 96365[1], 96366[1], 96367[1], 96368[1], 96372[1], 96374[1], 96375[1], 96376[1], 96377[1], 96523[0], 99155[0], 99156[0], 99157[0], 99211[1], 99212[1], 99213[1], 99214[1], 99215[1], 99217[1], 99218[1], 99219[1], 99220[1], 99221[1], 99222[1], 99223[1], 99231[1], 99232[1], 99233[1], 99234[1], 99235[1], 99236[1], 99238[1], 99239[1], 99241[1], 99242[1], 99243[1], 99244[1], 99245[1], 99251[1], 99252[1], 99253[1], 99254[1], 99255[1], 99291[1], 99292[1], 99304[1], 99305[1], 99306[1], 99307[1], 99308[1], 99309[1], 99310[1], 99315[1], 99316[1], 99334[1], 99335[1], 99336[1], 99337[1], 99347[1], 99348[1], 99349[1], 99350[1], 99374[1], 99375[1], 99377[1], 99378[1], 99446[0], 99447[0], 99448[0], 99449[0], 99451[0], 99452[0], 99495[0], 99496[0], G0463[1], G0471[1]
67345	0213T[0], 0216T[0], 0596T[1], 0597T[1], 0708T[1], 0709T[1], 12001[1], 12002[1], 12004[1], 12005[1], 12006[1], 12007[1], 12011[1], 12013[1], 12014[1], 12015[1], 12016[1], 12017[1], 12018[1], 12020[1], 12021[1], 12031[1], 12032[1], 12034[1], 12035[1], 12036[1], 12037[1], 12041[1], 12042[1], 12044[1], 12045[1], 12046[1], 12047[1], 12051[1], 12052[1], 12053[1], 12054[1], 12055[1], 12056[1], 12057[1], 13100[1], 13101[1], 13102[1], 13120[1], 13121[1], 13122[1], 13131[1], 13132[1], 13133[1], 13151[1], 13152[1], 13153[1], 36000[1], 36400[1], 36405[1], 36406[1], 36410[1], 36420[1], 36425[1], 36430[1], 36440[1], 36591[0], 36592[0], 36600[1], 36640[1], 43752[1], 51701[1], 51702[1], 51703[1], 62320[0], 62321[0], 62322[0], 62323[0], 62324[0], 62325[0], 62326[0], 62327[0], 64400[0], 64405[0], 64408[0], 64415[0], 64416[0], 64417[0], 64418[0], 64420[0], 64421[0], 64425[0], 64430[0], 64435[0], 64445[0], 64446[0], 64447[0], 64448[0], 64449[0], 64450[0], 64451[0], 64454[0], 64461[0], 64462[0], 64463[0], 64479[0], 64480[0], 64483[0], 64484[0], 64486[0], 64487[0], 64488[0], 64489[0], 64490[0], 64491[0], 64492[0], 64493[0], 64494[0], 64495[0], 64505[0], 64510[0], 64517[0], 64520[0], 64530[0], 67500[1], 69990[0], 92012[1], 92014[1], 92018[1], 92019[1], 93000[1], 93005[1], 93010[1], 93040[1], 93041[1], 93042[1], 93318[1], 93355[1], 94002[1], 94200[1], 94680[1], 94681[1], 94690[1], 95812[1], 95813[1], 95816[1], 95819[1], 95822[1], 95829[1], 95860[0], 95861[0], 95863[0], 95864[0], 95867[0], 95868[0], 95869[0], 95870[0], 95955[1], 96360[1], 96361[1], 96365[1], 96366[1], 96367[1], 96368[1], 96372[1], 96374[1], 96375[1], 96376[1], 96377[1], 96523[0], 99155[0], 99156[0], 99157[0], 99211[1], 99212[1], 99213[1], 99214[1], 99215[1], 99217[1], 99218[1], 99219[1], 99220[1], 99221[1], 99222[1], 99223[1], 99231[1], 99232[1], 99233[1], 99234[1], 99235[1], 99236[1], 99238[1], 99239[1], 99241[1], 99242[1], 99243[1], 99244[1], 99245[1], 99251[1], 99252[1], 99253[1], 99254[1], 99255[1], 99291[1], 99292[1], 99304[1], 99305[1], 99306[1], 99307[1], 99308[1], 99309[1], 99310[1], 99315[1], 99316[1], 99334[1], 99335[1], 99336[1], 99337[1], 99347[1], 99348[1], 99349[1], 99350[1], 99374[1], 99375[1], 99377[1], 99378[1], 99446[0], 99447[0], 99448[0], 99449[0], 99451[0], 99452[0], 99495[0], 99496[0], G0463[1], G0471[1]
67346	0213T[0], 0216T[0], 0596T[1], 0597T[1], 0708T[1], 0709T[1], 10005[1], 10007[1], 10009[1], 10011[1], 10021[1], 12001[1], 12002[1], 12004[1], 12005[1], 12006[1], 12007[1], 12011[1], 12013[1], 12014[1], 12015[1], 12016[1], 12017[1], 12018[1], 12020[1], 12021[1], 12031[1], 12032[1], 12034[1], 12035[1], 12036[1], 12037[1], 12041[1], 12042[1], 12044[1], 12045[1], 12046[1], 12047[1], 12051[1], 12052[1], 12053[1], 12054[1], 12055[1], 12056[1], 12057[1], 13100[1], 13101[1], 13102[1], 13120[1], 13121[1], 13122[1], 13131[1], 13132[1], 13133[1], 13151[1], 13152[1], 13153[1], 36000[1], 36400[1], 36405[1], 36406[1], 36410[1], 36420[1], 36425[1], 36430[1], 36440[1], 36591[0], 36592[0], 36600[1], 36640[1], 43752[1], 51701[1], 51702[1], 51703[1], 62320[0], 62321[0], 62322[0], 62323[0], 62324[0], 62325[0], 62326[0], 62327[0], 64400[0], 64405[0], 64408[0], 64415[0], 64416[0], 64417[0], 64418[0], 64420[0], 64421[0], 64425[0], 64430[0], 64435[0], 64445[0], 64446[0], 64447[0], 64448[0], 64449[0], 64450[0], 64451[0], 64454[0], 64461[0], 64462[0], 64463[0], 64479[0], 64480[0], 64483[0], 64484[0], 64486[0], 64487[0], 64488[0], 64489[0], 64490[0], 64491[0], 64492[0], 64493[0], 64494[0], 64495[0], 64505[0], 64510[0], 64517[0], 64520[0], 64530[0], 67500[1], 69990[0], 92012[1], 92014[1], 92018[1], 92019[1], 93000[1], 93005[1], 93010[1], 93040[1], 93041[1], 93042[1], 93318[1], 93355[1], 94002[1], 94200[1], 94680[1], 94681[1], 94690[1], 95812[1], 95813[1], 95816[1], 95819[1], 95822[1], 95829[1], 95955[1], 96360[1], 96361[1], 96365[1], 96366[1], 96367[1], 96368[1], 96372[1], 96374[1], 96375[1], 96376[1], 96377[1], 96523[0], 99155[0], 99156[0], 99157[0], 99211[1], 99212[1], 99213[1], 99214[1], 99215[1], 99217[1], 99218[1], 99219[1], 99220[1], 99221[1], 99222[1], 99223[1], 99231[1], 99232[1], 99233[1], 99234[1], 99235[1], 99236[1], 99238[1], 99239[1], 99241[1], 99242[1], 99243[1], 99244[1], 99245[1], 99251[1], 99252[1], 99253[1], 99254[1], 99255[1], 99291[1], 99292[1], 99304[1], 99305[1], 99306[1], 99307[1], 99308[1], 99309[1], 99310[1], 99315[1], 99316[1], 99334[1], 99335[1], 99336[1], 99337[1], 99347[1], 99348[1], 99349[1], 99350[1], 99374[1], 99375[1], 99377[1], 99378[1], 99446[0], 99447[0], 99448[0], 99449[0], 99451[0], 99452[0], 99495[1], 99496[1], G0463[1], G0471[1]
67400	0213T[0], 0216T[0], 0596T[1], 0597T[1], 0708T[1], 0709T[1], 10005[1], 10007[1], 10009[1], 10011[1], 10021[1], 11000[1], 11001[1], 11004[1], 11005[1], 11006[1], 11042[1], 11043[1], 11044[1], 11045[1], 11046[1], 11047[1], 12001[1], 12002[1], 12004[1], 12005[1], 12006[1], 12007[1], 12011[1], 12013[1], 12014[1], 12015[1], 12016[1], 12017[1], 12018[1], 12020[1], 12021[1], 12031[1], 12032[1], 12034[1], 12035[1], 12036[1], 12037[1], 12041[1], 12042[1], 12044[1], 12045[1], 12046[1], 12047[1], 12051[1], 12052[1], 12053[1], 12054[1], 12055[1], 12056[1], 12057[1], 13100[1], 13101[1], 13102[1], 13120[1], 13121[1], 13122[1], 13131[1], 13132[1], 13133[1], 13151[1], 13152[1], 13153[1], 36000[1], 36400[1], 36405[1], 36406[1], 36410[1], 36420[1], 36425[1], 36430[1], 36440[1], 36591[0], 36592[0], 36600[1], 36640[1], 43752[1], 51701[1], 51702[1], 51703[1], 62320[0], 62321[0], 62322[0], 62323[0], 62324[0], 62325[0], 62326[0], 62327[0], 64400[0], 64405[0], 64408[0], 64415[0], 64416[0], 64417[0], 64418[0], 64420[0], 64421[0], 64425[0], 64430[0], 64435[0], 64445[0], 64446[0], 64447[0], 64448[0], 64449[0], 64450[0], 64451[0], 64454[0], 64461[0], 64462[0], 64463[0], 64479[0], 64480[0], 64483[0], 64484[0], 64486[0], 64487[0], 64488[0], 64489[0], 64490[0], 64491[0], 64492[0], 64493[0], 64494[0], 64495[0], 64505[0], 64510[0], 64517[0], 64520[0], 64530[0], 67415[1], 67500[1], 69990[0], 92012[1], 92014[1], 92018[1], 92019[1], 93000[1], 93005[1], 93010[1], 93040[1], 93041[1], 93042[1], 93318[1], 93355[1], 94002[1], 94200[1], 94680[1], 94681[1], 94690[1], 95812[1], 95813[1], 95816[1], 95819[1], 95822[1], 95829[1], 95955[1], 96360[1], 96361[1], 96365[1], 96366[1], 96367[1], 96368[1], 96372[1], 96374[1], 96375[1], 96376[1], 96377[1], 96523[0], 97597[1], 97598[1], 97602[1], 99155[0], 99156[0], 99157[0], 99211[1], 99212[1], 99213[1], 99214[1], 99215[1], 99217[1], 99218[1], 99219[1], 99220[1], 99221[1], 99222[1], 99223[1], 99231[1], 99232[1], 99233[1], 99234[1], 99235[1], 99236[1], 99238[1], 99239[1], 99241[1], 99242[1], 99243[1], 99244[1], 99245[1], 99251[1], 99252[1], 99253[1], 99254[1], 99255[1], 99291[1], 99292[1], 99304[1], 99305[1], 99306[1], 99307[1], 99308[1], 99309[1], 99310[1], 99315[1], 99316[1], 99334[1], 99335[1], 99336[1], 99337[1], 99347[1], 99348[1], 99349[1], 99350[1], 99374[1], 99375[1], 99377[1], 99378[1], 99446[0], 99447[0], 99448[0], 99449[0], 99451[0], 99452[0], 99495[0], 99496[0], G0463[1], G0471[1], J0670[1], J2001[1]
67405	0213T[0], 0216T[0], 0596T[1], 0597T[1], 0708T[1], 0709T[1], 11000[1], 11001[1], 11004[1], 11005[1], 11006[1], 11042[1], 11043[1], 11044[1], 11045[1], 11046[1], 11047[1], 12001[1], 12002[1], 12004[1], 12005[1], 12006[1], 12007[1], 12011[1], 12013[1], 12014[1], 12015[1], 12016[1], 12017[1], 12018[1], 12020[1], 12021[1], 12031[1], 12032[1], 12034[1], 12035[1], 12036[1], 12037[1], 12041[1], 12042[1], 12044[1], 12045[1], 12046[1], 12047[1], 12051[1], 12052[1], 12053[1], 12054[1], 12055[1], 12056[1], 12057[1], 13100[1], 13101[1], 13102[1], 13120[1], 13121[1], 13122[1], 13131[1], 13132[1], 13133[1], 13151[1], 13152[1], 13153[1], 36000[1], 36400[1], 36405[1], 36406[1], 36410[1], 36420[1], 36425[1], 36430[1], 36440[1], 36591[0], 36592[0], 36600[1], 36640[1], 43752[1], 51701[1], 51702[1], 51703[1], 62320[0], 62321[0], 62322[0], 62323[0], 62324[0], 62325[0], 62326[0], 62327[0], 64400[0], 64405[0], 64408[0], 64415[0], 64416[0], 64417[0], 64418[0], 64420[0], 64421[0], 64425[0], 64430[0], 64435[0], 64445[0], 64446[0], 64447[0], 64448[0], 64449[0], 64450[0], 64451[0], 64454[0], 64461[0], 64462[0], 64463[0], 64479[0], 64480[0], 64483[0], 64484[0], 64486[0], 64487[0], 64488[0], 64489[0], 64490[0], 64491[0], 64492[0], 64493[0], 64494[0], 64495[0], 64505[0], 64510[0], 64517[0], 64520[0], 64530[0], 67400[1], 67415[1], 67500[1], 69990[0], 92012[1], 92014[1], 92018[1], 92019[1], 93000[1], 93005[1], 93010[1], 93040[1], 93041[1], 93042[1], 93318[1], 93355[1], 94002[1], 94200[1], 94680[1], 94681[1], 94690[1], 95812[1], 95813[1], 95816[1], 95819[1], 95822[1], 95829[1], 95955[1], 96360[1], 96361[1], 96365[1], 96366[1], 96367[1], 96368[1], 96372[1], 96374[1], 96375[1], 96376[1], 96377[1], 96523[0], 97597[1], 97598[1], 97602[1], 99155[0], 99156[0], 99157[0], 99211[1], 99212[1], 99213[1], 99214[1], 99215[1], 99217[1], 99218[1], 99219[1], 99220[1], 99221[1], 99222[1], 99223[1], 99231[1], 99232[1], 99233[1], 99234[1], 99235[1], 99236[1], 99238[1], 99239[1], 99241[1], 99242[1], 99243[1], 99244[1], 99245[1], 99251[1], 99252[1], 99253[1], 99254[1], 99255[1], 99291[1], 99292[1], 99304[1], 99305[1], 99306[1], 99307[1], 99308[1], 99309[1], 99310[1], 99315[1], 99316[1], 99334[1], 99335[1], 99336[1], 99337[1], 99347[1], 99348[1], 99349[1], 99350[1], 99374[1], 99375[1], 99377[1], 99378[1], 99446[0], 99447[0], 99448[0], 99449[0], 99451[0], 99452[0], 99495[0], 99496[0], G0463[1], G0471[1], J0670[1], J2001[1]

0 = Modifier usage not allowed or inappropriate 1 = Modifier usage allowed

Code 1	Code 2
67412	0213T[0], 0216T[0], 0596T[1], 0597T[1], 0708T[1], 0709T[1], 11000[1], 11001[1], 11004[1], 11005[1], 11006[1], 11042[1], 11043[1], 11044[1], 11045[1], 11046[1], 11047[1], 12001[1], 12002[1], 12004[1], 12005[1], 12006[1], 12007[1], 12011[1], 12013[1], 12014[1], 12015[1], 12016[1], 12017[1], 12018[1], 12020[1], 12021[1], 12031[1], 12032[1], 12034[1], 12035[1], 12036[1], 12037[1], 12041[1], 12042[1], 12044[1], 12045[1], 12046[1], 12047[1], 12051[1], 12052[1], 12053[1], 12054[1], 12055[1], 12056[1], 12057[1], 13100[1], 13101[1], 13102[1], 13120[1], 13121[1], 13122[1], 13131[1], 13132[1], 13133[1], 13151[1], 13152[1], 13153[1], 36000[1], 36400[1], 36405[1], 36406[1], 36410[1], 36420[1], 36425[1], 36430[1], 36440[1], 36591[0], 36592[0], 36600[1], 36640[1], 43752[1], 51701[1], 51702[1], 51703[1], 62320[0], 62321[0], 62322[0], 62323[0], 62324[0], 62325[0], 62326[0], 62327[0], 64400[0], 64405[0], 64408[0], 64415[0], 64416[0], 64417[0], 64418[0], 64420[0], 64421[0], 64425[0], 64430[0], 64435[0], 64445[0], 64446[0], 64447[0], 64448[0], 64449[0], 64450[0], 64451[0], 64454[0], 64461[0], 64462[0], 64463[0], 64479[0], 64480[0], 64483[0], 64484[0], 64486[0], 64487[0], 64488[0], 64489[0], 64490[0], 64491[0], 64492[0], 64493[0], 64494[0], 64495[0], 64505[0], 64510[0], 64517[0], 64520[0], 64530[0], 67400[1], 67405[1], 67415[1], 67500[1], 69990[0], 92012[1], 92014[1], 92018[1], 92019[1], 93000[1], 93005[1], 93010[1], 93040[1], 93041[1], 93042[1], 93318[1], 93355[1], 94002[1], 94200[1], 94680[1], 94681[1], 94690[1], 95812[1], 95813[1], 95816[1], 95819[1], 95822[1], 95829[1], 95955[1], 96360[1], 96361[1], 96365[1], 96366[1], 96367[1], 96368[1], 96372[1], 96374[1], 96375[1], 96376[1], 96377[1], 96523[0], 97597[1], 97598[1], 97602[1], 99155[0], 99156[0], 99157[0], 99211[1], 99212[1], 99213[1], 99214[1], 99215[1], 99217[1], 99218[1], 99219[1], 99220[1], 99221[1], 99222[1], 99223[1], 99231[1], 99232[1], 99233[1], 99234[1], 99235[1], 99236[1], 99238[1], 99239[1], 99241[1], 99242[1], 99243[1], 99244[1], 99245[1], 99251[1], 99252[1], 99253[1], 99254[1], 99255[1], 99291[1], 99292[1], 99304[1], 99305[1], 99306[1], 99307[1], 99308[1], 99309[1], 99310[1], 99315[1], 99316[1], 99334[1], 99335[1], 99336[1], 99337[1], 99347[1], 99348[1], 99349[1], 99350[1], 99374[1], 99375[1], 99377[1], 99378[1], 99446[0], 99447[0], 99448[0], 99449[0], 99451[0], 99452[0], 99495[0], 99496[0], G0463[1], G0471[1], J0670[1], J2001[1]
67413	0213T[0], 0216T[0], 0596T[1], 0597T[1], 0708T[1], 0709T[1], 11000[1], 11001[1], 11004[1], 11005[1], 11006[1], 11042[1], 11043[1], 11044[1], 11045[1], 11046[1], 11047[1], 12001[1], 12002[1], 12004[1], 12005[1], 12006[1], 12007[1], 12011[1], 12013[1], 12014[1], 12015[1], 12016[1], 12017[1], 12018[1], 12020[1], 12021[1], 12031[1], 12032[1], 12034[1], 12035[1], 12036[1], 12037[1], 12041[1], 12042[1], 12044[1], 12045[1], 12046[1], 12047[1], 12051[1], 12052[1], 12053[1], 12054[1], 12055[1], 12056[1], 12057[1], 13100[1], 13101[1], 13102[1], 13120[1], 13121[1], 13122[1], 13131[1], 13132[1], 13133[1], 13151[1], 13152[1], 13153[1], 36000[1], 36400[1], 36405[1], 36406[1], 36410[1], 36420[1], 36425[1], 36430[1], 36440[1], 36591[0], 36592[0], 36600[1], 36640[1], 43752[1], 51701[1], 51702[1], 51703[1], 62320[0], 62321[0], 62322[0], 62323[0], 62324[0], 62325[0], 62326[0], 62327[0], 64400[0], 64405[0], 64408[0], 64415[0], 64416[0], 64417[0], 64418[0], 64420[0], 64421[0], 64425[0], 64430[0], 64435[0], 64445[0], 64446[0], 64447[0], 64448[0], 64449[0], 64450[0], 64451[0], 64454[0], 64461[0], 64462[0], 64463[0], 64479[0], 64480[0], 64483[0], 64484[0], 64486[0], 64487[0], 64488[0], 64489[0], 64490[0], 64491[0], 64492[0], 64493[0], 64494[0], 64495[0], 64505[0], 64510[0], 64517[0], 64520[0], 64530[0], 67400[1], 67405[1], 67415[1], 67500[1], 69990[0], 92012[1], 92014[1], 92018[1], 92019[1], 93000[1], 93005[1], 93010[1], 93040[1], 93041[1], 93042[1], 93318[1], 93355[1], 94002[1], 94200[1], 94680[1], 94681[1], 94690[1], 95812[1], 95813[1], 95816[1], 95819[1], 95822[1], 95829[1], 95955[1], 96360[1], 96361[1], 96365[1], 96366[1], 96367[1], 96368[1], 96372[1], 96374[1], 96375[1], 96376[1], 96377[1], 96523[0], 97597[1], 97598[1], 97602[1], 99155[0], 99156[0], 99157[0], 99211[1], 99212[1], 99213[1], 99214[1], 99215[1], 99217[1], 99218[1], 99219[1], 99220[1], 99221[1], 99222[1], 99223[1], 99231[1], 99232[1], 99233[1], 99234[1], 99235[1], 99236[1], 99238[1], 99239[1], 99241[1], 99242[1], 99243[1], 99244[1], 99245[1], 99251[1], 99252[1], 99253[1], 99254[1], 99255[1], 99291[1], 99292[1], 99304[1], 99305[1], 99306[1], 99307[1], 99308[1], 99309[1], 99310[1], 99315[1], 99316[1], 99334[1], 99335[1], 99336[1], 99337[1], 99347[1], 99348[1], 99349[1], 99350[1], 99374[1], 99375[1], 99377[1], 99378[1], 99446[0], 99447[0], 99448[0], 99449[0], 99451[0], 99452[0], 99495[0], 99496[0], G0463[1], G0471[1], J0670[1], J2001[1]
67414	0213T[0], 0216T[0], 0596T[1], 0597T[1], 0708T[1], 0709T[1], 11000[1], 11001[1], 11004[1], 11005[1], 11006[1], 11042[1], 11043[1], 11044[1], 11045[1], 11046[1], 11047[1], 12001[1], 12002[1], 12004[1], 12005[1], 12006[1], 12007[1], 12011[1], 12013[1], 12014[1], 12015[1], 12016[1], 12017[1], 12018[1], 12020[1], 12021[1], 12031[1], 12032[1], 12034[1], 12035[1], 12036[1], 12037[1], 12041[1], 12042[1], 12044[1], 12045[1], 12046[1], 12047[1], 12051[1], 12052[1], 12053[1], 12054[1], 12055[1], 12056[1], 12057[1], 13100[1], 13101[1], 13102[1], 13120[1], 13121[1], 13122[1], 13131[1], 13132[1], 13133[1], 13151[1], 13152[1], 13153[1], 36000[1], 36400[1], 36405[1], 36406[1], 36410[1], 36420[1], 36425[1], 36430[1], 36440[1], 36591[0], 36592[0], 36600[1], 36640[1], 43752[1], 51701[1], 51702[1], 51703[1], 62320[0], 62321[0], 62322[0], 62323[0], 62324[0], 62325[0], 62326[0], 62327[0], 64400[0], 64405[0], 64408[0], 64415[0], 64416[0], 64417[0], 64418[0], 64420[0], 64421[0], 64425[0], 64430[0], 64435[0], 64445[0], 64446[0], 64447[0], 64448[0], 64449[0], 64450[0], 64451[0], 64454[0], 64461[0], 64462[0], 64463[0], 64479[0], 64480[0], 64483[0], 64484[0], 64486[0], 64487[0], 64488[0], 64489[0], 64490[0], 64491[0], 64492[0], 64493[0], 64494[0], 64495[0], 64505[0], 64510[0], 64517[0], 64520[0], 64530[0], 67400[1], 67405[1], 67500[1], 69990[0], 92012[1], 92014[1], 92018[1], 92019[1], 93000[1], 93005[1], 93010[1], 93040[1], 93041[1], 93042[1], 93318[1], 93355[1], 94002[1], 94200[1], 94680[1], 94681[1], 94690[1], 95812[1], 95813[1], 95816[1], 95819[1], 95822[1], 95829[1], 95955[1], 96360[1], 96361[1], 96365[1], 96366[1], 96367[1], 96368[1], 96372[1], 96374[1], 96375[1], 96376[1], 96377[1], 96523[0], 97597[1], 97598[1], 97602[1], 99155[0], 99156[0], 99157[0], 99211[1], 99212[1], 99213[1], 99214[1], 99215[1], 99217[1], 99218[1], 99219[1], 99220[1], 99221[1], 99222[1], 99223[1], 99231[1], 99232[1], 99233[1], 99234[1], 99235[1], 99236[1], 99238[1], 99239[1], 99241[1], 99242[1], 99243[1], 99244[1], 99245[1], 99251[1], 99252[1], 99253[1], 99254[1], 99255[1], 99291[1], 99292[1], 99304[1], 99305[1], 99306[1], 99307[1], 99308[1], 99309[1], 99310[1], 99315[1], 99316[1], 99334[1], 99335[1], 99336[1], 99337[1], 99347[1], 99348[1], 99349[1], 99350[1], 99374[1], 99375[1], 99377[1], 99378[1], 99446[0], 99447[0], 99448[0], 99449[0], 99451[0], 99452[0], 99495[0], 99496[0], G0463[1], G0471[1], J0670[1], J2001[1]
67415	0213T[0], 0216T[0], 0596T[1], 0597T[1], 0708T[1], 0709T[1], 10005[1], 10007[1], 10009[1], 10011[1], 10021[1], 12001[1], 12002[1], 12004[1], 12005[1], 12006[1], 12007[1], 12011[1], 12013[1], 12014[1], 12015[1], 12016[1], 12017[1], 12018[1], 12020[1], 12021[1], 12031[1], 12032[1], 12034[1], 12035[1], 12036[1], 12037[1], 12041[1], 12042[1], 12044[1], 12045[1], 12046[1], 12047[1], 12051[1], 12052[1], 12053[1], 12054[1], 12055[1], 12056[1], 12057[1], 13100[1], 13101[1], 13102[1], 13120[1], 13121[1], 13122[1], 13131[1], 13132[1], 13133[1], 13151[1], 13152[1], 13153[1], 36000[1], 36400[1], 36405[1], 36406[1], 36410[1], 36420[1], 36425[1], 36430[1], 36440[1], 36591[0], 36592[0], 36600[1], 36640[1], 43752[1], 51701[1], 51702[1], 51703[1], 62320[0], 62321[0], 62322[0], 62323[0], 62324[0], 62325[0], 62326[0], 62327[0], 64400[0], 64405[0], 64408[0], 64415[0], 64416[0], 64417[0], 64418[0], 64420[0], 64421[0], 64425[0], 64430[0], 64435[0], 64445[0], 64446[0], 64447[0], 64448[0], 64449[0], 64450[0], 64451[0], 64454[0], 64461[0], 64462[0], 64463[0], 64479[0], 64480[0], 64483[0], 64484[0], 64486[0], 64487[0], 64488[0], 64489[0], 64490[0], 64491[0], 64492[0], 64493[0], 64494[0], 64495[0], 64505[0], 64510[0], 64517[0], 64520[0], 64530[0], 67500[1], 69990[0], 92012[1], 92014[1], 92018[1], 92019[1], 93000[1], 93005[1], 93010[1], 93040[1], 93041[1], 93042[1], 93318[1], 93355[1], 94002[1], 94200[1], 94680[1], 94681[1], 94690[1], 95812[1], 95813[1], 95816[1], 95819[1], 95822[1], 95829[1], 95955[1], 96360[1], 96361[1], 96365[1], 96366[1], 96367[1], 96368[1], 96372[1], 96374[1], 96375[1], 96376[1], 96377[1], 96523[0], 99155[0], 99156[0], 99157[0], 99211[1], 99212[1], 99213[1], 99214[1], 99215[1], 99217[1], 99218[1], 99219[1], 99220[1], 99221[1], 99222[1], 99223[1], 99231[1], 99232[1], 99233[1], 99234[1], 99235[1], 99236[1], 99238[1], 99239[1], 99241[1], 99242[1], 99243[1], 99244[1], 99245[1], 99251[1], 99252[1], 99253[1], 99254[1], 99255[1], 99291[1], 99292[1], 99304[1], 99305[1], 99306[1], 99307[1], 99308[1], 99309[1], 99310[1], 99315[1], 99316[1], 99334[1], 99335[1], 99336[1], 99337[1], 99347[1], 99348[1], 99349[1], 99350[1], 99374[1], 99375[1], 99377[1], 99378[1], 99446[0], 99447[0], 99448[0], 99449[0], 99451[0], 99452[0], 99495[1], 99496[1], G0463[1], G0471[1]
67420	0213T[0], 0216T[0], 0596T[1], 0597T[1], 0708T[1], 0709T[1], 11000[1], 11001[1], 11004[1], 11005[1], 11006[1], 11042[1], 11043[1], 11044[1], 11045[1], 11046[1], 11047[1], 12001[1], 12002[1], 12004[1], 12005[1], 12006[1], 12007[1], 12011[1], 12013[1], 12014[1], 12015[1], 12016[1], 12017[1], 12018[1], 12020[1], 12021[1], 12031[1], 12032[1], 12034[1], 12035[1], 12036[1], 12037[1], 12041[1], 12042[1], 12044[1], 12045[1], 12046[1], 12047[1], 12051[1], 12052[1], 12053[1], 12054[1], 12055[1], 12056[1], 12057[1], 13100[1], 13101[1], 13102[1], 13120[1], 13121[1], 13122[1], 13131[1], 13132[1], 13133[1], 13151[1], 13152[1], 13153[1], 36000[1], 36400[1], 36405[1], 36406[1], 36410[1], 36420[1], 36425[1], 36430[1], 36440[1], 36591[0], 36592[0], 36600[1], 36640[1], 43752[1], 51701[1], 51702[1], 51703[1], 62320[0], 62321[0], 62322[0], 62323[0], 62324[0], 62325[0], 62326[0], 62327[0], 64400[0], 64405[0], 64408[0], 64415[0], 64416[0], 64417[0], 64418[0], 64420[0], 64421[0], 64425[0], 64430[0], 64435[0], 64445[0], 64446[0], 64447[0], 64448[0], 64449[0], 64450[0], 64451[0], 64454[0], 64461[0], 64462[0], 64463[0], 64479[0], 64480[0], 64483[0], 64484[0], 64486[0], 64487[0], 64488[0], 64489[0], 64490[0], 64491[0], 64492[0], 64493[0], 64494[0], 64495[0], 64505[0], 64510[0], 64517[0], 64520[0], 64530[0], 67412[1], 67415[1], 67440[1], 67450[1], 67500[1], 69990[0], 92012[1], 92014[1], 92018[1], 92019[1], 93000[1], 93005[1], 93010[1], 93040[1], 93041[1], 93042[1], 93318[1], 93355[1], 94002[1], 94200[1], 94680[1], 94681[1], 94690[1], 95812[1], 95813[1], 95816[1], 95819[1], 95822[1], 95829[1], 95955[1], 96360[1], 96361[1], 96365[1], 96366[1], 96367[1], 96368[1], 96372[1], 96374[1], 96375[1], 96376[1], 96377[1], 96523[0], 97597[1], 97598[1], 97602[1], 99155[0], 99156[0], 99157[0], 99211[1], 99212[1], 99213[1], 99214[1], 99215[1], 99217[1], 99218[1], 99219[1], 99220[1], 99221[1], 99222[1], 99223[1], 99231[1], 99232[1], 99233[1], 99234[1], 99235[1], 99236[1], 99238[1], 99239[1], 99241[1], 99242[1], 99243[1], 99244[1], 99245[1], 99251[1], 99252[1], 99253[1], 99254[1], 99255[1], 99291[1], 99292[1], 99304[1], 99305[1], 99306[1], 99307[1], 99308[1], 99309[1], 99310[1], 99315[1], 99316[1], 99334[1], 99335[1], 99336[1], 99337[1], 99347[1], 99348[1], 99349[1], 99350[1], 99374[1], 99375[1], 99377[1], 99378[1], 99446[0], 99447[0], 99448[0], 99449[0], 99451[0], 99452[0], 99495[0], 99496[0], G0463[1], G0471[1], J0670[1], J2001[1]
67430	0213T[0], 0216T[0], 0596T[1], 0597T[1], 0708T[1], 0709T[1], 11000[1], 11001[1], 11004[1], 11005[1], 11006[1], 11042[1], 11043[1], 11044[1], 11045[1], 11046[1], 11047[1], 12001[1], 12002[1], 12004[1], 12005[1], 12006[1], 12007[1], 12011[1], 12013[1], 12014[1], 12015[1], 12016[1], 12017[1], 12018[1], 12020[1], 12021[1], 12031[1], 12032[1], 12034[1], 12035[1], 12036[1], 12037[1], 12041[1], 12042[1], 12044[1], 12045[1], 12046[1], 12047[1], 12051[1], 12052[1], 12053[1], 12054[1], 12055[1], 12056[1], 12057[1], 13100[1], 13101[1], 13102[1], 13120[1], 13121[1], 13122[1], 13131[1], 13132[1], 13133[1], 13151[1], 13152[1], 13153[1], 36000[1], 36400[1], 36405[1], 36406[1], 36410[1], 36420[1], 36425[1], 36430[1], 36440[1], 36591[0], 36592[0], 36600[1], 36640[1], 43752[1], 51701[1], 51702[1], 51703[1],

0 = Modifier usage not allowed or inappropriate 1 = Modifier usage allowed

Code 1	Code 2
	62320[0], 62321[0], 62322[0], 62323[0], 62324[0], 62325[0], 62326[0], 62327[0], 64400[0], 64405[0], 64408[0], 64415[0], 64416[0], 64417[0], 64418[0], 64420[0], 64421[0], 64425[0], 64430[0], 64435[0], 64445[0], 64446[0], 64447[0], 64448[0], 64449[0], 64450[0], 64451[0], 64454[0], 64461[0], 64462[0], 64463[0], 64479[0], 64480[0], 64483[0], 64484[0], 64486[0], 64487[0], 64488[0], 64489[0], 64490[0], 64491[0], 64492[0], 64493[0], 64494[0], 64495[0], 64505[0], 64510[0], 64517[0], 64520[0], 64530[0], 67413[1], 67440[1], 67450[1], 67500[1], 69990[0], 92012[1], 92014[1], 92018[1], 92019[1], 93000[1], 93005[1], 93010[1], 93040[1], 93041[1], 93042[1], 93318[1], 93355[1], 94002[1], 94200[1], 94680[1], 94681[1], 94690[1], 95812[1], 95813[1], 95816[1], 95819[1], 95822[1], 95829[1], 95955[1], 96360[1], 96361[1], 96365[1], 96366[1], 96367[1], 96368[1], 96372[1], 96374[1], 96375[1], 96376[1], 96377[1], 96523[0], 97597[1], 97598[1], 97602[1], 99155[0], 99156[0], 99157[0], 99211[1], 99212[1], 99213[1], 99214[1], 99215[1], 99217[1], 99218[1], 99219[1], 99220[1], 99221[1], 99222[1], 99223[1], 99231[1], 99232[1], 99233[1], 99234[1], 99235[1], 99236[1], 99238[1], 99239[1], 99241[1], 99242[1], 99243[1], 99244[1], 99245[1], 99251[1], 99252[1], 99253[1], 99254[1], 99255[1], 99291[1], 99292[1], 99304[1], 99305[1], 99306[1], 99307[1], 99308[1], 99309[1], 99310[1], 99315[1], 99316[1], 99334[1], 99335[1], 99336[1], 99337[1], 99347[1], 99348[1], 99349[1], 99350[1], 99374[1], 99375[1], 99377[1], 99378[1], 99446[0], 99447[0], 99448[0], 99449[0], 99451[0], 99452[0], 99495[0], 99496[0], G0463[1], G0471[1], J0670[1], J2001[1]
67440	0213T[0], 0216T[0], 0596T[1], 0597T[1], 0708T[1], 0709T[1], 11000[1], 11001[1], 11004[1], 11005[1], 11006[1], 11042[1], 11043[1], 11044[1], 11045[1], 11046[1], 11047[1], 12001[1], 12002[1], 12004[1], 12005[1], 12006[1], 12007[1], 12011[1], 12013[1], 12014[1], 12015[1], 12016[1], 12017[1], 12018[1], 12020[1], 12021[1], 12031[1], 12032[1], 12034[1], 12035[1], 12036[1], 12037[1], 12041[1], 12042[1], 12044[1], 12045[1], 12046[1], 12047[1], 12051[1], 12052[1], 12053[1], 12054[1], 12055[1], 12056[1], 12057[1], 13100[1], 13101[1], 13102[1], 13120[1], 13121[1], 13122[1], 13131[1], 13132[1], 13133[1], 13151[1], 13152[1], 13153[1], 36000[1], 36400[1], 36405[1], 36406[1], 36410[1], 36420[1], 36425[1], 36430[1], 36440[1], 36591[0], 36592[0], 36600[1], 36640[1], 43752[1], 51701[1], 51702[1], 51703[1], 62320[0], 62321[0], 62322[0], 62323[0], 62324[0], 62325[0], 62326[0], 62327[0], 64400[0], 64405[0], 64408[0], 64415[0], 64416[0], 64417[0], 64418[0], 64420[0], 64421[0], 64425[0], 64430[0], 64435[0], 64445[0], 64446[0], 64447[0], 64448[0], 64449[0], 64450[0], 64451[0], 64454[0], 64461[0], 64462[0], 64463[0], 64479[0], 64480[0], 64483[0], 64484[0], 64486[0], 64487[0], 64488[0], 64489[0], 64490[0], 64491[0], 64492[0], 64493[0], 64494[0], 64495[0], 64505[0], 64510[0], 64517[0], 64520[0], 64530[0], 67405[1], 67450[1], 67500[1], 69990[0], 92012[1], 92014[1], 92018[1], 92019[1], 93000[1], 93005[1], 93010[1], 93040[1], 93041[1], 93042[1], 93318[1], 93355[1], 94002[1], 94200[1], 94680[1], 94681[1], 94690[1], 95812[1], 95813[1], 95816[1], 95819[1], 95822[1], 95829[1], 95955[1], 96360[1], 96361[1], 96365[1], 96366[1], 96367[1], 96368[1], 96372[1], 96374[1], 96375[1], 96376[1], 96377[1], 96523[0], 97597[1], 97598[1], 97602[1], 99155[0], 99156[0], 99157[0], 99211[1], 99212[1], 99213[1], 99214[1], 99215[1], 99217[1], 99218[1], 99219[1], 99220[1], 99221[1], 99222[1], 99223[1], 99231[1], 99232[1], 99233[1], 99234[1], 99235[1], 99236[1], 99238[1], 99239[1], 99241[1], 99242[1], 99243[1], 99244[1], 99245[1], 99251[1], 99252[1], 99253[1], 99254[1], 99255[1], 99291[1], 99292[1], 99304[1], 99305[1], 99306[1], 99307[1], 99308[1], 99309[1], 99310[1], 99315[1], 99316[1], 99334[1], 99335[1], 99336[1], 99337[1], 99347[1], 99348[1], 99349[1], 99350[1], 99374[1], 99375[1], 99377[1], 99378[1], 99446[0], 99447[0], 99448[0], 99449[0], 99451[0], 99452[0], 99495[0], 99496[0], G0463[1], G0471[1], J0670[1], J2001[1]
67445	0213T[0], 0216T[0], 0596T[1], 0597T[1], 0708T[1], 0709T[1], 11000[1], 11001[1], 11004[1], 11005[1], 11006[1], 11042[1], 11043[1], 11044[1], 11045[1], 11046[1], 11047[1], 12001[1], 12002[1], 12004[1], 12005[1], 12006[1], 12007[1], 12011[1], 12013[1], 12014[1], 12015[1], 12016[1], 12017[1], 12018[1], 12020[1], 12021[1], 12031[1], 12032[1], 12034[1], 12035[1], 12036[1], 12037[1], 12041[1], 12042[1], 12044[1], 12045[1], 12046[1], 12047[1], 12051[1], 12052[1], 12053[1], 12054[1], 12055[1], 12056[1], 12057[1], 13100[1], 13101[1], 13102[1], 13120[1], 13121[1], 13122[1], 13131[1], 13132[1], 13133[1], 13151[1], 13152[1], 13153[1], 36000[1], 36400[1], 36405[1], 36406[1], 36410[1], 36420[1], 36425[1], 36430[1], 36440[1], 36591[0], 36592[0], 36600[1], 36640[1], 43752[1], 51701[1], 51702[1], 51703[1], 62320[0], 62321[0], 62322[0], 62323[0], 62324[0], 62325[0], 62326[0], 62327[0], 64400[0], 64405[0], 64408[0], 64415[0], 64416[0], 64417[0], 64418[0], 64420[0], 64421[0], 64425[0], 64430[0], 64435[0], 64445[0], 64446[0], 64447[0], 64448[0], 64449[0], 64450[0], 64451[0], 64454[0], 64461[0], 64462[0], 64463[0], 64479[0], 64480[0], 64483[0], 64484[0], 64486[0], 64487[0], 64488[0], 64489[0], 64490[0], 64491[0], 64492[0], 64493[0], 64494[0], 64495[0], 64505[0], 64510[0], 64517[0], 64520[0], 64530[0], 67414[1], 67440[1], 67450[1], 67500[1], 69990[0], 92012[1], 92014[1], 92018[1], 92019[1], 93000[1], 93005[1], 93010[1], 93040[1], 93041[1], 93042[1], 93318[1], 93355[1], 94002[1], 94200[1], 94680[1], 94681[1], 94690[1], 95812[1], 95813[1], 95816[1], 95819[1], 95822[1], 95829[1], 95955[1], 96360[1], 96361[1], 96365[1], 96366[1], 96367[1], 96368[1], 96372[1], 96374[1], 96375[1], 96376[1], 96377[1], 96523[0], 97597[1], 97598[1], 97602[1], 99155[0], 99156[0], 99157[0], 99211[1], 99212[1], 99213[1], 99214[1], 99215[1], 99217[1], 99218[1], 99219[1], 99220[1], 99221[1], 99222[1], 99223[1], 99231[1], 99232[1], 99233[1], 99234[1], 99235[1], 99236[1], 99238[1], 99239[1], 99241[1], 99242[1], 99243[1], 99244[1], 99245[1], 99251[1], 99252[1], 99253[1], 99254[1], 99255[1], 99291[1], 99292[1], 99304[1], 99305[1], 99306[1], 99307[1], 99308[1], 99309[1], 99310[1], 99315[1], 99316[1], 99334[1], 99335[1], 99336[1], 99337[1], 99347[1], 99348[1], 99349[1], 99350[1], 99374[1], 99375[1], 99377[1], 99378[1], 99446[0], 99447[0], 99448[0], 99449[0], 99451[0], 99452[0], 99495[0], 99496[0], G0463[1], G0471[1], J0670[1], J2001[1]
67450	0213T[0], 0216T[0], 0596T[1], 0597T[1], 0708T[1], 0709T[1], 10005[1], 10007[1], 10009[1], 10011[1], 10021[1], 11000[1], 11001[1], 11004[1], 11005[1], 11006[1], 11042[1], 11043[1], 11044[1], 11045[1], 11046[1], 11047[1], 12001[1], 12002[1], 12004[1], 12005[1], 12006[1], 12007[1], 12011[1], 12013[1], 12014[1], 12015[1], 12016[1], 12017[1], 12018[1], 12020[1], 12021[1], 12031[1], 12032[1], 12034[1], 12035[1], 12036[1], 12037[1], 12041[1], 12042[1], 12044[1], 12045[1], 12046[1], 12047[1], 12051[1], 12052[1], 12053[1], 12054[1], 12055[1], 12056[1], 12057[1], 13100[1], 13101[1], 13102[1], 13120[1], 13121[1], 13122[1], 13131[1], 13132[1], 13133[1], 13151[1], 13152[1], 13153[1], 36000[1], 36400[1], 36405[1], 36406[1], 36410[1], 36420[1], 36425[1], 36430[1], 36440[1], 36591[0], 36592[0], 36600[1], 36640[1], 43752[1], 51701[1], 51702[1], 51703[1], 62320[0], 62321[0], 62322[0], 62323[0], 62324[0], 62325[0], 62326[0], 62327[0], 64400[0], 64405[0], 64408[0], 64415[0], 64416[0], 64417[0], 64418[0], 64420[0], 64421[0], 64425[0], 64430[0], 64435[0], 64445[0], 64446[0], 64447[0], 64448[0], 64449[0], 64450[0], 64451[0], 64454[0], 64461[0], 64462[0], 64463[0], 64479[0], 64480[0], 64483[0], 64484[0], 64486[0], 64487[0], 64488[0], 64489[0], 64490[0], 64491[0], 64492[0], 64493[0], 64494[0], 64495[0], 64505[0], 64510[0], 64517[0], 64520[0], 64530[0], 67400[1], 67500[1], 69990[0], 92012[1], 92014[1], 92018[1], 92019[1], 93000[1], 93005[1], 93010[1], 93040[1], 93041[1], 93042[1], 93318[1], 93355[1], 94002[1], 94200[1], 94680[1], 94681[1], 94690[1], 95812[1], 95813[1], 95816[1], 95819[1], 95822[1], 95829[1], 95955[1], 96360[1], 96361[1], 96365[1], 96366[1], 96367[1], 96368[1], 96372[1], 96374[1], 96375[1], 96376[1], 96377[1], 96523[0], 97597[1], 97598[1], 97602[1], 99155[0], 99156[0], 99157[0], 99211[1], 99212[1], 99213[1], 99214[1], 99215[1], 99217[1], 99218[1], 99219[1], 99220[1], 99221[1], 99222[1], 99223[1], 99231[1], 99232[1], 99233[1], 99234[1], 99235[1], 99236[1], 99238[1], 99239[1], 99241[1], 99242[1], 99243[1], 99244[1], 99245[1], 99251[1], 99252[1], 99253[1], 99254[1], 99255[1], 99291[1], 99292[1], 99304[1], 99305[1], 99306[1], 99307[1], 99308[1], 99309[1], 99310[1], 99315[1], 99316[1], 99334[1], 99335[1], 99336[1], 99337[1], 99347[1], 99348[1], 99349[1], 99350[1], 99374[1], 99375[1], 99377[1], 99378[1], 99446[0], 99447[0], 99448[0], 99449[0], 99451[0], 99452[0], 99495[0], 99496[0], G0463[1], G0471[1], J0670[1], J2001[1]
67500	0207T[1], 0213T[0], 0216T[0], 0563T[1], 0596T[1], 0597T[1], 0708T[1], 0709T[1], 12001[1], 12002[1], 12004[1], 12005[1], 12006[1], 12007[1], 12011[1], 12013[1], 12014[1], 12015[1], 12016[1], 12017[1], 12018[1], 12020[1], 12021[1], 12031[1], 12032[1], 12034[1], 12035[1], 12036[1], 12037[1], 12041[1], 12042[1], 12044[1], 12045[1], 12046[1], 12047[1], 12051[1], 12052[1], 12053[1], 12054[1], 12055[1], 12056[1], 12057[1], 13100[1], 13101[1], 13102[1], 13120[1], 13121[1], 13122[1], 13131[1], 13132[1], 13133[1], 13151[1], 13152[1], 13153[1], 36000[1], 36400[1], 36405[1], 36406[1], 36410[1], 36420[1], 36425[1], 36430[1], 36440[1], 36591[0], 36592[0], 36600[1], 36640[1], 43752[1], 51701[1], 51702[1], 51703[1], 62320[0], 62321[0], 62322[0], 62323[0], 62324[0], 62325[0], 62326[0], 62327[0], 64400[0], 64405[0], 64408[0], 64415[0], 64416[0], 64417[0], 64418[0], 64420[0], 64421[0], 64425[0], 64430[0], 64435[0], 64445[0], 64446[0], 64447[0], 64448[0], 64449[0], 64450[0], 64451[0], 64454[0], 64461[0], 64462[0], 64463[0], 64479[0], 64480[0], 64483[0], 64484[0], 64486[0], 64487[0], 64488[0], 64489[0], 64490[0], 64491[0], 64492[0], 64493[0], 64494[0], 64495[0], 64505[0], 64510[0], 64517[0], 64520[0], 64530[0], 69990[0], 92012[1], 92014[1], 92018[1], 92019[1], 93000[1], 93005[1], 93010[1], 93040[1], 93041[1], 93042[1], 93318[1], 93355[1], 94002[1], 94200[1], 94680[1], 94681[1], 94690[1], 95812[1], 95813[1], 95816[1], 95819[1], 95822[1], 95829[1], 95955[1], 96360[1], 96361[1], 96365[1], 96366[1], 96367[1], 96368[1], 96372[1], 96374[1], 96375[1], 96376[1], 96377[1], 96523[0], 99155[0], 99156[0], 99157[0], 99211[1], 99212[1], 99213[1], 99214[1], 99215[1], 99217[1], 99218[1], 99219[1], 99220[1], 99221[1], 99222[1], 99223[1], 99231[1], 99232[1], 99233[1], 99234[1], 99235[1], 99236[1], 99238[1], 99239[1], 99241[1], 99242[1], 99243[1], 99244[1], 99245[1], 99251[1], 99252[1], 99253[1], 99254[1], 99255[1], 99291[1], 99292[1], 99304[1], 99305[1], 99306[1], 99307[1], 99308[1], 99309[1], 99310[1], 99315[1], 99316[1], 99334[1], 99335[1], 99336[1], 99337[1], 99347[1], 99348[1], 99349[1], 99350[1], 99374[1], 99375[1], 99377[1], 99378[1], 99446[0], 99447[0], 99448[0], 99449[0], 99451[0], 99452[0], 99495[1], 99496[1], G0463[1], G0471[1], J0670[1], J2001[1]
67505	0213T[0], 0216T[0], 0596T[1], 0597T[1], 0708T[1], 0709T[1], 12001[1], 12002[1], 12004[1], 12005[1], 12006[1], 12007[1], 12011[1], 12013[1], 12014[1], 12015[1], 12016[1], 12017[1], 12018[1], 12020[1], 12021[1], 12031[1], 12032[1], 12034[1], 12035[1], 12036[1], 12037[1], 12041[1], 12042[1], 12044[1], 12045[1], 12046[1], 12047[1], 12051[1], 12052[1], 12053[1], 12054[1], 12055[1], 12056[1], 12057[1], 13100[1], 13101[1], 13102[1], 13120[1], 13121[1], 13122[1], 13131[1], 13132[1], 13133[1], 13151[1], 13152[1], 13153[1], 36000[1], 36400[1], 36405[1], 36406[1], 36410[1], 36420[1], 36425[1], 36430[1], 36440[1], 36591[0], 36592[0], 36600[1], 36640[1], 43752[1], 51701[1], 51702[1], 51703[1], 62320[0], 62321[0], 62322[0], 62323[0], 62324[0], 62325[0], 62326[0], 62327[0], 64400[0], 64405[0], 64408[0], 64415[0], 64416[0], 64417[0], 64418[0], 64420[0], 64421[0], 64425[0], 64430[0], 64435[0], 64445[0], 64446[0], 64447[0], 64448[0], 64449[0], 64450[0], 64451[0], 64454[0], 64461[0], 64462[0], 64463[0], 64479[0], 64480[0], 64483[0], 64484[0], 64486[0], 64487[0], 64488[0], 64489[0], 64490[0], 64491[0], 64492[0], 64493[0], 64494[0], 64495[0], 64505[0], 64510[0], 64517[0], 64520[0], 64530[0], 67500[1], 69990[0], 92012[1], 92014[1], 92018[1], 92019[1], 93000[1], 93005[1], 93010[1], 93040[1], 93041[1], 93042[1], 93318[1], 93355[1], 94002[1], 94200[1], 94680[1], 94681[1], 94690[1], 95812[1], 95813[1], 95816[1], 95819[1], 95822[1], 95829[1], 95955[1], 96360[1], 96361[1], 96365[1], 96366[1], 96367[1],

0 = Modifier usage not allowed or inappropriate 1 = Modifier usage allowed

Appendix A: NCCI - CPT Codes

Code 1	Code 2
	96368[1], 96372[1], 96374[1], 96375[1], 96376[1], 96377[1], 96523[0], 99155[0], 99156[0], 99157[0], 99211[1], 99212[1], 99213[1], 99214[1], 99215[1], 99217[1], 99218[1], 99219[1], 99220[1], 99221[1], 99222[1], 99223[1], 99231[1], 99232[1], 99233[1], 99234[1], 99235[1], 99236[1], 99238[1], 99239[1], 99241[1], 99242[1], 99243[1], 99244[1], 99245[1], 99251[1], 99252[1], 99253[1], 99254[1], 99255[1], 99291[1], 99292[1], 99304[1], 99305[1], 99306[1], 99307[1], 99308[1], 99309[1], 99310[1], 99315[1], 99316[1], 99334[1], 99335[1], 99336[1], 99337[1], 99347[1], 99348[1], 99349[1], 99350[1], 99374[1], 99375[1], 99377[1], 99378[1], 99446[0], 99447[0], 99448[0], 99449[0], 99451[0], 99452[0], 99495[1], 99496[1], G0463[1], G0471[1], J0670[1], J2001[1]
67515	0213T[0], 0216T[0], 0596T[1], 0597T[1], 0708T[1], 0709T[1], 12001[1], 12002[1], 12004[1], 12005[1], 12006[1], 12007[1], 12011[1], 12013[1], 12014[1], 12015[1], 12016[1], 12017[1], 12018[1], 12020[1], 12021[1], 12031[1], 12032[1], 12034[1], 12035[1], 12036[1], 12037[1], 12041[1], 12042[1], 12044[1], 12045[1], 12046[1], 12047[1], 12051[1], 12052[1], 12053[1], 12054[1], 12055[1], 12056[1], 12057[1], 13100[1], 13101[1], 13102[1], 13120[1], 13121[1], 13122[1], 13131[1], 13132[1], 13133[1], 13151[1], 13152[1], 13153[1], 36000[1], 36400[1], 36405[1], 36406[1], 36410[1], 36420[1], 36425[1], 36430[1], 36440[1], 36591[0], 36592[0], 36600[1], 36640[1], 43752[1], 51701[1], 51702[1], 51703[1], 62320[0], 62321[0], 62322[0], 62323[0], 62324[0], 62325[0], 62326[0], 62327[0], 64400[0], 64405[0], 64408[0], 64415[0], 64416[0], 64417[0], 64418[0], 64420[0], 64421[0], 64425[0], 64430[0], 64435[0], 64445[0], 64446[0], 64447[0], 64448[0], 64449[0], 64450[0], 64451[0], 64454[0], 64461[0], 64462[0], 64463[0], 64479[0], 64480[0], 64483[0], 64484[0], 64486[0], 64487[0], 64488[0], 64489[0], 64490[0], 64491[0], 64492[0], 64493[0], 64494[0], 64495[0], 64505[0], 64510[0], 64517[0], 64520[0], 64530[0], 67500[1], 67505[1], 69990[0], 92012[1], 92014[1], 92018[1], 92019[1], 93000[1], 93005[1], 93010[1], 93040[1], 93041[1], 93042[1], 93318[1], 93355[1], 94002[1], 94200[1], 94680[1], 94681[1], 94690[1], 95812[1], 95813[1], 95816[1], 95819[1], 95822[1], 95829[1], 95955[1], 96360[1], 96361[1], 96365[1], 96366[1], 96367[1], 96368[1], 96372[1], 96374[1], 96375[1], 96376[1], 96377[1], 96523[0], 99155[0], 99156[0], 99157[0], 99211[1], 99212[1], 99213[1], 99214[1], 99215[1], 99217[1], 99218[1], 99219[1], 99220[1], 99221[1], 99222[1], 99223[1], 99231[1], 99232[1], 99233[1], 99234[1], 99235[1], 99236[1], 99238[1], 99239[1], 99241[1], 99242[1], 99243[1], 99244[1], 99245[1], 99251[1], 99252[1], 99253[1], 99254[1], 99255[1], 99291[1], 99292[1], 99304[1], 99305[1], 99306[1], 99307[1], 99308[1], 99309[1], 99310[1], 99315[1], 99316[1], 99334[1], 99335[1], 99336[1], 99337[1], 99347[1], 99348[1], 99349[1], 99350[1], 99374[1], 99375[1], 99377[1], 99378[1], 99446[0], 99447[0], 99448[0], 99449[0], 99451[0], 99452[0], 99495[1], 99496[1], G0463[1], G0471[1], J0670[1], J2001[1]
67550	0213T[0], 0216T[0], 0596T[1], 0597T[1], 0708T[1], 0709T[1], 11000[1], 11001[1], 11004[1], 11005[1], 11006[1], 11042[1], 11043[1], 11044[1], 11045[1], 11046[1], 11047[1], 12001[1], 12002[1], 12004[1], 12005[1], 12006[1], 12007[1], 12011[1], 12013[1], 12014[1], 12015[1], 12016[1], 12017[1], 12018[1], 12020[1], 12021[1], 12031[1], 12032[1], 12034[1], 12035[1], 12036[1], 12037[1], 12041[1], 12042[1], 12044[1], 12045[1], 12046[1], 12047[1], 12051[1], 12052[1], 12053[1], 12054[1], 12055[1], 12056[1], 12057[1], 13100[1], 13101[1], 13102[1], 13120[1], 13121[1], 13122[1], 13131[1], 13132[1], 13133[1], 13151[1], 13152[1], 13153[1], 36000[1], 36400[1], 36405[1], 36406[1], 36410[1], 36420[1], 36425[1], 36430[1], 36440[1], 36591[0], 36592[0], 36600[1], 36640[1], 43752[1], 51701[1], 51702[1], 51703[1], 62320[0], 62321[0], 62322[0], 62323[0], 62324[0], 62325[0], 62326[0], 62327[0], 64400[0], 64405[0], 64408[0], 64415[0], 64416[0], 64417[0], 64418[0], 64420[0], 64421[0], 64425[0], 64430[0], 64435[0], 64445[0], 64446[0], 64447[0], 64448[0], 64449[0], 64450[0], 64451[0], 64454[0], 64461[0], 64462[0], 64463[0], 64479[0], 64480[0], 64483[0], 64484[0], 64486[0], 64487[0], 64488[0], 64489[0], 64490[0], 64491[0], 64492[0], 64493[0], 64494[0], 64495[0], 64505[0], 64510[0], 64517[0], 64520[0], 64530[0], 67500[1], 67560[1], 69990[0], 92012[1], 92014[1], 92018[1], 92019[1], 93000[1], 93005[1], 93010[1], 93040[1], 93041[1], 93042[1], 93318[1], 93355[1], 94002[1], 94200[1], 94680[1], 94681[1], 94690[1], 95812[1], 95813[1], 95816[1], 95819[1], 95822[1], 95829[1], 95955[1], 96360[1], 96361[1], 96365[1], 96366[1], 96367[1], 96368[1], 96372[1], 96374[1], 96375[1], 96376[1], 96377[1], 96523[0], 97597[1], 97598[1], 97602[1], 99155[0], 99156[0], 99157[0], 99211[1], 99212[1], 99213[1], 99214[1], 99215[1], 99217[1], 99218[1], 99219[1], 99220[1], 99221[1], 99222[1], 99223[1], 99231[1], 99232[1], 99233[1], 99234[1], 99235[1], 99236[1], 99238[1], 99239[1], 99241[1], 99242[1], 99243[1], 99244[1], 99245[1], 99251[1], 99252[1], 99253[1], 99254[1], 99255[1], 99291[1], 99292[1], 99304[1], 99305[1], 99306[1], 99307[1], 99308[1], 99309[1], 99310[1], 99315[1], 99316[1], 99334[1], 99335[1], 99336[1], 99337[1], 99347[1], 99348[1], 99349[1], 99350[1], 99374[1], 99375[1], 99377[1], 99378[1], 99446[0], 99447[0], 99448[0], 99449[0], 99451[0], 99452[0], 99495[0], 99496[0], G0463[1], G0471[1], J0670[1], J2001[1]
67560	0213T[0], 0216T[0], 0596T[1], 0597T[1], 0708T[1], 0709T[1], 11000[1], 11001[1], 11004[1], 11005[1], 11006[1], 11042[1], 11043[1], 11044[1], 11045[1], 11046[1], 11047[1], 12001[1], 12002[1], 12004[1], 12005[1], 12006[1], 12007[1], 12011[1], 12013[1], 12014[1], 12015[1], 12016[1], 12017[1], 12018[1], 12020[1], 12021[1], 12031[1], 12032[1], 12034[1], 12035[1], 12036[1], 12037[1], 12041[1], 12042[1], 12044[1], 12045[1], 12046[1], 12047[1], 12051[1], 12052[1], 12053[1], 12054[1], 12055[1], 12056[1], 12057[1], 13100[1], 13101[1], 13102[1], 13120[1], 13121[1], 13122[1], 13131[1], 13132[1], 13133[1], 13151[1], 13152[1], 13153[1], 36000[1], 36400[1], 36405[1], 36406[1], 36410[1], 36420[1], 36425[1], 36430[1], 36440[1], 36591[0], 36592[0], 36600[1], 36640[1], 43752[1], 51701[1], 51702[1], 51703[1], 62320[0], 62321[0], 62322[0], 62323[0], 62324[0], 62325[0], 62326[0], 62327[0], 64400[0], 64405[0], 64408[0], 64415[0], 64416[0], 64417[0], 64418[0], 64420[0], 64421[0], 64425[0], 64430[0], 64435[0], 64445[0], 64446[0], 64447[0], 64448[0], 64449[0], 64450[0], 64451[0], 64454[0], 64461[0], 64462[0], 64463[0], 64479[0], 64480[0], 64483[0], 64484[0], 64486[0], 64487[0], 64488[0], 64489[0], 64490[0], 64491[0], 64492[0], 64493[0], 64494[0], 64495[0], 64505[0], 64510[0], 64517[0], 64520[0], 64530[0], 67500[1], 69990[0], 92012[1], 92014[1], 92018[1], 92019[1], 93000[1], 93005[1], 93010[1], 93040[1], 93041[1], 93042[1], 93318[1], 93355[1], 94002[1], 94200[1], 94680[1], 94681[1], 94690[1], 95812[1], 95813[1], 95816[1], 95819[1], 95822[1], 95829[1], 95955[1], 96360[1], 96361[1], 96365[1], 96366[1], 96367[1], 96368[1], 96372[1], 96374[1], 96375[1], 96376[1], 96377[1], 96523[0], 97597[1], 97598[1], 97602[1], 99155[0], 99156[0], 99157[0], 99211[1], 99212[1], 99213[1], 99214[1], 99215[1], 99217[1], 99218[1], 99219[1], 99220[1], 99221[1], 99222[1], 99223[1], 99231[1], 99232[1], 99233[1], 99234[1], 99235[1], 99236[1], 99238[1], 99239[1], 99241[1], 99242[1], 99243[1], 99244[1], 99245[1], 99251[1], 99252[1], 99253[1], 99254[1], 99255[1], 99291[1], 99292[1], 99304[1], 99305[1], 99306[1], 99307[1], 99308[1], 99309[1], 99310[1], 99315[1], 99316[1], 99334[1], 99335[1], 99336[1], 99337[1], 99347[1], 99348[1], 99349[1], 99350[1], 99374[1], 99375[1], 99377[1], 99378[1], 99446[0], 99447[0], 99448[0], 99449[0], 99451[0], 99452[0], 99495[0], 99496[0], G0463[1], G0471[1], J0670[1], J2001[1]
67570	0213T[0], 0216T[0], 0596T[1], 0597T[1], 0708T[1], 0709T[1], 12001[1], 12002[1], 12004[1], 12005[1], 12006[1], 12007[1], 12011[1], 12013[1], 12014[1], 12015[1], 12016[1], 12017[1], 12018[1], 12020[1], 12021[1], 12031[1], 12032[1], 12034[1], 12035[1], 12036[1], 12037[1], 12041[1], 12042[1], 12044[1], 12045[1], 12046[1], 12047[1], 12051[1], 12052[1], 12053[1], 12054[1], 12055[1], 12056[1], 12057[1], 13100[1], 13101[1], 13102[1], 13120[1], 13121[1], 13122[1], 13131[1], 13132[1], 13133[1], 13151[1], 13152[1], 13153[1], 36000[1], 36400[1], 36405[1], 36406[1], 36410[1], 36420[1], 36425[1], 36430[1], 36440[1], 36591[0], 36592[0], 36600[1], 36640[1], 43752[1], 51701[1], 51702[1], 51703[1], 62320[0], 62321[0], 62322[0], 62323[0], 62324[0], 62325[0], 62326[0], 62327[0], 64400[0], 64405[0], 64408[0], 64415[0], 64416[0], 64417[0], 64418[0], 64420[0], 64421[0], 64425[0], 64430[0], 64435[0], 64445[0], 64446[0], 64447[0], 64448[0], 64449[0], 64450[0], 64451[0], 64454[0], 64461[0], 64462[0], 64463[0], 64479[0], 64480[0], 64483[0], 64484[0], 64486[0], 64487[0], 64488[0], 64489[0], 64490[0], 64491[0], 64492[0], 64493[0], 64494[0], 64495[0], 64505[0], 64510[0], 64517[0], 64520[0], 64530[0], 67311[1], 67312[1], 67400[1], 67405[1], 67440[1], 67450[1], 67500[1], 69990[0], 92012[1], 92014[1], 92018[1], 92019[1], 93000[1], 93005[1], 93010[1], 93040[1], 93041[1], 93042[1], 93318[1], 93355[1], 94002[1], 94200[1], 94680[1], 94681[1], 94690[1], 95812[1], 95813[1], 95816[1], 95819[1], 95822[1], 95829[1], 95955[1], 96360[1], 96361[1], 96365[1], 96366[1], 96367[1], 96368[1], 96372[1], 96374[1], 96375[1], 96376[1], 96377[1], 96523[0], 99155[0], 99156[0], 99157[0], 99211[1], 99212[1], 99213[1], 99214[1], 99215[1], 99217[1], 99218[1], 99219[1], 99220[1], 99221[1], 99222[1], 99223[1], 99231[1], 99232[1], 99233[1], 99234[1], 99235[1], 99236[1], 99238[1], 99239[1], 99241[1], 99242[1], 99243[1], 99244[1], 99245[1], 99251[1], 99252[1], 99253[1], 99254[1], 99255[1], 99291[1], 99292[1], 99304[1], 99305[1], 99306[1], 99307[1], 99308[1], 99309[1], 99310[1], 99315[1], 99316[1], 99334[1], 99335[1], 99336[1], 99337[1], 99347[1], 99348[1], 99349[1], 99350[1], 99374[1], 99375[1], 99377[1], 99378[1], 99446[0], 99447[0], 99448[0], 99449[0], 99451[0], 99452[0], 99495[0], 99496[0], G0463[1], G0471[1], J0670[1], J2001[1]
67700	0213T[0], 0216T[0], 0596T[1], 0597T[1], 0708T[1], 0709T[1], 11000[1], 11001[1], 11004[1], 11005[1], 11006[1], 11042[1], 11043[1], 11044[1], 11045[1], 11046[1], 11047[1], 12001[1], 12002[1], 12004[1], 12005[1], 12006[1], 12007[1], 12011[1], 12013[1], 12014[1], 12015[1], 12016[1], 12017[1], 12018[1], 12020[1], 12021[1], 12031[1], 12032[1], 12034[1], 12035[1], 12036[1], 12037[1], 12041[1], 12042[1], 12044[1], 12045[1], 12046[1], 12047[1], 12051[1], 12052[1], 12053[1], 12054[1], 12055[1], 12056[1], 12057[1], 13100[1], 13101[1], 13102[1], 13120[1], 13121[1], 13122[1], 13131[1], 13132[1], 13133[1], 13151[1], 13152[1], 13153[1], 36000[1], 36400[1], 36405[1], 36406[1], 36410[1], 36420[1], 36425[1], 36430[1], 36440[1], 36591[0], 36592[0], 36600[1], 36640[1], 43752[1], 51701[1], 51702[1], 51703[1], 62320[0], 62321[0], 62322[0], 62323[0], 62324[0], 62325[0], 62326[0], 62327[0], 64400[0], 64405[0], 64408[0], 64415[0], 64416[0], 64417[0], 64418[0], 64420[0], 64421[0], 64425[0], 64430[0], 64435[0], 64445[0], 64446[0], 64447[0], 64448[0], 64449[0], 64450[0], 64451[0], 64454[0], 64461[0], 64462[0], 64463[0], 64479[0], 64480[0], 64483[0], 64484[0], 64486[0], 64487[0], 64488[0], 64489[0], 64490[0], 64491[0], 64492[0], 64493[0], 64494[0], 64495[0], 64505[0], 64510[0], 64517[0], 64520[0], 64530[0], 67500[1], 69990[0], 92012[1], 92014[1], 92018[1], 92019[1], 93000[1], 93005[1], 93010[1], 93040[1], 93041[1], 93042[1], 93318[1], 93355[1], 94002[1], 94200[1], 94680[1], 94681[1], 94690[1], 95812[1], 95813[1], 95816[1], 95819[1], 95822[1], 95829[1], 95955[1], 96360[1], 96361[1], 96365[1], 96366[1], 96367[1], 96368[1], 96372[1], 96374[1], 96375[1], 96376[1], 96377[1], 96523[0], 97597[1], 97598[1], 97602[1], 99155[0], 99156[0], 99157[0], 99211[1], 99212[1], 99213[1], 99214[1], 99215[1], 99217[1], 99218[1], 99219[1], 99220[1], 99221[1], 99222[1], 99223[1], 99231[1], 99232[1], 99233[1], 99234[1], 99235[1], 99236[1], 99238[1], 99239[1], 99241[1], 99242[1], 99243[1], 99244[1], 99245[1], 99251[1], 99252[1], 99253[1], 99254[1], 99255[1], 99291[1], 99292[1], 99304[1], 99305[1], 99306[1], 99307[1], 99308[1], 99309[1], 99310[1], 99315[1], 99316[1], 99334[1], 99335[1], 99336[1], 99337[1], 99347[1], 99348[1], 99349[1], 99350[1], 99374[1], 99375[1], 99377[1], 99378[1], 99446[0], 99447[0], 99448[0], 99449[0], 99451[0], 99452[0], 99495[0], 99496[0], G0463[1], G0471[1], J0670[1], J2001[1]
67710	0213T[0], 0216T[0], 0596T[1], 0597T[1], 0708T[1], 0709T[1], 12001[1], 12002[1], 12004[1], 12005[1], 12006[1], 12007[1], 12011[1], 12013[1], 12014[1], 12015[1], 12016[1], 12017[1], 12018[1], 12020[1], 12021[1], 12031[1], 12032[1], 12034[1], 12035[1], 12036[1], 12037[1], 12041[1], 12042[1], 12044[1],

0 = Modifier usage not allowed or inappropriate 1 = Modifier usage allowed

Code 1	Code 2
	12045[1], 12046[1], 12047[1], 12051[1], 12052[1], 12053[1], 12054[1], 12055[1], 12056[1], 12057[1], 13100[1], 13101[1], 13102[1], 13120[1], 13121[1], 13122[1], 13131[1], 13132[1], 13133[1], 13151[1], 13152[1], 13153[1], 36000[1], 36400[1], 36405[1], 36406[1], 36410[1], 36420[1], 36425[1], 36430[1], 36440[1], 36591[0], 36592[0], 36600[1], 36640[1], 43752[1], 51701[1], 51702[1], 51703[1], 62320[0], 62321[0], 62322[0], 62323[0], 62324[0], 62325[0], 62326[0], 62327[0], 64400[0], 64405[0], 64408[0], 64415[0], 64416[0], 64417[0], 64418[0], 64420[0], 64421[0], 64425[0], 64430[0], 64435[0], 64445[0], 64446[0], 64447[0], 64448[0], 64449[0], 64450[0], 64451[0], 64454[0], 64461[0], 64462[0], 64463[0], 64479[0], 64480[0], 64483[0], 64484[0], 64486[0], 64487[0], 64488[0], 64489[0], 64490[0], 64491[0], 64492[0], 64493[0], 64494[0], 64495[0], 64505[0], 64510[0], 64517[0], 64520[0], 64530[0], 67500[1], 69990[0], 92012[1], 92014[1], 92018[1], 92019[1], 93000[1], 93005[1], 93010[1], 93040[1], 93041[1], 93042[1], 93318[1], 93355[1], 94002[1], 94200[1], 94680[1], 94681[1], 94690[1], 95812[1], 95813[1], 95816[1], 95819[1], 95822[1], 95829[1], 95955[1], 96360[1], 96361[1], 96365[1], 96366[1], 96367[1], 96368[1], 96372[1], 96374[1], 96375[1], 96376[1], 96377[1], 96523[0], 99155[0], 99156[0], 99157[0], 99211[1], 99212[1], 99213[1], 99214[1], 99215[1], 99217[1], 99218[1], 99219[1], 99220[1], 99221[1], 99222[1], 99223[1], 99231[1], 99232[1], 99233[1], 99234[1], 99235[1], 99236[1], 99238[1], 99239[1], 99241[1], 99242[1], 99243[1], 99244[1], 99245[1], 99251[1], 99252[1], 99253[1], 99254[1], 99255[1], 99291[1], 99292[1], 99304[1], 99305[1], 99306[1], 99307[1], 99308[1], 99309[1], 99310[1], 99315[1], 99316[1], 99334[1], 99335[1], 99336[1], 99337[1], 99347[1], 99348[1], 99349[1], 99350[1], 99374[1], 99375[1], 99377[1], 99378[1], 99446[0], 99447[0], 99448[0], 99449[0], 99451[0], 99452[0], 99495[0], 99496[0], G0463[1], G0471[1], J0670[1], J2001[1]
67715	0213T[0], 0216T[0], 0596T[1], 0597T[1], 0708T[1], 0709T[1], 11000[1], 11001[1], 11004[1], 11005[1], 11006[1], 11042[1], 11043[1], 11044[1], 11045[1], 11046[1], 11047[1], 12001[1], 12002[1], 12004[1], 12005[1], 12006[1], 12007[1], 12011[1], 12013[1], 12014[1], 12015[1], 12016[1], 12017[1], 12018[1], 12020[1], 12021[1], 12031[1], 12032[1], 12034[1], 12035[1], 12036[1], 12037[1], 12041[1], 12042[1], 12044[1], 12045[1], 12046[1], 12047[1], 12051[1], 12052[1], 12053[1], 12054[1], 12055[1], 12056[1], 12057[1], 13100[1], 13101[1], 13102[1], 13120[1], 13121[1], 13122[1], 13131[1], 13132[1], 13133[1], 13151[1], 13152[1], 13153[1], 36000[1], 36400[1], 36405[1], 36406[1], 36410[1], 36420[1], 36425[1], 36430[1], 36440[1], 36591[0], 36592[0], 36600[1], 36640[1], 43752[1], 51701[1], 51702[1], 51703[1], 62320[0], 62321[0], 62322[0], 62323[0], 62324[0], 62325[0], 62326[0], 62327[0], 64400[0], 64405[0], 64408[0], 64415[0], 64416[0], 64417[0], 64418[0], 64420[0], 64421[0], 64425[0], 64430[0], 64435[0], 64445[0], 64446[0], 64447[0], 64448[0], 64449[0], 64450[0], 64451[0], 64454[0], 64461[0], 64462[0], 64463[0], 64479[0], 64480[0], 64483[0], 64484[0], 64486[0], 64487[0], 64488[0], 64489[0], 64490[0], 64491[0], 64492[0], 64493[0], 64494[0], 64495[0], 64505[0], 64510[0], 64517[0], 64520[0], 64530[0], 67500[1], 69990[0], 92012[1], 92014[1], 92018[1], 92019[1], 93000[1], 93005[1], 93010[1], 93040[1], 93041[1], 93042[1], 93318[1], 93355[1], 94002[1], 94200[1], 94680[1], 94681[1], 94690[1], 95812[1], 95813[1], 95816[1], 95819[1], 95822[1], 95829[1], 95955[1], 96360[1], 96361[1], 96365[1], 96366[1], 96367[1], 96368[1], 96372[1], 96374[1], 96375[1], 96376[1], 96377[1], 96523[0], 97597[1], 97598[1], 97602[1], 99155[0], 99156[0], 99157[0], 99211[1], 99212[1], 99213[1], 99214[1], 99215[1], 99217[1], 99218[1], 99219[1], 99220[1], 99221[1], 99222[1], 99223[1], 99231[1], 99232[1], 99233[1], 99234[1], 99235[1], 99236[1], 99238[1], 99239[1], 99241[1], 99242[1], 99243[1], 99244[1], 99245[1], 99251[1], 99252[1], 99253[1], 99254[1], 99255[1], 99291[1], 99292[1], 99304[1], 99305[1], 99306[1], 99307[1], 99308[1], 99309[1], 99310[1], 99315[1], 99316[1], 99334[1], 99335[1], 99336[1], 99337[1], 99347[1], 99348[1], 99349[1], 99350[1], 99374[1], 99375[1], 99377[1], 99378[1], 99446[0], 99447[0], 99448[0], 99449[0], 99451[0], 99452[0], 99495[0], 99496[0], G0463[1], G0471[1], J0670[1], J2001[1]
67800	0207T[1], 0213T[0], 0216T[0], 0563T[1], 0596T[1], 0597T[1], 0708T[1], 0709T[1], 11000[1], 11001[1], 11004[1], 11005[1], 11006[1], 11042[1], 11043[1], 11044[1], 11045[1], 11046[1], 11047[1], 12001[1], 12002[1], 12004[1], 12005[1], 12006[1], 12007[1], 12011[1], 12013[1], 12014[1], 12015[1], 12016[1], 12017[1], 12018[1], 12020[1], 12021[1], 12031[1], 12032[1], 12034[1], 12035[1], 12036[1], 12037[1], 12041[1], 12042[1], 12044[1], 12045[1], 12046[1], 12047[1], 12051[1], 12052[1], 12053[1], 12054[1], 12055[1], 12056[1], 12057[1], 13100[1], 13101[1], 13102[1], 13120[1], 13121[1], 13122[1], 13131[1], 13132[1], 13133[1], 13151[1], 13152[1], 13153[1], 36000[1], 36400[1], 36405[1], 36406[1], 36410[1], 36420[1], 36425[1], 36430[1], 36440[1], 36591[0], 36592[0], 36600[1], 36640[1], 43752[1], 51701[1], 51702[1], 51703[1], 62320[0], 62321[0], 62322[0], 62323[0], 62324[0], 62325[0], 62326[0], 62327[0], 64400[0], 64405[0], 64408[0], 64415[0], 64416[0], 64417[0], 64418[0], 64420[0], 64421[0], 64425[0], 64430[0], 64435[0], 64445[0], 64446[0], 64447[0], 64448[0], 64449[0], 64450[0], 64451[0], 64454[0], 64461[0], 64462[0], 64463[0], 64479[0], 64480[0], 64483[0], 64484[0], 64486[0], 64487[0], 64488[0], 64489[0], 64490[0], 64491[0], 64492[0], 64493[0], 64494[0], 64495[0], 64505[0], 64510[0], 64517[0], 64520[0], 64530[0], 67500[1], 67700[1], 67810[1], 67840[1], 69990[0], 92012[1], 92014[1], 92018[1], 92019[1], 93000[1], 93005[1], 93010[1], 93040[1], 93041[1], 93042[1], 93318[1], 93355[1], 94002[1], 94200[1], 94680[1], 94681[1], 94690[1], 95812[1], 95813[1], 95816[1], 95819[1], 95822[1], 95829[1], 95955[1], 96360[1], 96361[1], 96365[1], 96366[1], 96367[1], 96368[1], 96372[1], 96374[1], 96375[1], 96376[1], 96377[1], 96523[0], 97597[1], 97598[1], 97602[1], 99155[0], 99156[0], 99157[0], 99211[1], 99212[1], 99213[1], 99214[1], 99215[1], 99217[1], 99218[1], 99219[1], 99220[1], 99221[1], 99222[1], 99223[1], 99231[1], 99232[1], 99233[1], 99234[1], 99235[1], 99236[1], 99238[1], 99239[1], 99241[1], 99242[1], 99243[1], 99244[1], 99245[1], 99251[1], 99252[1], 99253[1], 99254[1], 99255[1], 99291[1], 99292[1], 99304[1], 99305[1], 99306[1], 99307[1], 99308[1], 99309[1], 99310[1], 99315[1], 99316[1], 99334[1], 99335[1], 99336[1], 99337[1], 99347[1], 99348[1], 99349[1], 99350[1], 99374[1], 99375[1], 99377[1], 99378[1], 99446[0], 99447[0], 99448[0], 99449[0], 99451[0], 99452[0], 99495[0], 99496[0], G0463[1], G0471[1], J0670[1], J2001[1]
67801	0207T[1], 0213T[0], 0216T[0], 0563T[1], 0596T[1], 0597T[1], 0708T[1], 0709T[1], 11000[1], 11001[1], 11004[1], 11005[1], 11006[1], 11042[1], 11043[1], 11044[1], 11045[1], 11046[1], 11047[1], 12001[1], 12002[1], 12004[1], 12005[1], 12006[1], 12007[1], 12011[1], 12013[1], 12014[1], 12015[1], 12016[1], 12017[1], 12018[1], 12020[1], 12021[1], 12031[1], 12032[1], 12034[1], 12035[1], 12036[1], 12037[1], 12041[1], 12042[1], 12044[1], 12045[1], 12046[1], 12047[1], 12051[1], 12052[1], 12053[1], 12054[1], 12055[1], 12056[1], 12057[1], 13100[1], 13101[1], 13102[1], 13120[1], 13121[1], 13122[1], 13131[1], 13132[1], 13133[1], 13151[1], 13152[1], 13153[1], 36000[1], 36400[1], 36405[1], 36406[1], 36410[1], 36420[1], 36425[1], 36430[1], 36440[1], 36591[0], 36592[0], 36600[1], 36640[1], 43752[1], 51701[1], 51702[1], 51703[1], 62320[0], 62321[0], 62322[0], 62323[0], 62324[0], 62325[0], 62326[0], 62327[0], 64400[0], 64405[0], 64408[0], 64415[0], 64416[0], 64417[0], 64418[0], 64420[0], 64421[0], 64425[0], 64430[0], 64435[0], 64445[0], 64446[0], 64447[0], 64448[0], 64449[0], 64450[0], 64451[0], 64454[0], 64461[0], 64462[0], 64463[0], 64479[0], 64480[0], 64483[0], 64484[0], 64486[0], 64487[0], 64488[0], 64489[0], 64490[0], 64491[0], 64492[0], 64493[0], 64494[0], 64495[0], 64505[0], 64510[0], 64517[0], 64520[0], 64530[0], 67500[1], 67800[1], 67810[1], 67840[1], 69990[0], 92012[1], 92014[1], 92018[1], 92019[1], 93000[1], 93005[1], 93010[1], 93040[1], 93041[1], 93042[1], 93318[1], 93355[1], 94002[1], 94200[1], 94680[1], 94681[1], 94690[1], 95812[1], 95813[1], 95816[1], 95819[1], 95822[1], 95829[1], 95955[1], 96360[1], 96361[1], 96365[1], 96366[1], 96367[1], 96368[1], 96372[1], 96374[1], 96375[1], 96376[1], 96377[1], 96523[0], 97597[1], 97598[1], 97602[1], 99155[0], 99156[0], 99157[0], 99211[1], 99212[1], 99213[1], 99214[1], 99215[1], 99217[1], 99218[1], 99219[1], 99220[1], 99221[1], 99222[1], 99223[1], 99231[1], 99232[1], 99233[1], 99234[1], 99235[1], 99236[1], 99238[1], 99239[1], 99241[1], 99242[1], 99243[1], 99244[1], 99245[1], 99251[1], 99252[1], 99253[1], 99254[1], 99255[1], 99291[1], 99292[1], 99304[1], 99305[1], 99306[1], 99307[1], 99308[1], 99309[1], 99310[1], 99315[1], 99316[1], 99334[1], 99335[1], 99336[1], 99337[1], 99347[1], 99348[1], 99349[1], 99350[1], 99374[1], 99375[1], 99377[1], 99378[1], 99446[0], 99447[0], 99448[0], 99449[0], 99451[0], 99452[0], 99495[0], 99496[0], G0463[1], G0471[1], J0670[1], J2001[1]
67805	0207T[1], 0213T[0], 0216T[0], 0563T[1], 0596T[1], 0597T[1], 0708T[1], 0709T[1], 11000[1], 11001[1], 11004[1], 11005[1], 11006[1], 11042[1], 11043[1], 11044[1], 11045[1], 11046[1], 11047[1], 12001[1], 12002[1], 12004[1], 12005[1], 12006[1], 12007[1], 12011[1], 12013[1], 12014[1], 12015[1], 12016[1], 12017[1], 12018[1], 12020[1], 12021[1], 12031[1], 12032[1], 12034[1], 12035[1], 12036[1], 12037[1], 12041[1], 12042[1], 12044[1], 12045[1], 12046[1], 12047[1], 12051[1], 12052[1], 12053[1], 12054[1], 12055[1], 12056[1], 12057[1], 13100[1], 13101[1], 13102[1], 13120[1], 13121[1], 13122[1], 13131[1], 13132[1], 13133[1], 13151[1], 13152[1], 13153[1], 36000[1], 36400[1], 36405[1], 36406[1], 36410[1], 36420[1], 36425[1], 36430[1], 36440[1], 36591[0], 36592[0], 36600[1], 36640[1], 43752[1], 51701[1], 51702[1], 51703[1], 62320[0], 62321[0], 62322[0], 62323[0], 62324[0], 62325[0], 62326[0], 62327[0], 64400[0], 64405[0], 64408[0], 64415[0], 64416[0], 64417[0], 64418[0], 64420[0], 64421[0], 64425[0], 64430[0], 64435[0], 64445[0], 64446[0], 64447[0], 64448[0], 64449[0], 64450[0], 64451[0], 64454[0], 64461[0], 64462[0], 64463[0], 64479[0], 64480[0], 64483[0], 64484[0], 64486[0], 64487[0], 64488[0], 64489[0], 64490[0], 64491[0], 64492[0], 64493[0], 64494[0], 64495[0], 64505[0], 64510[0], 64517[0], 64520[0], 64530[0], 67500[1], 67800[1], 67801[1], 67810[1], 67840[1], 69990[0], 92012[1], 92014[1], 92018[1], 92019[1], 93000[1], 93005[1], 93010[1], 93040[1], 93041[1], 93042[1], 93318[1], 93355[1], 94002[1], 94200[1], 94680[1], 94681[1], 94690[1], 95812[1], 95813[1], 95816[1], 95819[1], 95822[1], 95829[1], 95955[1], 96360[1], 96361[1], 96365[1], 96366[1], 96367[1], 96368[1], 96372[1], 96374[1], 96375[1], 96376[1], 96377[1], 96523[0], 97597[1], 97598[1], 97602[1], 99155[0], 99156[0], 99157[0], 99211[1], 99212[1], 99213[1], 99214[1], 99215[1], 99217[1], 99218[1], 99219[1], 99220[1], 99221[1], 99222[1], 99223[1], 99231[1], 99232[1], 99233[1], 99234[1], 99235[1], 99236[1], 99238[1], 99239[1], 99241[1], 99242[1], 99243[1], 99244[1], 99245[1], 99251[1], 99252[1], 99253[1], 99254[1], 99255[1], 99291[1], 99292[1], 99304[1], 99305[1], 99306[1], 99307[1], 99308[1], 99309[1], 99310[1], 99315[1], 99316[1], 99334[1], 99335[1], 99336[1], 99337[1], 99347[1], 99348[1], 99349[1], 99350[1], 99374[1], 99375[1], 99377[1], 99378[1], 99446[0], 99447[0], 99448[0], 99449[0], 99451[0], 99452[0], 99495[0], 99496[0], G0463[1], G0471[1], J0670[1], J2001[1]
67808	0207T[1], 0213T[0], 0216T[0], 0563T[1], 0596T[1], 0597T[1], 0708T[1], 0709T[1], 11000[1], 11001[1], 11004[1], 11005[1], 11006[1], 11042[1], 11043[1], 11044[1], 11045[1], 11046[1], 11047[1], 12001[1], 12002[1], 12004[1], 12005[1], 12006[1], 12007[1], 12011[1], 12013[1], 12014[1], 12015[1], 12016[1], 12017[1], 12018[1], 12020[1], 12021[1], 12031[1], 12032[1], 12034[1], 12035[1], 12036[1], 12037[1], 12041[1], 12042[1], 12044[1], 12045[1], 12046[1], 12047[1], 12051[1], 12052[1], 12053[1], 12054[1], 12055[1], 12056[1], 12057[1], 13100[1], 13101[1], 13102[1], 13120[1], 13121[1], 13122[1], 13131[1], 13132[1], 13133[1], 13151[1], 13152[1], 13153[1], 36000[1], 36400[1], 36405[1], 36406[1], 36410[1], 36420[1], 36425[1], 36430[1], 36440[1], 36591[0], 36592[0], 36600[1], 36640[1], 43752[1], 51701[1], 51702[1], 51703[1], 62320[0], 62321[0], 62322[0], 62323[0], 62324[0], 62325[0], 62326[0], 62327[0], 64400[0], 64405[0], 64408[0], 64415[0], 64416[0], 64417[0], 64418[0], 64420[0], 64421[0], 64425[0], 64430[0], 64435[0], 64445[0], 64446[0], 64447[0], 64448[0], 64449[0], 64450[0], 64451[0], 64454[0], 64461[0], 64462[0], 64463[0], 64479[0], 64480[0], 64483[0], 64484[0], 64486[0], 64487[0], 64488[0],

0 = Modifier usage not allowed or inappropriate 1 = Modifier usage allowed

Appendix A: NCCI - CPT Codes

Code 1	Code 2
	64489[0], 64490[0], 64491[0], 64492[0], 64493[0], 64494[0], 64495[0], 64505[0], 64510[0], 64517[0], 64520[0], 64530[0], 67500[1], 67800[1], 67801[1], 67805[1], 67810[1], 67840[1], 69990[0], 92012[1], 92014[1], 92018[1], 92019[1], 93000[1], 93005[1], 93010[1], 93040[1], 93041[1], 93042[1], 93318[1], 93355[1], 94002[1], 94200[1], 94680[1], 94681[1], 94690[1], 95812[1], 95813[1], 95816[1], 95819[1], 95822[1], 95829[1], 95955[1], 96360[1], 96361[1], 96365[1], 96366[1], 96367[1], 96368[1], 96372[1], 96374[1], 96375[1], 96376[1], 96377[1], 96523[0], 97597[1], 97598[1], 97602[1], 99155[0], 99156[0], 99157[0], 99211[1], 99212[1], 99213[1], 99214[1], 99215[1], 99217[1], 99218[1], 99219[1], 99220[1], 99221[1], 99222[1], 99223[1], 99231[1], 99232[1], 99233[1], 99234[1], 99235[1], 99236[1], 99238[1], 99239[1], 99241[1], 99242[1], 99243[1], 99244[1], 99245[1], 99251[1], 99252[1], 99253[1], 99254[1], 99255[1], 99291[1], 99292[1], 99304[1], 99305[1], 99306[1], 99307[1], 99308[1], 99309[1], 99310[1], 99315[1], 99316[1], 99334[1], 99335[1], 99336[1], 99337[1], 99347[1], 99348[1], 99349[1], 99350[1], 99374[1], 99375[1], 99377[1], 99378[1], 99446[0], 99447[0], 99448[0], 99449[0], 99451[0], 99452[0], 99495[0], 99496[0], G0463[1], G0471[1], J2001[1]
67810	0213T[0], 0216T[0], 0596T[1], 0597T[1], 0708T[1], 0709T[1], 10005[1], 10007[1], 10009[1], 10011[1], 10021[1], 11102[1], 11104[1], 11106[1], 11310[1], 11311[1], 11312[1], 11313[1], 12001[1], 12002[1], 12004[1], 12005[1], 12006[1], 12007[1], 12011[1], 12013[1], 12014[1], 12015[1], 12016[1], 12017[1], 12018[1], 12020[1], 12021[1], 12031[1], 12032[1], 12034[1], 12035[1], 12036[1], 12037[1], 12041[1], 12042[1], 12044[1], 12045[1], 12046[1], 12047[1], 12051[1], 12052[1], 12053[1], 12054[1], 12055[1], 12056[1], 12057[1], 13100[1], 13101[1], 13102[1], 13120[1], 13121[1], 13122[1], 13131[1], 13132[1], 13133[1], 13151[1], 13152[1], 13153[1], 36000[1], 36400[1], 36405[1], 36406[1], 36410[1], 36420[1], 36425[1], 36430[1], 36440[1], 36591[0], 36592[0], 36600[1], 36640[1], 43752[1], 51701[1], 51702[1], 51703[1], 62320[0], 62321[0], 62322[0], 62323[0], 62324[0], 62325[0], 62326[0], 62327[0], 64400[0], 64405[0], 64408[0], 64415[0], 64416[0], 64417[0], 64418[0], 64420[0], 64421[0], 64425[0], 64430[0], 64435[0], 64445[0], 64446[0], 64447[0], 64448[0], 64449[0], 64450[0], 64451[0], 64454[0], 64461[0], 64462[0], 64463[0], 64479[0], 64480[0], 64483[0], 64484[0], 64486[0], 64487[0], 64488[0], 64489[0], 64490[0], 64491[0], 64492[0], 64493[0], 64494[0], 64495[0], 64505[0], 64510[0], 64517[0], 64520[0], 64530[0], 67500[1], 69990[0], 92012[1], 92014[1], 92018[1], 92019[1], 93000[1], 93005[1], 93010[1], 93040[1], 93041[1], 93042[1], 93318[1], 93355[1], 94002[1], 94200[1], 94680[1], 94681[1], 94690[1], 95812[1], 95813[1], 95816[1], 95819[1], 95822[1], 95829[1], 95955[1], 96360[1], 96361[1], 96365[1], 96366[1], 96367[1], 96368[1], 96372[1], 96374[1], 96375[1], 96376[1], 96377[1], 96523[0], 99155[0], 99156[0], 99157[0], 99211[1], 99212[1], 99213[1], 99214[1], 99215[1], 99217[1], 99218[1], 99219[1], 99220[1], 99221[1], 99222[1], 99223[1], 99231[1], 99232[1], 99233[1], 99234[1], 99235[1], 99236[1], 99238[1], 99239[1], 99241[1], 99242[1], 99243[1], 99244[1], 99245[1], 99251[1], 99252[1], 99253[1], 99254[1], 99255[1], 99291[1], 99292[1], 99304[1], 99305[1], 99306[1], 99307[1], 99308[1], 99309[1], 99310[1], 99315[1], 99316[1], 99334[1], 99335[1], 99336[1], 99337[1], 99347[1], 99348[1], 99349[1], 99350[1], 99374[1], 99375[1], 99377[1], 99378[1], 99446[0], 99447[0], 99448[0], 99449[0], 99451[0], 99452[0], 99495[1], 99496[1], G0463[1], G0471[1], J0670[1], J2001[1]
67820	0213T[0], 0216T[0], 0596T[1], 0597T[1], 0708T[1], 0709T[1], 12001[1], 12002[1], 12004[1], 12005[1], 12006[1], 12007[1], 12011[1], 12013[1], 12014[1], 12015[1], 12016[1], 12017[1], 12018[1], 12020[1], 12021[1], 12031[1], 12032[1], 12034[1], 12035[1], 12036[1], 12037[1], 12041[1], 12042[1], 12044[1], 12045[1], 12046[1], 12047[1], 12051[1], 12052[1], 12053[1], 12054[1], 12055[1], 12056[1], 12057[1], 13100[1], 13101[1], 13102[1], 13120[1], 13121[1], 13122[1], 13131[1], 13132[1], 13133[1], 13151[1], 13152[1], 13153[1], 36000[1], 36400[1], 36405[1], 36406[1], 36410[1], 36420[1], 36425[1], 36430[1], 36440[1], 36591[0], 36592[0], 36600[1], 36640[1], 43752[1], 51701[1], 51702[1], 51703[1], 62320[0], 62321[0], 62322[0], 62323[0], 62324[0], 62325[0], 62326[0], 62327[0], 64400[0], 64405[0], 64408[0], 64415[0], 64416[0], 64417[0], 64418[0], 64420[0], 64421[0], 64425[0], 64430[0], 64435[0], 64445[0], 64446[0], 64447[0], 64448[0], 64449[0], 64450[0], 64451[0], 64454[0], 64461[0], 64462[0], 64463[0], 64479[0], 64480[0], 64483[0], 64484[0], 64486[0], 64487[0], 64488[0], 64489[0], 64490[0], 64491[0], 64492[0], 64493[0], 64494[0], 64495[0], 64505[0], 64510[0], 64517[0], 64520[0], 64530[0], 67500[1], 69990[0], 92012[1], 92014[1], 92018[1], 92019[1], 93000[1], 93005[1], 93010[1], 93040[1], 93041[1], 93042[1], 93318[1], 93355[1], 94002[1], 94200[1], 94680[1], 94681[1], 94690[1], 95812[1], 95813[1], 95816[1], 95819[1], 95822[1], 95829[1], 95955[1], 96360[1], 96361[1], 96365[1], 96366[1], 96367[1], 96368[1], 96372[1], 96374[1], 96375[1], 96376[1], 96377[1], 96523[0], 99155[0], 99156[0], 99157[0], 99211[1], 99212[1], 99213[1], 99214[1], 99215[1], 99217[1], 99218[1], 99219[1], 99220[1], 99221[1], 99222[1], 99223[1], 99231[1], 99232[1], 99233[1], 99234[1], 99235[1], 99236[1], 99238[1], 99239[1], 99241[1], 99242[1], 99243[1], 99244[1], 99245[1], 99251[1], 99252[1], 99253[1], 99254[1], 99255[1], 99291[1], 99292[1], 99304[1], 99305[1], 99306[1], 99307[1], 99308[1], 99309[1], 99310[1], 99315[1], 99316[1], 99334[1], 99335[1], 99336[1], 99337[1], 99347[1], 99348[1], 99349[1], 99350[1], 99374[1], 99375[1], 99377[1], 99378[1], 99446[0], 99447[0], 99448[0], 99449[0], 99451[0], 99452[0], 99495[1], 99496[1], G0463[1], G0471[1]
67825	0213T[0], 0216T[0], 0596T[1], 0597T[1], 0708T[1], 0709T[1], 12001[1], 12002[1], 12004[1], 12005[1], 12006[1], 12007[1], 12011[1], 12013[1], 12014[1], 12015[1], 12016[1], 12017[1], 12018[1], 12020[1], 12021[1], 12031[1], 12032[1], 12034[1], 12035[1], 12036[1], 12037[1], 12041[1], 12042[1], 12044[1], 12045[1], 12046[1], 12047[1], 12051[1], 12052[1], 12053[1], 12054[1], 12055[1], 12056[1], 12057[1], 13100[1], 13101[1], 13102[1], 13120[1], 13121[1], 13122[1], 13131[1], 13132[1], 13133[1], 13151[1], 13152[1], 13153[1], 36000[1], 36400[1], 36405[1], 36406[1], 36410[1], 36420[1], 36425[1], 36430[1], 36440[1], 36591[0], 36592[0], 36600[1], 36640[1], 43752[1], 51701[1], 51702[1], 51703[1], 62320[0], 62321[0], 62322[0], 62323[0], 62324[0], 62325[0], 62326[0], 62327[0], 64400[0], 64405[0], 64408[0], 64415[0], 64416[0], 64417[0], 64418[0], 64420[0], 64421[0], 64425[0], 64430[0], 64435[0], 64445[0], 64446[0], 64447[0], 64448[0], 64449[0], 64450[0], 64451[0], 64454[0], 64461[0], 64462[0], 64463[0], 64479[0], 64480[0], 64483[0], 64484[0], 64486[0], 64487[0], 64488[0], 64489[0], 64490[0], 64491[0], 64492[0], 64493[0], 64494[0], 64495[0], 64505[0], 64510[0], 64517[0], 64520[0], 64530[0], 67500[1], 67820[1], 69990[0], 92012[1], 92014[1], 92018[1], 92019[1], 93000[1], 93005[1], 93010[1], 93040[1], 93041[1], 93042[1], 93318[1], 93355[1], 94002[1], 94200[1], 94680[1], 94681[1], 94690[1], 95812[1], 95813[1], 95816[1], 95819[1], 95822[1], 95829[1], 95955[1], 96360[1], 96361[1], 96365[1], 96366[1], 96367[1], 96368[1], 96372[1], 96374[1], 96375[1], 96376[1], 96377[1], 96523[0], 99155[0], 99156[0], 99157[0], 99211[1], 99212[1], 99213[1], 99214[1], 99215[1], 99217[1], 99218[1], 99219[1], 99220[1], 99221[1], 99222[1], 99223[1], 99231[1], 99232[1], 99233[1], 99234[1], 99235[1], 99236[1], 99238[1], 99239[1], 99241[1], 99242[1], 99243[1], 99244[1], 99245[1], 99251[1], 99252[1], 99253[1], 99254[1], 99255[1], 99291[1], 99292[1], 99304[1], 99305[1], 99306[1], 99307[1], 99308[1], 99309[1], 99310[1], 99315[1], 99316[1], 99334[1], 99335[1], 99336[1], 99337[1], 99347[1], 99348[1], 99349[1], 99350[1], 99374[1], 99375[1], 99377[1], 99378[1], 99446[0], 99447[0], 99448[0], 99449[0], 99451[0], 99452[0], 99495[0], 99496[0], G0463[1], G0471[1], J0670[1], J2001[1]
67830	0213T[0], 0216T[0], 0596T[1], 0597T[1], 0708T[1], 0709T[1], 12001[1], 12002[1], 12004[1], 12005[1], 12006[1], 12007[1], 12011[1], 12013[1], 12014[1], 12015[1], 12016[1], 12017[1], 12018[1], 12020[1], 12021[1], 12031[1], 12032[1], 12034[1], 12035[1], 12036[1], 12037[1], 12041[1], 12042[1], 12044[1], 12045[1], 12046[1], 12047[1], 12051[1], 12052[1], 12053[1], 12054[1], 12055[1], 12056[1], 12057[1], 13100[1], 13101[1], 13102[1], 13120[1], 13121[1], 13122[1], 13131[1], 13132[1], 13133[1], 13151[1], 13152[1], 13153[1], 36000[1], 36400[1], 36405[1], 36406[1], 36410[1], 36420[1], 36425[1], 36430[1], 36440[1], 36591[0], 36592[0], 36600[1], 36640[1], 43752[1], 51701[1], 51702[1], 51703[1], 62320[0], 62321[0], 62322[0], 62323[0], 62324[0], 62325[0], 62326[0], 62327[0], 64400[0], 64405[0], 64408[0], 64415[0], 64416[0], 64417[0], 64418[0], 64420[0], 64421[0], 64425[0], 64430[0], 64435[0], 64445[0], 64446[0], 64447[0], 64448[0], 64449[0], 64450[0], 64451[0], 64454[0], 64461[0], 64462[0], 64463[0], 64479[0], 64480[0], 64483[0], 64484[0], 64486[0], 64487[0], 64488[0], 64489[0], 64490[0], 64491[0], 64492[0], 64493[0], 64494[0], 64495[0], 64505[0], 64510[0], 64517[0], 64520[0], 64530[0], 67500[1], 67840[1], 69990[0], 92012[1], 92014[1], 92018[1], 92019[1], 93000[1], 93005[1], 93010[1], 93040[1], 93041[1], 93042[1], 93318[1], 93355[1], 94002[1], 94200[1], 94680[1], 94681[1], 94690[1], 95812[1], 95813[1], 95816[1], 95819[1], 95822[1], 95829[1], 95955[1], 96360[1], 96361[1], 96365[1], 96366[1], 96367[1], 96368[1], 96372[1], 96374[1], 96375[1], 96376[1], 96377[1], 96523[0], 99155[0], 99156[0], 99157[0], 99211[1], 99212[1], 99213[1], 99214[1], 99215[1], 99217[1], 99218[1], 99219[1], 99220[1], 99221[1], 99222[1], 99223[1], 99231[1], 99232[1], 99233[1], 99234[1], 99235[1], 99236[1], 99238[1], 99239[1], 99241[1], 99242[1], 99243[1], 99244[1], 99245[1], 99251[1], 99252[1], 99253[1], 99254[1], 99255[1], 99291[1], 99292[1], 99304[1], 99305[1], 99306[1], 99307[1], 99308[1], 99309[1], 99310[1], 99315[1], 99316[1], 99334[1], 99335[1], 99336[1], 99337[1], 99347[1], 99348[1], 99349[1], 99350[1], 99374[1], 99375[1], 99377[1], 99378[1], 99446[0], 99447[0], 99448[0], 99449[0], 99451[0], 99452[0], 99495[0], 99496[0], G0463[1], G0471[1], J0670[1], J2001[1]
67835	0213T[0], 0216T[0], 0596T[1], 0597T[1], 0708T[1], 0709T[1], 12001[1], 12002[1], 12004[1], 12005[1], 12006[1], 12007[1], 12011[1], 12013[1], 12014[1], 12015[1], 12016[1], 12017[1], 12018[1], 12020[1], 12021[1], 12031[1], 12032[1], 12034[1], 12035[1], 12036[1], 12037[1], 12041[1], 12042[1], 12044[1], 12045[1], 12046[1], 12047[1], 12051[1], 12052[1], 12053[1], 12054[1], 12055[1], 12056[1], 12057[1], 13100[1], 13101[1], 13102[1], 13120[1], 13121[1], 13122[1], 13131[1], 13132[1], 13133[1], 13151[1], 13152[1], 13153[1], 36000[1], 36400[1], 36405[1], 36406[1], 36410[1], 36420[1], 36425[1], 36430[1], 36440[1], 36591[0], 36592[0], 36600[1], 36640[1], 43752[1], 51701[1], 51702[1], 51703[1], 62320[0], 62321[0], 62322[0], 62323[0], 62324[0], 62325[0], 62326[0], 62327[0], 64400[0], 64405[0], 64408[0], 64415[0], 64416[0], 64417[0], 64418[0], 64420[0], 64421[0], 64425[0], 64430[0], 64435[0], 64445[0], 64446[0], 64447[0], 64448[0], 64449[0], 64450[0], 64451[0], 64454[0], 64461[0], 64462[0], 64463[0], 64479[0], 64480[0], 64483[0], 64484[0], 64486[0], 64487[0], 64488[0], 64489[0], 64490[0], 64491[0], 64492[0], 64493[0], 64494[0], 64495[0], 64505[0], 64510[0], 64517[0], 64520[0], 64530[0], 67500[1], 67830[1], 67840[1], 69990[0], 92012[1], 92014[1], 92018[1], 92019[1], 93000[1], 93005[1], 93010[1], 93040[1], 93041[1], 93042[1], 93318[1], 93355[1], 94002[1], 94200[1], 94680[1], 94681[1], 94690[1], 95812[1], 95813[1], 95816[1], 95819[1], 95822[1], 95829[1], 95955[1], 96360[1], 96361[1], 96365[1], 96366[1], 96367[1], 96368[1], 96372[1], 96374[1], 96375[1], 96376[1], 96377[1], 96523[0], 99155[0], 99156[0], 99157[0], 99211[1], 99212[1], 99213[1], 99214[1], 99215[1], 99217[1], 99218[1], 99219[1], 99220[1], 99221[1], 99222[1], 99223[1], 99231[1], 99232[1], 99233[1], 99234[1], 99235[1], 99236[1], 99238[1], 99239[1], 99241[1], 99242[1], 99243[1], 99244[1], 99245[1], 99251[1], 99252[1], 99253[1], 99254[1], 99255[1], 99291[1], 99292[1], 99304[1], 99305[1], 99306[1], 99307[1], 99308[1], 99309[1], 99310[1], 99315[1], 99316[1], 99334[1], 99335[1], 99336[1], 99337[1], 99347[1], 99348[1], 99349[1], 99350[1], 99374[1], 99375[1], 99377[1], 99378[1], 99446[0], 99447[0], 99448[0], 99449[0], 99451[0], 99452[0], 99495[0], 99496[0], G0463[1], G0471[1]

Appendix A: NCCI - CPT Codes

0 = Modifier usage not allowed or inappropriate 1 = Modifier usage allowed

Code 1	Code 2
67840	0207T[1], 0213T[0], 0216T[0], 0563T[1], 0596T[1], 0597T[1], 0708T[1], 0709T[1], 11000[1], 11001[1], 11004[1], 11005[1], 11006[1], 11042[1], 11043[1], 11044[1], 11045[1], 11046[1], 11047[1], 12001[1], 12002[1], 12004[1], 12005[1], 12006[1], 12007[1], 12011[1], 12013[1], 12014[1], 12015[1], 12016[1], 12017[1], 12018[1], 12020[1], 12021[1], 12031[1], 12032[1], 12034[1], 12035[1], 12036[1], 12037[1], 12041[1], 12042[1], 12044[1], 12045[1], 12046[1], 12047[1], 12051[1], 12052[1], 12053[1], 12054[1], 12055[1], 12056[1], 12057[1], 13100[1], 13101[1], 13102[1], 13120[1], 13121[1], 13122[1], 13131[1], 13132[1], 13133[1], 13151[1], 13152[1], 13153[1], 36000[1], 36400[1], 36405[1], 36406[1], 36410[1], 36420[1], 36425[1], 36430[1], 36440[1], 36591[0], 36592[0], 36600[1], 36640[1], 43752[1], 51701[1], 51702[1], 51703[1], 62320[0], 62321[0], 62322[0], 62323[0], 62324[0], 62325[0], 62326[0], 62327[0], 64400[0], 64405[0], 64408[0], 64415[0], 64416[0], 64417[0], 64418[0], 64420[0], 64421[0], 64425[0], 64430[0], 64435[0], 64445[0], 64446[0], 64447[0], 64448[0], 64449[0], 64450[0], 64451[0], 64454[0], 64461[0], 64462[0], 64463[0], 64479[0], 64480[0], 64483[0], 64484[0], 64486[0], 64487[0], 64488[0], 64489[0], 64490[0], 64491[0], 64492[0], 64493[0], 64494[0], 64495[0], 64505[0], 64510[0], 64517[0], 64520[0], 64530[0], 67500[1], 67850[1], 69990[0], 92012[1], 92014[1], 92018[1], 92019[1], 93000[1], 93005[1], 93010[1], 93040[1], 93041[1], 93042[1], 93318[1], 93355[1], 94002[1], 94200[1], 94680[1], 94681[1], 94690[1], 95812[1], 95813[1], 95816[1], 95819[1], 95822[1], 95829[1], 95955[1], 96360[1], 96361[1], 96365[1], 96366[1], 96367[1], 96368[1], 96372[1], 96374[1], 96375[1], 96376[1], 96377[1], 96523[0], 97597[1], 97598[1], 97602[1], 99155[0], 99156[0], 99157[0], 99211[1], 99212[1], 99213[1], 99214[1], 99215[1], 99217[1], 99218[1], 99219[1], 99220[1], 99221[1], 99222[1], 99223[1], 99231[1], 99232[1], 99233[1], 99234[1], 99235[1], 99236[1], 99238[1], 99239[1], 99241[1], 99242[1], 99243[1], 99244[1], 99245[1], 99251[1], 99252[1], 99253[1], 99254[1], 99255[1], 99291[1], 99292[1], 99304[1], 99305[1], 99306[1], 99307[1], 99308[1], 99309[1], 99310[1], 99315[1], 99316[1], 99334[1], 99335[1], 99336[1], 99337[1], 99347[1], 99348[1], 99349[1], 99350[1], 99374[1], 99375[1], 99377[1], 99378[1], 99446[0], 99447[0], 99448[0], 99449[0], 99451[0], 99452[0], 99495[0], 99496[0], G0463[1], G0471[1], J0670[1], J2001[1]
67850	0207T[1], 0213T[0], 0216T[0], 0563T[1], 0596T[1], 0597T[1], 0708T[1], 0709T[1], 12001[1], 12002[1], 12004[1], 12005[1], 12006[1], 12007[1], 12011[1], 12013[1], 12014[1], 12015[1], 12016[1], 12017[1], 12018[1], 12020[1], 12021[1], 12031[1], 12032[1], 12034[1], 12035[1], 12036[1], 12037[1], 12041[1], 12042[1], 12044[1], 12045[1], 12046[1], 12047[1], 12051[1], 12052[1], 12053[1], 12054[1], 12055[1], 12056[1], 12057[1], 13100[1], 13101[1], 13102[1], 13120[1], 13121[1], 13122[1], 13131[1], 13132[1], 13133[1], 13151[1], 13152[1], 13153[1], 36000[1], 36400[1], 36405[1], 36406[1], 36410[1], 36420[1], 36425[1], 36430[1], 36440[1], 36591[0], 36592[0], 36600[1], 36640[1], 43752[1], 51701[1], 51702[1], 51703[1], 62320[0], 62321[0], 62322[0], 62323[0], 62324[0], 62325[0], 62326[0], 62327[0], 64400[0], 64405[0], 64408[0], 64415[0], 64416[0], 64417[0], 64418[0], 64420[0], 64421[0], 64425[0], 64430[0], 64435[0], 64445[0], 64446[0], 64447[0], 64448[0], 64449[0], 64450[0], 64451[0], 64454[0], 64461[0], 64462[0], 64463[0], 64479[0], 64480[0], 64483[0], 64484[0], 64486[0], 64487[0], 64488[0], 64489[0], 64490[0], 64491[0], 64492[0], 64493[0], 64494[0], 64495[0], 64505[0], 64510[0], 64517[0], 64520[0], 64530[0], 67500[1], 69990[0], 92012[1], 92014[1], 92018[1], 92019[1], 93000[1], 93005[1], 93010[1], 93040[1], 93041[1], 93042[1], 93318[1], 93355[1], 94002[1], 94200[1], 94680[1], 94681[1], 94690[1], 95812[1], 95813[1], 95816[1], 95819[1], 95822[1], 95829[1], 95955[1], 96360[1], 96361[1], 96365[1], 96366[1], 96367[1], 96368[1], 96372[1], 96374[1], 96375[1], 96376[1], 96377[1], 96523[0], 99155[0], 99156[0], 99157[0], 99211[1], 99212[1], 99213[1], 99214[1], 99215[1], 99217[1], 99218[1], 99219[1], 99220[1], 99221[1], 99222[1], 99223[1], 99231[1], 99232[1], 99233[1], 99234[1], 99235[1], 99236[1], 99238[1], 99239[1], 99241[1], 99242[1], 99243[1], 99244[1], 99245[1], 99251[1], 99252[1], 99253[1], 99254[1], 99255[1], 99291[1], 99292[1], 99304[1], 99305[1], 99306[1], 99307[1], 99308[1], 99309[1], 99310[1], 99315[1], 99316[1], 99334[1], 99335[1], 99336[1], 99337[1], 99347[1], 99348[1], 99349[1], 99350[1], 99374[1], 99375[1], 99377[1], 99378[1], 99446[0], 99447[0], 99448[0], 99449[0], 99451[0], 99452[0], 99495[0], 99496[0], G0463[1], G0471[1], J0670[1], J2001[1]
67875	0213T[0], 0216T[0], 0596T[1], 0597T[1], 0708T[1], 0709T[1], 11000[1], 11001[1], 11004[1], 11005[1], 11006[1], 11042[1], 11043[1], 11044[1], 11045[1], 11046[1], 11047[1], 12001[1], 12002[1], 12004[1], 12005[1], 12006[1], 12007[1], 12011[1], 12013[1], 12014[1], 12015[1], 12016[1], 12017[1], 12018[1], 12020[1], 12021[1], 12031[1], 12032[1], 12034[1], 12035[1], 12036[1], 12037[1], 12041[1], 12042[1], 12044[1], 12045[1], 12046[1], 12047[1], 12051[1], 12052[1], 12053[1], 12054[1], 12055[1], 12056[1], 12057[1], 13100[1], 13101[1], 13102[1], 13120[1], 13121[1], 13122[1], 13131[1], 13132[1], 13133[1], 13151[1], 13152[1], 13153[1], 36000[1], 36400[1], 36405[1], 36406[1], 36410[1], 36420[1], 36425[1], 36430[1], 36440[1], 36591[0], 36592[0], 36600[1], 36640[1], 43752[1], 51701[1], 51702[1], 51703[1], 62320[0], 62321[0], 62322[0], 62323[0], 62324[0], 62325[0], 62326[0], 62327[0], 64400[0], 64405[0], 64408[0], 64415[0], 64416[0], 64417[0], 64418[0], 64420[0], 64421[0], 64425[0], 64430[0], 64435[0], 64445[0], 64446[0], 64447[0], 64448[0], 64449[0], 64450[0], 64451[0], 64454[0], 64461[0], 64462[0], 64463[0], 64479[0], 64480[0], 64483[0], 64484[0], 64486[0], 64487[0], 64488[0], 64489[0], 64490[0], 64491[0], 64492[0], 64493[0], 64494[0], 64495[0], 64505[0], 64510[0], 64517[0], 64520[0], 64530[0], 67500[1], 69990[0], 92012[1], 92014[1], 92018[1], 92019[1], 93000[1], 93005[1], 93010[1], 93040[1], 93041[1], 93042[1], 93318[1], 93355[1], 94002[1], 94200[1], 94680[1], 94681[1], 94690[1], 95812[1], 95813[1], 95816[1], 95819[1], 95822[1], 95829[1], 95955[1], 96360[1], 96361[1], 96365[1], 96366[1], 96367[1], 96368[1], 96372[1], 96374[1], 96375[1], 96376[1], 96377[1], 96523[0], 97597[1], 97598[1], 97602[1], 99155[0], 99156[0], 99157[0], 99211[1], 99212[1], 99213[1], 99214[1], 99215[1], 99217[1], 99218[1], 99219[1], 99220[1], 99221[1], 99222[1], 99223[1], 99231[1], 99232[1], 99233[1], 99234[1], 99235[1], 99236[1], 99238[1], 99239[1], 99241[1], 99242[1], 99243[1], 99244[1], 99245[1], 99251[1], 99252[1], 99253[1], 99254[1], 99255[1], 99291[1], 99292[1], 99304[1], 99305[1], 99306[1], 99307[1], 99308[1], 99309[1], 99310[1], 99315[1], 99316[1], 99334[1], 99335[1], 99336[1], 99337[1], 99347[1], 99348[1], 99349[1], 99350[1], 99374[1], 99375[1], 99377[1], 99378[1], 99446[0], 99447[0], 99448[0], 99449[0], 99451[0], 99452[0], 99495[1], 99496[1], G0463[1], G0471[1], J0670[1], J2001[1]
67880	0213T[0], 0216T[0], 0596T[1], 0597T[1], 0708T[1], 0709T[1], 12001[1], 12002[1], 12004[1], 12005[1], 12006[1], 12007[1], 12011[1], 12013[1], 12014[1], 12015[1], 12016[1], 12017[1], 12018[1], 12020[1], 12021[1], 12031[1], 12032[1], 12034[1], 12035[1], 12036[1], 12037[1], 12041[1], 12042[1], 12044[1], 12045[1], 12046[1], 12047[1], 12051[1], 12052[1], 12053[1], 12054[1], 12055[1], 12056[1], 12057[1], 13100[1], 13101[1], 13102[1], 13120[1], 13121[1], 13122[1], 13131[1], 13132[1], 13133[1], 13151[1], 13152[1], 13153[1], 21280[1], 36000[1], 36400[1], 36405[1], 36406[1], 36410[1], 36420[1], 36425[1], 36430[1], 36440[1], 36591[0], 36592[0], 36600[1], 36640[1], 43752[1], 51701[1], 51702[1], 51703[1], 62320[0], 62321[0], 62322[0], 62323[0], 62324[0], 62325[0], 62326[0], 62327[0], 64400[0], 64405[0], 64408[0], 64415[0], 64416[0], 64417[0], 64418[0], 64420[0], 64421[0], 64425[0], 64430[0], 64435[0], 64445[0], 64446[0], 64447[0], 64448[0], 64449[0], 64450[0], 64451[0], 64454[0], 64461[0], 64462[0], 64463[0], 64479[0], 64480[0], 64483[0], 64484[0], 64486[0], 64487[0], 64488[0], 64489[0], 64490[0], 64491[0], 64492[0], 64493[0], 64494[0], 64495[0], 64505[0], 64510[0], 64517[0], 64520[0], 64530[0], 67500[1], 67710[1], 67715[1], 69990[0], 92012[1], 92014[1], 92018[1], 92019[1], 93000[1], 93005[1], 93010[1], 93040[1], 93041[1], 93042[1], 93318[1], 93355[1], 94002[1], 94200[1], 94680[1], 94681[1], 94690[1], 95812[1], 95813[1], 95816[1], 95819[1], 95822[1], 95829[1], 95955[1], 96360[1], 96361[1], 96365[1], 96366[1], 96367[1], 96368[1], 96372[1], 96374[1], 96375[1], 96376[1], 96377[1], 96523[0], 99155[0], 99156[0], 99157[0], 99211[1], 99212[1], 99213[1], 99214[1], 99215[1], 99217[1], 99218[1], 99219[1], 99220[1], 99221[1], 99222[1], 99223[1], 99231[1], 99232[1], 99233[1], 99234[1], 99235[1], 99236[1], 99238[1], 99239[1], 99241[1], 99242[1], 99243[1], 99244[1], 99245[1], 99251[1], 99252[1], 99253[1], 99254[1], 99255[1], 99291[1], 99292[1], 99304[1], 99305[1], 99306[1], 99307[1], 99308[1], 99309[1], 99310[1], 99315[1], 99316[1], 99334[1], 99335[1], 99336[1], 99337[1], 99347[1], 99348[1], 99349[1], 99350[1], 99374[1], 99375[1], 99377[1], 99378[1], 99446[0], 99447[0], 99448[0], 99449[0], 99451[0], 99452[0], 99495[0], 99496[0], G0463[1], G0471[1], J0670[1], J2001[1]
67882	0213T[0], 0216T[0], 0596T[1], 0597T[1], 0708T[1], 0709T[1], 12001[1], 12002[1], 12004[1], 12005[1], 12006[1], 12007[1], 12011[1], 12013[1], 12014[1], 12015[1], 12016[1], 12017[1], 12018[1], 12020[1], 12021[1], 12031[1], 12032[1], 12034[1], 12035[1], 12036[1], 12037[1], 12041[1], 12042[1], 12044[1], 12045[1], 12046[1], 12047[1], 12051[1], 12052[1], 12053[1], 12054[1], 12055[1], 12056[1], 12057[1], 13100[1], 13101[1], 13102[1], 13120[1], 13121[1], 13122[1], 13131[1], 13132[1], 13133[1], 13151[1], 13152[1], 13153[1], 21280[1], 36000[1], 36400[1], 36405[1], 36406[1], 36410[1], 36420[1], 36425[1], 36430[1], 36440[1], 36591[0], 36592[0], 36600[1], 36640[1], 43752[1], 51701[1], 51702[1], 51703[1], 62320[0], 62321[0], 62322[0], 62323[0], 62324[0], 62325[0], 62326[0], 62327[0], 64400[0], 64405[0], 64408[0], 64415[0], 64416[0], 64417[0], 64418[0], 64420[0], 64421[0], 64425[0], 64430[0], 64435[0], 64445[0], 64446[0], 64447[0], 64448[0], 64449[0], 64450[0], 64451[0], 64454[0], 64461[0], 64462[0], 64463[0], 64479[0], 64480[0], 64483[0], 64484[0], 64486[0], 64487[0], 64488[0], 64489[0], 64490[0], 64491[0], 64492[0], 64493[0], 64494[0], 64495[0], 64505[0], 64510[0], 64517[0], 64520[0], 64530[0], 67500[1], 67710[1], 67715[1], 67880[1], 69990[0], 92012[1], 92014[1], 92018[1], 92019[1], 93000[1], 93005[1], 93010[1], 93040[1], 93041[1], 93042[1], 93318[1], 93355[1], 94002[1], 94200[1], 94680[1], 94681[1], 94690[1], 95812[1], 95813[1], 95816[1], 95819[1], 95822[1], 95829[1], 95955[1], 96360[1], 96361[1], 96365[1], 96366[1], 96367[1], 96368[1], 96372[1], 96374[1], 96375[1], 96376[1], 96377[1], 96523[0], 99155[0], 99156[0], 99157[0], 99211[1], 99212[1], 99213[1], 99214[1], 99215[1], 99217[1], 99218[1], 99219[1], 99220[1], 99221[1], 99222[1], 99223[1], 99231[1], 99232[1], 99233[1], 99234[1], 99235[1], 99236[1], 99238[1], 99239[1], 99241[1], 99242[1], 99243[1], 99244[1], 99245[1], 99251[1], 99252[1], 99253[1], 99254[1], 99255[1], 99291[1], 99292[1], 99304[1], 99305[1], 99306[1], 99307[1], 99308[1], 99309[1], 99310[1], 99315[1], 99316[1], 99334[1], 99335[1], 99336[1], 99337[1], 99347[1], 99348[1], 99349[1], 99350[1], 99374[1], 99375[1], 99377[1], 99378[1], 99446[0], 99447[0], 99448[0], 99449[0], 99451[0], 99452[0], 99495[0], 99496[0], G0463[1], G0471[1], J0670[1], J2001[1]
67900	0213T[0], 0216T[0], 0596T[1], 0597T[1], 0708T[1], 0709T[1], 12001[1], 12002[1], 12004[1], 12005[1], 12006[1], 12007[1], 12011[1], 12013[1], 12014[1], 12015[1], 12016[1], 12017[1], 12018[1], 12020[1], 12021[1], 12031[1], 12032[1], 12034[1], 12035[1], 12036[1], 12037[1], 12041[1], 12042[1], 12044[1], 12045[1], 12046[1], 12047[1], 12051[1], 12052[1], 12053[1], 12054[1], 12055[1], 12056[1], 12057[1], 13100[1], 13101[1], 13102[1], 13120[1], 13121[1], 13122[1], 13131[1], 13132[1], 13133[1], 13151[1], 13152[1], 13153[1], 36000[1], 36400[1], 36405[1], 36406[1], 36410[1], 36420[1], 36425[1], 36430[1], 36440[1], 36591[0], 36592[0], 36600[1], 36640[1], 43752[1], 51701[1], 51702[1], 51703[1], 62320[0], 62321[0], 62322[0], 62323[0], 62324[0], 62325[0], 62326[0], 62327[0], 64400[0], 64405[0], 64408[0], 64415[0], 64416[0], 64417[0], 64418[0], 64420[0], 64421[0], 64425[0], 64430[0], 64435[0], 64445[0], 64446[0], 64447[0], 64448[0], 64449[0], 64450[0], 64451[0], 64454[0], 64461[0], 64462[0], 64463[0], 64479[0], 64480[0], 64483[0], 64484[0], 64486[0], 64487[0], 64488[0], 64489[0], 64490[0], 64491[0], 64492[0], 64493[0], 64494[0], 64495[0], 64505[0], 64510[0], 64517[0], 64520[0], 64530[0], 67500[1], 69990[0], 92012[1], 92014[1], 92018[1], 92019[1], 93000[1], 93005[1], 93010[1], 93040[1], 93041[1],

0 = Modifier usage not allowed or inappropriate   1 = Modifier usage allowed

Code 1	Code 2
	93042[1], 93318[1], 93355[1], 94002[1], 94200[1], 94680[1], 94681[1], 94690[1], 95812[1], 95813[1], 95816[1], 95819[1], 95822[1], 95829[1], 95955[1], 96360[1], 96361[1], 96365[1], 96366[1], 96367[1], 96368[1], 96372[1], 96374[1], 96375[1], 96376[1], 96377[1], 96523[0], 99155[0], 99156[0], 99157[0], 99211[1], 99212[1], 99213[1], 99214[1], 99215[1], 99217[1], 99218[1], 99219[1], 99220[1], 99221[1], 99222[1], 99223[1], 99231[1], 99232[1], 99233[1], 99234[1], 99235[1], 99236[1], 99238[1], 99239[1], 99241[1], 99242[1], 99243[1], 99244[1], 99245[1], 99251[1], 99252[1], 99253[1], 99254[1], 99255[1], 99291[1], 99292[1], 99304[1], 99305[1], 99306[1], 99307[1], 99308[1], 99309[1], 99310[1], 99315[1], 99316[1], 99334[1], 99335[1], 99336[1], 99337[1], 99347[1], 99348[1], 99349[1], 99350[1], 99374[1], 99375[1], 99377[1], 99378[1], 99446[0], 99447[0], 99448[0], 99449[0], 99451[0], 99452[0], 99495[0], 99496[0], G0463[1], G0471[1], J0670[1], J2001[1]
67901	0213T[0], 0216T[0], 0565T[1], 0596T[1], 0597T[1], 0708T[1], 0709T[1], 12001[1], 12002[1], 12004[1], 12005[1], 12006[1], 12007[1], 12011[1], 12013[1], 12014[1], 12015[1], 12016[1], 12017[1], 12018[1], 12020[1], 12021[1], 12031[1], 12032[1], 12034[1], 12035[1], 12036[1], 12037[1], 12041[1], 12042[1], 12044[1], 12045[1], 12046[1], 12047[1], 12051[1], 12052[1], 12053[1], 12054[1], 12055[1], 12056[1], 12057[1], 13100[1], 13101[1], 13102[1], 13120[1], 13121[1], 13122[1], 13131[1], 13132[1], 13133[1], 13151[1], 13152[1], 13153[1], 15769[1], 15822[1], 15823[1], 20920[1], 20922[1], 36000[1], 36400[1], 36405[1], 36406[1], 36410[1], 36420[1], 36425[1], 36430[1], 36440[1], 36591[0], 36592[0], 36600[1], 36640[1], 43752[1], 51701[1], 51702[1], 51703[1], 62320[0], 62321[0], 62322[0], 62323[0], 62324[0], 62325[0], 62326[0], 62327[0], 64400[0], 64405[0], 64408[0], 64415[0], 64416[0], 64417[0], 64418[0], 64420[0], 64421[0], 64425[0], 64430[0], 64435[0], 64445[0], 64446[0], 64447[0], 64448[0], 64449[0], 64450[0], 64451[0], 64454[0], 64461[0], 64462[0], 64463[0], 64479[0], 64480[0], 64483[0], 64484[0], 64486[0], 64487[0], 64488[0], 64489[0], 64490[0], 64491[0], 64492[0], 64493[0], 64494[0], 64495[0], 64505[0], 64510[0], 64517[0], 64520[0], 64530[0], 67500[1], 67902[1], 69990[0], 92012[1], 92014[1], 92018[1], 92019[1], 92081[0], 92082[0], 92083[0], 93000[1], 93005[1], 93010[1], 93040[1], 93041[1], 93042[1], 93318[1], 93355[1], 94002[1], 94200[1], 94680[1], 94681[1], 94690[1], 95812[1], 95813[1], 95816[1], 95819[1], 95822[1], 95829[1], 95955[1], 96360[1], 96361[1], 96365[1], 96366[1], 96367[1], 96368[1], 96372[1], 96374[1], 96375[1], 96376[1], 96377[1], 96523[0], 99155[0], 99156[0], 99157[0], 99211[1], 99212[1], 99213[1], 99214[1], 99215[1], 99217[1], 99218[1], 99219[1], 99220[1], 99221[1], 99222[1], 99223[1], 99231[1], 99232[1], 99233[1], 99234[1], 99235[1], 99236[1], 99238[1], 99239[1], 99241[1], 99242[1], 99243[1], 99244[1], 99245[1], 99251[1], 99252[1], 99253[1], 99254[1], 99255[1], 99291[1], 99292[1], 99304[1], 99305[1], 99306[1], 99307[1], 99308[1], 99309[1], 99310[1], 99315[1], 99316[1], 99334[1], 99335[1], 99336[1], 99337[1], 99347[1], 99348[1], 99349[1], 99350[1], 99374[1], 99375[1], 99377[1], 99378[1], 99446[0], 99447[0], 99448[0], 99449[0], 99451[0], 99452[0], 99495[0], 99496[0], G0463[1], G0471[1], J0670[1], J2001[1]
67902	0213T[0], 0216T[0], 0565T[1], 0596T[1], 0597T[1], 0708T[1], 0709T[1], 12001[1], 12002[1], 12004[1], 12005[1], 12006[1], 12007[1], 12011[1], 12013[1], 12014[1], 12015[1], 12016[1], 12017[1], 12018[1], 12020[1], 12021[1], 12031[1], 12032[1], 12034[1], 12035[1], 12036[1], 12037[1], 12041[1], 12042[1], 12044[1], 12045[1], 12046[1], 12047[1], 12051[1], 12052[1], 12053[1], 12054[1], 12055[1], 12056[1], 12057[1], 13100[1], 13101[1], 13102[1], 13120[1], 13121[1], 13122[1], 13131[1], 13132[1], 13133[1], 13151[1], 13152[1], 13153[1], 15769[1], 15822[1], 15823[1], 20920[1], 20922[1], 36000[1], 36400[1], 36405[1], 36406[1], 36410[1], 36420[1], 36425[1], 36430[1], 36440[1], 36591[0], 36592[0], 36600[1], 36640[1], 43752[1], 51701[1], 51702[1], 51703[1], 62320[0], 62321[0], 62322[0], 62323[0], 62324[0], 62325[0], 62326[0], 62327[0], 64400[0], 64405[0], 64408[0], 64415[0], 64416[0], 64417[0], 64418[0], 64420[0], 64421[0], 64425[0], 64430[0], 64435[0], 64445[0], 64446[0], 64447[0], 64448[0], 64449[0], 64450[0], 64451[0], 64454[0], 64461[0], 64462[0], 64463[0], 64479[0], 64480[0], 64483[0], 64484[0], 64486[0], 64487[0], 64488[0], 64489[0], 64490[0], 64491[0], 64492[0], 64493[0], 64494[0], 64495[0], 64505[0], 64510[0], 64517[0], 64520[0], 64530[0], 67500[1], 69990[0], 92012[1], 92014[1], 92018[1], 92019[1], 92081[0], 92082[0], 92083[0], 93000[1], 93005[1], 93010[1], 93040[1], 93041[1], 93042[1], 93318[1], 93355[1], 94002[1], 94200[1], 94680[1], 94681[1], 94690[1], 95812[1], 95813[1], 95816[1], 95819[1], 95822[1], 95829[1], 95955[1], 96360[1], 96361[1], 96365[1], 96366[1], 96367[1], 96368[1], 96372[1], 96374[1], 96375[1], 96376[1], 96377[1], 96523[0], 99155[0], 99156[0], 99157[0], 99211[1], 99212[1], 99213[1], 99214[1], 99215[1], 99217[1], 99218[1], 99219[1], 99220[1], 99221[1], 99222[1], 99223[1], 99231[1], 99232[1], 99233[1], 99234[1], 99235[1], 99236[1], 99238[1], 99239[1], 99241[1], 99242[1], 99243[1], 99244[1], 99245[1], 99251[1], 99252[1], 99253[1], 99254[1], 99255[1], 99291[1], 99292[1], 99304[1], 99305[1], 99306[1], 99307[1], 99308[1], 99309[1], 99310[1], 99315[1], 99316[1], 99334[1], 99335[1], 99336[1], 99337[1], 99347[1], 99348[1], 99349[1], 99350[1], 99374[1], 99375[1], 99377[1], 99378[1], 99446[0], 99447[0], 99448[0], 99449[0], 99451[0], 99452[0], 99495[0], 99496[0], G0463[1], G0471[1], J2001[1]
67903	0213T[0], 0216T[0], 0596T[1], 0597T[1], 0708T[1], 0709T[1], 11000[1], 11001[1], 11004[1], 11005[1], 11006[1], 11042[1], 11043[1], 11044[1], 11045[1], 11046[1], 11047[1], 12001[1], 12002[1], 12004[1], 12005[1], 12006[1], 12007[1], 12011[1], 12013[1], 12014[1], 12015[1], 12016[1], 12017[1], 12018[1], 12020[1], 12021[1], 12031[1], 12032[1], 12034[1], 12035[1], 12036[1], 12037[1], 12041[1], 12042[1], 12044[1], 12045[1], 12046[1], 12047[1], 12051[1], 12052[1], 12053[1], 12054[1], 12055[1], 12056[1], 12057[1], 13100[1], 13101[1], 13102[1], 13120[1], 13121[1], 13122[1], 13131[1], 13132[1], 13133[1], 13151[1], 13152[1], 13153[1], 15822[1], 15823[1], 36000[1], 36400[1], 36405[1], 36406[1], 36410[1], 36420[1], 36425[1], 36430[1], 36440[1], 36591[0], 36592[0], 36600[1], 36640[1], 43752[1], 51701[1], 51702[1], 51703[1], 62320[0], 62321[0], 62322[0], 62323[0], 62324[0], 62325[0], 62326[0], 62327[0], 64400[0], 64405[0], 64408[0], 64415[0], 64416[0], 64417[0], 64418[0], 64420[0], 64421[0], 64425[0], 64430[0], 64435[0], 64445[0], 64446[0], 64447[0], 64448[0], 64449[0], 64450[0], 64451[0], 64454[0], 64461[0], 64462[0], 64463[0], 64479[0], 64480[0], 64483[0], 64484[0], 64486[0], 64487[0], 64488[0], 64489[0], 64490[0], 64491[0], 64492[0], 64493[0], 64494[0], 64495[0], 64505[0], 64510[0], 64517[0], 64520[0], 64530[0], 67500[1], 67904[1], 69990[0], 92012[1], 92014[1], 92018[1], 92019[1], 92081[0], 92082[0], 92083[0], 93000[1], 93005[1], 93010[1], 93040[1], 93041[1], 93042[1], 93318[1], 93355[1], 94002[1], 94200[1], 94680[1], 94681[1], 94690[1], 95812[1], 95813[1], 95816[1], 95819[1], 95822[1], 95829[1], 95955[1], 96360[1], 96361[1], 96365[1], 96366[1], 96367[1], 96368[1], 96372[1], 96374[1], 96375[1], 96376[1], 96377[1], 96523[0], 97597[1], 97598[1], 97602[1], 99155[0], 99156[0], 99157[0], 99211[1], 99212[1], 99213[1], 99214[1], 99215[1], 99217[1], 99218[1], 99219[1], 99220[1], 99221[1], 99222[1], 99223[1], 99231[1], 99232[1], 99233[1], 99234[1], 99235[1], 99236[1], 99238[1], 99239[1], 99241[1], 99242[1], 99243[1], 99244[1], 99245[1], 99251[1], 99252[1], 99253[1], 99254[1], 99255[1], 99291[1], 99292[1], 99304[1], 99305[1], 99306[1], 99307[1], 99308[1], 99309[1], 99310[1], 99315[1], 99316[1], 99334[1], 99335[1], 99336[1], 99337[1], 99347[1], 99348[1], 99349[1], 99350[1], 99374[1], 99375[1], 99377[1], 99378[1], 99446[0], 99447[0], 99448[0], 99449[0], 99451[0], 99452[0], 99495[0], 99496[0], G0463[1], G0471[1], J0670[1], J2001[1]
67904	0213T[0], 0216T[0], 0596T[1], 0597T[1], 0708T[1], 0709T[1], 11000[1], 11001[1], 11004[1], 11005[1], 11006[1], 11042[1], 11043[1], 11044[1], 11045[1], 11046[1], 11047[1], 12001[1], 12002[1], 12004[1], 12005[1], 12006[1], 12007[1], 12011[1], 12013[1], 12014[1], 12015[1], 12016[1], 12017[1], 12018[1], 12020[1], 12021[1], 12031[1], 12032[1], 12034[1], 12035[1], 12036[1], 12037[1], 12041[1], 12042[1], 12044[1], 12045[1], 12046[1], 12047[1], 12051[1], 12052[1], 12053[1], 12054[1], 12055[1], 12056[1], 12057[1], 13100[1], 13101[1], 13102[1], 13120[1], 13121[1], 13122[1], 13131[1], 13132[1], 13133[1], 13151[1], 13152[1], 13153[1], 15822[1], 15823[1], 36000[1], 36400[1], 36405[1], 36406[1], 36410[1], 36420[1], 36425[1], 36430[1], 36440[1], 36591[0], 36592[0], 36600[1], 36640[1], 43752[1], 51701[1], 51702[1], 51703[1], 62320[0], 62321[0], 62322[0], 62323[0], 62324[0], 62325[0], 62326[0], 62327[0], 64400[0], 64405[0], 64408[0], 64415[0], 64416[0], 64417[0], 64418[0], 64420[0], 64421[0], 64425[0], 64430[0], 64435[0], 64445[0], 64446[0], 64447[0], 64448[0], 64449[0], 64450[0], 64451[0], 64454[0], 64461[0], 64462[0], 64463[0], 64479[0], 64480[0], 64483[0], 64484[0], 64486[0], 64487[0], 64488[0], 64489[0], 64490[0], 64491[0], 64492[0], 64493[0], 64494[0], 64495[0], 64505[0], 64510[0], 64517[0], 64520[0], 64530[0], 67500[1], 67901[1], 69990[0], 92012[1], 92014[1], 92018[1], 92019[1], 92081[0], 92082[0], 92083[0], 93000[1], 93005[1], 93010[1], 93040[1], 93041[1], 93042[1], 93318[1], 93355[1], 94002[1], 94200[1], 94680[1], 94681[1], 94690[1], 95812[1], 95813[1], 95816[1], 95819[1], 95822[1], 95829[1], 95955[1], 96360[1], 96361[1], 96365[1], 96366[1], 96367[1], 96368[1], 96372[1], 96374[1], 96375[1], 96376[1], 96377[1], 96523[0], 97597[1], 97598[1], 97602[1], 99155[0], 99156[0], 99157[0], 99211[1], 99212[1], 99213[1], 99214[1], 99215[1], 99217[1], 99218[1], 99219[1], 99220[1], 99221[1], 99222[1], 99223[1], 99231[1], 99232[1], 99233[1], 99234[1], 99235[1], 99236[1], 99238[1], 99239[1], 99241[1], 99242[1], 99243[1], 99244[1], 99245[1], 99251[1], 99252[1], 99253[1], 99254[1], 99255[1], 99291[1], 99292[1], 99304[1], 99305[1], 99306[1], 99307[1], 99308[1], 99309[1], 99310[1], 99315[1], 99316[1], 99334[1], 99335[1], 99336[1], 99337[1], 99347[1], 99348[1], 99349[1], 99350[1], 99374[1], 99375[1], 99377[1], 99378[1], 99446[0], 99447[0], 99448[0], 99449[0], 99451[0], 99452[0], 99495[0], 99496[0], G0463[1], G0471[1], J0670[1], J2001[1]
67906	0213T[0], 0216T[0], 0596T[1], 0597T[1], 0708T[1], 0709T[1], 12001[1], 12002[1], 12004[1], 12005[1], 12006[1], 12007[1], 12011[1], 12013[1], 12014[1], 12015[1], 12016[1], 12017[1], 12018[1], 12020[1], 12021[1], 12031[1], 12032[1], 12034[1], 12035[1], 12036[1], 12037[1], 12041[1], 12042[1], 12044[1], 12045[1], 12046[1], 12047[1], 12051[1], 12052[1], 12053[1], 12054[1], 12055[1], 12056[1], 12057[1], 13100[1], 13101[1], 13102[1], 13120[1], 13121[1], 13122[1], 13131[1], 13132[1], 13133[1], 13151[1], 13152[1], 13153[1], 15822[1], 15823[1], 36000[1], 36400[1], 36405[1], 36406[1], 36410[1], 36420[1], 36425[1], 36430[1], 36440[1], 36591[0], 36592[0], 36600[1], 36640[1], 43752[1], 51701[1], 51702[1], 51703[1], 62320[0], 62321[0], 62322[0], 62323[0], 62324[0], 62325[0], 62326[0], 62327[0], 64400[0], 64405[0], 64408[0], 64415[0], 64416[0], 64417[0], 64418[0], 64420[0], 64421[0], 64425[0], 64430[0], 64435[0], 64445[0], 64446[0], 64447[0], 64448[0], 64449[0], 64450[0], 64451[0], 64454[0], 64461[0], 64462[0], 64463[0], 64479[0], 64480[0], 64483[0], 64484[0], 64486[0], 64487[0], 64488[0], 64489[0], 64490[0], 64491[0], 64492[0], 64493[0], 64494[0], 64495[0], 64505[0], 64510[0], 64517[0], 64520[0], 64530[0], 67500[1], 69990[0], 92012[1], 92014[1], 92018[1], 92019[1], 92081[0], 92082[0], 92083[0], 93000[1], 93005[1], 93010[1], 93040[1], 93041[1], 93042[1], 93318[1], 93355[1], 94002[1], 94200[1], 94680[1], 94681[1], 94690[1], 95812[1], 95813[1], 95816[1], 95819[1], 95822[1], 95829[1], 95955[1], 96360[1], 96361[1], 96365[1], 96366[1], 96367[1], 96368[1], 96372[1], 96374[1], 96375[1], 96376[1], 96377[1], 96523[0], 99155[0], 99156[0], 99157[0], 99211[1], 99212[1], 99213[1], 99214[1], 99215[1], 99217[1], 99218[1], 99219[1], 99220[1], 99221[1], 99222[1], 99223[1], 99231[1], 99232[1], 99233[1], 99234[1], 99235[1], 99236[1], 99238[1], 99239[1], 99241[1], 99242[1], 99243[1], 99244[1], 99245[1], 99251[1], 99252[1], 99253[1], 99254[1], 99255[1], 99291[1], 99292[1], 99304[1], 99305[1], 99306[1], 99307[1], 99308[1], 99309[1], 99310[1], 99315[1], 99316[1], 99334[1], 99335[1], 99336[1], 99337[1], 99347[1], 99348[1], 99349[1], 99350[1], 99374[1], 99375[1], 99377[1], 99378[1], 99446[0], 99447[0], 99448[0], 99449[0], 99451[0], 99452[0], 99495[0], 99496[0], G0463[1], G0471[1], J0670[1], J2001[1]

0 = Modifier usage not allowed or inappropriate 1 = Modifier usage allowed

Code 1	Code 2
67908	0213T[0], 0216T[0], 0596T[1], 0597T[1], 0708T[1], 0709T[1], 11000[1], 11001[1], 11004[1], 11005[1], 11006[1], 11042[1], 11043[1], 11044[1], 11045[1], 11046[1], 11047[1], 12001[1], 12002[1], 12004[1], 12005[1], 12006[1], 12007[1], 12011[1], 12013[1], 12014[1], 12015[1], 12016[1], 12017[1], 12018[1], 12020[1], 12021[1], 12031[1], 12032[1], 12034[1], 12035[1], 12036[1], 12037[1], 12041[1], 12042[1], 12044[1], 12045[1], 12046[1], 12047[1], 12051[1], 12052[1], 12053[1], 12054[1], 12055[1], 12056[1], 12057[1], 13100[1], 13101[1], 13102[1], 13120[1], 13121[1], 13122[1], 13131[1], 13132[1], 13133[1], 13151[1], 13152[1], 13153[1], 15822[1], 15823[1], 36000[1], 36400[1], 36405[1], 36406[1], 36410[1], 36420[1], 36425[1], 36430[1], 36440[1], 36591[0], 36592[0], 36600[1], 36640[1], 43752[1], 51701[1], 51702[1], 51703[1], 62320[0], 62321[0], 62322[0], 62323[0], 62324[0], 62325[0], 62326[0], 62327[0], 64400[0], 64405[0], 64408[0], 64415[0], 64416[0], 64417[0], 64418[0], 64420[0], 64421[0], 64425[0], 64430[0], 64435[0], 64445[0], 64446[0], 64447[0], 64448[0], 64449[0], 64450[0], 64451[0], 64454[0], 64461[0], 64462[0], 64463[0], 64479[0], 64480[0], 64483[0], 64484[0], 64486[0], 64487[0], 64488[0], 64489[0], 64490[0], 64491[0], 64492[0], 64493[0], 64494[0], 64495[0], 64505[0], 64510[0], 64517[0], 64520[0], 64530[0], 67500[1], 69990[0], 92012[1], 92014[1], 92018[1], 92019[1], 92081[0], 92082[0], 92083[0], 93000[1], 93005[1], 93010[1], 93040[1], 93041[1], 93042[1], 93318[1], 93355[1], 94002[1], 94200[1], 94680[1], 94681[1], 94690[1], 95812[1], 95813[1], 95816[1], 95819[1], 95822[1], 95829[1], 95955[1], 96360[1], 96361[1], 96365[1], 96366[1], 96367[1], 96368[1], 96372[1], 96374[1], 96375[1], 96376[1], 96377[1], 96523[0], 97597[1], 97598[1], 97602[1], 99155[0], 99156[0], 99157[0], 99211[1], 99212[1], 99213[1], 99214[1], 99215[1], 99217[1], 99218[1], 99219[1], 99220[1], 99221[1], 99222[1], 99223[1], 99231[1], 99232[1], 99233[1], 99234[1], 99235[1], 99236[1], 99238[1], 99239[1], 99241[1], 99242[1], 99243[1], 99244[1], 99245[1], 99251[1], 99252[1], 99253[1], 99254[1], 99255[1], 99291[1], 99292[1], 99304[1], 99305[1], 99306[1], 99307[1], 99308[1], 99309[1], 99310[1], 99315[1], 99316[1], 99334[1], 99335[1], 99336[1], 99337[1], 99347[1], 99348[1], 99349[1], 99350[1], 99374[1], 99375[1], 99377[1], 99378[1], 99446[0], 99447[0], 99448[0], 99449[0], 99451[0], 99452[0], 99495[0], 99496[0], G0463[1], G0471[1], J0670[1], J2001[1]
67909	0213T[0], 0216T[0], 0596T[1], 0597T[1], 0708T[1], 0709T[1], 12001[1], 12002[1], 12004[1], 12005[1], 12006[1], 12007[1], 12011[1], 12013[1], 12014[1], 12015[1], 12016[1], 12017[1], 12018[1], 12020[1], 12021[1], 12031[1], 12032[1], 12034[1], 12035[1], 12036[1], 12037[1], 12041[1], 12042[1], 12044[1], 12045[1], 12046[1], 12047[1], 12051[1], 12052[1], 12053[1], 12054[1], 12055[1], 12056[1], 12057[1], 13100[1], 13101[1], 13102[1], 13120[1], 13121[1], 13122[1], 13131[1], 13132[1], 13133[1], 13151[1], 13152[1], 13153[1], 15820[1], 15822[1], 36000[1], 36400[1], 36405[1], 36406[1], 36410[1], 36420[1], 36425[1], 36430[1], 36440[1], 36591[0], 36592[0], 36600[1], 36640[1], 43752[1], 51701[1], 51702[1], 51703[1], 62320[0], 62321[0], 62322[0], 62323[0], 62324[0], 62325[0], 62326[0], 62327[0], 64400[0], 64405[0], 64408[0], 64415[0], 64416[0], 64417[0], 64418[0], 64420[0], 64421[0], 64425[0], 64430[0], 64435[0], 64445[0], 64446[0], 64447[0], 64448[0], 64449[0], 64450[0], 64451[0], 64454[0], 64461[0], 64462[0], 64463[0], 64479[0], 64480[0], 64483[0], 64484[0], 64486[0], 64487[0], 64488[0], 64489[0], 64490[0], 64491[0], 64492[0], 64493[0], 64494[0], 64495[0], 64505[0], 64510[0], 64517[0], 64520[0], 64530[0], 67500[1], 69990[0], 92012[1], 92014[1], 92018[1], 92019[1], 93000[1], 93005[1], 93010[1], 93040[1], 93041[1], 93042[1], 93318[1], 93355[1], 94002[1], 94200[1], 94680[1], 94681[1], 94690[1], 95812[1], 95813[1], 95816[1], 95819[1], 95822[1], 95829[1], 95955[1], 96360[1], 96361[1], 96365[1], 96366[1], 96367[1], 96368[1], 96372[1], 96374[1], 96375[1], 96376[1], 96377[1], 96523[0], 99155[0], 99156[0], 99157[0], 99211[1], 99212[1], 99213[1], 99214[1], 99215[1], 99217[1], 99218[1], 99219[1], 99220[1], 99221[1], 99222[1], 99223[1], 99231[1], 99232[1], 99233[1], 99234[1], 99235[1], 99236[1], 99238[1], 99239[1], 99241[1], 99242[1], 99243[1], 99244[1], 99245[1], 99251[1], 99252[1], 99253[1], 99254[1], 99255[1], 99291[1], 99292[1], 99304[1], 99305[1], 99306[1], 99307[1], 99308[1], 99309[1], 99310[1], 99315[1], 99316[1], 99334[1], 99335[1], 99336[1], 99337[1], 99347[1], 99348[1], 99349[1], 99350[1], 99374[1], 99375[1], 99377[1], 99378[1], 99446[0], 99447[0], 99448[0], 99449[0], 99451[0], 99452[0], 99495[0], 99496[0], G0463[1], G0471[1], J0670[1], J2001[1]
67911	0213T[0], 0216T[0], 0596T[1], 0597T[1], 0708T[1], 0709T[1], 12001[1], 12002[1], 12004[1], 12005[1], 12006[1], 12007[1], 12011[1], 12013[1], 12014[1], 12015[1], 12016[1], 12017[1], 12018[1], 12020[1], 12021[1], 12031[1], 12032[1], 12034[1], 12035[1], 12036[1], 12037[1], 12041[1], 12042[1], 12044[1], 12045[1], 12046[1], 12047[1], 12051[1], 12052[1], 12053[1], 12054[1], 12055[1], 12056[1], 12057[1], 13100[1], 13101[1], 13102[1], 13120[1], 13121[1], 13122[1], 13131[1], 13132[1], 13133[1], 13151[1], 13152[1], 13153[1], 15260[1], 15820[1], 15822[1], 36000[1], 36400[1], 36405[1], 36406[1], 36410[1], 36420[1], 36425[1], 36430[1], 36440[1], 36591[0], 36592[0], 36600[1], 36640[1], 43752[1], 51701[1], 51702[1], 51703[1], 62320[0], 62321[0], 62322[0], 62323[0], 62324[0], 62325[0], 62326[0], 62327[0], 64400[0], 64405[0], 64408[0], 64415[0], 64416[0], 64417[0], 64418[0], 64420[0], 64421[0], 64425[0], 64430[0], 64435[0], 64445[0], 64446[0], 64447[0], 64448[0], 64449[0], 64450[0], 64451[0], 64454[0], 64461[0], 64462[0], 64463[0], 64479[0], 64480[0], 64483[0], 64484[0], 64486[0], 64487[0], 64488[0], 64489[0], 64490[0], 64491[0], 64492[0], 64493[0], 64494[0], 64495[0], 64505[0], 64510[0], 64517[0], 64520[0], 64530[0], 67500[1], 67830[1], 67882[1], 69990[0], 92012[1], 92014[1], 92018[1], 92019[1], 93000[1], 93005[1], 93010[1], 93040[1], 93041[1], 93042[1], 93318[1], 93355[1], 94002[1], 94200[1], 94680[1], 94681[1], 94690[1], 95812[1], 95813[1], 95816[1], 95819[1], 95822[1], 95829[1], 95955[1], 96360[1], 96361[1], 96365[1], 96366[1], 96367[1], 96368[1], 96372[1], 96374[1], 96375[1], 96376[1], 96377[1], 96523[0], 99155[0], 99156[0], 99157[0], 99211[1], 99212[1], 99213[1], 99214[1], 99215[1], 99217[1], 99218[1], 99219[1], 99220[1], 99221[1], 99222[1], 99223[1], 99231[1], 99232[1], 99233[1], 99234[1], 99235[1], 99236[1], 99238[1], 99239[1], 99241[1], 99242[1], 99243[1], 99244[1], 99245[1], 99251[1], 99252[1], 99253[1], 99254[1], 99255[1], 99291[1], 99292[1], 99304[1], 99305[1], 99306[1], 99307[1], 99308[1], 99309[1], 99310[1], 99315[1], 99316[1], 99334[1], 99335[1], 99336[1], 99337[1], 99347[1], 99348[1], 99349[1], 99350[1], 99374[1], 99375[1], 99377[1], 99378[1], 99446[0], 99447[0], 99448[0], 99449[0], 99451[0], 99452[0], 99495[0], 99496[0], G0463[1], G0471[1], J2001[1]
67912	0213T[0], 0216T[0], 0596T[1], 0597T[1], 0708T[1], 0709T[1], 12001[1], 12002[1], 12004[1], 12005[1], 12006[1], 12007[1], 12011[1], 12013[1], 12014[1], 12015[1], 12016[1], 12017[1], 12018[1], 12020[1], 12021[1], 12031[1], 12032[1], 12034[1], 12035[1], 12036[1], 12037[1], 12041[1], 12042[1], 12044[1], 12045[1], 12046[1], 12047[1], 12051[1], 12052[1], 12053[1], 12054[1], 12055[1], 12056[1], 12057[1], 13100[1], 13101[1], 13102[1], 13120[1], 13121[1], 13122[1], 13131[1], 13132[1], 13133[1], 13151[1], 13152[1], 13153[1], 15822[0], 36000[1], 36400[1], 36405[1], 36406[1], 36410[1], 36420[1], 36425[1], 36430[1], 36440[1], 36591[0], 36592[0], 36600[1], 36640[1], 43752[1], 51701[1], 51702[1], 51703[1], 62320[0], 62321[0], 62322[0], 62323[0], 62324[0], 62325[0], 62326[0], 62327[0], 64400[0], 64405[0], 64408[0], 64415[0], 64416[0], 64417[0], 64418[0], 64420[0], 64421[0], 64425[0], 64430[0], 64435[0], 64445[0], 64446[0], 64447[0], 64448[0], 64449[0], 64450[0], 64451[0], 64454[0], 64461[0], 64462[0], 64463[0], 64479[0], 64480[0], 64483[0], 64484[0], 64486[0], 64487[0], 64488[0], 64489[0], 64490[0], 64491[0], 64492[0], 64493[0], 64494[0], 64495[0], 64505[0], 64510[0], 64517[0], 64520[0], 64530[0], 67500[1], 69990[0], 92012[1], 92014[1], 92018[1], 92019[1], 93000[1], 93005[1], 93010[1], 93040[1], 93041[1], 93042[1], 93318[1], 93355[1], 94002[1], 94200[1], 94680[1], 94681[1], 94690[1], 95812[1], 95813[1], 95816[1], 95819[1], 95822[1], 95829[1], 95955[1], 96360[1], 96361[1], 96365[1], 96366[1], 96367[1], 96368[1], 96372[1], 96374[1], 96375[1], 96376[1], 96377[1], 96523[0], 99155[0], 99156[0], 99157[0], 99211[1], 99212[1], 99213[1], 99214[1], 99215[1], 99217[1], 99218[1], 99219[1], 99220[1], 99221[1], 99222[1], 99223[1], 99231[1], 99232[1], 99233[1], 99234[1], 99235[1], 99236[1], 99238[1], 99239[1], 99241[1], 99242[1], 99243[1], 99244[1], 99245[1], 99251[1], 99252[1], 99253[1], 99254[1], 99255[1], 99291[1], 99292[1], 99304[1], 99305[1], 99306[1], 99307[1], 99308[1], 99309[1], 99310[1], 99315[1], 99316[1], 99334[1], 99335[1], 99336[1], 99337[1], 99347[1], 99348[1], 99349[1], 99350[1], 99374[1], 99375[1], 99377[1], 99378[1], 99446[0], 99447[0], 99448[0], 99449[0], 99451[0], 99452[0], 99495[0], 99496[0], G0463[1], G0471[1], J0670[1], J2001[1]
67914	0213T[0], 0216T[0], 0596T[1], 0597T[1], 0708T[1], 0709T[1], 12001[1], 12002[1], 12004[1], 12005[1], 12006[1], 12007[1], 12011[1], 12013[1], 12014[1], 12015[1], 12016[1], 12017[1], 12018[1], 12020[1], 12021[1], 12031[1], 12032[1], 12034[1], 12035[1], 12036[1], 12037[1], 12041[1], 12042[1], 12044[1], 12045[1], 12046[1], 12047[1], 12051[1], 12052[1], 12053[1], 12054[1], 12055[1], 12056[1], 12057[1], 13100[1], 13101[1], 13102[1], 13120[1], 13121[1], 13122[1], 13131[1], 13132[1], 13133[1], 13151[1], 13152[1], 13153[1], 15820[1], 15822[1], 36000[1], 36400[1], 36405[1], 36406[1], 36410[1], 36420[1], 36425[1], 36430[1], 36440[1], 36591[0], 36592[0], 36600[1], 36640[1], 43752[1], 51701[1], 51702[1], 51703[1], 62320[0], 62321[0], 62322[0], 62323[0], 62324[0], 62325[0], 62326[0], 62327[0], 64400[0], 64405[0], 64408[0], 64415[0], 64416[0], 64417[0], 64418[0], 64420[0], 64421[0], 64425[0], 64430[0], 64435[0], 64445[0], 64446[0], 64447[0], 64448[0], 64449[0], 64450[0], 64451[0], 64454[0], 64461[0], 64462[0], 64463[0], 64479[0], 64480[0], 64483[0], 64484[0], 64486[0], 64487[0], 64488[0], 64489[0], 64490[0], 64491[0], 64492[0], 64493[0], 64494[0], 64495[0], 64505[0], 64510[0], 64517[0], 64520[0], 64530[0], 67500[1], 67916[1], 69990[0], 92012[1], 92014[1], 92018[1], 92019[1], 93000[1], 93005[1], 93010[1], 93040[1], 93041[1], 93042[1], 93318[1], 93355[1], 94002[1], 94200[1], 94680[1], 94681[1], 94690[1], 95812[1], 95813[1], 95816[1], 95819[1], 95822[1], 95829[1], 95955[1], 96360[1], 96361[1], 96365[1], 96366[1], 96367[1], 96368[1], 96372[1], 96374[1], 96375[1], 96376[1], 96377[1], 96523[0], 99155[0], 99156[0], 99157[0], 99211[1], 99212[1], 99213[1], 99214[1], 99215[1], 99217[1], 99218[1], 99219[1], 99220[1], 99221[1], 99222[1], 99223[1], 99231[1], 99232[1], 99233[1], 99234[1], 99235[1], 99236[1], 99238[1], 99239[1], 99241[1], 99242[1], 99243[1], 99244[1], 99245[1], 99251[1], 99252[1], 99253[1], 99254[1], 99255[1], 99291[1], 99292[1], 99304[1], 99305[1], 99306[1], 99307[1], 99308[1], 99309[1], 99310[1], 99315[1], 99316[1], 99334[1], 99335[1], 99336[1], 99337[1], 99347[1], 99348[1], 99349[1], 99350[1], 99374[1], 99375[1], 99377[1], 99378[1], 99446[0], 99447[0], 99448[0], 99449[0], 99451[0], 99452[0], 99495[0], 99496[0], G0463[1], G0471[1], J0670[1], J2001[1]
67915	0213T[0], 0216T[0], 0596T[1], 0597T[1], 0708T[1], 0709T[1], 12001[1], 12002[1], 12004[1], 12005[1], 12006[1], 12007[1], 12011[1], 12013[1], 12014[1], 12015[1], 12016[1], 12017[1], 12018[1], 12020[1], 12021[1], 12031[1], 12032[1], 12034[1], 12035[1], 12036[1], 12037[1], 12041[1], 12042[1], 12044[1], 12045[1], 12046[1], 12047[1], 12051[1], 12052[1], 12053[1], 12054[1], 12055[1], 12056[1], 12057[1], 13100[1], 13101[1], 13102[1], 13120[1], 13121[1], 13122[1], 13131[1], 13132[1], 13133[1], 13151[1], 13152[1], 13153[1], 15820[1], 15822[1], 36000[1], 36400[1], 36405[1], 36406[1], 36410[1], 36420[1], 36425[1], 36430[1], 36440[1], 36591[0], 36592[0], 36600[1], 36640[1], 43752[1], 51701[1], 51702[1], 51703[1], 62320[0], 62321[0], 62322[0], 62323[0], 62324[0], 62325[0], 62326[0], 62327[0], 64400[0], 64405[0], 64408[0], 64415[0], 64416[0], 64417[0], 64418[0], 64420[0], 64421[0], 64425[0], 64430[0], 64435[0], 64445[0], 64446[0], 64447[0], 64448[0], 64449[0], 64450[0], 64451[0], 64454[0], 64461[0], 64462[0], 64463[0], 64479[0], 64480[0], 64483[0], 64484[0], 64486[0], 64487[0], 64488[0], 64489[0], 64490[0], 64491[0], 64492[0], 64493[0], 64494[0], 64495[0], 64505[0], 64510[0], 64517[0], 64520[0], 64530[0], 67500[1], 67914[1], 67916[1], 69990[0], 92012[1], 92014[1], 92018[1], 92019[1], 93000[1], 93005[1], 93010[1], 93040[1], 93041[1], 93042[1], 93318[1], 93355[1], 94002[1], 94200[1], 94680[1],

0 = Modifier usage not allowed or inappropriate 1 = Modifier usage allowed

Code 1	Code 2
	94681[1], 94690[1], 95812[1], 95813[1], 95816[1], 95819[1], 95822[1], 95829[1], 95955[1], 96360[1], 96361[1], 96365[1], 96366[1], 96367[1], 96368[1], 96372[1], 96374[1], 96375[1], 96376[1], 96377[1], 96523[0], 99155[0], 99156[0], 99157[0], 99211[1], 99212[1], 99213[1], 99214[1], 99215[1], 99217[1], 99218[1], 99219[1], 99220[1], 99221[1], 99222[1], 99223[1], 99231[1], 99232[1], 99233[1], 99234[1], 99235[1], 99236[1], 99238[1], 99239[1], 99241[1], 99242[1], 99243[1], 99244[1], 99245[1], 99251[1], 99252[1], 99253[1], 99254[1], 99255[1], 99291[1], 99292[1], 99304[1], 99305[1], 99306[1], 99307[1], 99308[1], 99309[1], 99310[1], 99315[1], 99316[1], 99334[1], 99335[1], 99336[1], 99337[1], 99347[1], 99348[1], 99349[1], 99350[1], 99374[1], 99375[1], 99377[1], 99378[1], 99446[0], 99447[0], 99448[0], 99449[0], 99451[0], 99452[0], 99495[0], 99496[0], G0463[1], G0471[1], J0670[1], J2001[1]
67916	0213T[0], 0216T[0], 0596T[1], 0597T[1], 0708T[1], 0709T[1], 11000[1], 11001[1], 11004[1], 11005[1], 11006[1], 11042[1], 11043[1], 11044[1], 11045[1], 11046[1], 11047[1], 12001[1], 12002[1], 12004[1], 12005[1], 12006[1], 12007[1], 12011[1], 12013[1], 12014[1], 12015[1], 12016[1], 12017[1], 12018[1], 12020[1], 12021[1], 12031[1], 12032[1], 12034[1], 12035[1], 12036[1], 12037[1], 12041[1], 12042[1], 12044[1], 12045[1], 12046[1], 12047[1], 12051[1], 12052[1], 12053[1], 12054[1], 12055[1], 12056[1], 12057[1], 13100[1], 13101[1], 13102[1], 13120[1], 13121[1], 13122[1], 13131[1], 13132[1], 13133[1], 13151[1], 13152[1], 13153[1], 15820[1], 15822[1], 21280[1], 21282[1], 36000[1], 36400[1], 36405[1], 36406[1], 36410[1], 36420[1], 36425[1], 36430[1], 36440[1], 36591[0], 36592[0], 36600[1], 36640[1], 43752[1], 51701[1], 51702[1], 51703[1], 62320[0], 62321[0], 62322[0], 62323[0], 62324[0], 62325[0], 62326[0], 62327[0], 64400[0], 64405[0], 64408[0], 64415[0], 64416[0], 64417[0], 64418[0], 64420[0], 64421[0], 64425[0], 64430[0], 64435[0], 64445[0], 64446[0], 64447[0], 64448[0], 64449[0], 64450[0], 64451[0], 64454[0], 64461[0], 64462[0], 64463[0], 64479[0], 64480[0], 64483[0], 64484[0], 64486[0], 64487[0], 64488[0], 64489[0], 64490[0], 64491[0], 64492[0], 64493[0], 64494[0], 64495[0], 64505[0], 64510[0], 64517[0], 64520[0], 64530[0], 67500[1], 67950[1], 68320[1], 68326[1], 68330[1], 68705[1], 69990[0], 92012[1], 92014[1], 92018[1], 92019[1], 93000[1], 93005[1], 93010[1], 93040[1], 93041[1], 93042[1], 93318[1], 93355[1], 94002[1], 94200[1], 94680[1], 94681[1], 94690[1], 95812[1], 95813[1], 95816[1], 95819[1], 95822[1], 95829[1], 95955[1], 96360[1], 96361[1], 96365[1], 96366[1], 96367[1], 96368[1], 96372[1], 96374[1], 96375[1], 96376[1], 96377[1], 96523[0], 97597[1], 97598[1], 97602[1], 99155[0], 99156[0], 99157[0], 99211[1], 99212[1], 99213[1], 99214[1], 99215[1], 99217[1], 99218[1], 99219[1], 99220[1], 99221[1], 99222[1], 99223[1], 99231[1], 99232[1], 99233[1], 99234[1], 99235[1], 99236[1], 99238[1], 99239[1], 99241[1], 99242[1], 99243[1], 99244[1], 99245[1], 99251[1], 99252[1], 99253[1], 99254[1], 99255[1], 99291[1], 99292[1], 99304[1], 99305[1], 99306[1], 99307[1], 99308[1], 99309[1], 99310[1], 99315[1], 99316[1], 99334[1], 99335[1], 99336[1], 99337[1], 99347[1], 99348[1], 99349[1], 99350[1], 99374[1], 99375[1], 99377[1], 99378[1], 99446[0], 99447[0], 99448[0], 99449[0], 99451[0], 99452[0], 99495[0], 99496[0], G0463[1], G0471[1], J0670[1], J2001[1]
67917	0213T[0], 0216T[0], 0596T[1], 0597T[1], 0708T[1], 0709T[1], 12001[1], 12002[1], 12004[1], 12005[1], 12006[1], 12007[1], 12011[1], 12013[1], 12014[1], 12015[1], 12016[1], 12017[1], 12018[1], 12020[1], 12021[1], 12031[1], 12032[1], 12034[1], 12035[1], 12036[1], 12037[1], 12041[1], 12042[1], 12044[1], 12045[1], 12046[1], 12047[1], 12051[1], 12052[1], 12053[1], 12054[1], 12055[1], 12056[1], 12057[1], 13100[1], 13101[1], 13102[1], 13120[1], 13121[1], 13122[1], 13131[1], 13132[1], 13133[1], 13151[1], 13152[1], 13153[1], 15820[1], 15822[1], 21280[1], 21282[1], 36000[1], 36400[1], 36405[1], 36406[1], 36410[1], 36420[1], 36425[1], 36430[1], 36440[1], 36591[0], 36592[0], 36600[1], 36640[1], 43752[1], 51701[1], 51702[1], 51703[1], 62320[0], 62321[0], 62322[0], 62323[0], 62324[0], 62325[0], 62326[0], 62327[0], 64400[0], 64405[0], 64408[0], 64415[0], 64416[0], 64417[0], 64418[0], 64420[0], 64421[0], 64425[0], 64430[0], 64435[0], 64445[0], 64446[0], 64447[0], 64448[0], 64449[0], 64450[0], 64451[0], 64454[0], 64461[0], 64462[0], 64463[0], 64479[0], 64480[0], 64483[0], 64484[0], 64486[0], 64487[0], 64488[0], 64489[0], 64490[0], 64491[0], 64492[0], 64493[0], 64494[0], 64495[0], 64505[0], 64510[0], 64517[0], 64520[0], 64530[0], 67500[1], 67820[1], 67825[1], 67830[1], 67880[1], 67882[1], 67908[1], 67911[1], 67914[1], 67915[1], 67916[1], 67950[1], 67961[1], 68320[1], 68326[1], 68330[1], 68705[1], 69990[0], 92012[1], 92014[1], 92018[1], 92019[1], 93000[1], 93005[1], 93010[1], 93040[1], 93041[1], 93042[1], 93318[1], 93355[1], 94002[1], 94200[1], 94680[1], 94681[1], 94690[1], 95812[1], 95813[1], 95816[1], 95819[1], 95822[1], 95829[1], 95955[1], 96360[1], 96361[1], 96365[1], 96366[1], 96367[1], 96368[1], 96372[1], 96374[1], 96375[1], 96376[1], 96377[1], 96523[0], 99155[0], 99156[0], 99157[0], 99211[1], 99212[1], 99213[1], 99214[1], 99215[1], 99217[1], 99218[1], 99219[1], 99220[1], 99221[1], 99222[1], 99223[1], 99231[1], 99232[1], 99233[1], 99234[1], 99235[1], 99236[1], 99238[1], 99239[1], 99241[1], 99242[1], 99243[1], 99244[1], 99245[1], 99251[1], 99252[1], 99253[1], 99254[1], 99255[1], 99291[1], 99292[1], 99304[1], 99305[1], 99306[1], 99307[1], 99308[1], 99309[1], 99310[1], 99315[1], 99316[1], 99334[1], 99335[1], 99336[1], 99337[1], 99347[1], 99348[1], 99349[1], 99350[1], 99374[1], 99375[1], 99377[1], 99378[1], 99446[0], 99447[0], 99448[0], 99449[0], 99451[0], 99452[0], 99495[0], 99496[0], G0463[1], G0471[1], J0670[1], J2001[1]
67921	0213T[0], 0216T[0], 0596T[1], 0597T[1], 0708T[1], 0709T[1], 12001[1], 12002[1], 12004[1], 12005[1], 12006[1], 12007[1], 12011[1], 12013[1], 12014[1], 12015[1], 12016[1], 12017[1], 12018[1], 12020[1], 12021[1], 12031[1], 12032[1], 12034[1], 12035[1], 12036[1], 12037[1], 12041[1], 12042[1], 12044[1], 12045[1], 12046[1], 12047[1], 12051[1], 12052[1], 12053[1], 12054[1], 12055[1], 12056[1], 12057[1], 13100[1], 13101[1], 13102[1], 13120[1], 13121[1], 13122[1], 13131[1], 13132[1], 13133[1], 13151[1], 13152[1], 13153[1], 15820[1], 15822[1], 36000[1], 36400[1], 36405[1], 36406[1], 36410[1], 36420[1], 36425[1], 36430[1], 36440[1], 36591[0], 36592[0], 36600[1], 36640[1], 43752[1], 51701[1], 51702[1], 51703[1], 62320[0], 62321[0], 62322[0], 62323[0], 62324[0], 62325[0], 62326[0], 62327[0], 64400[0], 64405[0], 64408[0], 64415[0], 64416[0], 64417[0], 64418[0], 64420[0], 64421[0], 64425[0], 64430[0], 64435[0], 64445[0], 64446[0], 64447[0], 64448[0], 64449[0], 64450[0], 64451[0], 64454[0], 64461[0], 64462[0], 64463[0], 64479[0], 64480[0], 64483[0], 64484[0], 64486[0], 64487[0], 64488[0], 64489[0], 64490[0], 64491[0], 64492[0], 64493[0], 64494[0], 64495[0], 64505[0], 64510[0], 64517[0], 64520[0], 64530[0], 67500[1], 69990[0], 92012[1], 92014[1], 92018[1], 92019[1], 93000[1], 93005[1], 93010[1], 93040[1], 93041[1], 93042[1], 93318[1], 93355[1], 94002[1], 94200[1], 94680[1], 94681[1], 94690[1], 95812[1], 95813[1], 95816[1], 95819[1], 95822[1], 95829[1], 95955[1], 96360[1], 96361[1], 96365[1], 96366[1], 96367[1], 96368[1], 96372[1], 96374[1], 96375[1], 96376[1], 96377[1], 96523[0], 99155[0], 99156[0], 99157[0], 99211[1], 99212[1], 99213[1], 99214[1], 99215[1], 99217[1], 99218[1], 99219[1], 99220[1], 99221[1], 99222[1], 99223[1], 99231[1], 99232[1], 99233[1], 99234[1], 99235[1], 99236[1], 99238[1], 99239[1], 99241[1], 99242[1], 99243[1], 99244[1], 99245[1], 99251[1], 99252[1], 99253[1], 99254[1], 99255[1], 99291[1], 99292[1], 99304[1], 99305[1], 99306[1], 99307[1], 99308[1], 99309[1], 99310[1], 99315[1], 99316[1], 99334[1], 99335[1], 99336[1], 99337[1], 99347[1], 99348[1], 99349[1], 99350[1], 99374[1], 99375[1], 99377[1], 99378[1], 99446[0], 99447[0], 99448[0], 99449[0], 99451[0], 99452[0], 99495[0], 99496[0], G0463[1], G0471[1], J0670[1], J2001[1]
67922	0213T[0], 0216T[0], 0596T[1], 0597T[1], 0708T[1], 0709T[1], 12001[1], 12002[1], 12004[1], 12005[1], 12006[1], 12007[1], 12011[1], 12013[1], 12014[1], 12015[1], 12016[1], 12017[1], 12018[1], 12020[1], 12021[1], 12031[1], 12032[1], 12034[1], 12035[1], 12036[1], 12037[1], 12041[1], 12042[1], 12044[1], 12045[1], 12046[1], 12047[1], 12051[1], 12052[1], 12053[1], 12054[1], 12055[1], 12056[1], 12057[1], 13100[1], 13101[1], 13102[1], 13120[1], 13121[1], 13122[1], 13131[1], 13132[1], 13133[1], 13151[1], 13152[1], 13153[1], 15820[1], 15822[1], 36000[1], 36400[1], 36405[1], 36406[1], 36410[1], 36420[1], 36425[1], 36430[1], 36440[1], 36591[0], 36592[0], 36600[1], 36640[1], 43752[1], 51701[1], 51702[1], 51703[1], 62320[0], 62321[0], 62322[0], 62323[0], 62324[0], 62325[0], 62326[0], 62327[0], 64400[0], 64405[0], 64408[0], 64415[0], 64416[0], 64417[0], 64418[0], 64420[0], 64421[0], 64425[0], 64430[0], 64435[0], 64445[0], 64446[0], 64447[0], 64448[0], 64449[0], 64450[0], 64451[0], 64454[0], 64461[0], 64462[0], 64463[0], 64479[0], 64480[0], 64483[0], 64484[0], 64486[0], 64487[0], 64488[0], 64489[0], 64490[0], 64491[0], 64492[0], 64493[0], 64494[0], 64495[0], 64505[0], 64510[0], 64517[0], 64520[0], 64530[0], 67500[1], 67921[1], 69990[0], 92012[1], 92014[1], 92018[1], 92019[1], 93000[1], 93005[1], 93010[1], 93040[1], 93041[1], 93042[1], 93318[1], 93355[1], 94002[1], 94200[1], 94680[1], 94681[1], 94690[1], 95812[1], 95813[1], 95816[1], 95819[1], 95822[1], 95829[1], 95955[1], 96360[1], 96361[1], 96365[1], 96366[1], 96367[1], 96368[1], 96372[1], 96374[1], 96375[1], 96376[1], 96377[1], 96523[0], 99155[0], 99156[0], 99157[0], 99211[1], 99212[1], 99213[1], 99214[1], 99215[1], 99217[1], 99218[1], 99219[1], 99220[1], 99221[1], 99222[1], 99223[1], 99231[1], 99232[1], 99233[1], 99234[1], 99235[1], 99236[1], 99238[1], 99239[1], 99241[1], 99242[1], 99243[1], 99244[1], 99245[1], 99251[1], 99252[1], 99253[1], 99254[1], 99255[1], 99291[1], 99292[1], 99304[1], 99305[1], 99306[1], 99307[1], 99308[1], 99309[1], 99310[1], 99315[1], 99316[1], 99334[1], 99335[1], 99336[1], 99337[1], 99347[1], 99348[1], 99349[1], 99350[1], 99374[1], 99375[1], 99377[1], 99378[1], 99446[0], 99447[0], 99448[0], 99449[0], 99451[0], 99452[0], 99495[0], 99496[0], G0463[1], G0471[1], J0670[1], J2001[1]
67923	0213T[0], 0216T[0], 0596T[1], 0597T[1], 0708T[1], 0709T[1], 11000[1], 11001[1], 11004[1], 11005[1], 11006[1], 11042[1], 11043[1], 11044[1], 11045[1], 11046[1], 11047[1], 11442[1], 12001[1], 12002[1], 12004[1], 12005[1], 12006[1], 12007[1], 12011[1], 12013[1], 12014[1], 12015[1], 12016[1], 12017[1], 12018[1], 12020[1], 12021[1], 12031[1], 12032[1], 12034[1], 12035[1], 12036[1], 12037[1], 12041[1], 12042[1], 12044[1], 12045[1], 12046[1], 12047[1], 12051[1], 12052[1], 12053[1], 12054[1], 12055[1], 12056[1], 12057[1], 13100[1], 13101[1], 13102[1], 13120[1], 13121[1], 13122[1], 13131[1], 13132[1], 13133[1], 13151[1], 13152[1], 13153[1], 15820[1], 15822[1], 21280[1], 21282[1], 36000[1], 36400[1], 36405[1], 36406[1], 36410[1], 36420[1], 36425[1], 36430[1], 36440[1], 36591[0], 36592[0], 36600[1], 36640[1], 43752[1], 51701[1], 51702[1], 51703[1], 62320[0], 62321[0], 62322[0], 62323[0], 62324[0], 62325[0], 62326[0], 62327[0], 64400[0], 64405[0], 64408[0], 64415[0], 64416[0], 64417[0], 64418[0], 64420[0], 64421[0], 64425[0], 64430[0], 64435[0], 64445[0], 64446[0], 64447[0], 64448[0], 64449[0], 64450[0], 64451[0], 64454[0], 64461[0], 64462[0], 64463[0], 64479[0], 64480[0], 64483[0], 64484[0], 64486[0], 64487[0], 64488[0], 64489[0], 64490[0], 64491[0], 64492[0], 64493[0], 64494[0], 64495[0], 64505[0], 64510[0], 64517[0], 64520[0], 64530[0], 67500[1], 67825[1], 67840[1], 67904[1], 67921[1], 67922[1], 67950[1], 69990[0], 92012[1], 92014[1], 92018[1], 92019[1], 93000[1], 93005[1], 93010[1], 93040[1], 93041[1], 93042[1], 93318[1], 93355[1], 94002[1], 94200[1], 94680[1], 94681[1], 94690[1], 95812[1], 95813[1], 95816[1], 95819[1], 95822[1], 95829[1], 95955[1], 96360[1], 96361[1], 96365[1], 96366[1], 96367[1], 96368[1], 96372[1], 96374[1], 96375[1], 96376[1], 96377[1], 96523[0], 97597[1], 97598[1], 97602[1], 99155[0], 99156[0], 99157[0], 99211[1], 99212[1], 99213[1], 99214[1], 99215[1], 99217[1], 99218[1], 99219[1], 99220[1], 99221[1], 99222[1], 99223[1], 99231[1], 99232[1], 99233[1], 99234[1], 99235[1], 99236[1], 99238[1], 99239[1], 99241[1], 99242[1], 99243[1], 99244[1], 99245[1], 99251[1], 99252[1], 99253[1], 99254[1], 99255[1], 99291[1], 99292[1], 99304[1], 99305[1], 99306[1], 99307[1], 99308[1], 99309[1], 99310[1], 99315[1], 99316[1], 99334[1], 99335[1], 99336[1], 99337[1], 99347[1], 99348[1], 99349[1], 99350[1], 99374[1], 99375[1], 99377[1], 99378[1], 99446[0], 99447[0], 99448[0], 99449[0], 99451[0], 99452[0], 99495[0], 99496[0], G0463[1], G0471[1], J0670[1], J2001[1]

0 = Modifier usage not allowed or inappropriate 1 = Modifier usage allowed

Code 1	Code 2
67924	0213T[0], 0216T[0], 0596T[1], 0597T[1], 0708T[1], 0709T[1], 12001[1], 12002[1], 12004[1], 12005[1], 12006[1], 12007[1], 12011[1], 12013[1], 12014[1], 12015[1], 12016[1], 12017[1], 12018[1], 12020[1], 12021[1], 12031[1], 12032[1], 12034[1], 12035[1], 12036[1], 12037[1], 12041[1], 12042[1], 12044[1], 12045[1], 12046[1], 12047[1], 12051[1], 12052[1], 12053[1], 12054[1], 12055[1], 12056[1], 12057[1], 13100[1], 13101[1], 13102[1], 13120[1], 13121[1], 13122[1], 13131[1], 13132[1], 13133[1], 13151[1], 13152[1], 13153[1], 15820[1], 15822[1], 21280[1], 21282[1], 36000[1], 36400[1], 36405[1], 36406[1], 36410[1], 36420[1], 36425[1], 36430[1], 36440[1], 36591[0], 36592[0], 36600[1], 36640[1], 43752[1], 51701[1], 51702[1], 51703[1], 62320[0], 62321[0], 62322[0], 62323[0], 62324[0], 62325[0], 62326[0], 62327[0], 64400[0], 64405[0], 64408[0], 64415[0], 64416[0], 64417[0], 64418[0], 64420[0], 64421[0], 64425[0], 64430[0], 64435[0], 64445[0], 64446[0], 64447[0], 64448[0], 64449[0], 64450[0], 64451[0], 64454[0], 64461[0], 64462[0], 64463[0], 64479[0], 64480[0], 64483[0], 64484[0], 64486[0], 64487[0], 64488[0], 64489[0], 64490[0], 64491[0], 64492[0], 64493[0], 64494[0], 64495[0], 64505[0], 64510[0], 64517[0], 64520[0], 64530[0], 67500[1], 67904[1], 67917[1], 67921[1], 67922[1], 67923[1], 67930[1], 67950[1], 67961[1], 69990[0], 92012[1], 92014[1], 92018[1], 92019[1], 93000[1], 93005[1], 93010[1], 93040[1], 93041[1], 93042[1], 93318[1], 93355[1], 94002[1], 94200[1], 94680[1], 94681[1], 94690[1], 95812[1], 95813[1], 95816[1], 95819[1], 95822[1], 95829[1], 95955[1], 96360[1], 96361[1], 96365[1], 96366[1], 96367[1], 96368[1], 96372[1], 96374[1], 96375[1], 96376[1], 96377[1], 96523[0], 99155[0], 99156[0], 99157[0], 99211[1], 99212[1], 99213[1], 99214[1], 99215[1], 99217[1], 99218[1], 99219[1], 99220[1], 99221[1], 99222[1], 99223[1], 99231[1], 99232[1], 99233[1], 99234[1], 99235[1], 99236[1], 99238[1], 99239[1], 99241[1], 99242[1], 99243[1], 99244[1], 99245[1], 99251[1], 99252[1], 99253[1], 99254[1], 99255[1], 99291[1], 99292[1], 99304[1], 99305[1], 99306[1], 99307[1], 99308[1], 99309[1], 99310[1], 99315[1], 99316[1], 99334[1], 99335[1], 99336[1], 99337[1], 99347[1], 99348[1], 99349[1], 99350[1], 99374[1], 99375[1], 99377[1], 99378[1], 99446[0], 99447[0], 99448[0], 99449[0], 99451[0], 99452[0], 99495[0], 99496[0], G0463[1], G0471[1], J0670[1], J2001[1]
67930	0213T[0], 0216T[0], 0596T[1], 0597T[1], 0708T[1], 0709T[1], 11000[1], 11001[1], 11004[1], 11005[1], 11006[1], 11042[1], 11043[1], 11044[1], 11045[1], 11046[1], 11047[1], 12001[1], 12002[1], 12004[1], 12005[1], 12006[1], 12007[1], 12011[1], 12013[1], 12014[1], 12015[1], 12016[1], 12017[1], 12018[1], 12020[1], 12021[1], 12031[1], 12032[1], 12034[1], 12035[1], 12036[1], 12037[1], 12041[1], 12042[1], 12044[1], 12045[1], 12046[1], 12047[1], 12051[1], 12052[1], 12053[1], 12054[1], 12055[1], 12056[1], 12057[1], 13100[1], 13101[1], 13102[1], 13120[1], 13121[1], 13122[1], 13131[1], 13132[1], 13133[1], 13151[1], 13152[1], 13153[1], 36000[1], 36400[1], 36405[1], 36406[1], 36410[1], 36420[1], 36425[1], 36430[1], 36440[1], 36591[0], 36592[0], 36600[1], 36640[1], 43752[1], 51701[1], 51702[1], 51703[1], 62320[0], 62321[0], 62322[0], 62323[0], 62324[0], 62325[0], 62326[0], 62327[0], 64400[0], 64405[0], 64408[0], 64415[0], 64416[0], 64417[0], 64418[0], 64420[0], 64421[0], 64425[0], 64430[0], 64435[0], 64445[0], 64446[0], 64447[0], 64448[0], 64449[0], 64450[0], 64451[0], 64454[0], 64461[0], 64462[0], 64463[0], 64479[0], 64480[0], 64483[0], 64484[0], 64486[0], 64487[0], 64488[0], 64489[0], 64490[0], 64491[0], 64492[0], 64493[0], 64494[0], 64495[0], 64505[0], 64510[0], 64517[0], 64520[0], 64530[0], 67500[1], 67938[1], 69990[0], 92012[1], 92014[1], 92018[1], 92019[1], 93000[1], 93005[1], 93010[1], 93040[1], 93041[1], 93042[1], 93318[1], 93355[1], 94002[1], 94200[1], 94680[1], 94681[1], 94690[1], 95812[1], 95813[1], 95816[1], 95819[1], 95822[1], 95829[1], 95955[1], 96360[1], 96361[1], 96365[1], 96366[1], 96367[1], 96368[1], 96372[1], 96374[1], 96375[1], 96376[1], 96377[1], 96523[0], 97597[1], 97598[1], 97602[1], 99155[0], 99156[0], 99157[0], 99211[1], 99212[1], 99213[1], 99214[1], 99215[1], 99217[1], 99218[1], 99219[1], 99220[1], 99221[1], 99222[1], 99223[1], 99231[1], 99232[1], 99233[1], 99234[1], 99235[1], 99236[1], 99238[1], 99239[1], 99241[1], 99242[1], 99243[1], 99244[1], 99245[1], 99251[1], 99252[1], 99253[1], 99254[1], 99255[1], 99291[1], 99292[1], 99304[1], 99305[1], 99306[1], 99307[1], 99308[1], 99309[1], 99310[1], 99315[1], 99316[1], 99334[1], 99335[1], 99336[1], 99337[1], 99347[1], 99348[1], 99349[1], 99350[1], 99374[1], 99375[1], 99377[1], 99378[1], 99446[0], 99447[0], 99448[0], 99449[0], 99451[0], 99452[0], 99495[0], 99496[0], G0463[1], G0471[1], J0670[1], J2001[1]
67935	0213T[0], 0216T[0], 0596T[1], 0597T[1], 0708T[1], 0709T[1], 11000[1], 11001[1], 11004[1], 11005[1], 11006[1], 11042[1], 11043[1], 11044[1], 11045[1], 11046[1], 11047[1], 12001[1], 12002[1], 12004[1], 12005[1], 12006[1], 12007[1], 12011[1], 12013[1], 12014[1], 12015[1], 12016[1], 12017[1], 12018[1], 12020[1], 12021[1], 12031[1], 12032[1], 12034[1], 12035[1], 12036[1], 12037[1], 12041[1], 12042[1], 12044[1], 12045[1], 12046[1], 12047[1], 12051[1], 12052[1], 12053[1], 12054[1], 12055[1], 12056[1], 12057[1], 13100[1], 13101[1], 13102[1], 13120[1], 13121[1], 13122[1], 13131[1], 13132[1], 13133[1], 13151[1], 13152[1], 13153[1], 36000[1], 36400[1], 36405[1], 36406[1], 36410[1], 36420[1], 36425[1], 36430[1], 36440[1], 36591[0], 36592[0], 36600[1], 36640[1], 43752[1], 51701[1], 51702[1], 51703[1], 62320[0], 62321[0], 62322[0], 62323[0], 62324[0], 62325[0], 62326[0], 62327[0], 64400[0], 64405[0], 64408[0], 64415[0], 64416[0], 64417[0], 64418[0], 64420[0], 64421[0], 64425[0], 64430[0], 64435[0], 64445[0], 64446[0], 64447[0], 64448[0], 64449[0], 64450[0], 64451[0], 64454[0], 64461[0], 64462[0], 64463[0], 64479[0], 64480[0], 64483[0], 64484[0], 64486[0], 64487[0], 64488[0], 64489[0], 64490[0], 64491[0], 64492[0], 64493[0], 64494[0], 64495[0], 64505[0], 64510[0], 64517[0], 64520[0], 64530[0], 67500[1], 67938[1], 69990[0], 92012[1], 92014[1], 92018[1], 92019[1], 93000[1], 93005[1], 93010[1], 93040[1], 93041[1], 93042[1], 93318[1], 93355[1], 94002[1], 94200[1], 94680[1], 94681[1], 94690[1], 95812[1], 95813[1], 95816[1], 95819[1], 95822[1], 95829[1], 95955[1], 96360[1], 96361[1], 96365[1], 96366[1], 96367[1], 96368[1], 96372[1], 96374[1], 96375[1], 96376[1], 96377[1], 96523[0], 97597[1], 97598[1], 97602[1], 99155[0], 99156[0], 99157[0], 99211[1], 99212[1], 99213[1], 99214[1], 99215[1], 99217[1], 99218[1], 99219[1], 99220[1], 99221[1], 99222[1], 99223[1], 99231[1], 99232[1], 99233[1], 99234[1], 99235[1], 99236[1], 99238[1], 99239[1], 99241[1], 99242[1], 99243[1], 99244[1], 99245[1], 99251[1], 99252[1], 99253[1], 99254[1], 99255[1], 99291[1], 99292[1], 99304[1], 99305[1], 99306[1], 99307[1], 99308[1], 99309[1], 99310[1], 99315[1], 99316[1], 99334[1], 99335[1], 99336[1], 99337[1], 99347[1], 99348[1], 99349[1], 99350[1], 99374[1], 99375[1], 99377[1], 99378[1], 99446[0], 99447[0], 99448[0], 99449[0], 99451[0], 99452[0], 99495[0], 99496[0], G0463[1], G0471[1], J0670[1], J2001[1]
67938	0213T[0], 0216T[0], 0596T[1], 0597T[1], 0708T[1], 0709T[1], 11000[1], 11001[1], 11004[1], 11005[1], 11006[1], 11042[1], 11043[1], 11044[1], 11045[1], 11046[1], 11047[1], 12001[1], 12002[1], 12004[1], 12005[1], 12006[1], 12007[1], 12011[1], 12013[1], 12014[1], 12015[1], 12016[1], 12017[1], 12018[1], 12020[1], 12021[1], 12031[1], 12032[1], 12034[1], 12035[1], 12036[1], 12037[1], 12041[1], 12042[1], 12044[1], 12045[1], 12046[1], 12047[1], 12051[1], 12052[1], 12053[1], 12054[1], 12055[1], 12056[1], 12057[1], 13100[1], 13101[1], 13102[1], 13120[1], 13121[1], 13122[1], 13131[1], 13132[1], 13133[1], 13151[1], 13152[1], 13153[1], 36000[1], 36400[1], 36405[1], 36406[1], 36410[1], 36420[1], 36425[1], 36430[1], 36440[1], 36591[0], 36592[0], 36600[1], 36640[1], 43752[1], 51701[1], 51702[1], 51703[1], 62320[0], 62321[0], 62322[0], 62323[0], 62324[0], 62325[0], 62326[0], 62327[0], 64400[0], 64405[0], 64408[0], 64415[0], 64416[0], 64417[0], 64418[0], 64420[0], 64421[0], 64425[0], 64430[0], 64435[0], 64445[0], 64446[0], 64447[0], 64448[0], 64449[0], 64450[0], 64451[0], 64454[0], 64461[0], 64462[0], 64463[0], 64479[0], 64480[0], 64483[0], 64484[0], 64486[0], 64487[0], 64488[0], 64489[0], 64490[0], 64491[0], 64492[0], 64493[0], 64494[0], 64495[0], 64505[0], 64510[0], 64517[0], 64520[0], 64530[0], 67500[1], 69990[0], 92012[1], 92014[1], 92018[1], 92019[1], 93000[1], 93005[1], 93010[1], 93040[1], 93041[1], 93042[1], 93318[1], 93355[1], 94002[1], 94200[1], 94680[1], 94681[1], 94690[1], 95812[1], 95813[1], 95816[1], 95819[1], 95822[1], 95829[1], 95955[1], 96360[1], 96361[1], 96365[1], 96366[1], 96367[1], 96368[1], 96372[1], 96374[1], 96375[1], 96376[1], 96377[1], 96523[0], 97597[1], 97598[1], 97602[1], 99155[0], 99156[0], 99157[0], 99211[1], 99212[1], 99213[1], 99214[1], 99215[1], 99217[1], 99218[1], 99219[1], 99220[1], 99221[1], 99222[1], 99223[1], 99231[1], 99232[1], 99233[1], 99234[1], 99235[1], 99236[1], 99238[1], 99239[1], 99241[1], 99242[1], 99243[1], 99244[1], 99245[1], 99251[1], 99252[1], 99253[1], 99254[1], 99255[1], 99291[1], 99292[1], 99304[1], 99305[1], 99306[1], 99307[1], 99308[1], 99309[1], 99310[1], 99315[1], 99316[1], 99334[1], 99335[1], 99336[1], 99337[1], 99347[1], 99348[1], 99349[1], 99350[1], 99374[1], 99375[1], 99377[1], 99378[1], 99446[0], 99447[0], 99448[0], 99449[0], 99451[0], 99452[0], 99495[0], 99496[0], G0463[1], G0471[1], J0670[1], J2001[1]
67950	0213T[0], 0216T[0], 0596T[1], 0597T[1], 0708T[1], 0709T[1], 11000[1], 11001[1], 11004[1], 11005[1], 11006[1], 11042[1], 11043[1], 11044[1], 11045[1], 11046[1], 11047[1], 12001[1], 12002[1], 12004[1], 12005[1], 12006[1], 12007[1], 12011[1], 12013[1], 12014[1], 12015[1], 12016[1], 12017[1], 12018[1], 12020[1], 12021[1], 12031[1], 12032[1], 12034[1], 12035[1], 12036[1], 12037[1], 12041[1], 12042[1], 12044[1], 12045[1], 12046[1], 12047[1], 12051[1], 12052[1], 12053[1], 12054[1], 12055[1], 12056[1], 12057[1], 13100[1], 13101[1], 13102[1], 13120[1], 13121[1], 13122[1], 13131[1], 13132[1], 13133[1], 13151[1], 13152[1], 13153[1], 21280[1], 21282[1], 36000[1], 36400[1], 36405[1], 36406[1], 36410[1], 36420[1], 36425[1], 36430[1], 36440[1], 36591[0], 36592[0], 36600[1], 36640[1], 43752[1], 51701[1], 51702[1], 51703[1], 62320[0], 62321[0], 62322[0], 62323[0], 62324[0], 62325[0], 62326[0], 62327[0], 64400[0], 64405[0], 64408[0], 64415[0], 64416[0], 64417[0], 64418[0], 64420[0], 64421[0], 64425[0], 64430[0], 64435[0], 64445[0], 64446[0], 64447[0], 64448[0], 64449[0], 64450[0], 64451[0], 64454[0], 64461[0], 64462[0], 64463[0], 64479[0], 64480[0], 64483[0], 64484[0], 64486[0], 64487[0], 64488[0], 64489[0], 64490[0], 64491[0], 64492[0], 64493[0], 64494[0], 64495[0], 64505[0], 64510[0], 64517[0], 64520[0], 64530[0], 67500[1], 67715[1], 67880[1], 67882[1], 69990[0], 92012[1], 92014[1], 92018[1], 92019[1], 93000[1], 93005[1], 93010[1], 93040[1], 93041[1], 93042[1], 93318[1], 93355[1], 94002[1], 94200[1], 94680[1], 94681[1], 94690[1], 95812[1], 95813[1], 95816[1], 95819[1], 95822[1], 95829[1], 95955[1], 96360[1], 96361[1], 96365[1], 96366[1], 96367[1], 96368[1], 96372[1], 96374[1], 96375[1], 96376[1], 96377[1], 96523[0], 97597[1], 97598[1], 97602[1], 99155[0], 99156[0], 99157[0], 99211[1], 99212[1], 99213[1], 99214[1], 99215[1], 99217[1], 99218[1], 99219[1], 99220[1], 99221[1], 99222[1], 99223[1], 99231[1], 99232[1], 99233[1], 99234[1], 99235[1], 99236[1], 99238[1], 99239[1], 99241[1], 99242[1], 99243[1], 99244[1], 99245[1], 99251[1], 99252[1], 99253[1], 99254[1], 99255[1], 99291[1], 99292[1], 99304[1], 99305[1], 99306[1], 99307[1], 99308[1], 99309[1], 99310[1], 99315[1], 99316[1], 99334[1], 99335[1], 99336[1], 99337[1], 99347[1], 99348[1], 99349[1], 99350[1], 99374[1], 99375[1], 99377[1], 99378[1], 99446[0], 99447[0], 99448[0], 99449[0], 99451[0], 99452[0], 99495[0], 99496[0], G0463[1], G0471[1], J0670[1], J2001[1]
67961	0213T[0], 0216T[0], 0596T[1], 0597T[1], 0708T[1], 0709T[1], 11000[1], 11001[1], 11004[1], 11005[1], 11006[1], 11042[1], 11043[1], 11044[1], 11045[1], 11046[1], 11047[1], 11440[1], 11441[1], 11442[1], 11443[1], 11444[1], 11640[1], 11641[1], 11642[1], 11643[1], 11644[1], 11646[1], 12001[1], 12002[1], 12004[1], 12005[1], 12006[1], 12007[1], 12011[1], 12013[1], 12014[1], 12015[1], 12016[1], 12017[1], 12018[1], 12020[1], 12021[1], 12031[1], 12032[1], 12034[1], 12035[1], 12036[1], 12037[1], 12041[1], 12042[1], 12044[1], 12045[1], 12046[1], 12047[1], 12051[1], 12052[1], 12053[1], 12054[1], 12055[1], 12056[1], 12057[1], 13100[1], 13101[1], 13102[1], 13120[1], 13121[1], 13122[1], 13131[1], 13132[1], 13133[1], 13151[1], 13152[1], 13153[1], 14060[1], 14061[1], 14301[1], 14302[1], 15004[1], 21280[1], 36000[1], 36400[1], 36405[1], 36406[1], 36410[1], 36420[1], 36425[1], 36430[1], 36440[1], 36591[0], 36592[0], 36600[1], 36640[1], 43752[1], 51701[1], 51702[1], 51703[1], 62320[0], 62321[0], 62322[0],

0 = Modifier usage not allowed or inappropriate 1 = Modifier usage allowed

Code 1	Code 2
	62323[0], 62324[0], 62325[0], 62326[0], 62327[0], 64400[0], 64405[0], 64408[0], 64415[0], 64416[0], 64417[0], 64418[0], 64420[0], 64421[0], 64425[0], 64430[0], 64435[0], 64445[0], 64446[0], 64447[0], 64448[0], 64449[0], 64450[0], 64451[0], 64454[0], 64461[0], 64462[0], 64463[0], 64479[0], 64480[0], 64483[0], 64484[0], 64486[0], 64487[0], 64488[0], 64489[0], 64490[0], 64491[0], 64492[0], 64493[0], 64494[0], 64495[0], 64505[0], 64510[0], 64517[0], 64520[0], 64530[0], 67500[1], 67715[1], 67840[1], 67916[1], 67923[1], 67930[1], 67935[1], 67950[1], 67966[1], 68440[1], 69990[0], 92012[1], 92014[1], 92018[1], 92019[1], 93000[1], 93005[1], 93010[1], 93040[1], 93041[1], 93042[1], 93318[1], 93355[1], 94002[1], 94200[1], 94680[1], 94681[1], 94690[1], 95812[1], 95813[1], 95816[1], 95819[1], 95822[1], 95829[1], 95955[1], 96360[1], 96361[1], 96365[1], 96366[1], 96367[1], 96368[1], 96372[1], 96374[1], 96375[1], 96376[1], 96377[1], 96523[0], 97597[1], 97598[1], 97602[1], 99155[0], 99156[0], 99157[0], 99211[1], 99212[1], 99213[1], 99214[1], 99215[1], 99217[1], 99218[1], 99219[1], 99220[1], 99221[1], 99222[1], 99223[1], 99231[1], 99232[1], 99233[1], 99234[1], 99235[1], 99236[1], 99238[1], 99239[1], 99241[1], 99242[1], 99243[1], 99244[1], 99245[1], 99251[1], 99252[1], 99253[1], 99254[1], 99255[1], 99291[1], 99292[1], 99304[1], 99305[1], 99306[1], 99307[1], 99308[1], 99309[1], 99310[1], 99315[1], 99316[1], 99334[1], 99335[1], 99336[1], 99337[1], 99347[1], 99348[1], 99349[1], 99350[1], 99374[1], 99375[1], 99377[1], 99378[1], 99446[0], 99447[0], 99448[0], 99449[0], 99451[0], 99452[0], 99495[0], 99496[0], G0463[1], G0471[1], J0670[1], J2001[1]
67966	0213T[0], 0216T[0], 0596T[1], 0597T[1], 0708T[1], 0709T[1], 11000[1], 11001[1], 11004[1], 11005[1], 11006[1], 11042[1], 11043[1], 11044[1], 11045[1], 11046[1], 11047[1], 11440[1], 11441[1], 11442[1], 11443[1], 11444[1], 11446[1], 11640[1], 11641[1], 11642[1], 11643[1], 11644[1], 11646[1], 12001[1], 12002[1], 12004[1], 12005[1], 12006[1], 12007[1], 12011[1], 12013[1], 12014[1], 12015[1], 12016[1], 12017[1], 12018[1], 12020[1], 12021[1], 12031[1], 12032[1], 12034[1], 12035[1], 12036[1], 12037[1], 12041[1], 12042[1], 12044[1], 12045[1], 12046[1], 12047[1], 12051[1], 12052[1], 12053[1], 12054[1], 12055[1], 12056[1], 12057[1], 13100[1], 13101[1], 13102[1], 13120[1], 13121[1], 13122[1], 13131[1], 13132[1], 13133[1], 13151[1], 13152[1], 13153[1], 14060[1], 14061[1], 14301[1], 14302[1], 15004[1], 21280[1], 36000[1], 36400[1], 36405[1], 36406[1], 36410[1], 36420[1], 36425[1], 36430[1], 36440[1], 36591[0], 36592[0], 36600[1], 36640[1], 43752[1], 51701[1], 51702[1], 51703[1], 62320[0], 62321[0], 62322[0], 62323[0], 62324[0], 62325[0], 62326[0], 62327[0], 64400[0], 64405[0], 64408[0], 64415[0], 64416[0], 64417[0], 64418[0], 64420[0], 64421[0], 64425[0], 64430[0], 64435[0], 64445[0], 64446[0], 64447[0], 64448[0], 64449[0], 64450[0], 64451[0], 64454[0], 64461[0], 64462[0], 64463[0], 64479[0], 64480[0], 64483[0], 64484[0], 64486[0], 64487[0], 64488[0], 64489[0], 64490[0], 64491[0], 64492[0], 64493[0], 64494[0], 64495[0], 64505[0], 64510[0], 64517[0], 64520[0], 64530[0], 67500[1], 67715[1], 67916[1], 67917[1], 67923[1], 67924[1], 67930[1], 67935[1], 67950[1], 69990[0], 92012[1], 92014[1], 92018[1], 92019[1], 93000[1], 93005[1], 93010[1], 93040[1], 93041[1], 93042[1], 93318[1], 93355[1], 94002[1], 94200[1], 94680[1], 94681[1], 94690[1], 95812[1], 95813[1], 95816[1], 95819[1], 95822[1], 95829[1], 95955[1], 96360[1], 96361[1], 96365[1], 96366[1], 96367[1], 96368[1], 96372[1], 96374[1], 96375[1], 96376[1], 96377[1], 96523[0], 97597[1], 97598[1], 97602[1], 99155[0], 99156[0], 99157[0], 99211[1], 99212[1], 99213[1], 99214[1], 99215[1], 99217[1], 99218[1], 99219[1], 99220[1], 99221[1], 99222[1], 99223[1], 99231[1], 99232[1], 99233[1], 99234[1], 99235[1], 99236[1], 99238[1], 99239[1], 99241[1], 99242[1], 99243[1], 99244[1], 99245[1], 99251[1], 99252[1], 99253[1], 99254[1], 99255[1], 99291[1], 99292[1], 99304[1], 99305[1], 99306[1], 99307[1], 99308[1], 99309[1], 99310[1], 99315[1], 99316[1], 99334[1], 99335[1], 99336[1], 99337[1], 99347[1], 99348[1], 99349[1], 99350[1], 99374[1], 99375[1], 99377[1], 99378[1], 99446[0], 99447[0], 99448[0], 99449[0], 99451[0], 99452[0], 99495[0], 99496[0], G0463[1], G0471[1], J0670[1], J2001[1]
67971	0213T[0], 0216T[0], 0596T[1], 0597T[1], 0708T[1], 0709T[1], 12001[1], 12002[1], 12004[1], 12005[1], 12006[1], 12007[1], 12011[1], 12013[1], 12014[1], 12015[1], 12016[1], 12017[1], 12018[1], 12020[1], 12021[1], 12031[1], 12032[1], 12034[1], 12035[1], 12036[1], 12037[1], 12041[1], 12042[1], 12044[1], 12045[1], 12046[1], 12047[1], 12051[1], 12052[1], 12053[1], 12054[1], 12055[1], 12056[1], 12057[1], 13100[1], 13101[1], 13102[1], 13120[1], 13121[1], 13122[1], 13131[1], 13132[1], 13133[1], 13151[1], 13152[1], 13153[1], 14060[1], 14061[1], 14301[1], 14302[1], 15576[1], 15630[1], 21280[1], 21282[1], 36000[1], 36400[1], 36405[1], 36406[1], 36410[1], 36420[1], 36425[1], 36430[1], 36440[1], 36591[0], 36592[0], 36600[1], 36640[1], 43752[1], 51701[1], 51702[1], 51703[1], 62320[0], 62321[0], 62322[0], 62323[0], 62324[0], 62325[0], 62326[0], 62327[0], 64400[0], 64405[0], 64408[0], 64415[0], 64416[0], 64417[0], 64418[0], 64420[0], 64421[0], 64425[0], 64430[0], 64435[0], 64445[0], 64446[0], 64447[0], 64448[0], 64449[0], 64450[0], 64451[0], 64454[0], 64461[0], 64462[0], 64463[0], 64479[0], 64480[0], 64483[0], 64484[0], 64486[0], 64487[0], 64488[0], 64489[0], 64490[0], 64491[0], 64492[0], 64493[0], 64494[0], 64495[0], 64505[0], 64510[0], 64517[0], 64520[0], 64530[0], 67500[1], 67950[1], 69990[0], 92012[1], 92014[1], 92018[1], 92019[1], 93000[1], 93005[1], 93010[1], 93040[1], 93041[1], 93042[1], 93318[1], 93355[1], 94002[1], 94200[1], 94680[1], 94681[1], 94690[1], 95812[1], 95813[1], 95816[1], 95819[1], 95822[1], 95829[1], 95955[1], 96360[1], 96361[1], 96365[1], 96366[1], 96367[1], 96368[1], 96372[1], 96374[1], 96375[1], 96376[1], 96377[1], 96523[0], 99155[0], 99156[0], 99157[0], 99211[1], 99212[1], 99213[1], 99214[1], 99215[1], 99217[1], 99218[1], 99219[1], 99220[1], 99221[1], 99222[1], 99223[1], 99231[1], 99232[1], 99233[1], 99234[1], 99235[1], 99236[1], 99238[1], 99239[1], 99241[1], 99242[1], 99243[1], 99244[1], 99245[1], 99251[1], 99252[1], 99253[1], 99254[1], 99255[1], 99291[1], 99292[1], 99304[1], 99305[1], 99306[1], 99307[1], 99308[1], 99309[1], 99310[1], 99315[1], 99316[1], 99334[1], 99335[1], 99336[1], 99337[1], 99347[1], 99348[1], 99349[1], 99350[1], 99374[1], 99375[1], 99377[1], 99378[1], 99446[0], 99447[0], 99448[0], 99449[0], 99451[0], 99452[0], 99495[0], 99496[0], G0463[1], G0471[1]
67973	0213T[0], 0216T[0], 0596T[1], 0597T[1], 0708T[1], 0709T[1], 12001[1], 12002[1], 12004[1], 12005[1], 12006[1], 12007[1], 12011[1], 12013[1], 12014[1], 12015[1], 12016[1], 12017[1], 12018[1], 12020[1], 12021[1], 12031[1], 12032[1], 12034[1], 12035[1], 12036[1], 12037[1], 12041[1], 12042[1], 12044[1], 12045[1], 12046[1], 12047[1], 12051[1], 12052[1], 12053[1], 12054[1], 12055[1], 12056[1], 12057[1], 13100[1], 13101[1], 13102[1], 13120[1], 13121[1], 13122[1], 13131[1], 13132[1], 13133[1], 13151[1], 13152[1], 13153[1], 15576[1], 15630[1], 21280[1], 21282[1], 36000[1], 36400[1], 36405[1], 36406[1], 36410[1], 36420[1], 36425[1], 36430[1], 36440[1], 36591[0], 36592[0], 36600[1], 36640[1], 43752[1], 51701[1], 51702[1], 51703[1], 62320[0], 62321[0], 62322[0], 62323[0], 62324[0], 62325[0], 62326[0], 62327[0], 64400[0], 64405[0], 64408[0], 64415[0], 64416[0], 64417[0], 64418[0], 64420[0], 64421[0], 64425[0], 64430[0], 64435[0], 64445[0], 64446[0], 64447[0], 64448[0], 64449[0], 64450[0], 64451[0], 64454[0], 64461[0], 64462[0], 64463[0], 64479[0], 64480[0], 64483[0], 64484[0], 64486[0], 64487[0], 64488[0], 64489[0], 64490[0], 64491[0], 64492[0], 64493[0], 64494[0], 64495[0], 64505[0], 64510[0], 64517[0], 64520[0], 64530[0], 67500[1], 67950[1], 67971[1], 69990[0], 92012[1], 92014[1], 92018[1], 92019[1], 93000[1], 93005[1], 93010[1], 93040[1], 93041[1], 93042[1], 93318[1], 93355[1], 94002[1], 94200[1], 94680[1], 94681[1], 94690[1], 95812[1], 95813[1], 95816[1], 95819[1], 95822[1], 95829[1], 95955[1], 96360[1], 96361[1], 96365[1], 96366[1], 96367[1], 96368[1], 96372[1], 96374[1], 96375[1], 96376[1], 96377[1], 96523[0], 99155[0], 99156[0], 99157[0], 99211[1], 99212[1], 99213[1], 99214[1], 99215[1], 99217[1], 99218[1], 99219[1], 99220[1], 99221[1], 99222[1], 99223[1], 99231[1], 99232[1], 99233[1], 99234[1], 99235[1], 99236[1], 99238[1], 99239[1], 99241[1], 99242[1], 99243[1], 99244[1], 99245[1], 99251[1], 99252[1], 99253[1], 99254[1], 99255[1], 99291[1], 99292[1], 99304[1], 99305[1], 99306[1], 99307[1], 99308[1], 99309[1], 99310[1], 99315[1], 99316[1], 99334[1], 99335[1], 99336[1], 99337[1], 99347[1], 99348[1], 99349[1], 99350[1], 99374[1], 99375[1], 99377[1], 99378[1], 99446[0], 99447[0], 99448[0], 99449[0], 99451[0], 99452[0], 99495[0], 99496[0], G0463[1], G0471[1]
67974	0213T[0], 0216T[0], 0596T[1], 0597T[1], 0708T[1], 0709T[1], 12001[1], 12002[1], 12004[1], 12005[1], 12006[1], 12007[1], 12011[1], 12013[1], 12014[1], 12015[1], 12016[1], 12017[1], 12018[1], 12020[1], 12021[1], 12031[1], 12032[1], 12034[1], 12035[1], 12036[1], 12037[1], 12041[1], 12042[1], 12044[1], 12045[1], 12046[1], 12047[1], 12051[1], 12052[1], 12053[1], 12054[1], 12055[1], 12056[1], 12057[1], 13100[1], 13101[1], 13102[1], 13120[1], 13121[1], 13122[1], 13131[1], 13132[1], 13133[1], 13151[1], 13152[1], 13153[1], 15576[1], 15630[1], 21280[1], 21282[1], 36000[1], 36400[1], 36405[1], 36406[1], 36410[1], 36420[1], 36425[1], 36430[1], 36440[1], 36591[0], 36592[0], 36600[1], 36640[1], 43752[1], 51701[1], 51702[1], 51703[1], 62320[0], 62321[0], 62322[0], 62323[0], 62324[0], 62325[0], 62326[0], 62327[0], 64400[0], 64405[0], 64408[0], 64415[0], 64416[0], 64417[0], 64418[0], 64420[0], 64421[0], 64425[0], 64430[0], 64435[0], 64445[0], 64446[0], 64447[0], 64448[0], 64449[0], 64450[0], 64451[0], 64454[0], 64461[0], 64462[0], 64463[0], 64479[0], 64480[0], 64483[0], 64484[0], 64486[0], 64487[0], 64488[0], 64489[0], 64490[0], 64491[0], 64492[0], 64493[0], 64494[0], 64495[0], 64505[0], 64510[0], 64517[0], 64520[0], 64530[0], 67500[1], 67950[1], 67971[1], 67973[1], 69990[0], 92012[1], 92014[1], 92018[1], 92019[1], 93000[1], 93005[1], 93010[1], 93040[1], 93041[1], 93042[1], 93318[1], 93355[1], 94002[1], 94200[1], 94680[1], 94681[1], 94690[1], 95812[1], 95813[1], 95816[1], 95819[1], 95822[1], 95829[1], 95955[1], 96360[1], 96361[1], 96365[1], 96366[1], 96367[1], 96368[1], 96372[1], 96374[1], 96375[1], 96376[1], 96377[1], 96523[0], 99155[0], 99156[0], 99157[0], 99211[1], 99212[1], 99213[1], 99214[1], 99215[1], 99217[1], 99218[1], 99219[1], 99220[1], 99221[1], 99222[1], 99223[1], 99231[1], 99232[1], 99233[1], 99234[1], 99235[1], 99236[1], 99238[1], 99239[1], 99241[1], 99242[1], 99243[1], 99244[1], 99245[1], 99251[1], 99252[1], 99253[1], 99254[1], 99255[1], 99291[1], 99292[1], 99304[1], 99305[1], 99306[1], 99307[1], 99308[1], 99309[1], 99310[1], 99315[1], 99316[1], 99334[1], 99335[1], 99336[1], 99337[1], 99347[1], 99348[1], 99349[1], 99350[1], 99374[1], 99375[1], 99377[1], 99378[1], 99446[0], 99447[0], 99448[0], 99449[0], 99451[0], 99452[0], 99495[0], 99496[0], G0463[1], G0471[1]
67975	0213T[0], 0216T[0], 0596T[1], 0597T[1], 0708T[1], 0709T[1], 12001[1], 12002[1], 12004[1], 12005[1], 12006[1], 12007[1], 12011[1], 12013[1], 12014[1], 12015[1], 12016[1], 12017[1], 12018[1], 12020[1], 12021[1], 12031[1], 12032[1], 12034[1], 12035[1], 12036[1], 12037[1], 12041[1], 12042[1], 12044[1], 12045[1], 12046[1], 12047[1], 12051[1], 12052[1], 12053[1], 12054[1], 12055[1], 12056[1], 12057[1], 13100[1], 13101[1], 13102[1], 13120[1], 13121[1], 13122[1], 13131[1], 13132[1], 13133[1], 13151[1], 13152[1], 13153[1], 15576[1], 15630[1], 21280[1], 21282[1], 36000[1], 36400[1], 36405[1], 36406[1], 36410[1], 36420[1], 36425[1], 36430[1], 36440[1], 36591[0], 36592[0], 36600[1], 36640[1], 43752[1], 51701[1], 51702[1], 51703[1], 62320[0], 62321[0], 62322[0], 62323[0], 62324[0], 62325[0], 62326[0], 62327[0], 64400[0], 64405[0], 64408[0], 64415[0], 64416[0], 64417[0], 64418[0], 64420[0], 64421[0], 64425[0], 64430[0], 64435[0], 64445[0], 64446[0], 64447[0], 64448[0], 64449[0], 64450[0], 64451[0], 64454[0], 64461[0], 64462[0], 64463[0], 64479[0], 64480[0], 64483[0], 64484[0], 64486[0], 64487[0], 64488[0], 64489[0], 64490[0], 64491[0], 64492[0], 64493[0], 64494[0], 64495[0], 64505[0], 64510[0], 64517[0], 64520[0], 64530[0], 67500[1], 67950[1], 67971[1], 67973[1], 67974[1], 69990[0], 92012[1], 92014[1], 92018[1], 92019[1], 93000[1], 93005[1], 93010[1], 93040[1], 93041[1], 93042[1], 93318[1], 93355[1], 94002[1], 94200[1], 94680[1], 94681[1], 94690[1], 95812[1], 95813[1], 95816[1], 95819[1], 95822[1], 95829[1], 95955[1], 96360[1], 96361[1], 96365[1], 96366[1], 96367[1], 96368[1], 96372[1], 96374[1], 96375[1], 96376[1], 96377[1], 96523[0], 99155[0], 99156[0], 99157[0], 99211[1], 99212[1],

0 = Modifier usage not allowed or inappropriate 1 = Modifier usage allowed

Appendix A: NCCI - CPT Codes

Code 1	Code 2
	99213[1], 99214[1], 99215[1], 99217[1], 99218[1], 99219[1], 99220[1], 99221[1], 99222[1], 99223[1], 99231[1], 99232[1], 99233[1], 99234[1], 99235[1], 99236[1], 99238[1], 99239[1], 99241[1], 99242[1], 99243[1], 99244[1], 99245[1], 99251[1], 99252[1], 99253[1], 99254[1], 99255[1], 99291[1], 99292[1], 99304[1], 99305[1], 99306[1], 99307[1], 99308[1], 99309[1], 99310[1], 99315[1], 99316[1], 99334[1], 99335[1], 99336[1], 99337[1], 99347[1], 99348[1], 99349[1], 99350[1], 99374[1], 99375[1], 99377[1], 99378[1], 99446[0], 99447[0], 99448[0], 99449[0], 99451[0], 99452[0], 99495[0], 99496[0], G0463[1], G0471[1]
68020	0213T[0], 0216T[0], 0596T[1], 0597T[1], 0708T[1], 0709T[1], 12001[1], 12002[1], 12004[1], 12005[1], 12006[1], 12007[1], 12011[1], 12013[1], 12014[1], 12015[1], 12016[1], 12017[1], 12018[1], 12020[1], 12021[1], 12031[1], 12032[1], 12034[1], 12035[1], 12036[1], 12037[1], 12041[1], 12042[1], 12044[1], 12045[1], 12046[1], 12047[1], 12051[1], 12052[1], 12053[1], 12054[1], 12055[1], 12056[1], 12057[1], 13100[1], 13101[1], 13102[1], 13120[1], 13121[1], 13122[1], 13131[1], 13132[1], 13133[1], 13151[1], 13152[1], 13153[1], 36000[1], 36400[1], 36405[1], 36406[1], 36410[1], 36420[1], 36425[1], 36430[1], 36440[1], 36591[0], 36592[0], 36600[1], 36640[1], 43752[1], 51701[1], 51702[1], 51703[1], 62320[0], 62321[0], 62322[0], 62323[0], 62324[0], 62325[0], 62326[0], 62327[0], 64400[0], 64405[0], 64408[0], 64415[0], 64416[0], 64417[0], 64418[0], 64420[0], 64421[0], 64425[0], 64430[0], 64435[0], 64445[0], 64446[0], 64447[0], 64448[0], 64449[0], 64450[0], 64451[0], 64454[0], 64461[0], 64462[0], 64463[0], 64479[0], 64480[0], 64483[0], 64484[0], 64486[0], 64487[0], 64488[0], 64489[0], 64490[0], 64491[0], 64492[0], 64493[0], 64494[0], 64495[0], 64505[0], 64510[0], 64517[0], 64520[0], 64530[0], 67500[1], 69990[0], 92012[1], 92014[1], 92018[1], 92019[1], 93000[1], 93005[1], 93010[1], 93040[1], 93041[1], 93042[1], 93318[1], 93355[1], 94002[1], 94200[1], 94680[1], 94681[1], 94690[1], 95812[1], 95813[1], 95816[1], 95819[1], 95822[1], 95829[1], 95955[1], 96360[1], 96361[1], 96365[1], 96366[1], 96367[1], 96368[1], 96372[1], 96374[1], 96375[1], 96376[1], 96377[1], 96523[0], 99155[0], 99156[0], 99157[0], 99211[1], 99212[1], 99213[1], 99214[1], 99215[1], 99217[1], 99218[1], 99219[1], 99220[1], 99221[1], 99222[1], 99223[1], 99231[1], 99232[1], 99233[1], 99234[1], 99235[1], 99236[1], 99238[1], 99239[1], 99241[1], 99242[1], 99243[1], 99244[1], 99245[1], 99251[1], 99252[1], 99253[1], 99254[1], 99255[1], 99291[1], 99292[1], 99304[1], 99305[1], 99306[1], 99307[1], 99308[1], 99309[1], 99310[1], 99315[1], 99316[1], 99334[1], 99335[1], 99336[1], 99337[1], 99347[1], 99348[1], 99349[1], 99350[1], 99374[1], 99375[1], 99377[1], 99378[1], 99446[0], 99447[0], 99448[0], 99449[0], 99451[0], 99452[0], 99495[0], 99496[0], G0463[1], G0471[1], J2001[1]
68040	0213T[0], 0216T[0], 0596T[1], 0597T[1], 0708T[1], 0709T[1], 12001[1], 12002[1], 12004[1], 12005[1], 12006[1], 12007[1], 12011[1], 12013[1], 12014[1], 12015[1], 12016[1], 12017[1], 12018[1], 12020[1], 12021[1], 12031[1], 12032[1], 12034[1], 12035[1], 12036[1], 12037[1], 12041[1], 12042[1], 12044[1], 12045[1], 12046[1], 12047[1], 12051[1], 12052[1], 12053[1], 12054[1], 12055[1], 12056[1], 12057[1], 13100[1], 13101[1], 13102[1], 13120[1], 13121[1], 13122[1], 13131[1], 13132[1], 13133[1], 13151[1], 13152[1], 13153[1], 36000[1], 36400[1], 36405[1], 36406[1], 36410[1], 36420[1], 36425[1], 36430[1], 36440[1], 36591[0], 36592[0], 36600[1], 36640[1], 43752[1], 51701[1], 51702[1], 51703[1], 62320[0], 62321[0], 62322[0], 62323[0], 62324[0], 62325[0], 62326[0], 62327[0], 64400[0], 64405[0], 64408[0], 64415[0], 64416[0], 64417[0], 64418[0], 64420[0], 64421[0], 64425[0], 64430[0], 64435[0], 64445[0], 64446[0], 64447[0], 64448[0], 64449[0], 64450[0], 64451[0], 64454[0], 64461[0], 64462[0], 64463[0], 64479[0], 64480[0], 64483[0], 64484[0], 64486[0], 64487[0], 64488[0], 64489[0], 64490[0], 64491[0], 64492[0], 64493[0], 64494[0], 64495[0], 64505[0], 64510[0], 64517[0], 64520[0], 64530[0], 67500[1], 68020[1], 69990[0], 92012[1], 92014[1], 92018[1], 92019[1], 93000[1], 93005[1], 93010[1], 93040[1], 93041[1], 93042[1], 93318[1], 93355[1], 94002[1], 94200[1], 94680[1], 94681[1], 94690[1], 95812[1], 95813[1], 95816[1], 95819[1], 95822[1], 95829[1], 95955[1], 96360[1], 96361[1], 96365[1], 96366[1], 96367[1], 96368[1], 96372[1], 96374[1], 96375[1], 96376[1], 96377[1], 96523[0], 99155[0], 99156[0], 99157[0], 99211[1], 99212[1], 99213[1], 99214[1], 99215[1], 99217[1], 99218[1], 99219[1], 99220[1], 99221[1], 99222[1], 99223[1], 99231[1], 99232[1], 99233[1], 99234[1], 99235[1], 99236[1], 99238[1], 99239[1], 99241[1], 99242[1], 99243[1], 99244[1], 99245[1], 99251[1], 99252[1], 99253[1], 99254[1], 99255[1], 99291[1], 99292[1], 99304[1], 99305[1], 99306[1], 99307[1], 99308[1], 99309[1], 99310[1], 99315[1], 99316[1], 99334[1], 99335[1], 99336[1], 99337[1], 99347[1], 99348[1], 99349[1], 99350[1], 99374[1], 99375[1], 99377[1], 99378[1], 99446[0], 99447[0], 99448[0], 99449[0], 99451[0], 99452[0], 99495[1], 99496[1], G0463[1], G0471[1], J2001[1]
68100	0213T[0], 0216T[0], 0596T[1], 0597T[1], 0708T[1], 0709T[1], 10005[1], 10007[1], 10009[1], 10011[1], 10021[1], 11102[1], 11103[1], 11104[1], 11105[1], 11106[1], 11107[1], 12001[1], 12002[1], 12004[1], 12005[1], 12006[1], 12007[1], 12011[1], 12013[1], 12014[1], 12015[1], 12016[1], 12017[1], 12018[1], 12020[1], 12021[1], 12031[1], 12032[1], 12034[1], 12035[1], 12036[1], 12037[1], 12041[1], 12042[1], 12044[1], 12045[1], 12046[1], 12047[1], 12051[1], 12052[1], 12053[1], 12054[1], 12055[1], 12056[1], 12057[1], 13100[1], 13101[1], 13102[1], 13120[1], 13121[1], 13122[1], 13131[1], 13132[1], 13133[1], 13151[1], 13152[1], 13153[1], 36000[1], 36400[1], 36405[1], 36406[1], 36410[1], 36420[1], 36425[1], 36430[1], 36440[1], 36591[0], 36592[0], 36600[1], 36640[1], 43752[1], 51701[1], 51702[1], 51703[1], 62320[0], 62321[0], 62322[0], 62323[0], 62324[0], 62325[0], 62326[0], 62327[0], 64400[0], 64405[0], 64408[0], 64415[0], 64416[0], 64417[0], 64418[0], 64420[0], 64421[0], 64425[0], 64430[0], 64435[0], 64445[0], 64446[0], 64447[0], 64448[0], 64449[0], 64450[0], 64451[0], 64454[0], 64461[0], 64462[0], 64463[0], 64479[0], 64480[0], 64483[0], 64484[0], 64486[0], 64487[0], 64488[0], 64489[0], 64490[0], 64491[0], 64492[0], 64493[0], 64494[0], 64495[0], 64505[0], 64510[0], 64517[0], 64520[0], 64530[0], 67500[1], 68020[1], 68040[1], 69990[0], 92012[1], 92014[1], 92018[1], 92019[1], 93000[1], 93005[1], 93010[1], 93040[1], 93041[1], 93042[1], 93318[1], 93355[1], 94002[1], 94200[1], 94680[1], 94681[1], 94690[1], 95812[1], 95813[1], 95816[1], 95819[1], 95822[1], 95829[1], 95955[1], 96360[1], 96361[1], 96365[1], 96366[1], 96367[1], 96368[1], 96372[1], 96374[1], 96375[1], 96376[1], 96377[1], 96523[0], 99155[0], 99156[0], 99157[0], 99211[1], 99212[1], 99213[1], 99214[1], 99215[1], 99217[1], 99218[1], 99219[1], 99220[1], 99221[1], 99222[1], 99223[1], 99231[1], 99232[1], 99233[1], 99234[1], 99235[1], 99236[1], 99238[1], 99239[1], 99241[1], 99242[1], 99243[1], 99244[1], 99245[1], 99251[1], 99252[1], 99253[1], 99254[1], 99255[1], 99291[1], 99292[1], 99304[1], 99305[1], 99306[1], 99307[1], 99308[1], 99309[1], 99310[1], 99315[1], 99316[1], 99334[1], 99335[1], 99336[1], 99337[1], 99347[1], 99348[1], 99349[1], 99350[1], 99374[1], 99375[1], 99377[1], 99378[1], 99446[0], 99447[0], 99448[0], 99449[0], 99451[0], 99452[0], 99495[1], 99496[1], G0463[1], G0471[1], J0670[1], J2001[1]
68110	0213T[0], 0216T[0], 0596T[1], 0597T[1], 0708T[1], 0709T[1], 11000[1], 11001[1], 11004[1], 11005[1], 11006[1], 11042[1], 11043[1], 11044[1], 11045[1], 11046[1], 11047[1], 12001[1], 12002[1], 12004[1], 12005[1], 12006[1], 12007[1], 12011[1], 12013[1], 12014[1], 12015[1], 12016[1], 12017[1], 12018[1], 12020[1], 12021[1], 12031[1], 12032[1], 12034[1], 12035[1], 12036[1], 12037[1], 12041[1], 12042[1], 12044[1], 12045[1], 12046[1], 12047[1], 12051[1], 12052[1], 12053[1], 12054[1], 12055[1], 12056[1], 12057[1], 13100[1], 13101[1], 13102[1], 13120[1], 13121[1], 13122[1], 13131[1], 13132[1], 13133[1], 13151[1], 13152[1], 13153[1], 36000[1], 36400[1], 36405[1], 36406[1], 36410[1], 36420[1], 36425[1], 36430[1], 36440[1], 36591[0], 36592[0], 36600[1], 36640[1], 43752[1], 51701[1], 51702[1], 51703[1], 62320[0], 62321[0], 62322[0], 62323[0], 62324[0], 62325[0], 62326[0], 62327[0], 64400[0], 64405[0], 64408[0], 64415[0], 64416[0], 64417[0], 64418[0], 64420[0], 64421[0], 64425[0], 64430[0], 64435[0], 64445[0], 64446[0], 64447[0], 64448[0], 64449[0], 64450[0], 64451[0], 64454[0], 64461[0], 64462[0], 64463[0], 64479[0], 64480[0], 64483[0], 64484[0], 64486[0], 64487[0], 64488[0], 64489[0], 64490[0], 64491[0], 64492[0], 64493[0], 64494[0], 64495[0], 64505[0], 64510[0], 64517[0], 64520[0], 64530[0], 67500[1], 68040[1], 68100[1], 68115[1], 68135[1], 69990[0], 92012[1], 92014[1], 92018[1], 92019[1], 93000[1], 93005[1], 93010[1], 93040[1], 93041[1], 93042[1], 93318[1], 93355[1], 94002[1], 94200[1], 94680[1], 94681[1], 94690[1], 95812[1], 95813[1], 95816[1], 95819[1], 95822[1], 95829[1], 95955[1], 96360[1], 96361[1], 96365[1], 96366[1], 96367[1], 96368[1], 96372[1], 96374[1], 96375[1], 96376[1], 96377[1], 96523[0], 97597[1], 97598[1], 97602[1], 99155[0], 99156[0], 99157[0], 99211[1], 99212[1], 99213[1], 99214[1], 99215[1], 99217[1], 99218[1], 99219[1], 99220[1], 99221[1], 99222[1], 99223[1], 99231[1], 99232[1], 99233[1], 99234[1], 99235[1], 99236[1], 99238[1], 99239[1], 99241[1], 99242[1], 99243[1], 99244[1], 99245[1], 99251[1], 99252[1], 99253[1], 99254[1], 99255[1], 99291[1], 99292[1], 99304[1], 99305[1], 99306[1], 99307[1], 99308[1], 99309[1], 99310[1], 99315[1], 99316[1], 99334[1], 99335[1], 99336[1], 99337[1], 99347[1], 99348[1], 99349[1], 99350[1], 99374[1], 99375[1], 99377[1], 99378[1], 99446[0], 99447[0], 99448[0], 99449[0], 99451[0], 99452[0], 99495[0], 99496[0], G0463[1], G0471[1], J0670[1], J2001[1]
68115	0213T[0], 0216T[0], 0596T[1], 0597T[1], 0708T[1], 0709T[1], 11000[1], 11001[1], 11004[1], 11005[1], 11006[1], 11042[1], 11043[1], 11044[1], 11045[1], 11046[1], 11047[1], 12001[1], 12002[1], 12004[1], 12005[1], 12006[1], 12007[1], 12011[1], 12013[1], 12014[1], 12015[1], 12016[1], 12017[1], 12018[1], 12020[1], 12021[1], 12031[1], 12032[1], 12034[1], 12035[1], 12036[1], 12037[1], 12041[1], 12042[1], 12044[1], 12045[1], 12046[1], 12047[1], 12051[1], 12052[1], 12053[1], 12054[1], 12055[1], 12056[1], 12057[1], 13100[1], 13101[1], 13102[1], 13120[1], 13121[1], 13122[1], 13131[1], 13132[1], 13133[1], 13151[1], 13152[1], 13153[1], 36000[1], 36400[1], 36405[1], 36406[1], 36410[1], 36420[1], 36425[1], 36430[1], 36440[1], 36591[0], 36592[0], 36600[1], 36640[1], 43752[1], 51701[1], 51702[1], 51703[1], 62320[0], 62321[0], 62322[0], 62323[0], 62324[0], 62325[0], 62326[0], 62327[0], 64400[0], 64405[0], 64408[0], 64415[0], 64416[0], 64417[0], 64418[0], 64420[0], 64421[0], 64425[0], 64430[0], 64435[0], 64445[0], 64446[0], 64447[0], 64448[0], 64449[0], 64450[0], 64451[0], 64454[0], 64461[0], 64462[0], 64463[0], 64479[0], 64480[0], 64483[0], 64484[0], 64486[0], 64487[0], 64488[0], 64489[0], 64490[0], 64491[0], 64492[0], 64493[0], 64494[0], 64495[0], 64505[0], 64510[0], 64517[0], 64520[0], 64530[0], 67500[1], 68040[1], 68100[1], 68135[1], 69990[0], 92012[1], 92014[1], 92018[1], 92019[1], 93000[1], 93005[1], 93010[1], 93040[1], 93041[1], 93042[1], 93318[1], 93355[1], 94002[1], 94200[1], 94680[1], 94681[1], 94690[1], 95812[1], 95813[1], 95816[1], 95819[1], 95822[1], 95829[1], 95955[1], 96360[1], 96361[1], 96365[1], 96366[1], 96367[1], 96368[1], 96372[1], 96374[1], 96375[1], 96376[1], 96377[1], 96523[0], 97597[1], 97598[1], 97602[1], 99155[0], 99156[0], 99157[0], 99211[1], 99212[1], 99213[1], 99214[1], 99215[1], 99217[1], 99218[1], 99219[1], 99220[1], 99221[1], 99222[1], 99223[1], 99231[1], 99232[1], 99233[1], 99234[1], 99235[1], 99236[1], 99238[1], 99239[1], 99241[1], 99242[1], 99243[1], 99244[1], 99245[1], 99251[1], 99252[1], 99253[1], 99254[1], 99255[1], 99291[1], 99292[1], 99304[1], 99305[1], 99306[1], 99307[1], 99308[1], 99309[1], 99310[1], 99315[1], 99316[1], 99334[1], 99335[1], 99336[1], 99337[1], 99347[1], 99348[1], 99349[1], 99350[1], 99374[1], 99375[1], 99377[1], 99378[1], 99446[0], 99447[0], 99448[0], 99449[0], 99451[0], 99452[0], 99495[0], 99496[0], G0463[1], G0471[1], J0670[1], J2001[1]
68130	0213T[0], 0216T[0], 0596T[1], 0597T[1], 0708T[1], 0709T[1], 11000[1], 11001[1], 11004[1], 11005[1], 11006[1], 11042[1], 11043[1], 11044[1], 11045[1], 11046[1], 11047[1], 12001[1], 12002[1], 12004[1], 12005[1], 12006[1], 12007[1], 12011[1], 12013[1], 12014[1], 12015[1], 12016[1], 12017[1], 12018[1],

0 = Modifier usage not allowed or inappropriate 1 = Modifier usage allowed

Code 1	Code 2
	12020[1], 12021[1], 12031[1], 12032[1], 12034[1], 12035[1], 12036[1], 12037[1], 12041[1], 12042[1], 12044[1], 12045[1], 12046[1], 12047[1], 12051[1], 12052[1], 12053[1], 12054[1], 12055[1], 12056[1], 12057[1], 13100[1], 13101[1], 13102[1], 13120[1], 13121[1], 13122[1], 13131[1], 13132[1], 13133[1], 13151[1], 13152[1], 13153[1], 36000[1], 36400[1], 36405[1], 36406[1], 36410[1], 36420[1], 36425[1], 36430[1], 36440[1], 36591[0], 36592[0], 36600[1], 36640[1], 43752[1], 51701[1], 51702[1], 51703[1], 62320[0], 62321[0], 62322[0], 62323[0], 62324[0], 62325[0], 62326[0], 62327[0], 64400[0], 64405[0], 64408[0], 64415[0], 64416[0], 64417[0], 64418[0], 64420[0], 64421[0], 64425[0], 64430[0], 64435[0], 64445[0], 64446[0], 64447[0], 64448[0], 64449[0], 64450[0], 64451[0], 64454[0], 64461[0], 64462[0], 64463[0], 64479[0], 64480[0], 64483[0], 64484[0], 64486[0], 64487[0], 64488[0], 64489[0], 64490[0], 64491[0], 64492[0], 64493[0], 64494[0], 64495[0], 64505[0], 64510[0], 64517[0], 64520[0], 64530[0], 67500[1], 68040[1], 68100[1], 69990[0], 92012[1], 92014[1], 92018[1], 92019[1], 93000[1], 93005[1], 93010[1], 93040[1], 93041[1], 93042[1], 93318[1], 93355[1], 94002[1], 94200[1], 94680[1], 94681[1], 94690[1], 95812[1], 95813[1], 95816[1], 95819[1], 95822[1], 95829[1], 95955[1], 96360[1], 96361[1], 96365[1], 96366[1], 96367[1], 96368[1], 96372[1], 96374[1], 96375[1], 96376[1], 96377[1], 96523[0], 97597[1], 97598[1], 97602[1], 99155[0], 99156[0], 99157[0], 99211[1], 99212[1], 99213[1], 99214[1], 99215[1], 99217[1], 99218[1], 99219[1], 99220[1], 99221[1], 99222[1], 99223[1], 99231[1], 99232[1], 99233[1], 99234[1], 99235[1], 99236[1], 99238[1], 99239[1], 99241[1], 99242[1], 99243[1], 99244[1], 99245[1], 99251[1], 99252[1], 99253[1], 99254[1], 99255[1], 99291[1], 99292[1], 99304[1], 99305[1], 99306[1], 99307[1], 99308[1], 99309[1], 99310[1], 99315[1], 99316[1], 99334[1], 99335[1], 99336[1], 99337[1], 99347[1], 99348[1], 99349[1], 99350[1], 99374[1], 99375[1], 99377[1], 99378[1], 99446[0], 99447[0], 99448[0], 99449[0], 99451[0], 99452[0], 99495[0], 99496[0], G0463[1], G0471[1], J0670[1], J2001[1]
68135	0213T[0], 0216T[0], 0596T[1], 0597T[1], 0708T[1], 0709T[1], 12001[1], 12002[1], 12004[1], 12005[1], 12006[1], 12007[1], 12011[1], 12013[1], 12014[1], 12015[1], 12016[1], 12017[1], 12018[1], 12020[1], 12021[1], 12031[1], 12032[1], 12034[1], 12035[1], 12036[1], 12037[1], 12041[1], 12042[1], 12044[1], 12045[1], 12046[1], 12047[1], 12051[1], 12052[1], 12053[1], 12054[1], 12055[1], 12056[1], 12057[1], 13100[1], 13101[1], 13102[1], 13120[1], 13121[1], 13122[1], 13131[1], 13132[1], 13133[1], 13151[1], 13152[1], 13153[1], 36000[1], 36400[1], 36405[1], 36406[1], 36410[1], 36420[1], 36425[1], 36430[1], 36440[1], 36591[0], 36592[0], 36600[1], 36640[1], 43752[1], 51701[1], 51702[1], 51703[1], 62320[0], 62321[0], 62322[0], 62323[0], 62324[0], 62325[0], 62326[0], 62327[0], 64400[0], 64405[0], 64408[0], 64415[0], 64416[0], 64417[0], 64418[0], 64420[0], 64421[0], 64425[0], 64430[0], 64435[0], 64445[0], 64446[0], 64447[0], 64448[0], 64449[0], 64450[0], 64451[0], 64454[0], 64461[0], 64462[0], 64463[0], 64479[0], 64480[0], 64483[0], 64484[0], 64486[0], 64487[0], 64488[0], 64489[0], 64490[0], 64491[0], 64492[0], 64493[0], 64494[0], 64495[0], 64505[0], 64510[0], 64517[0], 64520[0], 64530[0], 67500[1], 68040[1], 69990[0], 92012[1], 92014[1], 92018[1], 92019[1], 93000[1], 93005[1], 93010[1], 93040[1], 93041[1], 93042[1], 93318[1], 93355[1], 94002[1], 94200[1], 94680[1], 94681[1], 94690[1], 95812[1], 95813[1], 95816[1], 95819[1], 95822[1], 95829[1], 95955[1], 96360[1], 96361[1], 96365[1], 96366[1], 96367[1], 96368[1], 96372[1], 96374[1], 96375[1], 96376[1], 96377[1], 96523[0], 99155[0], 99156[0], 99157[0], 99211[1], 99212[1], 99213[1], 99214[1], 99215[1], 99217[1], 99218[1], 99219[1], 99220[1], 99221[1], 99222[1], 99223[1], 99231[1], 99232[1], 99233[1], 99234[1], 99235[1], 99236[1], 99238[1], 99239[1], 99241[1], 99242[1], 99243[1], 99244[1], 99245[1], 99251[1], 99252[1], 99253[1], 99254[1], 99255[1], 99291[1], 99292[1], 99304[1], 99305[1], 99306[1], 99307[1], 99308[1], 99309[1], 99310[1], 99315[1], 99316[1], 99334[1], 99335[1], 99336[1], 99337[1], 99347[1], 99348[1], 99349[1], 99350[1], 99374[1], 99375[1], 99377[1], 99378[1], 99446[0], 99447[0], 99448[0], 99449[0], 99451[0], 99452[0], 99495[0], 99496[0], G0463[1], G0471[1], J2001[1]
68200	0213T[0], 0216T[0], 0596T[1], 0597T[1], 0708T[1], 0709T[1], 12001[1], 12002[1], 12004[1], 12005[1], 12006[1], 12007[1], 12011[1], 12013[1], 12014[1], 12015[1], 12016[1], 12017[1], 12018[1], 12020[1], 12021[1], 12031[1], 12032[1], 12034[1], 12035[1], 12036[1], 12037[1], 12041[1], 12042[1], 12044[1], 12045[1], 12046[1], 12047[1], 12051[1], 12052[1], 12053[1], 12054[1], 12055[1], 12056[1], 12057[1], 13100[1], 13101[1], 13102[1], 13120[1], 13121[1], 13122[1], 13131[1], 13132[1], 13133[1], 13151[1], 13152[1], 13153[1], 36000[1], 36400[1], 36405[1], 36406[1], 36410[1], 36420[1], 36425[1], 36430[1], 36440[1], 36591[0], 36592[0], 36600[1], 36640[1], 43752[1], 51701[1], 51702[1], 51703[1], 62320[0], 62321[0], 62322[0], 62323[0], 62324[0], 62325[0], 62326[0], 62327[0], 64400[0], 64405[0], 64408[0], 64415[0], 64416[0], 64417[0], 64418[0], 64420[0], 64421[0], 64425[0], 64430[0], 64435[0], 64445[0], 64446[0], 64447[0], 64448[0], 64449[0], 64450[0], 64451[0], 64454[0], 64461[0], 64462[0], 64463[0], 64479[0], 64480[0], 64483[0], 64484[0], 64486[0], 64487[0], 64488[0], 64489[0], 64490[0], 64491[0], 64492[0], 64493[0], 64494[0], 64495[0], 64505[0], 64510[0], 64517[0], 64520[0], 64530[0], 67500[1], 69990[0], 92012[1], 92014[1], 92018[1], 92019[1], 93000[1], 93005[1], 93010[1], 93040[1], 93041[1], 93042[1], 93318[1], 93355[1], 94002[1], 94200[1], 94680[1], 94681[1], 94690[1], 95812[1], 95813[1], 95816[1], 95819[1], 95822[1], 95829[1], 95955[1], 96360[1], 96361[1], 96365[1], 96366[1], 96367[1], 96368[1], 96372[1], 96374[1], 96375[1], 96376[1], 96377[1], 96523[0], 99155[0], 99156[0], 99157[0], 99211[1], 99212[1], 99213[1], 99214[1], 99215[1], 99217[1], 99218[1], 99219[1], 99220[1], 99221[1], 99222[1], 99223[1], 99231[1], 99232[1], 99233[1], 99234[1], 99235[1], 99236[1], 99238[1], 99239[1], 99241[1], 99242[1], 99243[1], 99244[1], 99245[1], 99251[1], 99252[1], 99253[1], 99254[1], 99255[1], 99291[1], 99292[1], 99304[1], 99305[1], 99306[1], 99307[1], 99308[1], 99309[1], 99310[1], 99315[1], 99316[1], 99334[1], 99335[1], 99336[1], 99337[1], 99347[1], 99348[1], 99349[1], 99350[1], 99374[1], 99375[1], 99377[1], 99378[1], 99446[0], 99447[0], 99448[0], 99449[0], 99451[0], 99452[0], 99495[1], 99496[1], G0463[1], G0471[1], J0670[1], J2001[1]
68320	0213T[0], 0216T[0], 0596T[1], 0597T[1], 0708T[1], 0709T[1], 11000[1], 11001[1], 11004[1], 11005[1], 11006[1], 11042[1], 11043[1], 11044[1], 11045[1], 11046[1], 11047[1], 12001[1], 12002[1], 12004[1], 12005[1], 12006[1], 12007[1], 12011[1], 12013[1], 12014[1], 12015[1], 12016[1], 12017[1], 12018[1], 12020[1], 12021[1], 12031[1], 12032[1], 12034[1], 12035[1], 12036[1], 12037[1], 12041[1], 12042[1], 12044[1], 12045[1], 12046[1], 12047[1], 12051[1], 12052[1], 12053[1], 12054[1], 12055[1], 12056[1], 12057[1], 13100[1], 13101[1], 13102[1], 13120[1], 13121[1], 13122[1], 13131[1], 13132[1], 13133[1], 13151[1], 13152[1], 13153[1], 36000[1], 36400[1], 36405[1], 36406[1], 36410[1], 36420[1], 36425[1], 36430[1], 36440[1], 36591[0], 36592[0], 36600[1], 36640[1], 43752[1], 51701[1], 51702[1], 51703[1], 62320[0], 62321[0], 62322[0], 62323[0], 62324[0], 62325[0], 62326[0], 62327[0], 64400[0], 64405[0], 64408[0], 64415[0], 64416[0], 64417[0], 64418[0], 64420[0], 64421[0], 64425[0], 64430[0], 64435[0], 64445[0], 64446[0], 64447[0], 64448[0], 64449[0], 64450[0], 64451[0], 64454[0], 64461[0], 64462[0], 64463[0], 64479[0], 64480[0], 64483[0], 64484[0], 64486[0], 64487[0], 64488[0], 64489[0], 64490[0], 64491[0], 64492[0], 64493[0], 64494[0], 64495[0], 64505[0], 64510[0], 64517[0], 64520[0], 64530[0], 67500[1], 67515[1], 68020[1], 68040[1], 68100[1], 68110[1], 68115[1], 68130[1], 68135[1], 68200[1], 68330[1], 68340[1], 68362[1], 68371[1], 69990[0], 92012[1], 92014[1], 92018[1], 92019[1], 93000[1], 93005[1], 93010[1], 93040[1], 93041[1], 93042[1], 93318[1], 93355[1], 94002[1], 94200[1], 94680[1], 94681[1], 94690[1], 95812[1], 95813[1], 95816[1], 95819[1], 95822[1], 95829[1], 95955[1], 96360[1], 96361[1], 96365[1], 96366[1], 96367[1], 96368[1], 96372[1], 96374[1], 96375[1], 96376[1], 96377[1], 96523[0], 97597[1], 97598[1], 97602[1], 99155[0], 99156[0], 99157[0], 99211[1], 99212[1], 99213[1], 99214[1], 99215[1], 99217[1], 99218[1], 99219[1], 99220[1], 99221[1], 99222[1], 99223[1], 99231[1], 99232[1], 99233[1], 99234[1], 99235[1], 99236[1], 99238[1], 99239[1], 99241[1], 99242[1], 99243[1], 99244[1], 99245[1], 99251[1], 99252[1], 99253[1], 99254[1], 99255[1], 99291[1], 99292[1], 99304[1], 99305[1], 99306[1], 99307[1], 99308[1], 99309[1], 99310[1], 99315[1], 99316[1], 99334[1], 99335[1], 99336[1], 99337[1], 99347[1], 99348[1], 99349[1], 99350[1], 99374[1], 99375[1], 99377[1], 99378[1], 99446[0], 99447[0], 99448[0], 99449[0], 99451[0], 99452[0], 99495[0], 99496[0], G0463[1], G0471[1], J0670[1], J2001[1]
68325	0213T[0], 0216T[0], 0596T[1], 0597T[1], 0708T[1], 0709T[1], 11000[1], 11001[1], 11004[1], 11005[1], 11006[1], 11042[1], 11043[1], 11044[1], 11045[1], 11046[1], 11047[1], 12001[1], 12002[1], 12004[1], 12005[1], 12006[1], 12007[1], 12011[1], 12013[1], 12014[1], 12015[1], 12016[1], 12017[1], 12018[1], 12020[1], 12021[1], 12031[1], 12032[1], 12034[1], 12035[1], 12036[1], 12037[1], 12041[1], 12042[1], 12044[1], 12045[1], 12046[1], 12047[1], 12051[1], 12052[1], 12053[1], 12054[1], 12055[1], 12056[1], 12057[1], 13100[1], 13101[1], 13102[1], 13120[1], 13121[1], 13122[1], 13131[1], 13132[1], 13133[1], 13151[1], 13152[1], 13153[1], 36000[1], 36400[1], 36405[1], 36406[1], 36410[1], 36420[1], 36425[1], 36430[1], 36440[1], 36591[0], 36592[0], 36600[1], 36640[1], 40818[1], 43752[1], 51701[1], 51702[1], 51703[1], 62320[0], 62321[0], 62322[0], 62323[0], 62324[0], 62325[0], 62326[0], 62327[0], 64400[0], 64405[0], 64408[0], 64415[0], 64416[0], 64417[0], 64418[0], 64420[0], 64421[0], 64425[0], 64430[0], 64435[0], 64445[0], 64446[0], 64447[0], 64448[0], 64449[0], 64450[0], 64451[0], 64454[0], 64461[0], 64462[0], 64463[0], 64479[0], 64480[0], 64483[0], 64484[0], 64486[0], 64487[0], 64488[0], 64489[0], 64490[0], 64491[0], 64492[0], 64493[0], 64494[0], 64495[0], 64505[0], 64510[0], 64517[0], 64520[0], 64530[0], 67500[1], 68020[1], 68040[1], 68100[1], 68110[1], 68115[1], 68130[1], 68135[1], 68200[1], 68320[1], 68326[1], 68330[1], 68335[1], 68340[1], 69990[0], 92012[1], 92014[1], 92018[1], 92019[1], 93000[1], 93005[1], 93010[1], 93040[1], 93041[1], 93042[1], 93318[1], 93355[1], 94002[1], 94200[1], 94680[1], 94681[1], 94690[1], 95812[1], 95813[1], 95816[1], 95819[1], 95822[1], 95829[1], 95955[1], 96360[1], 96361[1], 96365[1], 96366[1], 96367[1], 96368[1], 96372[1], 96374[1], 96375[1], 96376[1], 96377[1], 96523[0], 97597[1], 97598[1], 97602[1], 99155[0], 99156[0], 99157[0], 99211[1], 99212[1], 99213[1], 99214[1], 99215[1], 99217[1], 99218[1], 99219[1], 99220[1], 99221[1], 99222[1], 99223[1], 99231[1], 99232[1], 99233[1], 99234[1], 99235[1], 99236[1], 99238[1], 99239[1], 99241[1], 99242[1], 99243[1], 99244[1], 99245[1], 99251[1], 99252[1], 99253[1], 99254[1], 99255[1], 99291[1], 99292[1], 99304[1], 99305[1], 99306[1], 99307[1], 99308[1], 99309[1], 99310[1], 99315[1], 99316[1], 99334[1], 99335[1], 99336[1], 99337[1], 99347[1], 99348[1], 99349[1], 99350[1], 99374[1], 99375[1], 99377[1], 99378[1], 99446[0], 99447[0], 99448[0], 99449[0], 99451[0], 99452[0], 99495[0], 99496[0], G0463[1], G0471[1], J2001[1]
68326	0213T[0], 0216T[0], 0596T[1], 0597T[1], 0708T[1], 0709T[1], 11000[1], 11001[1], 11004[1], 11005[1], 11006[1], 11042[1], 11043[1], 11044[1], 11045[1], 11046[1], 11047[1], 12001[1], 12002[1], 12004[1], 12005[1], 12006[1], 12007[1], 12011[1], 12013[1], 12014[1], 12015[1], 12016[1], 12017[1], 12018[1], 12020[1], 12021[1], 12031[1], 12032[1], 12034[1], 12035[1], 12036[1], 12037[1], 12041[1], 12042[1], 12044[1], 12045[1], 12046[1], 12047[1], 12051[1], 12052[1], 12053[1], 12054[1], 12055[1], 12056[1], 12057[1], 13100[1], 13101[1], 13102[1], 13120[1], 13121[1], 13122[1], 13131[1], 13132[1], 13133[1], 13151[1], 13152[1], 13153[1], 36000[1], 36400[1], 36405[1], 36406[1], 36410[1], 36420[1], 36425[1], 36430[1], 36440[1], 36591[0], 36592[0], 36600[1], 36640[1], 43752[1], 51701[1], 51702[1], 51703[1], 62320[0], 62321[0], 62322[0], 62323[0], 62324[0], 62325[0], 62326[0], 62327[0], 64400[0], 64405[0], 64408[0], 64415[0], 64416[0], 64417[0], 64418[0], 64420[0], 64421[0], 64425[0], 64430[0], 64435[0], 64445[0], 64446[0], 64447[0], 64448[0], 64449[0], 64450[0], 64451[0], 64454[0], 64461[0], 64462[0],

Appendix A: NCCI - CPT Codes

0 = Modifier usage not allowed or inappropriate 1 = Modifier usage allowed

Code 1	Code 2
	64463[0], 64479[0], 64480[0], 64483[0], 64484[0], 64486[0], 64487[0], 64488[0], 64489[0], 64490[0], 64491[0], 64492[0], 64493[0], 64494[0], 64495[0], 64505[0], 64510[0], 64517[0], 64520[0], 64530[0], 67500[1], 68020[1], 68040[1], 68100[1], 68110[1], 68115[1], 68130[1], 68135[1], 68200[1], 68320[1], 68330[1], 68340[1], 68362[1], 68371[1], 69990[0], 92012[1], 92014[1], 92018[1], 92019[1], 93000[1], 93005[1], 93010[1], 93040[1], 93041[1], 93042[1], 93318[1], 93355[1], 94002[1], 94200[1], 94680[1], 94681[1], 94690[1], 95812[1], 95813[1], 95816[1], 95819[1], 95822[1], 95829[1], 95955[1], 96360[1], 96361[1], 96365[1], 96366[1], 96367[1], 96368[1], 96372[1], 96374[1], 96375[1], 96376[1], 96377[1], 96523[0], 97597[1], 97598[1], 97602[1], 99155[0], 99156[0], 99157[0], 99211[1], 99212[1], 99213[1], 99214[1], 99215[1], 99217[1], 99218[1], 99219[1], 99220[1], 99221[1], 99222[1], 99223[1], 99231[1], 99232[1], 99233[1], 99234[1], 99235[1], 99236[1], 99238[1], 99239[1], 99241[1], 99242[1], 99243[1], 99244[1], 99245[1], 99251[1], 99252[1], 99253[1], 99254[1], 99255[1], 99291[1], 99292[1], 99304[1], 99305[1], 99306[1], 99307[1], 99308[1], 99309[1], 99310[1], 99315[1], 99316[1], 99334[1], 99335[1], 99336[1], 99337[1], 99347[1], 99348[1], 99349[1], 99350[1], 99374[1], 99375[1], 99377[1], 99378[1], 99446[0], 99447[0], 99448[0], 99449[0], 99451[0], 99452[0], 99495[0], 99496[0], G0463[1], G0471[1], J2001[1]
68328	0213T[0], 0216T[0], 0596T[1], 0597T[1], 0708T[1], 0709T[1], 11000[1], 11001[1], 11004[1], 11005[1], 11006[1], 11042[1], 11043[1], 11044[1], 11045[1], 11046[1], 11047[1], 12001[1], 12002[1], 12004[1], 12005[1], 12006[1], 12007[1], 12011[1], 12013[1], 12014[1], 12015[1], 12016[1], 12017[1], 12018[1], 12020[1], 12021[1], 12031[1], 12032[1], 12034[1], 12035[1], 12036[1], 12037[1], 12041[1], 12042[1], 12044[1], 12045[1], 12046[1], 12047[1], 12051[1], 12052[1], 12053[1], 12054[1], 12055[1], 12056[1], 12057[1], 13100[1], 13101[1], 13102[1], 13120[1], 13121[1], 13122[1], 13131[1], 13132[1], 13133[1], 13151[1], 13152[1], 13153[1], 36000[1], 36400[1], 36405[1], 36406[1], 36410[1], 36420[1], 36425[1], 36430[1], 36440[1], 36591[0], 36592[0], 36600[1], 36640[1], 40818[1], 43752[1], 51701[1], 51702[1], 51703[1], 62320[0], 62321[0], 62322[0], 62323[0], 62324[0], 62325[0], 62326[0], 62327[0], 64400[0], 64405[0], 64408[0], 64415[0], 64416[0], 64417[0], 64418[0], 64420[0], 64421[0], 64425[0], 64430[0], 64435[0], 64445[0], 64446[0], 64447[0], 64448[0], 64449[0], 64450[0], 64451[0], 64454[0], 64461[0], 64462[0], 64463[0], 64479[0], 64480[0], 64483[0], 64484[0], 64486[0], 64487[0], 64488[0], 64489[0], 64490[0], 64491[0], 64492[0], 64493[0], 64494[0], 64495[0], 64505[0], 64510[0], 64517[0], 64520[0], 64530[0], 67500[1], 68020[1], 68040[1], 68100[1], 68110[1], 68115[1], 68130[1], 68135[1], 68200[1], 68320[1], 68325[1], 68326[1], 68330[1], 68335[1], 68340[1], 68362[1], 69990[0], 92012[1], 92014[1], 92018[1], 92019[1], 93000[1], 93005[1], 93010[1], 93040[1], 93041[1], 93042[1], 93318[1], 93355[1], 94002[1], 94200[1], 94680[1], 94681[1], 94690[1], 95812[1], 95813[1], 95816[1], 95819[1], 95822[1], 95829[1], 95955[1], 96360[1], 96361[1], 96365[1], 96366[1], 96367[1], 96368[1], 96372[1], 96374[1], 96375[1], 96376[1], 96377[1], 96523[0], 97597[1], 97598[1], 97602[1], 99155[0], 99156[0], 99157[0], 99211[1], 99212[1], 99213[1], 99214[1], 99215[1], 99217[1], 99218[1], 99219[1], 99220[1], 99221[1], 99222[1], 99223[1], 99231[1], 99232[1], 99233[1], 99234[1], 99235[1], 99236[1], 99238[1], 99239[1], 99241[1], 99242[1], 99243[1], 99244[1], 99245[1], 99251[1], 99252[1], 99253[1], 99254[1], 99255[1], 99291[1], 99292[1], 99304[1], 99305[1], 99306[1], 99307[1], 99308[1], 99309[1], 99310[1], 99315[1], 99316[1], 99334[1], 99335[1], 99336[1], 99337[1], 99347[1], 99348[1], 99349[1], 99350[1], 99374[1], 99375[1], 99377[1], 99378[1], 99446[0], 99447[0], 99448[0], 99449[0], 99451[0], 99452[0], 99495[0], 99496[0], G0463[1], G0471[1], J2001[1]
68330	0213T[0], 0216T[0], 0596T[1], 0597T[1], 0708T[1], 0709T[1], 11000[1], 11001[1], 11004[1], 11005[1], 11006[1], 11042[1], 11043[1], 11044[1], 11045[1], 11046[1], 11047[1], 12001[1], 12002[1], 12004[1], 12005[1], 12006[1], 12007[1], 12011[1], 12013[1], 12014[1], 12015[1], 12016[1], 12017[1], 12018[1], 12020[1], 12021[1], 12031[1], 12032[1], 12034[1], 12035[1], 12036[1], 12037[1], 12041[1], 12042[1], 12044[1], 12045[1], 12046[1], 12047[1], 12051[1], 12052[1], 12053[1], 12054[1], 12055[1], 12056[1], 12057[1], 13100[1], 13101[1], 13102[1], 13120[1], 13121[1], 13122[1], 13131[1], 13132[1], 13133[1], 13151[1], 13152[1], 13153[1], 36000[1], 36400[1], 36405[1], 36406[1], 36410[1], 36420[1], 36425[1], 36430[1], 36440[1], 36591[0], 36592[0], 36600[1], 36640[1], 43752[1], 51701[1], 51702[1], 51703[1], 62320[0], 62321[0], 62322[0], 62323[0], 62324[0], 62325[0], 62326[0], 62327[0], 64400[0], 64405[0], 64408[0], 64415[0], 64416[0], 64417[0], 64418[0], 64420[0], 64421[0], 64425[0], 64430[0], 64435[0], 64445[0], 64446[0], 64447[0], 64448[0], 64449[0], 64450[0], 64451[0], 64454[0], 64461[0], 64462[0], 64463[0], 64479[0], 64480[0], 64483[0], 64484[0], 64486[0], 64487[0], 64488[0], 64489[0], 64490[0], 64491[0], 64492[0], 64493[0], 64494[0], 64495[0], 64505[0], 64510[0], 64517[0], 64520[0], 64530[0], 67500[1], 68020[1], 68040[1], 68100[1], 68110[1], 68115[1], 68130[1], 68135[1], 68200[1], 68340[1], 69990[0], 92012[1], 92014[1], 92018[1], 92019[1], 93000[1], 93005[1], 93010[1], 93040[1], 93041[1], 93042[1], 93318[1], 93355[1], 94002[1], 94200[1], 94680[1], 94681[1], 94690[1], 95812[1], 95813[1], 95816[1], 95819[1], 95822[1], 95829[1], 95955[1], 96360[1], 96361[1], 96365[1], 96366[1], 96367[1], 96368[1], 96372[1], 96374[1], 96375[1], 96376[1], 96377[1], 96523[0], 97597[1], 97598[1], 97602[1], 99155[0], 99156[0], 99157[0], 99211[1], 99212[1], 99213[1], 99214[1], 99215[1], 99217[1], 99218[1], 99219[1], 99220[1], 99221[1], 99222[1], 99223[1], 99231[1], 99232[1], 99233[1], 99234[1], 99235[1], 99236[1], 99238[1], 99239[1], 99241[1], 99242[1], 99243[1], 99244[1], 99245[1], 99251[1], 99252[1], 99253[1], 99254[1], 99255[1], 99291[1], 99292[1], 99304[1], 99305[1], 99306[1], 99307[1], 99308[1], 99309[1], 99310[1], 99315[1], 99316[1], 99334[1], 99335[1], 99336[1], 99337[1], 99347[1], 99348[1], 99349[1], 99350[1], 99374[1], 99375[1], 99377[1], 99378[1], 99446[0], 99447[0], 99448[0], 99449[0], 99451[0], 99452[0], 99495[0], 99496[0], G0463[1], G0471[1], J0670[1], J2001[1]
68335	0213T[0], 0216T[0], 0596T[1], 0597T[1], 0708T[1], 0709T[1], 12001[1], 12002[1], 12004[1], 12005[1], 12006[1], 12007[1], 12011[1], 12013[1], 12014[1], 12015[1], 12016[1], 12017[1], 12018[1], 12020[1], 12021[1], 12031[1], 12032[1], 12034[1], 12035[1], 12036[1], 12037[1], 12041[1], 12042[1], 12044[1], 12045[1], 12046[1], 12047[1], 12051[1], 12052[1], 12053[1], 12054[1], 12055[1], 12056[1], 12057[1], 13100[1], 13101[1], 13102[1], 13120[1], 13121[1], 13122[1], 13131[1], 13132[1], 13133[1], 13151[1], 13152[1], 13153[1], 36000[1], 36400[1], 36405[1], 36406[1], 36410[1], 36420[1], 36425[1], 36430[1], 36440[1], 36591[0], 36592[0], 36600[1], 36640[1], 40818[1], 43752[1], 51701[1], 51702[1], 51703[1], 62320[0], 62321[0], 62322[0], 62323[0], 62324[0], 62325[0], 62326[0], 62327[0], 64400[0], 64405[0], 64408[0], 64415[0], 64416[0], 64417[0], 64418[0], 64420[0], 64421[0], 64425[0], 64430[0], 64435[0], 64445[0], 64446[0], 64447[0], 64448[0], 64449[0], 64450[0], 64451[0], 64454[0], 64461[0], 64462[0], 64463[0], 64479[0], 64480[0], 64483[0], 64484[0], 64486[0], 64487[0], 64488[0], 64489[0], 64490[0], 64491[0], 64492[0], 64493[0], 64494[0], 64495[0], 64505[0], 64510[0], 64517[0], 64520[0], 64530[0], 67500[1], 68020[1], 68040[1], 68100[1], 68110[1], 68115[1], 68130[1], 68135[1], 68200[1], 68320[1], 68326[1], 68330[1], 68340[1], 68362[1], 68371[1], 69990[0], 92012[1], 92014[1], 92018[1], 92019[1], 93000[1], 93005[1], 93010[1], 93040[1], 93041[1], 93042[1], 93318[1], 93355[1], 94002[1], 94200[1], 94680[1], 94681[1], 94690[1], 95812[1], 95813[1], 95816[1], 95819[1], 95822[1], 95829[1], 95955[1], 96360[1], 96361[1], 96365[1], 96366[1], 96367[1], 96368[1], 96372[1], 96374[1], 96375[1], 96376[1], 96377[1], 96523[0], 99155[0], 99156[0], 99157[0], 99211[1], 99212[1], 99213[1], 99214[1], 99215[1], 99217[1], 99218[1], 99219[1], 99220[1], 99221[1], 99222[1], 99223[1], 99231[1], 99232[1], 99233[1], 99234[1], 99235[1], 99236[1], 99238[1], 99239[1], 99241[1], 99242[1], 99243[1], 99244[1], 99245[1], 99251[1], 99252[1], 99253[1], 99254[1], 99255[1], 99291[1], 99292[1], 99304[1], 99305[1], 99306[1], 99307[1], 99308[1], 99309[1], 99310[1], 99315[1], 99316[1], 99334[1], 99335[1], 99336[1], 99337[1], 99347[1], 99348[1], 99349[1], 99350[1], 99374[1], 99375[1], 99377[1], 99378[1], 99446[0], 99447[0], 99448[0], 99449[0], 99451[0], 99452[0], 99495[0], 99496[0], G0463[1], G0471[1], J2001[1]
68340	0213T[0], 0216T[0], 0596T[1], 0597T[1], 0708T[1], 0709T[1], 11000[1], 11001[1], 11004[1], 11005[1], 11006[1], 11042[1], 11043[1], 11044[1], 11045[1], 11046[1], 11047[1], 12001[1], 12002[1], 12004[1], 12005[1], 12006[1], 12007[1], 12011[1], 12013[1], 12014[1], 12015[1], 12016[1], 12017[1], 12018[1], 12020[1], 12021[1], 12031[1], 12032[1], 12034[1], 12035[1], 12036[1], 12037[1], 12041[1], 12042[1], 12044[1], 12045[1], 12046[1], 12047[1], 12051[1], 12052[1], 12053[1], 12054[1], 12055[1], 12056[1], 12057[1], 13100[1], 13101[1], 13102[1], 13120[1], 13121[1], 13122[1], 13131[1], 13132[1], 13133[1], 13151[1], 13152[1], 13153[1], 36000[1], 36400[1], 36405[1], 36406[1], 36410[1], 36420[1], 36425[1], 36430[1], 36440[1], 36591[0], 36592[0], 36600[1], 36640[1], 43752[1], 51701[1], 51702[1], 51703[1], 62320[0], 62321[0], 62322[0], 62323[0], 62324[0], 62325[0], 62326[0], 62327[0], 64400[0], 64405[0], 64408[0], 64415[0], 64416[0], 64417[0], 64418[0], 64420[0], 64421[0], 64425[0], 64430[0], 64435[0], 64445[0], 64446[0], 64447[0], 64448[0], 64449[0], 64450[0], 64451[0], 64454[0], 64461[0], 64462[0], 64463[0], 64479[0], 64480[0], 64483[0], 64484[0], 64486[0], 64487[0], 64488[0], 64489[0], 64490[0], 64491[0], 64492[0], 64493[0], 64494[0], 64495[0], 64505[0], 64510[0], 64517[0], 64520[0], 64530[0], 67500[1], 67715[1], 68020[1], 68040[1], 68100[1], 68110[1], 68115[1], 68130[1], 68135[1], 68200[1], 69990[0], 92012[1], 92014[1], 92018[1], 92019[1], 93000[1], 93005[1], 93010[1], 93040[1], 93041[1], 93042[1], 93318[1], 93355[1], 94002[1], 94200[1], 94680[1], 94681[1], 94690[1], 95812[1], 95813[1], 95816[1], 95819[1], 95822[1], 95829[1], 95955[1], 96360[1], 96361[1], 96365[1], 96366[1], 96367[1], 96368[1], 96372[1], 96374[1], 96375[1], 96376[1], 96377[1], 96523[0], 97597[1], 97598[1], 97602[1], 99155[0], 99156[0], 99157[0], 99211[1], 99212[1], 99213[1], 99214[1], 99215[1], 99217[1], 99218[1], 99219[1], 99220[1], 99221[1], 99222[1], 99223[1], 99231[1], 99232[1], 99233[1], 99234[1], 99235[1], 99236[1], 99238[1], 99239[1], 99241[1], 99242[1], 99243[1], 99244[1], 99245[1], 99251[1], 99252[1], 99253[1], 99254[1], 99255[1], 99291[1], 99292[1], 99304[1], 99305[1], 99306[1], 99307[1], 99308[1], 99309[1], 99310[1], 99315[1], 99316[1], 99334[1], 99335[1], 99336[1], 99337[1], 99347[1], 99348[1], 99349[1], 99350[1], 99374[1], 99375[1], 99377[1], 99378[1], 99446[0], 99447[0], 99448[0], 99449[0], 99451[0], 99452[0], 99495[0], 99496[0], G0463[1], G0471[1], J0670[1], J2001[1]
68360	0213T[0], 0216T[0], 0596T[1], 0597T[1], 0708T[1], 0709T[1], 12001[1], 12002[1], 12004[1], 12005[1], 12006[1], 12007[1], 12011[1], 12013[1], 12014[1], 12015[1], 12016[1], 12017[1], 12018[1], 12020[1], 12021[1], 12031[1], 12032[1], 12034[1], 12035[1], 12036[1], 12037[1], 12041[1], 12042[1], 12044[1], 12045[1], 12046[1], 12047[1], 12051[1], 12052[1], 12053[1], 12054[1], 12055[1], 12056[1], 12057[1], 13100[1], 13101[1], 13102[1], 13120[1], 13121[1], 13122[1], 13131[1], 13132[1], 13133[1], 13151[1], 13152[1], 13153[1], 36000[1], 36400[1], 36405[1], 36406[1], 36410[1], 36420[1], 36425[1], 36430[1], 36440[1], 36591[0], 36592[0], 36600[1], 36640[1], 43752[1], 51701[1], 51702[1], 51703[1], 62320[0], 62321[0], 62322[0], 62323[0], 62324[0], 62325[0], 62326[0], 62327[0], 64400[0], 64405[0], 64408[0], 64415[0], 64416[0], 64417[0], 64418[0], 64420[0], 64421[0], 64425[0], 64430[0], 64435[0], 64445[0], 64446[0], 64447[0], 64448[0], 64449[0], 64450[0], 64451[0], 64454[0], 64461[0], 64462[0], 64463[0], 64479[0], 64480[0], 64483[0], 64484[0], 64486[0], 64487[0], 64488[0], 64489[0], 64490[0], 64491[0], 64492[0], 64493[0], 64494[0], 64495[0], 64505[0], 64510[0], 64517[0], 64520[0], 64530[0], 67500[1], 68020[1], 68040[1], 68100[1], 68110[1], 68115[1], 68130[1], 68135[1], 68200[1], 69990[0], 92012[1], 92014[1], 92018[1], 92019[1], 93000[1], 93005[1], 93010[1], 93040[1], 93041[1], 93042[1], 93318[1], 93355[1], 94002[1], 94200[1], 94680[1], 94681[1], 94690[1], 95812[1], 95813[1], 95816[1], 95819[1], 95822[1], 95829[1], 95955[1], 96360[1], 96361[1], 96365[1], 96366[1], 96367[1], 96368[1], 96372[1], 96374[1], 96375[1], 96376[1], 96377[1], 96523[0], 99155[0], 99156[0], 99157[0], 99211[1], 99212[1],

0 = Modifier usage not allowed or inappropriate 1 = Modifier usage allowed

Code 1	Code 2
	99213[1], 99214[1], 99215[1], 99217[1], 99218[1], 99219[1], 99220[1], 99221[1], 99222[1], 99223[1], 99231[1], 99232[1], 99233[1], 99234[1], 99235[1], 99236[1], 99238[1], 99239[1], 99241[1], 99242[1], 99243[1], 99244[1], 99245[1], 99251[1], 99252[1], 99253[1], 99254[1], 99255[1], 99291[1], 99292[1], 99304[1], 99305[1], 99306[1], 99307[1], 99308[1], 99309[1], 99310[1], 99315[1], 99316[1], 99334[1], 99335[1], 99336[1], 99337[1], 99347[1], 99348[1], 99349[1], 99350[1], 99374[1], 99375[1], 99377[1], 99378[1], 99446[0], 99447[0], 99448[0], 99449[0], 99451[0], 99452[0], 99495[0], 99496[0], G0463[1], G0471[1], J0670[1], J2001[1]
68362	0213T[0], 0216T[0], 0596T[1], 0597T[1], 0708T[1], 0709T[1], 12001[1], 12002[1], 12004[1], 12005[1], 12006[1], 12007[1], 12011[1], 12013[1], 12014[1], 12015[1], 12016[1], 12017[1], 12018[1], 12020[1], 12021[1], 12031[1], 12032[1], 12034[1], 12035[1], 12036[1], 12037[1], 12041[1], 12042[1], 12044[1], 12045[1], 12046[1], 12047[1], 12051[1], 12052[1], 12053[1], 12054[1], 12055[1], 12056[1], 12057[1], 13100[1], 13101[1], 13102[1], 13120[1], 13121[1], 13122[1], 13131[1], 13132[1], 13133[1], 13151[1], 13152[1], 13153[1], 36000[1], 36400[1], 36405[1], 36406[1], 36410[1], 36420[1], 36425[1], 36430[1], 36440[1], 36591[0], 36592[0], 36600[1], 36640[1], 43752[1], 51701[1], 51702[1], 51703[1], 62320[0], 62321[0], 62322[0], 62323[0], 62324[0], 62325[0], 62326[0], 62327[0], 64400[0], 64405[0], 64408[0], 64415[0], 64416[0], 64417[0], 64418[0], 64420[0], 64421[0], 64425[0], 64430[0], 64435[0], 64445[0], 64446[0], 64447[0], 64448[0], 64449[0], 64450[0], 64451[0], 64454[0], 64461[0], 64462[0], 64463[0], 64479[0], 64480[0], 64483[0], 64484[0], 64486[0], 64487[0], 64488[0], 64489[0], 64490[0], 64491[0], 64492[0], 64493[0], 64494[0], 64495[0], 64505[0], 64510[0], 64517[0], 64520[0], 64530[0], 67500[1], 68020[1], 68040[1], 68100[1], 68110[1], 68115[1], 68130[1], 68135[1], 68200[1], 68360[1], 69990[0], 92012[1], 92014[1], 92018[1], 92019[1], 93000[1], 93005[1], 93010[1], 93040[1], 93041[1], 93042[1], 93318[1], 93355[1], 94002[1], 94200[1], 94680[1], 94681[1], 94690[1], 95812[1], 95813[1], 95816[1], 95819[1], 95822[1], 95829[1], 95955[1], 96360[1], 96361[1], 96365[1], 96366[1], 96367[1], 96368[1], 96372[1], 96374[1], 96375[1], 96376[1], 96377[1], 96523[0], 99155[0], 99156[0], 99157[0], 99211[1], 99212[1], 99213[1], 99214[1], 99215[1], 99217[1], 99218[1], 99219[1], 99220[1], 99221[1], 99222[1], 99223[1], 99231[1], 99232[1], 99233[1], 99234[1], 99235[1], 99236[1], 99238[1], 99239[1], 99241[1], 99242[1], 99243[1], 99244[1], 99245[1], 99251[1], 99252[1], 99253[1], 99254[1], 99255[1], 99291[1], 99292[1], 99304[1], 99305[1], 99306[1], 99307[1], 99308[1], 99309[1], 99310[1], 99315[1], 99316[1], 99334[1], 99335[1], 99336[1], 99337[1], 99347[1], 99348[1], 99349[1], 99350[1], 99374[1], 99375[1], 99377[1], 99378[1], 99446[0], 99447[0], 99448[0], 99449[0], 99451[0], 99452[0], 99495[0], 99496[0], G0463[1], G0471[1]
68371	0213T[0], 0216T[0], 0596T[1], 0597T[1], 0708T[1], 0709T[1], 12001[1], 12002[1], 12004[1], 12005[1], 12006[1], 12007[1], 12011[1], 12013[1], 12014[1], 12015[1], 12016[1], 12017[1], 12018[1], 12020[1], 12021[1], 12031[1], 12032[1], 12034[1], 12035[1], 12036[1], 12037[1], 12041[1], 12042[1], 12044[1], 12045[1], 12046[1], 12047[1], 12051[1], 12052[1], 12053[1], 12054[1], 12055[1], 12056[1], 12057[1], 13100[1], 13101[1], 13102[1], 13120[1], 13121[1], 13122[1], 13131[1], 13132[1], 13133[1], 13151[1], 13152[1], 13153[1], 36000[1], 36400[1], 36405[1], 36406[1], 36410[1], 36420[1], 36425[1], 36430[1], 36440[1], 36591[0], 36592[0], 36600[1], 36640[1], 43752[1], 51701[1], 51702[1], 51703[1], 62320[0], 62321[0], 62322[0], 62323[0], 62324[0], 62325[0], 62326[0], 62327[0], 64400[0], 64405[0], 64408[0], 64415[0], 64416[0], 64417[0], 64418[0], 64420[0], 64421[0], 64425[0], 64430[0], 64435[0], 64445[0], 64446[0], 64447[0], 64448[0], 64449[0], 64450[0], 64451[0], 64454[0], 64461[0], 64462[0], 64463[0], 64479[0], 64480[0], 64483[0], 64484[0], 64486[0], 64487[0], 64488[0], 64489[0], 64490[0], 64491[0], 64492[0], 64493[0], 64494[0], 64495[0], 64505[0], 64510[0], 64517[0], 64520[0], 64530[0], 67500[1], 69990[0], 92012[1], 92014[1], 92018[1], 92019[1], 93000[1], 93005[1], 93010[1], 93040[1], 93041[1], 93042[1], 93318[1], 93355[1], 94002[1], 94200[1], 94680[1], 94681[1], 94690[1], 95812[1], 95813[1], 95816[1], 95819[1], 95822[1], 95829[1], 95955[1], 96360[1], 96361[1], 96365[1], 96366[1], 96367[1], 96368[1], 96372[1], 96374[1], 96375[1], 96376[1], 96377[1], 96523[0], 99155[0], 99156[0], 99157[0], 99211[1], 99212[1], 99213[1], 99214[1], 99215[1], 99217[1], 99218[1], 99219[1], 99220[1], 99221[1], 99222[1], 99223[1], 99231[1], 99232[1], 99233[1], 99234[1], 99235[1], 99236[1], 99238[1], 99239[1], 99241[1], 99242[1], 99243[1], 99244[1], 99245[1], 99251[1], 99252[1], 99253[1], 99254[1], 99255[1], 99291[1], 99292[1], 99304[1], 99305[1], 99306[1], 99307[1], 99308[1], 99309[1], 99310[1], 99315[1], 99316[1], 99334[1], 99335[1], 99336[1], 99337[1], 99347[1], 99348[1], 99349[1], 99350[1], 99374[1], 99375[1], 99377[1], 99378[1], 99446[0], 99447[0], 99448[0], 99449[0], 99451[0], 99452[0], 99495[0], 99496[0], G0463[1], G0471[1]
68400	0213T[0], 0216T[0], 0596T[1], 0597T[1], 0708T[1], 0709T[1], 12001[1], 12002[1], 12004[1], 12005[1], 12006[1], 12007[1], 12011[1], 12013[1], 12014[1], 12015[1], 12016[1], 12017[1], 12018[1], 12020[1], 12021[1], 12031[1], 12032[1], 12034[1], 12035[1], 12036[1], 12037[1], 12041[1], 12042[1], 12044[1], 12045[1], 12046[1], 12047[1], 12051[1], 12052[1], 12053[1], 12054[1], 12055[1], 12056[1], 12057[1], 13100[1], 13101[1], 13102[1], 13120[1], 13121[1], 13122[1], 13131[1], 13132[1], 13133[1], 13151[1], 13152[1], 13153[1], 36000[1], 36400[1], 36405[1], 36406[1], 36410[1], 36420[1], 36425[1], 36430[1], 36440[1], 36591[0], 36592[0], 36600[1], 36640[1], 43752[1], 51701[1], 51702[1], 51703[1], 62320[0], 62321[0], 62322[0], 62323[0], 62324[0], 62325[0], 62326[0], 62327[0], 64400[0], 64405[0], 64408[0], 64415[0], 64416[0], 64417[0], 64418[0], 64420[0], 64421[0], 64425[0], 64430[0], 64435[0], 64445[0], 64446[0], 64447[0], 64448[0], 64449[0], 64450[0], 64451[0], 64454[0], 64461[0], 64462[0], 64463[0], 64479[0], 64480[0], 64483[0], 64484[0], 64486[0], 64487[0], 64488[0], 64489[0], 64490[0], 64491[0], 64492[0], 64493[0], 64494[0], 64495[0], 64505[0], 64510[0], 64517[0], 64520[0], 64530[0], 67500[1], 69990[0], 92012[1], 92014[1], 92018[1], 92019[1], 93000[1], 93005[1], 93010[1], 93040[1], 93041[1], 93042[1], 93318[1], 93355[1], 94002[1], 94200[1], 94680[1], 94681[1], 94690[1], 95812[1], 95813[1], 95816[1], 95819[1], 95822[1], 95829[1], 95955[1], 96360[1], 96361[1], 96365[1], 96366[1], 96367[1], 96368[1], 96372[1], 96374[1], 96375[1], 96376[1], 96377[1], 96523[0], 99155[0], 99156[0], 99157[0], 99211[1], 99212[1], 99213[1], 99214[1], 99215[1], 99217[1], 99218[1], 99219[1], 99220[1], 99221[1], 99222[1], 99223[1], 99231[1], 99232[1], 99233[1], 99234[1], 99235[1], 99236[1], 99238[1], 99239[1], 99241[1], 99242[1], 99243[1], 99244[1], 99245[1], 99251[1], 99252[1], 99253[1], 99254[1], 99255[1], 99291[1], 99292[1], 99304[1], 99305[1], 99306[1], 99307[1], 99308[1], 99309[1], 99310[1], 99315[1], 99316[1], 99334[1], 99335[1], 99336[1], 99337[1], 99347[1], 99348[1], 99349[1], 99350[1], 99374[1], 99375[1], 99377[1], 99378[1], 99446[0], 99447[0], 99448[0], 99449[0], 99451[0], 99452[0], 99495[0], 99496[0], G0463[1], G0471[1], J0670[1], J2001[1]
68420	0213T[0], 0216T[0], 0596T[1], 0597T[1], 0708T[1], 0709T[1], 11000[1], 11001[1], 11004[1], 11005[1], 11006[1], 11042[1], 11043[1], 11044[1], 11045[1], 11046[1], 11047[1], 12001[1], 12002[1], 12004[1], 12005[1], 12006[1], 12007[1], 12011[1], 12013[1], 12014[1], 12015[1], 12016[1], 12017[1], 12018[1], 12020[1], 12021[1], 12031[1], 12032[1], 12034[1], 12035[1], 12036[1], 12037[1], 12041[1], 12042[1], 12044[1], 12045[1], 12046[1], 12047[1], 12051[1], 12052[1], 12053[1], 12054[1], 12055[1], 12056[1], 12057[1], 13100[1], 13101[1], 13102[1], 13120[1], 13121[1], 13122[1], 13131[1], 13132[1], 13133[1], 13151[1], 13152[1], 13153[1], 36000[1], 36400[1], 36405[1], 36406[1], 36410[1], 36420[1], 36425[1], 36430[1], 36440[1], 36591[0], 36592[0], 36600[1], 36640[1], 43752[1], 51701[1], 51702[1], 51703[1], 62320[0], 62321[0], 62322[0], 62323[0], 62324[0], 62325[0], 62326[0], 62327[0], 64400[0], 64405[0], 64408[0], 64415[0], 64416[0], 64417[0], 64418[0], 64420[0], 64421[0], 64425[0], 64430[0], 64435[0], 64445[0], 64446[0], 64447[0], 64448[0], 64449[0], 64450[0], 64451[0], 64454[0], 64461[0], 64462[0], 64463[0], 64479[0], 64480[0], 64483[0], 64484[0], 64486[0], 64487[0], 64488[0], 64489[0], 64490[0], 64491[0], 64492[0], 64493[0], 64494[0], 64495[0], 64505[0], 64510[0], 64517[0], 64520[0], 64530[0], 67500[1], 68530[1], 69990[0], 92012[1], 92014[1], 92018[1], 92019[1], 93000[1], 93005[1], 93010[1], 93040[1], 93041[1], 93042[1], 93318[1], 93355[1], 94002[1], 94200[1], 94680[1], 94681[1], 94690[1], 95812[1], 95813[1], 95816[1], 95819[1], 95822[1], 95829[1], 95955[1], 96360[1], 96361[1], 96365[1], 96366[1], 96367[1], 96368[1], 96372[1], 96374[1], 96375[1], 96376[1], 96377[1], 96523[0], 97597[1], 97598[1], 97602[1], 99155[0], 99156[0], 99157[0], 99211[1], 99212[1], 99213[1], 99214[1], 99215[1], 99217[1], 99218[1], 99219[1], 99220[1], 99221[1], 99222[1], 99223[1], 99231[1], 99232[1], 99233[1], 99234[1], 99235[1], 99236[1], 99238[1], 99239[1], 99241[1], 99242[1], 99243[1], 99244[1], 99245[1], 99251[1], 99252[1], 99253[1], 99254[1], 99255[1], 99291[1], 99292[1], 99304[1], 99305[1], 99306[1], 99307[1], 99308[1], 99309[1], 99310[1], 99315[1], 99316[1], 99334[1], 99335[1], 99336[1], 99337[1], 99347[1], 99348[1], 99349[1], 99350[1], 99374[1], 99375[1], 99377[1], 99378[1], 99446[0], 99447[0], 99448[0], 99449[0], 99451[0], 99452[0], 99495[0], 99496[0], G0463[1], G0471[1], J0670[1], J2001[1]
68440	0213T[0], 0216T[0], 0596T[1], 0597T[1], 0708T[1], 0709T[1], 12001[1], 12002[1], 12004[1], 12005[1], 12006[1], 12007[1], 12011[1], 12013[1], 12014[1], 12015[1], 12016[1], 12017[1], 12018[1], 12020[1], 12021[1], 12031[1], 12032[1], 12034[1], 12035[1], 12036[1], 12037[1], 12041[1], 12042[1], 12044[1], 12045[1], 12046[1], 12047[1], 12051[1], 12052[1], 12053[1], 12054[1], 12055[1], 12056[1], 12057[1], 13100[1], 13101[1], 13102[1], 13120[1], 13121[1], 13122[1], 13131[1], 13132[1], 13133[1], 13151[1], 13152[1], 13153[1], 36000[1], 36400[1], 36405[1], 36406[1], 36410[1], 36420[1], 36425[1], 36430[1], 36440[1], 36591[0], 36592[0], 36600[1], 36640[1], 43752[1], 51701[1], 51702[1], 51703[1], 62320[0], 62321[0], 62322[0], 62323[0], 62324[0], 62325[0], 62326[0], 62327[0], 64400[0], 64405[0], 64408[0], 64415[0], 64416[0], 64417[0], 64418[0], 64420[0], 64421[0], 64425[0], 64430[0], 64435[0], 64445[0], 64446[0], 64447[0], 64448[0], 64449[0], 64450[0], 64451[0], 64454[0], 64461[0], 64462[0], 64463[0], 64479[0], 64480[0], 64483[0], 64484[0], 64486[0], 64487[0], 64488[0], 64489[0], 64490[0], 64491[0], 64492[0], 64493[0], 64494[0], 64495[0], 64505[0], 64510[0], 64517[0], 64520[0], 64530[0], 67500[1], 69990[0], 92012[1], 92014[1], 92018[1], 92019[1], 93000[1], 93005[1], 93010[1], 93040[1], 93041[1], 93042[1], 93318[1], 93355[1], 94002[1], 94200[1], 94680[1], 94681[1], 94690[1], 95812[1], 95813[1], 95816[1], 95819[1], 95822[1], 95829[1], 95955[1], 96360[1], 96361[1], 96365[1], 96366[1], 96367[1], 96368[1], 96372[1], 96374[1], 96375[1], 96376[1], 96377[1], 96523[0], 99155[0], 99156[0], 99157[0], 99211[1], 99212[1], 99213[1], 99214[1], 99215[1], 99217[1], 99218[1], 99219[1], 99220[1], 99221[1], 99222[1], 99223[1], 99231[1], 99232[1], 99233[1], 99234[1], 99235[1], 99236[1], 99238[1], 99239[1], 99241[1], 99242[1], 99243[1], 99244[1], 99245[1], 99251[1], 99252[1], 99253[1], 99254[1], 99255[1], 99291[1], 99292[1], 99304[1], 99305[1], 99306[1], 99307[1], 99308[1], 99309[1], 99310[1], 99315[1], 99316[1], 99334[1], 99335[1], 99336[1], 99337[1], 99347[1], 99348[1], 99349[1], 99350[1], 99374[1], 99375[1], 99377[1], 99378[1], 99446[0], 99447[0], 99448[0], 99449[0], 99451[0], 99452[0], 99495[0], 99496[0], G0463[1], G0471[1], J2001[1]
68500	0213T[0], 0216T[0], 0596T[1], 0597T[1], 0708T[1], 0709T[1], 11000[1], 11001[1], 11004[1], 11005[1], 11006[1], 11042[1], 11043[1], 11044[1], 11045[1], 11046[1], 11047[1], 12001[1], 12002[1], 12004[1], 12005[1], 12006[1], 12007[1], 12011[1], 12013[1], 12014[1], 12015[1], 12016[1], 12017[1], 12018[1], 12020[1], 12021[1], 12031[1], 12032[1], 12034[1], 12035[1], 12036[1], 12037[1], 12041[1], 12042[1], 12044[1], 12045[1], 12046[1], 12047[1], 12051[1], 12052[1], 12053[1], 12054[1], 12055[1], 12056[1], 12057[1], 13100[1], 13101[1], 13102[1], 13120[1], 13121[1], 13122[1], 13131[1], 13132[1], 13133[1],

Appendix A: NCCI - CPT Codes

0 = Modifier usage not allowed or inappropriate 1 = Modifier usage allowed

Code 1	Code 2
	13151[1], 13152[1], 13153[1], 36000[1], 36400[1], 36405[1], 36406[1], 36410[1], 36420[1], 36425[1], 36430[1], 36440[1], 36591[0], 36592[0], 36600[1], 36640[1], 43752[1], 51701[1], 51702[1], 51703[1], 62320[0], 62321[0], 62322[0], 62323[0], 62324[0], 62325[0], 62326[0], 62327[0], 64400[0], 64405[0], 64408[0], 64415[0], 64416[0], 64417[0], 64418[0], 64420[0], 64421[0], 64425[0], 64430[0], 64435[0], 64445[0], 64446[0], 64447[0], 64448[0], 64449[0], 64450[0], 64451[0], 64454[0], 64461[0], 64462[0], 64463[0], 64479[0], 64480[0], 64483[0], 64484[0], 64486[0], 64487[0], 64488[0], 64489[0], 64490[0], 64491[0], 64492[0], 64493[0], 64494[0], 64495[0], 64505[0], 64510[0], 64517[0], 64520[0], 64530[0], 67500[1], 68400[1], 68505[1], 68510[1], 68550[1], 69990[0], 92012[1], 92014[1], 92018[1], 92019[1], 93000[1], 93005[1], 93010[1], 93040[1], 93041[1], 93042[1], 93318[1], 93355[1], 94002[1], 94200[1], 94680[1], 94681[1], 94690[1], 95812[1], 95813[1], 95816[1], 95819[1], 95822[1], 95829[1], 95955[1], 96360[1], 96361[1], 96365[1], 96366[1], 96367[1], 96368[1], 96372[1], 96374[1], 96375[1], 96376[1], 96377[1], 96523[0], 97597[1], 97598[1], 97602[1], 99155[0], 99156[0], 99157[0], 99211[1], 99212[1], 99213[1], 99214[1], 99215[1], 99217[1], 99218[1], 99219[1], 99220[1], 99221[1], 99222[1], 99223[1], 99231[1], 99232[1], 99233[1], 99234[1], 99235[1], 99236[1], 99238[1], 99239[1], 99241[1], 99242[1], 99243[1], 99244[1], 99245[1], 99251[1], 99252[1], 99253[1], 99254[1], 99255[1], 99291[1], 99292[1], 99304[1], 99305[1], 99306[1], 99307[1], 99308[1], 99309[1], 99310[1], 99315[1], 99316[1], 99334[1], 99335[1], 99336[1], 99337[1], 99347[1], 99348[1], 99349[1], 99350[1], 99374[1], 99375[1], 99377[1], 99378[1], 99446[0], 99447[0], 99448[0], 99449[0], 99451[0], 99452[0], 99495[0], 99496[0], G0463[1], G0471[1], J0670[1], J2001[1]
68505	0213T[0], 0216T[0], 0596T[1], 0597T[1], 0708T[1], 0709T[1], 11000[1], 11001[1], 11004[1], 11005[1], 11006[1], 11042[1], 11043[1], 11044[1], 11045[1], 11046[1], 11047[1], 12001[1], 12002[1], 12004[1], 12005[1], 12006[1], 12007[1], 12011[1], 12013[1], 12014[1], 12015[1], 12016[1], 12017[1], 12018[1], 12020[1], 12021[1], 12031[1], 12032[1], 12034[1], 12035[1], 12036[1], 12037[1], 12041[1], 12042[1], 12044[1], 12045[1], 12046[1], 12047[1], 12051[1], 12052[1], 12053[1], 12054[1], 12055[1], 12056[1], 12057[1], 13100[1], 13101[1], 13102[1], 13120[1], 13121[1], 13122[1], 13131[1], 13132[1], 13133[1], 13151[1], 13152[1], 13153[1], 36000[1], 36400[1], 36405[1], 36406[1], 36410[1], 36420[1], 36425[1], 36430[1], 36440[1], 36591[0], 36592[0], 36600[1], 36640[1], 43752[1], 51701[1], 51702[1], 51703[1], 62320[0], 62321[0], 62322[0], 62323[0], 62324[0], 62325[0], 62326[0], 62327[0], 64400[0], 64405[0], 64408[0], 64415[0], 64416[0], 64417[0], 64418[0], 64420[0], 64421[0], 64425[0], 64430[0], 64435[0], 64445[0], 64446[0], 64447[0], 64448[0], 64449[0], 64450[0], 64451[0], 64454[0], 64461[0], 64462[0], 64463[0], 64479[0], 64480[0], 64483[0], 64484[0], 64486[0], 64487[0], 64488[0], 64489[0], 64490[0], 64491[0], 64492[0], 64493[0], 64494[0], 64495[0], 64505[0], 64510[0], 64517[0], 64520[0], 64530[0], 67500[1], 68400[1], 68510[1], 68550[1], 69990[0], 92012[1], 92014[1], 92018[1], 92019[1], 93000[1], 93005[1], 93010[1], 93040[1], 93041[1], 93042[1], 93318[1], 93355[1], 94002[1], 94200[1], 94680[1], 94681[1], 94690[1], 95812[1], 95813[1], 95816[1], 95819[1], 95822[1], 95829[1], 95955[1], 96360[1], 96361[1], 96365[1], 96366[1], 96367[1], 96368[1], 96372[1], 96374[1], 96375[1], 96376[1], 96377[1], 96523[0], 97597[1], 97598[1], 97602[1], 99155[0], 99156[0], 99157[0], 99211[1], 99212[1], 99213[1], 99214[1], 99215[1], 99217[1], 99218[1], 99219[1], 99220[1], 99221[1], 99222[1], 99223[1], 99231[1], 99232[1], 99233[1], 99234[1], 99235[1], 99236[1], 99238[1], 99239[1], 99241[1], 99242[1], 99243[1], 99244[1], 99245[1], 99251[1], 99252[1], 99253[1], 99254[1], 99255[1], 99291[1], 99292[1], 99304[1], 99305[1], 99306[1], 99307[1], 99308[1], 99309[1], 99310[1], 99315[1], 99316[1], 99334[1], 99335[1], 99336[1], 99337[1], 99347[1], 99348[1], 99349[1], 99350[1], 99374[1], 99375[1], 99377[1], 99378[1], 99446[0], 99447[0], 99448[0], 99449[0], 99451[0], 99452[0], 99495[0], 99496[0], G0463[1], G0471[1], J0670[1], J2001[1]
68510	0213T[0], 0216T[0], 0596T[1], 0597T[1], 0708T[1], 0709T[1], 10005[1], 10007[1], 10009[1], 10011[1], 10021[1], 12001[1], 12002[1], 12004[1], 12005[1], 12006[1], 12007[1], 12011[1], 12013[1], 12014[1], 12015[1], 12016[1], 12017[1], 12018[1], 12020[1], 12021[1], 12031[1], 12032[1], 12034[1], 12035[1], 12036[1], 12037[1], 12041[1], 12042[1], 12044[1], 12045[1], 12046[1], 12047[1], 12051[1], 12052[1], 12053[1], 12054[1], 12055[1], 12056[1], 12057[1], 13100[1], 13101[1], 13102[1], 13120[1], 13121[1], 13122[1], 13131[1], 13132[1], 13133[1], 13151[1], 13152[1], 13153[1], 36000[1], 36400[1], 36405[1], 36406[1], 36410[1], 36420[1], 36425[1], 36430[1], 36440[1], 36591[0], 36592[0], 36600[1], 36640[1], 43752[1], 51701[1], 51702[1], 51703[1], 62320[0], 62321[0], 62322[0], 62323[0], 62324[0], 62325[0], 62326[0], 62327[0], 64400[0], 64405[0], 64408[0], 64415[0], 64416[0], 64417[0], 64418[0], 64420[0], 64421[0], 64425[0], 64430[0], 64435[0], 64445[0], 64446[0], 64447[0], 64448[0], 64449[0], 64450[0], 64451[0], 64454[0], 64461[0], 64462[0], 64463[0], 64479[0], 64480[0], 64483[0], 64484[0], 64486[0], 64487[0], 64488[0], 64489[0], 64490[0], 64491[0], 64492[0], 64493[0], 64494[0], 64495[0], 64505[0], 64510[0], 64517[0], 64520[0], 64530[0], 67500[1], 68400[1], 69990[0], 92012[1], 92014[1], 92018[1], 92019[1], 93000[1], 93005[1], 93010[1], 93040[1], 93041[1], 93042[1], 93318[1], 93355[1], 94002[1], 94200[1], 94680[1], 94681[1], 94690[1], 95812[1], 95813[1], 95816[1], 95819[1], 95822[1], 95829[1], 95955[1], 96360[1], 96361[1], 96365[1], 96366[1], 96367[1], 96368[1], 96372[1], 96374[1], 96375[1], 96376[1], 96377[1], 96523[0], 99155[0], 99156[0], 99157[0], 99211[1], 99212[1], 99213[1], 99214[1], 99215[1], 99217[1], 99218[1], 99219[1], 99220[1], 99221[1], 99222[1], 99223[1], 99231[1], 99232[1], 99233[1], 99234[1], 99235[1], 99236[1], 99238[1], 99239[1], 99241[1], 99242[1], 99243[1], 99244[1], 99245[1], 99251[1], 99252[1], 99253[1], 99254[1], 99255[1], 99291[1], 99292[1], 99304[1], 99305[1], 99306[1], 99307[1], 99308[1], 99309[1], 99310[1], 99315[1], 99316[1], 99334[1], 99335[1], 99336[1], 99337[1], 99347[1], 99348[1], 99349[1], 99350[1], 99374[1], 99375[1], 99377[1], 99378[1], 99446[0], 99447[0], 99448[0], 99449[0], 99451[0], 99452[0], 99495[1], 99496[1], G0463[1], G0471[1], J0670[1], J2001[1]
68520	0213T[0], 0216T[0], 0596T[1], 0597T[1], 0708T[1], 0709T[1], 11000[1], 11001[1], 11004[1], 11005[1], 11006[1], 11042[1], 11043[1], 11044[1], 11045[1], 11046[1], 11047[1], 12001[1], 12002[1], 12004[1], 12005[1], 12006[1], 12007[1], 12011[1], 12013[1], 12014[1], 12015[1], 12016[1], 12017[1], 12018[1], 12020[1], 12021[1], 12031[1], 12032[1], 12034[1], 12035[1], 12036[1], 12037[1], 12041[1], 12042[1], 12044[1], 12045[1], 12046[1], 12047[1], 12051[1], 12052[1], 12053[1], 12054[1], 12055[1], 12056[1], 12057[1], 13100[1], 13101[1], 13102[1], 13120[1], 13121[1], 13122[1], 13131[1], 13132[1], 13133[1], 13151[1], 13152[1], 13153[1], 36000[1], 36400[1], 36405[1], 36406[1], 36410[1], 36420[1], 36425[1], 36430[1], 36440[1], 36591[0], 36592[0], 36600[1], 36640[1], 43752[1], 51701[1], 51702[1], 51703[1], 62320[0], 62321[0], 62322[0], 62323[0], 62324[0], 62325[0], 62326[0], 62327[0], 64400[0], 64405[0], 64408[0], 64415[0], 64416[0], 64417[0], 64418[0], 64420[0], 64421[0], 64425[0], 64430[0], 64435[0], 64445[0], 64446[0], 64447[0], 64448[0], 64449[0], 64450[0], 64451[0], 64454[0], 64461[0], 64462[0], 64463[0], 64479[0], 64480[0], 64483[0], 64484[0], 64486[0], 64487[0], 64488[0], 64489[0], 64490[0], 64491[0], 64492[0], 64493[0], 64494[0], 64495[0], 64505[0], 64510[0], 64517[0], 64520[0], 64530[0], 67500[1], 68420[1], 68530[1], 69990[0], 92012[1], 92014[1], 92018[1], 92019[1], 93000[1], 93005[1], 93010[1], 93040[1], 93041[1], 93042[1], 93318[1], 93355[1], 94002[1], 94200[1], 94680[1], 94681[1], 94690[1], 95812[1], 95813[1], 95816[1], 95819[1], 95822[1], 95829[1], 95955[1], 96360[1], 96361[1], 96365[1], 96366[1], 96367[1], 96368[1], 96372[1], 96374[1], 96375[1], 96376[1], 96377[1], 96523[0], 97597[1], 97598[1], 97602[1], 99155[0], 99156[0], 99157[0], 99211[1], 99212[1], 99213[1], 99214[1], 99215[1], 99217[1], 99218[1], 99219[1], 99220[1], 99221[1], 99222[1], 99223[1], 99231[1], 99232[1], 99233[1], 99234[1], 99235[1], 99236[1], 99238[1], 99239[1], 99241[1], 99242[1], 99243[1], 99244[1], 99245[1], 99251[1], 99252[1], 99253[1], 99254[1], 99255[1], 99291[1], 99292[1], 99304[1], 99305[1], 99306[1], 99307[1], 99308[1], 99309[1], 99310[1], 99315[1], 99316[1], 99334[1], 99335[1], 99336[1], 99337[1], 99347[1], 99348[1], 99349[1], 99350[1], 99374[1], 99375[1], 99377[1], 99378[1], 99446[0], 99447[0], 99448[0], 99449[0], 99451[0], 99452[0], 99495[0], 99496[0], G0463[1], G0471[1], J0670[1], J2001[1]
68525	0213T[0], 0216T[0], 0596T[1], 0597T[1], 0708T[1], 0709T[1], 10005[1], 10007[1], 10009[1], 10011[1], 10021[1], 12001[1], 12002[1], 12004[1], 12005[1], 12006[1], 12007[1], 12011[1], 12013[1], 12014[1], 12015[1], 12016[1], 12017[1], 12018[1], 12020[1], 12021[1], 12031[1], 12032[1], 12034[1], 12035[1], 12036[1], 12037[1], 12041[1], 12042[1], 12044[1], 12045[1], 12046[1], 12047[1], 12051[1], 12052[1], 12053[1], 12054[1], 12055[1], 12056[1], 12057[1], 13100[1], 13101[1], 13102[1], 13120[1], 13121[1], 13122[1], 13131[1], 13132[1], 13133[1], 13151[1], 13152[1], 13153[1], 36000[1], 36400[1], 36405[1], 36406[1], 36410[1], 36420[1], 36425[1], 36430[1], 36440[1], 36591[0], 36592[0], 36600[1], 36640[1], 43752[1], 51701[1], 51702[1], 51703[1], 62320[0], 62321[0], 62322[0], 62323[0], 62324[0], 62325[0], 62326[0], 62327[0], 64400[0], 64405[0], 64408[0], 64415[0], 64416[0], 64417[0], 64418[0], 64420[0], 64421[0], 64425[0], 64430[0], 64435[0], 64445[0], 64446[0], 64447[0], 64448[0], 64449[0], 64450[0], 64451[0], 64454[0], 64461[0], 64462[0], 64463[0], 64479[0], 64480[0], 64483[0], 64484[0], 64486[0], 64487[0], 64488[0], 64489[0], 64490[0], 64491[0], 64492[0], 64493[0], 64494[0], 64495[0], 64505[0], 64510[0], 64517[0], 64520[0], 64530[0], 67500[1], 68420[1], 68440[1], 69990[0], 92012[1], 92014[1], 92018[1], 92019[1], 93000[1], 93005[1], 93010[1], 93040[1], 93041[1], 93042[1], 93318[1], 93355[1], 94002[1], 94200[1], 94680[1], 94681[1], 94690[1], 95812[1], 95813[1], 95816[1], 95819[1], 95822[1], 95829[1], 95955[1], 96360[1], 96361[1], 96365[1], 96366[1], 96367[1], 96368[1], 96372[1], 96374[1], 96375[1], 96376[1], 96377[1], 96523[0], 99155[0], 99156[0], 99157[0], 99211[1], 99212[1], 99213[1], 99214[1], 99215[1], 99217[1], 99218[1], 99219[1], 99220[1], 99221[1], 99222[1], 99223[1], 99231[1], 99232[1], 99233[1], 99234[1], 99235[1], 99236[1], 99238[1], 99239[1], 99241[1], 99242[1], 99243[1], 99244[1], 99245[1], 99251[1], 99252[1], 99253[1], 99254[1], 99255[1], 99291[1], 99292[1], 99304[1], 99305[1], 99306[1], 99307[1], 99308[1], 99309[1], 99310[1], 99315[1], 99316[1], 99334[1], 99335[1], 99336[1], 99337[1], 99347[1], 99348[1], 99349[1], 99350[1], 99374[1], 99375[1], 99377[1], 99378[1], 99446[0], 99447[0], 99448[0], 99449[0], 99451[0], 99452[0], 99495[1], 99496[1], G0463[1], G0471[1]
68530	0213T[0], 0216T[0], 0596T[1], 0597T[1], 0708T[1], 0709T[1], 11000[1], 11001[1], 11004[1], 11005[1], 11006[1], 11042[1], 11043[1], 11044[1], 11045[1], 11046[1], 11047[1], 12001[1], 12002[1], 12004[1], 12005[1], 12006[1], 12007[1], 12011[1], 12013[1], 12014[1], 12015[1], 12016[1], 12017[1], 12018[1], 12020[1], 12021[1], 12031[1], 12032[1], 12034[1], 12035[1], 12036[1], 12037[1], 12041[1], 12042[1], 12044[1], 12045[1], 12046[1], 12047[1], 12051[1], 12052[1], 12053[1], 12054[1], 12055[1], 12056[1], 12057[1], 13100[1], 13101[1], 13102[1], 13120[1], 13121[1], 13122[1], 13131[1], 13132[1], 13133[1], 13151[1], 13152[1], 13153[1], 36000[1], 36400[1], 36405[1], 36406[1], 36410[1], 36420[1], 36425[1], 36430[1], 36440[1], 36591[0], 36592[0], 36600[1], 36640[1], 43752[1], 51701[1], 51702[1], 51703[1], 62320[0], 62321[0], 62322[0], 62323[0], 62324[0], 62325[0], 62326[0], 62327[0], 64400[0], 64405[0], 64408[0], 64415[0], 64416[0], 64417[0], 64418[0], 64420[0], 64421[0], 64425[0], 64430[0], 64435[0], 64445[0], 64446[0], 64447[0], 64448[0], 64449[0], 64450[0], 64451[0], 64454[0], 64461[0], 64462[0], 64463[0], 64479[0], 64480[0], 64483[0], 64484[0], 64486[0], 64487[0], 64488[0], 64489[0], 64490[0], 64491[0], 64492[0], 64493[0], 64494[0], 64495[0], 64505[0], 64510[0], 64517[0], 64520[0], 64530[0], 67500[1], 68440[1], 68810[1], 68811[1], 68816[1], 68840[1], 69990[0], 92012[1], 92014[1], 92018[1], 92019[1], 93000[1], 93005[1], 93010[1], 93040[1], 93041[1], 93042[1], 93318[1], 93355[1], 94002[1],

0 = Modifier usage not allowed or inappropriate 1 = Modifier usage allowed

Code 1	Code 2
	94200[1], 94680[1], 94681[1], 94690[1], 95812[1], 95813[1], 95816[1], 95819[1], 95822[1], 95829[1], 95955[1], 96360[1], 96361[1], 96365[1], 96366[1], 96367[1], 96368[1], 96372[1], 96374[1], 96375[1], 96376[1], 96377[1], 96523[0], 97597[1], 97598[1], 97602[1], 99155[0], 99156[0], 99157[0], 99211[1], 99212[1], 99213[1], 99214[1], 99215[1], 99217[1], 99218[1], 99219[1], 99220[1], 99221[1], 99222[1], 99223[1], 99231[1], 99232[1], 99233[1], 99234[1], 99235[1], 99236[1], 99238[1], 99239[1], 99241[1], 99242[1], 99243[1], 99244[1], 99245[1], 99251[1], 99252[1], 99253[1], 99254[1], 99255[1], 99291[1], 99292[1], 99304[1], 99305[1], 99306[1], 99307[1], 99308[1], 99309[1], 99310[1], 99315[1], 99316[1], 99334[1], 99335[1], 99336[1], 99337[1], 99347[1], 99348[1], 99349[1], 99350[1], 99374[1], 99375[1], 99377[1], 99378[1], 99446[0], 99447[0], 99448[0], 99449[0], 99451[0], 99452[0], 99495[0], 99496[0], G0463[1], G0471[1], J0670[1], J2001[1]
68540	0213T[0], 0216T[0], 0596T[1], 0597T[1], 0708T[1], 0709T[1], 11000[1], 11001[1], 11004[1], 11005[1], 11006[1], 11042[1], 11043[1], 11044[1], 11045[1], 11046[1], 11047[1], 12001[1], 12002[1], 12004[1], 12005[1], 12006[1], 12007[1], 12011[1], 12013[1], 12014[1], 12015[1], 12016[1], 12017[1], 12018[1], 12020[1], 12021[1], 12031[1], 12032[1], 12034[1], 12035[1], 12036[1], 12037[1], 12041[1], 12042[1], 12044[1], 12045[1], 12046[1], 12047[1], 12051[1], 12052[1], 12053[1], 12054[1], 12055[1], 12056[1], 12057[1], 13100[1], 13101[1], 13102[1], 13120[1], 13121[1], 13122[1], 13131[1], 13132[1], 13133[1], 13151[1], 13152[1], 13153[1], 36000[1], 36400[1], 36405[1], 36406[1], 36410[1], 36420[1], 36425[1], 36430[1], 36440[1], 36591[0], 36592[0], 36600[1], 36640[1], 43752[1], 51701[1], 51702[1], 51703[1], 62320[0], 62321[0], 62322[0], 62323[0], 62324[0], 62325[0], 62326[0], 62327[0], 64400[0], 64405[0], 64408[0], 64415[0], 64416[0], 64417[0], 64418[0], 64420[0], 64421[0], 64425[0], 64430[0], 64435[0], 64445[0], 64446[0], 64447[0], 64448[0], 64449[0], 64450[0], 64451[0], 64454[0], 64461[0], 64462[0], 64463[0], 64479[0], 64480[0], 64483[0], 64484[0], 64486[0], 64487[0], 64488[0], 64489[0], 64490[0], 64491[0], 64492[0], 64493[0], 64494[0], 64495[0], 64505[0], 64510[0], 64517[0], 64520[0], 64530[0], 67500[1], 68440[1], 68500[1], 68505[1], 68510[1], 68550[1], 69990[0], 92012[1], 92014[1], 92018[1], 92019[1], 93000[1], 93005[1], 93010[1], 93040[1], 93041[1], 93042[1], 93318[1], 93355[1], 94002[1], 94200[1], 94680[1], 94681[1], 94690[1], 95812[1], 95813[1], 95816[1], 95819[1], 95822[1], 95829[1], 95955[1], 96360[1], 96361[1], 96365[1], 96366[1], 96367[1], 96368[1], 96372[1], 96374[1], 96375[1], 96376[1], 96377[1], 96523[0], 97597[1], 97598[1], 97602[1], 99155[0], 99156[0], 99157[0], 99211[1], 99212[1], 99213[1], 99214[1], 99215[1], 99217[1], 99218[1], 99219[1], 99220[1], 99221[1], 99222[1], 99223[1], 99231[1], 99232[1], 99233[1], 99234[1], 99235[1], 99236[1], 99238[1], 99239[1], 99241[1], 99242[1], 99243[1], 99244[1], 99245[1], 99251[1], 99252[1], 99253[1], 99254[1], 99255[1], 99291[1], 99292[1], 99304[1], 99305[1], 99306[1], 99307[1], 99308[1], 99309[1], 99310[1], 99315[1], 99316[1], 99334[1], 99335[1], 99336[1], 99337[1], 99347[1], 99348[1], 99349[1], 99350[1], 99374[1], 99375[1], 99377[1], 99378[1], 99446[0], 99447[0], 99448[0], 99449[0], 99451[0], 99452[0], 99495[0], 99496[0], G0463[1], G0471[1], J0670[1], J2001[1]
68550	0213T[0], 0216T[0], 0596T[1], 0597T[1], 0708T[1], 0709T[1], 11000[1], 11001[1], 11004[1], 11005[1], 11006[1], 11042[1], 11043[1], 11044[1], 11045[1], 11046[1], 11047[1], 12001[1], 12002[1], 12004[1], 12005[1], 12006[1], 12007[1], 12011[1], 12013[1], 12014[1], 12015[1], 12016[1], 12017[1], 12018[1], 12020[1], 12021[1], 12031[1], 12032[1], 12034[1], 12035[1], 12036[1], 12037[1], 12041[1], 12042[1], 12044[1], 12045[1], 12046[1], 12047[1], 12051[1], 12052[1], 12053[1], 12054[1], 12055[1], 12056[1], 12057[1], 13100[1], 13101[1], 13102[1], 13120[1], 13121[1], 13122[1], 13131[1], 13132[1], 13133[1], 13151[1], 13152[1], 13153[1], 36000[1], 36400[1], 36405[1], 36406[1], 36410[1], 36420[1], 36425[1], 36430[1], 36440[1], 36591[0], 36592[0], 36600[1], 36640[1], 43752[1], 51701[1], 51702[1], 51703[1], 62320[0], 62321[0], 62322[0], 62323[0], 62324[0], 62325[0], 62326[0], 62327[0], 64400[0], 64405[0], 64408[0], 64415[0], 64416[0], 64417[0], 64418[0], 64420[0], 64421[0], 64425[0], 64430[0], 64435[0], 64445[0], 64446[0], 64447[0], 64448[0], 64449[0], 64450[0], 64451[0], 64454[0], 64461[0], 64462[0], 64463[0], 64479[0], 64480[0], 64483[0], 64484[0], 64486[0], 64487[0], 64488[0], 64489[0], 64490[0], 64491[0], 64492[0], 64493[0], 64494[0], 64495[0], 64505[0], 64510[0], 64517[0], 64520[0], 64530[0], 67500[1], 68510[1], 69990[0], 92012[1], 92014[1], 92018[1], 92019[1], 93000[1], 93005[1], 93010[1], 93040[1], 93041[1], 93042[1], 93318[1], 93355[1], 94002[1], 94200[1], 94680[1], 94681[1], 94690[1], 95812[1], 95813[1], 95816[1], 95819[1], 95822[1], 95829[1], 95955[1], 96360[1], 96361[1], 96365[1], 96366[1], 96367[1], 96368[1], 96372[1], 96374[1], 96375[1], 96376[1], 96377[1], 96523[0], 97597[1], 97598[1], 97602[1], 99155[0], 99156[0], 99157[0], 99211[1], 99212[1], 99213[1], 99214[1], 99215[1], 99217[1], 99218[1], 99219[1], 99220[1], 99221[1], 99222[1], 99223[1], 99231[1], 99232[1], 99233[1], 99234[1], 99235[1], 99236[1], 99238[1], 99239[1], 99241[1], 99242[1], 99243[1], 99244[1], 99245[1], 99251[1], 99252[1], 99253[1], 99254[1], 99255[1], 99291[1], 99292[1], 99304[1], 99305[1], 99306[1], 99307[1], 99308[1], 99309[1], 99310[1], 99315[1], 99316[1], 99334[1], 99335[1], 99336[1], 99337[1], 99347[1], 99348[1], 99349[1], 99350[1], 99374[1], 99375[1], 99377[1], 99378[1], 99446[0], 99447[0], 99448[0], 99449[0], 99451[0], 99452[0], 99495[0], 99496[0], G0463[1], G0471[1], J0670[1], J2001[1]
68700	0213T[0], 0216T[0], 0596T[1], 0597T[1], 0708T[1], 0709T[1], 12001[1], 12002[1], 12004[1], 12005[1], 12006[1], 12007[1], 12011[1], 12013[1], 12014[1], 12015[1], 12016[1], 12017[1], 12018[1], 12020[1], 12021[1], 12031[1], 12032[1], 12034[1], 12035[1], 12036[1], 12037[1], 12041[1], 12042[1], 12044[1], 12045[1], 12046[1], 12047[1], 12051[1], 12052[1], 12053[1], 12054[1], 12055[1], 12056[1], 12057[1], 13100[1], 13101[1], 13102[1], 13120[1], 13121[1], 13122[1], 13131[1], 13132[1], 13133[1], 13151[1], 13152[1], 13153[1], 36000[1], 36400[1], 36405[1], 36406[1], 36410[1], 36420[1], 36425[1], 36430[1], 36440[1], 36591[0], 36592[0], 36600[1], 36640[1], 43752[1], 51701[1], 51702[1], 51703[1], 62320[0], 62321[0], 62322[0], 62323[0], 62324[0], 62325[0], 62326[0], 62327[0], 64400[0], 64405[0], 64408[0], 64415[0], 64416[0], 64417[0], 64418[0], 64420[0], 64421[0], 64425[0], 64430[0], 64435[0], 64445[0], 64446[0], 64447[0], 64448[0], 64449[0], 64450[0], 64451[0], 64454[0], 64461[0], 64462[0], 64463[0], 64479[0], 64480[0], 64483[0], 64484[0], 64486[0], 64487[0], 64488[0], 64489[0], 64490[0], 64491[0], 64492[0], 64493[0], 64494[0], 64495[0], 64505[0], 64510[0], 64517[0], 64520[0], 64530[0], 67500[1], 68440[1], 68720[1], 68750[1], 68770[1], 68840[1], 69990[0], 92012[1], 92014[1], 92018[1], 92019[1], 93000[1], 93005[1], 93010[1], 93040[1], 93041[1], 93042[1], 93318[1], 93355[1], 94002[1], 94200[1], 94680[1], 94681[1], 94690[1], 95812[1], 95813[1], 95816[1], 95819[1], 95822[1], 95829[1], 95955[1], 96360[1], 96361[1], 96365[1], 96366[1], 96367[1], 96368[1], 96372[1], 96374[1], 96375[1], 96376[1], 96377[1], 96523[0], 99155[0], 99156[0], 99157[0], 99211[1], 99212[1], 99213[1], 99214[1], 99215[1], 99217[1], 99218[1], 99219[1], 99220[1], 99221[1], 99222[1], 99223[1], 99231[1], 99232[1], 99233[1], 99234[1], 99235[1], 99236[1], 99238[1], 99239[1], 99241[1], 99242[1], 99243[1], 99244[1], 99245[1], 99251[1], 99252[1], 99253[1], 99254[1], 99255[1], 99291[1], 99292[1], 99304[1], 99305[1], 99306[1], 99307[1], 99308[1], 99309[1], 99310[1], 99315[1], 99316[1], 99334[1], 99335[1], 99336[1], 99337[1], 99347[1], 99348[1], 99349[1], 99350[1], 99374[1], 99375[1], 99377[1], 99378[1], 99446[0], 99447[0], 99448[0], 99449[0], 99451[0], 99452[0], 99495[0], 99496[0], G0463[1], G0471[1], J2001[1]
68705	0213T[0], 0216T[0], 0596T[1], 0597T[1], 0708T[1], 0709T[1], 12001[1], 12002[1], 12004[1], 12005[1], 12006[1], 12007[1], 12011[1], 12013[1], 12014[1], 12015[1], 12016[1], 12017[1], 12018[1], 12020[1], 12021[1], 12031[1], 12032[1], 12034[1], 12035[1], 12036[1], 12037[1], 12041[1], 12042[1], 12044[1], 12045[1], 12046[1], 12047[1], 12051[1], 12052[1], 12053[1], 12054[1], 12055[1], 12056[1], 12057[1], 13100[1], 13101[1], 13102[1], 13120[1], 13121[1], 13122[1], 13131[1], 13132[1], 13133[1], 13151[1], 13152[1], 13153[1], 36000[1], 36400[1], 36405[1], 36406[1], 36410[1], 36420[1], 36425[1], 36430[1], 36440[1], 36591[0], 36592[0], 36600[1], 36640[1], 43752[1], 51701[1], 51702[1], 51703[1], 62320[0], 62321[0], 62322[0], 62323[0], 62324[0], 62325[0], 62326[0], 62327[0], 64400[0], 64405[0], 64408[0], 64415[0], 64416[0], 64417[0], 64418[0], 64420[0], 64421[0], 64425[0], 64430[0], 64435[0], 64445[0], 64446[0], 64447[0], 64448[0], 64449[0], 64450[0], 64451[0], 64454[0], 64461[0], 64462[0], 64463[0], 64479[0], 64480[0], 64483[0], 64484[0], 64486[0], 64487[0], 64488[0], 64489[0], 64490[0], 64491[0], 64492[0], 64493[0], 64494[0], 64495[0], 64505[0], 64510[0], 64517[0], 64520[0], 64530[0], 67500[1], 68440[1], 68700[1], 68770[1], 69990[0], 92012[1], 92014[1], 92018[1], 92019[1], 93000[1], 93005[1], 93010[1], 93040[1], 93041[1], 93042[1], 93318[1], 93355[1], 94002[1], 94200[1], 94680[1], 94681[1], 94690[1], 95812[1], 95813[1], 95816[1], 95819[1], 95822[1], 95829[1], 95955[1], 96360[1], 96361[1], 96365[1], 96366[1], 96367[1], 96368[1], 96372[1], 96374[1], 96375[1], 96376[1], 96377[1], 96523[0], 99155[0], 99156[0], 99157[0], 99211[1], 99212[1], 99213[1], 99214[1], 99215[1], 99217[1], 99218[1], 99219[1], 99220[1], 99221[1], 99222[1], 99223[1], 99231[1], 99232[1], 99233[1], 99234[1], 99235[1], 99236[1], 99238[1], 99239[1], 99241[1], 99242[1], 99243[1], 99244[1], 99245[1], 99251[1], 99252[1], 99253[1], 99254[1], 99255[1], 99291[1], 99292[1], 99304[1], 99305[1], 99306[1], 99307[1], 99308[1], 99309[1], 99310[1], 99315[1], 99316[1], 99334[1], 99335[1], 99336[1], 99337[1], 99347[1], 99348[1], 99349[1], 99350[1], 99374[1], 99375[1], 99377[1], 99378[1], 99446[0], 99447[0], 99448[0], 99449[0], 99451[0], 99452[0], 99495[0], 99496[0], G0463[1], G0471[1], J0670[1], J2001[1]
68720	0213T[0], 0216T[0], 0596T[1], 0597T[1], 0708T[1], 0709T[1], 12001[1], 12002[1], 12004[1], 12005[1], 12006[1], 12007[1], 12011[1], 12013[1], 12014[1], 12015[1], 12016[1], 12017[1], 12018[1], 12020[1], 12021[1], 12031[1], 12032[1], 12034[1], 12035[1], 12036[1], 12037[1], 12041[1], 12042[1], 12044[1], 12045[1], 12046[1], 12047[1], 12051[1], 12052[1], 12053[1], 12054[1], 12055[1], 12056[1], 12057[1], 13100[1], 13101[1], 13102[1], 13120[1], 13121[1], 13122[1], 13131[1], 13132[1], 13133[1], 13151[1], 13152[1], 13153[1], 21280[1], 31239[1], 36000[1], 36400[1], 36405[1], 36406[1], 36410[1], 36420[1], 36425[1], 36430[1], 36440[1], 36591[0], 36592[0], 36600[1], 36640[1], 43752[1], 51701[1], 51702[1], 51703[1], 62320[0], 62321[0], 62322[0], 62323[0], 62324[0], 62325[0], 62326[0], 62327[0], 64400[0], 64405[0], 64408[0], 64415[0], 64416[0], 64417[0], 64418[0], 64420[0], 64421[0], 64425[0], 64430[0], 64435[0], 64445[0], 64446[0], 64447[0], 64448[0], 64449[0], 64450[0], 64451[0], 64454[0], 64461[0], 64462[0], 64463[0], 64479[0], 64480[0], 64483[0], 64484[0], 64486[0], 64487[0], 64488[0], 64489[0], 64490[0], 64491[0], 64492[0], 64493[0], 64494[0], 64495[0], 64505[0], 64510[0], 64517[0], 64520[0], 64530[0], 67500[1], 68440[1], 68525[1], 68530[1], 68770[1], 68810[1], 68811[1], 68816[1], 69990[0], 92012[1], 92014[1], 92018[1], 92019[1], 93000[1], 93005[1], 93010[1], 93040[1], 93041[1], 93042[1], 93318[1], 93355[1], 94002[1], 94200[1], 94680[1], 94681[1], 94690[1], 95812[1], 95813[1], 95816[1], 95819[1], 95822[1], 95829[1], 95955[1], 96360[1], 96361[1], 96365[1], 96366[1], 96367[1], 96368[1], 96372[1], 96374[1], 96375[1], 96376[1], 96377[1], 96523[0], 99155[0], 99156[0], 99157[0], 99211[1], 99212[1], 99213[1], 99214[1], 99215[1], 99217[1], 99218[1], 99219[1], 99220[1], 99221[1], 99222[1], 99223[1], 99231[1], 99232[1], 99233[1], 99234[1], 99235[1], 99236[1], 99238[1], 99239[1], 99241[1], 99242[1], 99243[1], 99244[1], 99245[1], 99251[1], 99252[1], 99253[1], 99254[1], 99255[1], 99291[1], 99292[1], 99304[1], 99305[1], 99306[1], 99307[1], 99308[1], 99309[1], 99310[1], 99315[1], 99316[1], 99334[1], 99335[1], 99336[1], 99337[1], 99347[1], 99348[1], 99349[1], 99350[1], 99374[1], 99375[1], 99377[1], 99378[1], 99446[0], 99447[0], 99448[0], 99449[0], 99451[0], 99452[0], 99495[0], 99496[0], G0463[1], G0471[1], J0670[1], J2001[1]

0 = Modifier usage not allowed or inappropriate 1 = Modifier usage allowed

Code 1	Code 2
68745	0213T[0], 0216T[0], 0596T[1], 0597T[1], 0708T[1], 0709T[1], 12001[1], 12002[1], 12004[1], 12005[1], 12006[1], 12007[1], 12011[1], 12013[1], 12014[1], 12015[1], 12016[1], 12017[1], 12018[1], 12020[1], 12021[1], 12031[1], 12032[1], 12034[1], 12035[1], 12036[1], 12037[1], 12041[1], 12042[1], 12044[1], 12045[1], 12046[1], 12047[1], 12051[1], 12052[1], 12053[1], 12054[1], 12055[1], 12056[1], 12057[1], 13100[1], 13101[1], 13102[1], 13120[1], 13121[1], 13122[1], 13131[1], 13132[1], 13133[1], 13151[1], 13152[1], 13153[1], 36000[1], 36400[1], 36405[1], 36406[1], 36410[1], 36420[1], 36425[1], 36430[1], 36440[1], 36591[0], 36592[0], 36600[1], 36640[1], 43752[1], 51701[1], 51702[1], 51703[1], 62320[0], 62321[0], 62322[0], 62323[0], 62324[0], 62325[0], 62326[0], 62327[0], 64400[0], 64405[0], 64408[0], 64415[0], 64416[0], 64417[0], 64418[0], 64420[0], 64421[0], 64425[0], 64430[0], 64435[0], 64445[0], 64446[0], 64447[0], 64448[0], 64449[0], 64450[0], 64451[0], 64454[0], 64461[0], 64462[0], 64463[0], 64479[0], 64480[0], 64483[0], 64484[0], 64486[0], 64487[0], 64488[0], 64489[0], 64490[0], 64491[0], 64492[0], 64493[0], 64494[0], 64495[0], 64505[0], 64510[0], 64517[0], 64520[0], 64530[0], 67500[1], 68440[1], 68525[1], 68530[1], 68770[1], 69990[0], 92012[1], 92014[1], 92018[1], 92019[1], 93000[1], 93005[1], 93010[1], 93040[1], 93041[1], 93042[1], 93318[1], 93355[1], 94002[1], 94200[1], 94680[1], 94681[1], 94690[1], 95812[1], 95813[1], 95816[1], 95819[1], 95822[1], 95829[1], 95955[1], 96360[1], 96361[1], 96365[1], 96366[1], 96367[1], 96368[1], 96372[1], 96374[1], 96375[1], 96376[1], 96377[1], 96523[0], 99155[0], 99156[0], 99157[0], 99211[1], 99212[1], 99213[1], 99214[1], 99215[1], 99217[1], 99218[1], 99219[1], 99220[1], 99221[1], 99222[1], 99223[1], 99231[1], 99232[1], 99233[1], 99234[1], 99235[1], 99236[1], 99238[1], 99239[1], 99241[1], 99242[1], 99243[1], 99244[1], 99245[1], 99251[1], 99252[1], 99253[1], 99254[1], 99255[1], 99291[1], 99292[1], 99304[1], 99305[1], 99306[1], 99307[1], 99308[1], 99309[1], 99310[1], 99315[1], 99316[1], 99334[1], 99335[1], 99336[1], 99337[1], 99347[1], 99348[1], 99349[1], 99350[1], 99374[1], 99375[1], 99377[1], 99378[1], 99446[0], 99447[0], 99448[0], 99449[0], 99451[0], 99452[0], 99495[0], 99496[0], G0463[1], G0471[1], J0670[1], J2001[1]
68750	0213T[0], 0216T[0], 0596T[1], 0597T[1], 0708T[1], 0709T[1], 11000[1], 11001[1], 11004[1], 11005[1], 11006[1], 11042[1], 11043[1], 11044[1], 11045[1], 11046[1], 11047[1], 12001[1], 12002[1], 12004[1], 12005[1], 12006[1], 12007[1], 12011[1], 12013[1], 12014[1], 12015[1], 12016[1], 12017[1], 12018[1], 12020[1], 12021[1], 12031[1], 12032[1], 12034[1], 12035[1], 12036[1], 12037[1], 12041[1], 12042[1], 12044[1], 12045[1], 12046[1], 12047[1], 12051[1], 12052[1], 12053[1], 12054[1], 12055[1], 12056[1], 12057[1], 13100[1], 13101[1], 13102[1], 13120[1], 13121[1], 13122[1], 13131[1], 13132[1], 13133[1], 13151[1], 13152[1], 13153[1], 36000[1], 36400[1], 36405[1], 36406[1], 36410[1], 36420[1], 36425[1], 36430[1], 36440[1], 36591[0], 36592[0], 36600[1], 36640[1], 43752[1], 51701[1], 51702[1], 51703[1], 62320[0], 62321[0], 62322[0], 62323[0], 62324[0], 62325[0], 62326[0], 62327[0], 64400[0], 64405[0], 64408[0], 64415[0], 64416[0], 64417[0], 64418[0], 64420[0], 64421[0], 64425[0], 64430[0], 64435[0], 64445[0], 64446[0], 64447[0], 64448[0], 64449[0], 64450[0], 64451[0], 64454[0], 64461[0], 64462[0], 64463[0], 64479[0], 64480[0], 64483[0], 64484[0], 64486[0], 64487[0], 64488[0], 64489[0], 64490[0], 64491[0], 64492[0], 64493[0], 64494[0], 64495[0], 64505[0], 64510[0], 64517[0], 64520[0], 64530[0], 67500[1], 68440[1], 68530[1], 68770[1], 69990[0], 92012[1], 92014[1], 92018[1], 92019[1], 93000[1], 93005[1], 93010[1], 93040[1], 93041[1], 93042[1], 93318[1], 93355[1], 94002[1], 94200[1], 94680[1], 94681[1], 94690[1], 95812[1], 95813[1], 95816[1], 95819[1], 95822[1], 95829[1], 95955[1], 96360[1], 96361[1], 96365[1], 96366[1], 96367[1], 96368[1], 96372[1], 96374[1], 96375[1], 96376[1], 96377[1], 96523[0], 97597[1], 97598[1], 97602[1], 99155[0], 99156[0], 99157[0], 99211[1], 99212[1], 99213[1], 99214[1], 99215[1], 99217[1], 99218[1], 99219[1], 99220[1], 99221[1], 99222[1], 99223[1], 99231[1], 99232[1], 99233[1], 99234[1], 99235[1], 99236[1], 99238[1], 99239[1], 99241[1], 99242[1], 99243[1], 99244[1], 99245[1], 99251[1], 99252[1], 99253[1], 99254[1], 99255[1], 99291[1], 99292[1], 99304[1], 99305[1], 99306[1], 99307[1], 99308[1], 99309[1], 99310[1], 99315[1], 99316[1], 99334[1], 99335[1], 99336[1], 99337[1], 99347[1], 99348[1], 99349[1], 99350[1], 99374[1], 99375[1], 99377[1], 99378[1], 99446[0], 99447[0], 99448[0], 99449[0], 99451[0], 99452[0], 99495[0], 99496[0], G0463[1], G0471[1], J0670[1], J2001[1]
68760	0213T[0], 0216T[0], 0596T[1], 0597T[1], 0708T[1], 0709T[1], 11000[1], 11001[1], 11004[1], 11005[1], 11006[1], 11042[1], 11043[1], 11044[1], 11045[1], 11046[1], 11047[1], 12001[1], 12002[1], 12004[1], 12005[1], 12006[1], 12007[1], 12011[1], 12013[1], 12014[1], 12015[1], 12016[1], 12017[1], 12018[1], 12020[1], 12021[1], 12031[1], 12032[1], 12034[1], 12035[1], 12036[1], 12037[1], 12041[1], 12042[1], 12044[1], 12045[1], 12046[1], 12047[1], 12051[1], 12052[1], 12053[1], 12054[1], 12055[1], 12056[1], 12057[1], 13100[1], 13101[1], 13102[1], 13120[1], 13121[1], 13122[1], 13131[1], 13132[1], 13133[1], 13151[1], 13152[1], 13153[1], 36000[1], 36400[1], 36405[1], 36406[1], 36410[1], 36420[1], 36425[1], 36430[1], 36440[1], 36591[0], 36592[0], 36600[1], 36640[1], 43752[1], 51701[1], 51702[1], 51703[1], 62320[0], 62321[0], 62322[0], 62323[0], 62324[0], 62325[0], 62326[0], 62327[0], 64400[0], 64405[0], 64408[0], 64415[0], 64416[0], 64417[0], 64418[0], 64420[0], 64421[0], 64425[0], 64430[0], 64435[0], 64445[0], 64446[0], 64447[0], 64448[0], 64449[0], 64450[0], 64451[0], 64454[0], 64461[0], 64462[0], 64463[0], 64479[0], 64480[0], 64483[0], 64484[0], 64486[0], 64487[0], 64488[0], 64489[0], 64490[0], 64491[0], 64492[0], 64493[0], 64494[0], 64495[0], 64505[0], 64510[0], 64517[0], 64520[0], 64530[0], 67500[1], 68440[1], 68705[1], 68770[1], 68801[1], 69990[0], 92012[1], 92014[1], 92018[1], 92019[1], 93000[1], 93005[1], 93010[1], 93040[1], 93041[1], 93042[1], 93318[1], 93355[1], 94002[1], 94200[1], 94680[1], 94681[1], 94690[1], 95812[1], 95813[1], 95816[1], 95819[1], 95822[1], 95829[1], 95955[1], 96360[1], 96361[1], 96365[1], 96366[1], 96367[1], 96368[1], 96372[1], 96374[1], 96375[1], 96376[1], 96377[1], 96523[0], 97597[1], 97598[1], 97602[1], 99155[0], 99156[0], 99157[0], 99211[1], 99212[1], 99213[1], 99214[1], 99215[1], 99217[1], 99218[1], 99219[1], 99220[1], 99221[1], 99222[1], 99223[1], 99231[1], 99232[1], 99233[1], 99234[1], 99235[1], 99236[1], 99238[1], 99239[1], 99241[1], 99242[1], 99243[1], 99244[1], 99245[1], 99251[1], 99252[1], 99253[1], 99254[1], 99255[1], 99291[1], 99292[1], 99304[1], 99305[1], 99306[1], 99307[1], 99308[1], 99309[1], 99310[1], 99315[1], 99316[1], 99334[1], 99335[1], 99336[1], 99337[1], 99347[1], 99348[1], 99349[1], 99350[1], 99374[1], 99375[1], 99377[1], 99378[1], 99446[0], 99447[0], 99448[0], 99449[0], 99451[0], 99452[0], 99495[0], 99496[0], G0463[1], G0471[1], J0670[1], J2001[1]
68761	0213T[0], 0216T[0], 0596T[1], 0597T[1], 0708T[1], 0709T[1], 11000[1], 11001[1], 11004[1], 11005[1], 11006[1], 11042[1], 11043[1], 11044[1], 11045[1], 11046[1], 11047[1], 12001[1], 12002[1], 12004[1], 12005[1], 12006[1], 12007[1], 12011[1], 12013[1], 12014[1], 12015[1], 12016[1], 12017[1], 12018[1], 12020[1], 12021[1], 12031[1], 12032[1], 12034[1], 12035[1], 12036[1], 12037[1], 12041[1], 12042[1], 12044[1], 12045[1], 12046[1], 12047[1], 12051[1], 12052[1], 12053[1], 12054[1], 12055[1], 12056[1], 12057[1], 13100[1], 13101[1], 13102[1], 13120[1], 13121[1], 13122[1], 13131[1], 13132[1], 13133[1], 13151[1], 13152[1], 13153[1], 36000[1], 36400[1], 36405[1], 36406[1], 36410[1], 36420[1], 36425[1], 36430[1], 36440[1], 36591[0], 36592[0], 36600[1], 36640[1], 43752[1], 51701[1], 51702[1], 51703[1], 62320[0], 62321[0], 62322[0], 62323[0], 62324[0], 62325[0], 62326[0], 62327[0], 64400[0], 64405[0], 64408[0], 64415[0], 64416[0], 64417[0], 64418[0], 64420[0], 64421[0], 64425[0], 64430[0], 64435[0], 64445[0], 64446[0], 64447[0], 64448[0], 64449[0], 64450[0], 64451[0], 64454[0], 64461[0], 64462[0], 64463[0], 64479[0], 64480[0], 64483[0], 64484[0], 64486[0], 64487[0], 64488[0], 64489[0], 64490[0], 64491[0], 64492[0], 64493[0], 64494[0], 64495[0], 64505[0], 64510[0], 64517[0], 64520[0], 64530[0], 67500[1], 68440[1], 68770[1], 68801[1], 68810[1], 68811[1], 69990[0], 92012[1], 92014[1], 92018[1], 92019[1], 93000[1], 93005[1], 93010[1], 93040[1], 93041[1], 93042[1], 93318[1], 93355[1], 94002[1], 94200[1], 94680[1], 94681[1], 94690[1], 95812[1], 95813[1], 95816[1], 95819[1], 95822[1], 95829[1], 95955[1], 96360[1], 96361[1], 96365[1], 96366[1], 96367[1], 96368[1], 96372[1], 96374[1], 96375[1], 96376[1], 96377[1], 96523[0], 97597[1], 97598[1], 97602[1], 99155[0], 99156[0], 99157[0], 99211[1], 99212[1], 99213[1], 99214[1], 99215[1], 99217[1], 99218[1], 99219[1], 99220[1], 99221[1], 99222[1], 99223[1], 99231[1], 99232[1], 99233[1], 99234[1], 99235[1], 99236[1], 99238[1], 99239[1], 99241[1], 99242[1], 99243[1], 99244[1], 99245[1], 99251[1], 99252[1], 99253[1], 99254[1], 99255[1], 99291[1], 99292[1], 99304[1], 99305[1], 99306[1], 99307[1], 99308[1], 99309[1], 99310[1], 99315[1], 99316[1], 99334[1], 99335[1], 99336[1], 99337[1], 99347[1], 99348[1], 99349[1], 99350[1], 99374[1], 99375[1], 99377[1], 99378[1], 99446[0], 99447[0], 99448[0], 99449[0], 99451[0], 99452[0], 99495[0], 99496[0], G0463[1], G0471[1], J2001[1]
68770	0213T[0], 0216T[0], 0596T[1], 0597T[1], 0708T[1], 0709T[1], 11000[1], 11001[1], 11004[1], 11005[1], 11006[1], 11042[1], 11043[1], 11044[1], 11045[1], 11046[1], 11047[1], 12001[1], 12002[1], 12004[1], 12005[1], 12006[1], 12007[1], 12011[1], 12013[1], 12014[1], 12015[1], 12016[1], 12017[1], 12018[1], 12020[1], 12021[1], 12031[1], 12032[1], 12034[1], 12035[1], 12036[1], 12037[1], 12041[1], 12042[1], 12044[1], 12045[1], 12046[1], 12047[1], 12051[1], 12052[1], 12053[1], 12054[1], 12055[1], 12056[1], 12057[1], 13100[1], 13101[1], 13102[1], 13120[1], 13121[1], 13122[1], 13131[1], 13132[1], 13133[1], 13151[1], 13152[1], 13153[1], 36000[1], 36400[1], 36405[1], 36406[1], 36410[1], 36420[1], 36425[1], 36430[1], 36440[1], 36591[0], 36592[0], 36600[1], 36640[1], 43752[1], 51701[1], 51702[1], 51703[1], 62320[0], 62321[0], 62322[0], 62323[0], 62324[0], 62325[0], 62326[0], 62327[0], 64400[0], 64405[0], 64408[0], 64415[0], 64416[0], 64417[0], 64418[0], 64420[0], 64421[0], 64425[0], 64430[0], 64435[0], 64445[0], 64446[0], 64447[0], 64448[0], 64449[0], 64450[0], 64451[0], 64454[0], 64461[0], 64462[0], 64463[0], 64479[0], 64480[0], 64483[0], 64484[0], 64486[0], 64487[0], 64488[0], 64489[0], 64490[0], 64491[0], 64492[0], 64493[0], 64494[0], 64495[0], 64505[0], 64510[0], 64517[0], 64520[0], 64530[0], 67500[1], 68440[1], 69990[0], 92012[1], 92014[1], 92018[1], 92019[1], 93000[1], 93005[1], 93010[1], 93040[1], 93041[1], 93042[1], 93318[1], 93355[1], 94002[1], 94200[1], 94680[1], 94681[1], 94690[1], 95812[1], 95813[1], 95816[1], 95819[1], 95822[1], 95829[1], 95955[1], 96360[1], 96361[1], 96365[1], 96366[1], 96367[1], 96368[1], 96372[1], 96374[1], 96375[1], 96376[1], 96377[1], 96523[0], 97597[1], 97598[1], 97602[1], 99155[0], 99156[0], 99157[0], 99211[1], 99212[1], 99213[1], 99214[1], 99215[1], 99217[1], 99218[1], 99219[1], 99220[1], 99221[1], 99222[1], 99223[1], 99231[1], 99232[1], 99233[1], 99234[1], 99235[1], 99236[1], 99238[1], 99239[1], 99241[1], 99242[1], 99243[1], 99244[1], 99245[1], 99251[1], 99252[1], 99253[1], 99254[1], 99255[1], 99291[1], 99292[1], 99304[1], 99305[1], 99306[1], 99307[1], 99308[1], 99309[1], 99310[1], 99315[1], 99316[1], 99334[1], 99335[1], 99336[1], 99337[1], 99347[1], 99348[1], 99349[1], 99350[1], 99374[1], 99375[1], 99377[1], 99378[1], 99446[0], 99447[0], 99448[0], 99449[0], 99451[0], 99452[0], 99495[0], 99496[0], G0463[1], G0471[1], J2001[1]
68801	0213T[0], 0216T[0], 0596T[1], 0597T[1], 0708T[1], 0709T[1], 12001[1], 12002[1], 12004[1], 12005[1], 12006[1], 12007[1], 12011[1], 12013[1], 12014[1], 12015[1], 12016[1], 12017[1], 12018[1], 12020[1], 12021[1], 12031[1], 12032[1], 12034[1], 12035[1], 12036[1], 12037[1], 12041[1], 12042[1], 12044[1], 12045[1], 12046[1], 12047[1], 12051[1], 12052[1], 12053[1], 12054[1], 12055[1], 12056[1], 12057[1], 13100[1], 13101[1], 13102[1], 13120[1], 13121[1], 13122[1], 13131[1], 13132[1], 13133[1], 13151[1], 13152[1], 13153[1], 36000[1], 36400[1], 36405[1], 36406[1], 36410[1], 36420[1], 36425[1], 36430[1], 36440[1], 36591[0], 36592[0], 36600[1], 36640[1], 43752[1], 51701[1], 51702[1], 51703[1], 62320[0], 62321[0], 62322[0], 62323[0], 62324[0], 62325[0], 62326[0], 62327[0], 64400[0], 64405[0], 64408[0], 64415[0], 64416[0], 64417[0], 64418[0], 64420[0], 64421[0], 64425[0], 64430[0], 64435[0], 64445[0],

0 = Modifier usage not allowed or inappropriate 1 = Modifier usage allowed

Code 1	Code 2
	64446[0], 64447[0], 64448[0], 64449[0], 64450[0], 64451[0], 64454[0], 64461[0], 64462[0], 64463[0], 64479[0], 64480[0], 64483[0], 64484[0], 64486[0], 64487[0], 64488[0], 64489[0], 64490[0], 64491[0], 64492[0], 64493[0], 64494[0], 64495[0], 64505[0], 64510[0], 64517[0], 64520[0], 64530[0], 67500[1], 68440[1], 69990[0], 92012[1], 92014[1], 92018[1], 92019[1], 93000[1], 93005[1], 93010[1], 93040[1], 93041[1], 93042[1], 93318[1], 93355[1], 94002[1], 94200[1], 94680[1], 94681[1], 94690[1], 95812[1], 95813[1], 95816[1], 95819[1], 95822[1], 95829[1], 95955[1], 96360[1], 96361[1], 96365[1], 96366[1], 96367[1], 96368[1], 96372[1], 96374[1], 96375[1], 96376[1], 96377[1], 96523[0], 99155[0], 99156[0], 99157[0], 99211[1], 99212[1], 99213[1], 99214[1], 99215[1], 99217[1], 99218[1], 99219[1], 99220[1], 99221[1], 99222[1], 99223[1], 99231[1], 99232[1], 99233[1], 99234[1], 99235[1], 99236[1], 99238[1], 99239[1], 99241[1], 99242[1], 99243[1], 99244[1], 99245[1], 99251[1], 99252[1], 99253[1], 99254[1], 99255[1], 99291[1], 99292[1], 99304[1], 99305[1], 99306[1], 99307[1], 99308[1], 99309[1], 99310[1], 99315[1], 99316[1], 99334[1], 99335[1], 99336[1], 99337[1], 99347[1], 99348[1], 99349[1], 99350[1], 99374[1], 99375[1], 99377[1], 99378[1], 99446[0], 99447[0], 99448[0], 99449[0], 99451[0], 99452[0], 99495[0], 99496[0], G0463[1], G0471[1]
68810	0213T[0], 0216T[0], 0596T[1], 0597T[1], 0708T[1], 0709T[1], 12001[1], 12002[1], 12004[1], 12005[1], 12006[1], 12007[1], 12011[1], 12013[1], 12014[1], 12015[1], 12016[1], 12017[1], 12018[1], 12020[1], 12021[1], 12031[1], 12032[1], 12034[1], 12035[1], 12036[1], 12037[1], 12041[1], 12042[1], 12044[1], 12045[1], 12046[1], 12047[1], 12051[1], 12052[1], 12053[1], 12054[1], 12055[1], 12056[1], 12057[1], 13100[1], 13101[1], 13102[1], 13120[1], 13121[1], 13122[1], 13131[1], 13132[1], 13133[1], 13151[1], 13152[1], 13153[1], 36000[1], 36400[1], 36405[1], 36406[1], 36410[1], 36420[1], 36425[1], 36430[1], 36440[1], 36591[0], 36592[0], 36600[1], 36640[1], 43752[1], 51701[1], 51702[1], 51703[1], 62320[0], 62321[0], 62322[0], 62323[0], 62324[0], 62325[0], 62326[0], 62327[0], 64400[0], 64405[0], 64408[0], 64415[0], 64416[0], 64417[0], 64418[0], 64420[0], 64421[0], 64425[0], 64430[0], 64435[0], 64445[0], 64446[0], 64447[0], 64448[0], 64449[0], 64450[0], 64451[0], 64454[0], 64461[0], 64462[0], 64463[0], 64479[0], 64480[0], 64483[0], 64484[0], 64486[0], 64487[0], 64488[0], 64489[0], 64490[0], 64491[0], 64492[0], 64493[0], 64494[0], 64495[0], 64505[0], 64510[0], 64517[0], 64520[0], 64530[0], 67500[1], 68801[1], 69990[0], 92012[1], 92014[1], 92018[1], 92019[1], 93000[1], 93005[1], 93010[1], 93040[1], 93041[1], 93042[1], 93318[1], 93355[1], 94002[1], 94200[1], 94680[1], 94681[1], 94690[1], 95812[1], 95813[1], 95816[1], 95819[1], 95822[1], 95829[1], 95955[1], 96360[1], 96361[1], 96365[1], 96366[1], 96367[1], 96368[1], 96372[1], 96374[1], 96375[1], 96376[1], 96377[1], 96523[0], 99155[0], 99156[0], 99157[0], 99211[1], 99212[1], 99213[1], 99214[1], 99215[1], 99217[1], 99218[1], 99219[1], 99220[1], 99221[1], 99222[1], 99223[1], 99231[1], 99232[1], 99233[1], 99234[1], 99235[1], 99236[1], 99238[1], 99239[1], 99241[1], 99242[1], 99243[1], 99244[1], 99245[1], 99251[1], 99252[1], 99253[1], 99254[1], 99255[1], 99291[1], 99292[1], 99304[1], 99305[1], 99306[1], 99307[1], 99308[1], 99309[1], 99310[1], 99315[1], 99316[1], 99334[1], 99335[1], 99336[1], 99337[1], 99347[1], 99348[1], 99349[1], 99350[1], 99374[1], 99375[1], 99377[1], 99378[1], 99446[0], 99447[0], 99448[0], 99449[0], 99451[0], 99452[0], 99495[0], 99496[0], G0463[1], G0471[1], J0670[1], J2001[1]
68811	0213T[0], 0216T[0], 0596T[1], 0597T[1], 0708T[1], 0709T[1], 12001[1], 12002[1], 12004[1], 12005[1], 12006[1], 12007[1], 12011[1], 12013[1], 12014[1], 12015[1], 12016[1], 12017[1], 12018[1], 12020[1], 12021[1], 12031[1], 12032[1], 12034[1], 12035[1], 12036[1], 12037[1], 12041[1], 12042[1], 12044[1], 12045[1], 12046[1], 12047[1], 12051[1], 12052[1], 12053[1], 12054[1], 12055[1], 12056[1], 12057[1], 13100[1], 13101[1], 13102[1], 13120[1], 13121[1], 13122[1], 13131[1], 13132[1], 13133[1], 13151[1], 13152[1], 13153[1], 36000[1], 36400[1], 36405[1], 36406[1], 36410[1], 36420[1], 36425[1], 36430[1], 36440[1], 36591[0], 36592[0], 36600[1], 36640[1], 43752[1], 51701[1], 51702[1], 51703[1], 62320[0], 62321[0], 62322[0], 62323[0], 62324[0], 62325[0], 62326[0], 62327[0], 64400[0], 64405[0], 64408[0], 64415[0], 64416[0], 64417[0], 64418[0], 64420[0], 64421[0], 64425[0], 64430[0], 64435[0], 64445[0], 64446[0], 64447[0], 64448[0], 64449[0], 64450[0], 64451[0], 64454[0], 64461[0], 64462[0], 64463[0], 64479[0], 64480[0], 64483[0], 64484[0], 64486[0], 64487[0], 64488[0], 64489[0], 64490[0], 64491[0], 64492[0], 64493[0], 64494[0], 64495[0], 64505[0], 64510[0], 64517[0], 64520[0], 64530[0], 67500[1], 68810[1], 69990[0], 92012[1], 92014[1], 92018[1], 92019[1], 93000[1], 93005[1], 93010[1], 93040[1], 93041[1], 93042[1], 93318[1], 93355[1], 94002[1], 94200[1], 94680[1], 94681[1], 94690[1], 95812[1], 95813[1], 95816[1], 95819[1], 95822[1], 95829[1], 95955[1], 96360[1], 96361[1], 96365[1], 96366[1], 96367[1], 96368[1], 96372[1], 96374[1], 96375[1], 96376[1], 96377[1], 96523[0], 99151[0], 99152[0], 99153[0], 99155[0], 99156[0], 99157[0], 99211[1], 99212[1], 99213[1], 99214[1], 99215[1], 99217[1], 99218[1], 99219[1], 99220[1], 99221[1], 99222[1], 99223[1], 99231[1], 99232[1], 99233[1], 99234[1], 99235[1], 99236[1], 99238[1], 99239[1], 99241[1], 99242[1], 99243[1], 99244[1], 99245[1], 99251[1], 99252[1], 99253[1], 99254[1], 99255[1], 99291[1], 99292[1], 99304[1], 99305[1], 99306[1], 99307[1], 99308[1], 99309[1], 99310[1], 99315[1], 99316[1], 99334[1], 99335[1], 99336[1], 99337[1], 99347[1], 99348[1], 99349[1], 99350[1], 99374[1], 99375[1], 99377[1], 99378[1], 99446[0], 99447[0], 99448[0], 99449[0], 99451[0], 99452[0], 99495[0], 99496[0], G0463[1], G0471[1]
68815	0213T[0], 0216T[0], 0596T[1], 0597T[1], 0708T[1], 0709T[1], 11000[1], 11001[1], 11004[1], 11005[1], 11006[1], 11042[1], 11043[1], 11044[1], 11045[1], 11046[1], 11047[1], 12001[1], 12002[1], 12004[1], 12005[1], 12006[1], 12007[1], 12011[1], 12013[1], 12014[1], 12015[1], 12016[1], 12017[1], 12018[1], 12020[1], 12021[1], 12031[1], 12032[1], 12034[1], 12035[1], 12036[1], 12037[1], 12041[1], 12042[1], 12044[1], 12045[1], 12046[1], 12047[1], 12051[1], 12052[1], 12053[1], 12054[1], 12055[1], 12056[1], 12057[1], 13100[1], 13101[1], 13102[1], 13120[1], 13121[1], 13122[1], 13131[1], 13132[1], 13133[1], 13151[1], 13152[1], 13153[1], 36000[1], 36400[1], 36405[1], 36406[1], 36410[1], 36420[1], 36425[1], 36430[1], 36440[1], 36591[0], 36592[0], 36600[1], 36640[1], 43752[1], 51701[1], 51702[1], 51703[1], 62320[0], 62321[0], 62322[0], 62323[0], 62324[0], 62325[0], 62326[0], 62327[0], 64400[0], 64405[0], 64408[0], 64415[0], 64416[0], 64417[0], 64418[0], 64420[0], 64421[0], 64425[0], 64430[0], 64435[0], 64445[0], 64446[0], 64447[0], 64448[0], 64449[0], 64450[0], 64451[0], 64454[0], 64461[0], 64462[0], 64463[0], 64479[0], 64480[0], 64483[0], 64484[0], 64486[0], 64487[0], 64488[0], 64489[0], 64490[0], 64491[0], 64492[0], 64493[0], 64494[0], 64495[0], 64505[0], 64510[0], 64517[0], 64520[0], 64530[0], 67500[1], 68810[1], 68811[1], 68816[1], 69990[0], 92012[1], 92014[1], 92018[1], 92019[1], 93000[1], 93005[1], 93010[1], 93040[1], 93041[1], 93042[1], 93318[1], 93355[1], 94002[1], 94200[1], 94680[1], 94681[1], 94690[1], 95812[1], 95813[1], 95816[1], 95819[1], 95822[1], 95829[1], 95955[1], 96360[1], 96361[1], 96365[1], 96366[1], 96367[1], 96368[1], 96372[1], 96374[1], 96375[1], 96376[1], 96377[1], 96523[0], 97597[1], 97598[1], 97602[1], 99155[0], 99156[0], 99157[0], 99211[1], 99212[1], 99213[1], 99214[1], 99215[1], 99217[1], 99218[1], 99219[1], 99220[1], 99221[1], 99222[1], 99223[1], 99231[1], 99232[1], 99233[1], 99234[1], 99235[1], 99236[1], 99238[1], 99239[1], 99241[1], 99242[1], 99243[1], 99244[1], 99245[1], 99251[1], 99252[1], 99253[1], 99254[1], 99255[1], 99291[1], 99292[1], 99304[1], 99305[1], 99306[1], 99307[1], 99308[1], 99309[1], 99310[1], 99315[1], 99316[1], 99334[1], 99335[1], 99336[1], 99337[1], 99347[1], 99348[1], 99349[1], 99350[1], 99374[1], 99375[1], 99377[1], 99378[1], 99446[0], 99447[0], 99448[0], 99449[0], 99451[0], 99452[0], 99495[0], 99496[0], G0463[1], G0471[1], J0670[1], J2001[1]
68816	0213T[0], 0216T[0], 0708T[1], 0709T[1], 12001[1], 12002[1], 12004[1], 12005[1], 12006[1], 12007[1], 12011[1], 12013[1], 12014[1], 12015[1], 12016[1], 12017[1], 12018[1], 12020[1], 12021[1], 12031[1], 12032[1], 12034[1], 12035[1], 12036[1], 12037[1], 12041[1], 12042[1], 12044[1], 12045[1], 12046[1], 12047[1], 12051[1], 12052[1], 12053[1], 12054[1], 12055[1], 12056[1], 12057[1], 13100[1], 13101[1], 13102[1], 13120[1], 13121[1], 13122[1], 13131[1], 13132[1], 13133[1], 13151[1], 13152[1], 13153[1], 36000[1], 36400[1], 36405[1], 36406[1], 36410[1], 36420[1], 36425[1], 36430[1], 36440[1], 36591[0], 36592[0], 36600[1], 36640[1], 43752[1], 62320[0], 62321[0], 62322[0], 62323[0], 62324[0], 62325[0], 62326[0], 62327[0], 64400[0], 64405[0], 64408[0], 64415[0], 64416[0], 64417[0], 64418[0], 64420[0], 64421[0], 64425[0], 64430[0], 64435[0], 64445[0], 64446[0], 64447[0], 64448[0], 64449[0], 64450[0], 64451[0], 64454[0], 64461[0], 64462[0], 64463[0], 64479[0], 64480[0], 64483[0], 64484[0], 64486[0], 64487[0], 64488[0], 64489[0], 64490[0], 64491[0], 64492[0], 64493[0], 64494[0], 64495[0], 64505[0], 64510[0], 64517[0], 64520[0], 64530[0], 67500[1], 68810[1], 68811[1], 69990[0], 92012[1], 92014[1], 92018[1], 92019[1], 93000[1], 93005[1], 93010[1], 93040[1], 93041[1], 93042[1], 93318[1], 93355[1], 94002[1], 94200[1], 94680[1], 94681[1], 94690[1], 95812[1], 95813[1], 95816[1], 95819[1], 95822[1], 95829[1], 95955[1], 96360[1], 96361[1], 96365[1], 96366[1], 96367[1], 96368[1], 96372[1], 96374[1], 96375[1], 96376[1], 96377[1], 96523[0], 99155[0], 99156[0], 99157[0], 99211[1], 99212[1], 99213[1], 99214[1], 99215[1], 99217[1], 99218[1], 99219[1], 99220[1], 99221[1], 99222[1], 99223[1], 99231[1], 99232[1], 99233[1], 99234[1], 99235[1], 99236[1], 99238[1], 99239[1], 99241[1], 99242[1], 99243[1], 99244[1], 99245[1], 99251[1], 99252[1], 99253[1], 99254[1], 99255[1], 99291[1], 99292[1], 99304[1], 99305[1], 99306[1], 99307[1], 99308[1], 99309[1], 99310[1], 99315[1], 99316[1], 99334[1], 99335[1], 99336[1], 99337[1], 99347[1], 99348[1], 99349[1], 99350[1], 99374[1], 99375[1], 99377[1], 99378[1], 99446[0], 99447[0], 99448[0], 99449[0], 99451[0], 99452[0], 99495[0], 99496[0], G0463[1], J0670[1], J2001[1]
68840	0213T[0], 0216T[0], 0596T[1], 0597T[1], 0708T[1], 0709T[1], 12001[1], 12002[1], 12004[1], 12005[1], 12006[1], 12007[1], 12011[1], 12013[1], 12014[1], 12015[1], 12016[1], 12017[1], 12018[1], 12020[1], 12021[1], 12031[1], 12032[1], 12034[1], 12035[1], 12036[1], 12037[1], 12041[1], 12042[1], 12044[1], 12045[1], 12046[1], 12047[1], 12051[1], 12052[1], 12053[1], 12054[1], 12055[1], 12056[1], 12057[1], 13100[1], 13101[1], 13102[1], 13120[1], 13121[1], 13122[1], 13131[1], 13132[1], 13133[1], 13151[1], 13152[1], 13153[1], 36000[1], 36400[1], 36405[1], 36406[1], 36410[1], 36420[1], 36425[1], 36430[1], 36440[1], 36591[0], 36592[0], 36600[1], 36640[1], 43752[1], 51701[1], 51702[1], 51703[1], 62320[0], 62321[0], 62322[0], 62323[0], 62324[0], 62325[0], 62326[0], 62327[0], 64400[0], 64405[0], 64408[0], 64415[0], 64416[0], 64417[0], 64418[0], 64420[0], 64421[0], 64425[0], 64430[0], 64435[0], 64445[0], 64446[0], 64447[0], 64448[0], 64449[0], 64450[0], 64451[0], 64454[0], 64461[0], 64462[0], 64463[0], 64479[0], 64480[0], 64483[0], 64484[0], 64486[0], 64487[0], 64488[0], 64489[0], 64490[0], 64491[0], 64492[0], 64493[0], 64494[0], 64495[0], 64505[0], 64510[0], 64517[0], 64520[0], 64530[0], 67500[1], 68440[1], 68801[1], 69990[0], 92012[1], 92014[1], 92018[1], 92019[1], 93000[1], 93005[1], 93010[1], 93040[1], 93041[1], 93042[1], 93318[1], 93355[1], 94002[1], 94200[1], 94680[1], 94681[1], 94690[1], 95812[1], 95813[1], 95816[1], 95819[1], 95822[1], 95829[1], 95955[1], 96360[1], 96361[1], 96365[1], 96366[1], 96367[1], 96368[1], 96372[1], 96374[1], 96375[1], 96376[1], 96377[1], 96523[0], 99155[0], 99156[0], 99157[0], 99211[1], 99212[1], 99213[1], 99214[1], 99215[1], 99217[1], 99218[1], 99219[1], 99220[1], 99221[1], 99222[1], 99223[1], 99231[1], 99232[1], 99233[1], 99234[1], 99235[1], 99236[1], 99238[1], 99239[1], 99241[1], 99242[1], 99243[1], 99244[1], 99245[1], 99251[1], 99252[1], 99253[1], 99254[1], 99255[1], 99291[1], 99292[1], 99304[1], 99305[1], 99306[1], 99307[1], 99308[1], 99309[1], 99310[1], 99315[1], 99316[1], 99334[1], 99335[1], 99336[1], 99337[1], 99347[1], 99348[1], 99349[1], 99350[1], 99374[1], 99375[1], 99377[1], 99378[1], 99446[0], 99447[0], 99448[0], 99449[0], 99451[0], 99452[0], 99495[0], 99496[0], G0463[1], G0471[1], J0670[1], J2001[1]

0 = Modifier usage not allowed or inappropriate 1 = Modifier usage allowed

Code 1	Code 2
68841	0213T[0], 0216T[0], 0596T[1], 0597T[1], 11000[1], 11001[1], 11004[1], 11005[1], 11006[1], 11042[1], 11043[1], 11044[1], 11045[1], 11046[1], 11047[1], 12001[1], 12002[1], 12004[1], 12005[1], 12006[1], 12007[1], 12011[1], 12013[1], 12014[1], 12015[1], 12016[1], 12017[1], 12018[1], 12020[1], 12021[1], 12031[1], 12032[1], 12034[1], 12035[1], 12036[1], 12037[1], 12041[1], 12042[1], 12044[1], 12045[1], 12046[1], 12047[1], 12051[1], 12052[1], 12053[1], 12054[1], 12055[1], 12056[1], 12057[1], 13100[1], 13101[1], 13102[1], 13120[1], 13121[1], 13122[1], 13131[1], 13132[1], 13133[1], 13151[1], 13152[1], 13153[1], 36000[1], 36400[1], 36405[1], 36406[1], 36410[1], 36420[1], 36425[1], 36430[1], 36440[1], 36591[0], 36592[0], 36600[1], 36640[1], 43752[1], 51701[1], 51702[1], 51703[1], 61650[1], 62320[0], 62321[0], 62322[0], 62323[0], 62324[0], 62325[0], 62326[0], 62327[0], 64400[0], 64405[0], 64408[0], 64415[0], 64416[0], 64417[0], 64418[0], 64420[0], 64421[0], 64425[0], 64430[0], 64435[0], 64445[0], 64446[0], 64447[0], 64448[0], 64449[0], 64450[0], 64451[0], 64454[0], 64461[0], 64462[0], 64463[0], 64479[0], 64480[0], 64483[0], 64484[0], 64486[0], 64487[0], 64488[0], 64489[0], 64490[0], 64491[0], 64492[0], 64493[0], 64494[0], 64495[0], 64505[0], 64510[0], 64517[0], 64520[0], 64530[0], 67500[1], 68440[1], 68530[1], 68700[1], 68770[1], 68801[1], 68810[1], 68811[1], 68815[1], 68816[1], 68840[1], 69990[0], 92012[1], 92014[1], 92018[1], 92019[1], 93000[1], 93005[1], 93010[1], 93040[1], 93041[1], 93042[1], 93318[1], 93355[1], 94002[1], 94200[1], 94680[1], 94681[1], 94690[1], 95812[1], 95813[1], 95816[1], 95819[1], 95822[1], 95829[1], 95955[1], 96360[1], 96361[1], 96365[1], 96366[1], 96367[1], 96368[1], 96372[1], 96374[1], 96375[1], 96376[1], 96377[1], 96523[0], 97597[1], 97598[1], 97602[1], 99155[0], 99156[0], 99157[0], 99211[1], 99212[1], 99213[1], 99214[1], 99215[1], 99217[1], 99218[1], 99219[1], 99220[1], 99221[1], 99222[1], 99223[1], 99231[1], 99232[1], 99233[1], 99234[1], 99235[1], 99236[1], 99238[1], 99239[1], 99241[1], 99242[1], 99243[1], 99244[1], 99245[1], 99251[1], 99252[1], 99253[1], 99254[1], 99255[1], 99291[1], 99292[1], 99304[1], 99305[1], 99306[1], 99307[1], 99308[1], 99309[1], 99310[1], 99315[1], 99316[1], 99334[1], 99335[1], 99336[1], 99347[1], 99348[1], 99349[1], 99350[1], 99374[1], 99375[1], 99377[1], 99378[1], 99446[0], 99447[0], 99448[0], 99449[0], 99451[0], 99452[0], 99495[0], 99496[0], G0463[1], G0471[1], J2001[1]
68850	0213T[0], 0216T[0], 0596T[1], 0597T[1], 0708T[1], 0709T[1], 12001[1], 12002[1], 12004[1], 12005[1], 12006[1], 12007[1], 12011[1], 12013[1], 12014[1], 12015[1], 12016[1], 12017[1], 12018[1], 12020[1], 12021[1], 12031[1], 12032[1], 12034[1], 12035[1], 12036[1], 12037[1], 12041[1], 12042[1], 12044[1], 12045[1], 12046[1], 12047[1], 12051[1], 12052[1], 12053[1], 12054[1], 12055[1], 12056[1], 12057[1], 13100[1], 13101[1], 13102[1], 13120[1], 13121[1], 13122[1], 13131[1], 13132[1], 13133[1], 13151[1], 13152[1], 13153[1], 36000[1], 36400[1], 36405[1], 36406[1], 36410[1], 36420[1], 36425[1], 36430[1], 36440[1], 36591[0], 36592[0], 36600[1], 36640[1], 43752[1], 51701[1], 51702[1], 51703[1], 62320[0], 62321[0], 62322[0], 62323[0], 62324[0], 62325[0], 62326[0], 62327[0], 64400[0], 64405[0], 64408[0], 64415[0], 64416[0], 64417[0], 64418[0], 64420[0], 64421[0], 64425[0], 64430[0], 64435[0], 64445[0], 64446[0], 64447[0], 64448[0], 64449[0], 64450[0], 64451[0], 64454[0], 64461[0], 64462[0], 64463[0], 64479[0], 64480[0], 64483[0], 64484[0], 64486[0], 64487[0], 64488[0], 64489[0], 64490[0], 64491[0], 64492[0], 64493[0], 64494[0], 64495[0], 64505[0], 64510[0], 64517[0], 64520[0], 64530[0], 67500[1], 69990[0], 76000[1], 77001[1], 77002[1], 92012[1], 92014[1], 92018[1], 92019[1], 93000[1], 93005[1], 93010[1], 93040[1], 93041[1], 93042[1], 93318[1], 93355[1], 94002[1], 94200[1], 94680[1], 94681[1], 94690[1], 95812[1], 95813[1], 95816[1], 95819[1], 95822[1], 95829[1], 95955[1], 96360[1], 96361[1], 96365[1], 96366[1], 96367[1], 96368[1], 96372[1], 96374[1], 96375[1], 96376[1], 96377[1], 96523[0], 99155[0], 99156[0], 99157[0], 99211[1], 99212[1], 99213[1], 99214[1], 99215[1], 99217[1], 99218[1], 99219[1], 99220[1], 99221[1], 99222[1], 99223[1], 99231[1], 99232[1], 99233[1], 99234[1], 99235[1], 99236[1], 99238[1], 99239[1], 99241[1], 99242[1], 99243[1], 99244[1], 99245[1], 99251[1], 99252[1], 99253[1], 99254[1], 99255[1], 99291[1], 99292[1], 99304[1], 99305[1], 99306[1], 99307[1], 99308[1], 99309[1], 99310[1], 99315[1], 99316[1], 99334[1], 99335[1], 99336[1], 99337[1], 99347[1], 99348[1], 99349[1], 99350[1], 99374[1], 99375[1], 99377[1], 99378[1], 99446[0], 99447[0], 99448[0], 99449[0], 99451[0], 99452[0], 99495[1], 99496[1], G0463[1], G0471[1], J0670[1], J1644[1], J2001[1]

0 = Modifier usage not allowed or inappropriate 1 = Modifier usage allowed

Code 1	Code 2
G0117	36591[0], 36592[0], 96523[0], 99446[0], 99447[0], 99448[0], 99449[0], 99451[0], 99452[0], G0118[0]
G0118	36591[0], 36592[0], 96523[0]

0 = Modifier usage not allowed or inappropriate 1 = Modifier usage allowed

Table of Risk

Level of Risk	Presenting Problem(s)	Diagnostic Procedure(s) Ordered	Management Options Selected
Minimal	One self-limited or minor problem, e.g., cold, insect bite, tinea corporis	Laboratory tests requiring venipuncture Chest X-rays EKG/EEG Urinalysis Ultrasound, e.g., echocardiography KOH prep	Rest Gargles Elastic bandages Superficial dressings
Low	Two or more self-limited or minor problems One stable chronic illness, e.g., well controlled hypertension, non-insulin dependent diabetes, cataract, BPH Acute uncomplicated illness or injury, e.g., cystitis, allergic rhinitis, simple sprain	Physiologic tests not under stress, e.g., pulmonary function test Non-cardiovascular imaging studies with contrast, e.g., barium enema Superficial needle biopsies Clinical laboratory tests requiring arterial puncture Skin biopsies	Over-the-counter drugs Minor surgery with no identified risk factors Physical therapy Occupational therapy IV fluids without additives
Moderate	One or more chronic illnesses with mild exacerbation, progression, or side effects of treatment Two or more stable chronic illnesses Undiagnosed new problem with uncertain prognosis, e.g., lump in breast Acute illness with systemic symptoms, e.g., pyelonephritis, pneumonitis, colitis Acute complicated injury, e.g., head injury with brief loss of consciousness	Physiologic tests under stress, e.g., cardio stress test, fetal contraction stress test Diagnostic endoscopies with no identified risk factors Deep needle or incisional biopsy Cardiovascular imaging studies with contrast and no identified risk factors, e.g., arteriogram, cardiac catheterization Obtain fluid from body cavity, e.g. lumbar puncture, thoracentesis, culdocentesis	Minor surgery with identified risk factors Elective major surgery (open, percutaneous or endoscopic) with no identified risk factors Prescription drug management Therapeutic nuclear medicine IV fluids with additives Closed treatment of fracture or dislocation without manipulation
High	One or more chronic illnesses with severe exacerbation, progression, or side effects of treatment Acute or chronic illnesses or injuries that pose a threat to life or bodily function, e.g., multiple trauma, acute MI, pulmonary embolus, severe respiratory distress, progressive severe rheumatoid arthritis, psychiatric illness with potential threat to self or others, peritonitis, acute renal failure An abrupt change in neurologic status, e.g., seizure, TIA, weakness, sensory loss	Cardiovascular imaging studies with contrast with identified risk factors Cardiac electrophysiological tests Diagnostic endoscopies with identified risk factors Discography	Elective major surgery (open, percutaneous or endoscopic) with identified risk factors Emergency major surgery (open, percutaneous or endoscopic) Parenteral controlled substances Drug therapy requiring intensive monitoring for toxicity Decision not to resuscitate or to deescalate care because of poor prognosis